ILLUSTRATED
ORTHOPEDIC
PHYSICAL ASSESSMENT

ILLUSTRATED

ORTHOPEDIC
PHYSICAL ASSESSMENT

RONALD C. EVANS, DC, FACO, FICC

Fellow, Academy of Chiropractic Orthopedists;
Fellow, International College of Chiropractic;
Senior Staff, Icon Whole Health;
Member and Chairman of the Iowa Board of
Chiropractic Examiners Iowa Department of
Public Health;
Chief Executive Officer,
ICPC;
Trustee, Foundation for Chiropractic Education
and Research, Des Moines, Iowa;
Examiner Emeritus, American Board of Chiropractic Orthopedists of
the American Chiropractic Association, Washington, DC;
Member of the Advisory Oversight Committee, Chiropractic Health Care Project,
Department of Defense of the United States of America

Photography by
Miriam C. Dunlap BA, MA

with 1546 illustrations
and 259 gamuts

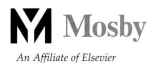

An Affiliate of Elsevier

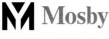

An Affiliate of Elsevier

Editor in Chief: John A. Schrefer
Acquisitions Editor: Kellie F. White
Associate Developmental Editor: Jennifer L. Watrous
Editorial Assistant: Becky Fuhrmann
Project Manager: Carol Sullivan Weis
Production Editor: Rachel E. Dowell
Design Coordinator: Mark A. Oberkrom
Designer: Rokusek Design
Cover Designer: Kathi Gosche
Cover Art: Greta Strief

SECOND EDITION

NOTICE

Medicine is an ever-changing field. Standard safety precautions must be followed, but as new research and clinical experience broaden our knowledge, changes in treatment and drug therapy may become necessary or appropriate. Readers are advised to check the most current product information provided by the manufacturer of each drug to be administered to verify the recommended dose, the method and duration of administration, and contraindications. It is the responsibility of the treating physician, relying on experience and knowledge of the patient, to determine dosages and the best treatment for each individual patient. Neither the publisher nor the editor assumes any liability for any injury and/or damage to persons or property arising from this publication.

Permissions may be sought directly from Elsevier's Health Sciences Rights Department in Philadelphia, USA: phone: (+1)215-238-7869, fax: (+1)215-238-2239, email: healthpermissions@elsevier.com. You may also complete your request on-line via the Elsevier Science homepage (http://www.elsevier.com), by selecting 'Customer Support' and then 'Obtaining Permissions'.

Mosby, Inc.
An Affiliate of Elsevier
11830 Westline Industrial Drive
St. Louis, Missouri 63146

Printed in United States of America

Library of Congress Cataloging in Publication Data

Evans, Ronald C.
    Illustrated orthopedic physical assessment / Ronald C. Evans ; photography by Miriam C. Dunlap.—2nd ed.
        p. ; cm.
    Includes bibliographical references and index.
    ISBN 0-323-00509-8 (alk. paper)
      1. Orthopedics—Diagnosis—Atlases. 2. Physical diagnosis—Atlases. 3. Physical orthopedic tests—Atlases. 4. Joints—Range of motion—Measurement—Atlases. I. Title.
    [DNLM: 1. Bone Diseases—diagnosis—Atlases. 2. Joint Diseases—diagnosis—Atlases. WE 17 E92i 2001]
RD734.E93 2001
616.7'075—dc21
                                                             00-045578

05 06 07 08 09 GW/MVY 9 8 7 6 5 4

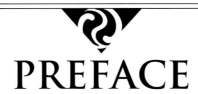

PREFACE

Although the first edition of *Illustrated Essentials in Orthopedic Physical Assessment* was an unqualified success—voted into the 1994-1995 Top 250 Books of the Year by *Doody's Health Sciences Book Review Journal*—it could be improved. Much of what made the first edition so successful has been retained in this second edition. Many major changes to the contents have been made, increasing the information on disease assessment, including more illustrations, and creating Orthopedic Gamuts. The book remains clinically relevant and useful for both the student and the practicing clinician.

The scope and organization of the second edition of the *Illustrated Orthopedic Physical Assessment* make it a suitable companion for the clinician at all levels of sophistication, progressing from the initial procedures of orthopedic diagnosis to the requirements of the advanced student and the experienced practitioner. Included in the 13 chapters are diagnostic facts in orthopedics, which are organized in a manner most likely to be useful during the examination of patients. This book's functional internal design with liberal use of Orthopedic Gamuts offers a convenient vehicle for refreshing the memory about clinical orthopedic phenomenon that are seldom encountered and easily forgotten.

Only the unusual reader and clinician could master the contents of the *Illustrated Orthopedic Physical Assessment* by studying it in sequence, from beginning to end. Rather, the student or clinician should digest the principles and procedures in segments as general diagnostic knowledge progresses. First, the reader should become familiar with Chapters 1 and 2 and the descriptions of the cardinal signs and symptoms. From these chapters the clinician should explore the regional chapters. As contact with patients increases and specific questions arise, the reader should become familiar with the comments for each diagnostic procedure. The comments section of each test or sign amplifies the knowledge of each underlying pathologic condition that can be discovered with the pertinent test or procedure.

Chapter 13 presents rationale and procedures for investigating malingering or nonorganically based complaints. Included with Chapter 13 are numerous medical record forms, outcomes assessment forms, and pain-scale analogs.

Each chapter of *Illustrated Orthopedic Physical Assessment* has a specific format. The format lends to the quick referencing of tests and maneuvers and cross-referencing of associated procedures.

Each chapter begins with indexing of the tests found therein. Each chapter also begins with cross-reference tables by assessment procedure and by the syndrome or tissue suspected. Furthermore, each chapter presents the separate protocols for the regional joint assessment procedures and for assessment of pain in the particular joint or region.

Each chapter begins with a set of axioms. Axioms are self-evident or universally recognized truths. Axioms are also established rules, principles, or laws. An axiom used in this text is also a principle that is accepted as true without proof as the basis for argument.

Each chapter introduction addresses the various unique considerations or pathologic conditions of the focal joint. The introductory section contains the index of the tests presented and illustrated in the chapter.

Laced throughout each chapter are **Orthopedic Gamuts.** The various gamuts present a range or spectrum of facts or concepts in assessing orthopedic disease. The gamuts in each chapter may represent both universal orthopedic precepts and specific regional principles and maxims. The gamuts serve as diagnostic rubric in examining a patient.

Essential anatomy is presented in each chapter. The essential anatomy section is not all encompassing but rather discusses only the typical tissues that can be examined in orthopedic physical procedures. Essential motion assessment for the joint is included. These illustrations depict the expected full ranges of movement for the joint. The discussion further identifies the amount of lost motion that can affect the activities of daily living. Essential muscle function for each joint is also included. This section identifies the musculature that is the prime mover of the joint, the innervation and the action of the muscle, and limited discussion of the muscular anatomy. Essential plain film imaging elements are addressed in each chapter, specific for the region or joint discussed.

Each test, maneuver, sign, law, or phenomenon is presented separately. The common usage name for the test, as identified in Stedman's, Dorland's, or Churchill's medical dictionaries, is used as the heading for the test. This name is followed by equally common synonyms and eponyms. Eponyms for certain examinations vary from locale to locale or among institutions within the same area. Such observations are a reflection of the training center's influence. This is especially true where the names of prominent local physicians are commonly used for these examinations. Occasionally, the same test is given two or more names, or the name can apply to more than one test or sign. In a problem-oriented situation, eponyms are routinely used in the physical evaluation process. Familiarity with the terms and techniques used in determining regional problems enables the physician and assistant to record and clarify an orthopedic examination. After the name of the test, maneuver, or sign, the specific pathologic condition the test is suited to elicit is identified.

A *test* is part of the physical examination in which direct contact with the patient is made. It also may be a chemical test, radiograph, or other study. All tests described in this book relate to the physical examination.

A *sign* is elucidated by a test or a particular maneuver. A sign can be simply a visual observation (e.g., antalgia) and is an indication of the existence of a problem perceived by the examiner.

A *maneuver* is a complex motion or series of movements, used either as a test or treatment. A maneuver is also a method or technique.

A *phenomenon* is any sign or objective symptom or any observable occurrence or fact.

A *law* is a description of a phenomenon so thoroughly tested and accepted that it is regarded as a principle governing like phenomena.

For each testing procedure in this book, a general comment is presented about the pathologic condition targeted by the test. This comment is followed by a bulleted discussion of how the test is conducted. Each procedure is supported by photo illustrations and legends. Each test is cross-referenced with other supportive tests and procedures. An accurate documentation or diagnostic statement format is suggested for each test. When possible, a **Clinical Pearl** identifies the subtle nuances or finesse of the tests that the author has gleaned from empirical practice.

At the close of most chapters, a **Critical Thinking** section is included. The critical thinking section is a range of questions germane to the specific region or joint of the chapter. The questions largely pertain to information contained in this text but may occasionally require the reader to cross-reference with other literature or current scientific journals. The answers for each question are contained in this reference as well.

In some instances, the bibliography reflects older volumes or works than are commonly found in scientific literature today. These older references are the original work of the creators of various tests or procedures in this book. Preserving the books in these reference lists is an attempt to preserve a continuum in the developments of orthopedic investigation.

In an effort to accurately depict tissue and pathology involved in orthopedic disease and injury, numerous new illustrations have been included in this edition of *Illustrated Orthopedic Physical Assessment.* The new illustrations are mostly from the outstanding and benchmark works of selected authors. Their works are exemplary in great scientific writing, strongly contributing to the fund of knowledge of modern physicians. The artwork and line drawings used in these works are unsurpassed. Special credit is due to their creators.

Although the various tests and procedures in this book are presented in an anatomic or regional format, the application of the tests are accomplished in a more natural flow of examination procedures. The natural flow of the examination usually moves the patient from the standing position, through sitting, supine, and side-lying positions, to the prone position. Appendix A is a listing of tests, alphabetically and anatomically; Appendix B is a listing of tests according to the position of the patient.

A picture shows me at a glance what it takes dozens of pages of a book to expound.
Turgenev, 1883

One picture is worth more than a thousand words.
Chinese Proverb

RONALD C. EVANS

PREFACE TO THE FIRST EDITION

The basic observation of a patient's antalgia and exacerbative movements allows the formulation of the presenting signs and symptoms into a recognizable disease syndrome. The essence of diagnosis is the clinically demonstrable or reproducible signs of disease.

Many physicians associate an aura of mysticism with the ease and speed with which the orthopedic specialist arrives at a diagnosis. It is in fact, the specialist's development of interviewing, observation, and physical testing skills that allows proceeding directly to the heart of the patient's problem.

I have been privileged in private practice to be challenged by myriad orthopedic health problems presented by my patients. I believe that my early and fumbling years were well tolerated by these patients. They may have become well in spite of my efforts. They have remained loyal indeed. In later years of practice, many of the early patients return with new diseases. These diseases are often much more difficult to diagnose and to treat. My skills as an orthopedic specialist have been honed to a fine edge out of

necessity. Some of these patients will not outlive me to give me yet another chance to get it right.

The perspective of the role of the physician in modern medicine has changed. Physicians are no longer viewed as the omnipotent beings they were formerly thought to be. The physician is expected to recognize personal skill limitations and make appropriate consultations and referrals. Patients expect the correct diagnosis the first time around. At the least, they deserve that.

This book is created to relieve the frustration and discomfort for two parties in their quest for wellness. First are the physicians and orthopedic specialists, who labor mightily in pushing, pulling, poking, bending, and twisting patients' body parts as they search for the cause of the suffering. Second are the patients, who have been not-so-gently pushed, pulled, poked, bent, and twisted into inhuman configurations, as they wait furtively for the discovery of the cause of their anguish. I salute both parties for their endurance in seeking the origin of disease.

ACKNOWLEDGMENTS

One of the richest resources for this revision continues to be the physicians who attend my classes and take the time to tell me about various orthopedic cases and procedures. Without their continued interest in scientific rationale, *Illustrated Orthopedic Physical Assessment* would not have come to be.

My peers and colleagues, Dr. James R. Brandt and Dr. Gregory R. Norton, again participated tirelessly in revisions for *Illustrated Orthopedic Physical Assessment.* I am grateful for their willingness to contribute time and guidance in this second round of academic exercise.

Two individuals, Mrs. Pamela Schwartz and Mrs. Lori Vann, have been inexhaustible in their efforts to keep up with my revisions of the second edition manuscript. I am indebted to their zeal to make this edition of *Illustrated Orthopedic Physical Assessment* as successful as the first. They each made the task of revision more interesting and less heavy. I must also thank Ms. Joy R. Woodworth for her diligence in preparing numerous computer-generated charts and tables found throughout this edition. Her insight and creativity added immeasurably to the quality of this text.

Ms. Amy Christopher and Ms. Leslie Mosby, developmental editors for the second edition, are the finest. With great professionalism and enthusiasm each has redirected this edition of *Illustrated Essentials in Orthopedic Physical Assessment* into a much more meaningful work of medical literature. Ms. Christopher oversaw the beginning of the revision and Ms. Mosby guided its middle work. At completion, Ms. Suzanne Kastner, production editor, and Ms. Jennifer Watrous, associate developmental editor, made the critical and elegant decisions for the structure of this edition. Both have been immensely encouraging at the most difficult deadlines. I am grateful for their expertise, patience, and acumen and would work with each again.

Last, but certainly not least, I thank Ms. Martha Sasser and Ms. Kellie F. White, acquisitions editors. Harcourt Health Sciences continues to be a great and growing publishing company. Ms. Sasser nurtured the first edition to the hands of readers and had confidence that the second edition could go further. Ms. Sasser became not only a compassionate editor but a great friend and visionary. I am ever grateful for her editorial acumen and positive, reassuring spirit. Ms. White, also engaged in the first and second editions, provided exceptional encouragement at the most difficult times. *Illustrated Orthopedic Physical Assessment* would not exist without her persistence and patience. I look forward to our next collaboration.

INTRODUCTION

Solving a patient's health problem can be a demanding exercise of orthopedic medical detection and logical deduction. Each health problem is a new diagnostic jigsaw puzzle for which the pieces must be found and fitted together in a carefully organized manner.

ORTHOPEDIC GAMUT

Success requires an organized thought process in approaching the patient's problem. There must be a clear plan to follow and a particular aim in each stage of the investigation.

First, it must be determined whether a lesion of the musculoskeletal system is present. This determination is accomplished by analysis of the history and physical examination.

Second, the location of the lesion must be determined. Is it possible to locate the lesion at one site, or are multiple sites involved? The examiner must develop a system to relate the signs and symptoms to a basic knowledge of musculoskeletal anatomy.

Third, what pathologic conditions are capable of producing the lesions?

Fourth, from careful analysis of the history and examination and by intelligent use of ancillary tests, which of these suspected conditions is most likely to be present?

Each examination or investigation should have a plan for including or excluding a specific member of a "short list" of suspected conditions. It is always the failure to have such an organized plan or approach that makes the diagnosis of orthopedic health problems so artificially difficult. Routine steps must be followed but not blind routine or blunderbuss investigations.

Diagnosis purely by comparison with previous cases is reserved for the physician or orthopedic specialist who is very experienced and remembers the cases very accurately, but this combination is not the norm. The entry-level physician or orthopedic specialist will come nearer to diagnostic accuracy by logically progressing through the medical investigation paradigm.

Despite all this, however, the right approach will never be achieved until one misconception is laid to rest. This misconception is that the exact solution of an orthopedic problem does not matter very much and that such a solution will be of academic interest only, with no useful nonsurgical treatment. Such a view is nonsense. It is true that health science is frustrated in treating motor neuron disease; no cure exists for hereditary ataxia, and no reliable method exists to prevent relapses in disseminated sclerosis. Contrary to many beliefs, these diseases occupy only a small part of the orthopedist's time.

Think for a moment of the transformation in the last 30 years in the treatment of cervical spine trauma, intervertebral disc prolapse, carpal tunnel syndrome, and deficiency neuropathies. Think of the influence of physiologic therapeutics in hypersensitivity states and in acute episodes of soft-tissue disease, of the continuing progress of manipulative therapy in certain facets of the migraine headache process, mechanical lower-back disorders, and trigeminal neuralgia. Consider the advances of chiropractic orthopedics in treating various forms of benign spinal compression.

Finally, the solution of an orthopedic problem takes time. A solution cannot be rushed, and the examiner must never allow the approach to be influenced by the exhortations of optimistic colleagues to "just glance at this case while passing" or to "just run over the musculoskeletal system, it won't take 5 minutes." It will, it always does, and so it should.

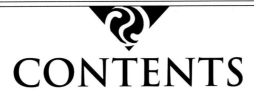

CONTENTS

ILLUSTRATED
ORTHOPEDIC
PHYSICAL ASSESSMENT

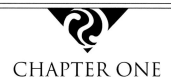

CHAPTER ONE

ASSESSMENT OF MUSCULOSKELETAL DISORDERS

AXIOMS IN ASSESSMENT OF MUSCULOSKELETAL DISORDERS

- Eliciting the patient's history is the quintessential skill in orthopedics.
- An examiner needs to learn about major presenting symptoms, the chronology of the disorder, and its impact on the patient.
- The orthopedic examination is the focal activity in the assessment of the patient.

INTRODUCTION

The orthopedic evaluation process can be divided into three phases: history taking, examination, and diagnosis.

From the moment of the first encounter with a patient, the examiner is simultaneously observing and examining the movements and mannerisms of the patient as well as listening to what is being said. The diagnostic process is complex; the examiner needs to establish the physical issues that are of greatest importance to the patient (those most disrupting to the activities of daily living) and try to differentiate the anatomic and pathologic aspects of any disease or injury that might be present.

The history provides much information about what the patient is experiencing and the impact of the condition on the patient. Orthopedic examination is essential to define the structures involved; together, these processes allow differentiation of orthopedic disorders into various diagnostic categories (Box 1-1).

BOX 1-1

Precis in Orthopedic Diagnosis

1. History
2. Examination
3. Determination of disability (PILS):
   P Preventable causes of disability
   I   Independent living
   L Lifestyle
   S Social support

HISTORY TAKING

A carefully elicited history is a most crucial element in orthopedic assessment. An experienced examiner can form an idea of the extent and magnitude simply from the patient's history.

The complaint history of a musculoskeletal condition should cover certain essential points. History of trauma may help differentiate between inherent laxity and past instability. If an injury caused the problem, the examiner should determine whether the patient stopped the injurious activity immediately and self-treated the resulting condition. It is not uncommon to find injured joints and adjacent structures neglected, deconditioned, weakened, or atrophied because of prolonged periods of protection.

An accurate description of the injury event, including the exact position of the injured part at the time of injury, is essential.

ORTHOPEDIC GAMUT 1-1

WORKING DIAGNOSIS

Essential steps in drawing a working diagnosis about a patient's complaint include the following:
1. History taking
2. Observation
3. Palpation
4. Orthopedic testing
5. Clinical, laboratory, and imaging procedures

The exact site of the pain is also important. Patients often identify pain in one location, such as the hip, but point somewhere else, such as the sacroiliac joint. The more distal the pain, the more accurately patients define its location.

Chief Complaint

Patients who have more than one complaint, such as those with pain of spinal origin, should rank the complaints in priority. Although patients occasionally seek attention for stiffness or some other joint-related complaint, most patients with musculoskeletal conditions do so for reasons of pain.

The basic elements of examining the patient include observation and inspection, palpation, neurologic evaluation, vital signs, range-of-motion studies, clinical laboratory studies, orthopedic tests, and diagnostic imaging.

OBSERVATION AND INSPECTION

ORTHOPEDIC GAMUT 1-2

OBSERVATION AND INSPECTION

Observation and inspection of the patient occur anytime during the examination or history interview, especially when the patient is not aware of the observation. In this way, the examiner notes the following:

1. Antalgia or deformities of posture
2. Gait disturbances, especially if the patient needs assistance
3. Spinal symmetry, which includes prominences or elevations, flattening or depressions, scoliosis, or abnormalities of the anteroposterior curvature
4. Surface scars and wounds

The first impressions—observations made while taking the patient's history—are often the most revealing.

A useful approach in clinical examination of the human locomotor system is to seek answers to the "Critical 5" questions in orthopedics. Once all five questions have been answered, a differential diagnosis can usually be established (Box 1-2).

A rapid joint screening examination suffices initially. Abnormal joints are subjected to a more focused orthopedic regional examination procedure.

The examiner must determine the presence of active or current inflammation, the presence of irreversible joint damage from past injury or inflammation, and existing mechanical defects. These findings are not mutually exclusive.

BOX 1-2

Critical Questions in Orthopedic Physical Examination

1. Are any joints abnormal?
2. What is the nature of the abnormality?
3. What is the extent of the involvement?
4. Are other features of diagnostic importance present?

The distribution of joint involvement is important in reaching a diagnosis. Certain patterns characterize specific disorders. The number of involved joints may also be of diagnostic significance.

ORTHOPEDIC GAMUT 1-3

FEATURES OF DIAGNOSTIC IMPORTANCE

Other characteristic features of diagnostic importance in determining the extent of the disease or injury include the joint or regional involvement:

1. Is involvement symmetric or asymmetric?
2. Are large or small joints affected?
3. Is the distribution of the condition peripheral or axial?
4. Does the condition affect upper versus lower limbs, or vice versa?

It is important to learn what exacerbates or relieves the symptom pattern. Equally important is knowing how long the complaints have existed (Table 1-1).

A number of other features may be of diagnostic importance. Many of these features present as skin signs or nodules. Examples include rheumatoid nodules (Fig. 1-1), gouty tophi (Fig. 1-2), dermatomyositis (Fig. 1-3), and psoriatic arthritis (Fig. 1-4).

The answers to the Critical 5 questions provide sufficient information to establish a differential diagnosis. They must. If not, the examiner must retrace each examination step until a logical and credible diagnosis can be reached.

TABLE 1-1

JOINT PATTERNS IN ORTHOPEDIC/RHEUMATIC DISORDERS

Diagnosis	Symmetry	Number of Joints Involved*	Large/Small Joints	Peripheral/ Central Distribution	Upper/ Lower Limb	Predilection
Rheumatoid arthritis	Symmetric	Mono/oligo/ polyarthritis	Large/small	Peripheral	Upper/lower	MCPs, PIPs, MTPs, DIPs
Ankylosing spondylitis				Central		Sacroiliac joints, hip, shoulder
Psoriatic arthritis	Asymmetric	Polyarthritis	Large/small	Peripheral	Upper/lower	DIPs, sacroiliac joints
Reactive arthritis	Asymmetric	Oligoarthritis/ polyarthritis	Large	Peripheral	Lower	Sacroiliac joints, DIPs (toes)
Gout	Asymmetric	Monoarthritis/ oligoarthritis	Large/small	Peripheral	Lower > upper	First MTP, knee, hip

MCPs, Metacarpophalangeal joints; *PIPs,* proximal interphalangeal joints; *MTPs,* metatarsophalangeals; *DIPs,* distal interphalangeal joints.
Monoarthritis denotes inflammation in a single joint, *oligoarthritis* denotes 2 to 4 joints, *polyarthritis* denotes 5 or more joints.

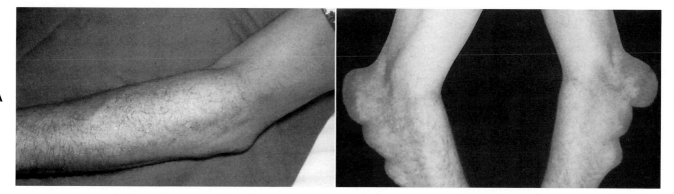

A   B

FIG. 1-1   **A,** Rheumatoid nodules. **B,** Large nodules may develop in the olecranon bursa as well as in the subcutaneous tissue.   *(From Klippel JH, Dieppe PA:* Rheumatology, *vol 1-2, ed 2, London, 1998, Mosby.)*

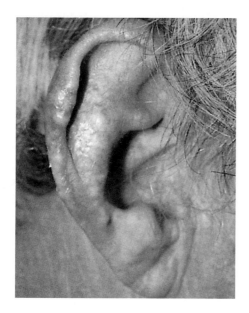

FIG. 1-2   Gouty tophi represent deposits of urate crystals.
(From Klippel JH, Dieppe PA: Rheumatology, *vol 1-2, ed 2, London, 1998, Mosby.)*

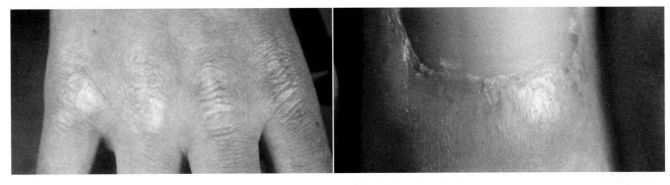

FIG. 1-3   Skin and nailfold lesions seen in dermatomyositis. Patches **(A)** and periungual edema and nailfold **(B)**. *(From Klippel JH, Dieppe PA:* Rheumatology, *vol 1-2, ed 2, London, 1998, Mosby.)*

PALPATION

Palpation is the process of assessing the physical characteristics of joints and contiguous structures by touching or feeling the patient's body. The purpose of palpation is to locate and substantiate areas of tenderness, swelling, and abnormal muscle tone. Palpation allows the examiner to identify a localized increase or decrease in surface temperature and the presence of induration and mass. Palpation can be performed with the fingertips, by percussion (gently tapping with a reflex hammer), with vibration (using a C-128 tuning fork), or with the blunt end of a cotton-tip applicator. Palpation examination procedures can be accomplished with the patient in the standing, sitting, or prone position.

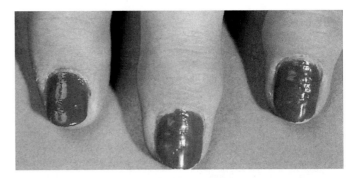

FIG. 1-4   Psoriatic arthritis, with swelling of the distal interphalangeal joint and pitting in the adjacent fingernails. *(From Klippel JH, Dieppe PA:* Rheumatology, *vol 1-2, ed 2, London, 1998, Mosby.)*

deficits, and tenderness. Palpation also aids in establishing the integrity of local circulation.

NEUROLOGIC EVALUATION

The neurologic evaluation involves locating the lesion; testing deep tendon, superficial, and pathologic reflexes (Fig. 1-5); testing cranial nerve and brainstem function; measuring body parts (mensuration); grading muscular strength; and testing the gross sensory modalities (Fig. 1-6).

Cerebral dysfunction is determined during the consultation by noting the patient's mannerisms and orientation to time, space, and body parts (oriented ×3). Further evaluations of lesions in the cerebrum require advanced imaging procedures and electroneurodiagnostic testing.

Cerebellar lesions are characterized by repeated cogwheel-type muscle actions while the patient's eyes are open. The posterior columns of the spinal cord are the source of the dysfunction when repeated muscle actions are smooth and occur while the patient's eyes are open. However, these same muscular actions cannot be repeated with the eyes closed. This is known as *Romberg's sign* and is easily demonstrated by having the patient stand with feet together and eyes closed. Brainstem dysfunction is discerned through testing of the cranial nerves. The type and

---

ORTHOPEDIC GAMUT 1-4

PALPATION

Effective spinal palpation is also accomplished with the patient in the sitting or kneeling Adam's position:

1. In palpating various structures, the examiner assesses the skin and subcutaneous tissue. Rolling of the skin (Kibler's test) can be accomplished. The examiner observes for surface temperature, hypesthesia, hyperhidrosis, and muscle splinting.
2. Tenderness of muscles and tendons and their attachments is assessed, in both the anatomic rest position and through various ranges of motion.

Tendon sheaths and bursae are palpated for thickness, crepitus (especially silken/snowball crepitus), and tenderness. The joints are palpated for all anatomic components to include bones, capsule, ligaments, any specialized structures, swelling, a change of shape or deformity, positional

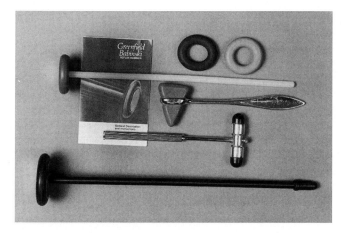

FIG. 1-5   From top to bottom, the Greenfield Babinski reflex hammer, Taylor reflex hammer, Buck's neurologic hammer, and Babinski reflex hammer.

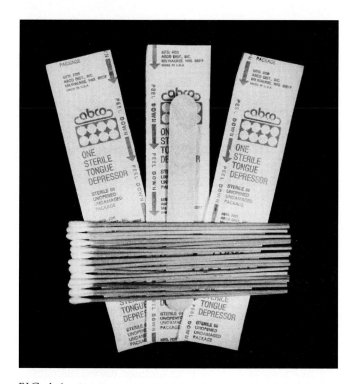

FIG. 1-6   Single-tipped cotton applicators are both economical and versatile and can be used in the following settings: in emergency rooms, examining rooms, outpatient clinics, and laboratories and on dressing carts. Sterile tongue depressors are usually made from white birchwood that is ¹⁄₁₆″ thick. These tongue depressors are evenly cut and highly polished for smooth and clean edges, ends, and surfaces.

quality of paralysis, reflexes, muscle tone, clonus, atrophy, fasciculation, and reactions of degeneration can differentiate spinal cord lesions from lower motor neuron disorders.

Deep tendon reflexes help the examiner locate the lower motor neuron lesion and differentiate it from an upper motor neuron lesion.

ORTHOPEDIC GAMUT 1-5

DEEP TENDON REFLEXES

1.	Scapulohumeral C5-C6	6.	Ulnar C8-T1
2.	Biceps C5-C6	7.	Patellar L2-L4
3.	Radial C5-C6	8.	Hamstring L4-S1
4.	Triceps C7-C8	9.	Achilles S1-S2
5.	Wrist C7-C8		

Superficial reflexes differentiate lower motor neuron lesions from upper motor neuron lesions.

ORTHOPEDIC GAMUT 1-6

SUPERFICIAL REFLEXES

1. Corneal III, V
2. Upper abdominal T7-T9
3. Lower abdominal T10-T12
4. Cremasteric
5. Gluteal
6. Plantar
7. T12-L2
8. L4-L5
9. S1-S2

Pathologic reflexes determine the presence of upper motor neuron lesions.

ORTHOPEDIC GAMUT 1-7

PATHOLOGIC REFLEXES

1. Hoffmann
2. Babinski
3. Chaddock
4. Oppenheim
5. Bechterew-Mendel
6. Rossolimo
7. Gordon
8. Schaeffer

Cranial nerve function is determined by testing brainstem activity.

ORTHOPEDIC GAMUT 1-8

CRANIAL NERVES AND BASIC FUNCTION

I: Smell
II: Vision
III: Light accommodation
III, IV, VI: Eye movement
V: Sensation (wink)
VII: Facial muscle (taste)
VIII: Auditory (balance)
IX: Taste (gag)
X: Voice (swallow)
XI: Shoulder (shrug)
XII: Tongue (motor)

On occasion, eliciting a particular reflex is difficult; distraction techniques are helpful in such situations. If less-than-normal reactivity is encountered in the upper or lower extremities, the patient is directed to perform an isometric contraction in the opposite upper or lower extremities (Jendrassik's maneuver).

ORTHOPEDIC GAMUT 1-9

COMMONLY ACCEPTED DEEP TENDON REFLEX GRADING SCHEME

0 = Absent
1 = Diminished or hyporeactive
2 = Average
2+ = Slightly exaggerated (hyperreactive)
3 = Exaggerated (hyperreactive)
4 = Associated with myoclonus

Mensuration of body parts is used to determine atrophy and functional and anatomic abnormalities (Fig. 1-7).

ORTHOPEDIC GAMUT 1-10

COMMON AREAS OF MENSURATION

1. Excursion of the chest during inspiration and expiration
2. Upper extremity circumference (brachium and antebrachium); measured in the noncontracted and contracted state
3. Lower extremity circumferences (thigh and calf); measured in the noncontracted and contracted states
4. Leg length (measured standing versus supine or prone); differentiates a functional short leg from an anatomic short leg

Grip strength testing examines the function of the ulnar nerve and can help differentiate myoneural dysfunction from malingering activity (Fig. 1-8). Cervical intrinsic muscle testing relates to the cervical spine functions of flexion, extension, lateral flexion, and rotation.

Thoracolumbar intrinsic muscle function is associated with trunk flexion and extension and lateral flexion and rotation.

Testing of the gross sensory modalities allows for evaluation of the dermatomes involved in superficial and deep sensations and proprioception (Fig. 1-9).

The superficial sensations include light touch, pain, and temperature. Light touch is mediated by the dorsal columns and is easily examined with a cotton ball. Pain receptors are mediated by the lateral spinothalamic tracts and are tested by a pinprick and hot and cold temperatures. Temperature, or thermal sensation, mediated by the dorsal

FIG. 1-7 Soft linen tape is marked in inches on one side and centimeters on the other. The fast-reading clinical thermometer is made of heat-tempered, fully aged Corning glass and has permanent markings. A break-resistant bulb encloses triple-distilled mercury, and a precise constriction chamber allows for softer, easier shakedown.

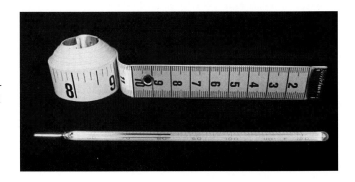

ORTHOPEDIC GAMUT 1-11

CERVICAL SPINE EXTRINSIC MUSCULATURE WITH SPECIFIC NERVE ROOTS NOTED

1. Deltoid C5
2. Biceps C6
3. Wrist extensors C6
4. Triceps C7
5. Wrist flexors C7
6. Finger extensors C7
7. Finger flexors C8
8. Finger abductors T1

ORTHOPEDIC GAMUT 1-12

THORACOLUMBAR EXTRINSIC MUSCULATURE AND SPECIFIC ASSOCIATED NERVE ROOT LEVELS

1. Hip flexors L2-L3
2. Knee extensors L3-L4
3. Ankle extensors L4-L5
4. Hip extensors L4-L5
5. Knee flexors L5-S1
6. Ankle flexors S1-S2

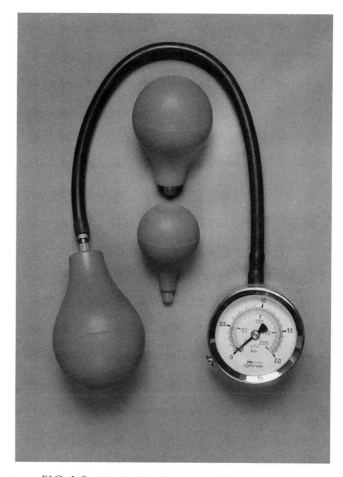

FIG. 1-8   Martin Vigorimeter aneroid dynamometer.

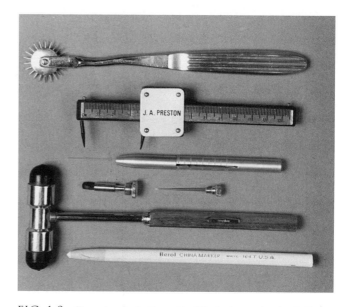

FIG. 1-9   From top to bottom, the Wartenberg pinwheel; Boley two-point discrimination gauge; von Frey anesthesimeter; Buck's camel hair brush, pin, and neurological hammer; and a Berol China Marker.

columns, is tested with warm (not hot) and cool (not cold) temperatures.

The deep sensations are vibration and deep pressure perception. Vibration is tested with a C-128 or lower-frequency tuning fork and is mediated by the dorsal columns of the spinal cord (Fig. 1-10). Deep pressure is tested by squeezing any muscular part of the body and is mediated in the dorsal columns.

Proprioception, or joint position sense, is mediated by the dorsal columns and can be tested by having the patient point to a particular part of the body while keeping the eyes closed.

Pain and Patterns of Pain

Pain that arises with activity and decreases with rest is likely to have a mechanical cause. The pain may be positional;

most cases of mechanical spinal pain have both a provocative and palliative arc of motion.

Patterns of pain originating in the spine appear similar. Spinal pain is the most difficult to differentially diagnose. There are three primary patterns: dermatogenous, myogenous, and scleratogenous (Fig. 1-11).

A dermatome is the area of sensation attributed to a particular nerve root level. Dermatomal pain is often described as sharp, stabbing, and well demarcated. Dermatomal pain may result from herniated discs, stretch injuries, and tumors.

Pain referral within muscular or fascial tissue is myogenous pain. Areas known as *trigger points* refer pain to a distant site. Trigger points are evident in patients with myofascial pain syndromes. Specific sites of tenderness that do not result from referred pain are termed *tender points*. Tender points develop in patients with varied soft-tissue, rheumatic, and collagen-vascular disorders. These disorders include systemic lupus erythematosus and fibromyalgia.

Pain referred from somatic structures, such as cartilage, ligament, joint capsule, or bone, may not follow a dermatome pattern as does nerve root pain. This pain is known as *scleratogenous pain.* Patients may describe this type of pain as dull, achy, diffuse, and difficult to pinpoint. Scleratogenous pain is one of the more common spinal pain patterns.

Local versus Referred Pain

Patients with referred pain often point to large generalized areas. Patients with localized lesions can be more specific. A patient complaining of unrelenting spinal pain who demonstrates full, pain-free range of motion presents a problem. This patient has either viscerosomatic pain, which mandates further diagnostic testing, or pain resulting from a psychosocial cause. If referred pain from a diseased organ system is mimicking a local orthopedic problem, the examiner should not hesitate to order appropriate tests.

Every effort should be made to objectify the patient's report of pain and discomfort. Measurement instruments such as the Visual Analog Scale (Fig. 1-12) have

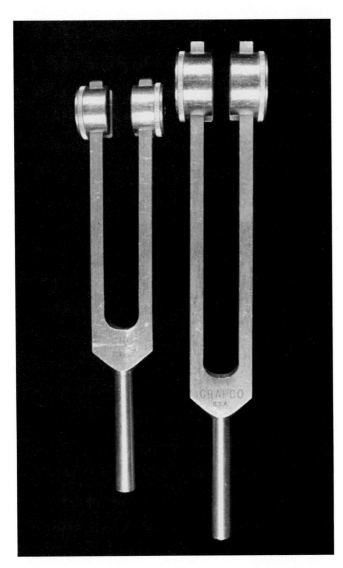

FIG. 1-10 Aluminum alloy tuning forks, available in C-64, C-128, C-256, C-512, C-1024, C-2048, and C-4096 vibrations. The lower-frequency tuning forks are the usual choices for bone vibration conduction studies.

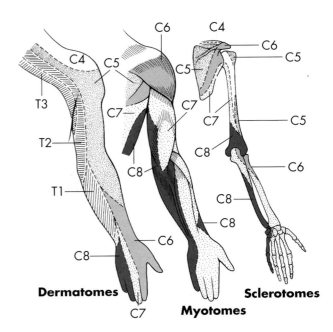

FIG. 1-11 Primary patterns of pain originating in the spine: dermatomes, myotomes, and sclerotomes. Demonstrated for the right upper extremity. *(From Saidoff DC, McDonough A: Critical pathways in therapeutic interventions: upper extremities, St Louis, 1997, Mosby.)*

been shown to be both reliable and valid for examining a patient's pain. The McGill Short Form Questionnaire (Fig. 1-13) has been helpful for pain measurement in a clinical setting.

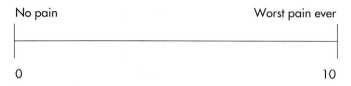

FIG. 1-12   Visual Analog Scale for objective pain measurement. *(From Malone TR, McPoil TG, Nitz AJ: Orthopedic and sports physical therapy, ed 3, St Louis, 1997, Mosby.)*

VITAL SIGNS

Vital signs include the brachial blood pressure, peripheral pulse rate, respiration rate, height, weight, and vital capacity. The instruments used in these measurements include stethoscopes, spirometers, scales, tape measures, and blood pressure cuffs (Fig. 1-14).

RANGE OF MOTION

Of all the orthopedic tests that an examiner performs on a patient, none is more crucial than the range-of-motion testing of the affected area. Range-of-motion testing provides information about the origin of the patient's pain, because movement may reproduce the pain. The patient should be examined symmetrically for active motion of all the joints that may be involved in the dysfunction or injury

Check only one item for each category to describe your pain today.

1	2	3	4
1 Flickering	1 Jumping	1 Pricking	1 Sharp
2 Quivering	2 Flashing	2 Boring	2 Cutting
3 Pulsing	3 Shooting	3 Drilling	3 Lacerating
4 Throbbing		4 Stabbing	
5 Beating		5 Lancinating	
6 Pounding			

5	6	7	8
1 Pinching	1 Tugging	1 Hot	1 Tingling
2 Pressing	2 Pulling	2 Burning	2 Itchy
3 Gnawing	3 Wrenching	3 Scalding	3 Smarting
4 Cramping		4 Searing	4 Stinging
5 Crushing			

9	10	11	12
1 Dull	1 Tender	1 Tiring	1 Sickening
2 Sore	2 Taut	2 Exhausting	2 Suffocating
3 Hurting	3 Rasping		
4 Aching	4 Splitting		
5 Heavy			

13	14	15	16
1 Fearful	1 Punishing	1 Wretched	1 Annoying
2 Frightful	2 Grueling	2 Blinding	2 Troublesome
3 Terrifying	3 Cruel		3 Miserable
	4 Vicious		4 Intense
	5 Killing		5 Unbearable

17	18	19	20
1 Spreading	1 Tight	1 Cool	1 Nagging
2 Radiating	2 Numb	2 Cold	2 Nauseating
3 Penetrating	3 Drawing	3 Freezing	3 Agonizing
4 Piercing	4 Squeezing		4 Dreadful
	5 Tearing		5 Torturing

FIG. 1-13   McGill Short Form Pain Questionnaire.   *(From Malone TR, McPoil TG, Nitz AJ: Orthopedic and sports physical therapy, ed 3, St Louis, 1997, Mosby; from Melzacker R: The McGill Pain Questionnaire: major properties and scoring methods, Pain 1:277, 1975.)*

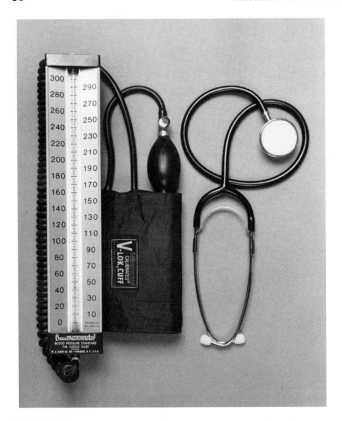

FIG. 1-14 Wall-mounted sphygmomanometer and stethoscope. Most significant heart sounds occur in the frequency range of 200 to 500 Hz, but human auditory sensitivity is limited to those sounds below 1000 Hz. Stethoscopes amplify the lower frequencies.

(Fig. 1-15). The examiner then takes the patient through passive range of motion. In this process, the examiner evaluates the "end-feel" (i.e., springiness) of the joint in question.

ORTHOPEDIC GAMUT 1-13

PASSIVE RANGE OF MOTION

In passive joint motion assessment, the end-feel is important. The accepted end-feel categories are as follows:

1. *Bone-to-bone:* an abrupt halt to movement when two hard surfaces meet
2. *Capsular end feel:* a "leathery" resistance to movement with a slight amount of give at the very end of the range
3. *Springy block:* a usually pathologic end-feel, generally representing an intraarticular displacement
4. *Tissue approximation:* no further joint movement available
5. *Empty feel:* usually pathologic

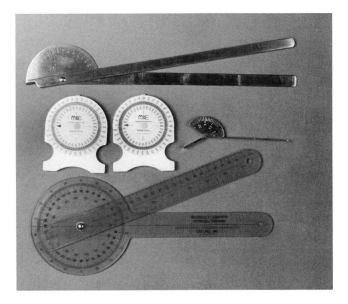

FIG. 1-15 From top to bottom, stainless steel goniometer measures movement of joints from 0 to 180 degrees. Inclinometers measure the angular motion from 0 to 360 degrees. Finger or small joint goniometer measures the movement of interphalangeal joints of fingers and toes. Plastic radiographic goniometer provides standard orthopedic measurements of joint motion and neutral position.

Any movable joint in the body, including the spine, can be tested for range of motion. Range of motion is assessed bilaterally by comparing findings with a given set of normal values. Normal values can vary dramatically depending on the reference source used. An examiner must exercise careful professional judgment to ensure objectivity. Any range of motion that is less than normal may indicate or be the result of muscle spasm, sprain, strain, joint subluxation, general arthritic degeneration, postsurgical condition, or obesity.

STABILITY TESTING

Because clinical examination reveals the degree of ligamentous or joint sprain (Table 1-2), the examiner must be able to test accurately for joint instability. Stability testing moves joint and periarticular structures through arcs and end-range motions. Stability testing involves stressing ligamentous tissues and joint capsules (Fig. 1-16).

MUSCULAR ASSESSMENT

Movement restrictions in a joint's passive range of motion are not exclusively articular. Muscular hypertonicity limits passive movement and often occurs in association with articular lesions (joint dysfunction). Chronic joint problems are also commonly associated with myofascitis.

ORTHOPEDIC GAMUT 1-14

MUSCLE TESTING

When assessing muscle tissue, resisted movements are the most revealing. Standard interpretation of resisted muscle testing movement findings include the following:

1. Painful and strong is equated with a minor lesion of muscle or tendon.

2. Painful and weak equates with a major lesion of the muscle or tendon.

3. Painless and weak equates with neurologic injury or complete rupture of the muscular attachment.

4. Painless and strong is normal.

TABLE 1-2

INJURED LIGAMENT RESIDUAL FUNCTION

Extent of Failure	Sprain	Damage*	Joint Motion, Subluxation	Residual Strength	Residual Functional Length	Residual Functional Capacity
Minimal	First degree	Less than one third of fibers failed; includes most sprains with few to some fibers failed. Microtears also exist.	None	Retained or slightly decreased	Normal	Retained
Partial	Second degree	One-third to two-thirds ligament damage; significant damage, but parts of the ligament are still functional. Microtears may exist.	In general, minimal or no increased motion Remaining fibers in ligament resist opening	Marked decrease At risk for complete failure	Increased, still within functional range but may later act as a check rein rather than subtle control of joint motions	Marked compromise; requires healing to regain function
Complete	Third degree	More than two-thirds to complete failure; continuity remains in part.	Depends on secondary restraints	Little to none	Lost	Severely compromised or lost
		Continuity lost and gross separation between fibers.	Depends on secondary restraints	None	Lost	Lost

From Feagin JA, editor: *The crucial ligaments,* New York, 1988, Churchill Livingstone.

*Estimate of damage is often difficult; however, the different types listed can usually be differentiated. Note: Anterior and posterior cruciate tears commonly exist with little to no abnormal laxity. The examination for medial and lateral ligamentous injury is usually more accurate.

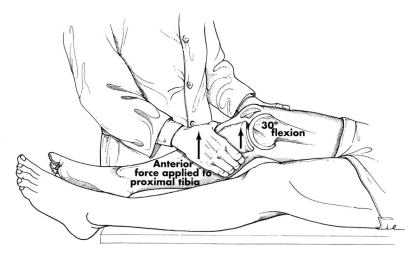

30° flexion

Anterior force applied to proximal tibia

FIG. 1-16   Lachman's test of the anterior cruciate ligament. *(From Scuderi GR, McCann PD, Bruno PJ: Sports medicine: principles of primary care, St Louis, 1997, Mosby.)*

TABLE 1-3

LABORATORY STUDIES USEFUL IN DIAGNOSING LOW BACK SYNDROMES

Test	Measurement	Low Back Implication
Complete Blood Count Hematocrit hemaglobin	A measure of volume of circulating red blood cells	May be diminished in systemic diseases (i.e., neoplasm) and in chronic spinal infections.
White blood count and differential	Amount and type of circulating white blood cells	Total white blood cell and shifts in differential may be present in spinal infections or occasionally in spondyloarthropathies.
Sedimentation Rate	Nonspecific test of inflammation	Increased in spinal infections, may be increased in neoplasms and spondyloarthropathies.
Chemistry Calcium Phosphorus	A measure of circulating calcium and phosphorus	Calcium is elevated in hyperparathyroidism, may be elevated with primary and secondary osseous tumors, alterations in the distribution of calcium and phosphorus accompany many metabolic disorders but are normal in osteoporosis.
Alkaline Phosphatase	Enzyme associated with bone formation; therefore elevation implies increased bone formation	May be elevated in primary or secondary osseous neoplasms.
Acid Phosphatase	An enzyme associated with tumors metastatic to bone	Increased in prostatic tumors.
Serum Proteins (albumin globulin protein electrophoresis) protein	Measurement of amount and type circulating	Elevations of one fraction of globulin is associated with multiple myeloma.
HLA 27-B Antigen	A circulating antigen	Usually individuals with spondyloarthropathies are HLA 27-B positive. Note 6%-8% of males have this antigen and therefore its presence is not confirmatory of a spondyloarthropathy.

Adapted from Pope ML: *Occupational low back pain, assessment, treatment and prevention,* St Louis, 1991, Mosby.

CLINICAL LABORATORY

For the examiner concerned with musculoskeletal disorders, differential diagnosis becomes a challenge. Complete blood and urine tests can help determine a diagnosis. Diseases of the heart, liver, kidney, pancreas, and prostate can mimic back pain of spinal origin.

Most laboratory testing has limited utility for orthopedic diagnosis (Table 1-3). As an example, in rheumatoid arthritis, the diagnosis is often established from the history and physical examination; for systemic lupus erythematosus, from the laboratory test antinuclear antibody (ANA); for gout, from a synovial fluid examination; and for ankylosing spondylitis, from a radiograph. In common disorders such as osteoarthritis, fibromyalgia, or muscular strains and sprains, there is essentially no diagnostic role for laboratory tests except to exclude other diagnostic possibilities.

The simplest orthopedic screen includes rheumatoid factor, ANA, and uric acid, although more elaborate screens are available, which may include erythrocyte sedimentation rate, C-reactive protein, antistreptolysin O titer, protein electrophoresis, quantitative immunoglobulins, and ANA subsets such as anti-Ro and anti-LA, anti-Sm, and anticentromere antibodies.

ORTHOPEDIC GAMUT 1-15

LABORATORY TESTING

For laboratory testing in orthopedic evaluations, results interpretation errors usually involve one of four areas:

1. False-positive results
2. False-negative results
3. Measurement error
4. Differences in groups of patients compared with individual patients

SYNOVIAL FLUID

Normal synovial fluid is a hypocellular, avascular connective tissue. In disease, the synovial fluid increases in volume and can be aspirated. Synovial fluid is a transudate of plasma supplemented with high-molecular-weight, saccharide-rich molecules. The most notable of these is hyaluronans, which is produced by fibroblast-derived type B

BOX 1-3

Normal Synovial Fluid

Osmolarity	296 mOsm/L	Total protein	~25 g/L
pH	7.44	Albumin	~8 g/L
Pco_2	6.0 kPa (range 4.7-7.3)	α_1-antitrypsin	0.78 µg/L
		Ceruloplasmin	~43 mg/L
Po_2	<4.0 kPa	Haptoglobin	~90 mg/L
Potassium	4.0 mmol/L	α_2-macroglobin	0.31 g/L
Sodium	136 mmol/L	Lactoferrin	0.44 mg/L
Calcium	1.8 mmol/L	IgG	2.62 g/L
Urea	2.5 mmol/L	IgA	0.85 g/L
Uric acid	0.23 mmol/L	IgM	0.14 g/L
Glucose	100 mmol/L	IL-1β	20 pg/ml
Chondroitin sulfate	40 mg/L	IL-2	15.1 U/ml
		TNF-α	1.38 hg/ml
Hyaluronate	2.14 g/L	INF-α	350 U/ml
Cholesterol	Small amounts	INF-δ	13.7 U/ml

Adapted from Klippel JH, Dieppe PA: *Rheumatology,* vol 1-2, ed 2, London, 1998, Mosby.
IL, Interleukin; *TNF,* tumor necrosis factor; *INF,* interferon.

synoviocytes (Box 1-3). Variation in the volume and composition of synovial fluid reflects pathologic processes within the joint.

ORTHOPEDIC GAMUT 1-16

ANALYSIS OF SYNOVIAL FLUID

For three significant aspects, analysis of synovial fluid differs from other body fluids:

1. Synovial joints are rarely affected by neoplastic processes.
2. Recognition of noncellular particulate material, such as microorganisms and crystals and cartilage fragments, is essential for defining the disease process affecting the joint.
3. Diagnostic information comes not only from recognition of cell types but also from their quantification.

ORTHOPEDIC TESTS

Orthopedic tests are positive, or a sign is present, when the procedure duplicates the patient's complaint or symptom. Tests are based on joint, muscle, or nerve function. If testing causes different pain or symptoms, it may indeed be significant, but the result is not positive for the findings the test was designed to elicit. A subjective complaint, when

consistent with an objective finding, becomes another objective finding.

During an examination, the examiner must use techniques that defeat the human tendency of exaggeration. The examiner must conduct many tests so that the patient is not aware of which specific tissue function is being examined. With time and exposure to myriad orthopedic disorders, examiners develop the skill and accuracy necessary to reach diagnoses efficiently. However, interpreting the results of examination processes in a clinically meaningful way requires the examiner to consider the reliability of the clinical measurements and tests.

Interpretation and analysis of examination procedures depend not only on the reliability and validity of such measures but also on the sensitivity and specificity of the "signs" elicited by the test procedures.

DIAGNOSTIC IMAGING MODALITIES IN ORTHOPEDICS

Diagnostic imaging procedures are important to the diagnosis and management of an orthopedic condition. The decision to use any diagnostic imaging procedure, especially ionizing imaging procedures, should be based on a demonstrated need and should be used only after an adequate medical history is obtained and a physical examination conducted. The decision to use any imaging procedure must also be based on the assumption that the results of the examination, even if negative, will significantly affect the treatment of the patient. The value of the information gained from the imaging examination must be worth the possible detrimental effects of the procedure. In imaging modalities that use ionizing radiation (plain film radiography, fluoroscopy, and computed tomography [CT]), the possible effect of radiation on the patient or future offspring must be considered (Fig. 1-17).

Plain Film Radiography (Conventional Radiography)

Plain film radiography, or conventional radiography, provides a wide and diverse array of diagnostic data about musculoskeletal problems, such as soft-tissue injury, bony malalignment, loss of integrity of the osseous structures, and joint space abnormality.

Plain film x-ray examination is an efficient way to discover dislocations, fractures, the static component of anatomic subluxations, certain types of stress injuries, metastatic disease, some types of primary tumors, metabolic disease, degenerative arthropathic diseases (Table 1-4), and abnormalities in the growth plate.

Soft-tissue structures require careful scrutiny on film because they may offer subtle clues to serious or underlying pathologic abnormalities.

A radiologic evaluation of the traumatized sites should include films of the adjacent joints. If there is a need for

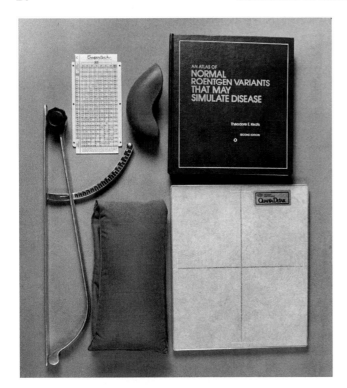

FIG. 1-17   From left to right and top to bottom, Supertech x-ray factoring computer, gonadal shielding, *An atlas of normal roentgen variants that may simulate disease* (by Theodore E. Keats), radiographic calipers, sandbag, DuPont Quanta Detail Rare Earth x-ray cassette screens and compatible film.

ORTHOPEDIC GAMUT 1-17

ASSESSMENT ABILITIES OF PLAIN FILM RADIOGRAPHY

1. Plain film radiography is the least expensive and most widely available imaging technique.
2. Radiography offers higher spatial resolution than any other modality, providing extremely high contrast for cortical and trabecular bone.
3. Radiography affords only a projectional viewing perspective.
4. Projection of three-dimensional anatomy onto a two-dimensional film results in morphologic distortion and superimposition of overlapping structures.
5. The sensitivity for trabecular bone loss is relatively poor.
6. As much as 30% to 50% of trabecular bone must be removed before the change becomes perceptible on conventional radiographs.
7. The contrast for soft tissues that are not calcified or fatty is relatively poor.
8. Radiography cannot directly visualize the articular cartilage, inflamed synovial tissue, joint effusion, bone marrow edema, or intraarticular fat pads.

TABLE 1-4

PLAIN FILM EVALUATION IN DEGENERATIVE ARTHROPATHIC DISORDERS

Diagnosis	Site of Plain Film Findings
Psoriatic arthritis	Hand, sacroiliac joints (common); pubis symphysis, hip, knee (less common)
Rheumatoid arthritis	Wrist and hand, shoulder, knee, cervical spine, hip
Spondyloarthropathy	Sacroiliac joints, thoracolumbar spine
Osteoarthritis	Lumbosacral spine, hip, knee, foot and ankle, hand

special projections, other radiologic investigation may be necessary (Table 1-5).

Care must be taken to investigate the possibility of associated injuries in trauma victims (Table 1-6). Patients may not realize that such injuries have occurred.

The patient's history and clinical evaluation are guides that help determine which portion(s) of the body should be radiographed and how many different views should be produced (Fig. 1-18).

Tomography

Conventional tomography is also known as *thin section radiography, planigraphy,* and *linear tomography.* Conventional tomography is largely replaced by CT. However, some circumstances, such as evaluating subtle alterations of bone density and ruling out fracture, necessitate conventional tomography. CT scans are used for more detailed appreciation of skeletal pathologic processes, which can help evaluate suspected intervertebral disc protrusions or herniations, facet disease, or central canal and lateral recess stenosis. If spinal disease is suspected and is not well identified on plain films and the patient is not responding to care, a CT scan is indicated. A CT scan is especially useful for the appreciation of bone and calcifications and surpasses magnetic resonance imaging (MRI) in this regard.

CT has been useful in a wide variety of musculoskeletal disorders, including those related to trauma (Fig. 1-19), back pain (e.g., herniated nucleus pulposus) (Fig. 1-20), and metabolic bone disease (e.g., osteoporosis, tumor [e.g., soft-tissue masses]).

Clinicians may use the noninvasive technique of quantitative CT to measure bone mineral density.

TABLE 1-5

PREFERRED RADIOGRAPHIC VIEWS IN SKELETAL TRAUMA

Area	Specific Views	Area	Specific Views
Skull	Posteroanterior or anteroposterior Caldwell	Sternum, sterno-clavicular joints	Posteroanterior
	Townes		Right and left anterior obliques with cephalad angle of tube
	Lateral (one lateral should be upright)		Lateral
Facial bones	Waters	Elbow	Anteroposterior
	Modified Waters		Lateral
	Caldwell		Capitellum
	Lateral	Radioulnar joints (forearm)	Anteroposterior or posteroanterior
Cervical spine	Anteroposterior		Lateral
	Coned odontoid or orthopantogram	Wrist and hand	Posteroanterior
	Odontoid		Oblique internal, external, or both
	Lateral (cross-table or upright)		Lateral
	Swimmer's lateral (cross-table)		Navicular views, if needed
	Both obliques, when possible	Pelvis, acetabulum	Anteroposterior
Thoracic spine	Anteroposterior		Obliques (Judet)
	Lateral (cross-table or routine)	Hip, proximal part of femur	Anteroposterior pelvis
	Swimmer's (coned to upper thoracic spine)		Frog-leg or cross-table lateral
Lumbar spine	Anteroposterior		Obliques
	Lateral (cross-table or upright)	Femur	Anteroposterior (to include hip and knee)
	Lateral (coned to L5-S1)		Lateral (to include hip and knee)
Sacrum	Anteroposterior (tube-angled cephalad)	Distal part of femur and knee	Anteroposterior
	Lateral		Lateral
Chest	Posteroanterior or anteroposterior		Tunnel
	Left lateral (may not be possible in trauma)		Internal oblique
	Lateral decubitus (pneumothorax, pleural fluid)	Tibia, fibula	Anteroposterior (to include ankle and knee)
Ribs	Anteroposterior or posteroanterior		Lateral (to include both joints)
	Oblique	Ankle	Anteroposterior
Shoulder	Anteroposterior (internal rotation)		Oblique (mortise)
	Anteroposterior (neutral)		Lateral
	Transscapular lateral (Neer)	Calcaneus	Tangential
	Axillary		Lateral
Humerus	Anteroposterior (to include elbow and shoulder)	Foot	Lateral
	Lateral (to include both joints)		Anteroposterior
Clavicle	Anteroposterior or posteroanterior (to include both joints with and without weight bearing)		Oblique
			Lateral

From Gustilo RB, Kyle RF, Templeman DC: *Fractures and dislocations,* vol 1, St Louis, 1993, Mosby.

TABLE 1-6

INJURIES ASSOCIATED WITH SKELETAL TRAUMA

Fracture	Associated Injury	Fracture	Associated Injury
Bone and bone		**Bone and vascular**	
Spine	Remote additional spinal fracture	Ribs 1, 2, or 3	Ruptured aorta
Chest wall	Scapula fracture	Sternum	Myocardial contusion
Anterior pelvic arch	Sacrum fracture or dislocated sacroiliac joint	Pelvis	Laceration of pelvic arterial tree
Femoral shaft	Fracture or fracture-dislocation of hip	Distal third femur	Laceration of femoral artery
Tibia (severe)	Dislocated hip	Knee dislocation	Popliteal artery laceration
Calcaneus	Fractured thoracolumbar spine		
Bone and viscera			
Chance fracture of spine	Ruptured mesentery or small bowel		
Lower ribs	Laceration of liver, spleen, kidney, or diaphragm		
Pelvis	Ruptured bladder or urethra		
Pelvis	Ruptured diaphragm		

Adapted from Rogers LF, Hendrix RW: Evaluating the multiple injured patient radiographically, *Orthop Clin North Am* 21(3):444, 1990.

ORTHOPEDIC GAMUT 1-18

ASSESSMENT ABILITIES OF COMPUTED TOMOGRAPHY

1. The greatest advantage of CT over conventional radiography is its tomographic nature.
2. CT provides high contrast between bone and adjacent tissues and is excellent for evaluating osseous structures.
3. CT offers slightly greater soft-tissue contrast than does radiography.
4. Image contrast is insufficient to visualize the articular cartilage or synovial tissue or to discriminate between tendonitis and tendon rupture.
5. CT reveals only the surfaces of these structures; it does not disclose intrasubstance changes that may precede gross morphologic disruption.

Discography

Although effective, discography has been a controversial imaging modality for spinal disc disease. Clinicians use discography for specific cases of spinal pain that are recalcitrant to conventional therapy.

ORTHOPEDIC GAMUT 1-19

DISCOGRAPHY

Discography is used to do the following:

1. Rule out disc involvement, especially as a cause of postoperative pain
2. Determine the appropriate level for spinal fusion
3. Test the potential effectiveness of chemonucleolysis
4. Visualize internal disc anatomy

Magnetic Resonance Imaging

MRI is a computerized, thin-section imaging procedure that uses a magnetic field and radio frequency waves rather than ionizing radiation. MRI can produce thin-section images in the sagittal, coronal, or axial planes, as well as any other oblique plane desired. The MRI can image neurologic structures and other soft tissues and can reveal disc degeneration before any other imaging method. Indications for MRI are similar to those for CT. MRI is superior for the evaluation of suspected spinal cord tumors or damage, intracranial disease, and various types of central nervous system disease (e.g., multiple sclerosis). MRI is especially useful in the identification of small differences among similar soft tissues and surpasses CT in this regard.

For patients who have sustained head trauma with skull fractures, MRI is an efficient way to identify the early signs of cerebral edema. The test procedure of choice for diagnosing metastatic disease is an MRI scan (Table 1-7).

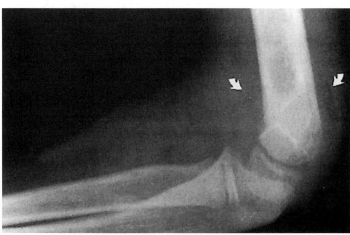

FIG. 1-18   Displacement of fat pads in the elbow by joint effusion.   *(From Klippel JH, Dieppe PA:* Rheumatology, *vol 1-2, ed 2, London, 1998, Mosby.)*

ORTHOPEDIC GAMUT 1-20

MAGNETIC RESONANCE IMAGING

For certain pathologic conditions, MRI is the diagnostic procedure of choice:

1. Spinal disc disease
2. Medullary tumor
3. Multiple sclerosis
4. Cerebral edema
5. Spinal stenosis
6. Metastatic disease
7. Herniated disc
8. Discitis (or infection)
9. Meniscal tear (fibrocartilage abnormalities)
10. Central nervous system tumor
11. Soft-tissue tumor

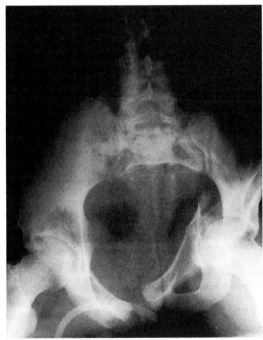

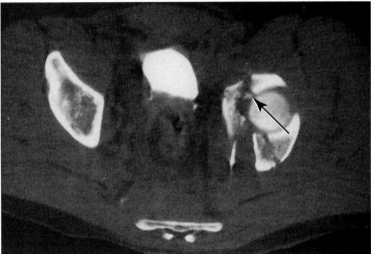

FIG. 1-19   Complex acetabular fracture. **A,** Anteroposterior plain film. **B,** Axial computed tomography scan. *(From Gustilo RB, Kyle RF, Templeman DC:* Fractures and dislocations, *vol 1, St Louis, 1993, Mosby.)*

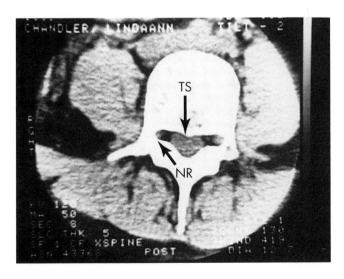

FIG. 1-20   Axial image showing a right paracentral herniation of the nucleus pulposus. *(From Brier SR:* Primary care orthopedics, *St Louis, Mosby, 1999.)*

TABLE 1-7

MAGNETIC RESONANCE IMAGING VERSUS COMPUTED TOMOGRAPHY

Anatomic Area	Indications	Recommended Procedure	Anatomic Area	Indications	Recommended Procedure
Brain (including brainstem)	Initial evaluation (e.g., demyelination disease seizures)	MRI	Musculo-skeletal spine (cont'd)	Lower back or radicular pain in older person	MRI or CT*
	Previous normal CT	MRI		Cervical disk disease	MRI
	Previous abnormal CT	CT or MRI*		Spinal stenosis	
	Unchanged abnormal CT with increase in symptoms	MRI		Cervical	MRI
				Lumbar	CT or MRI*
	Contrast allergy	MRI		Tumors	MRI
	Acute trauma	CT		Metastatic disease	MRI
	Pituitary tumors	MRI	Hips	Early detection of aseptic necrosis	MRI
Ear, nose, throat, and eye	Neurosensory hearing loss (e.g., to rule out acoustic neuroma)	CT		Congenital hip dislocation or reduction	US
	Conductive hearing loss	CT	Extremities	Tumors, disease, or injury to muscle, ligaments, or cartilage	MRI
	Cancer staging (including laryngeal cancer)	MRI or CT*			
	Cholesteatoma of temporal bone	CT		Confirmation of calcification or fracture	CT
	Fractures of facial bones	CT	Chest	Diseases of the hila	MRI
	Thyroid or parathyroid dysfunction (after US)	MRI		Diseases of the mediastinum	MRI or CT*
				Lung disease	CT
	Sinus conditions	CT or MRI*	Abdomen and pelvis	General survey (e.g., to rule out tumor)	CT
	Orbital disease	MRI or CT*		Liver disease	CT or MRI*
	Disease of optic tracts and chiasm	MRI		Renal cell cancer staging	MRI
				Prostate disease	MRI, CT, or US
	Internal derangement of temporomandibular joint	MRI		Bladder disease	MRI or CT
				Abdominal aortic aneurysm	MRI
Musculoskel-etal spine	Lower back or radicular pain in younger person	MRI		Other	*

From Brier SR: *Primary care orthopedics,* St Louis, 1999, Mosby; originally courtesy of Robert Goodman, MD, South Suffolk MRI, PC, Bayshore, New York.
CT, Computed tomography; *MRI,* magnetic resonance imaging; *US,* ultrasonography.
*Consult radiologist for imaging options.

ORTHOPEDIC GAMUT 1-21

ASSESSMENT ABILITIES OF MAGNETIC RESONANCE IMAGING

1. Diarthrodial joints are particularly suitable for MRI.
2. MRI is unparalleled in its ability to depict soft-tissue detail.
3. MRI is the only modality that can examine all components of the joint simultaneously.

Contrast Arthrography

The conventional use of arthrography in musculoskeletal disease involves the use of air to distend a synovial joint and a radiopaque contrast agent to outline anatomic structures. The injection of contrast material into the joint space results in a radiographic outline of the cartilage, menisci, ligaments, or synovium. Conventional arthrography is used in diagnosis of the scope and magnitude of orthopedic trauma to the shoulder, wrist, knee, and ankle (Table 1-8).

Radionuclide Scanning

Examinations conducted with the use of nuclear medicine techniques, including bone scans, positron emission tomography (PET) scans, and single-photon emission computed tomography (SPECT) scans, are valuable in diagnostic imaging because of their highly sensitive and non-invasive nature. Whole-body scanning for metastatic and infectious diseases, as well as inflammatory and ischemic processes, is possible with scintigraphy (Fig. 1-21).

Highly active individuals (e.g., competitive athletes) are prime candidates for bone scanning when the diagnosis is uncertain. A bone scan may show increased uptake of the radioactive isotope consistent with a stress fracture (Fig. 1-22).

Bone scanning has become common in the evaluation of child abuse. Very young children typically do not develop stress fractures of multiple fracture sites in normal living situations (Fig. 1-23).

Video Fluoroscopy

Video fluoroscopy is used when a function study of the joint is warranted. Video fluoroscopy should be used when a

ORTHOPEDIC GAMUT 1-22

ASSESSMENT ABILITIES OF RADIONUCLIDE SCANNING

1. The principal advantage of scintigraphy over other imaging modalities is its ability to identify tissues or organs with abnormal physiologic or biochemical properties.

2. Increased skeletal uptake can be seen at sites of elevated blood flow or increased bone metabolism.
3. Scintigraphy is a convenient way of surveying the entire skeleton for multifocal processes.

TABLE 1-8

JOINTS TYPICALLY STUDIED WITH COMPUTED TOMOGRAPHIC ARTHROGRAPHY FOLLOWING TRAUMA

Joint	To Observe
Knee	Meniscus, cruciate and collateral ligaments, hyaline cartilage tears, osteochondral defects
Shoulder	Rotator cuff, glenoid labrum disruption
Hip	Hyaline cartilage integrity and tears, prosthetic joint loosening
Wrist	Triangular fibrocartilage, intercarpal ligament integrity
Elbow	Hyaline cartilage integrity, osteochondral defects
Ankle	Ligamentous tears, osteochondral defects
Temporomandibular	Disc and condylar integrity

Adapted from Gustilo RB, Kyle RF, Templeman DC: *Fractures and dislocations,* vol 1, St Louis, 1993, Mosby.

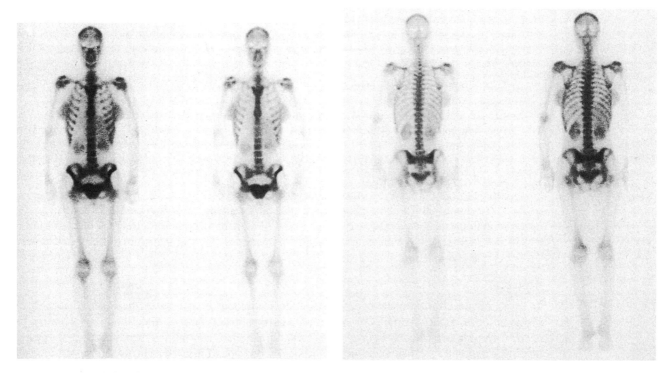

FIG. 1-21   Normal bone scans.   *(From Early PJ, Sodel DB:* Principles and practice of nuclear medicine, *St Louis, 1995, Mosby.)*

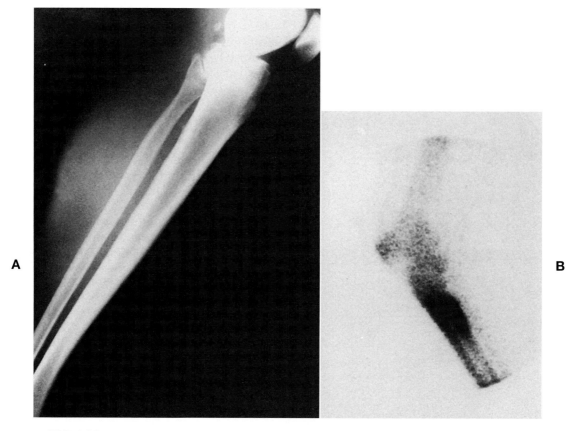

FIG. 1-22   Radiographic film **(A)** and bone scan **(B)** demonstrating stress fracture.   *(From Nicholas JA, Hershman EB:* The lower extremity and spine in sports medicine, *ed 4, St Louis, 1995, Mosby.)*

biomechanical abnormality is present but is not adequately demonstrated by plain film stress surveys or other examination methods.

Diagnostic Ultrasound

Diagnostic ultrasound, a sound wave echo study, is particularly useful for the evaluation of soft tissues. The diagnostic ultrasound does not provide the same quality of image as CT or MRI.

Diagnostic ultrasound requires high-resolution equipment, including a high-frequency transducer. Diagnostic ultrasound performs well in the detection of rotator cuff tears and other tendon abnormalities, as well as in the identification of some metabolic disease. In cases of suspected pediatric hip disease, diagnostic ultrasound is the recommended primary imaging technique.

Myelography

Traditional myelographic techniques involve the introduction of small amounts of water-soluble contrast medium into the subarachnoid space, either through a lumbar approach below the level of the conus medullaris or at the level of C1-C2 through a posterolateral approach. Standard films of the spinal canal are made to determine the presence or absence of a filling defect. In cases of acute spinal trauma, myelography may be used in conjunction with CT (Fig. 1-24). Myelography remains valuable in the evaluation

of intrinsic spinal cord lesions, nerve root lesions, and dural tears associated with severe trauma (Box 1-4).

Thermography

Using temperature differentials in the body, thermography illustrates nerve fiber involvement in injury or disease. Thermograms do not provide specific information regarding the cause of nerve fiber irritation. In addition, they cannot

---

ORTHOPEDIC GAMUT 1-23

ASSESSMENT ABILITIES OF ULTRASONOGRAPHY

1. Ultrasonography offers direct multiplanar tomography without any need for image reformatting.
2. Ultrasonography can also provide images in real time, without any exposure to ionizing radiation.
3. The modality is inexpensive and widely available.
4. Ultrasonography offers relatively good soft-tissue contrast and is particularly effective at identifying fluid collections such as bursitis and abscesses.
5. Ultrasound waves cannot penetrate bone.

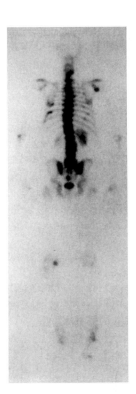 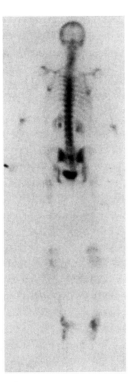

A   **B**

FIG. 1-23 **A,** Whole-body scintigraphy. **B,** Normal bone scan is shown for comparison. *(From Klippel JH, Dieppe PA: Rheumatology, vol 1-2, ed 2, London, 1998, Mosby.)*

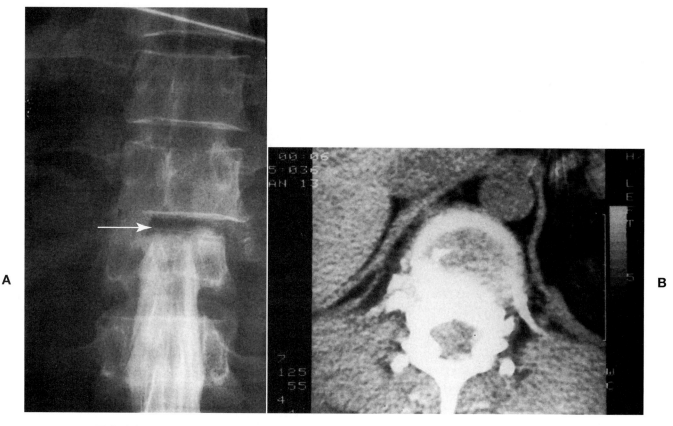

FIG. 1-24   Lumbar myelogram **(A)**, with computed tomography axial image **(B)** through the T12 body.   *(From Gustilo RB, Kyle RF: Fractures and dislocations, vol 1, St Louis, 1993, Mosby.)*

BOX 1-4

Strengths and Limitations of Myelographic Studies

Strengths
Studies of the subarachnoid space are possible.
Intraarachnoid lesions are shown.
Demarcation of multidisc levels is shown.
Information on surgical scars is provided.
Assessment of flexion and extension dynamic are possible.

Limitations
Lesions removed from outside of the thecal sac can be missed.
Study variations are problematic.
Detail shown in the dorsal spine is poor.
Postoperative studies are impossible to read with accuracy.
Testing procedure is invasive.

From Brier SR: *Primary care orthopedics,* St Louis, 1999, Mosby.

differentiate between cervical causes of neural pain (e.g., herniated disc, scar tissue, or muscle spasm).

Reflex sympathetic dystrophy is part of a spectrum of sympathetically mediated pain syndromes that usually occur in an extremity after a seemingly minor injury or surgical procedure.

ELECTRODIAGNOSTIC TESTING

Although electrodiagnostic testing provides valuable information, it does not stand alone as a diagnostic entity (Table 1-9). The data obtained must be correlated with the physical examination findings and case history.

With surface measurement of motor nerve conduction, velocity provides a valuable ancillary procedure in the diagnosis of various peripheral nerve lesions in both the upper and lower extremities. This form of testing involves stimulating a peripheral nerve at two separate positions along its course and recording the action potentials observed on an oscilloscopic screen. Slow conduction times indicate nerve entrapment syndromes across the point at which the impulses are delayed.

ORTHOPEDIC GAMUT 1-24

ASSESSMENT ABILITIES OF THERMOGRAPHY

1. The thermographic examination is conducted with the use of contact liquid crystal detectors or electronic infrared sensors.
2. Thermography is extremely sensitive to microvascular changes in the skin.
3. Thermography is excellent for differentiating between a neurologic and vascular abnormality.

4. Thermography has a greater degree of sensitivity in documenting neurovascular abnormality than any other imaging system.
5. Thermography has a greater degree of specificity of image than radionuclide bone scan.
6. Thermography has a lesser degree of specificity of image resolution than CT or MRI.

TABLE 1-9

STRENGTHS AND LIMITATIONS OF ELECTRODIAGNOSTIC TESTING

Testing Modality	Strengths	Limitations
Nerve conduction velocity	Helpful in ruling out peripheral entrapment neuropathic conditions (e.g., prolonged latencies exhibited in carpal tunnel syndrome, tarsal tunnel syndrome) and ulnar neuropathic variations	Provides imperfect sensitivity; limited localization and determination of injury severity; timing of study is an important factor
F waves	Provides screening for late motor response with distal sweeps starting at the foot	Evaluates motor reflex only; possibly evaluates abnormal findings only in the presence of multiple-level injury
H reflex	Equivalent of ankle joint reflex; evaluates monosynaptic reflex with sensory and motor S1 function	Provides assessment of S1 nerve root only
SSEPs	Helpful in documenting sensory pathway disturbances in proximal neural injury and central conduction delays, as in myopathies and multiple sclerosis	Offers imperfect localization; findings are rarely abnormal if results of other electrodiagnostic tests are within normal limits
Needle EMG	Useful in assessing conductivity of neural tissues; helpful in determining site and severity of lesion; may be helpful in early assessment of recovery, screening for fibrillation potentials, and signs of denervation from nerve root compression disorders	Unable to detect denervation potentials for 14-28 days after injury; provides imperfect sensitivity; study timing is an important factor; proximal lesions are sometimes inaccessible anatomically; effectiveness is reduced after surgery

Adapted from Brier SR: *Primary care orthopedics,* St Louis, 1999, Mosby.
SSEPs, Somatosensory-evoked potentials; *EMG,* electromyography.

The electrical responses of nervous system sensory tracks are known as *somatosensory-evoked potentials* (SSEPs). SSEPs are useful in the evaluation of various pathologic variations from the peripheral nerve through the spinal cord to the somatosensory region of the brain. SSEPs are used to assess diseases of the spinal cord, trauma to the spine, neuromuscular disease, and demyelinating disorders.

Using needle electrodes, needle electromyography (EMG) is widely used to diagnose nerve root lesions at the level of the spine. It also is used to differentiate a central spinal lesion from a peripheral neuropathic condition. Results of the procedure are accurate in differentiating disease of a neuromuscular origin.

DOPPLER ULTRASONIC VASCULAR TESTING

Doppler vascular testing allows the assessment of pulses in noisy environments or when pulses are weak. This is also efficient when palpation of a pulse is questionable or not possible. The Doppler instrument also aids in the assessment of circulation distal to fracture sites, burns, and other injuries that potentially compromise vascular tissue. The Doppler instrument can aid in the quick determination of the extent of injury (Fig. 1-25).

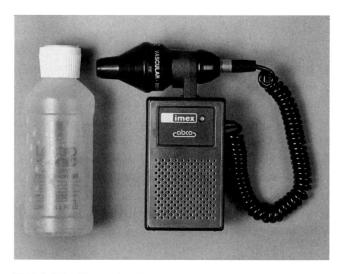

FIG. 1-25   The pocket Doppler *(right)* audibly monitors pulses in noisy environments when palpation is questionable or not possible or when the pulse is especially weak or rapid. The Doppler also aids in the assessment of circulation distal to fractures, burns, and other injuries to quickly determine the extent of injury. Transmission gel *(left)* is used to couple the Doppler head to the skin surface and eliminate air gaps that can degrade sound transmission.

BIBLIOGRAPHY

American Medical Association: *Guides to the evaluation of permanent impairment,* ed 4, Chicago, 1993, American Medical Association.

Anderson KN, Anderson LE: *Mosby's pocket dictionary of medicine, nursing, & allied health,* ed 2, St Louis, 1994, Mosby.

Ballou SP, Kushner I: C-reactive protein and the acute phase response, *Adv Intern Med* 37:313, 1992.

Barkauskas VH, Stoltenberg-Allen K, Baumann LC, Darling-Fisher C: *Health & physical assessment,* ed 2, St Louis, 1998, Mosby.

Bechman H, Markakis K, Suchman A, Frankel R: Getting the most from a 20 minute visit, *Am J Gastroenterol* 89:662, 1994.

Bogduk N, Aprill C, Derby R: Discography. In White AH, Schofferman JA, editors: *Spine care,* vol 1, St Louis, 1995, Mosby.

Brier SR: *Primary care orthopedics,* St Louis, 1999, Mosby.

Bushong SC: *Radiologic science for technologist: physics, biology, and protection,* ed 5, St Louis, 1993, Mosby.

Canale T: *Campbell's operative orthopaedics,* vol 1-4, ed 9, St Louis, 1998, Mosby.

Cardinal E, Lafortune M, Burns P: Power Doppler US in synovitis: reality or artifact? *Radiology* 200:868, 1996.

Chandnani VP, et al: Knee hyaline cartilage evaluated with MR imaging: a cadaveric study involving multiple imaging sequences and intraarticular injection of gadolinium and saline solution, *Radiology* 178:557, 1991.

Cipriano JJ: *Photographic manual of regional orthopaedic and neurological test,* ed 3, Baltimore, 1997, Williams & Wilkins.

Conwell TD: *Documenting patient progress "daily office charting seminar" thorough accurate quick procedures,* ed 11, Lakewood, Colo, 1990, Clinical Advancement Plus Seminars.

Dambro MR, Griffith JA: *Griffith's 5 minute clinical consult,* Baltimore, 1997, Williams & Wilkins.

Datz FL: *Handbook of nuclear medicine,* ed 2, St Louis, 1993, Mosby.

Delitto A, Snyder-Mackler L: The diagnostic process: examples in orthopedic physical therapy, *Phys Ther* 75:203, 1995.

Dickenson AH: Spinal cord pharmacology of pain, *Br J Anaesth* 75:193, 1995.

Disler DG, et al: Fat-suppressed three-dimensional spoiled gradient-echo MR imaging of hyaline cartilage defects in the knee: comparison with standard MR imaging and arthroscopy, *AJR* 167:127, 1996.

Doherty M: *Color atlas and text of osteoarthritis,* London, 1994, Wolfe.

Doherty M, Doherty J: *Clinical examination in rheumatology,* London, 1992, Wolfe.

Doherty M, George E: *Self-assessment picture tests in rheumatology,* London, 1995, Mosby-Wolfe.

Dray A: Inflammatory mediators of pain, *Br J Anaesth* 75:125, 1995.

Early PJ, Sodee DB: *Principles and practice of nuclear medicine,* St Louis, 1995, Mosby.

Epstein O, Perkin GD, deBono DP, Cookson J: *Clinical examination,* ed 2, London, 1997, Mosby.

Feldmann E: *Current diagnosis in neurology,* St Louis, 1994, Mosby.

Freemont AJ, Denton J: *Atlas of synovial fluid cytopathology,* vol 18, Dordrecht, 1991, Kluwer Academic.

Freemont FJ, et al: The diagnostic value of synovial fluid cytoanalysis: a reassessment, *Ann Rheum Dis* 50:101, 1991.

Goldie BS: *Orthopaedic diagnosis and management a guide to the care of orthopaedic patients,* ed 2, Oxford, 1998, ISIS Medical Media.

Greenstein GM: *Clinical assessment of neuromusculoskeletal disorders,* St Louis, 1997, Mosby.

Gustilo RB, Kyle RF, Templeman DC: *Fractures and dislocations,* vol 1, St Louis, 1993, Mosby.

Haack E, Tkach J: Fast MR imaging: techniques and clinical applications, *AJR* 155:951, 1990.

Hall LD, Tyler JA: Can quantitative magnetic resonance imaging detect and monitor the progression of early osteoarthritis? In Kuetner KE, Goldberg VM, editors: *Osteoarthritic disorders,* Rosemont, Ill, 1995, American Academy of Orthopaedic Surgeons.

Hartley A: *Practical joint assessment lower quadrant,* ed 2, St Louis, 1995, Mosby.

Hawkins RJ: *An organized approach to musculoskeletal examination and history taking,* St Louis, 1995, Mosby.

Hayes KW, Petersen C, Falconer J: An examination of Cyriax's passive motion tests with patients having osteoarthritis of the knee, *Phys Ther* 74:697, 1994.

Herndon WA: Acute and chronic injury: its effect on growth in the young athlete. In Frana WA, et al, editors: *Advances in sports medicine fitness,* vol 3, Chicago, 1990, Year-Book Medical.

Hinkle CZ: *Fundamentals of anatomy & movement a workbook and guide,* St Louis, 1997, Mosby.

Jablonski S: *Dictionary of medical acronyms & abbreviations,* ed 3, Philadelphia, 1998, Hanley & Belfus.

Jones MA: Clinical reasoning in manual therapy, *Phys Ther* 72:875, 1992.

Katirji B: *Electromyography in clinical practice a case study approach,* St Louis, 1998, Mosby.

Kessler RM, Herling D: Assessment of musculoskeletal disorders. In Kessler RM, Herling D, editors: *Management of common musculoskeletal disorders,* ed 2, Philadelphia, 1990, JB Lippincott.

Kettenbach G: *Writing s.o.a.p. notes,* Philadelphia, 1990, FA Davis.

Klippel JH, Dieppe PA: *Rheumatology,* vol 1-2, ed 2, London, 1998, Mosby.

Konowitz KB: Reflex sympathy dystrophy syndrome sometimes misdiagnosed, often misunderstood, *J Am Chiro Assoc* 35:58, 1998.

Lewis CB, Knortz KA: *Orthopedic assessment and treatment of the geriatric patient,* St Louis, 1993, Mosby.

Magee DJ: *Orthopedic physical assessment,* ed 3, Philadelphia, 1997, WB Saunders.

Maher C, Adams R: Reliability of pain and stiffness assessments in clinical manual lumbar spine examination, *Phys Ther* 74:801, 1994.

Malone TR, McPoil TG, Nitz AJ: *Orthopedic and sports physical therapy,* ed 3, St Louis, 1997, Mosby.

McKinnis LN: Fundamentals of radiology for physical therapists. In Richardson JK, Iglarsh ZA, editors: *Clinical orthopedic physical therapy,* Philadelphia, 1994, WB Saunders.

McRae R: *Clinical orthopaedic examination,* ed 3, Edinburgh, 1990, Churchill Livingstone.

Mengel MB, Schwiebert LP: *Ambulatory medicine the primary care of families,* ed 2, Stamford, Conn, 1996, Appleton & Lange.

Mennell JM: *The musculoskeletal system differential diagnosis from symptoms and physical signs,* Gaithersburg, Md, 1992, Aspen.

Mercier LR, Pettid FJ: *Practical orthopedics,* ed 5, St Louis, 2000, Mosby.

Micheli LJ: Reflex sympathetic dystrophy may stem from sports (news brief), *Physician Sports Med* 18:35, 1990.

Middleton GD, McFarlin JE, Lipsky PE: Prevalence and clinical impact of fibromyalgia in systemic lupus erythematous, *Arthritis Rheum* 8:1181, 1994.

Mosby-Year Book, Inc: *Expert 10-minute physical examination,* St Louis, 1997, Mosby.

Nardone DA, et al: A model for the diagnostic medical interview: nonverbal, verbal and cognitive assessments, *J Gen Intern Med* 7:437, 1992.

Nettina SM: *The Lippincott manual of nursing practice,* ed 6, Philadelphia, 1996, Lippincott.

Newman JS, Laing TJ, McCarthy CJ, Adler RS: Power Doppler sonography of synovitis: assessment of therapeutic response—preliminary observations, *Radiology* 198:582, 1996.

Pagana KD, Pagana TJ: *Mosby's manual of diagnostic and laboratory tests,* St Louis, 1998, Mosby.

Peterfy CG, Genant HK: Emerging applications of magnetic resonance imaging for evaluating the articular cartilage, *Radiol Clin North Am* 34:195, 1996.

Peterfy CG, et al: MR imaging of the arthritic knee: improved discrimination of cartilage, synovium and effusion with pulsed saturation transfer and fat-suppressed T1-weighted sequences, *Radiology* 191:413, 1994.

Raspe HH: Back pain. In Silman AJ, Hochberg M, editors: *Epidemiology of the rheumatic diseases,* Oxford, 1993, Oxford University Press.

Ravel R: *Clinical laboratory medicine clinical application of laboratory data,* ed 6, St Louis, 1995, Mosby.

Rogers LF, Hendrix RW: Evaluating the multiple injured patients radiographically, *Orthop Clin North Am* 21:437, 1990.

Saidoff DC, McDonough AL: *Critical pathways in therapeutic intervention: lower extremity,* St Louis, 1997, Mosby.

St. Claire SM: Diagnosis and treatment of fibromyalgia syndrome, *J Neuromusc Syst* 2:3, 1994.

Schumacher HR, Klippel JH, Koopman WJ: *Primer on the rheumatic diseases,* ed 10, Atlanta, 1993, Arthritis Foundation.

Shankman GA: *Fundamental orthopedic management for the physical therapist assistant,* St Louis, 1997, Mosby.

Smith RC, Hoppe RB: The patient's story: integrating the patient and physician centered approaches to interviewing, *Ann Intern Med* 115:470, 1991.

Stamford JA: Descending control of pain, *Br J Anaesth* 75:217, 1995.

Sugimoto H, Takeda A, Masuyama J, Furuse M: Early-stage rheumatoid arthritis: diagnostic accuracy of MR imaging, *Radiology* 198:185, 1996.

Tamai K, Yamato M, Yamaguchi T, Ohno W: Dynamic magnetic resonance imaging for the evaluation of synovitis in patients with rheumatoid arthritis, *Arthritis Rheum* 37:1151, 1994.

Thibodeau GA, Patton KT: *Pocket reference to accompany anatomy & physiology,* ed 3, St Louis, 1996, Mosby.

Thompson JM: *Clinical outlines for health assessment,* St Louis, 1997, Mosby.

Toghill PJ: *Examining patients an introduction to clinical medicine,* London, 1990, Edward Arnold.

Torg JS, Shepard RJ: *Current therapy in sports medicine,* ed 3, St Louis, 1995, Mosby.

Weinstein SL, Buckwalter JA: *Turek's orthopaedics principles and their application,* ed 5, Philadelphia, 1994, JB Lippincott.

White KP, Speechley M, Harth M, Ostbye T: Fibromyalgia in rheumatology practice: a survey of Canadian rheumatologists, *J Rheumatol* 22:722, 1995.

Wolfe F, et al: The prevalence and characteristics of fibromyalgia in the general population, *Arthritis Rheum* 38:19, 1995.

Woolf CJ: Somatic pain-pathogenesis and prevention, *Br J Anaesth* 75:169, 1995.

Zatouroff M: *Diagnosis in color physical signs in general medicine,* ed 2, London, 1996, Mosby-Wolfe.

Zitelli BJ, Davis HW: *Atlas of pediatric physical diagnosis,* ed 2, London, 1992, Wolfe.

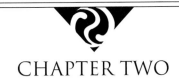

CHAPTER TWO

CARDINAL SYMPTOMS AND SIGNS

AXIOMS IN ASSESSMENT OF CARDINAL SYMPTOMS AND SIGNS

- The important presenting symptoms in neuromusculoskeletal disease or injury include pain, stiffness, locking, swelling, weakness or difficulty moving, and fatigue
- Pain is the most common presenting symptom.

The actual technique of examination varies according to individual preference. Nevertheless, it is useful to develop and adhere to a particular routine. Familiarity with such a routine ensures that no step in the examination is overlooked.

The part to be examined should be adequately exposed and in good light. Many mistakes are made simply because the examiner does not insist on the removal of enough clothing to allow proper examination. When an extremity is being examined, the uninvolved extremity should always be used for comparison.

ORTHOPEDIC GAMUT 2-1

VISUAL INSPECTION

Visual inspection should be carried out systematically, with attention to four areas:

1. *Bones:* Observe the general alignment and position of the parts to detect any deformity, shortening, or unusual posture.
2. *Soft tissues:* Observe the soft-tissue contours, comparing bilaterally and noting any visible evidence of general or local swelling or muscle wasting.
3. *Color and texture of the skin:* Look for rubor, cyanosis, pigmentation, shininess, loss of hair, or other changes.
4. *Scars or sinuses:* If a scar is present, determine from its appearance whether it was caused by operation (linear scar with suture marks), injury (irregular scar), or suppuration (broad, adherent, puckered scar).

ORTHOPEDIC GAMUT 2-2

PALPATION

Four points should be considered in palpation:

1. *Skin temperature:* By careful bilateral comparison, determine whether there is an area of increased warmth or of unusual coolness. An increase in local temperature denotes increased blood flow; the usual cause is an inflammatory reaction. A rapidly growing tumor also may cause marked local hyperemia.
2. *Bones:* Investigate the general shape and outline of the bone. Palpate in particular for thickening, abnormal prominence, or disturbed relationship of the normal landmarks.
3. *Soft tissue:* Direct attention to the muscle (spasm, atrophy), joint tissue (synovial membrane, joint distension), and the detection of any local or general swelling of the part.
4. *Local tenderness:* The exact borders of any local tenderness should be delineated. An attempt should be made to relate this tenderness to a particular structure.

ORTHOPEDIC GAMUT 2-3

PRESENTING SYMPTOMS AND SIGNS

Presenting symptoms and signs will differentiate musculoskeletal complaints into five main types:

1. Inflammatory disease
2. Mechanical articular or periarticular disorder
3. Systemic disease presenting with musculoskeletal symptoms or signs
4. Functional disorder
5. Idiopathic

CARDINAL SYMPTOMS

Pain and Sensibility

Of symptoms, pain is usually most important for the patient. Of signs, swelling of a joint or periarticular tissue is important. With regard to pain, the examiner must be certain of the site and distribution. The patient's verbal description may be misleading. The patient should be able to point to or define the site of maximum intensity and map out the area over which pain is experienced.

Articular or periarticular pain may radiate widely and may be felt in a spot distant from the originating tissues. Such referred pain is a perceptual error occurring at the sensory cortex and reflects shared innervation by structures derived from the same embryonic segment. Cortical cells most commonly receive stimuli from the skin. When the same cells receive an initial painful stimulus from a deeply situated myotomal/sclerotomal structure, they interpret the signal based on experience. The patient feels pain in the area of the skin (dermatome) that shares the connection. An important distinction for dermatomal pain is that referred pain is felt deeply, rather than in the skin itself, and its boundaries are indistinct. Referred pain radiates segmentally without crossing the midline. Because the dermatome often extends more distally than the myotome, the pain is mainly referred distally. The more distal the originating structure from the spinal cord, the more accurate the pain localization is likely to be. In addition to pain referral, tenderness also may be experienced at a distant site. Dermatomes are variable between individuals. For example, the precise area of pain referral may differ between patients with the same musculoskeletal problem. The more superficial a soft-tissue structure, the more precise its pain localization. Massage over the area of referred pain may improve rather than worsen the pain, and pressure over the originating tissue may reproduce the pain.

The quality of musculoskeletal pain sometimes provides important diagnostic clues. For example, nerve entrapment may produce pain that is described as being similar to an electric shock and of a shooting type. In contrast, vascular pain may be throbbing, and joint pains are often described as severe aching sensations.

The patient's description of the quality of the pain is often not helpful in diagnosis. Pain descriptions are based on the patient's frame of reference and shaded by his or her emotional state. Helpful descriptions include sharp, shooting pain that travels a distance and is characteristic of root entrapment or extreme pain, typical of crystal deposition synovitis. Although topographic localization occurs at the sensory cortex level, pain appreciation and severity are determined by cells in the supraorbital region of the frontal lobe. This is why the patient's emotional state has such an influence over the severity of the pain. The memory of pain is retained in the temporal lobe.

Factors that exacerbate or ameliorate the pain are important. Pain during use suggests a mechanical problem, particularly if it worsens during use and quickly improves when resting. Pain while at rest and pain that is worse at the beginning rather than at the end of use implies a marked inflammatory component. Night pain is a distressing symptom that reflects intraosseous hypertension and accompanies serious problems, such as avascular necrosis, bone neoplastic activity, or bone collapse adjacent to a severely arthritic joint. Persistent bony pain is characteristic of neoplastic invasion. The activities that create a mechanical pain may provide clues as to the appropriate diagnosis. Periarticular problems are often induced by a specific type of activity but are also divided by region (Table 2-1).

It is appropriate to test sensibility to both light touch and pinprick throughout the affected area. In unilateral afflictions, the opposite side should be similarly tested.

TABLE 2-1

REGIONAL PERIARTICULAR SYNDROMES

Region	Periarticular Syndrome
Jaw	Temporomandibular joint dysfunction (myofascial pain syndrome)
Shoulder	Subacromial bursitis
	Long-head bicipital tendinitis
	Rotator cuff tear
Elbow	Olecranon bursitis
	Epicondylitis
Wrist	Extensor tendinitis (including de Quervain's tenosynovitis)
	Gonococcal tenosynovitis
Hand	Palmar fasciitis (Dupuytren's contracture)
	Ligamentous or capsular injury
Hip	Greater trochanteric bursitis
	Adductor syndrome
	Ischial bursitis
	Fascia lata syndrome
Knee	Anserine bursitis
	Prepatellar bursitis
	Meniscal injury
	Ligamentous tear-laxity
	Baker's cyst
Ankle	Peroneal tendinitis
	Achilles tendinitis
	Retrocalcaneal bursitis
	Calcaneal fasciitis
	Sprain
	Erythema nodosum
Foot	Plantar fasciitis
	Pes planus ("fallen arches")

Adapted from Kelley WN, et al: *Textbook of rheumatology*, ed 5, Philadelphia, 1997, WB Saunders.

From knowledge of the cutaneous distribution of the peripheral nerves, the particular nerves may be identified.

The sense of pain is served by free nerve endings located in the skin and certain visceral tissues. Pain can be caused by stimuli of different natures. Strong mechanical stimuli (intense pressure) and very hot and very cold stimuli (thermal and certain chemical stimuli, such as acidic substances) all can cause pain. Pain receptors have a high threshold of stimulation. These receptors are usually acti-

vated when stimulus strength is very high. Because such strong stimuli are usually noxious, the evoked sensation is also called *nociception* (pain sense). The pain receptors activated by noxious stimuli are called *nociceptors*.

Tissue damage results in the local release of certain internal nociceptive substances such as serotonin, pressor substance (substance P), histamine, and kinin peptides (bradykinin) in the injured area. These substances then act on the free nerve endings, activating pain signals. Sharp pain is conveyed by thin, myelinated, fast, type A delta fibers. Dull, aching, and hurting pain is conveyed by unmyelinated, slow, conducting type C fibers.

Peripheral Nociceptors

The skin, joint structures, arterial walls, and periosteum are richly supplied with nociceptors that are activated by a variety of mechanical (stretching), thermal (heat and cold), and chemical stimuli (Fig. 2-1). The main neurotransmitters involved in pain inhibitory pathways are serotonin, norepinephrine, and the endogenous opioids (Fig. 2-2).

Weakness

Weakness of limbs or of the whole body can be an important clue. The pattern of asymmetric or symmetric muscle weakness and its central or peripheral distribution may give vital clues to the diagnosis. *Weakness* may describe the difficulty that the patient has with movement because of joint disease, or the feeling of insecurity that is associated with a loss of proprioception that accompanies many forms of joint disease. Patients may also use the term *weakness* to describe general fatigue rather than loss of muscle power.

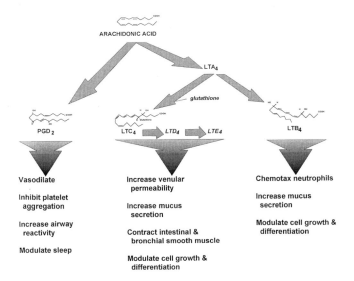

FIG. 2-1 Major leukotriene and prostaglandin products of mast cells and basophils. *LT,* Leukotriene; *PG,* prostaglandin. *(From Kelley WN, et al:* Textbook of rheumatology, *ed 5, Philadelphia, 1997, WB Saunders.)*

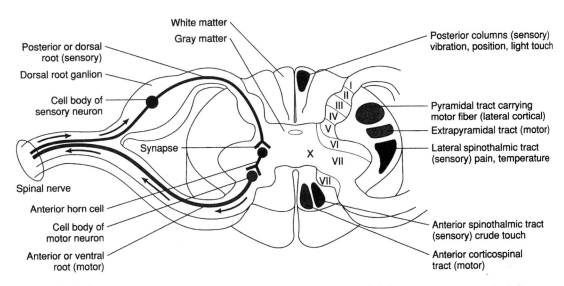

FIG. 2-2 Cross section of the spinal cord. Spinal nerve roots and their neurons appear on the left side. Spinal nerve tracts appear in white matter on right side. All tracts and nerves are bilateral.
(From Barkauskas VH, et al: Health and physical assessment, *ed 2, St Louis, 1998, Mosby.)*

Stiffness

Stiffness is a subjective sensation of resistance to movement that probably reflects fluid distension of the limiting boundary of the inflamed tissue. Stiffness resulting from this phenomenon is most noticeable when arising from bed and after inactivity or rest. As normal use resumes, fluid clears from the inflamed structures and stiffness wears off. The duration and severity of early morning stiffness and inactivity stiffness reflect the degree of local inflammation.

Locking of a joint, a limb, or the spine is less common. *Locking* may be used to describe very severe stiffness, but more commonly, it is used to describe a specific mechanical event in which some internal derangement of a joint actually causes it to lock in one position. The mechanical locking continues until the patient initiates a "trick" movement or gets help from someone else who frees it up. Such mechanical locking experienced in spinal elements is typical in many patients with ankylosing spondylitis (Fig. 2-3). This can also be seen in advance kyphoscoliosis (Fig. 2-4).

Disability and Handicap

Disability is present when a tissue, organ, or system cannot function adequately. A handicap exists when disability interferes with a patient's daily activities or social/occupational performance. A marked disability does not necessarily cause a handicap. Conversely, minor disability may produce a major handicap. Both conditions require separate assessment. Patients' perception of their problems will be molded by their adaptation to the depreciated tissue as well as aspirations for recovery (Box 2-1).

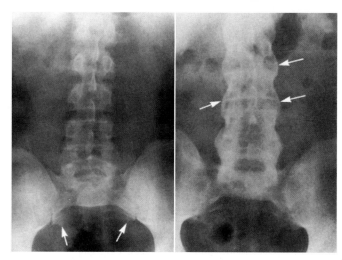

FIG. 2-3   Ankylosing spondylitis presenting with bilateral symmetric sacroiliitis **(A)** *(arrows)*. Ten years later, sacroiliac joint appears similar to previous film **(B),** but the spine exhibits advanced syndesmophytes not noted on previous film *(arrows)*. *(From Marchiori DM:* Clinical imaging, *St Louis, 1998, Mosby.)*

injury on the patient's ability to perform activities of daily living and on the patient's capacity to carry out a normal daily routine, including work, leisure, and other social activities.

ORTHOPEDIC GAMUT 2-4

ASSESSING DISABILITY

An aide in assessing the more important aspects of disability is the *PILS* mnemonic, which considers four issues:

1. P Preventable causes of disability (e.g., falls, direct trauma)
2. I Independence (e.g., self-care)
3. L Lifestyle (roles, goals)
4. S Social factors (e.g., family, friends, shelter)

ORTHOPEDIC GAMUT 2-5

FUNCTIONAL ASSESSMENT

A complete functional assessment includes evaluation of the following:

1. *Self-care:* ability to wash, bath, attend to toilet needs, dress, cook, and feed oneself
2. *Mobility:* ability to stand, transfer, walk, negotiate stairs, drive, and use public transportation
3. *Lifestyle:* nature of occupation, work capacity, and Social Security benefits

---

Assessment of a disorder affecting the locomotor system, local or generalized, is not complete without evaluation of the patient's functional status and quality of life. This includes assessing the impact of the condition or

Systemic Illness

Inflammatory musculoskeletal disease may trigger a marked acute-phase response and cause nonspecific symptoms of systemic upset. Symptoms may include fever, reduced appetite, weight loss, fatigue, lethargy, and irritability. The patient might not volunteer specific complaints but might

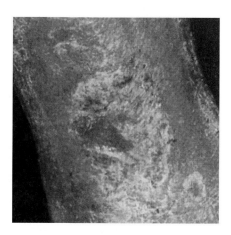

FIG. 2-13   Statis ulcer.   *(From Habif TP:* Clinical dermatology, *ed 3, St Louis, 1996, Mosby.)*

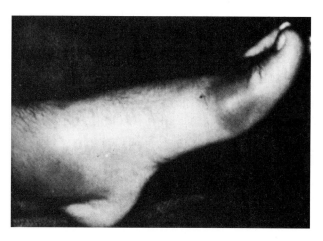

FIG. 2-14   Inflammatory response of acute gout of the great toe. *(From Prior JA, Silberstein JS, Stang FM:* Physical diagnosis: the history and examination of the patient, *ed 6, St Louis, 1981, Mosby.)*

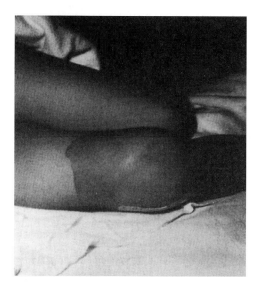

FIG. 2-15   Septic arthritis.   *(From* Mosby's medical, nursing, & allied health dictionary, *St Louis, 1998, Mosby.)*

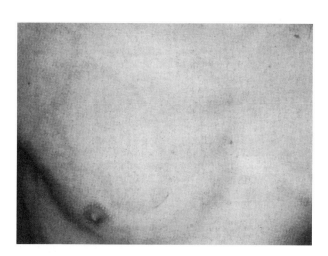

FIG. 2-16   Erythema migrans.   *(From* Mosby's medical, nursing, & allied health dictionary, *St Louis, 1998, Mosby.)*

require histopathology and immunofluorescence studies (Fig. 2-17).

Misdiagnosis of acute lupus may occur in patients expressing other photosensitive eruptions and in patients with conditions that produce vascular dilation (Table 2-5). A clinical history and examination are usually sufficient to discriminate acute lupus from other photosensitive eruptions.

Features of dermatomyositis rash (Fig. 2-18) allow discrimination from lupus. These features include occasional nasolabial fold involvement, prominent heliotrope and extrafacial involvement (Fig. 2-19), erythema following the course of extensor tendons, and scaling and fissuring of lateral aspects of the fingers (mechanic's hands). Gottron's papules with erythema over the interphalangeal joints are pathognomonic for dermatomyositis.

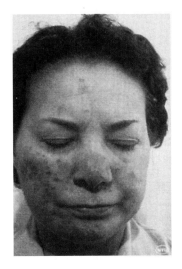

FIG. 2-17   Acne rosacea. *(From Barkauskas VH, et al:* Health and physical assessment, *ed 2, St Louis, 1998, Mosby.)*

TABLE 2-4

FACIAL DISEASES CONFUSED WITH LUPUS

Polymorphous light eruption (occasional)
Benign lymphocytic infiltration of Jessner (rare)
Seborrheic dermatitis (common)
Acne rosacea (common)
Tinea faciei (occasional)
Lupus vulgaris tuberculous (rare)
Lupus pernio sarcoid (rare)

TABLE 2-5

REVISED CRITERIA FOR THE CLASSIFICATION OF SYSTEMIC LUPUS ERYTHEMATOSUS (1982)

Criterion	Definition
1. Malar rash	Fixed erythema, flat or raised, over the eminences, tending to spare the nasolabial folds
2. Discoid rash	Erythematous raised patches with adherent keratotic scaling and follicular plugging; atrophic scarring may occur in older lesions
3. Photosensitivity	Skin rash as a result of unusual reaction to sunlight, by patient history or physician observation
4. Oral ulcers	Oral or nasopharyngeal ulceration, usually painless, observed by a physician
5. Arthritis	Nonerosive arthritis involving two or more peripheral joints, characterized by tenderness, swelling, or effusion
6. Serositis	(a) Pleuritis—convincing history of pleuritic pain or rub heard by a physician or evidence of pleural effusion *or*
	(b) Pericarditis—documented by ECG or rub or evidence of pericardial effusion
7. Renal disorder	(a) Persistent proteinuria greater than 0.5 grams per day or greater than 3+ if quantification not performed *or*
	(b) Cellular casts—may be red cell, hemoglobin, granular, tubular, or mixed
8. Neurologic disorder	(a) Seizures—in the absence of offending drugs or known metabolic derangements, e.g., uremia, ketoacidosis, or electrolyte imbalance *or*
	(b) Psychosis—in the absence of offending drugs or known metabolic derangements, e.g., uremia, ketoacidosis, or electrolyte imbalance
9. Hematologic disorders	(a) Hemolytic anemia—with reticulocytosis *or*
	(b) Leukopenia—less than 4000/mm^3 total on two or more occasions *or*
	(c) Lymphopenia—less than 1500/mm^3 on two or more occasions *or*
	(d) Thrombocytopenia—less than 100,000/mm^3 in the absence of offending drugs
10. Immunologic disorder	(a) Positive LE cell preparation *or*
	(b) Anti-DNA; antibody to native DNA in abnormal titer *or*
	(c) Anti-Sm: presence of antibody to Sm nuclear antigen *or*
	(d) False-positive serologic test for syphilis known to be positive for at least 6 months and confirmed by *Treponema pallidum* immobilization or fluorescent treponemal antibody absorption test
11. Antinuclear antibody	An abnormal titer of antinuclear antibody by immunofluorescence or an equivalent assay at any point in time and in the absence of drugs known to be associated with "drug-induced lupus" syndrome

From Tan EM, et al: The 1982 revised criteria for the classification of SLE, *Arthritis Rheum* 25:1271, 1982.

Tenderness

Precise localization of tenderness is the most useful sign in determining the cause of the problem. Joint line/capsular tenderness signifies arthropathy or capsular disease around the whole margin. Localized joint line tenderness suggests intracapsular pathologic processes. Periarticular point tenderness, away from the joint line, usually signifies bursitis or enthesopathy.

The only reliable finding on examination in fibromyalgia is the presence of multiple tender points. The diagnostic utility of a tender point evaluation has been objectively documented with the use of a dolorimeter or algometer, pressure-loaded gauges that accurately measure force per area, and with manual palpation. The criteria of at least 11 of 18 tender points are recommended for classification purposes but should not be considered essential in individual patient diagnoses. Patients with fewer than 11 tender points can be diagnosed with fibromyalgia provided other symptoms and signs are present. An investigation must be made to determine whether the fibromyalgia is primary or secondary.

Warmth

Warmth is one of the cardinal signs of inflammation. The back of the examiner's hand is a sensitive thermometer for comparing skin temperature above, over, and below an inflamed structure (Fig. 2-20).

Painful Arc of Movement

Ligament injuries are detected by eliciting tenderness over that damaged portion of the affected tendon. Injuries are also detected in attempting to distract the bony structures held together by the ligament.

When the tendon is subject to disease or excessive load, it may rupture. In tendon disease or injury less than rupture, tendinitis usually results. Tendinitis is detected by eliciting a "painful arc" of active movement in the plane of action of the affected tendon. Passive movement in the same plane is almost pain free (Table 2-6).

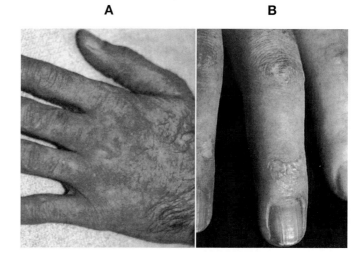

FIG. 2-19 **A,** Systemic lupus erythematosus. **B,** Dermatomyositis. *(From Soter NA, Franks AG Jr: Cutaneous manifestations of rheumatic diseases: an update. In Kelley WN, et al:* Textbook of rheumatology, *ed 4, Philadelphia, 1995, WB Saunders. Update No. 15, pp 1-24.)*

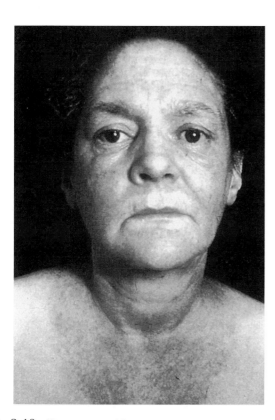

FIG. 2-18 Dermatomyositis. *(From Soter NA, Franks AG Jr: Cutaneous manifestations of rheumatic diseases: an update. In Kelley WN, et al:* Textbook of rheumatology, *ed 4, Philadelphia, 1995, WB Saunders. Update No. 15, pp 1-24.)*

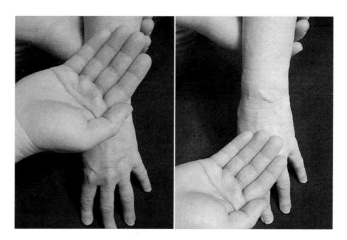

FIG. 2-20 Testing for warmth.

TABLE 2-6

DIAGNOSTICALLY USEFUL CLINICAL FEATURES IN THE INITIAL EVALUATION OF THE PATIENT WITH ACUTE MUSCULOSKELETAL SYMPTOMS

	Tendinitis/Bursitis	Noninflammatory Joint Problems*	Systemic Rheumatic Disease
Symptoms			
AM stiffness	Focal, brief	Focal, brief	Significant, prolonged
Constitutional symptoms	Absent	Absent	Present
Peak period of discomfort	With use	After prolonged use	After prolonged inactivity
Locking or instability	Unusual, except rotator cuff tear, trigger finger	Implies loose body, internal derangement, or weakness	Uncommon
Symmetry	Uncommon	Occasional	Common
Signs			
Tenderness	Focal, periarticular, or tender points (fibromyalgia)	Unusual	Over entire exposed joint spaces
Inflammation (fluid, pain, warmth, erythema)	Over tendon or bursa	Unusual	Common
Instability	Uncommon	Occasional	Uncommon
Multisystem disease	No	No	Often

From Kelley WN, et al: *Textbook of rheumatology,* ed 5, Philadelphia, 1997, WB Saunders.
*For example, osteoarthritis or internal derangement.

TABLE 2-7

SPECIFIC MUSCULOSKELETAL DEFORMITIES

Lower Limb
Hallux abductovalgus
Genu varum
Genu valgum
Dislocation of the patella
Valgus deformity of the heel
Coxa vara
Pes planovalgus
Fixed flexion of the knee
Fixed flexion of the hip
Upper Limb
Fixed flexion of DIPs/PIPs/MCPs ("prayer sign")
Ulnar deviation
Swan neck deformity of finger
Boutonnière deformity
Z-shaped thumb
Volar subluxation of wrist
Dorsal subluxation of inferior radioulnar joint
Fixed flexion of elbow
Cubitus valgus
Upward subluxation of shoulder
Anterior dislocation of shoulder
Posterior dislocation of shoulder

DIPs, Distal interphalangeal joints; *PIP,* proximal interphalangeal joints; *MCPs,* metacarpophalangeal joints; *IP,* interphalangeal.

Fixed Deformity

ORTHOPEDIC GAMUT 2-7

COMMON TERMS TO DESCRIBE PERIPHERAL JOINT DEFORMITIES

1. *Dislocation:* articulating surfaces are displaced to the degree that they are no longer in contact with each other
2. *Fixed flexion:* loss of joint extension, resulting in permanent flexion
3. *Valgus:* the distal part of the joint is directed laterally from the midline
4. *Varus:* the distal part of the joint is directed medially toward the midline

Although deformity may be observed at rest, most deformities become more apparent when the limb is bearing weight or being used. The examiner should determine whether the deformity is correctable or noncorrectable. Many conditions are associated with characteristic deformities, but no deformity is pathognomonic of one disease (Table 2-7). Shorthand terms are used for combined deformities, such as *swan-neck* finger deformity for hyperextension at the proximal and fixed flexion at the distal interphalangeal joints.

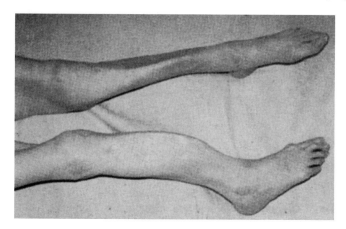

FIG. 2-21 Paget's disease causing deformities in the legs. *(From Mosby's medical, nursing, & allied health dictionary, St Louis, 1998, Mosby.)*

TABLE 2-8

Joint Plane Motion Characteristics

Type	Planes	Joints
Hinge	1	Elbow, knee, ankle, MCP, PIP, DIP, MTP
Two-way hinge	2 (circumduction)	Wrist, trapezio-metacarpal
Ball and socket	All planes	Shoulder, hip

MCP, Metacarpophalangeal; *PIP,* proximal interphalangeal; *DIP,* distal interphalangeal; *MTP,* metatarsophalangeal.

Fixed deformity exists when a joint cannot be placed in the neutral (anatomic) position. The degree of fixed deformity at a joint is determined by moving the joint, as near as it will come, to the neutral position and then measuring the remaining angle. In valgus deformity the distal part of the extremity is deviated laterally (outward) in relation to the proximal part. In hallux valgus the first metatarsal is deviated outward in relation to the foot. In genu valgum the lower leg is deviated outward in relation to the thigh. Varus deformity is the opposite. The distal part of an extremity is deviated medially (inward) in relation to the proximal part (Fig. 2-21).

Movement

For every joint there is a normal range of motion. Ranges vary with age, gender, and ethnic origin. A range that is considered outside the upper limit is deemed to be hypermobile. Ranges below the lower limit are deemed hypomobile. The normal joint range of motion is diminished by joint inflammation or by irreversible damage to the joint structures. In trauma or disease, movement is first lost from the extremes of the range. Increasing joint damage results in more profound loss of range of motion. When movement is lost completely, it is known as *ankylosis.* This is further complicated by the involvement of multiple planes of motion (Table 2-8).

Synovitis reduces most or all joint movements, but tenosynovitis and periarticular lesions affect movement in only one plane. Synovitis and arthropathy cause a similar reduction of active and passive movement. The pattern of pain during movement is of diagnostic significance. Pain that is absent or minimal in the midrange but increases toward the extremes of restricted movement is stress pain. Universal stress pain is the most sensitive sign of synovitis. Selective stress pain, occurring in one plane of movement only, is characteristic of a localized intraarticular or periarticular lesion. Pain uniformly present throughout a range of movement reflects mechanical rather than inflammatory problems.

A useful method for demonstrating periarticular problems is resisted, active (isometric) movement. This method requires the patient to push against the examiner's restraining hand to contract the muscle of interest without moving the adjacent joints. If the patient's pain is reproduced and no joint has moved, the pain probably arises from muscle, tendon, or tendon insertion. Conversely, passive stress tests produce pain by stretching the responsible ligament or tendon.

ORTHOPEDIC GAMUT 2-8

RANGE OF MOTION

Range of motion is assessed as follows:

1. Range of active movement
2. Passive versus active movement
3. Pain during movement
4. Movement crepitation

The normal range of motion varies from patient to patient. Limitation of movement in all directions suggests some form of arthritis. Selective limitation of movement in some directions with free movement in others suggests a mechanical derangement.

Passive movement range is usually equal to the active range. The passive range will exceed the active range only when the muscles responsible for movement are paralyzed and when the muscles or their tendons are torn, severed, or unduly slack.

Hypermobility is recognized by a series of passive maneuvers collectively known as the *9-point scale of Beighton.* The recognition of joint hypermobility rests on the ability of the patient to perform a series of passive joint maneuvers (Box 2-2 and Figs. 2-22 and 2-23).

Stability

Localized ligamentous or capsular instability may result from traumatic or inflammatory lesions. Arthropathy, particularly inflammatory, may produce instability via cartilage loss and capsular inflammation, as well as by ligamentous rupture. Stability is determined by demonstration of excessive movement on stressing the joint. Comparison with the unaffected side is helpful.

The stability of a joint depends partly on the integrity of its articulating surfaces and partly on intact ligaments. When a joint is unstable, mobility is abnormal. When testing for abnormal mobility, the examiner must ensure that the muscles controlling the joint are relaxed. A muscle in strong contraction can often conceal ligamentous instability (Table 2-9).

BOX 2-2

Modified Beighton Joint Laxity Index

1. Hyperextension of the elbows
2. Hyperextension of the knees
3. Apposition of the thumb to the flexor aspect of the forearm
4. Passive dorsiflexion of the metacarpophalangeal joints to 90 degrees
5. Passive dorsiflexion of the ankle past 90 degrees
6. Dorsolumbar flexion, placing hands flat on floor with knees fully extended

1 point is awarded for each side of the body for each extremity clinically involved.
1 point is awarded for dorsolumbar flexion hypermobility.
Total points available for indexing is 11.

TABLE 2-9

JOINT INSTABILITY

Finding

Passive side-to-side movement of the tibia on the femur (collateral knee ligaments)
Passive anteroposterior movement of the tibia on the femur (cruciate ligaments)
Gross genu recurvatum
Positive Trendelenburg's sign
"Arthritis mutilans"—flail interphalangeal joints
Spontaneous dislocation of the shoulder or patella
Pes planus (collapse of the longitudinal arch)

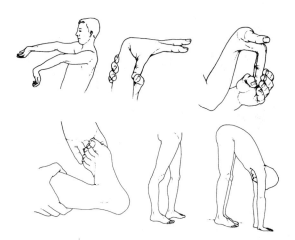

FIG. 2-22 Maneuvers that may be used to establish the presence of clinically significant joint laxity. It is not unusual to find extreme laxity of the small joints and less laxity in large joints. Laxity decreases with age. *(Redrawn and modified from Wynne-Davies R: Acetabular dysplasia and familial joint laxity: two etiological factors in congenital dislocation of the hip. A review of 589 patients and their families,* J Bone Joint Surg *52B:704, 1970.)*

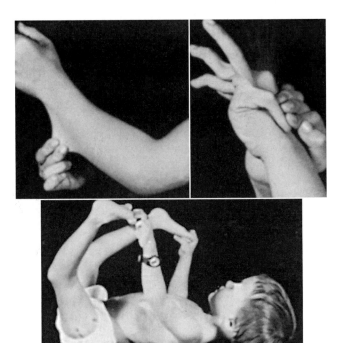

FIG. 2-23 Joint hypermobility. Recurrent dislocations may require surgical repair. *(From Kelley WN, et al:* Textbook of rheumatology, *ed 5, Philadelphia, 1997, WB Saunders.)*

Crepitation

Crepitation is palpable crunching present throughout the movement of the involved structure. Fine crepitation may be audible by stethoscope and is not transmitted through the adjacent bone. Fine crepitation may accompany inflammation of the tendon sheath, bursa, or synovium. Coarse crepitation may be audible at a distance and is palpable through the bone. Coarse crepitation usually reflects cartilage or bone damage.

ORTHOPEDIC GAMUT 2-9

CREPITUS NOISES (OTHER THAN FINE OR COARSE)

1. Ligamentous snaps—usually single, loud, and painless—that are common around the upper femur as a clicking hip
2. Cracking by joint distraction, which is common at the finger joints and is caused by production of an intraarticular gas bubble (such cracking cannot be repeated until the bubble has reformed)
3. Reproducible clunking noises that occur at irregular surfaces, such as when the scapula moves on the ribs

---

Muscular Atrophy

Muscle atrophy is a common sign but can be difficult to detect, particularly in the elderly. Synovitis quickly produces local spinal reflex inhibition of muscles acting across the joint. Atrophy can be rapid (within several days) in septic arthritis. Severe arthropathy produces widespread periarticular wasting. Localized atrophy is more characteristic of a mechanical tendon or muscle problem or nerve entrapment.

Fasciculations

Fasciculations are the visible, spontaneous contractions of muscle fibers supplied by a single motor nerve filament. Visible dimpling or twitching may occur. Fasciculations that occur during muscular contraction (twitching) are associated with conditions of irritability that result in poorly coordinated contraction of small and large motor units (spasmophilia). Benign fasciculation occurs in the normal individual and is characterized by normal muscle strength and size. Fascicular twitches noted during rest in a patient with exaggerated muscular weakness and atrophy are characteristic of a peripheral motor neuron disorder.

Cramps and Spasm

Muscular spasm, or tremor (Table 2-10), may occur at rest or with movement. Spasms and tremors occur in the normal individual with metabolic and electrolyte alterations. Cramping is a common complaint following excessive sweating and subsequent hyponatremia, hypocalcemia, hypomagnesemia, and hyperuricemia.

Tetany

Hypocalcemia and hypomagnesemia often cause the involuntary spasms of skeletal muscle, which resemble cramping. Tetanic cramps can be elicited by percussing the motor nerve leading to a muscle group at frequencies of 15 to 20 per second. Chvostek's sign is the spasm of facial muscles

---

TABLE 2-10

Tremor Classification

Cause	Type and Rate of Movement	Description
Anxiety	Fine, rapid, 10 to 12/sec	Irregular, variable Increased by attempts to move part; decreased by relaxation of part
Parkinsonism	Fine, regular, or coarse, 2 to 5/sec	Occurs at rest May be inhibited by movement Involves flexion of finger and thumb "pill rolling" Accompanied by rigidity, "cogwheel" phenomena, bradykinesia
Cerebellar tremor	Variable rate	Evident only on movement (most prominent on finger-to-nose test) Dysmetria (seen when patient is asked to pat rapidly; pats are of unequal force and do not all arrive at same point)
Essential or senile Metabolic	Coarse, 3 to 7/sec	Involves the jaw, sometimes the tongue, and sometimes the entire head Disappears on complete relaxation or in response to alcohol Variable Patient is obviously ill; if illness is a result of hepatic failure, patient will have other signs, such as palpable liver, spider nevi

From Barkauskas VH, Stoltenberg-Allen K, Baumann LC, Darling-Fisher C: *Health & physical assessment,* ed 2, St Louis, 1998, Mosby.

produced by tapping over the facial nerve near its foramen of exit.

Impairment of Gait

It is difficult to find a spinal or lower extremity orthopedic or neurologic disorder that does not produce abnormalities of gait at some time during its course.

ORTHOPEDIC GAMUT 2-10

GAIT

Gait impairments of predominant neurologic origin include the following (in descending order of frequency):

1. Disorders of the corticospinal pathways (spasticity)
2. Basal ganglia (parkinsonism)
3. Cerebellum and connections (ataxia)
4. Cerebral cortex (gait apraxia)
5. Neuromuscular system (weakness)
6. Sensation (ataxia)

Bladder Control

Incontinence and other disturbances of urinary bladder function are occasionally the first manifestation of disease of the spinal cord, as well as the rest of the nervous system. The physiology of micturition is complex. The terms *atonic bladder* and *spastic bladder* are no longer useful in describing different levels of neurologic involvement because they are related mainly to local factors in the bladder wall.

ORTHOPEDIC GAMUT 2-11

IMPAIRED MICTURITION

Localization of impaired micturition depends on the following:

1. Loss of bladder sensation
2. Perineal sensory loss
3. Patulous anal sphincter
4. Absence of the bulbocavernous and anocutaneous reflexes
5. Sensory, motor, and reflex changes in the lower extremities

---

An associated history of erectile dysfunction or rectal incontinence should clearly suggest the presence of a common neurogenic cause for urinary incontinence. The additional presence of sacral pain should suggest tumor in the sacral region.

BIBLIOGRAPHY

Abrams WB, Berkow R: *The Merck manual of geriatrics,* Rahway, NJ, 1990, Merck Sharp & Dohme Research Laboratories.

Adams JC, Hamblen DL: *Outline of orthopaedics,* ed 11, Edinburgh, 1990, Churchill Livingstone.

Alario AJ: *Practical guide to the care of the pediatric patient,* St Louis, 1997, Mosby.

Anderson KN, Anderson LE: *Mosby's pocket dictionary of medicine, nursing, & allied health,* ed 2, St Louis, 1994, Mosby.

Barkauskas VH, Stoltenberg-Allen K, Baumann LC, Darling-Fisher C: *Health & physical assessment,* ed 2, St Louis, 1998, Mosby.

Bechman H, Markakis K, Suchman A, Frankel R: Getting the most from a 20 minute visit, *Am J Gastroenterol* 89:662, 1994.

Brotzman SB: *Clinical orthopaedic rehabilitation,* St Louis, 1996, Mosby.

Brown DE, Neumann RD: *Orthopedic secrets,* Philadelphia, 1995, Hanley & Belfus.

Bucholz RW: *Orthopaedic decision making,* ed 2, St Louis, 1996, Mosby.

Bunker TD, Schranz PJ: *Clinical challenges in orthopaedics: the shoulder,* Oxford, 1998, ISIS Medical Media.

Campbell JB, Campbell JM: *Mosby's survival guide to medical abbreviations & acronyms prefixes & suffixes symbols Greek alphabet,* St Louis, 1995, Mosby.

Canale ST: *Campbell's operative orthopaedics,* vol 1-4, ed 9, St Louis, 1998, Mosby.

Cardinal E, Lafortune M, Burns P: Power Doppler US in synovitis: reality or artifact? *Radiology* 200:868, 1996.

Chard MD, et al: Shoulder disorders in the elderly: a community survey, *Arthritis Rheum* 34:766, 1991.

Cipriano JJ: *Photographic manual of regional orthopaedic and neurological test,* ed 3, Baltimore, 1997, Williams & Wilkins.

Cohn RE: *Impairment rating examination and disability evaluation,* ed 3, Wilkesboro, NC, 1994, R Ernest Cohn.

Conwell TD: *Documenting patient progress "daily office charting seminar" thorough accurate quick procedures,* ed 11, Lakewood, Colo, 1990, Clinical Advancement Plus Seminars.

Copeland SA, Gschwend N, Landi A, Saffar P: *Joint stiffness of the upper limb,* St Louis, 1997, Mosby.

Craik RL, Oatis CA: *Gait analysis theory and application,* St Louis, 1995, Mosby.

Dambro MR, Griffith JA: *Griffith's 5 minute clinical consult,* Baltimore, 1997, Williams & Wilkins.

Demeter SL, Andersson GBJ, Smith GM: *Disability evaluation,* St Louis, 1996, Mosby.

Dickenson AH: Spinal cord pharmacology of pain, *Br J Anaesth* 75:193, 1995.

Doherty M: *Color atlas and text of osteoarthritis,* London, 1994, Wolfe.

Doherty M, Dacre J, Dieppe P, Snaith M: The "GALS" locomotor screen, *Ann Rheum Dis* 51:1165, 1992.

Doherty M, Doherty J: *Clinical examination in rheumatology,* London, 1992, Wolfe.

Doherty M, George E: *Self-assessment picture tests in rheumatology,* London, 1995, Mosby-Wolfe.

Dray A: Inflammatory mediators of pain, *Br J Anaesth* 75:125, 1995.

Epstein O, Perkin GD, deBono DP, Cookson J: *Clinical examination,* ed 2, London, 1997, Mosby.

Feldmann E: *Current diagnosis in neurology,* St Louis, 1994, Mosby.

Ferezy JS: *The chiropractic neurological examination,* Gaithersburg, Md, 1992, Aspen.

Fitzpatrick TB, et al: *Color atlas and synopsis of clinical dermatology common and serious diseases,* ed 2, New York, 1992, McGraw-Hill.

Goldie BS: *Orthopaedic diagnosis and management a guide to the care of orthopaedic patients,* ed 2, Oxford, 1998, ISIS Medical Media.

Greenstein GM: *Clinical assessment of neuromusculoskeletal disorders,* St Louis, 1997, Mosby.

Haack E, Tkach J: Fast MR imaging: techniques and clinical applications, *AJR* 155:951, 1990.

Hartley A: *Practical joint assessment lower quadrant,* ed 2, St Louis, 1995, Mosby.

Hassell AB, et al: The relationship between serial measures of disease activity and outcome in rheumatoid arthritis, *Q J Med* 86:601, 1995.

Hawkins RJ: *An organized approach to musculoskeletal examination and history taking,* St Louis, 1995, Mosby.

Hinkle CZ: *Fundamentals of anatomy & movement a workbook and guide,* St Louis, 1997, Mosby.

Katirji B: *Electromyography in clinical practice a case study approach,* St Louis, 1998, Mosby.

Klippel JH, Dieppe PA: *Rheumatology,* vol 1-2, ed 2, London, 1998, Mosby.

Lewis CB, Knortz KA: *Orthopedic assessment and treatment of the geriatric patient,* St Louis, 1993, Mosby.

Magee DJ: *Orthopedic physical assessment,* ed 3, Philadelphia, 1997, WB Saunders.

Malone TR, McPoil TG, Nitz AJ: *Orthopedic and sports physical therapy,* ed 3, St Louis, 1997, Mosby.

Mathews DA, Suchman AL, Branch WT: Making "connexions": enhancing the therapeutic potential of patient-clinician relationships, *Ann Intern Med* 118:973, 1993.

McRae R: *Clinical orthopaedic examination,* ed 3, Edinburgh, 1990, Churchill Livingstone.

Mengel MB, Schwiebert LP: *Ambulatory medicine the primary care of families,* ed 2, Stamford, Conn, 1996, Appleton & Lange.

Mennell JM: *The musculoskeletal system differential diagnosis from symptoms and physical signs,* Gaithersburg, Md, 1992, Aspen.

Mercier LR, Pettid FJ: *Practical orthopedics,* ed 5, St Louis, 2000, Mosby.

Mosby-Year Book, Inc: *Expert 10-minute physical examination,* St Louis, 1997, Mosby.

Nardone DA, et al: A model for the diagnostic medical interview: nonverbal, verbal and cognitive assessments, *J Gen Intern Med* 7:437, 1992.

Nettina SM: *The Lippincott manual of nursing practice,* ed 6, Philadelphia, 1996, Lippincott.

Newton RW: *Color atlas of pediatric neurology,* St Louis, 1995, Mosby-Wolfe.

Ogilvie-Harris DJ, Saleh K: Generalized synovial chondromatosis of the knee: a comparison of removal of the loose bodies alone with arthroscopic synovectomy, *Arthroscopy* 10:166, 1994.

Olson WH, Brumback RA, Gascon G, Iyer V: *Handbook of symptom-oriented neurology,* ed 2, St Louis, 1994, Mosby.

Perhala RS, Wilke WS, Clough JD, Segal AM: Local infectious complications following large joint replacement in rheumatoid arthritis patients treated with methotrexate versus those not treated with methotrexate, *Arthritis Rheum* 34:146, 1991.

Peterfy CG, Genant HK: Emerging applications of magnetic resonance imaging for evaluating the articular cartilage, *Radiol Clin North Am* 34:195, 1996.

Peterfy CG, et al: MR imaging of the arthritic knee: improved discrimination of cartilage, synovium and effusion with pulsed saturation transfer and fat-suppressed T1-weighted sequences, *Radiology* 191: 413, 1994.

Rachlin ES: *Myofascial pain and fibromyalgia trigger point management,* St Louis, 1994, Mosby.

Raspe HH: Back pain. In Silman AJ, Hochberg M, editors: *Epidemiology of the rheumatic diseases,* Oxford, 1993, Oxford University Press.

Rubens DJ, Blebea JS, Totterman SMS, Hooper MM: Rheumatoid arthritis: evaluation of wrist extensor tendons with clinical examination versus MR imaging—a preliminary report, *Radiology* 187:831, 1993.

Schumacher HR, Klippel JH, Koopman WJ: *Primer on the rheumatic diseases,* ed 10, Atlanta, 1993, Arthritis Foundation.

Smith RC, Hoppe RB: The patient's story: integrating the patient and physician centered approaches to interviewing, *Ann Intern Med* 115:470, 1991.

Stamford JA: Descending control of pain, *Br J Anaesth* 75:217, 1995.

Stein C: The control of pain in peripheral tissue by opioids, *N Engl J Med* 332:1685, 1995.

Stevens JC, Beard CM, O'Fallon WM, Kurland LT: Conditions associated with carpal tunnel syndrome, *Mayo Clin Proc* 67:541, 1992.

Sugimoto H, Takeda A, Masuyama J, Furuse M: Early-stage rheumatoid arthritis: diagnostic accuracy of MR imaging, *Radiology* 198:185, 1996.

Tan JC, Horn SE: *Practical manual of physical medicine and rehabilitation,* St Louis, 1998, Mosby.

Thibodeau GA, Patton KT: *Anatomy & physiology,* ed 3, St Louis, 1996, Mosby.

Thibodeau GA, Patton KT: *Pocket reference to accompany anatomy & physiology,* ed 3, St Louis, 1996, Mosby.

Thompson JM: *Clinical outlines for health assessment,* St Louis, 1997, Mosby.

Toghill PJ: *Examining patients an introduction to clinical medicine,* London, 1990, Edward Arnold.

Wakefield TS, Frank RG: *The clinician's guide to neuromusculoskeletal practice,* Abbotsford, Wisc, 1995, Allied Health of Wisconsin, S.C.

Weinstein SL, Buckwalter JA: *Turek's orthopaedics principles and their application,* ed 5, Philadelphia, 1994, JB Lippincott.

White G: *Levene's color atlas of dermatology,* ed 2, London, 1997, Mosby-Wolfe.

White G: *Regional dermatology,* London, 1994, Mosby-Wolfe.

White KP, Speechley M, Harth M, Ostbye T: Fibromyalgia in rheumatology practice: a survey of Canadian rheumatologists, *J Rheumatol* 22:722, 1995.

Windsor RE, Lox DM: *Soft tissue injuries: diagnosis and treatment,* Philadelphia, 1998, Hanley & Belfus.

Wolfe F, et al: The prevalence and characteristics of fibromyalgia in the general population, *Arthritis Rheum* 38:19, 1995.

Woolf CJ: Somatic pain-pathogenesis and prevention, *Br J Anaesth* 75:169, 1995.

Zatouroff M: *Diagnosis in color physical signs in general medicine,* ed 2, London, 1996, Mosby-Wolfe.

Zitelli BJ, Davis HW: *Atlas of pediatric physical diagnosis,* ed 2, London, 1992, Wolfe.

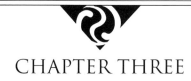

THE CERVICAL SPINE

vertebral arteries, the spinal cord, and the spinal nerves, all of which require great protection.

Normal function of the cervical spine requires that all movements are accomplished without injury to the spinal cord and the millions of nerve fibers that pass through it. The spinal cord has the capacity to adapt itself to marked alteration in the length of the cervical spinal canal. Flexion of the neck lengthens the spinal canal, and extension shortens it. The thickness of the cervical spinal cord and the diameter of the spinal canal vary considerably from person to person.

The nerve roots in the neck are particularly vulnerable to injury because of their relatively horizontal position in comparison with those of the lumbar spine (Fig. 3-2). Stretching of the spinal cord itself is greatest at the cervical spine, which also predisposes the cord and nerve roots to trauma.

Differential diagnostic possibilities include cardiovascular disease, myocardial infarction, aortic dissection, meningitis, cervical osteoarthritis, hypertension, temporal arteritis, polymyalgia rheumatica, a spectrum of neurologic diseases and syndromes, various metabolic bone diseases, primary and metastatic cancer, infection, lymphoma, and myeloma.

AXIOMS OF CERVICAL SPINE ASSESSMENT

- Cervical spine syndromes are extremely common and are probably the fourth most common cause of pain.
- At any given time, 9% of men and 12% of women have neck pain with or without arm and hand pain, and 35% of the population can remember having had neck pain at some time.
- The cervical spine is the origin of a large proportion of shoulder, elbow, hand, and wrist disorders.
- Most people who develop pain in the neck do not seek medical attention because they regard such pain as a part of life, so they simply wait for it to disappear.

INTRODUCTION

Neck discomfort commonly appears following sudden and unusual motion of the neck because the neck is the most mobile segment of the spine. Many delicate and vital structures pass through the neck, including the carotid and

ORTHOPEDIC GAMUT 3-1

ORTHOPEDIC EXAMINATION

An orthopedic examination of the cervical spine includes the following:

1. History
2. Vital signs
3. Inspection
4. Palpation of superficial and deep tissues, and joint play
5. Percussion
6. Instrumentation (other physical measurement)
7. Range-of-motion evaluation
8. Orthopedic maneuvers
9. Neurologic examination
10. Imaging
11. Laboratory evaluation

There are many provocative tests for the cervical spine. The anatomic structures commonly tested are dural tension; foraminal and vertebral canal patency; and muscle, tendon, or ligamentous injuries (Table 3-3). During investigation of the upper extremity the examiner must differentiate between canal or nerve root lesions by physical examination and, if necessary, electrodiagnostic studies. Cervical spine canal stenosis, whether of bony or soft-tissue origins, can present with lower extremity signs and symptoms. Most notable is long tract pain, or rhizalgia, appearing in an ipsilateral leg with a cervical nerve root lesion.

ESSENTIAL CLINICAL ANATOMY

The atlas consists of a pair of strong lateral masses that are linked by the anterior arch and the posterior arch (Fig. 3-4). The posterior arch of the atlas is attached to the posterior rim of the foramen magnum by the atlantooccipital membrane (Fig. 3-5).

Children often have lax ligaments, which increases spinal motion. This most commonly occurs in the cervical region. Increased motion seen during physical or x-ray

Text continued on p. 51

TABLE 3-1

CERVICAL SPINE CROSS-REFERENCE TABLE BY SYNDROME OR TISSUE

Cervical Spine	Nerve Root	VBA Syndrome	Brachial Plexus	Meningitis	IVD Syndrome	Tumor	Fracture	Dural Irritation	Sprain	Facet	Myospasm	Subluxation	Arthritis
Test/Sign													
Bakody sign	●												
Barre-Lieou sign		●											
Bikele's sign			●	●									
Brachial plexus tension test	●		●		●	●	●						
Dejerine's sign	●												
DeKleyn's test		●											
Distraction test	●									●	●		
Foraminal compression test	●												
Hallpike maneuver		●											
Hautant's test		●											
Jackson compression test					●	●				●		●	●
Lhermitte's sign								●					
Maximum cervical compression test	●									●	●		
Naffziger's test	●					●			●		●		
O'Donoghue maneuver									●		●		
Rust's sign							●			●		●	●
Shoulder depression test	●							●		●			
Soto-Hall sign				●	●		●			●		●	●
Spinal percussion test					●		●				●		
Spurling's test	●												
Swallowing test					●	●							●
Underburg's test		●											
Valsalva maneuver					●	●							
Vertebrobasilar artery functional maneuver		●											

VBA, Vertebrobasilar artery; *IVD*, intervertebral disc.

ORTHOPEDIC GAMUT 3-2

NEURAL RESPONSES

Pathologic neural responses to cervical injury can be grouped into four categories:

1. Transient neurologic deficit (lasting less than 8 weeks) involving the nerve roots, trunk or the brachial plexus, or motor unit

2. Longstanding, consistent neurologic deficit (lasting more than 8 weeks)
3. Cervical myelopathy (clonus, lower or upper limb findings)
4. Gross spinal cord impairment (quadriplegia) (Fig. 3-3)

TABLE 3-2

CERVICAL SPINE CROSS-REFERENCE TABLE BY SYNDROME OR TISSUE

Arthritis	Jackson cervical compression test	Nerve root	Bakody sign
	Rust's sign		Brachial plexus tension test
	Soto-Hall sign		Dejerine's sign
	Swallowing test		Distraction test
Brachial plexus	Bikele's sign		Maximum cervical compression test
	Brachial plexus tension test		Naffziger's test
Dural irritation	Lhermitte's sign		Shoulder depression test
	Shoulder depression test		Spurling's test
Facet	Distraction test	Sprain	Naffziger's test
	Jackson cervical compression test		O'Donoghue maneuver
	Maximum cervical compression test		Rust's sign
	Shoulder depression test		Soto-Hall sign
Fracture	Brachial plexus tension test	Subluxation	Jackson cervical compression test
	Rust's sign		Rust's sign
	Soto-Hall sign		Soto-Hall sign
	Spinal percussion test	Tumor	Brachial plexus tension test
Intervertebral disc syndrome	Brachial plexus tension test		Jackson cervical compression test
	Jackson cervical compression test		Swallowing test
	Naffziger's test		Valsalva maneuver
	Soto-Hall sign	Vertebrobasilar artery syndrome	Barre-Lieou sign
	Spinal percussion test		DeKleyn's test
	Swallowing test		Hallpike maneuver
	Valsalva maneuver		Hautant's test
Meningitis	Brachial plexus tension test		Underburg's test
	Soto-Hall sign		Vertebrobasilar artery functional maneuver
Myospasm	Distraction test		
	Maximum cervical compression test		
	Naffziger's test		
	O'Donoghue maneuver		
	Soto-Hall sign		
	Spinal percussion test		

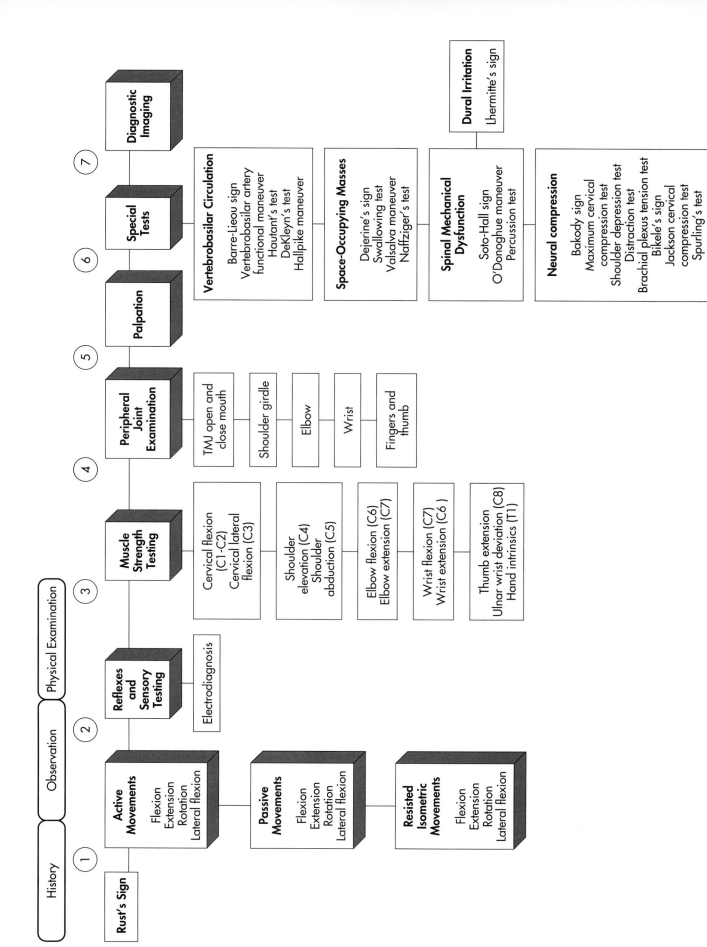

FIG. 3-1 Cervical spine assessment chart. *TMJ*, Temporomandibular joint.

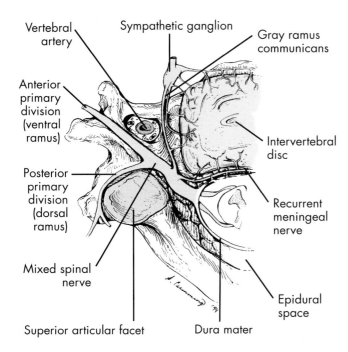

FIG. 3-2 Typical cervical segment demonstrating the neural elements. *(From Cramer GD, Darby SA: Basic and clinical anatomy of the spine, spinal cord, and ANS, St Louis, 1995, Mosby.)*

TABLE 3-3

COMMON PROVOCATIVE TESTS TO EVALUATE THE SPINE

Provocative Test	Anatomic Structures Being Tested	Positive Finding(s)
Cervical spine		
Jackson's compression test	Dural sheath, nerve root, spinal nerve	Radicular pain
Spurling's compression test	Dural sheath, nerve root, spinal nerve	Radicular pain
Maximal foraminal compression test	Dural sheath, nerve root, spinal nerve	Radicular pain
Distraction test	Dural sheath, nerve root, spinal nerve	Relief of radicular pain
Shoulder depression test	Dural sheath, nerve root, spinal nerve, brachial plexus	Radicular pain to one or more dermatomes
E.A.S.T. test	Subclavian artery	Vascular compromise
Eden's test	Scalene musculature	Radiculopathy to multiple dermatomes or vascular compromise
Thoracic spine		
Wright's hyperabduction test	Pectoralis minor	Vascular compromise, subclavian artery, TOS
Tests for anterior thoracic wall	Peripheral nerve, muscles	Radicular pain, dull ache
Lumbar spine		
Straight leg raise (SLR)	Dural sheath, nerve root, spinal nerve	Radiculopathy to one dermatome usually
Braggard's test	Dural sheath, nerve root, spinal nerve	Radiculopathy to one dermatome usually
Bekhterev's test (Bechterew)	Dural sheath, nerve root, spinal nerve	Radiculopathy to one dermatome usually
Neri's bow string test	Dural sheath, nerve root, spinal nerve	Radiculopathy to one dermatome usually

From Greenstein GM: *Clinical assessment of neuromusculoskeletal disorders,* St Louis, 1997, Mosby.
E.A.S.T., Elevated arm stress test; *TOS,* thoracic outlet syndrome.

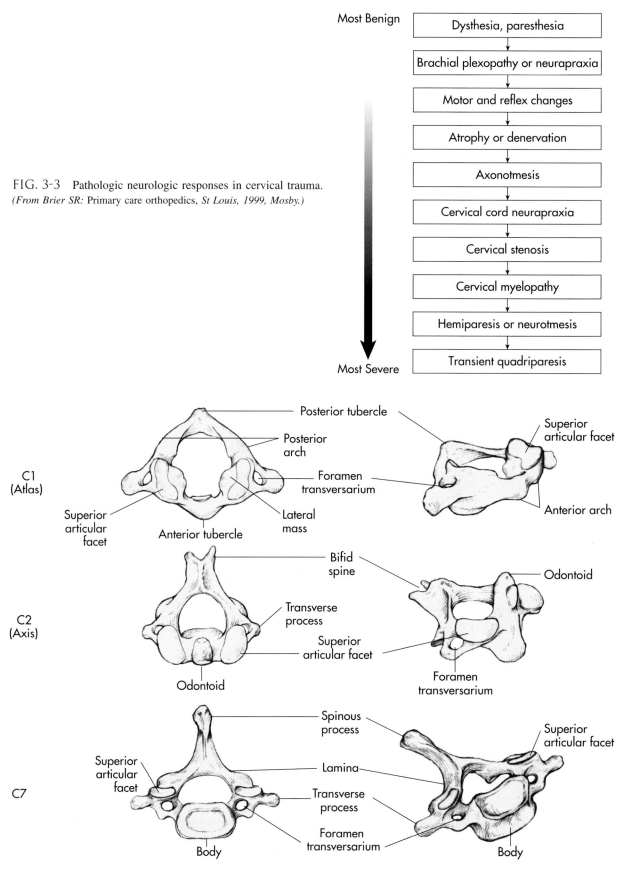

Most Benign

| Dysthesia, paresthesia |
| Brachial plexopathy or neurapraxia |
| Motor and reflex changes |
| Atrophy or denervation |
| Axonotmesis |
| Cervical cord neurapraxia |
| Cervical stenosis |
| Cervical myelopathy |
| Hemiparesis or neurotmesis |
| Transient quadriparesis |

Most Severe

FIG. 3-3 Pathologic neurologic responses in cervical trauma. *(From Brier SR:* Primary care orthopedics, *St Louis, 1999, Mosby.)*

C1 (Atlas)

Posterior tubercle
Posterior arch
Foramen transversarium
Lateral mass
Anterior tubercle
Superior articular facet
Superior articular facet
Anterior arch

C2 (Axis)

Bifid spine
Transverse process
Superior articular facet
Odontoid
Odontoid
Foramen transversarium

C7

Spinous process
Lamina
Transverse process
Foramen transversarium
Superior articular facet
Superior articular facet
Body
Body

FIG. 3-4 Cervical vertebrae C1, C2, and C7. *(From Mathers LH, et al:* Clinical anatomy principles, *St Louis, 1996, Mosby.)*

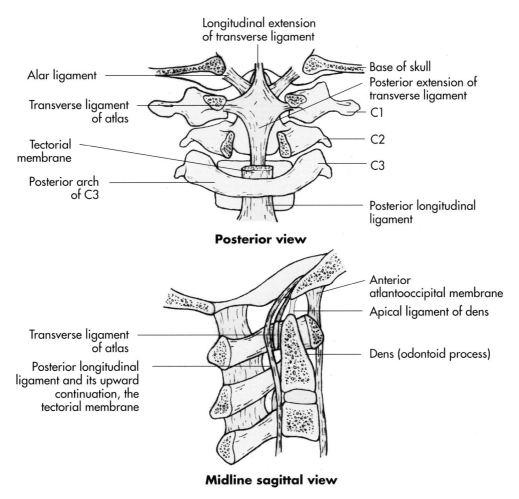

FIG. 3-5   Ligaments connecting the skull and vertebral column. *(From Mathers LH, et al:* Clinical anatomy principles, *St Louis, 1996, Mosby.)*

examination should be differentiated from pathologic subluxation. On imaging of the cervical spine, the predental space should not exceed 3 mm. A predental space greater than 3 mm has been found in 20% of normal patients younger than 8 years of age and can be followed on patients into early adulthood.

Pathologic subluxation of the atlas on the axis that compromises the spinal cord (compressive myelopathy) is associated with rheumatoid arthritis and ankylosing spondylitis. The common characteristic of these disorders is the destructive weakening of the atlantooccipital ligament system, with resultant translation of the structures.

The costal element in C7 is one of the most common from which accessory ribs may form (e.g., a "cervical rib"). Abnormal positioning of a cervical rib heightens the risk of compression of the nerves and vessels (Fig. 3-6).

The articulations of the vertebral column are of great importance. The vertebral column supports much weight; serves as an axis for movement of the limbs, trunk, head, and neck; and protects the spinal cord from trauma (Fig. 3-7).

The intervertebral discs are fibrocartilaginous flattened structures interposed between adjacent vertebral bodies (Fig. 3-8). Each disc consists of a gelatinous inner region (i.e., the nucleus pulposus), surrounded by a solid ring of stiffer material (i.e., the annulus fibrosus) (Fig. 3-9).

The vertebral artery is closely related to the cervical spine and is the first branch of the subclavian artery. It enters the foramen of the transverse process of C6 and ascends through the remaining foramina of the tops of the cervical vertebrae (Fig. 3-10). The vertebral artery passes beneath the posterior atlantooccipital membrane (Fig. 3-11). The union of the two vertebral arteries forms the basilar artery.

ESSENTIAL MOTION ASSESSMENT

During a cervical spine range-of-motion assessment, the examiner should examine active then passive movements. For flexion, the patient brings the chin onto the chest; for extension, the patient bends the head backward as far as

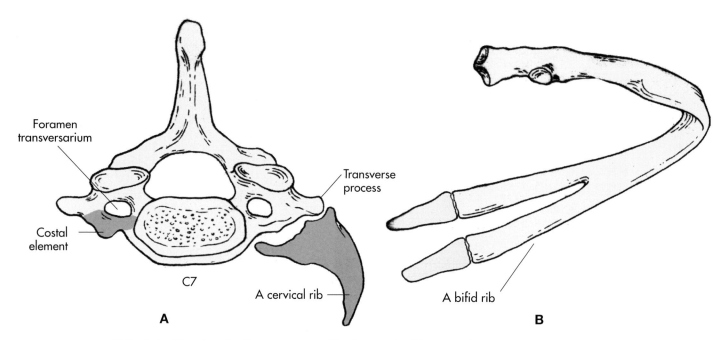

Foramen
transversarium

Transverse
process

Costal
element

C7

A cervical rib

A

A bifid rib

B

FIG. 3-6   Variations in rib structures. **A,** Cervical rib. **B,** Bifid rib with two costal cartilages.
(From Mathers LH, et al: Clinical anatomy principles, *St Louis, 1996, Mosby.)*

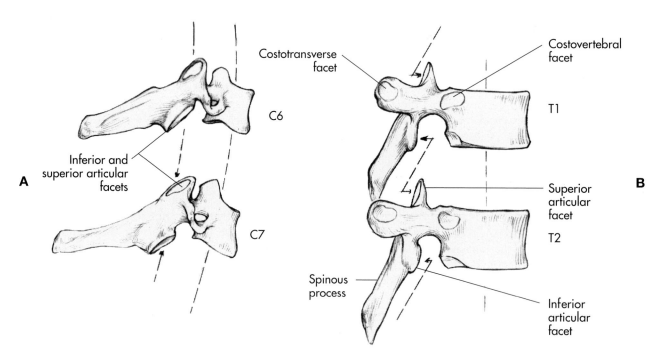

Costotransverse
facet

Costovertebral
facet

C6

T1

Inferior and
superior articular
facets

A

C7

Superior
articular
facet

T2

B

Spinous
process

Inferior
articular
facet

FIG. 3-7   Vertebral articulations. **A,** Cervical vertebrae. **B,** Thoracic vertebrae.   *(From Mathers LH,
et al:* Clinical anatomy principles, *St Louis, 1996, Mosby.)*

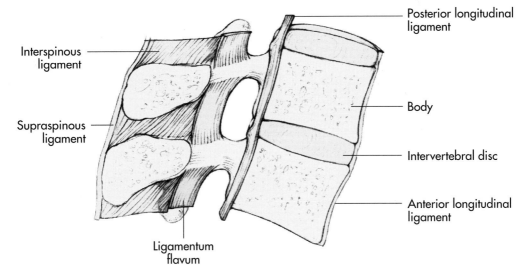

FIG. 3-8   Midsagittal section through a typical vertebra.   *(From Mathers LH, et al:* Clinical anatomy principles, *St Louis, 1996, Mosby.)*

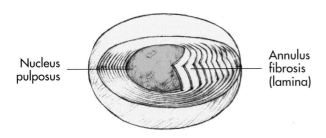

FIG. 3-9   Intervertebral disc.   *(From Mathers LH, et al:* Clinical anatomy principles, *St Louis, 1996, Mosby.)*

possible (Fig. 3-12). For lateral flexion, the patient brings an ear toward the shoulder, first on one side and then on the other. For rotation, the patient looks over one shoulder and then the other. Repeating the movements while applying gentle pressure over the vertex of the skull may trigger pain or paresthesia in the arm if there is a critical degree of narrowing at an intervertebral foramen (Fig. 3-13). In evaluating cervical spine range of motion, the examiner observes not only the total range of movement but also the smoothness and comfort with which the patient accomplishes the motions (Figs. 3-14 to 3-21).

ESSENTIAL MUSCLE FUNCTION ASSESSMENT

The muscles of the vertebral column are often in an increased state of contraction. This stiffens the vertebral column to serve as a platform for movement of the head or limbs (Fig. 3-22, p. 60).

ORTHOPEDIC GAMUT 3-3

VERTEBRAL MUSCLES

The vertebral muscles are divided into two large groups:

1. Extrinsic muscles, which are important in the attachment of limbs and limb girdles to the vertebrae and contribute to motions of the trunk
2. Intrinsic muscles, which stabilize and carry out motions of the vertebral column itself

---

ORTHOPEDIC GAMUT 3-4

CERVICAL SPINE MUSCLE STRENGTH

To evaluate cervical spine muscle strength, the patient does the following:

1. Pushes a cheek against the examiner's hand (This maneuver also tests the motor function of cranial nerve XI [sternocleidomastoid muscle]) (Fig. 3-25, p. 62)
2. Pushes the back of the head against the examiner's hand (Fig. 3-29, p. 64)
3. Pushes the forehead against the examiner's hand (Figs. 3-26 to 3-28, p. 63)

Text continued on p. 61

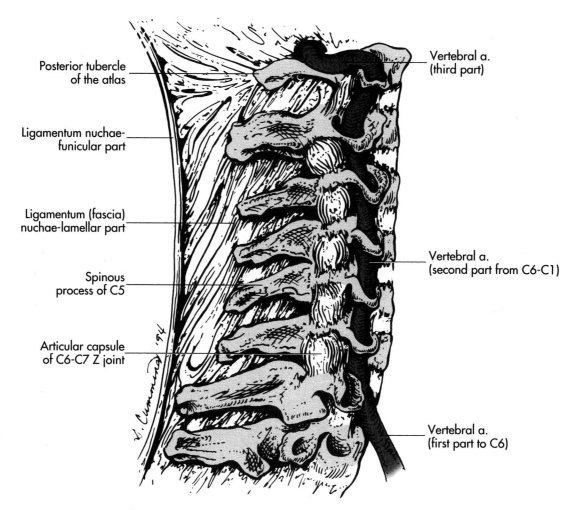

Posterior tubercle
of the atlas

Ligamentum nuchae-
funicular part

Ligamentum (fascia)
nuchae-lamellar part

Spinous
process of C5

Articular capsule
of C6-C7 Z joint

Vertebral a.
(third part)

Vertebral a.
(second part from C6-C1)

Vertebral a.
(first part to C6)

FIG. 3-10   Lateral view of the cervical portion of the vertebral column.   *(From Cramer GD, Darby SA: Basic and clinical anatomy of the spine, spinal cord, and ANS, St Louis, 1995, Mosby.)*

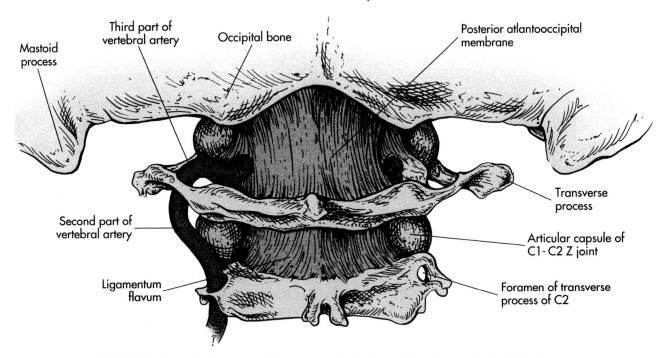

FIG. 3-11   Posterior ligaments of the upper cervical region.   *(From Cramer GD, Darby SA:* Basic and clinical anatomy of the spine, spinal cord, and ANS, *St Louis, 1995, Mosby.)*

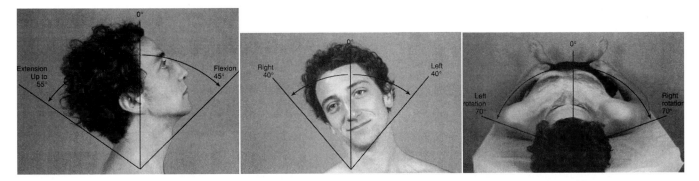

FIG. 3-12   Range of motion of the cervical spine.   *(From Barkauskas VH, Stoltenberg-Allen K, Baumann LC, Darling-Fisher C:* Health & physical assessment, *ed 2, St Louis, 1998, Mosby.)*

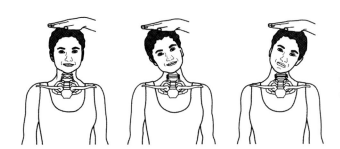

FIG. 3-13   Compression of the vertex of the skull to reproduce cervical root pain.   *(From Epstein O, Perkin GD, deBono DP, Cookson J:* Clinical examination, *ed 2, London, 1997, Mosby.)*

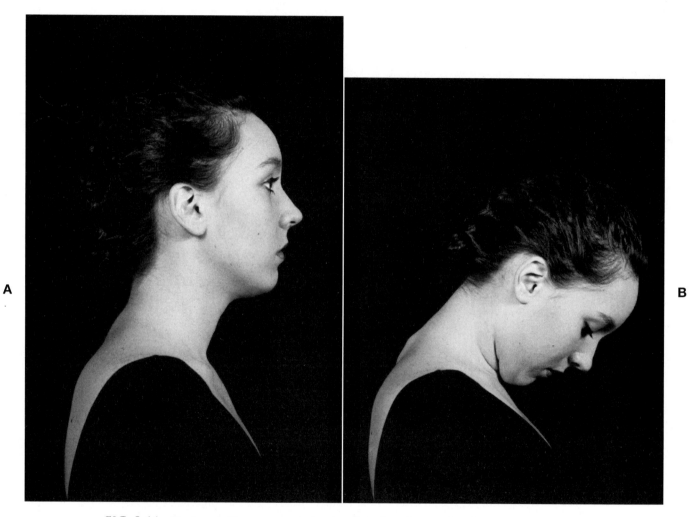

A

B

FIG. 3-14   Flexion. **A,** To assess cervical range of motion, the examiner has the patient sit with the head upright. **B,** The examiner then instructs the patient to tuck the chin in toward the chest. The expected range of motion is 80 to 90 degrees. Excessive range is when the chin can reach the chest while the patient's mouth is closed. Two finger widths' distance between the chin and the chest can be considered normal. Forty degrees or less of retained cervical flexion is an impairment of neck function in the activities of daily living.

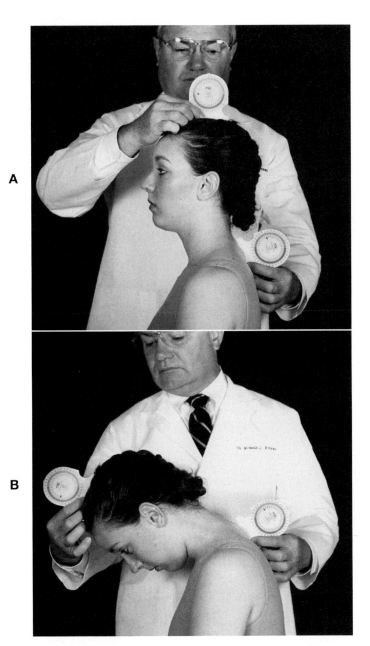

A

B

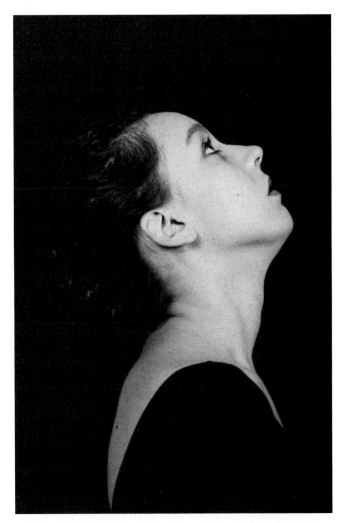

FIG. 3-15 Flexion assessed with an inclinometer. **A,** With the patient seated and the cervical spine in the neutral position, the examiner places one inclinometer over the T1 spinous process in the sagittal plane. The second inclinometer is placed at the superior aspect of the occiput, or on top of the head, also in the sagittal plane. Both inclinometers are zeroed in these positions. **B,** The patient flexes the head and neck forward. The examiner records both angles. The T1 inclination is subtracted from the cranial inclination to determine the cervical flexion angle. The expected range of motion is 60 degrees or greater from the neutral position.

FIG. 3-16 Extension. Extension range of motion is 70 degrees. In extension the plane of the nose and forehead should be nearly horizontal. Fifty degrees or less of retained cervical extension is an impairment of neck function in the activities of daily living.

FIG. 3-17 Extension assessed with an inclinometer. The patient is seated with the cervical spine in the neutral position. The examiner places one inclinometer slightly lateral to the T1 spinous process in the sagittal plane. The second inclinometer is placed at the superior aspect of the occiput, or on top of the head, in the sagittal plane. Both inclinometers are zeroed in these positions. The patient extends the head and neck, and the examiner records the angle of both inclinometers. The T1 inclination is subtracted from the occipital inclination to determine the cervical extension angle. The expected range of motion is 75 degrees or greater from the neutral position.

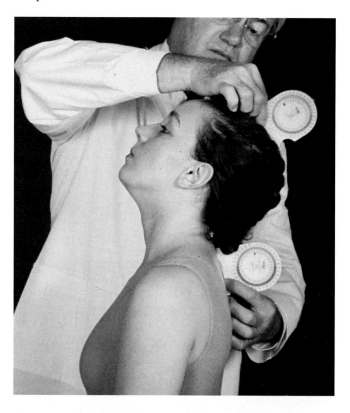

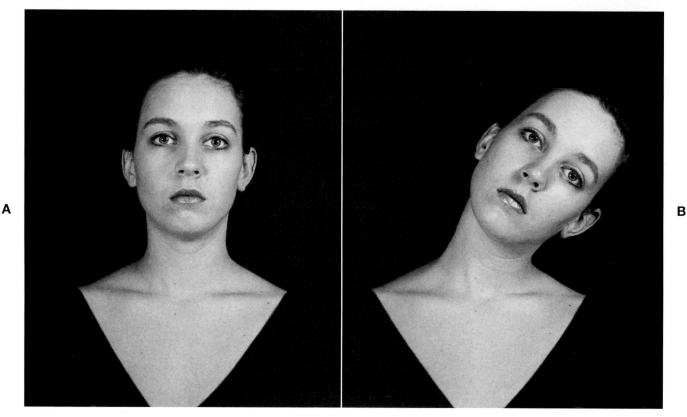

A

B

FIG. 3-18 Lateral flexion. **A,** The patient begins with the cervical spine in the neutral position. **B,** Lateral flexion of the cervical spine is normally about 20 to 45 degrees to the right and left. Most lateral flexion occurs between the occiput and C1 and between C1 and C2. Thirty degrees or less of retained lateral flexion is an impairment of neck function in the activities of daily living.

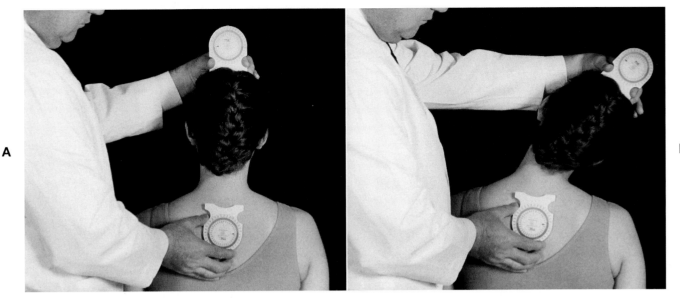

FIG. 3-19 Lateral flexion assessed with an inclinometer. **A,** With the patient seated and the cervical spine in a neutral position, the examiner places one inclinometer on the T1 spinous process in the coronal plane. The examiner places the second inclinometer at the superior aspect of the occiput, or on top of the head, also in the coronal plane. Both instruments are then zeroed. **B,** The patient laterally flexes the head and neck to one side. The examiner records the angles of both instruments. The T1 inclination is subtracted from the occipital inclination to determine the cervical lateral flexion angle. The expected range of motion is 45 degrees or greater from the neutral position. The procedure should be repeated for the opposite side.

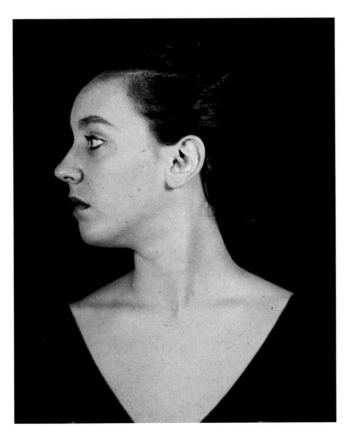

FIG. 3-20 Rotation. Normal rotation of the cervical spine is 70 to 90 degrees. Often, the patient's chin does not reach the plane of the shoulder. Sixty degrees or less of retained cervical rotation is an impairment of the cervical spine in the activities of daily living.

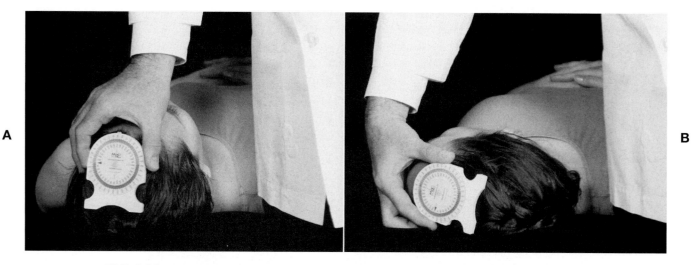

FIG. 3-21   Rotation assessed with an inclinometer. **A,** With the patient in a supine position, the examiner places the inclinometer at the crown of the head in the coronal plane. The instrument is zeroed. **B,** The patient rotates the head to one side, and the examiner records the angle indicated on the instrument. This angle is the cervical spine rotation angle. Repeat the procedure for the opposite side. The expected range of motion is 80 degrees or greater from the neutral position.

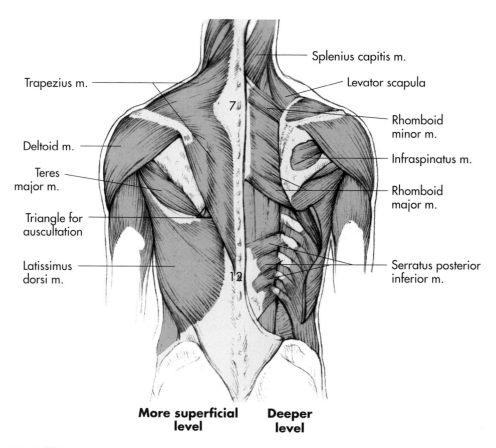

FIG. 3-22   Superficial back muscles. *(From Mathers LH, et al: Clinical anatomy principles, St Louis, 1996, Mosby.)*

The intrinsic longitudinal vertebral muscles, placed more superficially, are collectively called the *erector spinae* (Fig. 3-23). The cervical region contains elongated muscles originating from the spinous process (the splenius muscles) and others from the transverse processes (the semispinalis muscles). The suboccipital muscles are a special group of muscles linking the atlas, the axis, and the base of the skull (Fig. 3-24).

ESSENTIAL IMAGING

PLAIN FILM IMAGING

The minimum set of films for the cervical spine includes the anteroposterior (AP), lateral, open-mouth, and odontoid views. The vertebra C7 must be visualized on the lateral projection when the cervical spine is being examined because many fracture-dislocations occur in the lower cervical spine or at the cervicothoracic junction (Fig. 3-29).

The open-mouth view is vital in assessing the normal articulation of the lateral masses of the atlas (C1) with those of the axis (C2). This is especially true when assessing a possible Jefferson burst fracture with disruption of the normal neural ring of C1, causing lateral displacement of its lateral masses.

Of equal importance is the articulation between the anterior arch of C1 and the odontoid process of C2 on the lateral projection. Laxity or disruption of the transverse ligament may result in an unstable atlantoaxial joint (Fig. 3-30). In the lower cervical spine the translation of a single vertebra over the inferior vertebral segment greater than 3 or 3.5 mm signifies instability.

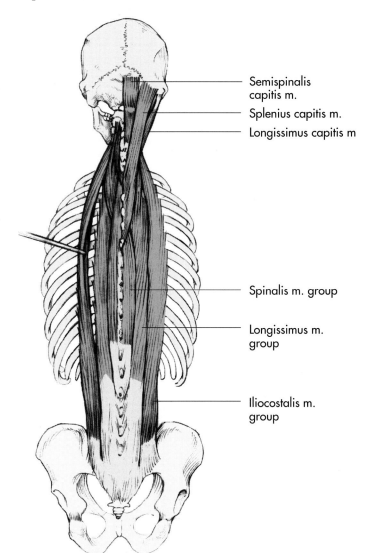

FIG. 3-23 Erector spinae muscles. *(From Mathers LH, et al: Clinical anatomy principles, St Louis, 1996, Mosby.)*

Semispinalis capitis m.
Splenius capitis m.
Longissimus capitis m
Spinalis m. group
Longissimus m. group
Iliocostalis m. group

Oblique views of the cervical spine aid in evaluating the neural foramina and the posterior elements (Fig. 3-31).

The pillar view is another special-view plain film. Using 20 to 30 degrees of caudal angulation of the x-ray beam enables a more precise inspection of the lateral masses when pillar fractures and facet dislocations are suspected in hyperextension and rotational injuries.

MAGNETIC RESONANCE IMAGING

Magnetic resonance imaging (MRI) has gained recognition based on its high soft-tissue contrast, lack of ionizing radiation, and direct multiplanar acquisition. In many institutions it has become the most widely used screening method for evaluating the spine. A wide variety of specialized surface coils have been produced. With each of these,

---

ORTHOPEDIC GAMUT 3-5

CERVICAL SPINE INSTABILITY

Plain film, lateral, flexion, or extension views reveal evidence of cervical spine instability, which includes the following:

1. Anterolisthesis (sagittal displacement of vertebral body more than 3.5 mm)
2. Increased spinous spacing
3. Subluxation of facet joints
4. Acute angular deformity at level of injury (11-degree angulation of adjacent vertebral bodies)
5. Sagittal diameter of spinal canal less than 13 mm
6. Fracture or dislocation
7. Atlantodental interval (ADI) greater than 3 mm in adults and 4 mm in children

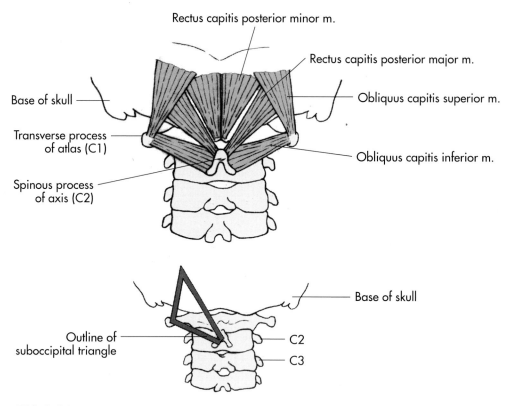

FIG. 3-24   Suboccipital triangle.   *(From Mathers LH, et al:* Clinical anatomy principles, *St Louis, 1996, Mosby.)*

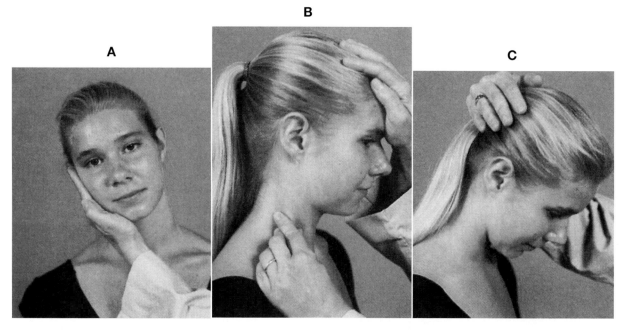

FIG. 3-25   Examining the strength of the sternocleidomastoid and trapezius muscles. **A,** Rotation against resistance. **B,** Flexion with palpation of the sternocleidomastoid muscle. **C,** Extension against resistance.   *(From Barkauskas VH, Stoltenberg-Allen K, Baumann LC, Darling-Fisher C:* Health & physical assessment, *ed 2, St Louis, 1998, Mosby.)*

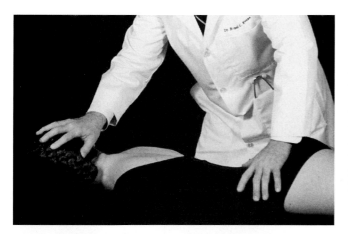

FIG. 3-26   Posterolateral head and neck extensors. The muscles included in this test are chiefly the splenius capitis and cervicis, semispinalis capitis and cervicis, and cervical erector spinae. The patient is prone on the examining table. Slight fixation is necessary. The patient tries a posterolateral extension with the face turned toward the side tested. The upper trapezius, also a posterolateral neck extensor, is tested in a similar manner with the face turned away from the side examined. The examiner applies pressure in an anterior direction against the posterolateral aspect of the head.

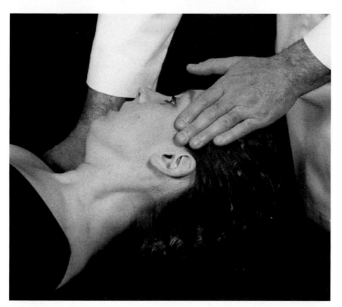

FIG. 3-27   Anterolateral head and neck flexors. The muscles acting in this test are chiefly the sternocleidomastoid and scaleni. The patient is supine on the examination table. If the patient's anterior abdominal muscles are weak, the examiner can give fixation by firm downward pressure on the thorax. The patient attempts anterolateral neck flexion. The examiner applies pressure to the temporal region of the head in an obliquely posterior direction. If the neck muscles are strong enough to hold the head but not strong enough to flex completely, the patient may try to lift the head from the table by raising the shoulders. This occurs especially in the tests for right and left neck flexors because the patient attempts to aid the maneuver by taking some weight on the elbow or hand, allowing the shoulder to rise from the table. To prevent this, the examiner holds the patient's shoulder flat on the table.

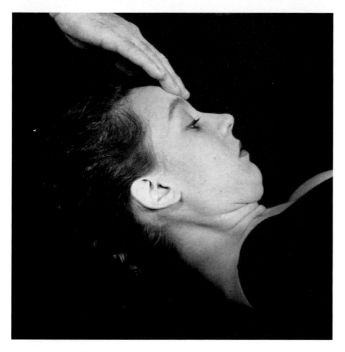

FIG. 3-28   Anterior head and neck flexors. The patient is resting on the examination table in the supine position with elbows bent and hands over the head. The anterior abdominal muscles must be strong enough to give anterior fixation of the thorax to the pelvis. This strength allows the head to be raised by the neck flexors. If the abdominal muscles are weak, the examiner can provide fixation by applying firm, downward pressure on the thorax. Children 5 years or younger should always have fixation of the thorax provided by the examiner. The patient tries to flex the cervical spine by lifting the head from the table toward the sternum while keeping the mouth closed and the chin depressed. The examiner applies pressure to the forehead in a posterior direction.

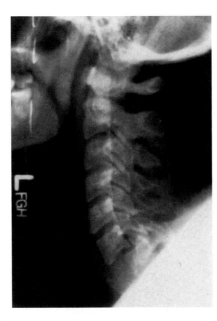

FIG. 3-29 Lateral x-ray film demonstrating significant anterior subluxation of C6 on C7 with depression of the shoulders. *(From Watkins RG:* The spine in sports, *St Louis, 1996, Mosby.)*

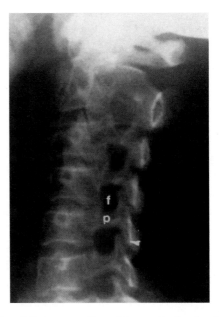

FIG. 3-31 Oblique x-ray film of the cervical spine demonstrating patent normal foramina. *(From Watkins RG:* The spine in sports, *St Louis, 1996, Mosby.)*

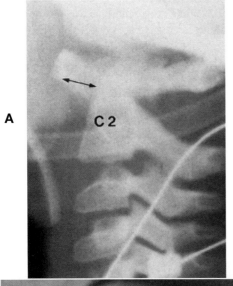

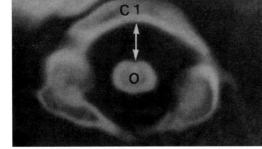

FIG. 3-30 Lateral x-ray film **(A)** and axial computed tomography scan **(B)** demonstrating widening between the anterior arch of C1 and the odontoid process of C2. *(From Watkins RG:* The spine in sports, *St Louis, 1996, Mosby.)*

either the entire cervical, lumbar, or most of the thoracic spine may be imaged in one acquisition. Improvements in coil technology consisting of phased-array coils have allowed imaging of most of the spinal column in one acquisition with no additional scanning time (Fig. 3-32).

ORTHOPEDIC GAMUT 3-6

CERVICAL SPINE PLAIN FILM SERIES

The typical cervical spine plain film series consists of the following:

1. AP open-mouth (APOM) view (Figs. 3-33 to 3-35)
2. AP lower cervical (APLC) view (Figs. 3-36 to 3-38)
3. Lateral cervical view (Figs. 3-39 and 3-40)
4. Oblique views (Figs. 3-41 to 3-43)

Specific views are used to evaluate complex regions of anatomy or spinal placement at extremes of motion (Box 3-1).

In assessing the sagittal diameter of the spinal canal, on a lateral view, the shortest distance from the posterior aspect of the vertebral body to the spinolaminar line is measured. The distance between the posterior aspect of the dens and the posterior cervical line is measured at C1. The ranges for diameter by level are listed in Table 3-4.

Text continued on p. 70

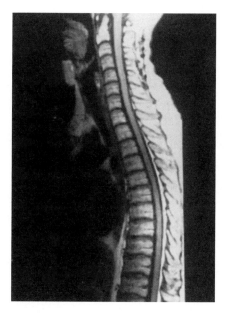

FIG. 3-32   Sagittal T1-weighted image of the entire cervical and thoracic spine.   *(From Watkins RG: The spine in sports, St Louis, 1996, Mosby.)*

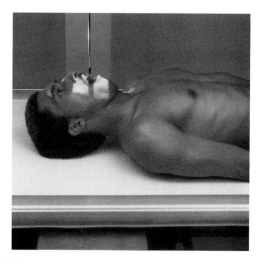

FIG. 3-33   AP atlas and axis.   *(From Ballinger PW: Merrill's atlas of radiographic positions and radiologic procedures, vol 1-3, ed 8, St Louis, 1995, Mosby.)*

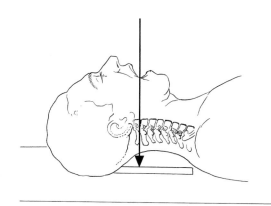

FIG. 3-34   Open-mouth spine alignment.   *(From Ballinger PW: Merrill's atlas of radiographic positions and radiologic procedures, vol 1-3, ed 8, St Louis, 1995, Mosby.)*

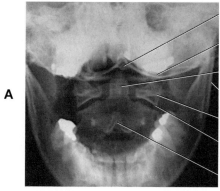

A

Occipital base

Occlusal surface of teeth

Dens (odontoid process)

Mandibular ramus

Lateral mass of atlas

Inferior articular process of atlas

Spinous process of axis

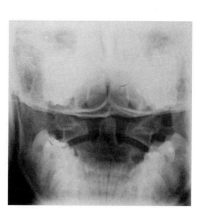

B

FIG. 3-35   **A** and **B,** Open-mouth atlas and axis.   *(From Ballinger PW: Merrill's atlas of radiographic positions and radiologic procedures, vol 1-3, ed 8, St Louis, 1995, Mosby.)*

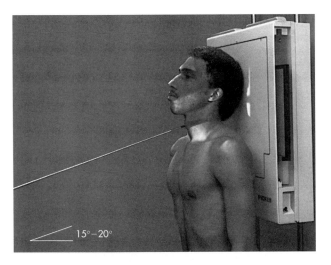

FIG. 3-36   AP axial cervical vertebrae, upright. *(From Ballinger PW:* Merrill's atlas of radiographic positions and radiologic procedures, *vol 1-3, ed 8, St Louis, 1995, Mosby.)*

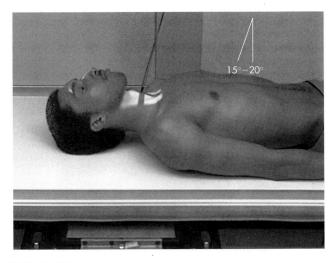

FIG. 3-37   AP axial cervical vertebrae, recumbent. *(From Ballinger PW:* Merrill's atlas of radiographic positions and radiologic procedures, *vol 1-3, ed 8, St Louis, 1995, Mosby.)*

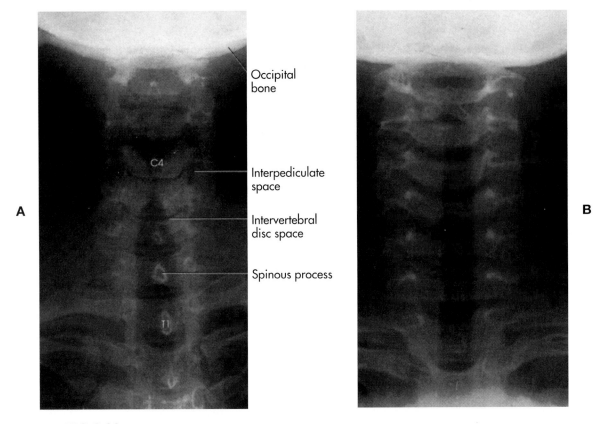

FIG. 3-38   **A** and **B,** AP axial cervical vertebrae.   *(From Ballinger PW:* Merrill's atlas of radiographic positions and radiologic procedures, *vol 1-3, ed 8, St Louis, 1995, Mosby.)*

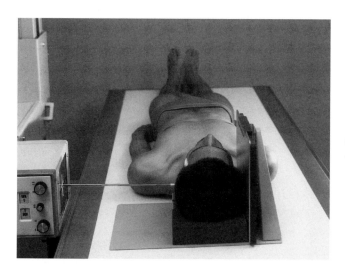

FIG. 3-39 Lateral atlas and axis. *(From Ballinger PW:* Merrill's atlas of radiographic positions and radiologic procedures, *vol 1-3, ed 8, St Louis, 1995, Mosby.)*

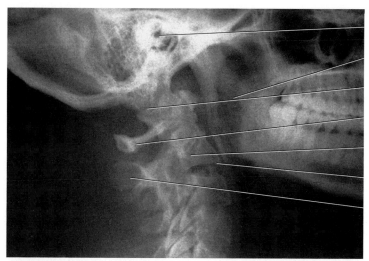

External acoustic meatus

Superimposed mandibular rami

Atlantooccipital articulation

Posterior arch, atlas

Transverse process, axis

Body of axis

Spinous process, axis

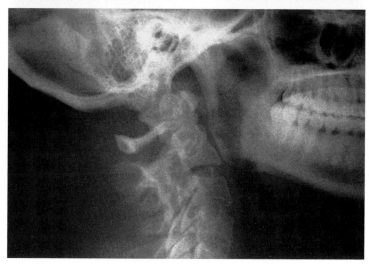

FIG. 3-40 Lateral atlas and axis. *(From Ballinger PW:* Merrill's atlas of radiographic positions and radiologic procedures, *vol 1-3, ed 8, St Louis, 1995, Mosby.)*

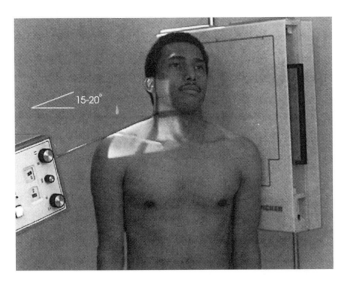

FIG. 3-41 Upright AP axial oblique intervertebral foramina, LPO. *(From Ballinger PW: Merrill's atlas of radiographic positions and radiologic procedures, vol 1-3, ed 8, St Louis, 1995, Mosby.)*

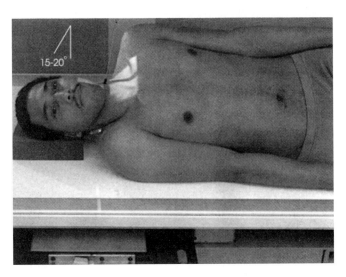

FIG. 3-42 Recumbent AP axial oblique left intervertebral foramina, RPO. *(From Ballinger PW: Merrill's atlas of radiographic positions and radiologic procedures, vol 1-3, ed 8, St Louis, 1995, Mosby.)*

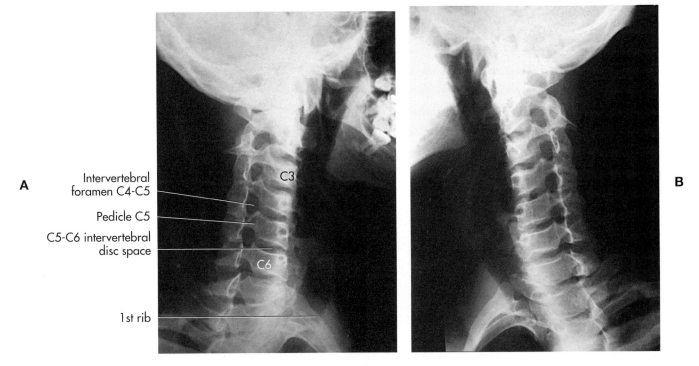

A

Intervertebral foramen C4-C5

Pedicle C5

C5-C6 intervertebral disc space

1st rib

C3

C6

B

FIG. 3-43 AP axial oblique intervertebral foramina. **A,** LPO position. **B,** RPO position. *(From Ballinger PW: Merrill's atlas of radiographic positions and radiologic procedures, vol 1-3, ed 8, St Louis, 1995, Mosby.)*

BOX 3-1

Accepted Cervical Spine Imaging

Anteroposterior lower cervical view (APLC)
Anteroposterior open-mouth view (APOM)
Lateral view

Anterior oblique views (right and left)
Additional views
   Flexion and extension lateral view
   Fuch's view
   Pillar or Boyleston view

Data from Greenstein GM, *Clinical assessment of neuromusculoskeletal disorders,* St Louis, 1997, Mosby.

TABLE 3-4

ACCEPTED SAGITTAL CANAL DIAMETER OF THE CERVICAL SPINE

Level	Diameter (mm)	
	Minimum	**Maximum**
C1	16	31
C2	14	27
C3	13	23
C4 to C7	12	22

Adapted from Greenstein GM: *Clinical assessment of neuromusculoskeletal disorders,* St Louis, 1997, Mosby.

BAKODY SIGN

SHOULDER ABDUCTION TEST
CERVICAL FORAMINAL COMPRESSION TEST

Assessment for Cervical Nerve Root Compression

Comment

Annular fissures, or rents, develop in the degenerating disc and may coalesce, ultimately allowing nuclear material to extrude into the neural canals. When the extruded nucleus pulposus forms a broad-based extension of the disc beyond the peripheral confines of the vertebral end-plate, it is bulging. When focal asymmetric nuclear material extends beyond the end-plate but is still contained by the posterior longitudinal ligament, the nucleus is protruding. With further expulsion of nuclear material, disc extrusion occurs. With disc extrusion, free or sequestered disc fragments may migrate away from the parent disc level (Fig. 3-44).

Cervical radiculopathy is more common than cervical myelopathy. Cervical radiculopathy consists of pain and neurologic dysfunction produced by irritation or injury to a spinal nerve. The injury may be caused by a herniated cervical disc, cervical foraminal stenosis, tumors, fractures, or dislocations. The pathognomic characteristic of cervical radiculopathy is pain in the distribution of nerve (Table 3-5).

Although cervical nerve root compression is a part of the syndrome of cervical osteoarthritis, particularly with zygapophyseal and Luschka joint involvement, faulty posture of the cervical spine may contribute to the cervical nerve root compression, or it may be the primary cause of compression.

Hyperextension of the cervical spine, performed with the chin in a forward position, compresses the zygapophyseal joints and Luschka joints on the posterior surfaces of the cervical vertebrae. Hyperextension is the cause and pathogenesis of the compression.

There are neither specific genetic and environmental factors nor specific epidemiologic factors for cervical compression. In cervical hyperextension syndromes, radiographic characteristics may include those typical of cervical osteoarthritis in addition to other postural factors.

TABLE 3-5

CLINICAL FINDINGS ASSOCIATED WITH THE CERVICAL NERVE ROOTS

Root	Disc	Muscle	Reflex	Sensation	Myelogram/CT/MR Deficit
C5	C4-C5	Deltoid Biceps	Biceps	Lateral arm Deltoid area Axillary nerve	C4-C5
C6	C5-C6	Biceps Wrist extensors	Brachioradialis	Thumb, index, ring fingers Lateral forearm Musculocutaneous nerve	C5-C6
C7	C6-C7	Triceps Wrist flexors Finger extensors	Triceps	Middle finger and/or ring finger	C6-C7
C8	C7-T1	Hand intrinsics Finger flexors		Ring and fifth fingers Medial forearm Medial anterior brachial cutaneous nerve	C7-T1
T1	T1-T2	Hand intrinsics		Medial arm Medial brachial cutaneous nerve	

Adapted from Watkins RG: *The spine in sports,* St Louis, 1996, Mosby.
CT, Computed tomography; *MR,* magnetic resonance.

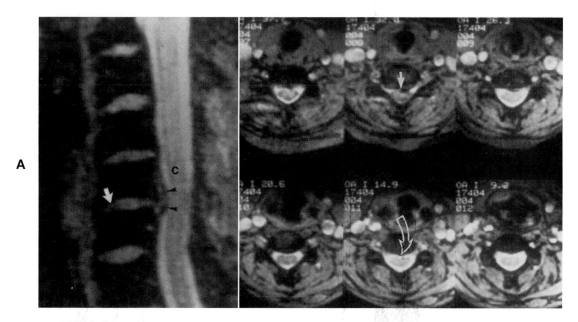

FIG. 3-44   Sagittal (**A**) and axial gradient-recalled (**B**) magnetic resonance imaging scans of the cervical spine showing central disc extrusion effacing ventral subarachnoid space in contrast to normal subarachnoid space.   *(From Watkins RG:* The spine in sports, *St Louis, 1996, Mosby.)*

A cervical nerve root compression syndrome may result from direct trauma to the nerve roots from the pincerlike action of the foraminal architecture during an acute hyperextension trauma, from chronic irritation from hypertrophic spurring, or from disc disease. This latter source may be a traumatic aggravation of chronic disc disease or an acute herniation or prolapse of disc material. Symptoms of nerve root compression are distinctly different from those of neurovascular compression syndromes or reflex sympathetic dystrophy. The symptoms of nerve root compression include proximal (root) pain and neck pain, distal paresthesia in dermatome patterns, muscle weakness in one or several muscles supplied by a single root, loss of deep tendon reflexes, muscle fasciculation, and radiating pains that are further aggravated by movements of the neck.

Irritation of the cervical nerve roots may cause pain, sensory changes, muscle atrophy, or spasm and alteration of the tendon reflexes anywhere along the segmental distribution. Any condition causing a narrowing of the intervertebral canals may cause compression of the nerve roots and the spinal branches of the vertebral arteries, venous congestion and irritation, and compression of the recurrent meningeal nerves.

Encroachment, or narrowing, of the intervertebral canals may be the result of some involvement of the proximate soft-tissue structures or bony structures. Any condition that causes inflammation and swelling of the dural sleeves of the nerve roots may also cause neural compression.

PROCEDURE

- While in the seated position, the patient actively places the palm of the affected extremity on top of the head, raising the elbow to a height approximately level with the head (Fig. 3-45).
- By elevating the suprascapular nerve, traction of the lower trunk of the brachial plexus is relieved (Fig. 3-46).
- Overall, this maneuver decreases stretching of the compressed nerve root.
- The sign is present when the radiating pain is lessened or disappears with this maneuver.
- The test is as reliable as Spurling's test and is less painful for the patient to endure.

Confirmation Procedures

Dejerine's sign, Valsalva maneuver, Naffziger's test, reflexes, maximum foraminal compression test, distraction test, brachial plexus tension test, Bikele's sign, Jackson cervical compression test, Spurling's test, electrodiagnosis, and diagnostic imaging

DIAGNOSTIC STATEMENT

A cervical nerve root compression is indicated by a positive Bakody sign on the right. A cervical nerve root compression syndrome is suspected in the presence of Bakody sign on the right.

CLINICAL PEARL

Patients with moderate to severe radicular symptoms usually do not have to be directed into the Bakody sign position because it also is an antalgic pain-relieving posture. The more difficult it is for the patient to lower the arm, the more difficult the condition will be to treat conservatively. If the patient cannot lower the arm without severe exacerbation of pain, surgery is probably indicated. Patients with moderate to severe cervical nerve root compression find the most comfortable sleeping positions to be those that involve abduction and elevation of the arm. Again, this position relieves the traction of the neural elements and is an antalgic position for someone experiencing cervical nerve root compression. A patient often voluntarily assumes the Bakody sign position while in the examination room.

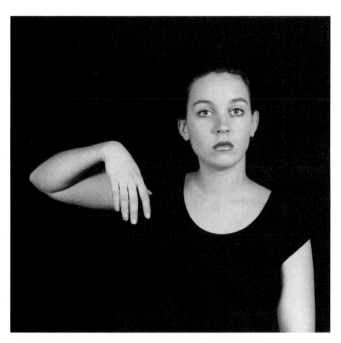

FIG. 3-45 The patient abducts and externally rotates the ipsilateral shoulder by moving the hand toward the head.

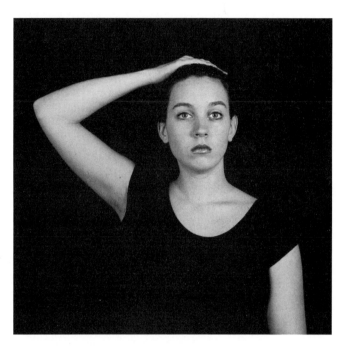

FIG. 3-46 The hand is placed on top of the head. If this position relieves radicular pain, this is a positive sign that indicates a nerve root syndrome.

BARRE-LIEOU SIGN

Assessment for Vertebral Artery Syndrome

Comment

Rotation of the neck to one side usually decreases the circulation in the atlantoaxial portion of the contralateral vertebral artery. When there is kinking of the artery, atheromata, or osteoarthritis, such movement reduces the circulation even more. Other mechanisms that could alter the blood supply to the brainstem are carotid sinus compression, use of a surgical collar, pugilistic activities, manipulation of the neck that causes the release of emboli from atheromatous plaques in the great vessels, and thrombosis with infarction of the cerebellum or brainstem.

Vertebral artery insufficiency, whether permanent or transitory, has been identified as the explanation for some of the symptoms seen with hyperextension/hyperflexion injuries. The course of the vertebral artery in the cervical spine is tortuous, and the artery passes through, over, and around structures that may become malaligned after trauma (Fig. 3-47). Abnormal pressures or tractional stresses may impede circulation through these arteries. The vertebral arteries also may be compressed as a result of chronic degenerative disease of the cervical spine. This compression may occur at any point along its usual course from C6 to C2 and may become symptomatic after cervical spine trauma.

Increased tissue pressures from myospasm, edema, or hemorrhage may also compromise the blood flow through the vertebral artery. This is especially true when patency is already compromised because of atherosclerosis or a congenital anomaly. Arterial spasm may also occur.

ORTHOPEDIC GAMUT 3-8

TRAUMA TO THE VERTEBRAL ARTERY

Three areas in which the vertebral artery is most susceptible to trauma are as follows:

1. The posterior atlantooccipital membrane, which is dense and inelastic and may become calcified (firmly attached to the artery)
2. The space between the occiput and posterior arch of the atlas, especially during extension
3. Between the lateral mass of the atlas and the transverse process of the axis, especially during extension and rotation

---

ORTHOPEDIC GAMUT 3-7

VERTEBRAL ARTERY COMPRESSION

Three mechanisms of vertebral artery compression have been described:

1. Osteophytes from the lateral disc margin
2. Anteriorly extending osteophytes from the facet joint
3. Compression from the inferior facet as a result of posterior subluxation and a scissoring effect by the adjacent superior facet

---

Older patients with preexisting atherosclerotic disease are at a greater risk of injury that results in vertebral artery syndrome, or vertebrobasilar artery insufficiency.

The history is important in patients with carotid artery stenosis or occlusion. The symptoms may range from a minor problem, such as blurring of vision in one eye, to profound obtundation, aphasia, and hemiparesis.

In midbasilar artery occlusion, the effect is profound ("locked-in" syndrome). Locked-in syndrome is a condition of total consciousness, with or without impaired sensation, and no voluntary movement except vertical eye movement and convergence. The syndrome results from interference of basilar artery blood flow in the region of the midpons, producing bilateral ventral pontine infarction. This serves as a transection of the brainstem at the midpons region.

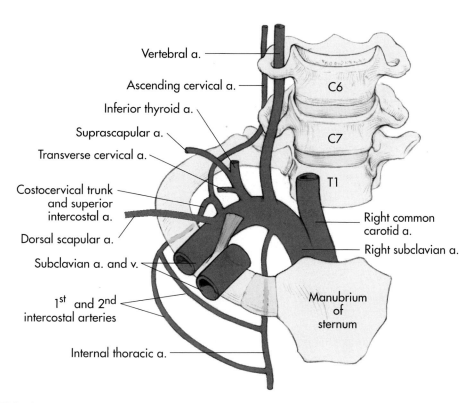

Vertebral a.

Ascending cervical a.

Inferior thyroid a.

Suprascapular a.

Transverse cervical a.

Costocervical trunk and superior intercostal a.

Dorsal scapular a.

Subclavian a. and v.

1st and 2nd intercostal arteries

Internal thoracic a.

C6

C7

T1

Right common carotid a.

Right subclavian a.

Manubrium of sternum

FIG. 3-47 Vertebral artery and cervical vertebrae. *(From Mathers LH, et al: Clinical anatomy principles, St Louis, 1996, Mosby.)*

ORTHOPEDIC GAMUT 3-9

LOCKED-IN SYNDROME

Locked-in syndrome characteristics include the following:

1. Retained consciousness
2. No volitional movement of the body
3. Nuclei of cranial nerves V to XII destroyed, resulting in their paralysis
4. Loss of sensations carried in the medial lemniscus
5. Normal hearing
6. Sparing of cranial nerve IV nucleus and the superior colliculus of the quadrigeminal plate

PROCEDURE

- The examiner instructs the patient to slowly rotate the head from side to side while in a seated position (Fig. 3-48).

- Rotating the head causes compression of the vertebral arteries (Fig. 3-49).
- Vertigo, dizziness, visual disturbances, nausea, syncope, and nystagmus are signs of a positive test (Fig. 3-50).
- A positive finding strongly indicates a buckling of the ipsilateral vertebral artery.

Confirmation Procedures

Vertebrobasilar artery functional maneuver, Hautant's test, DeKleyn's test, Hallpike maneuver, Underburg's test, Doppler vascular investigation, carotid auscultation, and diagnostic imaging

DIAGNOSTIC STATEMENT

Barre-Lieou sign is present on the left. This finding indicates vertebrobasilar insufficiency on the right side.

CLINICAL PEARL

The patient with a positive Barre-Lieou sign is a poor risk for aggressive cervical spine manipulation. Such manipulation should not be undertaken until all vascular causes have been investigated. Aggravation of the *sympathetic ganglia* of the cervical spine can produce many, if not all, of these symptoms (vertigo, dizziness, visual disturbances, nausea, syncope, and nystagmus), in which case cervical spinal manipulation is not contraindicated. It is critical that the examiner distinguish between vascular and neural origins before manipulation is performed.

In 1926, Barre studied and established a syndrome that was further described in 1928 by his student Lieou. So diverse and widespread is the combination of symptoms and signs that some people no longer regard the syndrome as a disorder associated with the cervical spine; rather, they view the syndrome as one caused by vertebral artery insufficiency and its multivariate characteristics. The symptoms of this syndrome include pain in the head, neck, eyes, ears, face, sinuses, and throat; sensory disturbances in the pharynx and larynx; paroxysmal hoarseness and aphonia; tinnitus that is synchronous with the pulse; various auditory hallucinations, such as whistling and humming; deafness; visual disturbances, such as blurring, scintillating scotomata, photophobia, blepharospasm, squinting sensations, and a peculiar pulling at the back of the eyes; flushing; sweating; salivation; lacrimation; nausea; vomiting; and rhinorrhea.

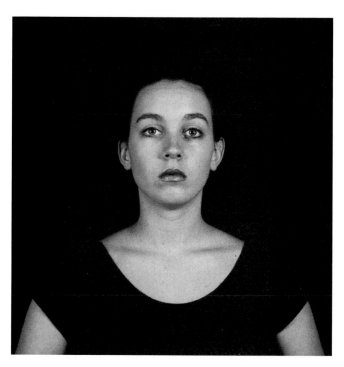

FIG. 3-48 The patient is seated as comfortably and as erect as possible. Blood pressure and pulse are examined and recorded before starting the test.

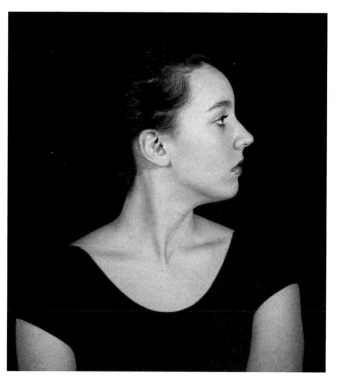

FIG. 3-49 The patient rotates the head maximally from side to side. This movement is performed slowly at first and then accelerated until the patient's tolerance is reached.

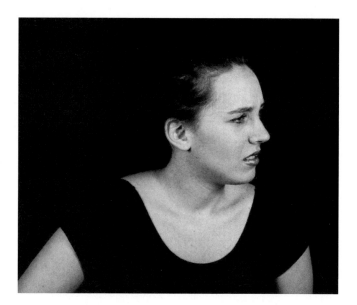

FIG. 3-50 A vertebral artery syndrome is indicated by vertigo, blurred vision, nausea, syncope, or nystagmus. These symptoms may occur singly or in combination.

BIKELE'S SIGN

Assessment for Brachial Plexus Neuritis and Meningitis

Comment

The most common and least understood cervical injury is neurapraxia of the nerve roots and brachial plexus. Brachial plexus lesions result in motor and sensory syndromes of muscles of the upper extremities. The brachial plexus is made up of the anterior primary rami of the four lower cervical nerves, C5 through C8, and the greater part of T1. The C5 and C6 rami form the upper trunk, the C7 ramus forms the middle trunk, and the C8 and T1 rami form the lower trunk. Trunks are placed in the supraclavicular fossa distal to the anterior scalene muscle. Each trunk splits into an anterior and posterior division, with derivation of three cords from them. The lateral cord is formed by the anterior division of the upper and middle trunks, the medial cord by the anterior division of the lower trunk (C8 and T1), and the posterior cord by the posterior divisions of all three trunks and nerves. The upper trunk branches to the supraclavicular nerve, innervating the supraspinatus and infraspinatus muscles, as well as the subclavius muscles. The lateral cord branches to the lateral anterior thoracic nerve, innervating the greater pectoral muscle. The medial cord becomes the medial anterior thoracic cord, which goes to the pectoral muscles and the medial antebrachial and brachiocutaneous nerves. The posterior cord branches to the subscapular nerve, which innervates the subscapular and teres major muscle, and the thoracodorsal nerve, which innervates the latissimus dorsi muscles. Terminal branches of the posterior cord are the axillary and radial nerves, and the terminal branches of the lateral cord are the musculocutaneous (biceps) component and the lateral component of the median nerve. The terminal branches of the medial cord are the ulnar nerve and the medial component of the median nerve.

Brachial plexopathy (sometimes called a *stinger, burner,* or *dead* arm) is also a possible result of a lateral flexion traction injury. The neurologic deficit may last for only a few seconds, or it may occur intermittently for several days. Swelling at the nerve root or distal to the spine can combine with traction to the nerve sleeves, making the deficit more severe.

PROCEDURE

- With the arm held upward and backward and the elbow fully flexed, the patient extends the elbow (Fig. 3-51).
- If such movement meets with resistance and increases radicular pain from the cervicodorsal region, the test is positive (Fig. 3-52).
- This finding indicates brachial plexus neuritis or meningitis because this maneuver stretches the brachial plexus nerve roots or coverings.

Confirmation Procedures

Reflexes, sensory testing, Bakody sign, Dejerine's sign, Valsalva maneuver, maximum foraminal encroachment testing, shoulder depression test, distraction test, brachial plexus tension test, Jackson cervical compression test, Spurling's test, electrodiagnosis, and diagnostic imaging

When reflex sympathetic symptoms are present, additional tests may be indicated. These tests include matchstick testing, pilomotor response testing, and thermography.

DIAGNOSTIC STATEMENT

Bikele's sign is present on the right. This result suggests brachial plexus neuritis.

CLINICAL PEARL

Injury to the C8 and T1 roots, the lower trunk, or the medial cord of the brachial plexus may be caused by tumors, disease of the pulmonary apex, or a fractured clavicle or cervical rib. Aneurysm of the arch of the aorta, fracture or dislocation of the humeral head, or unusually abrupt and severe upward traction of the arm may also injure the nerves.

Although Bikele's sign does not usually produce a profound finding in minor cervical nerve root compression syndromes, the maneuver often produces startling results in lower brachial plexopathy in the thoracic outlet. Reflex sympathetic changes may be present with the plexopathy and should be correlated with other physiologic findings.

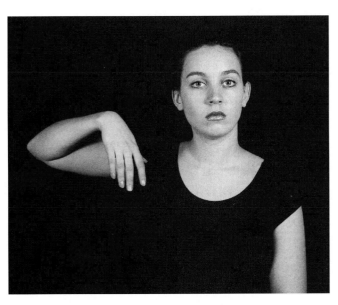

FIG. 3-51 The patient is seated and abducts the shoulder to 90 degrees. The shoulder is externally rotated.

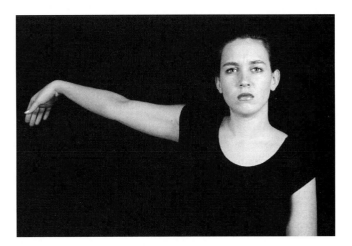

FIG. 3-52 The arm is fully extended at the elbow, and the patient attempts to reach behind. In the presence of radiculopathy or plexopathy, this maneuver produces the radicular pain.

BRACHIAL PLEXUS TENSION TEST

Assessment for Cervical
Nerve Root Syndrome or Compression (C5)

Comment

A direct traumatic insult to the nerve roots causes inflammation in the dural sleeves and perineural tissues, which may result in fibrosis. Adhesions may occur between the dural sleeves and the adjacent capsular tissues. Normally, the nerve roots are free in the intervertebral canals and can move 1/4 to 1/2 of an inch. Nerve roots that are injured or compressed by capsular thickening or bony encroachments cannot move within the intervertebral canals. Nerve roots subjected to compressive forces by osteophytic encroachments have varying amounts of distortion and perineural fibrosis.

In many instances at least one fiber of a nerve root fails to continue in that particular nerve root. This fiber descends to join the adjacent distal nerve root. For instance, one of the fourth cervical nerve root fibers that leaves the cord at that level may actually leave the spinal canal with fibers of the fifth cervical nerve root. If the fourth cervical nerve root is irritated within the foramen of the fifth cervical nerve root, the examiner may find that the fourth cervical nerve is also involved.

The fifth cervical nerve root is the root irritated most often, and the sixth, fourth, third, second, and seventh roots become irritated in that order of frequency. Irritation or compression of a nerve root may cause pain-sensory changes anywhere along its distribution. Localized areas of tenderness and muscle spasm will be found at the site of the pain. The examiner often finds some areas of segmental tenderness of which the patient is not aware. These myalgic areas are found only by deep palpation because hyperalgesia, or superficial tenderness, is not present.

In cases affecting the fifth cervical root, the pain extends from the scapular area to the front of the arm and forearm and can extend as far as the radial side of the hand. However, the pain does not reach the thumb, and the pins-and-needles sensation is absent. The weak muscles are the supraspinatus, the infraspinatus, the deltoid, and the biceps. The biceps reflex may be sluggish or absent, and the brachioradialis reflex is sluggish, absent, or inverted.

From its position at the thoracic outlet, the brachial plexus is the neurologic switchboard responsible for transferring the sensory and motor impulses from the cervical nerve roots to the peripheral nerves of the first thoracic nerve root contributing to the plexus.

The examination of a person with a brachial plexopathy should begin with observation for round shoulders, forward neck, or obvious swelling. The examiner should palpate the paraspinal region for spasm or hypertonicity in the musculature. Similarly, the examiner should palpate the supraclavicular area for swelling, spasm, or masses that can adversely affect the brachial plexus.

The individual with brachial plexopathy usually has transient paresis of the upper limb because of an excessive lateral flexion injury of the cervical spine, with or without shoulder depression. Paresthesia generally emanates from the middle or lower cord of the plexus, reproducing the usual distribution of the dysthetic response seen in contact sports injuries called *burners* or *stingers*. Sometimes, the entire hand goes numb and weak, and the individual tries to shake the limb to reduce the pain.

Brachial neurapraxia involves demyelination of the axon sheath without disruption. In some neuronal injuries the axon is interrupted, but the surrounding tissues remain intact. Degeneration of the affected muscles (axonotmesis) appears on electrodiagnostic studies 2 to 3 weeks after sustaining the neural injury. Patterns of reinnervation often develop. In contrast, recovery from neurotmesis, a severe injury that destroys the axon and supporting structures, is unlikely.

PROCEDURE

- The examiner passively elevates the patient's shoulders through abduction (Figs. 3-53 and 3-54).
- The elbows are extended to a point just short of the onset of pain and are maintained in that position.
- The shoulders are externally rotated to the point just short of the onset of pain and maintained (Fig. 3-55).
- The examiner supports the shoulders and forearms in this position as the patient flexes the elbows (Fig. 3-56).
- Reproduction of symptoms suggests cervical spine disorders, most likely the C5 nerve root.
- In addition, from this challenge position, symptoms increase when the cervical spine is flexed.

Confirmation Procedures

Dejerine's sign, Valsalva maneuver, reflex testing, Bakody sign, maximum foraminal encroachment test, shoulder depression test, distraction test, Bikele's sign, Jackson cervical compression test, Spurling's test, and diagnostic imaging

---

DIAGNOSTIC STATEMENT

The brachial plexus tension test is positive on the right. This result suggests a C5 nerve root syndrome.

CLINICAL PEARL

Although the brachial plexus tension test involves shoulder joint movement, it also provides maximum stretch on the brachial plexus, which affects the lower branches of the cervical spine (C5) the most. If this test is positive, the early stages of a C5 nerve root disorder may be present along with the subtle signs of a positive doorbell sign (pain that occurs at the superior scapuloverteberal border and radiates with the use of deep palpation of the C5 segment) and pain in the deltoid area. The deltoid pain is often misconstrued as an articular problem of the shoulder.

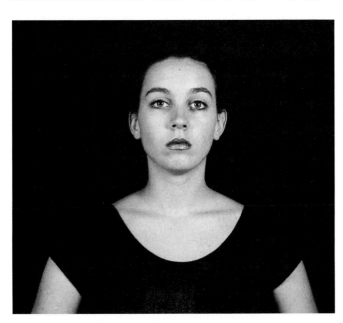

FIG. 3-53 The patient is sitting erect. An alternative is to have the patient assume the supine position on the examination table.

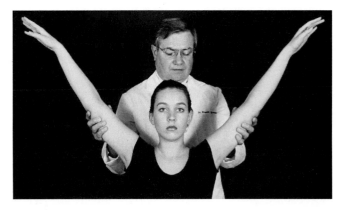

FIG. 3-54 The patient fully elevates the shoulders through abduction to the end-point of joint play. The elbows are fully extended. The examiner supports the patient's arms in this position.

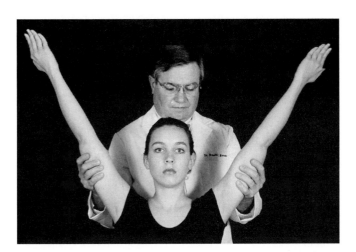

FIG. 3-55 The patient externally rotates the shoulders to the end-point of joint play or to the onset of discomfort. The examiner supports the patient's arms in this position.

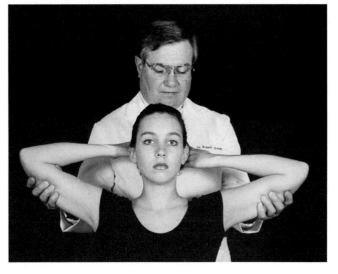

FIG. 3-56 As the shoulders are supported in this position, the patient flexes the elbows. Reproduction of the radicular symptoms suggests a nerve root syndrome that probably involves C5. If symptoms do not appear, a final maneuver is the flexion of the cervical spine.

DEJERINE'S SIGN

DEJERINE'S TRIAD
TRIAD OF DEJERINE

Assessment for Herniated or Protruding Intervertebral Disc and Spinal Cord Tumor or Spinal Compression Fracture

Comments

The symptoms of a cervical disc injury vary according to the status and site of the injury. Acute disc protrusions typically have radicular symptoms down one arm; the pain can be bilateral if the spinal canal is compromised and the protrusion is central or large. Motor, reflex, or sensory changes are a distinct possibility, and the examiner should examine the patient regularly for such changes during the first 2 weeks of care. The presence of Dejerine's sign (pain on coughing, sneezing, or straining) suggests a space-occupying lesion. Compression tests with the patient in various positions are helpful. The position of the disc bulge or the site of the canal-nerve root compromise of the cervical spine causes pain in patients with disc and nerve root lesions; distraction maneuvers are usually palliative.

Referred pain to the arm, hand, and scapula is common. Injury to the C5 nerve root level often causes scapular pain. During the acute phase the patient experiences muscle spasm and guarding, local or referred pain from annular nerve fiber stimulation, or posterior joint dysfunction. There is a distinct loss of range of motion, and some swelling may be present. Patients often complain of instability, such as difficulty rising from the recumbent position.

Infections and tumors, benign or malignant, are rare occurrences in the cervical spine. The cervical spine is unique, anatomically and physiologically, with its concentration of crowded, critical structures. Rapid clinical catastrophe is a constant threat unless early diagnosis of tumor and infection is instituted. Neurologic structures have little tolerance to mechanical compression. The possibilities of quadriplegia, spinal cord stroke, and death are always in the background. The close anatomic and physiologic relationships among the spinal cord, nerve roots, and peripheral nervous system and the structurally confining implications of the skeletal and soft tissues make early diagnosis mandatory in these cervical spinal disorders.

Space-occupying lesions in or around the spinal canal cause a broad spectrum of clinical syndromes, ranging from neck pain, radiculitis, and paresthesia to quadriparesis and death. Cervical cord compression can be caused by the gross space occupation of an expanding abscess; a rapidly growing vertebral, medullary, or extramedullary tumor; or the fracture, collapse, and dislocation of the supporting structures. These structures include the bones, discs, joints, ligaments, and tendons. Critical structures that are at risk when tumors and infections of the cervical spine are present include the lower brainstem, cervical spinal cord, nerve roots and rootlets, ganglia and common spinal nerves, vertebral arteries, carotid artery, trachea, and esophagus.

Radiating pain in the cervical spine, shoulder, and arm that is accompanied by tenderness, muscle spasms, and decreased cervical spine movements may be the only clinical manifestations of a benign, space-occupying mass. Torticollis is more common in masses involving the upper cervical spine. Mass enlargement or bony displacement may cause clinical symptoms and signs of radiculitis or spinal cord compression. Spinal stroke occurs when the radicular arteries, the end arteries in the cord itself, or the anterior and posterior spinal arteries are constricted.

Clinical manifestations of cervical disc disease are highly variable. Patients may have many complaints and physical findings. Generally, signs and symptoms can be categorized as neurogenic or discogenic. *Neurogenic* symptoms result from pressure on the cervical nerve roots or the spinal cord by disc material or by posterior or posterolateral osteophytes. Patients may have radicular symptoms alone, or they may have signs and symptoms of nerve root and spinal cord compression simultaneously.

Patients with *discogenic* symptoms have no objective dermatomal neurologic findings. Patients complain of intermittent, chronic pain in the posterior cervical region and the shoulder, chest wall, and scapular region. Occipital headaches are common. The pain experienced by patients with discogenic symptoms results from the stimulation of the sensory receptors of the sinuvertebral nerve. The sinuvertebral nerve is located in the fibrous ring of the intervertebral disc and in the posterior and anterior longitudinal ligament.

Root pain is often produced or aggravated by coughing, sneezing, or straining, such as during defecation or any other measures that suddenly increase intrathoracic and intraabdominal pressure. Because the intervertebral veins do not contain valves, such pressure increases block the venous flow from the epidural space through the intervertebral veins or permit a retrograde flow of blood. This pressure increase causes distension of the veins in the epidural space, which in turn forces the dura, which envelops the nerve roots, toward the spinal cord. Because the nerve roots are fixed to the spinal cord proximally and peripherally at the intervertebral foramen, the displacement of the dura results in a stretching of the involved nerve root, which may result in pain. In addition, distension of the intervertebral vein may result in direct compression of the nerve root.

PROCEDURE

- Coughing, sneezing, and straining during defecation may aggravate radiculitis symptoms (Fig. 3-57).
- This aggravation results from the mechanical obstruction of spinal fluid flow.
- Dejerine's sign is present when one of the following exists: herniated or protruding intervertebral disc, spinal cord tumor, or spinal compression fracture.

- The course of the radiculitis helps identify the location of the lesion.

Confirmation Procedures

Swallowing test, Valsalva maneuver, Naffziger's test, vascular assessment, and diagnostic imaging (e.g., MRI)

DIAGNOSTIC STATEMENT

Dejerine's sign is present. This finding suggests a space-occupying mass at the C5 level.

Dejerine's sign is present with reproduced radicular symptoms on the right in the C5 dermatome. This result suggests a space-occupying mass at that vertebral level.

CLINICAL PEARL

Patients with radicular symptoms and pronounced Dejerine's sign, especially if it is in the lumbar spine, should be told to bend the knees and lean into a wall during a cough or sneeze. This maneuver reduces intradiscal pressure and minimizes the effect of the cough or sneeze on the nerve root. A more worrisome situation is the sudden, unexpected absence of Dejerine's sign when all other clinical findings indicate an active nerve root compression. The loss of the sign indicates fragmentation of the disc with momentary decompression of the nerve.

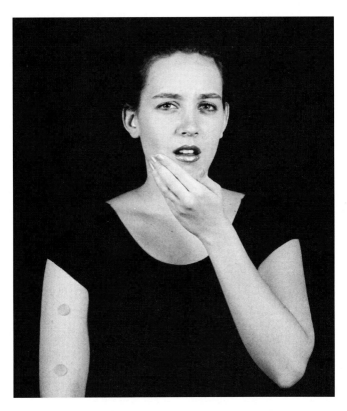

FIG. 3-57 Coughing, sneezing, or straining during defecation causes a reproduction of radicular symptoms, which suggests a space-occupying mass that is creating neurologic compression.

DEKLEYN'S TEST

Assessment for Vertebral Artery Syndrome

Comment

The vertebral artery is often the first and largest branch of the subclavian artery. It passes upward to enter the foramen in the sixth cervical transverse process. It continues to course upward, encased by the bony rings formed by the transverse foramina. After emerging from the transverse foramen of the atlas, the vertebral artery proceeds to wind posteriorly and medially around the lateral mass of the atlas. The vertebral artery then passes through the foramen magnum and at the lower border of the pons unites with the vertebral artery of the opposite side to form the basilar artery. The posterior inferior cerebellar arteries (PICA) leave the vertebral arteries just before they join each other (Fig. 3-58).

Vertebral artery syndrome (also called *vertebral artery compression syndrome* or *vertebrobasilar artery insufficiency*) is characterized by recurring transient episodes of cerebral symptoms (Fig. 3-59). The notable cerebral symptoms include vertigo, nystagmus, and sudden postural collapse without unconsciousness. These symptoms are precipitated by rotation and hyperextension of the neck and are caused by temporary occlusion of the vertebral artery. This mechanical action produces ischemia at the base of the brain. A combination of cerebrovascular arteriosclerosis and cervical spondylosis is fundamental in this syndrome.

The main tributaries to the basilar artery at the base of the brain are the internal carotid and vertebral arteries. Occlusive arterial disease gradually reduces blood flow to a certain critical point. Any further reduction in the caliber of the vessel, unless an adequate collateral supply has developed, will result in ischemia and cerebral symptoms.

Normally, hyperextension and rotation of the neck compresses and may occlude the vertebral artery on the contralateral side at the level of the atlas and axis. However, symptoms do not develop because collateral circulation is adequate. When vessels are occluded by atheromatous plaques and compressed by osteophytes, collateral blood flow may be insufficient and symptoms may develop as the vertebral artery becomes blocked momentarily during the rotation and hyperextension movement of the cervical spine.

Various causes of dizziness must first be ruled out, particularly those caused by labyrinthine or cerebellar disease. The drop attack must be differentiated from epilepsy, syncope, and Stokes-Adams syndrome. Carotid sinus sensitivity, with its cardioinhibitory and vasodepressor reflexes, can be identified by an electrocardiogram (ECG) that is conducted while the carotid sinus is massaged.

The subclavian steal syndrome must be ruled out because its symptoms are caused by basilar artery insufficiency. However, syncopal episodes are precipitated by exertion of the upper extremity. With the subclavian steal syndrome, occlusion occurs at the portion of the subclavian artery that is proximal to the origin of the vertebral artery. Because of this occlusion, blood flow is diverted from the opposite vertebral artery into the artery on the obstructed side, which results in perfusion of the distal subclavian bed with blood that was intended for cerebral circulation.

ORTHOPEDIC GAMUT 3-10

VERTEBRAL ARTERY PATENCY TESTS

There are several variations of the vertebral artery patency tests:

1. Houle's test
2. DeKleyn's test
3. Smith and Estridge's maneuver *(see Note 1 below)*
4. Modified Adson's maneuver
5. Extension rotation test
6. Maigne's test *(see Note 1 below)*
7. Wallenberg test
8. Reclination test *(see Note 2 below)*

Note 1: Maigne's, Smith and Estridge's Maneuver

The patient's head is maintained for several seconds in a position of rotation and extension. The patient is asked to comment on the development of any symptoms of vertebrobasilar insufficiency, and the examiner observes for nystagmus. If vertebrobasilar insufficiency signs or symptoms occur, the head is immediately returned to a neutral position.

Note 2: Reclination Test (Sitting)

With the patient sitting, the examiner moves the patient's head into extreme positions of extension and rotation. If threatening signs or symptoms occur, the head is returned to the neutral position.

Normally, even if these maneuvers occlude one vertebral artery, no symptoms occur because adequate brainstem

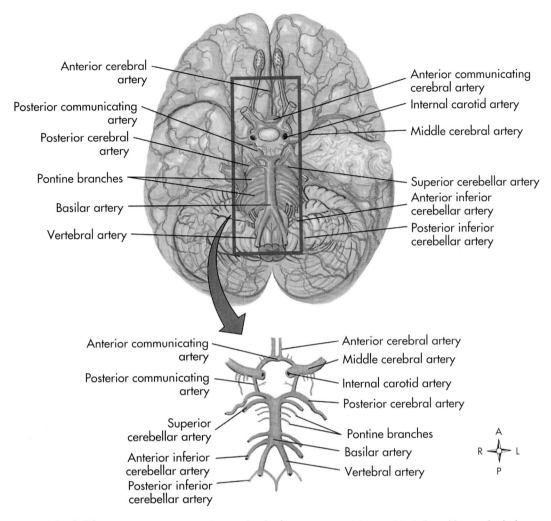

FIG. 3-58 Arterial blood supply to the brain. *(From Seidel HM:* Mosby's guide to physical examination, *ed 4, St Louis, 1999, Mosby.)*

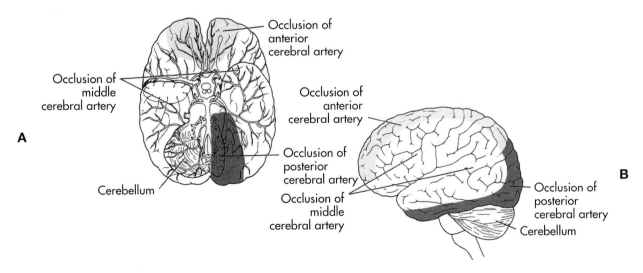

FIG. 3-59 Areas of the brain affected by occlusion of the anterior, middle, and posterior cerebral artery branches. **A,** Inferior view. **B,** Lateral view. *(From Seidel HM:* Mosby's guide to physical examination, *ed 4, St Louis, 1999, Mosby.)*

blood flow occurs through the opposite vertebral artery (VA). These tests, when positive, indicate only that rotation has produced brainstem ischemia, possibly resulting from compression of one vertebral artery, and inadequate patency of the opposite artery. These tests do not necessarily indicate any underlying arteriopathy that would predispose the patient to arterial wall damage and vertebrobasilar syndrome.

PROCEDURE

- With the patient in the supine position and the patient's head off the table, the examiner instructs the patient to hyperextend and rotate the head and hold this position for 15 to 45 seconds (Fig. 3-60).
- The patient repeats this maneuver with the head rotated and extended to the opposite side.

- Vertigo, blurred vision, nausea, syncope, and nystagmus are signs of a positive test.

Confirmation Procedures

Hautant's test, George's screening procedure, Underburg's test, Hallpike maneuver, vertebrobasilar artery functional maneuver, Barre-Lieou sign, vascular assessment, vascular imaging, and MRI

DIAGNOSTIC STATEMENT

DeKleyn's test is positive following cervical rotation to the right with hyperextension. This result suggests vertebral artery syndrome on the ipsilateral side.

ORTHOPEDIC GAMUT 3-11

POTENTIAL SITES OF COMPRESSION OR INJURY DURING SPINAL MOVEMENT

There are at least eight potential sites in the cervical spine at which arterial structures can be compressed or injured by spinal movement:

1. Between C1-C2 transverse processes (Rotation tends to produce stretching of the vertebral artery at this site.)
2. At the level C2-C3 as a result of compression of the vertebral artery by the superior articular facet of C3 on the ipsilateral side to head rotation
3. By the C1 transverse process compressing the internal carotid artery
4. At the C4-C5 or C5-C6 levels as a result of osteoarthrosis of the uncovertebral joints, which can displace the vertebral artery anteriorly and laterally (Compression of the artery is ipsilateral to the side of head rotation.)

5. As a result of compression before entering the C6 transverse process, by traction over a prominent longus colli muscle, or by tissue communicating between the longus colli and scalenus anticus muscles
6. By constriction of the vertebral artery by the ventral ramus of the second cervical nerve during head rotation
7. At the atlantooccipital aperture, on extension:
   - By compression between the posterior arch of atlas and the foramen magnum
   - By folding of the atlantooccipital joint capsule anteriorly and the atlantooccipital membrane posteriorly
8. By compression by the oblique capitis inferior muscle or intertransversarii muscle between the transverse foramina of C1 and C2

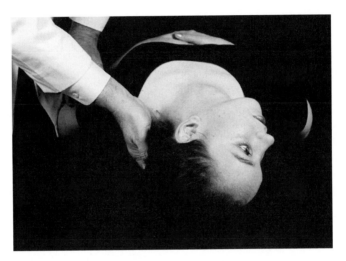

FIG. 3-60   The patient is supine with the head extending off the end of the examination table. The patient rotates and hyperextends the neck to one side and holds this position for 15 to 45 seconds. The examiner may provide minimal support for the weight of the skull. The maneuver is repeated for the opposite side. The production of vertigo, visual disturbance, nausea, syncope, or nystagmus indicates vertebrobasilar circulation compromise.

DISTRACTION TEST

Assessment for Cervical Nerve Root Compression, Intervertebral Foraminal Encroachment, and Facet Capsulitis

Comment

Synovial folds (menisci) from Z joints project into the Z joints at all levels of the cervical spine.

ORTHOPEDIC GAMUT 3-12

Z JOINT MENISCI

Four distinct types of cervical Z joint menisci exist (Fig. 3-61):

Type I: Menisci are thin and protrude far into the Z joints, covering approximately 50% of the joint surface (found only in children).

Type II: Menisci are relatively large wedges that protrude a significant distance into the joint space (found almost exclusively at the lateral C1-C2 Z joints).

Type III: Folds are rather small nubs (found throughout the C2-C3 to C6-C7 cervical Z joints of most healthy adults).

Type IV: Menisci are quite large and thick (found in degenerative Z joints).

When the individual vertebrae are united, the articular process of each side of the cervical spine forms an articular pilar that bulges laterally at the pediculolaminar junction (Fig. 3-62).

The cervical articular pillars support the weight of the head and neck. Therefore weight bearing in the cervical region is carried out by a series of three longitudinal columns: one anterior column, which runs through the vertebral bodies, and two posterior columns, which run through the right and left articular pillars.

Articular pillar fracture is fairly common in the cervical spine and often goes undetected. This type of fracture is usually a chip fracture of a superior articular facet. The patient often experiences transient radicular pain, which is usually followed by mild to intense neck pain. Persistent radiculopathy in such patients indicates displacement of the fractured facet onto the dorsal root as it exits the intervertebral foramen.

The complaints of patients with chronic or degenerative conditions of the cervical disc are quite different from those of patients with acute conditions. Patients with chronic conditions experience intermittent episodes of pain, discomfort, and muscle spasm. Exacerbations come from exertion. Pain and stiffness may result from weather changes or unexplained causes. Radiculopathy is not always present. Hyporeflexia, motor weakness, and sensory disturbance (especially paresthesia) are common (Table 3-6).

In cervical spine hyperflexion or hyperextension injuries, there are significant indirect signs of trauma. These signs are evident on typical plain radiographic studies.

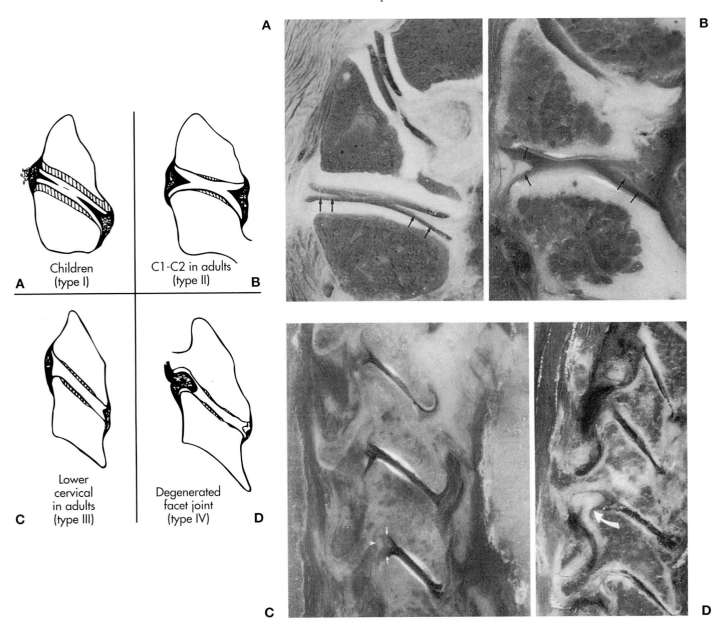

FIG. 3-61 Four types of menisci (*left* and *right*). **A,** Type I. **B,** Type II. **C,** Type III. **D,** Type IV.
(From Yu et al: Brain, *109:259-278, England, 1987, Oxford University Press.)*

ORTHOPEDIC GAMUT 3-13

INDIRECT SIGNS OF CERVICAL TRAUMA OR INJURY

Abnormal Soft Tissue

Hemorrhage caused by injury of the paracervical soft tissues displaces certain physiologic spaces that are appreciated radiographically, representing a space-occupying lesion:

1. Widened retropharyngeal space (in excess of 7 mm)
2. Widened retrotracheal space (in excess of 21 mm)
3. Displacement of the prevertebral fat stripe
4. Tracheal deviation and laryngeal dislocation

Abnormal Vertebral Alignment

Injury of soft tissue (a strain or sprain of muscle, tendon, ligament, and capsule) produces spasm, identified by the following:

1. Loss of lordosis
2. Acute kyphotic hyperangulation
3. Torticollis
4. Widened interspinous space
5. Rotation of vertebral bodies (one spinous process significantly rotated, suggests unilateral facet dislocation)
6. Widened middle atlantoaxial joint (the atlantodental interspace [ADI]) (in excess of 2 mm in adults or 5 mm in children)
7. Abnormal intervertebral disc
8. Widening of apophyseal joints

TABLE 3-6

COMMON CLINICAL FEATURES OF CERVICAL DISC SYNDROMES

Disc	Pain	Sensory Change	Motor Weakness, Atrophy	Reflex Change
C4-C5 (C5 root)	Base of neck, shoulder, anterolateral aspect of arm	Numbness in deltoid region	Deltoid, biceps	Biceps
C5-C6 (C6 root)	Neck, shoulder, medial border of scapula, lateral aspect of arm, dorsum of forearm	Dorsolateral aspect of thumb and index finger	Biceps, extensor pollicus longus	Biceps, brachioradialis
C6-C7 (C7 root)	Neck, shoulder, medial border of scapula, lateral aspect of arm, dorsum of forearm	Index and middle fingers, dorsum of hand	Triceps	Triceps

Adapted from Mercier LR: *Practical Orthopedics,* ed 4, St Louis, 1995, Mosby.

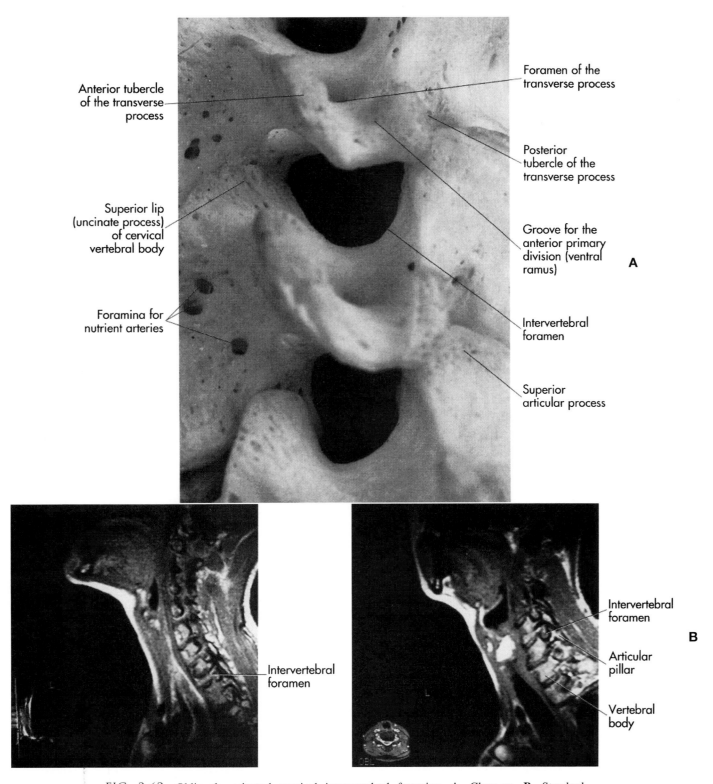

Anterior tubercle of the transverse process

Superior lip (uncinate process) of cervical vertebral body

Foramina for nutrient arteries

Foramen of the transverse process

Posterior tubercle of the transverse process

Groove for the anterior primary division (ventral ramus)

Intervertebral foramen

Superior articular process

A

Intervertebral foramen

Intervertebral foramen

Articular pillar

Vertebral body

B

FIG. 3-62 Obliquely oriented cervical intervertebral foramina. **A,** Close-up. **B,** Standard magnetic resonance imaging scans. *(From Cramer GD, Darby SA: Basic and clinical anatomy of the spine, spinal cord, and ANS, St Louis, 1995, Mosby.)*

PROCEDURE

- With the patient seated, the examiner exerts upward pressure on the patient's head (Figs. 3-63 and 3-64).
- This removes the weight of the patient's head from the neck.
- Generalized, increased pain indicates muscle spasm.
- Relief of pain indicates intervertebral foraminal encroachment or facet capsulitis.
- The examiner continues the distraction for up to 30 to 60 seconds to completely relax the involved tissues (Fig. 3-65).
- This test provides some prediction of the effect of cervical spine traction in relieving pain or paresthesia.
- Nerve root compression may be relieved, with disappearance of the symptoms and signs, if the intervertebral foramina are opened or the disc spaces extended.

- Pressure on the joint capsules of the apophyseal joints is also decreased by distraction.

Confirmation Procedures

Bakody sign, maximum foraminal encroachment test, shoulder depression test, brachial plexus tension test, Bikele's sign, Jackson cervical compression test, Spurling's test, reflexes, and diagnostic imaging

DIAGNOSTIC STATEMENT

Distraction test is positive in relieving the C5 radicular pain on the right. This result suggests nerve root compression syndrome at that level, on the right.

CLINICAL PEARL

The distraction test not only indicates the nature of the patient's complaint but also identifies the merit of cervical traction in the treatment regimen. It should also be noted that the higher the poundage of *static* cervical traction required for relief, the more unstable the nerve compression syndrome. Indeed, the higher poundage requirement is often an indicator of the need for surgical resolution.

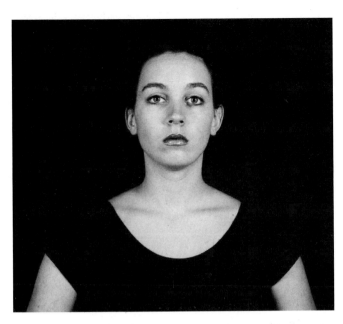

FIG. 3-63   The patient is seated comfortably, with the spine erect and the head and neck in a neutral position.

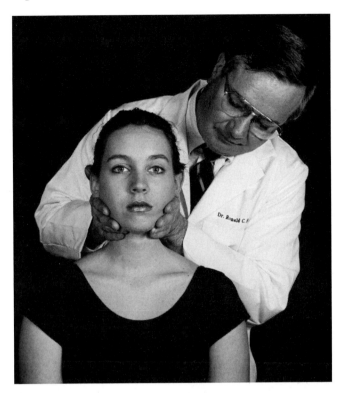

FIG. 3-64   With the hands cupping the patient's mandible and occiput, the examiner lifts the patient's head. A positive finding is the relief of the patient's localized or radicular pain. The sign is confirmed if the symptoms return when the weight of the head is returned to the neck.

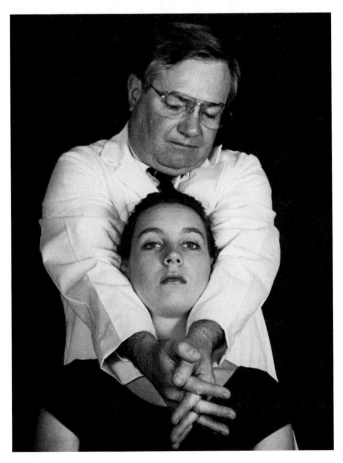

FIG. 3-65   Alternatively, the examiner can lift the patient's head by clasping the forearms under the patient's mandible. In this procedure the back of the patient's head is fixed against the examiner's chest. In both methods the lift or distraction is maintained for as many seconds as possible but not beyond patient tolerance.

FORAMINAL COMPRESSION TEST

Assessment for Cervical Nerve Root Encroachment

Comment

Radiculopathy can result from disc or osteophyte encroachment on one or several cervical nerve roots, especially C6 (C5-C6 disc) and C7 (C6-C7 disc). Such encroachment may result in pain or paresthesias affecting the upper limb dermatomes at the involved levels, with weakness and hyporeflexia (Fig. 3-66).

Approximately one fifth of the intervertebral foramen in the cervical region is filled by the dorsal and ventral roots (medially) or the spinal nerve (laterally). When the spine is in the neutral position, the dorsal and ventral roots are located in the inferior portion of the foramen at or below the disc level. Hypertrophy of the superior and inferior articular processes secondary to degeneration (osteoarthritis) of the Z joints may result in compression of the dorsal rootlets, dorsal root, or dorsal root ganglion.

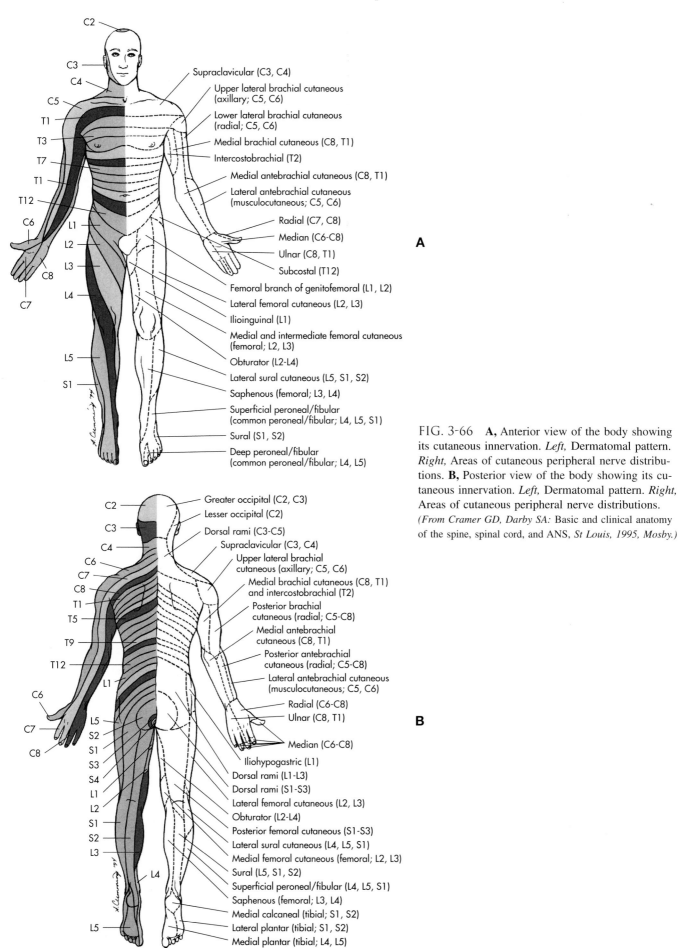

A, Anterior view:

Supraclavicular (C3, C4)
Upper lateral brachial cutaneous (axillary; C5, C6)
Lower lateral brachial cutaneous (radial; C5, C6)
Medial brachial cutaneous (C8, T1)
Intercostobrachial (T2)
Medial antebrachial cutaneous (C8, T1)
Lateral antebrachial cutaneous (musculocutaneous; C5, C6)
Radial (C7, C8)
Median (C6-C8)
Ulnar (C8, T1)
Subcostal (T12)
Femoral branch of genitofemoral (L1, L2)
Lateral femoral cutaneous (L2, L3)
Ilioinguinal (L1)
Medial and intermediate femoral cutaneous (femoral; L2, L3)
Obturator (L2-L4)
Lateral sural cutaneous (L5, S1, S2)
Saphenous (femoral; L3, L4)
Superficial peroneal/fibular (common peroneal/fibular; L4, L5, S1)
Sural (S1, S2)
Deep peroneal/fibular (common peroneal/fibular; L4, L5)

B, Posterior view:

Greater occipital (C2, C3)
Lesser occipital (C2)
Dorsal rami (C3-C5)
Supraclavicular (C3, C4)
Upper lateral brachial cutaneous (axillary; C5, C6)
Medial brachial cutaneous (C8, T1) and intercostobrachial (T2)
Posterior brachial cutaneous (radial; C5-C8)
Medial antebrachial cutaneous (C8, T1)
Posterior antebrachial cutaneous (radial; C5-C8)
Lateral antebrachial cutaneous (musculocutaneous; C5, C6)
Radial (C6-C8)
Ulnar (C8, T1)
Median (C6-C8)
Iliohypogastric (L1)
Dorsal rami (L1-L3)
Dorsal rami (S1-S3)
Lateral femoral cutaneous (L2, L3)
Obturator (L2-L4)
Posterior femoral cutaneous (S1-S3)
Lateral sural cutaneous (L4, L5, S1)
Medial femoral cutaneous (femoral; L2, L3)
Sural (L5, S1, S2)
Superficial peroneal/fibular (L4, L5, S1)
Saphenous (femoral; L3, L4)
Medial calcaneal (tibial; S1, S2)
Lateral plantar (tibial; S1, S2)
Medial plantar (tibial; L4, L5)

FIG. 3-66 **A,** Anterior view of the body showing its cutaneous innervation. *Left,* Dermatomal pattern. *Right,* Areas of cutaneous peripheral nerve distributions. **B,** Posterior view of the body showing its cutaneous innervation. *Left,* Dermatomal pattern. *Right,* Areas of cutaneous peripheral nerve distributions. *(From Cramer GD, Darby SA: Basic and clinical anatomy of the spine, spinal cord, and ANS, St Louis, 1995, Mosby.)*

The outer fibers of the annulus fibrosis of the cervical intervertebral discs are richly supplied with sensory receptors from which impulses are transmitted by way of the sinuvertebral nerve. When the anterior fibers of each of the cervical discs from C3 to C7 are stimulated on one side of the midline, pain is referred to the vertebral border of the scapula on the ipsilateral side (doorbell sign). Pain from the upper cervical discs develops a more cephalad level along the inner border of the scapula. Pain from the lower disc develops at a more caudad level. When the anterior peripheral fibers are stimulated in the midline, pain develops in the interscapular area.

If the disc is ruptured in a posterior or posterolateral direction, the resulting pain is of three types: discogenic, neurogenic, or myelogenic.

In discogenic pain, the disc rupture extends to but not through the peripheral fibers. Pain develops first at the medial scapular border and then spreads to the shoulder and down the posterior surface of the arm as far as the elbow. This produces a sometimes severe deep, dull, aching sensation that usually subsides in 5 to 10 minutes.

In neurogenic pain, the peripheral fibers of the disc are lacerated with or without herniation of disc fragments into the spinal canal. Fluid pressure is transmitted through the defect resting against the nerve root and spinal cord. Neurogenic pain that is the result of nerve root irritation has a sharper, more intense quality that is described as an electric shock or a hot burning sensation. This type of pain shoots into the arm, forearm, and hand along a dermatome distribution.

Myelogenic pain results from a central posterior defect, which permits a midline protrusion and spinal cord compression, allowing the pressure of the disc to be transmitted to the spinal cord. This pain produces a momentary shocklike sensation (Lhermitte's sign) that shoots downward along the spine and that may spread into one or several extremities.

PROCEDURE

- With the patient in the seated position, the examiner rotates the patient's neck while exerting strong downward pressure on the head (Figs. 3-67 to 3-69).
- The test is then repeated bilaterally with the head in a neutral position (Fig. 3-70).
- When the neck is rotated and downward pressure is applied, closure of the intervertebral foramen occurs.
- Localized pain indicates foraminal encroachment.
- Radicular pain indicates pressure on the nerve root.
- If nerve root involvement is suspected, the neurologic level must be evaluated.

Confirmation Procedures

Bakody sign, maximum foraminal encroachment test, shoulder depression test, distraction test, brachial plexus tension test, Bikele's sign, Jackson cervical compression test, Spurling's test, reflex and sensory testing, electrodiagnosis, and diagnostic imaging

---

DIAGNOSTIC STATEMENT

Foraminal compression testing is positive on the right, in the C5 dermatome. This result suggests nerve root encroachment.

CLINICAL PEARL

This test, as well as other compression maneuvers, often produces a cervical collapse sign in addition to radicular complaints. In the presence of capsular sprain with radicular components, compression overcomes the modicum of muscular strength that remains in the neck and is required for postural control. This condition means that the neck will collapse or buckle during the test. This collapse is found in grade II or greater sprain syndromes.

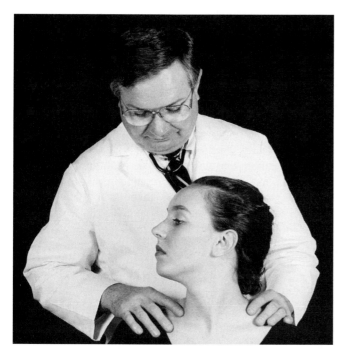

FIG. 3-67   The seated patient actively rotates the head from side to side. Localization of any discomfort is noted.

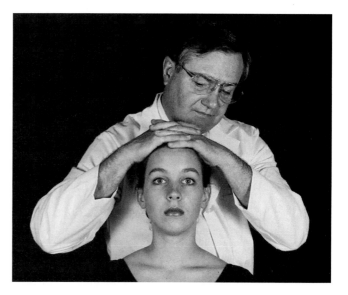

FIG. 3-68   With the patient seated and the head and neck returned to a neutral position, the examiner exerts progressively increasing downward pressure (compression) on the head and neck. Symptoms may lateralize and localize at this point.

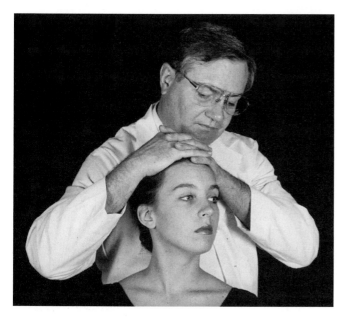

FIG. 3-69   The head is rotated toward the side of complaint and similar compression is applied. Reproduction of the complaint is a positive finding and indicates foraminal encroachment.

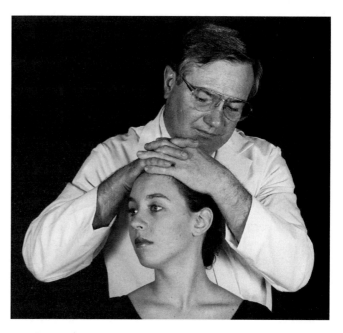

FIG. 3-70   The maneuver is repeated for the opposite side.

HALLPIKE MANEUVER

Assessment for Vertebrobasilar Artery Insufficiency

Comment

Rotation of the cervical spine to the extent of 45 to 50 degrees occurs chiefly at the atlantoaxial joint. This is about half of total cervical spine rotation. The vertebral artery is held fast at the C1 and C2 transverse foramina by fibrous tissue. During head rotation, the vertebral artery is stretched, compressed, and torqued. Decreased flow or even cessation of flow through one vertebral artery can occur when the head is turned. The atlantoaxial joint is the probable site of vessel compression.

The blood flow in the vertebral arteries fluctuates during normal daily activities, but symptoms do not occur because of adequate circulation from the opposite vertebral artery. Occlusion of one vertebral artery does not necessarily reduce the arterial supply to the posterior fossa via the basilar or posterior cerebellar arteries. Compression or spasm of a vertebral artery from C1-C2 rotation will induce symptoms only if flow in the contralateral vertebral artery is already compromised.

In cerebral transient ischemic attacks the symptoms vary according to which area of the brain is ischemic. There are two main groups of symptoms: those associated with partial or total ischemia of a cerebral hemisphere and those associated with ischemia of the brainstem. The symptoms most often include transient contralateral weakness of the lower face, fingers, hand, arm, or leg. Such patients may also experience fleeting sensory symptoms, such as tingling, paresthesia, or numbness, in parts of the body contralateral to the ischemia. Ischemia in the dominant hemisphere may cause dysphasia, with impairment of speech and, at times, a transient lack of understanding.

Patients with ischemia in the portion of the brain that is supplied by the posterior cerebral artery may experience blurred vision or may notice transient hemianopic or altitudinal visual field defects or impairment of visual acuity.

Ischemia or insufficiency resulting from internal carotid artery stenosis often produces transient retinal ischemia, which results in monocular blindness or reduced acuity on the side of the stenosis combined with contralateral weakness of the face, arm, or leg.

Ischemic attacks that involve the section of the brain that is supplied by the vertebral and basilar arteries have an extremely wide range of symptoms. Common symptoms include vertigo, tinnitus, diplopia, dysarthria, dysphagia, and dysphonia. Patients may complain of unilateral or bilateral face, arm, and leg weakness and unilateral or bilateral sensations of numbness and tingling in the face, arms, or legs. Tinnitus, hearing loss, and ataxia may be present. In addition, patients with brainstem ischemia experience drop attacks in which they suddenly lose postural tone and fall to the ground without losing consciousness; they then immediately regain postural control and rise quickly. Dizziness is the most common complaint with transient ischemic attacks that are caused by vertebrobasilar insufficiency. However, dizziness is commonly associated with other physiologic disturbances and is rarely the only symptom of brainstem ischemia.

Although the symptoms of vertebrobasilar artery ischemia vary, they tend to occur in combinations that aid in diagnosis. Vertigo, ataxia, dysarthria, paresthesia, diplopia, tinnitus, and dysphagia, as well as focal weakness of the face, jaw, or pharynx tend to coexist, although not always in the same sequence or combination. Another grouping of symptoms is that of unilateral or bilateral weakness of the extremities with drop attacks and diplopia. The reason for these differences in symptom combinations can be found by referring to any diagram of the blood supply of the brainstem. Ischemia of the dorsal and lateral portions of the brainstem, which are supplied by the circumferential arteries, produces the first group of symptoms. Ischemia of the more ventral portions, supplied by the medial perforating arteries, causes the second group of symptoms.

PROCEDURE

- The Hallpike maneuver is an enhanced DeKleyn's test and must be performed with extreme caution.
- The patient lies in the supine position, with the head extending off the end of the examination table.
- The examiner provides support for the weight of the skull (Fig. 3-71).
- The examiner brings the patient's head into positions of reclination (extension), rotation, and lateral flexion (Fig. 3-72).

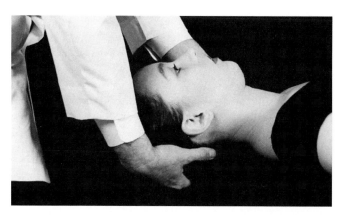

FIG. 3-71   The patient is lying supine with the head extending off the end of the examination table. The examiner provides support for the weight of the skull.

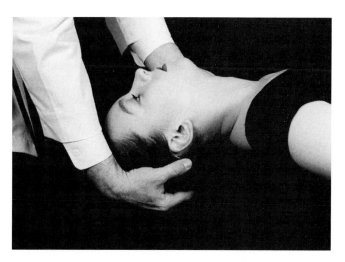

FIG. 3-72   The examiner brings the patient's head into the reclination (extension) position.

- The patient's eyes are open so that the examiner may look for nystagmus and other neurovascular signs (Fig. 3-73).
- The test is repeated for the opposite side (Fig. 3-74).
- These positions are held for 15 to 45 seconds.
- In a final maneuver the patient's head is allowed to hang freely in extreme extension (hyperextension) off the end of the examination table (Fig. 3-75).
- Vertigo, blurred vision, nausea, syncope, and nystagmus are signs of a positive test.

Confirmation Procedures

Barre-Lieou sign, vertebrobasilar artery functional maneuver, Hautant's test, DeKleyn's test, Underburg's test, vascular assessment, and vascular imaging (MRI)

DIAGNOSTIC STATEMENT

Hallpike maneuver is positive. This result suggests vertebrobasilar arterial insufficiency.

CLINICAL PEARL

Cervical spine manipulation and adjunctive therapeutic techniques are safe to use. Nevertheless, the patient's welfare is always of prime concern, and screening tests will help identify patients who may be predisposed to cerebrovascular problems. During these procedures symptoms of vertigo, nystagmus, dizziness, fainting, nausea, vomiting, visual blurring, headache (onset), or other sensory disturbances may identify a possible vertebrobasilar insufficiency. Problems in the cervical spine apart from the vertebral arteries may cause the same signs and symptoms. In suspected vertebral artery constriction, resisted neck extension may be painful and prolonged cervical extension may produce a feeling of faintness. The transverse processes of the atlas are often tender on the side of involvement. These symptoms may improve significantly by using manipulative procedures. Therefore manipulation should not necessarily be abandoned; rather, the manipulative technique should be modified so that simultaneous extension and rotation are not used.

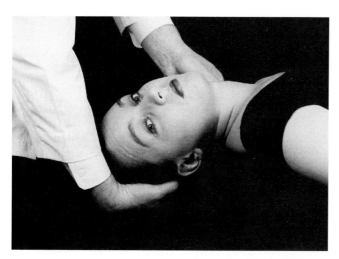

FIG. 3-73   The examiner then moves the patient's head into rotation and lateral flexion. The patient's eyes are open so that the examiner may look for nystagmus and other neurovascular signs.

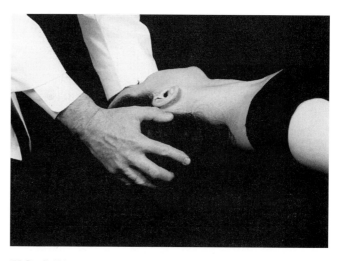

FIG. 3-74   The test is repeated for the opposite side. These positions are held for 15 to 45 seconds.

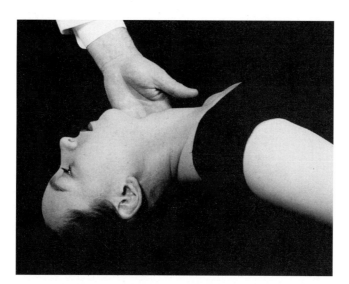

FIG. 3-75   In a final maneuver the patient's head is allowed to hang freely in extreme extension (hyperextension) off the end of the examination table. Vertigo, blurred vision, nausea, syncope, and nystagmus are signs of a positive test. The test indicates vertebral, basilar, or carotid artery stenosis or compression.

HAUTANT'S TEST

Assessment for Vertebral Artery Syndrome

Comment

Vertebral artery syndrome often occurs as a result of spondylotic changes in the cervical spine. Osteophyte formation in combination with reduced cervical height and a forward head position may cause encroachment on the vertebral foramina. This encroachment, which may be further irritated by cervical position, results in decreased blood flow through the vertebral artery to the brain.

The atlantoaxial joints (C1-C2) constitute the most mobile articulations of the spine. Flexion and extension involve a move of approximately 10 degrees, and lateral flexion involves a move of approximately 5 degrees. Rotation, which involves a move of approximately 50 degrees, is the primary movement of these joints. During rotation the height of the cervical spine decreases (because of the shape of the facet joints) as the vertebrae approximate. The odontoid process of C2 acts as a pivot point for the rotation. This middle, or median, joint is classified as a pivot (trochoidal) type of joint. The lateral atlantoaxial, or facet, joints are classed as plane joints. If a patient can talk and chew, some motion is probably occurring at C1-C2. Rotation of the cervical spine past 50 degrees to one side may lead to kinking of the contralateral vertebral artery. The ipsilateral vertebral artery may kink at 45 degrees of rotation. This kinking of the ipsilateral vertebral artery may lead to vertigo, nausea, tinnitus, drop attacks, visual disturbances, stroke, or death.

If an osteophyte developing on the neurocentral joint extends laterally, the vertebral artery foramen may be encroached and the vertebral artery may become significantly compressed. Minor degrees of vertebral artery compromise may be responsible for the so-called vertebral artery syndrome. Occasionally, a neurocentral osteophyte may produce severe kinking of the artery, which eventually results in vertebral artery thrombosis. Thrombosis may extend superiorly and involve the posteroinferior cerebellar artery. Occlusion of this artery leads to the development of Wallenberg's syndrome.

ORTHOPEDIC GAMUT 3-15

WALLENBERG'S SYNDROME

Wallenberg's syndrome is characterized by the following:

1. Dysphagia, ipsilateral palatal weakness, and vocal cord paralysis (involvement of the nucleus ambiguous of the vagus)
2. Impairment of sensation to pain and temperature on the same side of the face (involvement of the descending root and nucleus of the fifth cranial nerve)
3. Horner's syndrome in the homolateral eye (involvement of the descending sympathetic fibers)
4. Nystagmus (involvement of the vestibular nuclei)
5. Cerebellar dysfunction in the ipsilateral arm and leg (interference of the function of the midbrain and cerebellum)
6. Impairment of sensation to pain and temperature on the side of the body opposite (involvement of the spinothalamic tract)

Injury to a vertebral artery can occur anywhere along its path, by stretching, compression, or torquing forces. For older patients objective evaluation for vertebral artery syndrome is accomplished by modifying the common tests (Figs. 3-76 and 3-77).

Dizziness, nystagmus, nausea, and unilateral pupil dilation are positive indicators that vertebral artery syndrome can be differentially diagnosed from vestibular dysfunction if the provocative posture, rather than movement, of the head reproduces the symptoms.

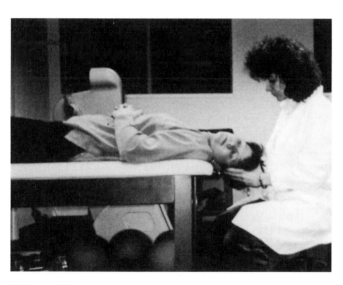

FIG. 3-76 Evaluation for vertebral artery syndrome. *(From Lewis CB, Knortz KA:* Orthopedic assessment and treatment of the geriatric patient, *St Louis, 1993, Mosby.)*

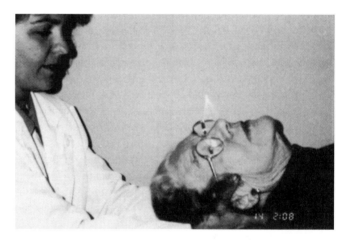

FIG. 3-77 Modification of test for vertebral artery syndrome for older persons. *(From Lewis CB, Knortz KA:* Orthopedic assessment and treatment of the geriatric patient, *St Louis, 1993, Mosby.)*

PROCEDURE

- While seated the patient extends the arms out in front with the palms up (Figs. 3-78 and 3-79).
- With eyes closed, the patient extends and rotates the head to one side (Fig. 3-80).
- The patient repeats this maneuver with the head extended and rotated to the opposite side.
- Drifting of the arms, vertigo, blurred vision, nausea, syncope, and nystagmus are signs of a positive test.
- The test indicates vertebral, basilar, or carotid artery stenosis or compression.

Confirmation Procedures

Barre-Lieou sign, vertebrobasilar artery functional maneuver, DeKleyn's test, Hallpike maneuver, Underburg's test, vascular testing or imaging, and diagnostic imaging

DIAGNOSTIC STATEMENT

Hautant's test is positive on the right. This result suggests vertebral artery syndrome on the ipsilateral side.

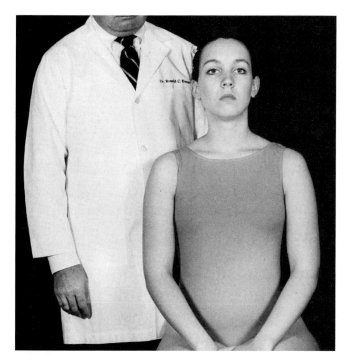

FIG. 3-78   The patient is seated comfortably with the head and neck in a neutral position.

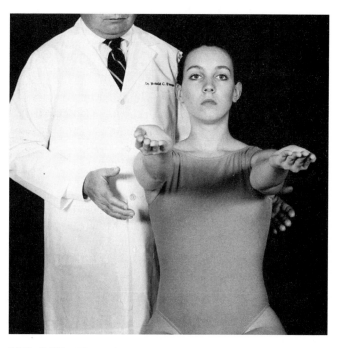

FIG. 3-79   The patient extends the arms forward and elevates them to shoulder level. The hands are supinated. The patient maintains this position for a few seconds.

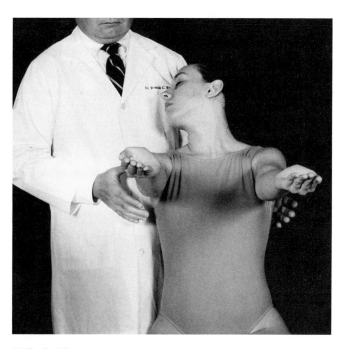

FIG. 3-80   The patient closes the eyes, rotates the head to one side, and hyperextends the neck. The examiner observes for any significant drifting of the arms from their original position. Drifting of the arms is a positive sign for vertebrobasilar vascular compromise.

Assessment for Cervical
Nerve Root Compression Resulting
from a Space-Occupying Lesion, Subluxation,
Inflammatory Edema, Exostosis
of Degenerative Joint Disease, Tumor,
or Intervertebral Disc Herniation

Comment

Patients who are symptomatic for cervical disc degeneration usually have compression of a nearby nerve root or the spinal cord. Acute herniation of degenerated disc material produces such compression and resembles an acute lumbar disc herniation. The various syndromes related to chronic disc degeneration, with herniation and insidious compression or degenerative subluxation, make the condition difficult to diagnose during clinical presentation. Typical of the confusion surrounding the problem of chronic disc degeneration are its many partial synonyms: osteoarthritis, chronic herniated disc, chondroma, spur formation, and others. The term *cervical spondylosis* has recently gained favor and may be used interchangeably for *chronic cervical disc degeneration.*

From C3 through C7 the average AP measurement of the cervical canal is 17 mm. Spinal cord compression will occur only if the canal is reduced to 11 mm or less. In cervical spondylosis some reduction will usually take place in the AP diameter of the spinal canal, and when associated with a canal that is initially small, myelopathy can occur.

The dorsal and ventral nerve roots pass through the subarachnoid space and converge to form the spinal nerve at approximately the level of its respective intervertebral foramen.

Root pain may awaken the patient after several hours of sleep and may be relieved approximately 15 to 30 minutes after the patient sits up. The patient may learn to prevent the pain by sleeping in a chair. However, in contrast to peripheral neuritis, the antalgic position is the important determining factor. If the patient lies down for awhile during the day, the pain would occur as it does during the night. This feature of root pain occurs because the spinal column lengthens when the patient lies down and shortens when the patient sits up. Because the length of the spinal cord remains the same regardless of the patient's position, the lengthening of the spinal column results in a tensing of, or traction on, the nerve roots.

At each intervertebral foramen, a mixed spinal nerve is formed by the fusion of the dorsal (afferent, sensory) and ventral (efferent motor, sympathetic) roots (Fig. 3-81).

In the cervical spine each cervical root exits above the vertebra that shares the same numeric designation. That is, the C5 root exits above the C5 vertebra (i.e., between the C4 and C5 vertebrae). Because there are seven cervical vertebrae but eight cervical roots, the C8 roots exist between the C7 and T1 vertebrae (Fig. 3-82).

Cervical radiculopathy often is the result of a herniated intervertebral disc, or it can be caused by osteophytic spondylitic changes that result in mechanical compression of the cervical root.

ORTHOPEDIC GAMUT 3-16

CERVICAL NERVE ROOT
COMPRESSION SYNDROME

Clinical axioms regarding cervical nerve root compression syndrome include the following:

1. When sensory manifestations occur in C7 radiculopathy, the index or middle finger always is involved.
2. When sensory manifestations occur in C8 radiculopathy, the little or ring finger always is involved.
3. The thumb is never involved exclusively in C7 radiculopathy.
4. Significant triceps weakness is seen only in C7 radiculopathy.
5. Significant supraspinatus and infraspinatus weakness is seen only in C5 radiculopathy.
6. Significant interossei and hand intrinsic weakness is seen only in C8 radiculopathy.

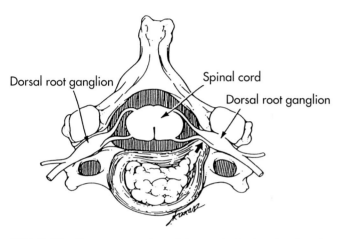

FIG. 3-81 Transverse section of the cervical spine showing the usual site of root injury in cervical radiculopathy due to disc herniation. *(From Brown WF, Bolton CF: Clinical electromyography, ed 2, Boston, 1993, Butterworth-Heinemann.)*

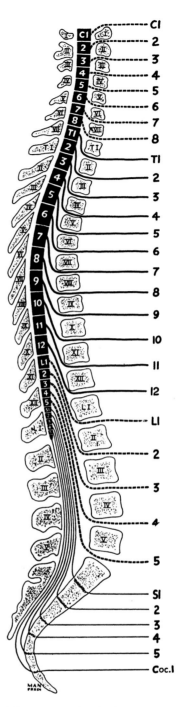

FIG. 3-82 Alignments of spinal segments and roots to vertebrae. *(From Katirji B: Electromyography in clinical practice: a case study approach, St Louis, 1998, Mosby.)*

Despite the variability in sensory and motor presentations of cervical radiculopathies, certain classic symptoms and signs exist and are extremely helpful in localizing the compressed root (Table 3-7).

PROCEDURE

- Cervical compression is commonly performed by having the patient sit up and bend the head obliquely backward while the examiner applies downward pressure on the vertex (Figs. 3-83 and 3-84).
- However, with the Jackson cervical compression test, the head is only slightly rotated to the involved side (Fig. 3-85).
- In either case, the sign is positive if localized pain radiates down the arm.
- A positive sign indicates nerve involvement from a space-occupying lesion, subluxation, inflammatory

swelling, exostosis of degenerative joint disease, tumor, or disc herniation.

Confirmation Procedures
Bakody sign, maximum foraminal encroachment test, shoulder depression test, distraction test, brachial plexus tension test, Bikele's sign, Spurling's test, foraminal compression test, reflexes, sensory testing, and diagnostic imaging

---

DIAGNOSTIC STATEMENT

Jackson cervical compression is positive on the right and elicits pain in the C5 dermatome. This suggests a nerve-compressing space-occupying lesion near the C5 nerve root.

TABLE 3-7

CLINICAL PRESENTATIONS IN CERVICAL RADICULOPATHIES

	C5	C6	C7	C8
Pain	To parascapular area, shoulder, and upper arm	To shoulder, arm, forearm, and thumb/index finger	To posterior arm, forearm, and index/middle fingers	To medial arm, forearm, and little/ring fingers
Sensory	Upper arm	Lateral arm, forearm, and thumb/index fingers	Index and middle fingers	Medial arm, forearm, and little finger
Motor	Scapular fixators, shoulder abduction, and elbow flexion	Shoulder abduction, elbow flexion, and forearm pronation	Elbow extension, wrist and fingers extension	Hand intrinsics, long flexors and extensors of fingers
Hyporeflexia/areflexia	Biceps and/or brachioradialis reflexes	Biceps and/or brachioradialis reflexes	Triceps reflex	None

Adapted from Katirji B: *Electromyography in clinical practice: a case study approach,* St Louis, 1998, Mosby.

CLINICAL PEARL

Closure of the intervertebral foramina occurs on the side of flexion in this maneuver. This test should be performed without excessive discomfort. The collapse sign may be present.

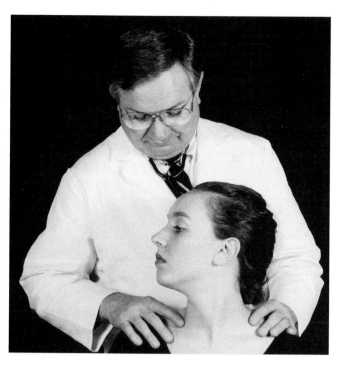

FIG. 3-83 While seated, the patient rotates the head from side to side. Localization of any complaint is noted.

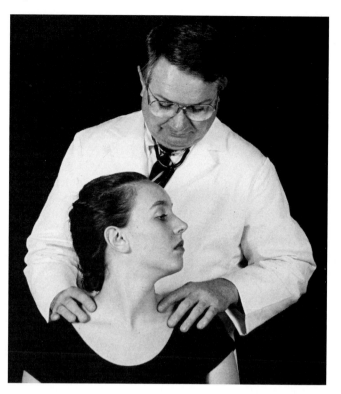

FIG. 3-84 Pain on the side opposite of rotation suggests muscular strain, whereas pain on the side of rotation suggests facet or nerve root involvement.

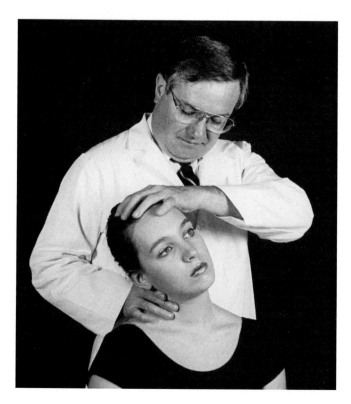

FIG. 3-85 The head is laterally flexed in an attempt to approximate the ear to the shoulder. This position is held, and the examiner exerts downward pressure on the patient's head. An exacerbation of the local or radicular pain indicates a positive test.

Assessment for Myelopathy of the Cervical Spine

Comment

Cervical myelopathy results from spinal cord injury caused by a cervical spine pathologic condition, such as spondylitic spurs, central disc herniation, tumors, and dislocation of the cervical spine.

Examining for cervical myelopathy is of paramount importance in evaluating every patient with a spinal problem. Key historical and physical examination factors should be noted. During the history every patient should be asked about a gait disturbance. Questioning patients about sports activities can reveal the key aspects of loss of balance and control, potentially pointing to cervical myelopathy. Questions concerning numbness and tingling in the legs, numbness in the hands, loss of agility in the hands, inability to fasten small buttons, deterioration in handwriting, loss of ability to stand on one foot, and a decrease in bowel, bladder, or sexual function should be asked of every patient with cervical pain.

When the history and physical examination suggest the presence of cervical myelopathy, the appropriate diagnostic tests with indication of abnormality are MRI or a contrast computed tomography (CT) scan of the cervical spine. With significant neurologic symptoms, an electromyogram (EMG) and nerve conduction study can also be ordered to rule out radiculopathy.

Peripheral neuropathy is a disorder that affects the peripheral motor, sensory, or autonomic nerves to a variable degree. If only one nerve is affected, it is considered a mononeuropathy. If several nerves are involved in a distal symmetric or asymmetric fashion, it is considered a polyneuropathy. If multiple, single-peripheral nerves or their branches are involved, this pattern is considered mononeuritis multiplex.

Patients with any form of peripheral neuropathy often describe their symptoms similarly, using words such as *prickling, burning,* or *jabbing.* These symptoms often indicate whether disease exists in the peripheral nerves.

In most patients with polyneuropathy, distal weakness is more prominent than proximal weakness, and an accompanying sensory abnormality is usually present. With mononeuropathy, muscles innervated by a single peripheral nerve are weak and atrophic. This pattern must be differentiated from that in a patient with a radiculopathy, in which only the muscles supplied by a single root are affected. The pattern must also be differentiated from that of a patient with a plexopathy, in which the pattern of motor and sensory dysfunction is in a multiple root or peripheral nerve distribution.

Neuropathies that develop abruptly and that are associated with pain are usually of an ischemic origin, such as in rheumatoid arthritis and polyarteritis nodosa. Neuropathies that evolve over a few days may be caused by industrial intoxications, such as those associated with the use of thallium or triorthocresyl phosphate.

ORTHOPEDIC GAMUT 3-17

NEUROPATHY

Neuropathy evolving over many weeks or months suggests several possibilities:

1. Exposure to toxic agents or drugs
2. Nutritional deficiencies
3. Chronically abnormal metabolic state
4. Remote effect of a malignant disease
5. Genetic polyneuropathy (which may have an insidious onset at any age)

The spinal canal can be compromised in many ways. The canal may be congenitally stenotic; anomalies in the canal or even a smaller-than-usual canal can leave the person vulnerable to later injury. Cervical spine stenosis can also occur as a result of trauma or repetitive injury.

The signs and symptoms of cervical canal stenosis range from simple paresthesia to myelopathy to transient quadriplegia.

Developmental stenosis of the cervical spine has been associated with cervical cord neurapraxia, transient quadriplegia, chronic intervertebral disc disease, and ligamentous instability. Secondary myelopathy of the cervical cord may follow severe neck injury in patients with a stenotic cervical canal.

The Torg ratio is the ratio of the width of the canal to the AP width at the midpoint of the corresponding vertebral body; a ratio of less than 4:5 (i.e., 0.80) indicates spinal stenosis (Fig. 3-86). An AP dimension of 13 mm or less may be indicative of cord compression. The interpediculate spacing is less significant in the cervical region than in the dorsolumbar spine.

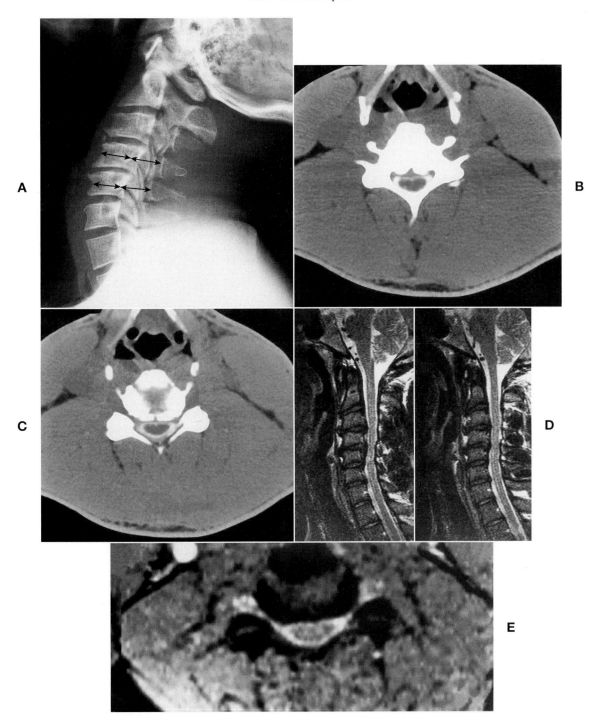

FIG. 3-86 **A,** Lateral cervical spinal radiograph in transient quadriplegia. **B,** Postcontrast computed tomography (CT) scan at C5. **C,** Postcontrast CT scan opposite C4-C5 disc space. **D,** Sagittal T2-weighted magnetic resonance imaging (MRI) scans. **E,** Axial MRI scan opposite C4-C5. *(From Nicholas JA, Hershman EB: The lower extremity and spine in sports medicine, vol 2, St Louis, 1995, Mosby.)*

Primary diseases of muscle are not usually confused with peripheral neuropathies, but in some cases electrophysiologic studies are required for differentiation. Distal symmetric or asymmetric paresthesia in the extremities without a significant component of muscle weakness should be differentiated from multiple sclerosis, cervical spondylitic myelopathy, or occasionally, extradural tumors of the cervical cord. Constant and severe pain in the neck or pain while flexing the neck (Lhermitte's sign) usually indicates cervical cord disease. Symptoms or signs of spasticity may occur later in these myelopathies, which can create a problem in diagnosis. Electrophysiologic testing usually resolves the issue.

PROCEDURE

- The patient is seated on the examining table (Fig. 3-87).
- The patient's head is passively flexed (Fig. 3-88).

- A sharp pain radiating down the spine and into the upper or lower limbs is a positive finding (Fig. 3-89).
- Dural irritation in the spine is indicated.
- The test is similar to a combination of other meningeal irritation challenges.

Confirmation Procedures
Soto-Hall sign, reflexes and sensory testing, electrodiagnosis, and MRI

DIAGNOSTIC STATEMENT

Lhermitte's sign is present. This result suggests myelopathy of the cervical spine.

CLINICAL PEARL

Although Lhermitte's sign is often construed as a pathognomonic test for multiple sclerosis, it is not. However, Lhermitte's sign does reveal or suggest myelopathy resulting from multiple sclerosis, stenosis, tumor, or disc herniation.

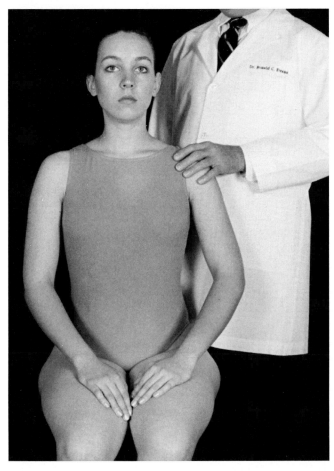

FIG. 3-87   The patient sits comfortably but erect with the head and neck in the neutral position.

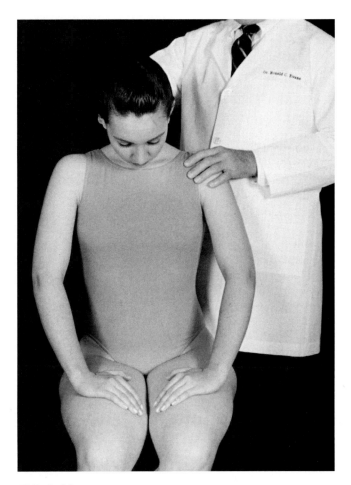

FIG. 3-88   The head and neck are passively flexed toward the patient's chest.

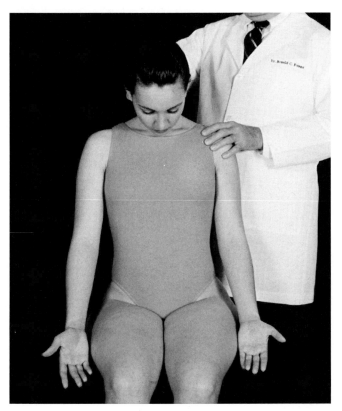

FIG. 3-89   The patient may experience a sharp, radiating pain or paresthesia along the spine and into one or more extremities. The presence of these symptoms suggests myelopathy and constitutes a positive test.

MAXIMUM CERVICAL COMPRESSION TEST

**Assessment for Cervical
Nerve Root Syndrome or Facet Syndrome
(Concave Testing) and Cervical Muscular
Strain (Convex Testing)**

Comment

Often associated with cervical muscular strain, myofascial trigger points refer dull, aching pain. This deep pain ranges from uncomfortable to incapacitating. Active trigger points are hyperirritable areas of skeletal muscle tissue that cause pain. Latent trigger points cause weakness and restriction of movement but are not painful.

Active trigger points demonstrate a "jump sign." Stimulation of the affected trigger point will cause the musculature to react.

ORTHOPEDIC GAMUT 3-18

MYOFASCIAL INVOLVEMENT

There are two common areas of myofascial involvement of the cervical spine:

1. Levator scapulae
2. Scalenes

The anterior, middle, and posterior scalene muscles act to stabilize the cervical spine against lateral movement and elevate the first and second ribs during inspiration. Tightness in these muscles may occlude nerves and blood vessels and compress nerves to the proximal and distal part of the arm.

Physical symptoms include morning edema specifically on the radial and dorsal aspect of the hand.

The vulnerability to injury of the cervical region is so great that even low- to moderate-intensity trauma can compromise a multitude of systems. As a result, a variety of signs and symptoms may develop. As is known the secondary effects of whiplash are sometimes as disabling, if not more so, than the soreness and muscular stiffness of the initial symptoms (Table 3-8 and Fig. 3-90).

ORTHOPEDIC GAMUT 3-19

TESTS OF DIFFERENTIATION

Three tests help in differentiating other thoracic outlet syndrome causes from the scalene trigger point hyperirritability:

1. *The cramp test:* The patient fully rotates the head to the affected side and drops the chin to the clavicle. The test is positive if a firm contraction or cramp of the scalene muscles occurs.
2. *The finger-flexion test:* A positive finding is present when all of the medial fingertips cannot press tightly against the metacarpophalangeal joints when the proximal phalanges are extended.
3. *The scalene relief test:* Elevation of the arm and clavicle lifts the clavicle from the underlying scalenes. To do this the patient places the forearm of the involved side across the forehead (similar to reverse Bakody sign); this produces pain relief within minutes.

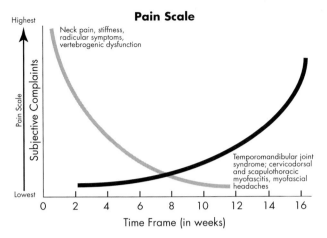

FIG. 3-90   Clinical picture of moderate to severe whiplash trauma. *(From Brier SR: Primary care orthopedics, St Louis, 1999, Mosby.)*

TABLE 3-8

SYMPTOMS EXPERIENCED WITH CERVICAL ACCELERATION/DECELERATION SYNDROMES

Symptom	Lesion Site
Headache	Suboccipital muscles, greater occipital nerve, myofascial trigger points, facet point irritation
Disorientation, irritability	Brain
Visual disturbances	Vertebrobasilar artery network, brainstem, cervical spinal cord
Memory and concentration disturbances	Brain
Vertigo	Cervical sympathetic nerves, vertebral artery, inner ear
Arm and hand numbness	Brachial plexus, scalenes
Thumb, index finger, middle finger numbness; weakness; temperature changes	Median nerve, carpal tunnel
Difficulty swallowing	Pharynx
Ringing in ears	Temporomandibular joint, vertebral and basilar arteries, cervical sympathetic chain, inner ear
Dizziness, light-headedness	Cervical sympathetic nerves, brain, inner ear
Neck and shoulder pain	Paravertebral muscles, apophyseal joints, cervical nerve roots, cervical disc
Poor balance, proprioception, and posture	Inner ear

Adapted from Brier SR: *Primary care orthopedics,* St Louis, 1999, Mosby.

Acute injury (sprain) of a joint produces synovial effusion, histamine release, capsular or ligamentous stretching or tearing, bleeding, and associated clinical disabilities. Some of these conditions are visible and palpable in joints of the extremities but not the spine. With repetition of the traumatic process or with chronic stress on the joint from shearing and other forces, a chronic synovial reaction is established. This reaction extends to the underlying articular cartilage. The cartilage softens and then becomes rough and eroded. Stresses in the capsule and periosteum result in marginal osteophytosis, which may encroach on the underlying nerve root. A loose body may develop in the joint cavity, or an osteophytic process may fracture and lie free or loosely attached in or near the foramen. The facetal bone may thicken or become hypertrophic, and the laminae may do so as well. Degenerative enlargement of facets with irritative compression of one or more cervical roots may also occur.

Trauma to the cervical spine may injure the nervous tissue and related structures in several ways. During the hyperextension phase of an injury, nerve roots may suffer a compression injury at the point of exit from the neural foramina. The nerve root may become contused enough to produce actual disruption of axons and resulting axonotmesis. However, because the internal structure is fairly well preserved, recovery is spontaneous. Neurapraxic injury is more common and is clinically manifested as the transient paresthesia that is seen most often approximately a week after the trauma occurred. The spinal cord, dura, and arachnoid may also be contused. During the hyperflexion phase traction injury may occur.

The nerve supply to the capsular and ligamentous structures of the cervical spine is of significance in the interpretation of painful conditions. The capsules of the atlantoaxial joints and those of the posterior or apophyseal joints are supplied by the capsular branches of the medial divisions of the posterior primary rami of the cervical spine nerves. The posterior longitudinal ligament and the capsular structures of the lateral interbody joints receive their nerve supply from the recurrent spinal meningeal nerves (the sinuvertebral nerves), which contain afferent somatic sensory fibers and efferent sympathetic fibers.

Chronic cervical strain is the most common cause of neck pain that mimics cervical spondylosis. This mimicry has led to unnecessary myelography because the associated patterns of referred pain and neuralgia are so similar between the two conditions.

PROCEDURE

While in the seated position, the patient is instructed to approximate the chin to the shoulder and extend the neck (Figs. 3-91 to 3-93).

- The test is performed bilaterally.
- Pain on the concave side indicates nerve root or facet involvement.
- Pain on the convex side indicates muscular strain.

Confirmation Procedures

Dejerine's sign, swallowing test, Valsalva maneuver, Naffziger's test, Bakody sign, shoulder depression test, distraction test, brachial plexus tension test, Bikele's sign, Jackson cervical compression test, Spurling's test, foraminal compression test, reflexes, sensory testing, and diagnostic imaging

---

DIAGNOSTIC STATEMENT

Maximum cervical compression on the left is positive on the right. This result suggests neural compression at C5.

Maximum cervical compression on the left is positive on the left. This result is consistent with muscular strain of the cervical paraspinals.

CLINICAL PEARL

The patient with lower cervical nerve root compression syndrome has already discovered that looking up or down with the head rotated is uncomfortable and produces neck and arm pain. If these positions are already producing pain, then attempts to use manipulative procedures incorporating these positions will be difficult for the patient to tolerate.

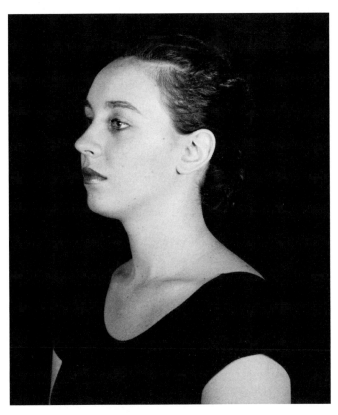

FIG. 3-91   The patient is seated comfortably with the head and neck in the neutral position.

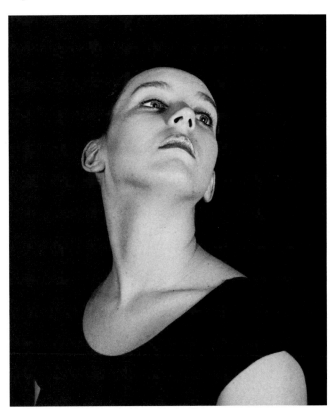

FIG. 3-92   The patient actively rotates the head and hyperextends the neck toward the side of radicular complaint. Reproduction of symptoms suggests foraminal encroachment. The maneuver is repeated for the opposite side.

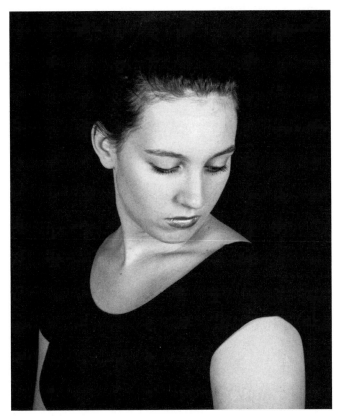

FIG. 3-93   A slight variation of this test requires rotation and maximum flexion of the neck toward the side of radicular complaint, as if looking into a shirt pocket. Reproduction of the radicular complaint suggests foraminal encroachment of a nerve root.

NAFFZIGER'S TEST

Assessment for Space-Occupying Mass in the Cervical Spine or Canal

Comment

A herniated cervical disc causing nerve root compression not responsive to conservative treatment may require surgery. Disc herniation commonly occurs at the high-motion segments of C4-C5, C5-C6, and C6-C7. As the intradiscal contents leave the annulus, they may migrate around the adjacent nerve root, resulting in radiculopathy. If the herniated disc displaces into the epidural space, cord compression may result. Free fragments of disc material occasionally may be found in the epidural space. Patients usually present with severe radicular pain involving the upper extremity and shoulder girdle area. Disc herniation of C4-C5 results in numbness around the shoulder and weakness of the deltoid muscle. Deep tendon reflexes are not altered. With C5-C6 disc herniation, the patient loses the biceps reflex and biceps muscle strength. Numbness along the dorsal aspect of the thumb and index finger is typical. Herniations of the C6-C7 disc cause depression of the triceps reflex, weakness of the triceps muscle, and numbness of the long and ring fingers.

Although spinal cord tumors are rare, they are always a part of the differential diagnosis of neck pain. These tumors arise within the spinal cord from cells that may be metastatic. Such tumors can be primary or secondary, and extradural or intradural. Intradural tumors require further sorting into extramedullary or intramedullary.

Of the intradural tumors, 71% are extramedullary; 32% of these are meningiomas, and 38% are schwannomas. The remaining tumors found in this location are sarcomas, angiomas, chordomas, lymphomas, lipomas, epidermoids, melanomas, and neuroblastomas. Other kinds of lesions occur very rarely. Virtually any kind of tumor may metastasize to the intradural space, but such spread is distinctly unusual.

Of meningiomas, 15% are either completely extradural or both intradural and extradural, and 85% are intradural and extramedullary. Meningiomas are found in the cervical region in about 13% of the patients. The tumors are usually nodular, well circumscribed, and less well encapsulated than neurofibromas. The histology of cervical meningiomas is not different from that of meningiomas elsewhere, and malignant tumors are very rare. The tumors begin growing at the dorsal root entry zone and are clinically indistinguishable from neurofibromatosis. It is uncommon for the pain to be localized. An unusual meningioma involves the upper cervical area as well as the intracranial cavity and is called a *foramen magnum tumor*. Tumors in this area are difficult to diagnose and are most commonly meningiomas.

Symptoms of meningiomas are bizarre and often variable. Patients with these tumors often have their complaints dismissed as psychiatric. A nondescript headache is an early complaint. Weakness and paresthesia in the lower extremities may occur, but the complaints and locations often vary from examination to examination. Muscular atrophy and fibrillation in the hands and forearms are common and probably result from compression of the anterior spinal arteries. A mistaken diagnosis of lower motor neuron disease in the cervical region is common. The course of the illness is relentlessly progressive, and the nature of the disease often becomes apparent only when quadriparesis is evident.

Changing position, coughing, or sneezing or a rise in cerebrospinal fluid pressure results in increased pain.

PROCEDURE

- Naffziger's compression test is performed by having the patient sit erect while the examiner holds digital pressure over the jugular veins for 30 to 40 seconds (Fig. 3-94).
- The patient is then instructed to cough deeply.
- Pain along the distribution of a nerve may indicate nerve root compression (Fig. 3-95).
- Although this test is more commonly used for lower back involvement, cervical or thoracic root compression may also be aggravated.
- Local pain in the spine does not positively indicate nerve compression but may indicate the site of a strain or sprain injury or other lesion.
- The sign is always positive in the presence of cord tumors, particularly spinal meningiomas.
- The resulting increased spinal fluid pressure above the tumor causes the growth to compress or pull on certain sensory nerve structures, which produces radicular pain.
- **The test is contraindicated for a geriatric patient, and extreme care should be taken when performing this test on anyone suspected of having atherosclerosis.**
- In all cases, the patient should be alerted that jugular pressure may result in light-headedness or dizziness.

Confirmation Procedures

Dejerine's sign, swallowing test, Valsalva maneuver, Barre-Lieou sign, vertebrobasilar artery functional maneuver, Hautant's test, DeKleyn's test, Hallpike maneuver, Underburg's test, and vascular assessment

---

DIAGNOSTIC STATEMENT

Naffziger's test is positive. This result suggests a space-occupying mass in the cervical spine.

CLINICAL PEARL

This is not a good test for a geriatric or atheromatous patient to endure. The resulting increase in cerebrospinal fluid pressure is uncomfortable, and the momentary circulatory obstruction may result in significant syncope.

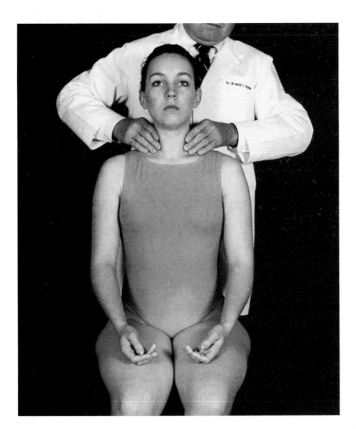

FIG. 3-94 With the patient seated comfortably, the examiner occludes the jugular veins bilaterally for 30 to 40 seconds.

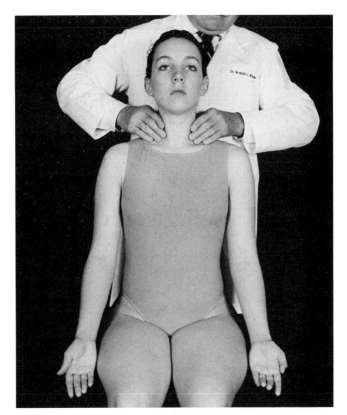

FIG. 3-95 The patient may experience radicular pain or localized pain in the spine. The finding is nonspecific but suggests a space-occupying mass in the spinal column.

Assessment for Cervical Muscular Strain (Isometric) and Cervical Ligamentous Sprain (Passive Range of Motion)

Comment

Examination of whiplash injuries requires evaluation of entities such as fracture, instability, and spinal cord or nerve root compression. These are readily apparent on routine clinical and radiologic assessment. However, many more serious bony, articular, and ligamentous injuries can occur in whiplash (Fig. 3-96). These injuries may be undetectable on plain films, CT, or MRI. This is especially true of injuries to the cervical zygapophyseal joints. Furthermore, the intervertebral discs have the potential to cause chronic symptoms with no obvious clinical or radiologic findings.

Most patients with cervical strain complain of paraspinal muscular aches and stiffness that may extend as far cephalad as the suboccipital region (Table 3-9). Chronic muscular strain of the cervical spine can affect distant organ systems. Pain may be referred to the head, orbits, or scapula.

A strain is damage to a muscle or tendon as a direct result of a sudden forcible contraction or violent stretching. Muscle strain includes those cases of overuse and overstretching that are just short of actual muscular rupture.

ORTHOPEDIC GAMUT 3-21

STRAINS

Strains are divided into three categories according to the degree of muscle tissue damage:

1. A *mild* strain is a low-grade inflammatory reaction accompanied by no appreciable hemorrhage, minimal amounts of swelling and edema, and some disruption of adjacent fibers.
2. A *moderate* strain involves laceration of fibers and appreciable hemorrhaging into the surrounding tissue (hematoma), followed by an inflammatory reaction with swelling and edema.
3. A *severe* strain is the consequence of a single, violent incident that results in complete disruption of the muscle unit. These strains occur when a tendon is torn from the bone or pulled apart, when the musculotendinous junction ruptures, or when the muscle ruptures through its belly.

ORTHOPEDIC GAMUT 3-20

CERVICAL SPINE MUSCULAR INJURY

The mechanism of cervical spine muscular injury is usually one of the following:

1. Athletic participation (which is by far the most frequent means of sustaining a strain injury)
2. Overuse
3. Overstretching
4. Contraction of the muscle against resistance
5. Direct blow

In all varieties of strain, contraction of the muscle against resistance will increase pain. This response is a characteristic finding of strains and differentiates the injury from sprains. A sprain is an injury to a ligamentous tissue that results in some degree of damage to the fibers of the ligament or its attachments.

Fundamentally, motion that exceeds the tolerance of a ligament is sufficient to produce a sprain. The extent of damage depends on the amount and duration of the applied force. As the abnormal force is applied, the ligament becomes tense and gives way at one or more of its attachments or at a point within its substance. A sprain also may involve injury to the periosteum, muscles, tendons, blood vessels, supporting soft tissue, and nerves in the adjacent area.

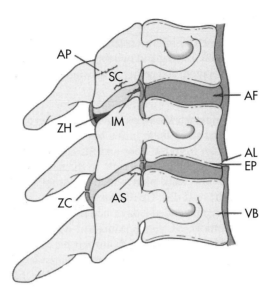

FIG. 3-96   Sites for clinical consideration following cervical spine acceleration/deceleration trauma. *AF,* Annulus fibrosus tear; *AL,* articular longitudinal tear; *AP,* articular pillar fracture; *AS,* articular surface fracture; *EP,* end-plate avulsion; *IM,* intraarticular meniscus contusion; *SC,* subchoronal plate fracture; *VB,* vertebral body fracture; *ZC,* zygapophyseal capsule tear; *ZH,* zygapophyseal hemarthrosis. *(Adapted from* Spine, state of the art reviews, *1993:7.)*

TABLE 3-9

CERVICAL STRAIN ASSESSMENT

Physical examination findings	Paravertebral muscle tenderness
	Intermittent stiffness
	Loss of cervical mobility
	Headaches and alterations of postural reflexes in chronic sufferers
	Normal neurologic signs
	No instability; screening for postural distortion
	Intersegmental posterior joint dysfunction
X-ray finding	Findings generally normal
	Possible decrease in cervical lordosis

Adapted from Brier SR: *Primary care orthopedics,* St Louis, 1999, Mosby.

ORTHOPEDIC GAMUT 3-22

SPRAINS

Sprains are divided into four categories according to the severity of the ligamentous injury:

1. A *mild* sprain describes an injury in which only a few of the ligamentous fibers are severed.
2. A *moderate* sprain is a more severe tearing but less than a complete separation of the ligament.
3. A *severe* sprain is a complete tearing of a ligament from its attachments or a complete separation within its substance.
4. A *sprain-fracture* has occurred when the ligamentous attachment pulls loose with a fragment of bone (avulsion).

The examination of a sprain initially will reveal discomfort when an attempt is made to stretch the ligament or the mechanism of injury is repeated. This one maneuver, when positive, will differentiate a sprain from a strain.

It is possible to separate various grades of cervical whiplash injury according to the degree of external trauma, orthopedic, and neurologic findings, as well as patient disability (Table 3-10).

PROCEDURE

- While the patient is sitting, the cervical spine is actively moved through resisted range of motion and then through passive range of motion (Fig. 3-97).
- Pain during resisted range of motion, or isometric contraction, signifies muscle strain (Fig. 3-98).
- Pain during passive range of motion signifies ligamentous sprain (Fig. 3-99).

Confirmation Procedures
Soto-Hall sign, spinal percussion test, and diagnostic imaging

DIAGNOSTIC STATEMENT

O'Donoghue maneuver is positive for sprain of the cervical spine.

O'Donoghue maneuver is positive for muscular strain of the cervical spine.

ORTHOPEDIC GAMUT 3-23

CERVICAL ACCELERATION-DECELERATION INJURY

There are five types of cervical acceleration-deceleration injury:

Type I: Patients can have severe injuries as a result of seemingly small degrees of acceleration trauma. The symptoms include mild discomfort and stiffness of the cervical spine and loss of small increments in range of motion.

Type II: Injury palpable muscle splinting, restriction of motion, and mild to moderate spasm. There is no neurologic deficits or evidence of radiculopathy.

Type III: Injury symptoms include moderate ligamentous sprain, advanced muscle swelling, and muscle spasm. There is loss of range of motion in all planes.

Type IV: Injury produces radicular symptoms that may be bilateral or unilateral. Motor and reflex changes are common.

Type V: Injury usually presents signs of neurologic instability. Cervical fracture or facet dislocation are common. Myelopathy and frank disc herniation commonly occur. Swelling and disc fragmentation are possible at the level of the spinal canal.

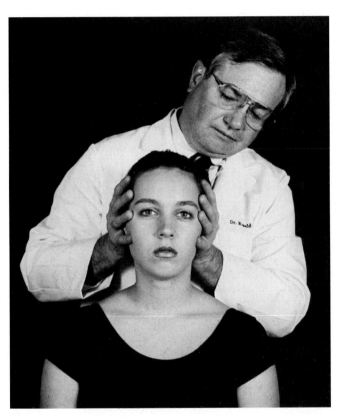

FIG. 3-97   The patient is seated comfortably, with the head and neck in the neutral position. The examiner grasps the patient's head with both hands.

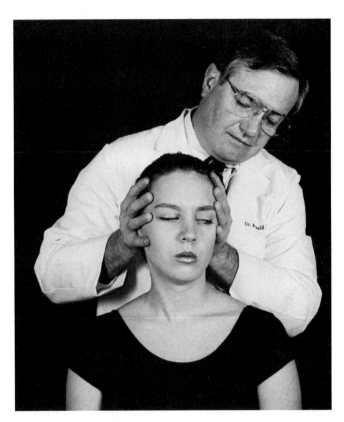

FIG. 3-98   The patient actively attempts rotation of the head to one side against isometric resistance. Pain production at this stage suggests muscular strain of the activated musculature. The test is repeated for the opposite side.

TABLE 3-10

CERVICAL ACCELERATION/DECELERATION INJURY TYPES

	Type I	Type II	Type III	Type IV	Type V
Physical examination findings	Cervical stiffness or discomfort No motor or sensory deficits No nerve root traction signs No instability Intersegmental fixation, spinal subluxation Results of compression tests normal	Palpable tenderness and muscle guarding No motor or sensory deficits Sympathetic nerve irritation (mild) consisting of headache, dizziness, or light-headedness intermittent for the first week Mild instability Mild to moderate muscle spasm	Swelling and spasm Loss of range of motion in all planes Sympathetic nerve injury with deficit for 7-10 days Moderate signs of instability Possible radiculopathy without motor or reflex loss Results of orthopedic testing abnormal Evaluation for cervical disc lesion and craniomandibular injury	Pain, spasm, and disability Severe restriction of motion in all planes Sympathetic nerve injury involving head, face, and eye disturbances Moderate to severe instability Concomitant disk and articular and soft-tissue injury Severe generalized pain and spasm produced by orthopedic testing; abnormal nerve root traction signs Unilateral or bilateral radicular symptoms	Severe spinal trauma, frank disc herniation with fragmentation common Loss of motor function common Myelopathy and spinal cord compromise Multiple injury sites, often with deformity
X-ray findings	Normal	Unremarkable, except for hypolordosis	Soft-tissue swelling and loss of lordotic curve No osseous abnormality	Secondary soft-tissue swelling Loss of lordotic curve Need to rule out ligamentous disruption, fracture, and anatomic subluxation (anterior vertebral translation)	Ligamentous instability usually seen on lateral projection Need to rule out fracture or facet dislocation Immediate follow-up with CT scan to evaluate for occult fractures, disc injury, and spinal cord compromise

Adapted from Brier SR: *Primary care orthopedics,* St Louis, 1999, Mosby.

CLINICAL PEARL

This maneuver can be applied to any joint or series of joints to determine ligamentous or muscular movement. By remembering that resisted range of motion stresses mainly muscles and passive range of motion stresses mainly ligaments, the examiner should be able to differentiate between strain and sprain and should be able to determine whether a combination of both is present.

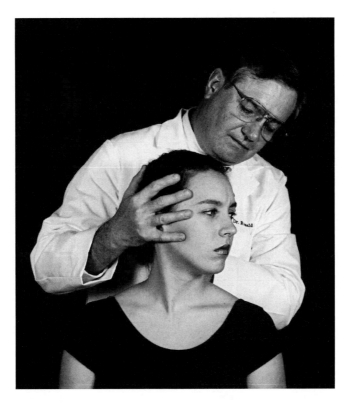

FIG. 3-99 If isometric testing is negative, the examiner passively rotates the patient's head and neck to one side to the limit of joint play. Pain produced in this maneuver suggests ligamentous injury. The maneuver is performed bilaterally.

RUST'S SIGN

Assessment for Severe Cervical Spine Sprain, Upper Cervical Rheumatoid Arthritis, Upper Cervical Spine Fracture, and Severe Upper Cervical Spine Subluxation

Comment

Of the three areas in the upper cervical spine in which fractures can be identified, the most common is the odontoid fracture, followed by the so-called hangman's fracture and by Jefferson's fracture. Anatomic areas, such as transverse processes, spinous processes, and lamina and lateral masses, may also be injured. Compression fractures of the upper three vertebral bodies occur, but these fractures are uncommon. Upper cervical fractures are usually associated with injury to the head or face and not to the neck itself. Most patients with upper cervical vertebral fractures sustain minimal neurologic damage because a severe spinal cord injury results in death from respiratory arrest before the patient can be treated. Pathologic fractures of the upper cervical spine occur in osteomyelitis, tuberculosis, osteogenic sarcoma, and metastatic carcinoma, as well as in association with nasopharyngeal infections (Grisel's disease). Untreated fractures of the upper cervical spine may produce serious neurologic sequelae.

A lateral radiograph of the upper cervical spine (C-spine) should be obtained in all trauma patients who complain of neck pain; have evidence of head, fascial, or neck trauma; or have altered consciousness. A lateral C-spine radiograph will detect approximately 85% of injuries to the cervical spine and should be adequate to assess alignment from the skull to the T1 vertebral body.

Type II odontoid process fractures may be displaced anteriorly or posteriorly. There is greater potential for neurologic injury with posterior displacement. Type III odontoid process fractures may be displaced or undisplaced.

A quick and accurate diagnosis in the traumatized spinal patient is essential. It is vital to assess whether the injury is stable or unstable. Because 5% to 10% of spinal cord injuries occur in the postinjury period because of patient mishandling, any cervical spine motion should be limited until proper examination is performed to exclude any catastrophic fracture. This is usually accomplished with plain film radiography in the AP, lateral, and open-mouth projections. Because there may be spasm or voluntary guarding as a result of pain, significant ligamentous injury may be masked on the initial x-ray films, thereby necessitating further evaluation with flexion and extension views.

An acute flexion injury may result in a fracture of the dens with the ligament remaining intact (Fig. 3-101). CT and MRI can easily demonstrate the fracture on images in the coronal projection.

Flexion fractures in the lower cervical spine occur typically at the C5-C6 intervertebral disc level, the most mobile segment of the cervical spine. The common "teardrop" fracture refers to a triangular piece of bone from the anterosuperior end-plate of the compressed vertebral body. With more significant force, the posterior ligamentous complex may be disrupted, resulting in complete bony failure with severe compression and comminution of the vertebral body (Fig. 3-102). This "burst" type of fracture usually involves a sagittal component of the vertebral body, as well as fractures of the posterior arch. Bony fragments are

---

ORTHOPEDIC GAMUT 3-24

ODONTOID PROCESS FRACTURES

The Anderson/D'Alonzo classification of odontoid process fractures:

Type I: Fractures of the odontoid are thought to represent an avulsion injury of the tip of the dens by the alar ligament. This injury is very rare, and because it is located above the transverse ligament, there is no associated atlantoaxial instability (Fig. 3-100).

Type II: Fractures through the body or base of the odontoid have a reported prevalence of nonunion of up to 64%.

Type III: Fractures that extend into the cancellous bone of the axis have an excellent prognosis with adequate reduction and external immobilization.

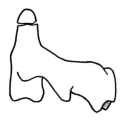
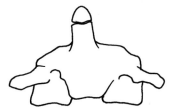

Type I

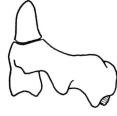
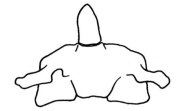

FIG. 3-100 Fractures of the odontoid are classified into three types depending on the line of the fracture through the odontoid. *(From Bucholz RW:* Orthopaedic decision making, *ed 2, St Louis, 1996, Mosby.)*

Type II

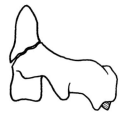
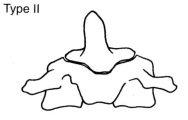

Type III

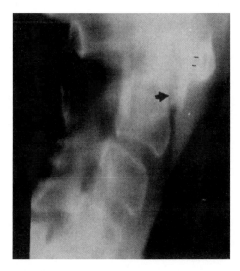

FIG. 3-101 Lateral x-ray film of C1-C2 showing displaced fracture at the base of the odontoid process with a normal atlantoaxial space, suggesting integrity of the transverse ligament. *(From Watkins RG:* The spine in sports, *St Louis, 1996, Mosby.)*

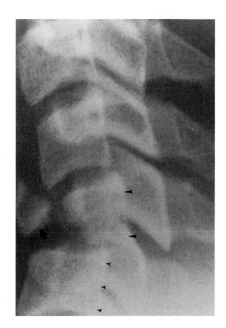

FIG. 3-102 Lateral view of a cervical teardrop fracture with posterior displacement of the remaining body into the spinal canal. *(From Watkins RG:* The spine in sports, *St Louis, 1996, Mosby.)*

often displaced posteriorly into the spinal canal, resulting in spinal cord compression and causing severe neurologic damage. CT is excellent in demonstrating any retropulsed bony fragments within the spinal canal (Fig. 3-103).

Most patients with upper cervical spine fractures have sustained the trauma from automobile accidents, diving injuries, or falls. A large percentage of patients exhibit neck rigidity and complain of painful torticollis that is sometimes out of proportion to the injury. Such complaints, either immediately following an injury or as long as several weeks later, should alert the physician to the possibility of an upper cervical spine fracture. Examination reveals neck rigidity, and there is often tenderness over the upper cervical spine and occasionally paraparesis or quadriparesis. The symptoms and signs may be puzzling and atypical. For instance, sleep attacks have been described.

Atlantoaxial subluxation is the most common and significant manifestation of rheumatoid involvement of the cervical spine. Long duration of disease, advanced patient age, and peripheral joint erosive instability are associated with more common and severe C1-C2 instabilities.

The instability pattern of rheumatoid involvement of the atlantoaxial joint complex is usually one of two types: anterior atlantoaxial subluxation or upward translocation of the odontoid (which is also called *superior migration, vertical subluxation,* and *downward luxation of the atlas on the axis*). Posterior subluxation of the atlantoaxial joint does not occur in rheumatoid arthritis unless there is an associated fracture of the odontoid or nearly complete arthritic erosion and destruction of the odontoid. The anterior and posterior contact points of the odontoid are true synovial joints. Synovitis destruction of the front or back of the odontoid on the anterior arch of C1 produces some instability.

ORTHOPEDIC GAMUT 3-25

ATLANTOAXIAL INSTABILITY

Atlantoaxial instability caused by rheumatoid arthritis results from a combination of the following:

1. Local arthritic and mechanical instability and pain
2. Neurologic dysfunction of brainstem, cord, and peripheral nerve (root)
3. Vertebral artery insufficiency

In atlantoaxial instability caused by rheumatoid arthritis, pain in the cervical area is common and usually of moderate severity. Subjective symptoms include paresthesia in the hands, "electric shock" sensations, and feelings of weakness. Joint crepitus and instability in the upper cervical spine may be felt upon palpation. The crepitus is often in the form of a "clunk" as C1 subluxation forward on C2. This produces an increased prominence of C2 posteriorly. Described as the *Sharp and Purser test,* this "clunk test" or phenomenon is to be avoided in early examination of the patient.

PROCEDURE

- If the patient spontaneously grasps the head with both hands when lying down or when arising from a recumbent position, this is a positive sign that indicates severe sprain, rheumatoid arthritis, fracture, or severe cervical subluxation (Figs. 3-104 and 3-105).

Confirmation Procedure
Diagnostic imaging

DIAGNOSTIC STATEMENT

Rust's sign is present. This result suggests severe upper cervical (atlantoaxial) instability.

CLINICAL PEARL

No other physical finding is as important or as revealing as Rust's sign. The presence of this sign mandates that (1) no further passive or active testing be undertaken, (2) imaging be performed immediately, and (3) the neck be adequately supported by using a cervical collar. Rust's sign has never been observed in conditions of minor consequence.

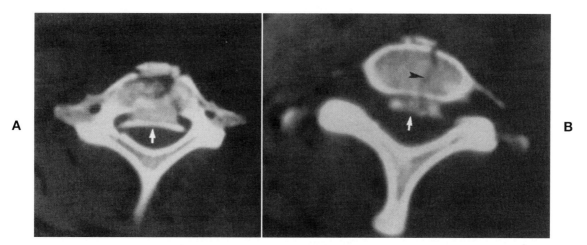

FIG. 3-103 Axial computed tomography images demonstrating the posteriorly displaced bony fragments as well as a sagittal cleavage fracture through the vertebral body. *(From Watkins RG: The spine in sports, St Louis, 1996, Mosby.)*

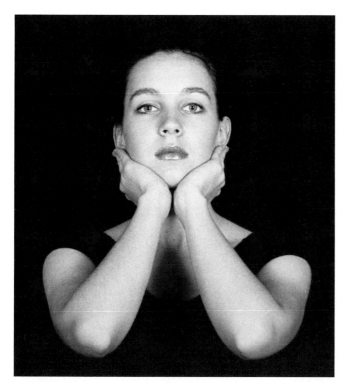

FIG. 3-104 The patient presents with a markedly splinted cervical spine and holds the weight of the head with both hands. Removal of this support cannot be tolerated. This implies gross instability of the upper cervical spine as a result of fracture or severe sprain.

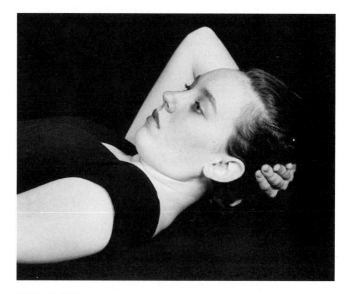

FIG. 3-105 No less significant is the patient who cannot rise from the supine position without lifting the head manually. This suggests gross upper cervical spine instability as a result of fracture or severe sprain.

SHOULDER DEPRESSION TEST

Assessment for Cervical Dural Sleeve Adhesion (Nerve Root) and Shoulder Adhesive Capsulitis

Comment

Following trauma, scar formation will occur with regularity around the dura and nerve roots. The reasons this will cause symptoms in one patient and not in others are not well understood. One explanation is that the scar tissue can act as a tethering force as well as a constricting force around the nerve roots. A direct traumatic insult to the nerve roots causes inflammation in the dural sleeves and perineural tissues. This inflammation may result in fibrosis, and adhesions may occur between the dural sleeves and the adjacent capsular structures. Normally, the nerve roots are free in the intervertebral canals and can be moved approximately ¼ to ½ of an inch. Nerve roots that have been injured or compressed by capsular thickening or bony encroachments cannot move within the intervertebral canals.

Nerve roots subjected to compressive forces by osteophytic encroachments have varying degrees of distortion and perineural fibrosis.

The typical "burner" or "stinger" can result from different injury mechanisms. History, physical examination, and appropriate diagnostic studies help differentiate brachial plexus from cervical nerve root lesions.

Brachial plexus injuries are more likely to occur in younger patients with less-well-developed neck musculature. Brachial plexus injuries usually are traction injuries resulting from lateral neck flexion away from the side of involvement. Ipsilateral shoulder depression is also a component. Pain and paresthesias involving the arm and shoulder are transient. In this injury Spurling's test is negative (Fig. 3-106). Weakness involves the deltoid, supraspinatus, infraspinatus, and biceps.

Root lesions result from compression of the nerve root and/or dorsal root ganglion in the intervertebral foramen. Hyperextension or hyperextension with lateral neck flexion are the common mechanisms of injury. Neck pain and a decreased cervical range of motion may be present. Spurling's test is positive.

PROCEDURE

- With the patient seated, the examiner depresses the patient's shoulder on the affected side and laterally flexes the cervical spine away from that shoulder (Figs. 3-107 and 3-108).
- This sign is positive if radicular pain is produced or aggravated.
- A positive sign indicates adhesions of the dural sleeves, spinal nerve roots, or adjacent structures of the joint capsule of the shoulder.

Confirmation Procedures

Bakody sign, maximum foraminal encroachment test, distraction test, brachial plexus tension test, Bikele's sign, Jackson cervical compression test, Spurling's test, foraminal compression test, reflexes, sensory testing, and diagnostic imaging

---

DIAGNOSTIC STATEMENT

Shoulder depression testing is positive on the right. This result suggests dural sleeve adhesion at C5.

CLINICAL PEARL

As with cervical distraction testing, this maneuver helps predict the viability of cervical traction in therapy. A sharply positive finding usually means that the patient will not tolerate cervical traction. The traction may aggravate the dural sleeve adhesion instead of relieving it.

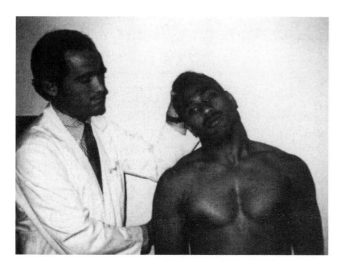

FIG. 3-106 Spurling's maneuver. *(From Torg JS, Shepard RJ: Current therapy in sports medicine, ed 3, St Louis, 1995, Mosby.)*

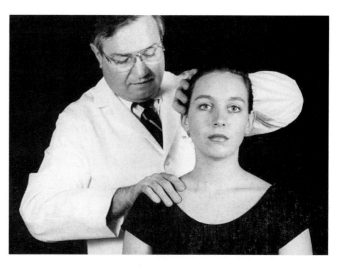

FIG. 3-107 The patient is seated, and the head and neck are in the neutral position. On the side of complaint, the examiner uses the contact points of the lateral skull and superior shoulder.

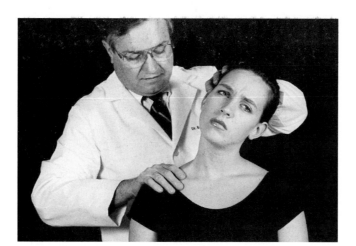

FIG. 3-108 In a slow, controlled fashion, the examiner depresses the shoulder while flexing the head toward the opposite shoulder. Reproduction of symptoms suggests a brachial plexitis or dural sleeve adhesion.

SOTO-HALL SIGN

Assessment for Cervical Spine Subluxation, Exostoses, Intervertebral Disc Lesion, Muscular Strain, Ligamentous Sprain, Vertebral Fracture, or Meningeal Irritation (Febrile)

Comment

The neck is at risk for injury in contact sports because of the inability to pad, brace, or protect the cervical spine while maintaining its function. The cervical spine must be flexible enough to allow the head and eyes to move to the right place at the right time. The spine also serves as a conduit for the central nervous system. The spinal cord and the cervical nerve roots pass through the cervical spine, making injury to the neck a potentially catastrophic event.

Even noncontact sports can be responsible for traumatic spinal injuries. Although fractures with spinal cord injuries are common, fractures without neurologic deficits are more common (Figs. 3-109 and 3-110).

Most local cervical spinal pain is secondary to involvement of the vertebral bodies, intervertebral discs, and ligamentous structures and the associated spasms of the paravertebral muscles. Too often, the symptoms of neck pain are translated into evidence for diagnosis of arthritis or disc disease without adequate examination of the patient or full consideration of the various possible causes of this symptom.

During infancy and childhood, neck pain is uncommon, but when it occurs, the possibilities are intriguing. Discitis is an important consideration when it occurs as a local bacterial infection of the disc space in the cervicothoracic region and is accompanied by x-ray changes that are characteristic but late to develop. Meningismus, or meningitis, particularly in infants and very young children (whose sensorium may be difficult to evaluate) can present as neck pain caused by meningeal inflammation and associated muscle spasm. Lymphomatous infiltration or an abscess in the epidural space may become painful well before neurologic symptoms are evident. A herniated disc may also be symptomatic.

Although infections in the cervical spine are rare, the consequences of failing to diagnose such infections are so ominous that infection is a necessary consideration even in instances of slightly aberrant cervical spine syndromes. About 15% of bone infections involve the spine, but the spine is the most common site of tuberculosis of bone. Of the entire spine—cervical, thoracic, lumbar, and sacral—the cervical spine is the most uncommon site for infection. Although all age groups may have infections in the spine, people in their teens or 40s and older have the highest rates of incidence.

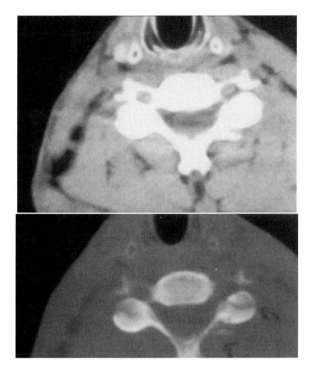

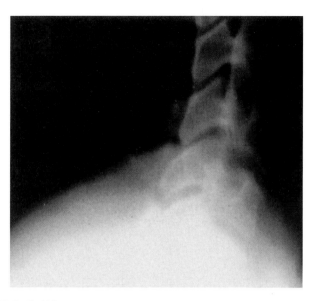

FIG. 3-109   A fractured lamina and facet of this kind can occur with head trauma.   *(From Watkins RG: The spine in sports, St Louis, 1996, Mosby.)*

FIG. 3-110   A facet fracture healed with nonoperative care and produced a stiff but stable segment.   *(From Watkins RG: The spine in sports, St Louis, 1996, Mosby.)*

PROCEDURE

- The patient is placed supine (Fig. 3-111).
- The examiner places one hand on the sternum of the patient and exerts slight pressure so that no flexion can take place at either the lumbar or thoracic regions of the spine (Fig. 3-112).
- The examiner places the other hand under the patient's occiput and flexes the head toward the chest (Fig. 3-113).
- The test is primarily used when fracture of a vertebra is suspected.
- The flexion of the head and neck on the sternum progressively produces a pull on the posterior spinous ligaments.
- When the spinous process of the injured vertebra is reached, the patient experiences a noticeable local pain.
- A positive result indicates subluxation, exostoses, disc lesion, sprain or strain, vertebral fracture, or meningeal irritation (there must be an elevated temperature for corroboration) (Fig. 3-114).

Confirmation Procedures

O'Donoghue maneuver, spinal percussion, Lhermitte's sign, Dejerine's sign, swallowing test, Valsalva maneuver, Naffziger's test, reflexes, sensory testing, and diagnostic imaging

---

DIAGNOSTIC STATEMENT

Soto-Hall (afebrile) sign is positive with pain elicited at the C5 level.

Soto-Hall (febrile) sign is positive with nuchal rigidity noted and positive Kernig's or Brudzinski's sign, which suggests meningeal irritation or inflammation.

CLINICAL PEARL

Soto-Hall sign is often misapplied in the assessment of fractures and sprains for the entire spine. The sign is a nonspecific test with limited capacity to localize conditions of the cervical and upper thoracic spine. The use of this sign to draw conclusions below T8 is largely guesswork.

With the Kernig/Brudzinski phenomena in this test, the patient's temperature must be assessed. A febrile patient with Kernig's or Brudzinski's sign—a variation of Soto-Hall sign—is a high-risk candidate for meningitis.

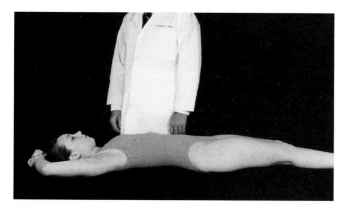

FIG. 3-111   The patient rests on the examining table in a supine position with the legs fully extended and the arms extended over the head.

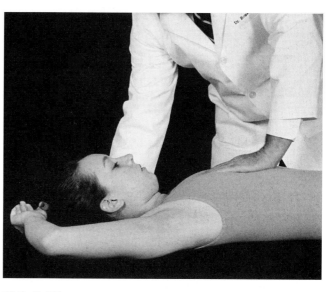

FIG. 3-112   The examiner supports the patient's head with one hand while stabilizing the patient's chest with the other hand.

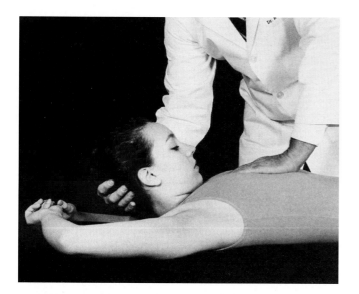

FIG. 3-113   The head and neck are sharply and passively flexed, approximating the patient's chin to the chest. Any tendency for the shoulders to rise from the table is countered with downward sternal pressure. Pain that is localized to the cervicothoracic spine suggests subluxation, exostoses, disc lesion, sprain, strain, or fracture of vertebrae.

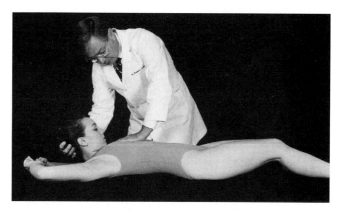

FIG. 3-114   While the head is flexed toward the chest, a reflex flexion of the knees and thighs may be produced. This reflex is equivalent to a Kernig's or Brudzinski's sign and suggests meningitis.

Assessment for Osseous or Soft-Tissue Injury

Comment

Compression fractures resulting from axial loading may be stable or unstable. Stability depends on the degree of displacement and associated soft-tissue injury. Axial cervical burst fractures are usually unstable and result in neurologic damage. Dislocation of the cervical facet joints may occur unilaterally or bilaterally in association with forward displacement of a vertebral body on the one below. Injuries to the upper cervical spine may result in C1-C2 instabilities as a result of rupture to the transverse and alar ligaments. These ligaments stabilize or fix the odontoid process to C1.

ORTHOPEDIC GAMUT 3-26

ATLANTOAXIAL INJURIES

The radiographic signs of atlantoaxial injuries are often subtle:

1. The prevertebral soft-tissue shadow on the lateral radiograph should be less than 5 mm wide at C2 and 5 to 10 mm wide in front of the ring of the atlas.
2. The lateral C-spine view will reveal fractures of the posterior ring of the atlas.
3. The open-mouth odontoid view helps in detecting subtle displacement of the lateral masses in relation to the facets of the axis.

ORTHOPEDIC GAMUT 3-27

CERVICAL SPINE FLEXION-EXTENSION RADIOGRAPHS

The following are prerequisites for cervical spine flexion-extension radiographs:

1. A neurologically intact patient
2. Performance of all movements actively by the patient
3. No altered state of consciousness (including intoxication)
4. Direct physician supervision of the radiographic study

TABLE 3-11

REFERRAL ZONES ASSOCIATED WITH TRIGGER POINTS IN MYOFASCIAL PAIN SYNDROME

Localized Trigger Points	Referral Zone
Suboccipital muscles	Temporal region
	Vertex of head
	Temporalis muscle via greater occipital nerve
Levator scapula	Inferior or superior scapula border, occiput
Greater or lesser rhomboid muscles	Cervical spine, shoulder, or scapula region
Infraspinous or teres minor muscles	Arm, shoulder, hand
Sternocleidomastoid muscles	Supraorbital region
	Temporal region
	Forehead, ear
Scalene muscles	Shoulder, arm or hand, chest, scapula
Masseter muscle	Ear, suboccipital region, temporal region
Trapezius muscle	Suboccipital region, shoulder, orbit or temporal area

From Brier SR: *Primary care orthopedics,* St Louis, 1999, Mosby.

Isolated fractures of the posterior arch of the atlas are secondary to hyperextension with or without axial loading of the upper cervical spine. In this there is approximately a 50% chance that some other cervical injury is also present.

The Jefferson (or burst) fracture may involve four fractures: two anterior and two posterior to the lateral masses. Because of the spreading of the lateral masses and the arch, neurologic compromise rarely occurs.

Transverse ligament ruptures occur from direct blows to the occiput. If the distance between the anterior ring of C1 and the anterior cortex of the odontoid process on the lateral flexion radiograph is more than 5 mm, a transverse ligament rupture is present. If the distance is more than 9 to 10 mm, additional ruptures of the alar ligaments and apical ligaments of the odontoid process are present.

Pain or discomfort that is nonarticular may be myofascial in origin. The patient with myofascial pain typically has multiple sites of trigger points that refer pain to a distant site (Table 3-11).

Vehicular accidents are a common source of trauma to the lower cervical spine and may cause a wide variety of fractures and dislocations. Compression fractures at the anterior edge of the vertebral bodies may be caused by a hyperflexion motion alone or in combination with a vertical compression. The stability of these fractures depends on the degree of vertebral compression and the presence of posterior ligamentous damage.

Traumatic injuries of the cervical spine are among the most common causes of severe disability and death after trauma. These injuries often are not diagnosed in the emergency room situation. Approximately one third of the injuries to the cervical spine result from motor vehicle accidents, one third from falling, and the remaining one third from some type of athletic injury or wound inflicted by a missile or falling object.

The incidence of cervical spine injuries peaks during adolescence, young adulthood, and again during the sixth and seventh decades. Because of the nature of accidents resulting in cervical spine injuries, most involve young, healthy persons who are very active. This includes those who engage in physically dangerous activities and occasionally those who exhibit sociopathic personality traits. People in their fifth and sixth decades make up the second largest group of cervical spinal injury patients. Cervical spondylosis and a preexisting narrow spinal canal are closely associated with injury in this age group. Lesser forces may result in severe spine and spinal cord injury in this group.

PROCEDURE

- With the patient seated and the head slightly flexed, the examiner percusses the spinous processes and associated musculature of each of the cervical vertebra with a neurologic reflex hammer (Fig. 3-115).

- Evidence of localized pain indicates a possible fractured vertebra.
- Evidence of radicular pain indicates a possible disc lesion.
- Because of the nonspecific nature of this test, other conditions will also elicit a positive pain response.
- A ligamentous sprain will cause pain when the spinous processes are percussed.
- Percussing the paraspinal musculature will elicit a positive sign for muscular strain (Fig. 3-116).

Confirmation Procedures
Soto-Hall sign, O'Donoghue test, Dejerine's sign, swallowing test, Valsalva maneuver, Naffziger's test, Lhermitte's sign, and diagnostic imaging

---

DIAGNOSTIC STATEMENT

Spinal percussion elicits pain on the spinous process of C5. This result suggests osseous injury or ligamentous sprain at that level.

Spinal percussion elicits pain at the paraspinal muscle on the right at C5. This result suggests soft-tissue injury at that level.

CLINICAL PEARL

When soft-tissue percussion reproduces the pain, the examiner may expect the same phenomenon from applications of ultrasound to the tissue. This pain represents spasmophilia, and the uses of such therapies may need to be delayed until the soft tissue is no longer reactive to percussion.

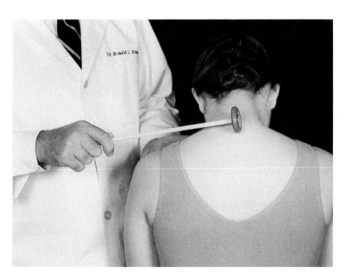

FIG. 3-115 In the seated position, the patient flexes the cervical spine forward, exposing the spinous processes as much as possible. The examiner percusses the spinous processes of each vertebra. Localized pain is evidence of a fracture or severe sprain. Radiating pain suggests an intervertebral disc syndrome.

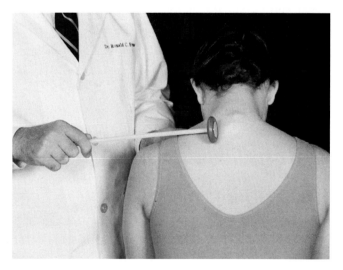

FIG. 3-116 The paravertebral tissues are percussed. Pain elicited in the soft tissues suggests muscular strain and highly sensitive myofascial trigger points.

SPURLING'S TEST

Assessment for Cervical Nerve Root Compression Syndrome

Comment

Narrowing of the intervertebral foramina, pressure and shearing forces on the zygapophyseal joint surfaces, intervertebral disc compression, and pressure on stiff ligamentous and muscular structures may all cause pain. A pain pattern may be perfectly reproduced, which allows for identification of the neurologic level. If radicular pain or paresthesia with referral to the upper extremity occurs, nerve root irritation is present. If the pain is confined to the neck, soft, connective tissues or joints are more likely to be the pain-sensitive structures.

Root pain may be aggravated by spinal motions that narrow the intervertebral foramen through which the diseased nerve root passes. In cervical nerve root disease, simultaneous extension and lateral flexion of the neck toward the affected side or a blow to the vertex of the head (Spurling's test) may result in sudden aggravation of neck and dermatomal arm pain, paresthesia, or both.

This test is sometimes of value in the diagnosis of a laterally herniated intervertebral disc in the cervical spine.

All patients who sustain sufficient injury to the cervical spine to make the examiner suspect cervical disc compromise should have a standard three-view plain x-ray film series (Table 3-12).

Patients with persistent radiculopathy with or without motor loss for at least 4 to 8 weeks should undergo electrodiagnostic testing after MRI. Electrodiagnostic tests can document any central denervating disorder or concomitant peripheral entrapment neuropathy.

PROCEDURE

- The test is performed with the patient seated (Fig. 3-117).
- The examiner places one hand on top of the patient's head and gradually increases downward pressure (Fig. 3-118).

ORTHOPEDIC GAMUT 3-28

MRI SCANS

Follow-up with an MRI scan of the cervical spine is appropriate for the following patients:

1. Patients who do not respond to conservative measures of care within 2 to 4 weeks and have abnormal neurologic findings
2. Those who have persistent radiculopathy and loss of motion in multiple planes
3. Those who exhibit signs of myelopathy and stenosis
4. Those who have progressive symptoms with motor or sensory deficits
5. Patients who have a cervical spinal canal of questionable patency
6. Patients who have equivocal findings on routine radiography

---

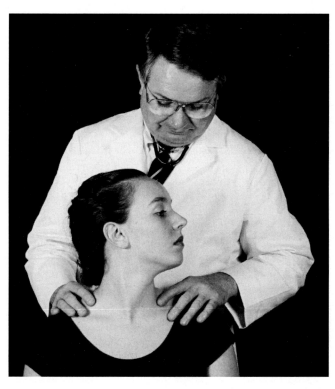

FIG. 3-117   While seated comfortably and with an erect posture, the patient actively rotates the head from side to side. Localization of pain is noted.

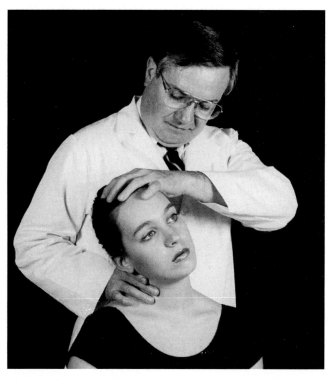

FIG. 3-118   The patient's head is laterally flexed toward the side of complaint. The examiner applies gradually progressive downward pressure to the head and neck. Reproduction of symptoms or collapse sign at this point constitutes a positive test. The balance of the test should not be completed.

TABLE 3-12

CERVICAL DISC SYNDROMES

	Acute	Chronic
Type	Herniated cervical disc	Degenerative disc disease
Physical examination findings	Paravertebral myospasm	Chronic cervical stiffness, hypertonicity
	Limited range of motion with signs of instability	Upper extremity referral
	Radicular signs with possible arm, hand, or scapula referral	Possible bilateral or unilateral intermittent radiculopathy, progressive motor changes or atrophy, prolonged cervical instability
	Often motor, sensory, or reflex changes	
	Nerve root traction signs	Possible nerve root traction signs
	Abnormal results on compression tests	Abnormal results on compression tests
X-ray findings	Standard three-view series (i.e., anteroposterior, open-mouth, lateral), if antecedent trauma	Same as for acute conditions, plus oblique films, if neuroforaminal pathologic abnormality or fracture suspected
	Decreased intervertebral disc spacing or spondylosis possible	Decreased intervertebral disc space, osteophytes, possible anterior subluxation secondary to anterior longitudinal ligament buckling
	Altered cervical lordosis	Hypolordosis
Secondary diagnoses	Cervical radiculopathy, radiculitis; cervical myelopathy; cervical spinal stenosis; acute cervical myospasm	Cervical radiculopathy, radiculitis; cervical myelopathy; cervical spinal stenosis; acute cervical myospasm

Adapted from Brier SR: *Primary care orthopedics,* St Louis, 1999, Mosby.

- The patient notes any pain or paresthesia and the distribution thereof.
- Pressure may also be applied while the head is laterally flexed to either side and extended (Fig. 3-119).
- Pressure should be maintained.
- This maneuver closes the intervertebral foramina on the side of the flexion and reproduces the familiar pain or paresthesia (Fig. 3-120).

Confirmation Procedures
Bakody sign, maximum foraminal encroachment test, shoulder depression test, distraction test, brachial plexus tension test, Bikele's sign, Jackson cervical compression test, foraminal compression test, reflex and sensory testing, electrodiagnosis, and diagnostic imaging

---

DIAGNOSTIC STATEMENT

Spurling's test is positive on the right with pain and paresthesia elicited in the C5 dermatome. This suggests nerve root compression of the C5 nerve root.

CLINICAL PEARL

Spurling's test is an aggressive cervical compression test, and the patient should be informed of each step as it is introduced. However, the examiner should not cue the patient for pain responses. Spurling's test elicits collapse sign quite easily.

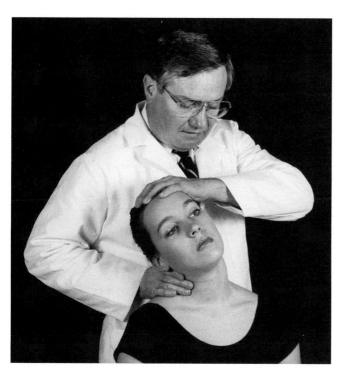

FIG. 3-119   From the laterally flexed position, the neck is extended as far as the patient can tolerate. The examiner applies progressive downward pressure. Reproduction of radicular symptoms suggests nerve root compression. Localized spinal pain suggests facet involvement.

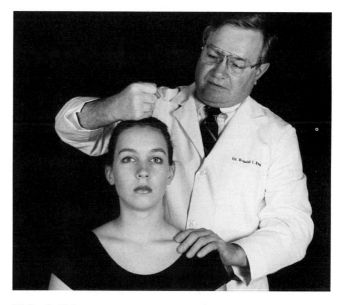

FIG. 3-120   A vertical blow is delivered to the uppermost portion of the cranium. The examiner may wish to interpose a hand between the concussing hand and the patient's skull. The head and neck are first in a neutral position for this procedure and then positioned into lateral flexion and extension for a repeated procedure. The test will stimulate any nerve root irritation or other pain-sensitive structures related to disc disease and cervical spondylosis. Use of this modification should not be a surprise to the patient.

SWALLOWING TEST

Assessment for Space-Occupying Mass, Ligamentous Sprain, Muscular Strain, Fracture, Cervical Intervertebral Disc Lesion, Tumor, or Osteophyte at the Anterior Portion of the Cervical Spine

Comment

Dysphagia may be of prognostic significance and is often indicative of esophageal injury, pharyngeal hemorrhage or edema, or retropharyngeal hemorrhage. Dysphagia may also result from severe muscle spasm.

When dysphagia is present, the examiner should look for ligamentous disruption, dislocation, subluxation, or fracture and should make careful use of cineradiography, tomography, and CT or bone scanning to uncover the true nature and extent of the injuries.

Anterior osteophytes from the cervical vertebrae, particularly C5, C6, and C7, may compress the posterior wall of the esophagus and irritate the tissues and smooth muscle. The symptom may be either dysphagia or simply an annoying awareness of swallowing.

True disc herniation is relatively uncommon in the elderly because of the decreased water content of the nucleus pulposus. When disc herniation does occur, it is usually triggered by some form of trauma. Symptoms may include sudden and severe neck and arm pain as well as paresthesia along the involved nerve root. Neck movements, especially lateral flexion toward the affected side, will typically aggravate the pain.

PROCEDURE

- While seated, the patient is instructed to swallow (Fig. 3-121).
- Presence of pain or difficulty swallowing indicates a space-occupying lesion, ligamentous sprain, muscular strain, or fracture, such as disc protrusion, tumor, or osteophyte at the anterior portion of the cervical spine.

Confirmation Procedures

Dejerine's sign, Valsalva maneuver, Naffziger's test, Lhermitte's sign, reflexes and sensory testing, and diagnostic imaging

---

DIAGNOSTIC STATEMENT

A positive swallowing test indicates that dysphagia is present. This result suggests esophageal irritation.

CLINICAL PEARL

Dysphagia is often observed after hyperextension trauma of the cervical spine. Coupled with other sympathetic nervous system phenomena, the patient attributes the sore throat or hoarseness to a cold. The dysphagia is fleeting but serves as a more conclusive sign as to the extent of soft-tissue involvement in the injury.

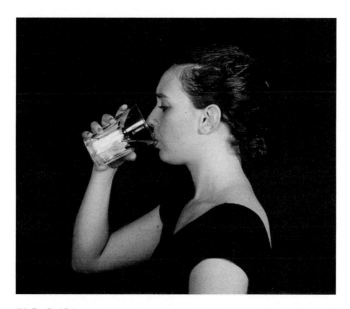

FIG. 3-121   The patient is seated and instructed to swallow. A beverage or small food item may be needed to induce this activity. The presence of pain indicates esophageal irritation caused by direct trauma or a retroesophageal space-occupying mass.

UNDERBURG'S TEST

Assessment for Vertebrobasilar Artery Syndrome

Comment

The blood supply of the vital neck structures, including bony spine, spinal cord, nerve roots, coverings, and posterior cranial fossa and cerebral visual cortex, is derived from the vertebral arteries. The tortuous course these arteries take and the susceptibility of their intimate coverings to structural change places them in a vulnerable position. In most instances the protective mechanism is amazingly adequate. However, when changes, such as atheromatous cracks, develop within the vessels, circulation may be compromised or temporarily obstructed.

The artery is intimately related to the Luschka joints medially and the apophyseal joint posterolaterally, so osteophyte formation at either site may encroach on the artery's usual course. The efficiency of the vertebral artery system is related to the anastomosis at the circle of Willis with the internal carotid system. A weak point in one area may influence the other.

Contrast studies have been used to show that head and neck movement, primarily involving rotation, may alter blood flow in the vertebral artery. Pathologic changes in the vertebral artery may favor ischemia. The flow between C6 and C2 may be diminished on the side to which the head and neck is turned, and the flow may be increased in the opposite vessel at the point where the artery twists over the arch of the atlas. Changes in such a mechanism would explain transient attacks of vertigo that are attributed to vertebrobasilar ischemia.

ORTHOPEDIC GAMUT 3-29

BRAINSTEM ISCHEMIA

In vertebrobasilar artery brainstem ischemia is caused by the following:

1. Trauma to the arterial wall producing damage to the arterial wall
2. Trauma to the arterial wall producing vasospasm

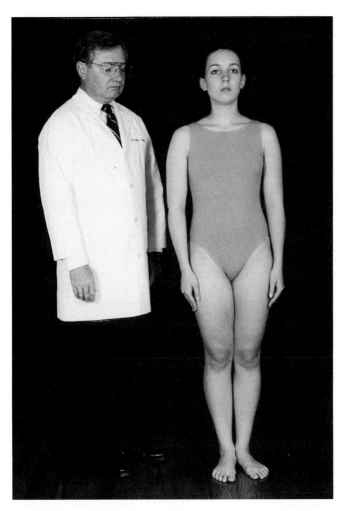

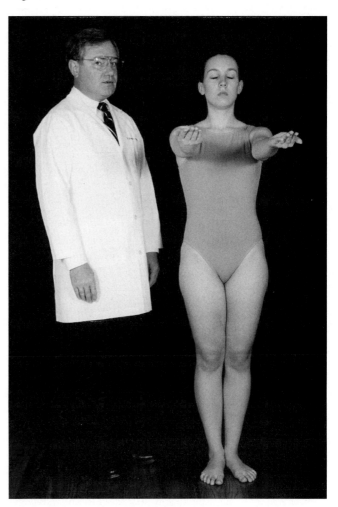

FIG. 3-122 The patient stands with the eyes open and the arms resting at the sides. The postural base is narrowed. The examiner observes for any equilibrium difficulty. It is important for the examiner to remain close to the patient throughout this procedure.

FIG. 3-123 The patient closes the eyes and elevates the extended arms forward to shoulder level. The patient's hands are fully supinated. While the patient maintains this position with the narrowed postural base, the examiner observes for loss of equilibrium or drift of the arms and pronation of the hands.

ORTHOPEDIC GAMUT 3-30

DAMAGE TO THE ARTERY WALL

In vertebrobasilar syndrome, damage to the artery wall is caused by the following:

1. Compression and/or stretching of the vertebral artery wall that applies enough force to disrupt the vasovasorum, resulting in subintimal hematoma. Vertebral artery blood flow is decreased by occlusion of the lumen.
2. The intima is the most likely tissue to tear when the vessel is stretched and/or compressed. Exposure of the subendothelial tissue leads to the cascade mechanism, resulting in clot formation (thrombosis). The clot remains adherent to the tear and may lead to vessel occlusion.
3. The propagating clot extends into the lumen. The blood flow may "break off" part of the clot and form an embolus. The embolus causes arterial occlusion distally, leading to infarction.
4. When blood dissects the intima and the internal elastica, a dissecting aneurysm is formed.

ORTHOPEDIC GAMUT 3-31

VASOSPASM

Arterial wall trauma producing vasospasm follows Virchow's triad:

1. Change in vessel wall: In VBA neck rotation causes the artery to be momentarily compressed or stretched. This may result in spasm, without vertebral artery damage.
2. Change in blood flow: In VBA, even after the removal of the arterial compression, the spasm may persist. This reduces the blood supply to tissue. Blood flow may stagnate within the involved vessel.
3. Change in blood constituents: Within the vertebrobasilar system the vertebral arteries can be sufficiently compromised (stasis) to initiate a propagating thrombus and subsequent embolism.

PROCEDURE

- The patient is standing and is instructed to outstretch the arms, supinate the hands, and close the eyes (Figs. 3-122 to 3-124).
- The patient marches in place and extends and rotates the head while continuing to march (Fig. 3-125).
- The test is repeated with the head rotated and extended to the opposite side.
- The examiner watches for a loss of balance, dropping of the arms, and pronation of the hands.
- If this occurs, the examiner should suspect vertebral, basilar, or carotid artery stenosis or compression.

Confirmation Procedures

Barre-Lieou sign, vertebrobasilar artery function test, Hautant's test, DeKleyn's test, Hallpike maneuver, vascular diagnosis, and diagnostic imaging

DIAGNOSTIC STATEMENT

Underburg's test is positive. This result suggests vertebrobasilar artery syndrome.

CLINICAL PEARL

If the patient loses equilibrium at any time while the eyes are closed, cerebellar circulation must be evaluated. In this procedure the patient may lose equilibrium as soon as the head is rotated to one side. The examiner must be prepared to prevent the patient from falling.

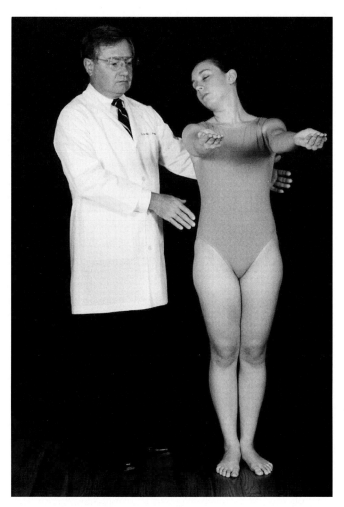

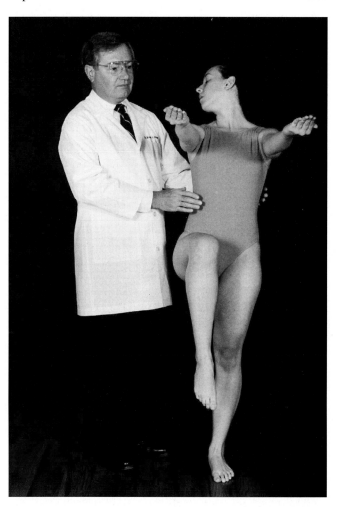

FIG. 3-124   The patient extends the neck and rotates the head to one side while maintaining a narrowed postural base, elevating the arms, and supinating the hands. The eyes remain closed. The examiner observes for difficulty in the performance of each segment of the test.

FIG. 3-125   The patient attempts to maintain the head and neck rotation or extension, arm elevation, and hand supination while marching in place. Loss of balance, dropping or drifting of the arms, or pronation of the hands is indicative of vertebrobasilar or carotid artery stenosis or compression. The test is repeated with the head and neck rotated to the opposite side.

VALSALVA MANEUVER

NEURO-ORTHOPEDIC APPLICATION

Assessment for Space-Occupying Lesion, Tumor, Intervertebral Disc Herniation, or Osteophytes

Comment

More than 90% of disc lesions in the cervical spine occur at the C5 and C6 levels. As degeneration of a disc occurs, two different types of lesions can produce very similar symptoms. The first is the soft disc protrusion or nuclear herniation. In this lesion a mass of nucleus pulposus bulges outward, commonly posterolaterally (Fig. 3-126). Complete extrusion of disc material may occur. With acute rupture of a cervical disc, immediate compression of the nerve root occurs. Compression results in nerve root symptoms and radicular pain.

The second lesion results from chronic disc degeneration with subsequent narrowing of the disc space. This is cervical "spondylosis" and occurs primarily in the older age group. As narrowing and collapse of the disc proceeds, the vertebrae become more closely approximated, which leads to spur formation along the disc edges and at the joints of Luschka. Mild subluxation of the facet joint may also occur. All of these changes decrease the size of the intervertebral foramen, which results in pressure on the nerve root. Mild inflammation and swelling are usually present in conjunction with osteophyte formation, which further contributes to the narrowing of the foramen and nerve root compression. Coughing, sneezing, and straining can accentuate the pain, which may radiate into the shoulder and arm and along the radial aspect of the forearm (Fig. 3-127).

Spondylosis in the cervical spine may occasionally produce symptoms referable to the lower extremities (cervical spondylotic myelopathy). These symptoms occur as a result of pressure of posterior osteophytes on the anterior portion of the cervical spinal cord. The symptom complex appears as a combination of cervical root and cord symptoms (rhizalgia).

In most cases the diagnosis is clear without further testing. Neck, interscapular, and/or arm pain that is aggravated by neck motion is typical (Figs. 3-128 and 3-129).

ORTHOPEDIC GAMUT 3-32

CERVICAL SPINE SPONDYLOSIS

Assessment of cervical spine spondylosis includes the following:

1. Plain roentgenograms are usually performed first, within the first few weeks of onset of symptoms. AP and lateral views are sufficient.
2. Myelography, sometimes followed by CT, will demonstrate loss of the normal root "sleeve," and indentation of the dural sac is often seen.
3. MRI is performed.
4. Electromyography and discography are performed. However, the diagnosis can usually be well established on the basis of the history, physical examination, and myelogram alone.

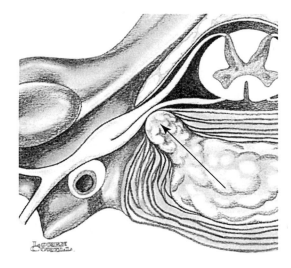

FIG. 3-126   Disc herniation causing nerve root compression. *(From Mercier LR, Pettid FJ: Practical orthopedics, ed 4, St Louis, 1995, Mosby.)*

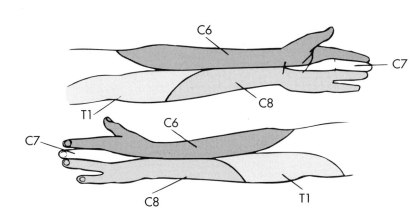

FIG. 3-127   Volar and dorsal dermatome pattern of the forearm and hand.   *(From Mercier LR, Pettid FJ: Practical orthopedics, ed 4, St Louis, 1995, Mosby.)*

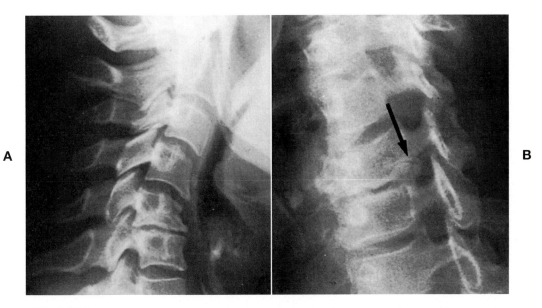

FIG. 3-128   Lateral **(A)** and oblique **(B)** radiographs showing degenerative disc disease at the C5-C6 level.   *(From Mercier LR, Pettid FJ: Practical orthopedics, ed 4, St Louis, 1995, Mosby.)*

Disc compression of the nerve root is influenced by changes in volume and consistency of the disc as well as changes in position of the motion segment. These factors form the basis for a number of diagnostic measures. During infantile and adult stages, the intervertebral disc is not stiff and inflexible; rather, the disc is a connective tissue structure, which can physiologically change its form and volume by loading and unloading. The remaining parts of the motion segment, including the nerve fibers, adjust themselves to these changes. There is sufficient space between the dural sac and its nerve roots in relation to the posterior part of the intervertebral disc. Changes in the form of the disc as well as changes in the position of the nerve roots during spinal movement will not influence the spinal nerves. The epidural space, which is filled with fatty tissue and venous plexus, varies in width. As a rule, the intervertebral foramen is large enough to allow ample space for the passage of nerves. When the spinal space becomes diminished by disc protrusions, osteophytes, engorged vessels, or stenosis (a narrowing of the spinal canal), the nerve roots come under pressure. When the nerve roots come in contact with a disc surface that has undergone physiologic changes, the nerve roots can no longer alter their position, making them more sensitive to the mechanical influence.

Symptoms of extramedullary lesions may include local tissue destruction, radicular involvement by space-occupying mass or bony compression, or spinal cord compression secondary to bony collapse or tumor. Radicular pain is common, and the spinal cord level is usually discrete. Sensory loss is uniform, and motor loss is often uniform also.

Radicular complaints follow the roots involved and are similar to those associated with disc herniation.

PROCEDURE

- The patient takes a deep breath and holds it while bearing down abdominally (Figs. 3-130 and 3-131).
- A positive test is indicated by increased pain caused by increased intrathecal pressure.
- Increased intrathecal pressure is usually caused by a space-occupying lesion (herniated disc, tumor, osteophytes).
- The test should be done with care and caution because the patient may become dizzy and pass out while or shortly after performing this test because the procedure can block the blood supply to the brain.

Confirmation Procedures

Dejerine's sign, swallowing test, Naffziger's test, Bakody sign, maximum foraminal encroachment test, shoulder depression test, distraction test, brachial plexus tension test, Bikele's sign, Jackson cervical compression test, Spurling's test, foraminal compression test, reflexes and sensory testing, and diagnostic imaging

---

DIAGNOSTIC STATEMENT

Valsalva maneuver is positive. This result elicits radicular pain on the right in the C5 dermatome.

ORTHOPEDIC GAMUT 3-33

NERVE ROOT INVOLVEMENT

Guidelines for quick localization of nerve root involvement are as follows:

1. If the deltoid muscle is spared, the lesion is likely to be at C4-C5.
2. If the biceps are spared, the lesion is likely to be at C5-C6.
3. If the triceps are spared, the lesion is likely to be at C6-C7.
4. If the hands are spared, the level is likely to be C7-T1 or below.

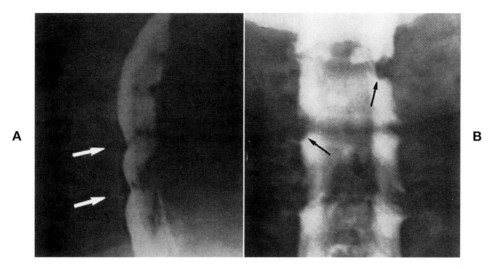

FIG. 3-129   Myelographic findings in cervical disc disease. **A,** Lateral view. **B,** Anteroposterior view. *(From Mercier LR, Pettid FJ:* Practical orthopedics, *ed 4, St Louis, 1995, Mosby.)*

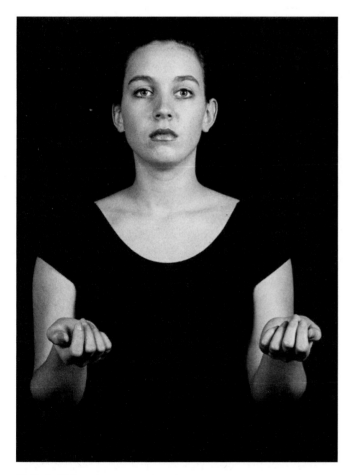

FIG. 3-130   The patient is seated comfortably. The arms may be slightly flexed at the elbows. The patient is instructed to take a deep breath and hold it.

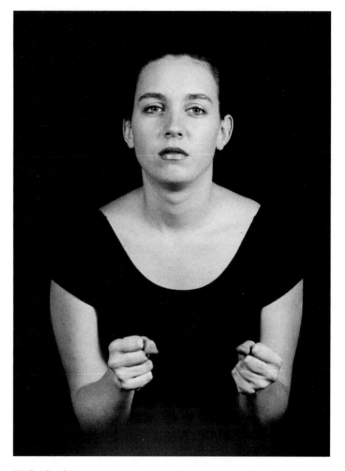

FIG. 3-131   While holding the deep breath, the patient bears down to create greater intraabdominal pressure. Reproduction of radicular pain is indicative of nerve root compression by a space-occupying mass in the spine.

VERTEBROBASILAR ARTERY FUNCTIONAL MANEUVER

Assessment for Vertebral, Basilar, or Carotid Artery Stenosis or Compression

Comment

The vertebral arteries are vulnerable to injury in the foramina of the lower cervical vertebra, at the junction between C1 and C2, and as they pass over the arch of C1 through the atlantooccipital membrane. Intimal disruption may lead to acute, complete thrombotic occlusion, subintimal hematoma, dissection of the artery, or pseudoaneurysm formation. Obviously, atlantooccipital dislocation usually causes total disruption of the vertebrobasilar system and results in death.

The mechanism of injury seems to be cervical hyperextension accompanied by excessive rotation. Severely diminished flow in one of the vertebral arteries may lead to occlusion of the posterior inferior cerebellar artery on that side, resulting in a lateral medullary infarction (Wallenberg's syndrome). This syndrome is characterized by the ipsilateral loss of cranial nerves V, IX, X, and XI and by cerebellar ataxia, Horner's syndrome, and contralateral loss of pain and temperature sensation.

With increasing severity of injury, vascular involvement can ascend to the basilar, superior cerebellar, and posterior cerebral arteries. Sudden death, quadriplegia, or locked-in syndrome (quadriplegia accompanied by the loss of lower cranial nerves, which allows eye blinking only) can ensue. These symptoms should alert the examiner to the possibility of vascular injury, which means that immediate cerebral arteriography is recommended to obtain an accurate diagnosis.

Symptoms of vertebrobasilar insufficiency include paroxysmal symptoms induced by certain head movements, mainly rotation, extension, and lateral flexion. Dizziness, diplopia, drop attack, syncope, and spinal stroke increase in frequency and intensity with increasing magnitudes of cervical osteoarthritis, atheromatosis in vessels, and advanced age. Manipulation of the neck in patients with these characteristics is hazardous.

The time between the vertebral artery trauma and the onset of ischemic symptoms and signs can vary from immediate to several days later. The interval is probably related to the mechanism of injury. When brainstem ischemia is caused by vasoconstriction, symptoms are immediate; ischemia symptoms (other than the pain of dissection) resulting from thrombus embolus become symptomatic only after some time.

ORTHOPEDIC GAMUT 3-34

VERTEBROBASILAR INSUFFICIENCY

The major signs and symptoms of vertebrobasilar insufficiency are as follows:

1. Dizziness, vertigo, giddiness, light-headedness
2. Drop attacks, loss of consciousness
3. Diplopia (or other visual problems/amaurosis fugax)
4. Dysarthria (speech difficulties)
5. Dysphagia
6. Ataxia of gait (walking difficulties, incoordination of the extremities, ataxia, falling to one side)
7. Nausea (with possible vomiting)
8. Numbness on one side of the face and/or body
9. Nystagmus

Dizziness is the most common symptom of vertebrobasilar insufficiency and may be unaccompanied by any other symptoms or signs.

There is marked pathophysiologic involvement of the Luschka and zygapophyseal joints when encroachment of the vertebral artery occurs, especially at the occipitoatlantoaxial level, but this involvement may occur at any level. Atheromatous plaques with calcification may be noted in the carotid artery (specifically at the siphon) and in the walls of the vertebral artery. There is occasionally a rare aneurysm of the vertebral or carotid artery in the cervical spine. Angiography discloses varying magnitudes of obstruction or complete obstruction such as that caused by thrombosis.

In patients suspected of having carotid occlusive disease, a thorough physical examination that includes blood pressure measurements in both arms and careful auscultation of the heart should be performed. In the absence of a precordial murmur a bruit at the carotid bifurcation suggests carotid bifurcation arthrosclerosis either in the internal or external artery or both. No physical finding differentiates which of these sites is involved (Fig. 3-132). It is important to listen over the supraclavicular region, where a bruit suggests subclavian or innominate artery stenosis. A significant difference in blood pressure between the two extremities confirms the presence of subclavian artery obstruction.

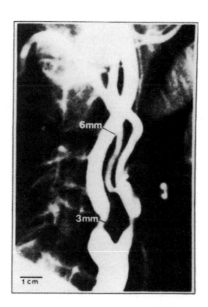

FIG. 3-132 Stenosis of carotid diameter. *(From Lynch TG, Hobson RW: Vascular surgery: principles and practice, New York, 1987, McGraw-Hill.)*

ORTHOPEDIC GAMUT 3-35

VERTEBROBASILAR ISCHEMIA

There are three types of vertebrobasilar ischemia:

1. Transient ischemic attacks (TIAs) are brief episodes of neurologic dysfunction most commonly caused by embolic showers from an atheromatous carotid artery to the ipsilateral cerebral hemisphere. Patients experience paresthesia or anesthesia in an arm or leg. When a motor abnormality is prominent, weakness, paralysis, or incoordination on the involved side of the body is present. Brief aphasic or dysphasic symptoms occur with involvement of the dominant hemisphere. Attacks are brief, lasting for a few seconds to minutes. Rarely do the attacks extend beyond 3 hours. TIAs occur on the side opposite the involved area of the brain and carotid artery.
2. Reversible ischemia neurologic deficits (RINDs) persist for longer than 24 hours and disappear completely. When the symptoms of RINDs occur and are identical to those of TIA, the patient may have sustained a small area of cerebral infarction. Neurologic symptoms that persist for long periods are diagnosed as a completed stroke.
3. "Stroke in evolution" and crescendo TIAs may occur. A patient with a stroke in evolution experiences acute neurologic deficit, which progresses over hours or days and ultimately results in a fixed deficit caused by cerebral infarction. Crescendo carotid TIAs is a syndrome of multiple TIAs occurring within a short time. Each attack is followed by complete recovery. These syndromes indicate high-grade carotid artery stenosis with embolization and are an urgent indication for further evaluation.

ORTHOPEDIC GAMUT 3-36

RESIDUAL EFFECT OF CAROTID OCCLUSION

When serious residual effects of carotid occlusion occur, the symptoms will conform to one of the following syndromes:

1. Wallenberg (occlusion of the posterior inferior cerebral artery)
2. Locked-in (occlusion of the basilar artery)
3. Other brainstem syndromes
4. Occipital lobe injury
5. Cerebellar injury
6. Thalamus injury

- This second maneuver should be performed only if initial palpation and auscultation did not reveal bruits or pulsations.
- The test is considered positive if either maneuver reveals pulsations or bruits.
- The rotation and hyperextension portion of this test places motion-induced compression on the vertebral arteries.
- Vertigo, dizziness, visual blurring, nausea, faintness, and nystagmus are all signs of a positive test, which indicates vertebral, basilar, or carotid artery stenosis or compression.

Confirmation Procedures
Barre-Lieou sign, Hautant's test, DeKleyn's test, Hallpike maneuver, Underburg's test, reflex and sensory testing, vascular assessment, vascular imaging, and MRI

PROCEDURE

- With the patient in a seated position, the examiner palpates the carotid and subclavian arteries and auscultates for pulsations and bruits (Fig. 3-133).
- If neither of these exist, the patient is instructed to rotate and hyperextend the head to one side and then the other (Fig. 3-134).

DIAGNOSTIC STATEMENT

The vertebrobasilar artery functional maneuver is positive. This result suggests arterial stenosis or compression at the upper cervical level.

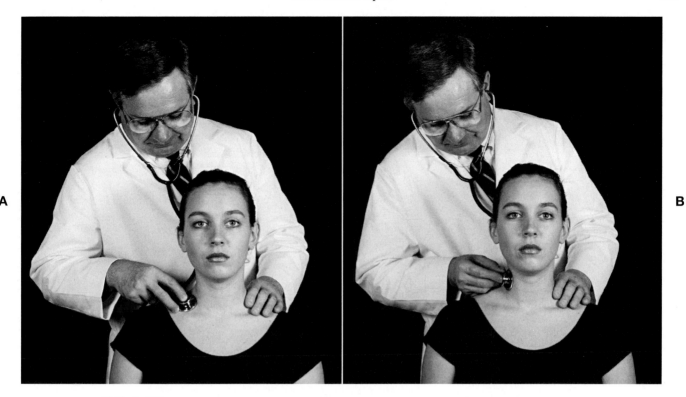

FIG. 3-133   While the patient is in a seated position, the subclavian (**A**) and then the carotid (**B**) arteries are auscultated for bruits. This is followed by palpation of the arteries for pulse assessment. If bruits are present, the balance of the test is not completed, and the test is considered positive.

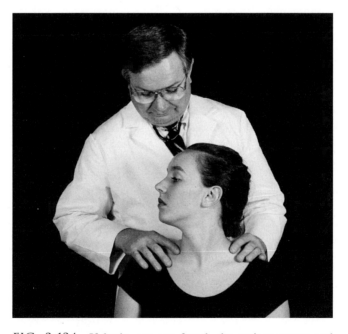

FIG. 3-134   If bruits are not found, the patient rotates and hyperextends the head and neck, both to the right and left. The production of vertigo, visual disturbances, nausea, syncope, or nystagmus is indicative of vertebral, basilar, or carotid artery stenosis or compression.

CRITICAL THINKING

What artery serves as the major source of blood to the cervical cord and cervical spine?

The vertebral artery

Is the atlantoaxial joint (C1, C2) a stable joint?

No, the atlantoaxial joint is unstable because of a small contact area between the joint surfaces.

The teardrop fracture of the cervical spine is caused by what type of injury?

The mechanism of injury is hyperflexion.

In cervical trauma, what radiograph should be obtained before anything else is done?

The initial radiograph is a lateral radiograph of the cervical spine, preferably made with the patient still on a stretcher or gurney.

When fracture is not obvious on a lateral radiograph of the cervical spine, what else is evaluated to determine whether fracture has occurred?

The prevertebral fat stripe at C3, 3.5 mm is standard; at C4, 5.0 mm; and at C5, C6, and C7, approximately 15 mm, with up to 20 mm at the distal portion. If abnormal widening is noted at any area along the anterior cervical spine, fracture should be suspected.

What is the most common cervical spine congenital abnormality associated with traumatic quadriplegia?

The most common congenital abnormality is stenosis of the cervical spine canal, with the quadriplegia occurring at the stenotic level.

Name the six most common types of forces that cause cervical spine fracture.

1. Compressive flexion
2. Vertical compression
3. Distractive flexion
4. Compressive extension
5. Distractive extension
6. Lateral flexion

What is the most common imaging finding associated with compressive extension injuries?

Unilateral vertebral arch fracture that involves the articular process

What are the most common signs and symptoms of Hangman's fracture?

Marked apprehension and fear with a sense of subjective instability; Rust's sign; pain radiating along the course of the greater occipital nerve (C2); occipital neuralgia (frequent) that leads to marked guarding of neck motion

What vertebral level is the most common injury site in children?

The most common site of injury is from the occiput to C3. Lesions at the atlantoaxial joint are noted in 70% of children younger than 15 years of age but in only 16% of adults

What changes in motor function, sensory function, or reflexes are expected in C4 quadriplegia?

Spontaneous breathing; shrugging of the shoulders independently; loss of functional abdominal muscles; sensation in the upper anterior chest wall but not in the upper extremities; absence of all reflexes

What motor, sensation, and reflex changes are expected in C5 quadriplegia?

The deltoid muscle and a portion of the biceps muscle are functioning. Shoulder abduction and flexion/extension can be performed. Elbow flexion is present. All of these functions are weak. Sensation is normal over the upper portion of the anterior chest wall and the lateral aspect of the arm from the shoulder to the elbow crease. The biceps reflex may be normal or slightly decreased.

What motor functions, sensations, and reflexes would remain intact in C6 quadriplegia?

Both the biceps and rotator cuff muscles continue to function. The extensor carpi radialis longus and brevis and extensor carpi ulnaris may not be functioning. Almost full function of the shoulder is retained, as well as full flexion of the elbow. Full supination and partial pronation of the forearm is seen, with partial extension of the wrist. The strength of wrist extension is normal. The lateral side of the entire upper extremity as well as the thumb, index, and half of the middle finger have normal sensory power. Both the biceps and the brachioradialis reflexes are normal.

What motor functions, sensations, and reflexes remain intact in C7 quadriplegia?

The triceps, wrist flexors, and long-finger extensors are functional. The patient can hold objects, but the grasp is extremely weak. The patient may be able to attempt parallel bar and brace function for general exercise.

What is the most common pain pattern of herniated cervical disc?

The most common pain pattern for the cervical disc is radiation into the scapular area and down the lateral aspect of the arm into the forearm and hand.

BIBLIOGRAPHY

Abrams WB, Berkow R: *The Merck manual of geriatrics,* Rahway, NJ, 1990, Merck Sharp & Dohme Research Laboratories.

Adams JC, Hamblen DL: *Outline of orthopaedics,* ed 11, Edinburgh, 1990, Churchill Livingstone.

Alario AJ: *Practical guide to the care of the pediatric patient,* St Louis, 1997, Mosby.

Alexander E Jr, Davis CH: Reduction and fusion of fracture of the odontoid process, *J Neurosurg* 31:580, 1969.

Allen BL, Ferguson RL, Lehmann TR, O'Brien RP: A mechanistic classification of closed indirect fractures and dislocations of the lower cervical spine, *Spine* 7:1, 1982.

Allison D, Strickland N: *Acronyms & synonyms in medical imaging,* Oxford, 1996, ISIS Medical Media.

American Medical Association: *Guides to the evaluation of permanent impairment,* ed 4, Chicago, 1993, American Medical Association.

American Medical Association: *How to use guides to the evaluation of permanent impairment,* ed 4, Falmouth, Colo, 1993, SEAK.

Ames MD, Schut L: Results of treatment of 171 consecutive myelomeningoceles, *Pediatrics* 50:466, 1972.

Amyes EW, Anderson FM: Fracture of the odontoid process of the axis, *J Bone Joint Surg* 56A:1663, 1974.

Anderson KN, Anderson LE: *Mosby's pocket dictionary of medicine, nursing, & allied health,* ed 2, St Louis, 1994, Mosby.

Apley AG, Solomon L: *Concise system of orthopaedics and fractures,* London, 1988, Butterworth-Heinemann.

Askenasy HM, Braham MJ, Kosary IZ: Delayed spinal myelopathy after atlanto-axial fracture dislocation, *J Neurosurg* 17:1100, 1960.

Bailey RW, Badgley CE: Stabilization of the cervical spine by anterior fusion, *J Bone Joint Surg* 42A:565, 1960.

Ballinger PW: *Merrill's atlas of radiographic positions and radiologic procedures,* vol 1-3, ed 8, St Louis, 1995, Mosby.

Barkauskas VH, Stoltenberg-Allen K, Baumann LC, Darling-Fisher C: *Health & physical assessment,* ed 2, St Louis, 1998, Mosby.

Barnsley L, Lord S, Bogduk N: Whiplash injury, *Pain* 59:283, 1994.

Barnsley L, Lord SM, Wallis BJ, Bogduk N: The prevalence of chronic cervical zygapophyseal joint pain after whiplash, *Spine* 10:20, 1995.

Barre JA: Le syndrome sympathique cervical posterieur et sa cause frequente, l'artherite cervicale, *Rev Neurol (Paris)* 33:1246, 1926.

Bateman JE: *The shoulder and neck,* Philadelphia, 1972, WB Saunders.

Bernstein EF: *Vascular diagnosis,* ed 4, St Louis, 1993, Mosby.

Berquist T: *MRI of the musculoskeletal system,* ed 3, Philadelphia, 1996, JB Lippincott.

Bettmane EH, Neudorfer RJ: Cervical disc pathology resulting in dysphagia in an adolescent boy, *NY State J Med* 60:2465, 1960.

Bland JH: Rheumatoid arthritis of the cervical spine, *J Rheumatol* 1:319, 1974.

Bland JH: *Disorders of the cervical spine diagnosis and medical management,* Philadelphia, 1987, WB Saunders.

Bocchi L, Orso CA: Whiplash injuries of the cervical spine, *Ital J Orthop Traumatol* 9:171, 1983.

Bohlman HH: The neck. In D'Ambrosia R, editor: *Regional examination and differential diagnosis of musculoskeletal disorders,* Philadelphia, 1977, JB Lippincott.

Bohlman HH: Late anterior decompression and fusion for the spinal cord injuries: review of 100 cases with long term results, *Orthopaedic Transactions* 4:42, 1980.

Bohlman HH: Indications for late anterior decompression and fusion for cervical spinal cord injuries. In Tator CH, editor: *Early management of acute cervical spinal cord injury,* New York, 1982, Raven Press.

Bohlman HH, Bahniuk E, Field G, Raskulinecz G: Spinal cord monitoring of experimental incomplete cervical spinal cord injury, *Spine* 6:428, 1981.

Bohlman HH, Ducker TB, Lucas JT: Spine and spinal cord injuries. In Rothman RH, Simeone FA, editors: *The spine,* ed 2, Philadelphia, 1982, WB Saunders.

Bohlman HH, Eismont FJ: Surgical techniques of anterior decompression and fusion for spinal cord injuries, *Clin Orthop* 138:154, 1981.

Bohlman HH, Riley L Jr, Robinson RA: Anterolateral approaches to the cervical spine. In Ruge D, Wiltse LL, editors: *Spinal disorders,* Philadelphia, 1977, Lea & Febiger.

Bradley JP, Tibone JE, Watkins RC: History, physical examination, and diagnostic tests for neck and upper extremity problems. In Watkins RG, editor: *The spine in sports,* St Louis, 1996, Mosby.

Brain WR: Some unsolved problems in cervical spondylosis, *Br Med Bull* 1:711, 1963.

Brieg A: *Biomechanics of the central nervous system,* Chicago, 1960, Mosby.

Brieg A, Turnbull IM, Hassler O: Effects of mechanical stresses in the spinal cord in cervical spondylosis, *J Neurosurg* 25:45, 1966.

Brier SR: *Primary care orthopedics,* St Louis, 1999, Mosby.

Brooks M, Evans R, Fairclough J: *Sports injuries,* ed 2, London, 1992, Gower Medical.

Brotzman SB: *Clinical orthopaedic rehabilitation,* St Louis, 1996, Mosby.

Brown DE, Neumann RD: *Orthopedic secrets,* Philadelphia, 1995, Hanley & Belfus.

Bucholz RW: *Orthopaedic decision making,* ed 2, St Louis, 1996, Mosby.

Bunker TD, Schranz PJ: *Clinical challenges in orthopaedics: the shoulder,* Oxford, 1998, ISIS Medical Media.

Cailliet R: *Head and face pain syndromes,* Philadelphia, 1992, FA Davis.

Campbell JB, Campbell JM: *Mosby's survival guide to medical abbreviations & acronyms prefixes & suffixes symbols Greek alphabet,* St Louis, 1995, Mosby.

Canale ST: *Campbell's operative orthopaedics,* vol 1-4, ed 9, St Louis, 1998, Mosby.

Carver G, Willits J: Comparative study and risk factors of a CVA, *J Am Chiropractic Assoc* 32:65, 1996.

Cashley MAP: Basilar artery migraine or cerebral vascular accident? *J Manip Physiol Ther* 16:112, 1993.

Cervical Spine Research Society: *The cervical spine,* Philadelphia, 1983, JB Lippincott.

Chapman S, Nakielyn R: *Aids to radiological differential diagnosis,* ed 3, London, 1995, Bailliere Tindall.

Chobanian AV, Gavras H: *Hypertension,* Summit, 1990, CIBA Pharmaceutical.

Cipriano JJ: *Photographic manual of regional orthopaedic and neurological test,* ed 3, Baltimore, 1997, Williams & Wilkins.

Cloward RB: The clinical significance of the sinu-vertebral nerve or the cervical spine in relation to the cervical disc syndrome, *J Neurol Neurosurg Psychiatry* 23:321, 1960.

Cohn RE: *Impairment rating examination and disability evaluation,* ed 3, Wilkesboro, NC, 1994, R Ernest Cohn.

Conlon PW, Isdale IC, Rose BS: Rheumatoid arthritis of the cervical spine: an analysis of 333 cases, *Ann Rheum Dis* 25:120, 1966.

Cramer GD, Darby SA: *Basic and clinical anatomy of the spine, spinal cord, and ANS,* St Louis, 1995, Mosby.

Crellin RQ, MacCabe JJ, Hamilton EB: Surgical management of the cervical spine in rheumatoid arthritis, *J Bone Joint Surg* 52B:244, 1970.

Dambro MR, Griffith JA: *Griffith's 5 minute clinical consult,* Baltimore, 1997, Williams & Wilkins.

D'Ambrogio KJ, Roth GB: *Positional release therapy assessment & treatment of musculoskeletal dysfunction,* St Louis, 1997, Mosby.

D'Ambrosia RD: *Musculoskeletal disorders: regional examination and differential diagnosis,* Philadelphia, 1977, JB Lippincott.

Dandy DJ: *Essential orthopaedics and trauma,* Edinburgh, 1989, Churchill Livingstone.

Daniels L, Worthington C: *Muscle testing: techniques of manual examination,* Philadelphia, 1980, WB Saunders.

Darby S, Cramer G: Pain generators and pathways of the head and neck. In Curl D, editor: *Chiropractic approach to head pain,* Baltimore, 1994, Williams & Wilkins.

Davidson RI, Dunn EJ, Metzmaker W: The shoulder abduction test in the diagnosis of radicular pain in cervical extradural compressive monoradiculopathies, *Spine* 6:441, 1981.

de Kleyn A, Nieuwenhuyse P: Schwindelanfaelle und nystagmus bei einer bestimmten stellung des dopfes, *Acta Otolaryng* 11:155, 1927.

de Kleyn A, Versteegh C: Uber verschledene formen von nemieres syndrome, *Dtsch Z Nervenheilkd* 132:157, 1933.

DeJong RH: *The neurologic examination,* ed 3, New York, 1967, Harper & Row.

Deltoff MN, Kogon PL: *The portable skeletal x-ray library,* St Louis, 1998, Mosby.

Demeter SL, Andersson GBJ, Smith GM: *Disability evaluation,* St Louis, 1996, Mosby.

Deshpande JK, Tobias JD: *The pediatric pain handbook,* St Louis, 1996, Mosby.

Dettenmeier PA: *Radiographic assessment for nurses,* St Louis, 1995, Mosby.

Doherty M: *Color atlas and text of osteoarthritis,* London, 1994, Wolfe.

Doherty M, Doherty J: *Clinical examination in rheumatology,* London, 1992, Wolfe.

Doherty M, George E: *Self-assessment picture tests in rheumatology,* London, 1995, Mosby-Wolfe.

Dossett AB, Watkins RG: Stinger injuries in football. In Watkins RG, editor: *The spine in sports,* St Louis, 1996, Mosby.

Dreyfus P, Michaelsen M, Fletcher D: Atlanto-occipital and atlantoaxial joint pain patterns, *Spine* 19:1125, 1994.

Durrett LC: Management of patients with vertebrobasilar ischemia, *Chiro Technique* 6:95, 1994.

Elster AD: *Questions and answers in magnetic resonance imaging,* St Louis, 1994, Mosby.

Epstein O, Perkin GD, deBono DP, Cookson J: *Clinical examination,* ed 2, London, 1997, Mosby.

Esposito MD, et al: Thoracic outlet syndrome in a throwing athlete diagnosed with MRI and MRA, *J Magn Reson Imaging* 7:598, 1997.

Farrar WE: *Atlas of infections of the nervous system,* London, 1993, Wolfe.

Feldmann E: *Current diagnosis in neurology,* St Louis, 1994, Mosby.

Ferezy JS: *The chiropractic neurological examination,* Gaithersburg, Md, 1992, Aspen.

Fisher M: Basilar artery embolism after surgery under general anesthesia: a case report, *Neurology* 43:1856, 1993.

Ford JS: *Posttraumatic headache,* Chicago, 1985, Med Recertification Associates.

Foreman SM, Croft AC: *Whiplash injuries: the cervical acceleration/ deceleration syndrome,* Baltimore, 1992, Williams & Wilkins.

Fornage B: *Musculoskeletal ultrasound,* New York, 1995, Churchill Livingstone.

Ganguly DN, Roy KKS: A study on the craniovertebral joint in man, *Anat Anz* 114:433, 1964.

Gowers WR: *Diseases of the nervous system,* ed 2, London, 1969, Churchill.

Garcia JH: *Neuropathology the diagnostic approach,* St Louis, 1997, Mosby.

Gargan MF, Fairbank JCT: Anatomy of the spine. In Watkins RG, editor: *The spine in sports,* St Louis, 1996, Mosby.

Goldie BS: *Orthopaedic diagnosis and management: a guide to the care of orthopaedic patients,* ed 2, Oxford, 1998, ISIS Medical Media.

Gracovetsky S: Biomechanics of the spine. In White A, Scholfferman JA, editors: *Spine care: diagnosis and treatment,* St Louis, 1994, Mosby.

Greenspan A, Montesano P: *Imaging of the spine in clinical practice,* London, 1993, Wolfe.

Greenstein GM: *Clinical assessment of neuromusculoskeletal disorders,* St Louis, 1997, Mosby.

Grossman ZD, et al: *Cost-effective diagnostic imaging the examiner's guide,* ed 3, St Louis, 1995, Mosby.

Hall CW, Danoff D: Sleep attacks-apparent relationship to atlantoaxial dislocation, *Arch Neurol* 32:57, 1975.

Hammer WI: *Functional soft tissue examination and treatment by manual methods the extremities,* Gaithersburg, Md, 1991, Aspen.

Hann CL: Retropharyngeal-tendinitis, *AJR Am J Roentgenol* 130:1137, 1978.

Hartley A: *Practical joint assessment upper quadrant,* ed 2, St Louis, 1995, Mosby.

Hastings D, McNab I, Lawson V: Neoplasms of the atlas and axis, *Can J Surg* 11:290, 1968.

Hawkins RJ: *An organized approach to musculoskeletal examination and history taking,* St Louis, 1995, Mosby.

Helliwell PS, Evans PF, Wright V: The straight cervical spine: does it indicate muscle spasm? *J Bone Joint Surg (Br)* 76:103, 1994.

Hinkle CZ: *Fundamentals of anatomy & movement a workbook and guide,* St Louis, 1997, Mosby.

Howe JR, Taren JA: Foramen magnum tumors: pitfalls in diagnosis, *JAMA* 225:1060, 1973.

Isdale IC, Corrigan B: Backward luxation of the atlas, *Ann Rheum Dis* 29:6, 1970.

Jablonski S: *Dictionary of medical acronyms & abbreviations,* ed 3, Philadelphia, 1998, Hanley & Belfus.

Jackson R: *The cervical syndrome,* ed 3, Springfield, Ill, 1966, Charles C Thomas.

Jonsson HJ, Cesarini K, Sahlstedt B, Rauschning W: Findings and outcome in whiplash-type neck distortions, *Spine* 19:2733, 1994.

Kanner R: *Pain management secrets,* Philadelphia, 1997, Hanley & Belfus.

Katirji B: *Electromyography in clinical practice: a case study approach,* St Louis, 1998, Mosby.

Katz WA: *Rheumatic diseases diagnosis and management,* Philadelphia, 1977, JB Lippincott.

Keats TE: *Atlas of roentgenographic measurement,* ed 6, St Louis, 1990, Mosby.

Keats TH: *Atlas of normal roentgen variants,* ed 6, St Louis, 1996, Mosby.

Keiser RP, Grimes HA: Intervertebral disc space infections in children, *Clin Orthop* 30:163, 1963.

Kendall HO, Kendall FP, Wadsworth GE: *Muscles testing and function,* ed 2, Baltimore, 1971, Williams & Wilkins.

Kettenbach G: *Writing s.o.a.p. notes,* Philadelphia, 1990, FA Davis.

Keuter EJW: Non-traumatic atlanto-axial dislocation associated with nasopharyngeal infections (Grisel's disease), *Acta Neurochirurg* 21:11, 1969.

Klippel JH, Dieppe PA: *Rheumatology,* vol 1-2, ed 2, London, 1998, Mosby.

Koenigsberg R: *Churchill's illustrated medical dictionary,* New York, 1989, Churchill Livingstone.

Kramer J: *Intervertebral disc diseases,* Chicago, 1981, Mosby.

Kumar R, Berger RJ, Dunsker SB, Keller JT: Innervation of the spinal dura, myth or reality? *Spine* 21:18, 1996.

Lambert EH, Rooke ED: Myasthenic state and lung cancer. In Brain RL, Norris FH, editors: *The remote effects of cancer on the nervous system,* New York, 1965, Grune & Stratton.

Lavy CBD, Barrett DS: *Questions and answers on Apley's concise system of orthopaedics and fractures,* Oxford, 1991, Butterworth-Heinemann.

Lerner AJ: *The little black book of neurology,* ed 3, St Louis, 1995, Mosby.

Levick JR: An investigation into the validity of subatmospheric pressure recordings from synovial fluid and their dependence on joint angle, *J Physiol* 289:55, 1979.

Lewis CB, Knortz KA: *Orthopedic assessment and treatment of the geriatric patient,* St Louis, 1993, Mosby.

Lhermitte J: Etude de la commotion de la moelle, *Rev Neurol (Paris)* 1:210, 1932.

Lhermitte J, Bollak P, Nicholas M: Les douleurs a type de decharge electrique dans la sclerose en plaques, un cas e forme sensitive de la sclerose multiple, *Rev Neurol (Paris)* 2:56, 1924.

Lieou YC: *Syndrome sympathique cervical posterieur et arthrite cervicale chronique: etude clinique et radiologique,* Strasbourg, 1928, Schuler and Minh.

Lipson SJ: Fractures of the atlas associated with fractures of the odontoid process and transverse ligament ruptures, *J Bone Joint Surg* 59A:940, 1977.

Lorber J: Spina bifida cystica, *Arch Dis Child* 47:854, 1972.

Loth TS: *Orthopedic boards review II: a case study approach,* St Louis, 1996, Mosby.

Macnab I: Acceleration extension injuries of the cervical spine. In Rothmann RH, Simeone FA, editors: *The spine,* vol 2, ed 2, Philadelphia, 1982, WB Saunders.

Magee DJ: *Orthopedic physical assessment,* ed 3, Philadelphia, 1997, WB Saunders.

Maitland GD: *Vertebral manipulation,* London, 1973, Butterworths.

Malone TR, McPoil TG, Nitz AJ: *Orthopedic and sports physical therapy,* ed 3, St Louis, 1997, Mosby.

Marchiori DM: *Clinical imaging with skeletal, chest, and abdomen pattern differentials,* St Louis, 1999, Mosby.

Markhashov AM: Variations in the arterial blood supply of the spine, *Vestn Khir* 94:64, 1965.

Martel W: The occipito-atlanto-axial joints in rheumatoid arthritis and ankylosing spondylitis, *AJR Am J Roentgenol* 86:233, 1961.

Martin JH: *Neuroanatomy text and atlas,* ed 2, Stamford, Conn, 1996, Appleton & Lange.

Mathers LH, et al: *Clinical anatomy principles,* St Louis, 1996, Mosby.

Mayo Clinic & Mayo Foundation: *Clinical examination in neurology,* Philadelphia, 1981, WB Saunders.

Mazion JM: *Illustrated manual of neurological reflexes/signs/tests, part I orthopedic signs/tests/maneuvers for office procedure, part II,* Orlando, 1980, Daniels.

McRae R: *Clinical orthopaedic examination,* ed 3, Edinburgh, 1990, Churchill Livingstone.

Medical Economics Books: *Patient care flow chart manual,* ed 3, Ordell, NJ, 1982, Medical Economics Books.

Mellion MB: *Sports medicine secrets,* Philadelphia, 1994, Hanley & Belfus.

Mellion MB: *Office sports medicine,* ed 2, St Louis, 1996, Mosby.

Mengel MB, Schwiebert LP: *Ambulatory medicine the primary care of families,* ed 2, Stamford, Conn, 1996, Appleton & Lange.

Mennell JM: *The musculoskeletal system differential diagnosis from symptoms and physical signs,* Gaithersburg, Md, 1992, Aspen.

Mercier LR, Pettid FJ: *Practical orthopedics,* ed 4, St Louis, 1995, Mosby.

Michelow BJ, et al: The natural history of obstetrical brachial plexus palsy, *Plast Reconstr Surg* 93:675, 1994.

Miller B: Manual therapy treatment of myofascial pain and dysfunction. In Rachlin ES, editor: *Myofascial pain and fibromyalgia,* St Louis, 1994, Mosby.

Modic MT, Masaryk TJ, Ross JS: *Magnetic resonance imaging of the spine,* ed 2, St Louis, 1994, Mosby.

Mosby-Year Book, Inc: *Expert 10-minute physical examination,* St Louis, 1997, Mosby.

Nettina SM: *The Lippincott manual of nursing practice,* ed 6, Philadelphia, 1996, Lippincott.

Newton RW: *Color atlas of pediatric neurology,* St Louis, 1995, Mosby-Wolfe.

Nicholas JA, Hershman EB: *The lower extremity & spine in sports medicine,* vol 1-2, ed 2, St Louis, 1995, Mosby.

Nordin M, Andersson GBJ, Pope MH: *Musculoskeletal disorders in the workplace: principles and practice,* St Louis, 1997, Mosby.

Norris SH, Watt I: The prognosis of neck injuries resulting from rear-end vehicle collisions, *J Bone Joint Surg* 65B:608, 1983.

O'Connor CE, Pekow PS, Klingersmith MT: Brachial plexus injury (burners) incidence and risk factors in collegiate football players: a prospective study, *J Athletic Training* 33:(suppl)5, 1998.

O'Donoghue DH: *Treatment of injuries to athletes,* ed 3, Philadelphia, 1976, WB Saunders.

Oh VMS: Brain infarction and neck calisthenics, *Lancet* 342:739, 1993.

Olson WH, Brumback RA, Gascon G, Iyer V: *Handbook of symptom-oriented neurology,* ed 2, St Louis, 1994, Mosby.

Omer GE, Spinner M: *Management of peripheral nerve problems,* Philadelphia, 1981, WB Saunders.

O'Young B, Young MA, Stiens SA: *PM&R secrets,* Philadelphia, 1997, Hanley & Belfus.

Pagana KD, Pagana TJ: *Mosby's manual of diagnostic and laboratory tests,* St Louis, 1998, Mosby.

Patten J: *Neurological differential diagnosis,* ed 2, London, 1996, Springer.

Payne EE, et al: The cervical spine, *Brain* 80:571, 1957.

Pheasant S: *Ergonomics, work and health,* Gaithersburg, Md, 1991, Aspen.

Prineas J: Polyneuropathies of undetermined cause, *Acta Neurol Scand* 46(suppl 44):1, 1970.

Przybylski G, Marion DW: Injury to the vertebrae and spinal cord. In Moore EE, Mattox KL, Feliziano DV, editors: *Trauma,* ed 3, Stanford, Conn, 1996, Appleton & Lange.

Rachlin ES: *Myofascial pain and fibromyalgia trigger point management,* St Louis, 1994, Mosby.

Radnovc BP, Sturzenegger M, Stefano GD: Long-term outcome after whiplash injury: a two-year follow-up considering features of injury mechanism and somatic, radiologic, and psychosocial factors, *Medicine* 74:281, 1995.

Rana NA, et al: Upward translocation of the dens in rheumatoid arthritis, *J Bone Joint Surg* 55B:471, 1973.

Ranawat CS, et al: Cervical spine fusion in rheumatoid arthritis, *J Bone Joint Surg* 61A:1003, 1979.

Ravel R: *Clinical laboratory medicine clinical application of laboratory data,* ed 6, St Louis, 1995, Mosby.

Resnick D, Niwayama G: *Diagnosis of bone and joint disorders,* Philadelphia, ed 3, 1995, WB Saunders.

Robbins SL: Blood vessels. In Robbins SL, editor: *Pathologic basis of disease,* Philadelphia, 1974, WB Saunders.

Rolak LA: *Neurology secrets,* ed 2, Philadelphia, 1998, Hanley & Belfus.

Rothman RH, Simeone FA: *The spine,* vol 1, Philadelphia, 1975, WB Saunders.

Rumack CM, Wilson SR, Charboneau JW: *Diagnostic ultrasound,* vol 1-2, ed 2, St Louis, 1998, Mosby.

Saal JA, Dillingham MF: Nonoperative treatment and rehabilitation of disc, facet, and soft tissue injuries. In Nicholas JA, Hershman EB, editors: *The lower extremity and spine in sports medicine,* vol 2, St Louis, 1995, Mosby.

Saidoff DC, McDonough AL: *Critical pathways in therapeutic intervention,* St Louis, 1997, Mosby.

Schneider RC, Livingston KE, Cave AJE: "Hangman's fracture" of the cervical spine, *J Meirpsirg* 22:141, 1965.

Schumacher HR, Klippel JH, Koopman WJ: *Primer on the rheumatic diseases,* ed 10, Atlanta, 1993, Arthritis Foundation.

Scott NW: Office Orthopedic Practice: *The orthopedic clinics of North America,* vol 13, Philadelphia, 1982, WB Saunders.

Seidel HM: *Mosby's guide to physical examination,* ed 4, St Louis, 1999, Mosby.

Shankman GA: *Fundamental orthopedic management for the physical therapist assistant,* St Louis, 1997, Mosby.

Sharp J, Purser DW: Spontaneous atlanto-axial dislocation in ankylosing spondylitis and rheumatoid arthritis, *Ann Rheum Dis* 20:47, 1961.

Silberstein SD, Lipton RB, Goadsby PJ: *Headache in clinical practice,* Oxford, 1998, Isis Medical Media.

Simons DG: Clinical and etiological update of myofascial pain from trigger points, *J Musculoskel Pain* 4:93, 1996.

Sledge CB, Poss R: *The year book of orthopedics 1997,* St Louis, 1997, Mosby.

Smith PH, Benn RT, Sharp J: Natural history of rheumatoid cervical luxations, *Ann Rheum Dis* 31:431, 1972.

Specht NT, Russo RD: *Practical guide to diagnostic imaging,* St Louis, 1998, Mosby.

Sprou G: Basilar artery insufficiency secondary to obstruction of left subclavian artery, *Circulation* 28:259, 1963.

Spurling RG, Scoville WB: Lateral rupture of the cervical intervertebral discs, *Syn Gyn Obstet* 78:350, 1944.

Starlanyl D, Copeland ME: *Fibromyalgia & chronic myofascial pain syndrome: a survival manual,* Oakland, 1996, New Harbinger.

Stedman TL: *Stedman's medical dictionary,* ed 25, Baltimore, 1990, Williams & Wilkins.

Stewart DL, Abeln SH: *Documenting functional outcomes in physical therapy,* St Louis, 1993, Mosby.

Stoller DW: *Magnetic resonance imaging in orthopaedics & sports medicine,* Philadelphia, 1993, JB Lippincott.

Sutton D, Young JWR: *A concise textbook of clinical imaging,* ed 2, St Louis, 1995, Mosby.

Tan JC, Horn SE: *Practical manual of physical medicine and rehabilitation,* St Louis, 1998, Mosby.

Tan JC, Nordin M: The role of physical therapy in the treatment of cervical disc disease, *Orthop Clin North Am* 23:435, 1992.

Taybi H, Lachman RS: *Radiology of syndromes, metabolic disorders, and skeletal dysplasias,* ed 4, St Louis, 1996, Mosby.

Terrett AGJ: *Malpractice avoidance for chiropractors,* West Des Moines, 1996, National Chiropractic Mutual Insurance Company.

Tettenborn B, et al: Postoperative brainstem and cerebellar infarcts, *Neurology* 43:471, 1993.

Theisler CW: *Migraine headache disease diagnostic and management strategies,* Gaithersburg, Md, 1990, Aspen.

Thibodeau GA, Patton KT: *Anatomy & physiology,* ed 3, St Louis, 1996, Mosby.

Thibodeau GA, Patton KT: *Pocket reference to accompany anatomy & physiology,* ed 3, St Louis, 1996, Mosby.

Thompson AJ, Polman C, Hohlfeld R: *Multiple sclerosis: clinical challenges and controversies,* St Louis, 1997, Mosby.

Thompson JM: *Clinical outlines for health assessment,* St Louis, 1997, Mosby.

Thurston SE: *The little black book of neurology,* Chicago, 1987, Mosby.

Toghill PJ: *Examining patients: an introduction to clinical medicine,* London, 1990, Edward Arnold.

Tollison CD, Satterthwaite JR, Tollison JW: *Handbook of pain management,* ed 2, Baltimore, 1994, Williams & Wilkins.

Torg JS, Shepard RJ: *Current therapy in sports medicine,* ed 3, St Louis, 1995, Mosby.

Torg JS, et al: The relationship of development narrowing of the cervical spinal canal to reversible and irreversible injury of the cervical spinal cord in football players, *J Sone Joint Surg Am* 78:1308, 1996.

Turek SL: *Orthopaedics principles and their applications,* ed 3, Philadelphia, 1977, JP Lippincott.

Van Beusekom GT: The neurological syndrome associated with cervical luxations in rheumatoid arthritis, *Acta Orthop Belg* 58:38, 1972.

Van Holsbeeck M, Introcaso JH: *Musculoskeletal ultrasound,* St Louis, 1991, Mosby.

Wakefield TS, Frank RG: *The examiner's guide to neuromusculoskeletal practice,* Abbotsford, Wisc, 1995, Allied Health of Wisconsin, S.C.

Watkins RG: *The spine in sports,* St Louis, 1996, Mosby.

Weineck J: *Functional anatomy in sports,* ed 2, St Louis, 1990, Mosby.

Weinstein SL, Buckwalter JA: *Turek's orthopaedics principles and their application,* ed 5, Philadelphia, 1994, JB Lippincott.

White A: Biomechanical stability of the cervical spine, *Clin Orthop* 109:85, 1975.

White AH, Schofferman JA: *Spine care,* vol 1-2, St Louis, 1995, Mosby.

White G: *Regional dermatology,* London, 1994, Mosby-Wolfe.

White G: *Levene's color atlas of dermatology,* ed 2, London, 1997, Mosby-Wolfe.

Whitmore I, Willan PLT: *Multiple choice questions in human anatomy,* London, 1995, Mosby.

Wickstrom J, LaRocca H: Trauma: head and neck injuries from acceleration-deceleration forces. In Ruge D, Wiltse LL, editors: *Spinal disorders: diagnosis and treatment,* Philadelphia, 1977, Lea & Febiger.

Wilkinson M: The anatomy and pathology of cervical spondylosis, *Proc Roy Soc Lond (Belg)* 57:159, 1964.

Windsor RE, Lox DM: *Soft tissue injuries: diagnosis and treatment,* Philadelphia, 1998, Hanley & Belfus.

Yashon D: *Spinal injury,* New York, 1978, Appleton-Century-Crofts.

Yochum T, Rowe L: *Essentials of skeletal radiology,* ed 2, Baltimore, 1996, Williams & Wilkins.

Yousem DM: *Case review head and neck imaging,* St Louis, 1998, Mosby.

Zatouroff M: *Diagnosis in color physical signs in general medicine,* ed 2, London, 1996, Mosby-Wolfe.

Zitelli BJ, Davis HW: *Atlas of pediatric physical diagnosis,* ed 2, London, 1992, Wolfe.

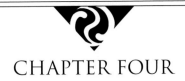

THE SHOULDER

Abbott-Saunders test
Adson's test
Allen maneuver
Apley's test
Apprehension test
Bryant's sign
Calloway's test
Codman's sign
Costoclavicular maneuver
Dawbarn's sign
Dugas' test
George's screening procedure
Halstead maneuver
Hamilton's test
Impingement sign
Ludington's test
Mazion's shoulder maneuver
Reverse Bakody maneuver
Roos' test
Shoulder compression test
Speed's test
Subacromial push-button sign
Supraspinatus press test
Transverse humeral ligament test
Wright's test
Yergason's test

AXIOMS IN SHOULDER ASSESSMENT

- Shoulder motion involves four primary articulations: the glenohumeral, acromioclavicular, sternoclavicular, and scapulothoracic.
- Common shoulder disorders include rotator cuff tendinitis, rotator cuff tears, capsulitis (frozen shoulder), glenohumeral arthritis, and acromioclavicular syndromes.
- In early capsulitis and glenohumeral arthritis, all active and passive motions are painful, there is no pain on resisted motion, and passive motion is decreased.

INTRODUCTION

The shoulder is a system of joints, and many movements of this system involve the neck. Completely independent action of the shoulder is possible, but independent, simultaneous action of the shoulder and neck is not.

The glenohumeral joint may be affected as part of widespread joint disease (i.e., a polyarthropathy such as rheumatoid arthritis, crystal deposition disease arthropathy, other inflammatory arthropathies, or generalized osteoarthritis). Periarticular conditions can be grouped into categories with and without capsulitis. In the absence of capsular involvement, passive joint motion is largely unaffected, whereas active movement may be limited by pain and/or weakness. In the presence of capsulitis, multidirectional restriction of passive motion is seen. Clinical and radiologic studies are used to differentiate these conditions from articular conditions.

Referred pain to the shoulder can occur with cervical disorders, Pancoast's tumor of the lung, a subphrenic pathologic condition, entrapment neuropathies, myofascial pain syndromes, and brachial neuritis (Table 4-3).

Identification of the primary cause of shoulder pain is not always easy. Referred pain to the shoulder girdle region occurs from multiple sources other than the neck. With diaphragmatic irritation, pain is referred along the phrenic nerve to the supraclavicular region, the trapezius, and the superomedial angle of the scapula. Gastric and pancreatic diseases may refer pain to the interscapular region. The rare superior sulcus lung tumor, or Pancoast's tumor, occasionally coincident with Horner's syndrome, may have shoulder pain as its initial symptom (Fig. 4-2).

TABLE 4-1

SHOULDER JOINT CROSS-REFERENCE TABLE BY ASSESSMENT PROCEDURE

Test/Sign	Biceps Tendon	Scalenus Anticus Syndrome	Thoracic Outlet Syndrome	Rotator Cuff	Anterior Dislocation	Posterior Dislocation	Supraspinatus Tendon	Subacromial Bursa	Subclavian Arterial Stenosis	Adhesive Capsulitis	Transverse Humeral Ligament
Abbott-Saunders test	●										
Adson's test		●	●								
Allen maneuver			●								
Apley's test				●							
Apprehension test					●	●					
Bryant's sign					●	●					
Calloway's test					●	●					
Codman's sign				●			●				
Costoclavicular maneuver			●								
Dawbarn's sign								●			
Dugas' test					●	●					
George's screening procedure									●		
Halstead maneuver			●								
Hamilton's test					●	●					
Impingement sign	●						●				
Ludington's test	●										
Mazion's shoulder maneuver					●	●	●			●	
Reverse Bakody maneuver		●	●								
Roos' test			●								
Shoulder compression test			●							●	
Speed's test	●										
Subacromial push-button sign				●			●				
Supraspinatus press test							●				
Transverse humeral ligament test	●										●
Wright's test			●								
Yergason's test	●										●

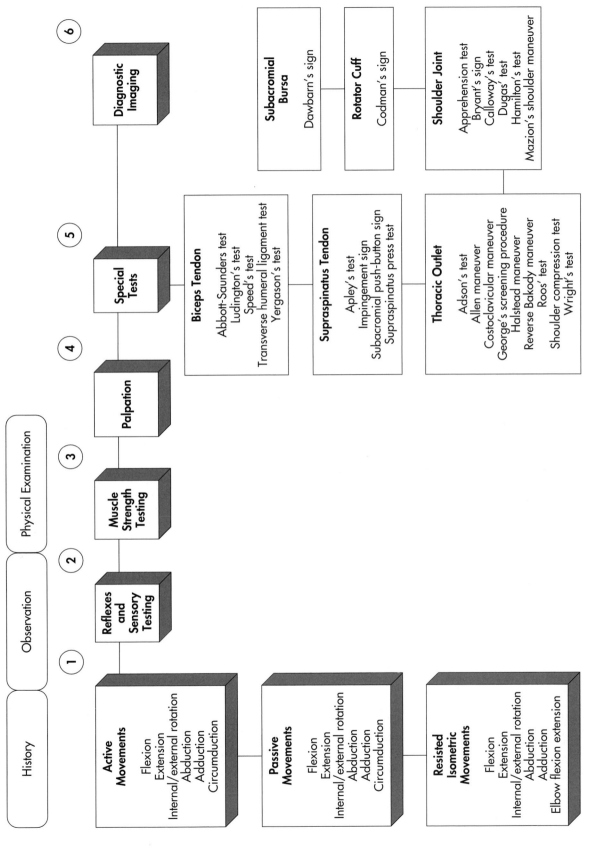

FIG. 4-1   Shoulder joint assessment.

TABLE 4-2

SHOULDER JOINT CROSS-REFERENCE TABLE BY SYNDROME OR TISSUE

Adhesive capsulitis	Mazion's shoulder maneuver	Scalenus anticus syndrome	Adson's test
Anterior dislocation	Apprehension test		Reverse Bakody maneuver
	Bryant's sign	Subcromial bursa	Dawbarn's sign
	Calloway's test	Subclavian arterial stenosis	George's screening procedure
	Dugas' test		Shoulder compression test
	Hamilton's test	Supraspinatus tendon	Codman's sign
	Mazion's shoulder maneuver		Impingement sign
Biceps tendon	Abbott-Saunders test		Subacromial push-button sign
	Impingement sign		Supraspinatus press test
	Ludington's test	Thoracic outlet syndrome	Adson's test
	Speed's test		Allen maneuver
	Transverse humeral ligament test		Costoclavicular maneuver
	Yergason's test		Halstead maneuver
Posterior dislocation	Apprehension test		Reverse Bakody maneuver
	Bryant's sign		Roos' test
	Calloway's test		Shoulder compression test
	Dugas' test		Wright's test
	Hamilton's test	Transverse humeral ligament	Transverse humeral ligament test
	Mazion's shoulder maneuver		Yergason's test
Rotator cuff	Apley's test		
	Codman's sign		
	Mazion's shoulder maneuver		
	Subacromial push-button sign		

The arm as a lever is useless unless it has a fixed base. The fixed base comes largely from the layers of flat muscles piled one on top of another and attached to all surfaces of the scapula.

Paralytic disorders implicating these muscles come into clinical focus when weakness in the fixation mechanism is demonstrated. The serratus anterior, when paralyzed, allows the scapula to swing backward and loosen its attachment to the chest. The trapezius allows the scapula to spin like a pinwheel, which contributes to the loss of fixation.

The mobility of this part of the body results from the configuration of the bony parts and the mechanically advantageous attachment of the multiple muscles. The shallow socket and ball head favor frictionless spinning, and the main joint has four accessory articulating zones that compliment and enhance the action of the shoulder.

Everyday activities are made up of acts such as lifting, holding, pushing, turning, and shoving. It is through such common and accepted motions that clinical disorders are manifested. These are combined pattern motions with contributions from many parts of the shoulder complex. Individual joint and muscle contribution may be analyzed in these acts to aid localization and understanding of injury and disease. Consideration must also be given to the part that the elbow and hand play in shoulder function. Shoulders are used unconsciously during actions of the hand, wrist, and elbow. Injury or disease may hamper normal action of any of these areas, so increased replacement effort is sought from the shoulder. For example, loss of rotatory range, as in

TABLE 4-3

COMMON CAUSES OF SHOULDER PAIN

Periarticular Disorders
- Rotator cuff tendinitis/impingement syndrome
- Calcific tendinitis
- Rotator cuff tear
- Bicipital tendinitis
- Acromioclavicular arthritis

Glenohumeral Disorders
- Inflammatory arthritis
- Osteoarthritis
- Osteonecrosis
- Cuff arthropathy
- Septic arthritis
- Glenoid labrum tears
- Adhesive capsulitis
- Glenohumeral instability

Regional Disorders
- Cervical radiculopathy
- Brachial neuritis
- Nerve entrapment syndromes
- Sternoclavicular arthritis
- Reflex sympathetic dystrophy
- Fibrositis
- Neoplasms
- Miscellaneous
  - Gallbladder disease
  - Splenic trauma
  - Subphrenic abscess
  - Myocardial infarction
  - Thyroid disease
  - Diabetes mellitus
  - Renal osteodystrophy

From Kelley WN, et al: *Textbook of rheumatology,* ed 5, Philadelphia, 1997, WB Saunders.

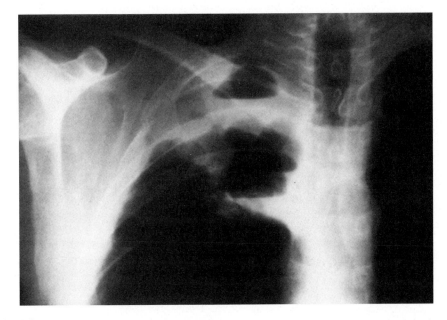

FIG. 4-2   Pancoast's tumor.   *(From Nicholas JA, Hershman EB, editor:* The upper extremity in sports medicine, *St Louis, 1990, Mosby.)*

arthrodesis of the wrist or elbow, unconsciously results in increased rotation at the shoulder. Weakness or disorder of one muscle group evokes replacement effort in another group. For example, the hunching motion by the trapezius that follows attempted abduction is a replacement effort associated with paralysis of the deltoid. Scrutiny of these purposeful patterns is of great help in understanding disability in this region.

Chronic overuse syndromes with repetitive stretching, as in rowing, swimming, or throwing, are injuries of repetitive microtrauma. Atraumatic disorders generally result from ligamentous laxity or congenital hypoplasia of the glenoid. Impact injuries may be divided into direct and indirect trauma. For direct trauma, the injury force is in direct contact with the shoulder complex. Indirect forces injuring the shoulder usually pass up through the hand, wrist, or elbow and result in a rotational or longitudinal force directed along the humerus.

ORTHOPEDIC GAMUT 4-1

DIRECT TRAUMA

Direct trauma to the shoulder includes the following:

1. Posterior dislocations of the sternoclavicular joint
2. Acromioclavicular subluxations or dislocations after a fall on the posterior superior shoulder
3. Direct blows to the supraclavicular brachial plexus at the base of the neck or axillary nerve as it courses under the deltoid
4. Clavicular fractures
5. Muscle contusions

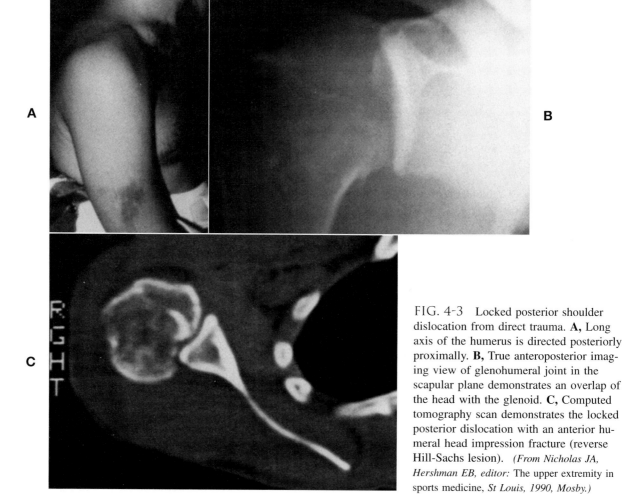

A   **B**   **C**

FIG. 4-3 Locked posterior shoulder dislocation from direct trauma. **A,** Long axis of the humerus is directed posteriorly proximally. **B,** True anteroposterior imaging view of glenohumeral joint in the scapular plane demonstrates an overlap of the head with the glenoid. **C,** Computed tomography scan demonstrates the locked posterior dislocation with an anterior humeral head impression fracture (reverse Hill-Sachs lesion). *(From Nicholas JA, Hershman EB, editor:* The upper extremity in sports medicine, *St Louis, 1990, Mosby.)*

Indirect trauma results in muscle, tendon, ligament, and brachial plexus stretch, strain, rupture, and bony fractures. Glenohumeral subluxations are usually caused by indirect forces (Fig. 4-3).

ESSENTIAL ANATOMY

The shoulder joint is a ball-and-socket joint that is the articulation of the humerus and the glenoid fossa of the scapula (Fig. 4-4). To describe the anatomy of the shoulder joint, it may be more accurate to use the term *shoulder joint complex*. The shoulder joint complex really consists of four joints: the glenohumeral, the acromioclavicular, the sterno-clavicular, and the scapulothoracic articulation (Fig. 4-5). The acromioclavicular joint is formed by the lateral end of the clavicle and acromion. The acromioclavicular joint is reinforced by the surrounding capsule and ligaments, containing an anterior, posterior, superior, and inferior component, in addition to the coracoclavicular ligaments, which are made up of two individual ligaments: the coracoid and trapezoid ligaments (Fig. 4-6). The short head of the biceps arises with the coracobrachialis from the scapular coracoid process and runs down the medial side of the long head of the biceps.

The two bellies join as a common distal tendon just above the elbow joint as a flattened tendon, only to separate into two distal insertions (Fig. 4-7).

The serratus anterior muscle extends from the deep surface of the scapula to the upper eight or nine ribs. When this muscle does not function, the scapula is not held tightly against the chest wall and protrudes outward or "wings." The most common cause is injury to the long thoracic nerve, which innervates the serratus anterior.

Like most parts of the body, the shoulder region has a set of deep veins, usually accompanying the major arterial trunks, and a set of superficial veins, draining the skin and subcutaneous tissues (Fig. 4-8). The brachial and axillary

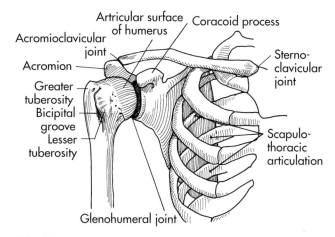

FIG. 4-5   Shoulder joint complex: the acromioclavicular joint, sternoclavicular joint, glenohumeral joint, and scapulothoracic articulation. *(From Nicholas JA, Hershman EB, editors:* The upper extremity in sports medicine, *St Louis, 1990, Mosby.)*

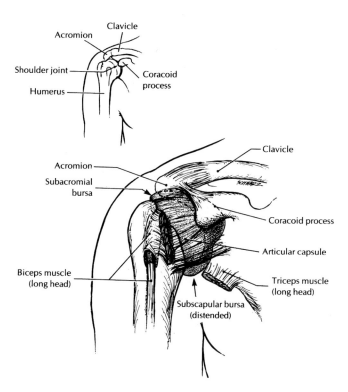

FIG. 4-4   Shoulder joint.   *(From Barkauskas VH, Stoltenberg-Allen K, Baumann LC, Darling-Fisher C:* Health & physical assessment, *ed 2, St Louis, 1998, Mosby.)*

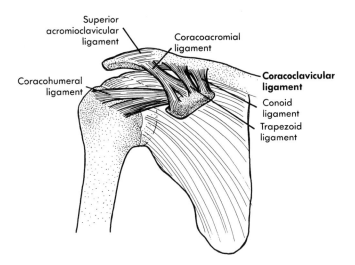

FIG. 4-6   Acromioclavicular joint with surrounding ligaments, including the coracoclavicular, coracoacromial, and coracohumeral.   *(From Nicholas JA, Hershman EB, editor:* The upper extremity in sports medicine, *St Louis, 1990, Mosby.)*

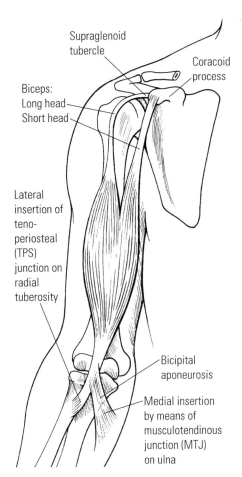

FIG. 4-7 Biceps brachii. *(From Saidoff DC, McDonough AL: Critical pathways in therapeutic intervention, St Louis, 1997, Mosby.)*

Supraglenoid tubercle

Coracoid process

Biceps: Long head / Short head

Lateral insertion of teno-periosteal (TPS) junction on radial tuberosity

Bicipital aponeurosis

Medial insertion by means of musculotendinous junction (MTJ) on ulna

ORTHOPEDIC GAMUT 4-2

SHOULDER MOVEMENTS

Shoulder movements are as follows:

1. Elevation in the coronal (frontal) plane (abduction and adduction)
2. Flexion and extension in the sagittal plane (Figs. 4-14 and 4-15)
3. Horizontal adduction and abduction in the transverse (horizontal) plane (Figs. 4-16 and 4-17)
4. Internal and external rotation (torque around the humerus) (Figs. 4-18 and 4-19)

The shoulder's total range of external and internal rotation is described as 180 degrees (external rotation 108 degrees [60%] and internal rotation 72 degrees [40%]) with the arm placed at anatomic position. With the arm at 90 degrees of abduction, the total rotational arc is 120 degrees (more internal rotation), and at full flexion, minimal internal and external rotation is possible.

Inflammation caused by injury to any of the anatomic structures located between the acromion and the ascending humeral head during shoulder abduction will cause a painful arc between 60 to 120 degrees (Fig. 4-20).

The deltoid muscle is hinged at its origin and therefore exerts a shear force that forces the humerus upward on the glenoid labrum at abduction. In elevation to 90 degrees, the deltoid's shear forces are converted to a compressive force that places the humerus directly into the glenoid cavity (Fig. 4-21). With a weak or damaged supraspinatus tendon, the loss of the rotational force component results in painful impingement attributable to the imbalance of normal compressive forces (Fig. 4-22).

Adhesive capsulitis, also called *frozen shoulder,* is characterized by decreased shoulder range of motion, pain, capsular inflammation, fibrous synovial adhesions, and reduction of the joint cavity (Fig. 4-23).

veins and their tributaries represent the deep veins of the shoulder.

The nerve supply to the shoulder joint complex (Fig. 4-9) arises mainly from the fifth through the seventh cervical nerve roots via its formation into the brachial plexus.

The brachial plexus is the major structure for innervation of the shoulder area (Fig. 4-10).

On the lateral aspect of the shoulder, extending inferiorly from acromion to midhumerus, the skin is innervated by a cutaneous branch of the axillary nerve (C5 to C6) (Fig. 4-11).

The axillary artery is the central structure of the axilla (Fig. 4-12).

ESSENTIAL MOTION ASSESSMENT

Shoulder motion is interpreted through excursion of the arm from the body and is recorded according to the anatomic planes (Fig. 4-13).

ESSENTIAL MUSCLE FUNCTION ASSESSMENT

The muscles surrounding the shoulder joint complex provide the ability to generate motion while simultaneously providing dynamic stability to the glenohumeral joint.

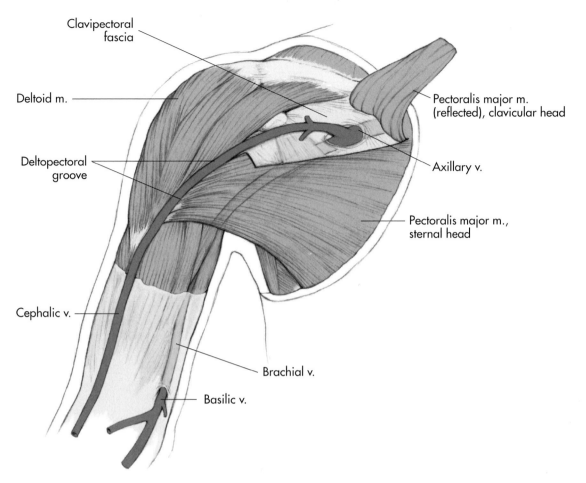

Clavipectoral fascia

Deltoid m.

Deltopectoral groove

Cephalic v.

Basilic v.

Brachial v.

Pectoralis major m. (reflected), clavicular head

Axillary v.

Pectoralis major m., sternal head

FIG. 4-8 Superficial veins of the arm and axilla. *(From Mathers LH, et al:* Clinical anatomy principles, *St Louis, 1996, Mosby.)*

ORTHOPEDIC GAMUT 4-3

MUSCLES OF THE SHOULDER JOINT COMPLEX

Muscles of the shoulder joint complex can be divided into three categories:

1. Those attaching to the scapula with their origin from the axial skeleton
2. Those that have their origin from the scapula and insert onto the humerus
3. Those that have their origin from the axial skeleton and insert onto the humerus

---

ORTHOPEDIC GAMUT 4-4

MUSCLE ATTACHMENTS

The scapula to spine muscle attachments are as follows:

1. Trapezius
2. Levator scapula
3. Rhomboid major
4. Rhomboid minor
5. Serratus anterior

Muscles, particularly those attaching to the scapula with their origin from the axial skeleton, include the trapezius, levator scapula, rhomboid major and minor, and serratus anterior (Fig. 4-24).

The trapezius is innervated by the spinal accessory nerve, which travels along its undersurface. The levator scapula originates from the posterior tubercles of the transverse processes of the first through fourth cervical vertebrae. It receives its innervation from the cervical plexus and occasionally from the dorsal scapular nerve.

Text continued on p. 180

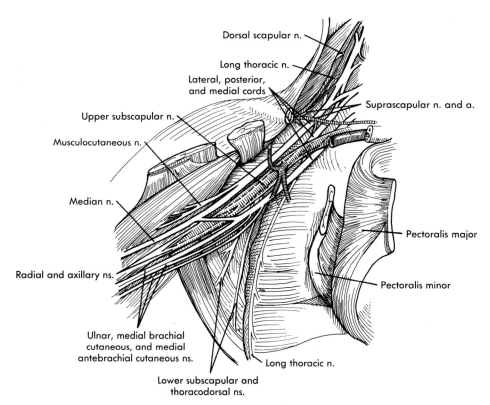

FIG. 4-9   Neurovascular supply to the shoulder joint complex.   *(From Nicholas JA, Hershman EB, editors:* The upper extremity in sports medicine, *St Louis, 1990, Mosby.)*

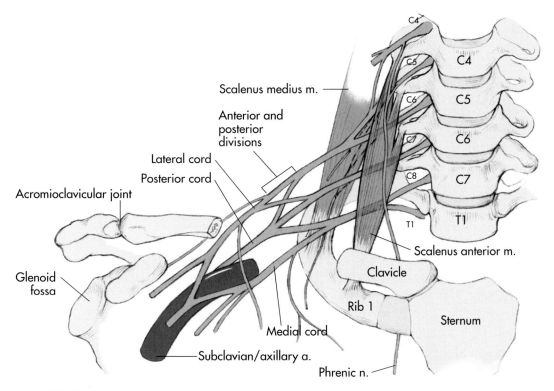

FIG. 4-10 Brachial plexus with relationships of nearby structures. *(From Mathers LH, et al: Clinical anatomy principles, St Louis, 1996, Mosby.)*

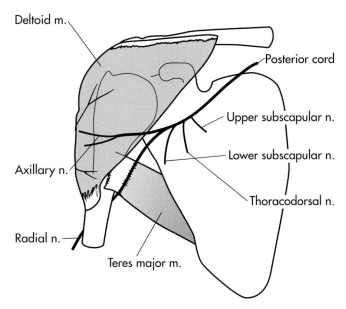

FIG. 4-11 Branches of the posterior cord of the brachial plexus. *(From Mathers LH, et al: Clinical anatomy principles, St Louis, 1996, Mosby.)*

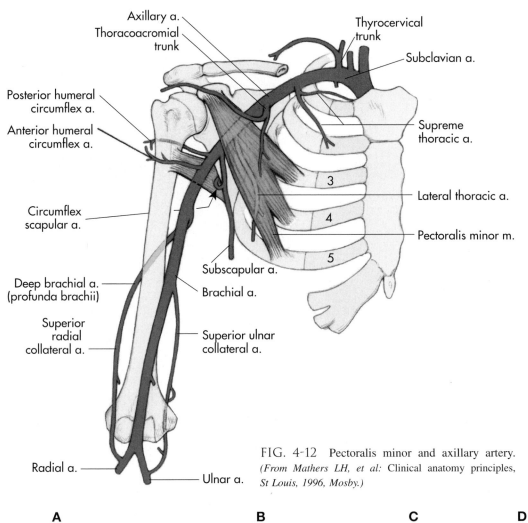

FIG. 4-12   Pectoralis minor and axillary artery. *(From Mathers LH, et al:* Clinical anatomy principles, *St Louis, 1996, Mosby.)*

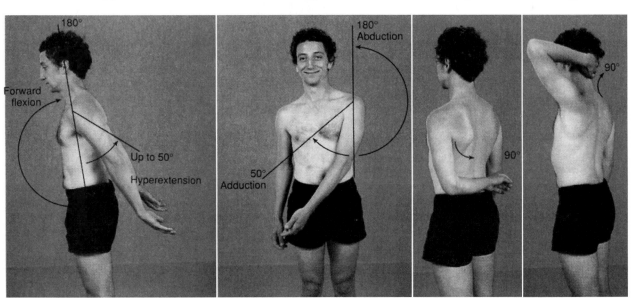

FIG. 4-13   Range of motion of the shoulder. **A,** Forward flexion and hyperextension. **B,** Abduction and adduction. **C,** Internal rotation. **D,** External rotation.   *(From Barkauskas VH, Stoltenberg-Allen K, Baumann LC, Darling-Fisher C:* Health & physical assessment, *ed 2, St Louis, 1998, Mosby.)*

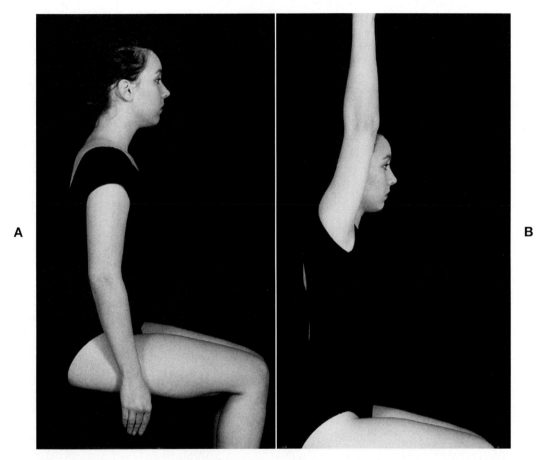

FIG. 4-14 **A,** The patient sits with the shoulder in a neutral position and the arm hanging straight at the side. **B,** The arm may be flexed 110 degrees at the shoulder and carried on up to 180 degrees in circumduction flexion. In this movement, the head of the humerus does not encounter the same obstructions from the coracoacromial arch that occurs during abduction. The scapula is fixed to the chest initially and then moves forward around the chest wall during the 90 degrees of elevation, ending up farther in front than during the motion of abduction. Flexion is accomplished by the anterior deltoid, pectoralis major, coracobrachialis, and biceps. A retained flexion range of motion that is 160 degrees or less is an impairment of the shoulder in the activities of daily living.

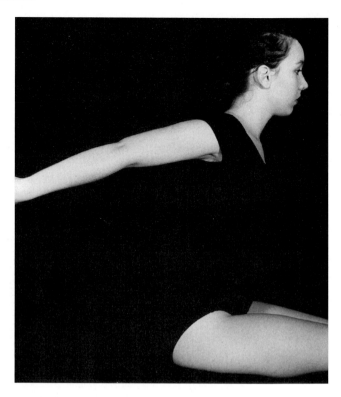

FIG. 4-15 The arm may be extended at the shoulder behind the line of the body for 50 degrees. In this action, the clavicle rotates downward a little on its long axis and moves backward, with the sternoclavicular joint as the fulcrum. The scapula shifts backward and tilts upward a little on the chest wall. Extension is accomplished by the posterior deltoid, latissimus, teres major and minor, infraspinatus, and triceps muscles. Adhesive joint disorders and arthritis in the glenohumeral joint interfere with extension. Forty degrees or less of retained extension range of motion is an impairment of the shoulder in the activities of daily living.

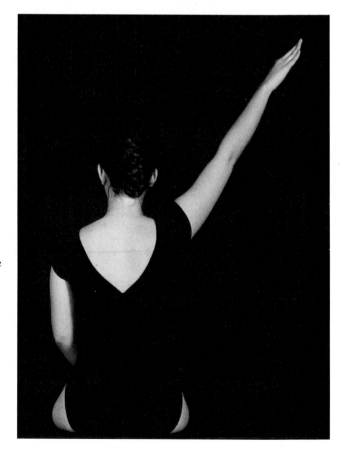

FIG. 4-16 Abducting the arm from the side of the body to over the head is a complex procedure. The normal range of motion is 180 degrees and is accomplished largely at the glenohumeral joint, but all of the axillary joints contribute. The muscles chiefly concerned are the trapezius, the serratus anterior, and the deltoid and rotator cuff group. Less than 160 degrees of retained abduction range of motion is an impairment of the shoulder in the activities of daily living.

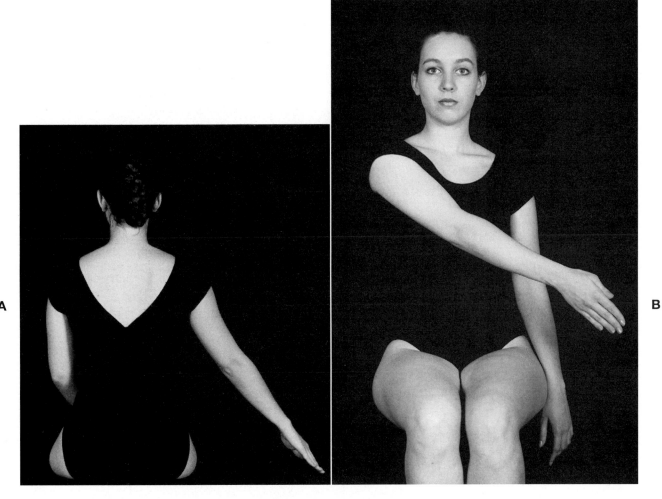

FIG. 4-17 From 180 degrees circumduction, the arm may be pulled down to the side **(A)**, and at the end of the excursion the arm can be adducted in front of the chest 50 degrees farther **(B).** This action takes place with the assistance of gravity, and when resistance is added, the latissimus dorsi, teres major, and pectoralis major are the movers. As the arm descends from 180 degrees circumduction, the clavicle rotates downward on its long axis. The scapula moves on the chest wall during the middle 90 degrees, starting at 45 degrees from the top and stopping at 45 degrees from the bottom. The motion is largely at the glenohumeral joint, as the head of the humerus rotates internally and follows a linear arc from the bottom to the top of the glenoid. This motion reverses the route taken during abduction. A retained adduction range of motion of 30 degrees or less is an impairment of the shoulder in the activities of daily living.

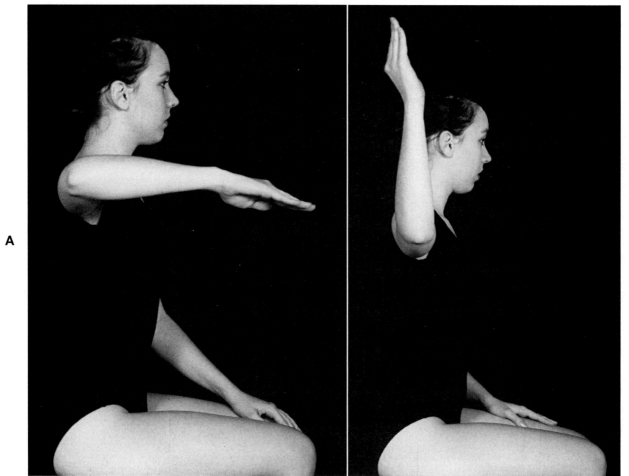

A   **B**

FIG. 4-18   From the midposition, which involves horizontal abduction of the arm at the side
(A), the shoulder may be externally rotated almost 90 degrees **(B).** Nearly all of this movement
occurs at the glenohumeral joint. When the arm is at the side, this action is accomplished by the
infraspinatus, teres minor, and posterior deltoid. When the arm is horizontal, the supraspinatus also
contributes. External rotation is the most important action, and when this rotation is lost, shoulder
action is seriously compromised. Sixty degrees or less of retained external rotation is an impairment
of the shoulder in the activities of daily living.

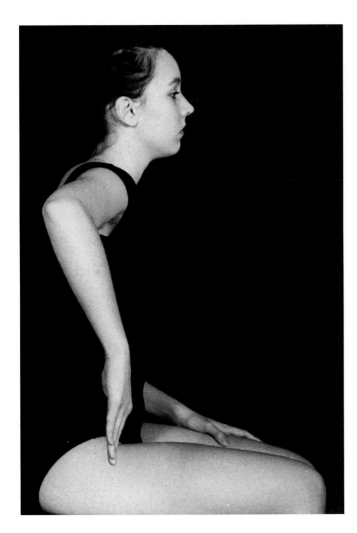

FIG. 4-19   The arm may be turned inward a little more than 90 degrees in both horizontal and vertical planes. This movement occurs chiefly at the glenohumeral joint and is powered by the subscapularis, pectoralis major, latissimus dorsi, and teres major muscles. The motion is an action that synchronizes with adduction as a striking blow and is hindered mainly by paralytic deformities. Sixty degrees or less of retained internal rotation is an impairment of the shoulder in the activities of daily living.

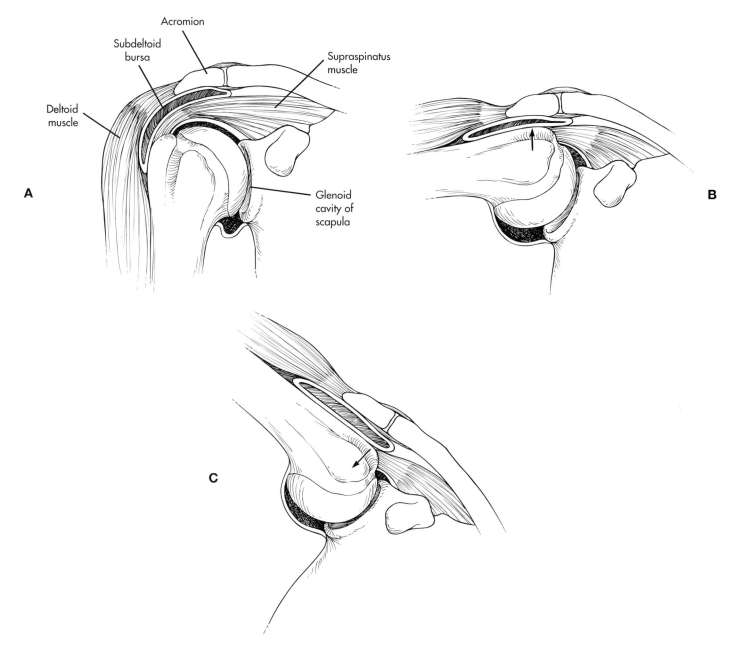

FIG. 4-20   The translatory motion of the glenohumeral joint during shoulder abduction. **A,** The shoulder in anatomic position. **B,** At 90 degrees. **C,** At 170 degrees.   *(From Greenstein GM:* Clinical assessment of neuromusculoskeletal disorders, *St Louis, 1997, Mosby.)*

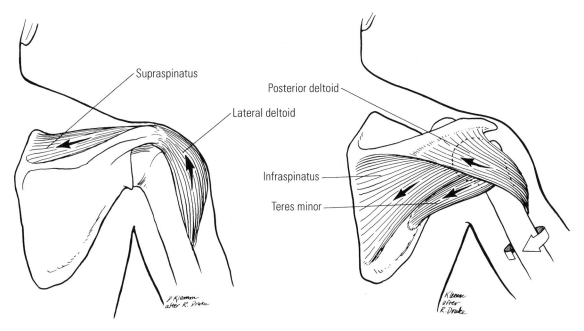

FIG. 4-21   The rotator cuff and deltoid muscle forces at the onset of abduction (0 degrees) and with the arm elevated 90 degrees.   *(From Saidoff DC, McDonough AL:* Critical pathways in therapeutic intervention, *St Louis, 1997, Mosby.)*

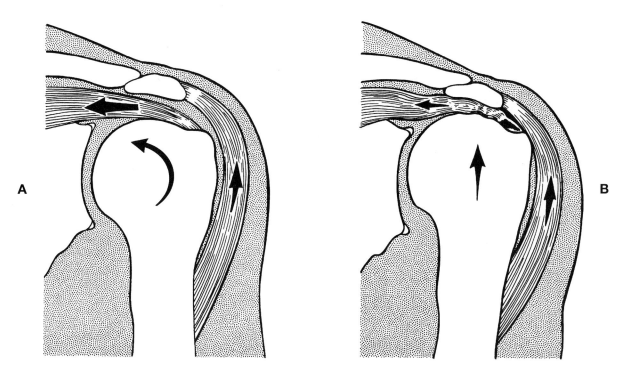

FIG. 4-22   Supraspinatus, exerting a rotational force, works in synergy with the deltoid, which yields a compressive force. **A,** Working together, both muscles facilitate shoulder elevation. **B,** Deep surface tearing of the supraspinatus weakens the cuff's ability to hold the humeral head down and away from the underside of the acromion, resulting in impingement.   *(From Saidoff DC, McDonough AL:* Critical pathways in therapeutic intervention, *St Louis, 1997, Mosby.)*

The rhomboids also lie deep to the trapezius, with the rhomboid minor arising from the spinous processes of the seventh cervical and thoracic vertebrae and the intervening supraspinous ligament. Both rhomboids are supplied by the dorsal scapular nerve.

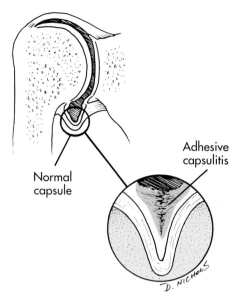

FIG. 4-23   Adhesive capsulitis or "frozen shoulder." *(From Shankman GA:* Fundamental orthopedic management for the physical therapist assistant, *St Louis, 1997, Mosby.)*

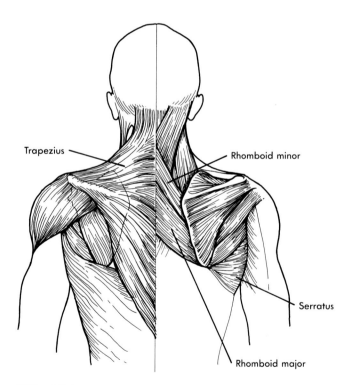

FIG. 4-24   Posterior view of superficial and deep muscles connecting the axial skeleton to the scapula. *(From Nicholas JA, Hershman EB, editors:* The upper extremity in sports medicine, *St Louis, 1990, Mosby.)*

The serratus anterior arises from the outer surface of the first eight ribs and follows the curvature of the ribs to insert along the medial aspect of the scapula on its costal surface. The serratus anterior is supplied by the long thoracic nerve.

The subscapularis muscle arises from the costal surface of the scapula, with its muscles converging into an anterior tendon that inserts onto the lesser tuberosity of the humerus. It is innervated by the subscapularis nerve.

The supraspinatus muscle arises from the supra-spinous fossa and passes laterally under the coracoacro-mial arch to attach to the greater tuberosity. It is supplied by the suprascapular nerve and vessels that travel on its undersurface.

The infraspinatus muscle arises from the infraspinous fossa and travels laterally to insert on the posterior aspect of the greater tuberosity. It is also supplied by the suprascapular nerve and vessels.

The teres minor muscle arises from the central third of the lateral border of the scapula below the scapular neck to pass behind the long head of the triceps and insert onto the lower posterior aspect of the greater tuberosity.

The teres major muscle arises from the lower third of the lateral border of the scapula and travels around the anterior aspect of the humerus and in front of the long head of the triceps to insert onto the crest of the lesser tubercle (Fig. 4-25). The teres minor and deltoid receive their innervation by the axillary nerve, whereas the teres major is supplied by the lower subscapular nerve (Figs. 4-26 to 4-31).

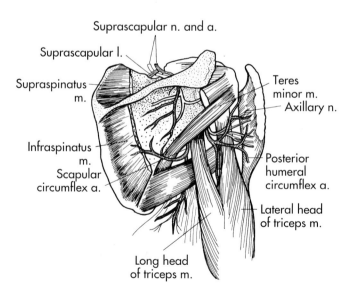

FIG. 4-25   Posterior view of shoulder with quadrangular space containing the axillary nerve and posterior humeral circumflex artery and the triangular space containing the scapular circumflex artery. *(From Nicholas JA, Hershman EB, editors:* The upper extremity in sports medicine, *St Louis, 1990, Mosby.)*

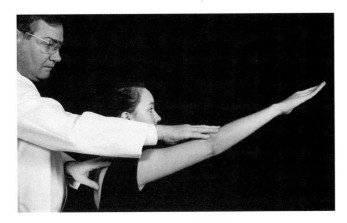

FIG. 4-26 The prime movers of flexion of the shoulder are the anterior portion of the deltoid muscle (axillary nerve, C5, and C6) and the coracobrachialis muscle (musculocutaneous nerve, C5, and C6). The accessory muscles to flexion are the middle fibers of the deltoid, the clavicular fibers of the pectoralis major, and the biceps brachii. To test flexion of the shoulder, the examiner immobilizes the patient's scapula on the side being tested. The examiner achieves immobilization by grasping and holding the lower border with one hand. The patient flexes the arm anteriorly to 90 degrees while the forearm is pronated and the elbow slightly flexed. The examiner's free hand provides graded resistance just above the elbow. Rotation, adduction, or abduction of the arm should be prevented while flexion is being tested.

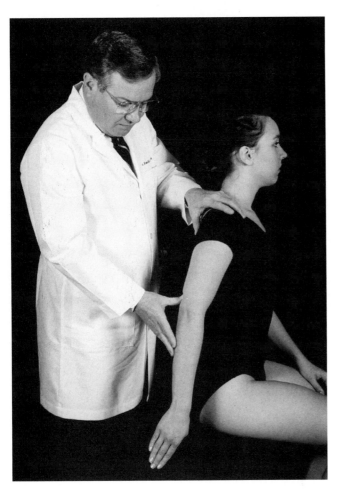

FIG. 4-27 The prime movers involved in shoulder extension are the latissimus dorsi (thoracodorsal nerve and C6 through C8), teres major (lowest subscapular nerve, C5, and C6), and deltoid (axillary nerve, C5, and C6) muscles. The teres minor and the long head of the triceps muscles are accessory to this motion. Extension of the shoulder is tested with the patient's elbow straightened and the forearm fully pronated (palm posterior) to prevent lateral rotation and adduction. The examiner fixes the scapula as described for testing flexion, and the patient extends the arm posteriorly through the range of motion. The examiner's other hand, which is placed just above the elbow, provides graded resistance.

FIG. 4-28   The prime movers involved in abduction are the middle fibers of the deltoid (axillary nerve, C5, and C6) and the supraspinatus (suprascapular nerve and C5) muscles. The accessory muscles involved in abduction are the anterior and posterior fibers of the deltoid and serratus anterior muscles. The latter muscle functions by direct action of the scapula. Abduction of the shoulder is tested while the patient's arm is at the side, while the forearm is between pronation and supination (palm medial), and while the elbow is flexed a few degrees. The examiner stabilizes the scapula as described for flexion. The patient abducts the arm to 90 degrees. This abduction occurs against graded resistance applied by the examiner's other hand, which is placed proximal to the patient's elbow.

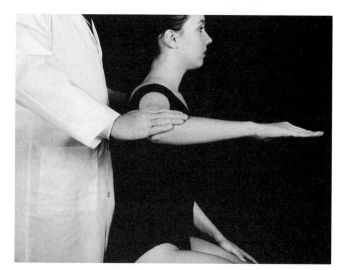

FIG. 4-29   The prime mover involved in adduction of the shoulder is the pectoralis major muscle (medial and lateral pectoral nerves, C5 through C8, and T1). The anterior fibers of the deltoid muscle are accessory to this motion. Adduction also occurs mainly at the glenohumeral joint and is assessed with the patient's arm abducted to 90 degrees. The patient adducts the arm anteriorly through the horizontal plane of motion and against graded resistance. This resistance is applied by the examiner's other hand, which is placed over the front of the arm and proximal to the patient's elbow.

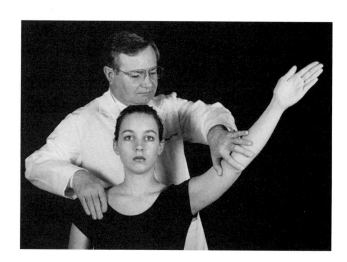

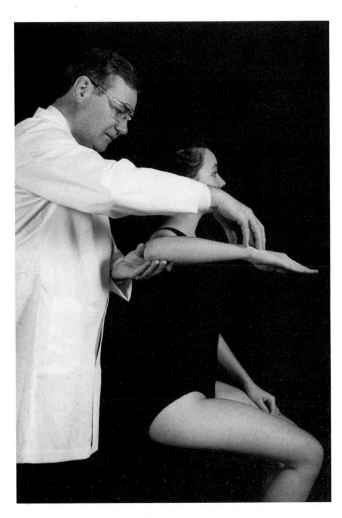

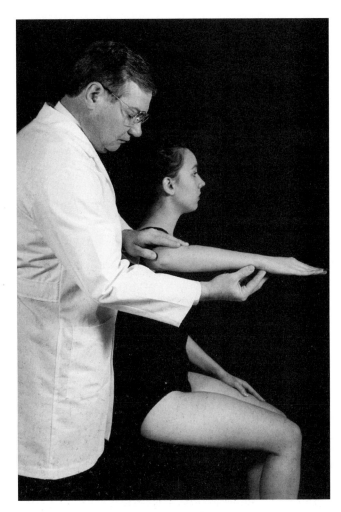

FIG. 4-30 The prime movers involved in external rotation are the infraspinatus (suprascapular nerve, C5, and C6) and teres minor (axillary nerve and C5). The posterior fibers of the deltoid muscle are accessory to this motion. The external rotation of the shoulder is assessed with the patient's arm abducted to 90 degrees (or at the patient's side if abduction is not possible), with the elbow flexed to 90 degrees, and with the hand and fingers pointing forward. The examiner supports the patient's elbow by holding it with one hand while the patient rotates the arm upward (or outward if shoulder abduction is not possible) against graded resistance that is applied by the examiner's other hand, which is placed on the patient's forearm proximal to the wrist.

FIG. 4-31 The prime movers of internal rotation of the shoulder are the subscapularis (upper and lower subscapular nerves, C5, and C6), pectoralis major (medial and lateral pectoral nerves, C5 through C8, and T1), and teres major (lowest subscapular nerve, C5, and C6) muscles. The anterior fibers of the deltoid muscle are accessory to this motion. Internal rotation of the shoulder is tested with the arm abducted to 90 degrees (or at the side if abduction is not possible), the elbow flexed to 90 degrees, and the hand pointed forward. The examiner supports the patient's elbow with one hand, as described previously, while the patient rotates the arm downward (or inward if the shoulder abduction is not possible) against graded resistance that is applied by the examiner's other hand, which is placed on the patient's forearm proximal to the wrist.

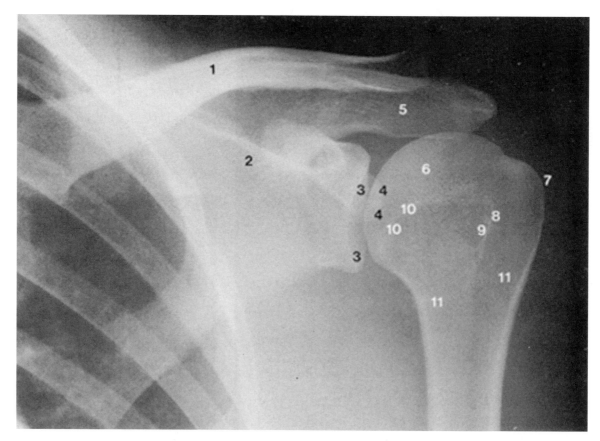

FIG. 4-32   Shoulder joint. Anteroposterior plain film. *1*, Clavicle; *2*, scapula; *3*, glenoid fossa; *4*, humeral head, articular surface; *5*, acromion; *6*, head of humerus; *7*, greater tubercle of humerus; *8*, intertubercular groove; *9*, lesser tubercle of humerus; *10*, anatomic neck; *11*, surgical neck.   *(From Mathers LH, et al:* Clinical anatomy principles, *St Louis, 1996, Mosby.)*

ESSENTIAL IMAGING

The shoulder girdle consists of the two bones that attach the upper limb to the thoracic wall: the scapula and clavicle. The glenoid fossa of the scapula forms the articulation of the shoulder girdle with the head of the humerus (Figs. 4-32 and 4-33).

The most important films to obtain are the true anteroposterior (AP) (Figs. 4-34 and 4-35) and the modified West Point views (Figs. 4-36 to 4-39). Both of these projections provide an excellent view of a glenohumeral joint. The examiner is able to appreciate the characteristic posterior glenoid wear (Fig. 4-40). The acromioclavicular joint can be radiographically evaluated and correlated with the physical examination. The AP view should include the proximal two thirds of the humeral shaft so that the physician can safely estimate the appropriate humeral component diameter (Figs. 4-41 and 4-42). When clinically indicated, the radiographic examination of the shoulder must include a cervical spine series.

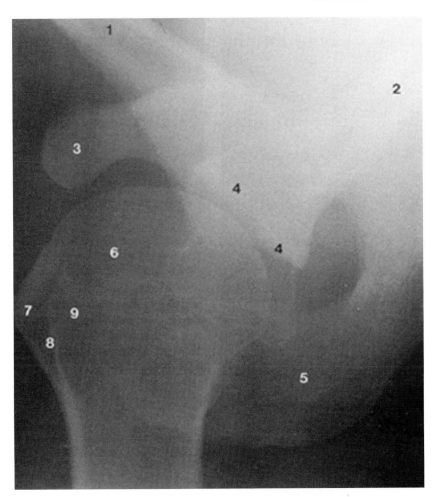

FIG. 4-33   Glenohumeral joint plain film of the left shoulder from cephalad. *1,* Clavicle; *2,* spine of scapula; *3,* coracoid process; *4,* glenoid fossa; *5,* acromion; *6,* head of humerus; *7,* lesser tubercle; *8,* intertubercular groove; *9,* greater tubercle. *(From Mathers LH, et al:* Clinical anatomy principles, *St Louis, 1996, Mosby.)*

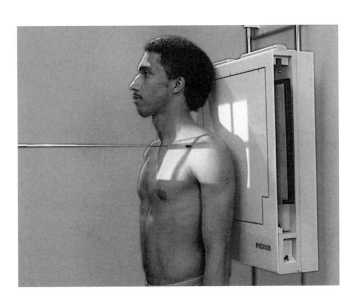

FIG. 4-34   Anteroposterior shoulder with neutral rotation of the humerus. *(From Ballinger PW:* Merrill's atlas of radiographic positions and radiologic procedures, *vol 1-3, ed 8, St Louis, 1995, Mosby.)*

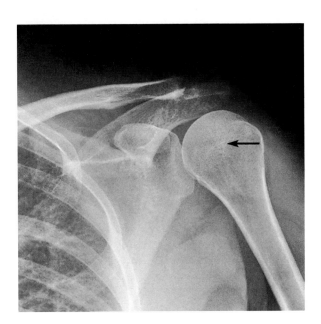

FIG. 4-35   Anteroposterior shoulder in neutral rotation of the humerus. *(From Ballinger PW:* Merrill's atlas of radiographic positions and radiologic procedures, *vol 1-3, ed 8, St Louis, 1995, Mosby.)*

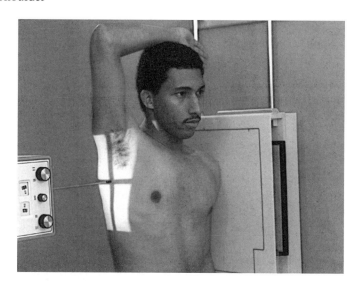

FIG. 4-36   Upright transthoracic lateral shoulder.   *(From Ballinger PW:* Merrill's atlas of radiographic positions and radiologic procedures, *vol 1-3, ed 8, St Louis, 1995, Mosby.)*

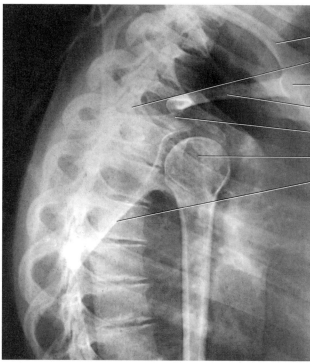

Unaffected clavicle

Scapula (superior border)

Sternum

Clavicle

Acromion process

Humeral head

Scapula (lateral border)

FIG. 4-37   Transthoracic lateral shoulder.   *(From Ballinger PW:* Merrill's atlas of radiographic positions and radiologic procedures, *vol 1-3, ed 8, St Louis, 1995, Mosby.)*

FIG. 4-38   Radiographic appearance of the modified West Point view.   *(From Nicholas JA, Hershman EB, editors:* The upper extremity in sports medicine, *St Louis, 1990, Mosby.)*

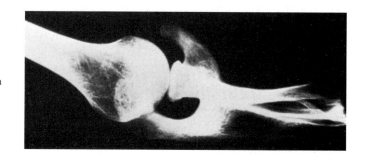

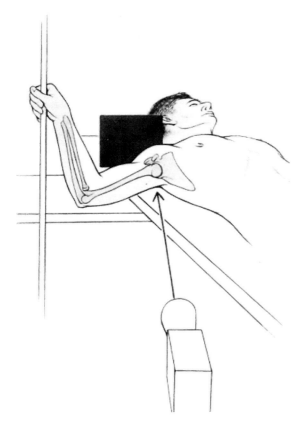

FIG. 4-39 Technique of obtaining the supine modified West Point view. With the patient laying supine and holding onto a support, the x-ray tube is angled 20 degrees upward from the floor and 20 degrees away from the long axis of the patient's body. *(From Nicholas JA, Hershman EB, editors:* The upper extremity in sports medicine, *St Louis, 1990, Mosby.)*

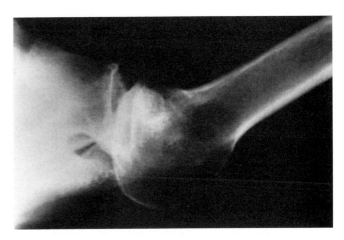

FIG. 4-40 Modified West Point view shows the marked posterior subluxation and migration. *(From Nicholas JA, Hershman EB, editors:* The upper extremity in sports medicine, *St Louis, 1990, Mosby.)*

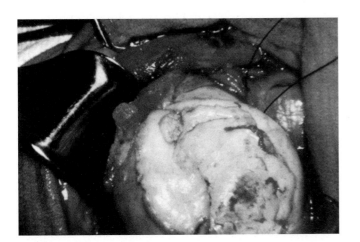

FIG. 4-41 Intraoperative view demonstrating the circumferential nature of the osteophytes on the humeral head. *(From Nicholas JA, Hershman EB, editors:* The upper extremity in sports medicine, *St Louis, 1990, Mosby.)*

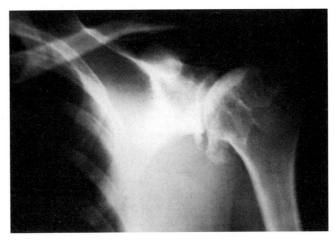

FIG. 4-42 Characteristic inferior glenoid osteophyte seen with loss of sphericity of the humeral head. *(From Nicholas JA, Hershman EB, editors:* The upper extremity in sports medicine, *St Louis, 1990, Mosby.)*

ABBOTT-SAUNDERS TEST

Assessment for Biceps Tendinitis

Comment

Rotator cuff tears may be acute or chronic, partial or full thickness. Partial tears may occur in any age group following trauma. A full-thickness (or complete) tear is rarely seen in individuals younger than 40 years of age. A partial tear can result from a fall or explosive shoulder movement and presents very much as a rotator cuff tendinitis. Full active range of motion may be preserved. The acute complete rupture after trauma should be easily diagnosed. Chronic full-thickness tears are found incidentally in approximately 27% of patients at autopsy.

Examination of rotator cuff tears reveals many of the features of rotator cuff tendinitis. The patient often is unable to maintain the arm in abduction when lowering it from the elevated position. Subacromial crepitus and pain on impingement testing are present. A common clinical finding is atrophy of the infraspinatus.

Subluxation of the tendon of the long head may be isolated and result from attrition but is often concomitant with moderate to massive tears extending into the anterior portion of the cuff.

When an excessive load is applied to the arm in the position of abduction and external rotation, the line of pull of the long bicipital tendon is placed in the coronal plane and presses against the medial wall of the groove but is restrained from bowstringing by the lesser tuberosity acting as a simple pulley.

ORTHOPEDIC GAMUT 4-5

BICEPS TENDON

The biceps tendon may luxate medially out of the groove and over the lesser medial tuberosity in one of two patterns:

1. Rupture of the transverse ligament and subluxation of the biceps tendon out of the groove, with the tendon lying anterior to the subscapularis muscle
2. Tendon subluxation beneath the subscapularis muscle belly (Fig. 4-43)

The long tendon returns into the groove once the upper arm is rotated medially and then laterally while the forearm is flexed at the elbow (Yergason's test) (Fig. 4-44).

Rupture or stretching of the fascial covering of the bicipital groove permits the tendon to subluxate from the groove. This may occur as an acute injury. The predisposing factor for this condition is a congenitally shallow bicipital groove. The intertubercular groove not only may be shallow but may be broader than normal. This permits the tendon to flatten out and slide back and forth within the groove itself. The patient complains of a snap that occurs anteriorly in the shoulder and is accompanied by pain. The pain is followed by residual soreness along the bicipital groove. The soreness is elicited by the same motions that cause pain with tenosynovitis. Rupture or stretching of the fascial covering of the bicipital groove is indistinguishable from tenosynovitis. In a muscular patient, it may be difficult to palpate the subluxing tendon. If the condition becomes chronic, as a result of a defect in the roof of the groove with redundant tissue, chronic synovitis usually occurs. Movement of the shoulder results in painful snapping as the tendon slips back and forth out of the groove, particularly during rotation of the arm.

PROCEDURE

- With the patient in the seated position, the examiner fully abducts and externally rotates the patient's arm (Figs. 4-45 and 4-46).
- The examiner then lowers the arm to the patient's side (Fig. 4-47).
- A palpable or audible click indicates a subluxation or dislocation of the biceps tendon.

Alternatively, DeAnquin's test can be performed.
- While the examiner's finger(s) palpate for the point of maximal tenderness within the bicipital groove, the shoulder is alternately rotated.
- A positive test occurs in biceps tendinitis when the patient feels pain as the tendon glides beneath the examiner's finger.

Confirmation Procedures

Ludington's test, Speed's test, transverse humeral ligament test, and Yergason's test

---

DIAGNOSTIC STATEMENT

Abbott-Saunders test is positive for the right shoulder. This result indicates subluxation or dislocation of the biceps tendon.

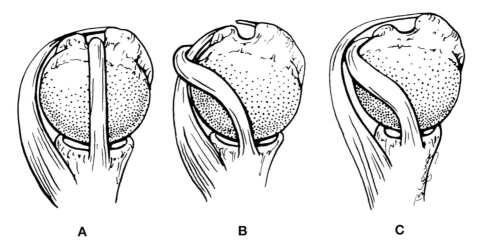

FIG. 4-43 **A,** The normal relationship of the biceps tendon in the groove covered by the transverse humeral ligament. **B,** Rupture of the transverse ligament and subluxation of the biceps tendon out of the groove with the tendon lying anterior to the subscapularis muscle. **C,** Intertendinous disruption of the subscapularis commonly occurs when the subscapularis insertion degenerates and the tendon subluxates beneath the muscle-tendon belly. *(From Saidoff DC, McDonough AL:* Critical pathways in therapeutic intervention, *St Louis, 1997, Mosby.)*

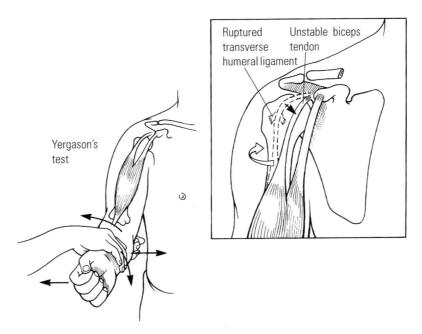

FIG. 4-44 Yergason's test for long biceps tendon stability. The examiner resists supination as the patient simultaneously externally rotates the shoulder against resistance. *(From Saidoff DC, McDonough AL:* Critical pathways in therapeutic intervention, *St Louis, 1997, Mosby.)*

CLINICAL PEARL

The biceps tendon will not rupture or dislocate under ordinary stresses unless it is already weak. The predisposing factor to rupture or dislocation is age degeneration, which is probably accelerated by oft-repeated friction and angulation at the point where the tendon enters the bicipital groove of the humerus.

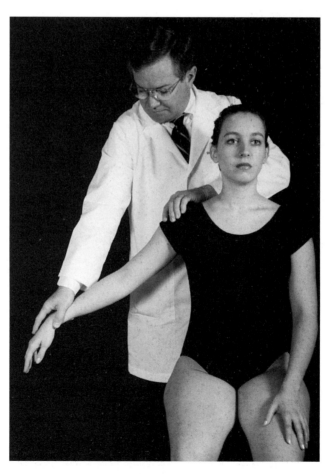

FIG. 4-45   With the patient in the seated position, the examiner fully abducts the patient's arm.

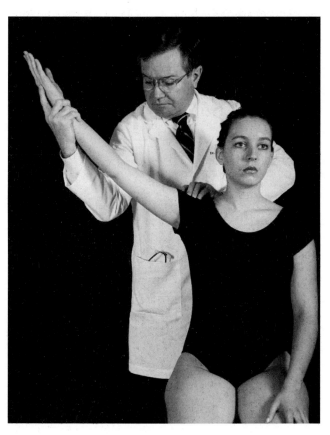

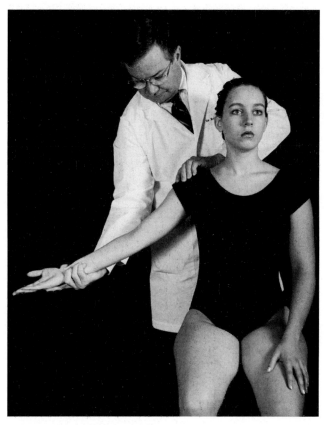

FIG. 4-46 The examiner externally rotates the patient's arm when the arm is at the top of the abduction maneuver.

FIG. 4-47 While maintaining the arm in external rotation, the examiner then lowers the arm to the patient's side. A palpable or audible click is a positive finding, which indicates a subluxation or dislocation of the biceps tendon.

ADSON'S TEST

Assessment for Neurovascular Compression of the Subclavian Artery and Brachial Plexus Caused by Scalenus Anticus or Cervical Rib Thoracic Outlet Syndromes

Comment

Anatomic anomalies of cervicothoracic structures include the presence of a cervical rib (Fig. 4-48), unusually long transverse processes of the seventh cervical vertebra, and an anomalous fibrous band. Cervical ribs, which articulate with the seventh cervical vertebra (Fig. 4-49) are present in 1% of the population.

The brachial plexus and the subclavian artery can be compressed as they pass between the anterior and medial scalene muscles and the first rib, yielding a characteristic neurovascular syndrome, the anterior scalene syndrome.

All three scalene muscles originate from the transverse processes of the cervical vertebrae and insert on the first and second ribs. The anterior and medial scalene muscles insert on the respective tubercles on the first rib and sandwich the subclavian artery into a sulcus. The posterior scalenus muscle is fixed to the second rib. A variable scalenus minimus muscle may exist and insert between the anterior and medial scalenus muscles. The scalene muscles raise the first and second rib during inspiration. Unilateral contraction inclines the head to the side of action and turns the face to the opposite side. Bilateral contraction flexes the cervical spine. The anterior and medial scalene muscles form one side of the scalene foramen, with the sternocleidomastoid muscle and the first rib forming the other sides. Bounded by the anterior scalene muscle, the first rib, and the medial scalene muscle, the posterior scalene foramen admits the brachial plexus and the subclavian artery to the costoclavicular space. The posterior foramen can range from 0.4 to 3.5 cm in width.

The subclavian artery bends over and passes through a sulcus in the first rib. Made up of nerve roots from C5 to C8 and T1, the brachial plexus represents the innervation of the entire upper extremity and lies tautly stretched and without bony protection in this region.

Neurovascular compression can occur when disease or anatomic variations narrow a tight foramen. In the development of the anterior scalene syndrome, some anatomic variations are very important.

The anterior scalene syndrome has many similarities with the costoclavicular syndrome, also known as the *syndrome of the cervical rib.*

Under normal circumstances, there is enough room in the posterior scalene foramen of the brachial plexus and the subclavian artery. However, many anatomic variations and consequent changes in the functional anatomy of the shoulder and upper extremity can cause the development of the clinical symptoms. Many embryologic, anatomic, and physiologic factors create a disposition for development of compression in the posterior scalene foramen.

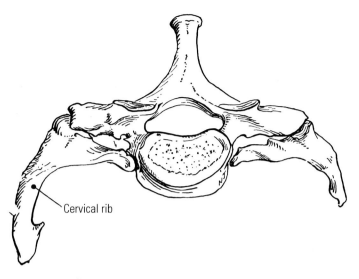

FIG. 4-48 Cervical rib. *(From Saidoff DC, McDonough AL:* Critical pathways in therapeutic intervention, *St Louis, 1997, Mosby.)*

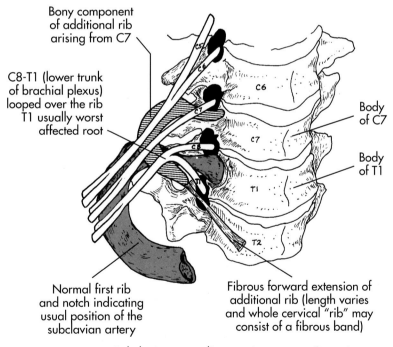

FIG. 4-49   Relation of the cervical rib to its surrounding structures.   *(From Saidoff DC, McDonough AL:* Critical pathways in therapeutic intervention, *St Louis, 1997, Mosby.)*

The neurovascular symptoms depend on the frequency, duration, and degree of compression of the subclavian artery and the brachial plexus. The lower roots of the brachial plexus (C8-T1) are at higher risk than the more superior roots because of their location in the plexus. The symptoms include pain in the fingers, hand, forearm, arm, and shoulder and paresthesia and hyperesthesia, especially in the eighth cervical and first thoracic nerve root dermatomes. Numbness occurs most often in the fingers, hand, and forearm. Depending on the degree of arterial compression, ischemic symptoms of numbness, cold, weakness, and skin color changes appear.

PROCEDURE

- The examiner locates the radial pulse of the involved extremity (Fig. 4-50).
- The patient's head is rotated to the involved extremity (Fig. 4-51).
- The patient extends the neck as the examiner externally rotates and extends the shoulder.

- The patient takes a deep breath and holds it (Fig. 4-52).
- Loss of the pulse is a positive test.
- If the test is negative, it is repeated by having the patient rotate the head to the uninvolved extremity.

Confirmation Procedures

Allen maneuver, costoclavicular maneuver, George's screening procedure, Halstead maneuver, reverse Bakody maneuver, Roos' test, shoulder compression test, and Wright's test

DIAGNOSTIC STATEMENT

Adson's test is positive on the right. This result indicates thoracic outlet syndrome caused by scalenus anticus syndrome or cervical rib syndrome.

CLINICAL PEARL

Radiographic demonstration of a cervical rib does not prove that it is the cause of the symptoms. The condition has to be distinguished (1) from other causes of pain and paresthesia in the forearm and hand, (2) from other causes of muscle atrophy in the hand, and (3) from other causes of peripheral vascular changes in the upper extremity.

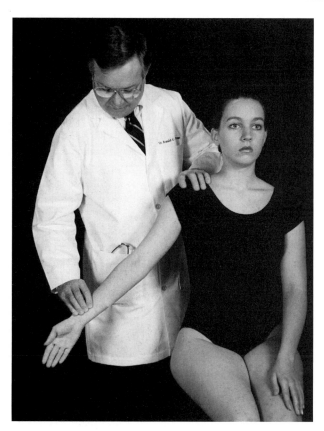

FIG. 4-50 The patient is seated comfortably with the arms at the sides. The examiner slightly abducts the affected arm and palpates the radial pulse.

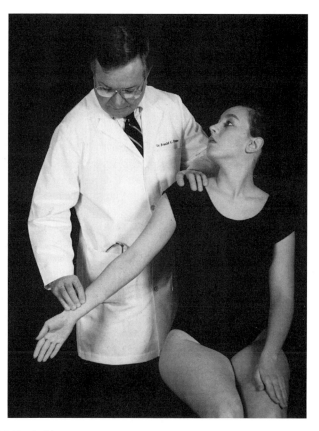

FIG. 4-51 The patient rotates the head toward the affected shoulder. The patient then extends the head, and the examiner externally rotates and extends the shoulder slightly.

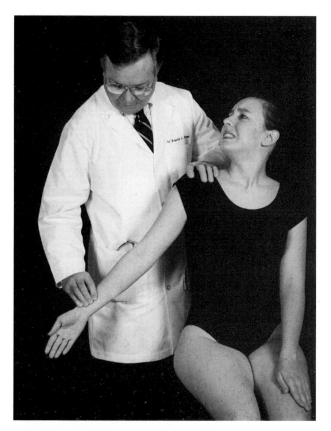

FIG. 4-52 The patient takes a deep breath and holds it. Loss of the pulse is a positive test. If the test is negative, it is repeated with the patient turning the head to the uninvolved side (modified Adson's test).

Assessment for Thoracic Outlet Syndrome

Comment

Multiple etiologic possibilities, complex anatomic considerations, and a variety of neurogenic and vascular symptoms engage the interest of many disciplines that encounter the thoracic outlet neurovascular compression syndromes. Static and dynamic anatomic relationships within the thoracic outlet dictate morbid aberrations in blood perfusion and neural function.

Usually, a contributory anatomic element that underlies each of the compression syndromes can be identified. Therefore the usual clinical maneuvers used to bracket the level of compression can be equivocal. Patients often do not have one single complaint or set of complaints that unfailingly point to a compression syndrome. In fact, symptoms of several compression syndromes may be similar.

The anatomic areas of potential neurovascular compression are the interscalene space, near the thoracic rib; the costoclavicular space; and the axilla between the coracoid process and pectoralis minor tendon.

Sensory disturbances can occur in either a dermatomal (root) distribution or in the distribution of peripheral nerves (Fig. 4-53). If spinal cord lesions are suspected, it is important to evaluate all sensory functions, including light touch, temperature, vibration, position sense, and pain (pinprick).

Pulses can be evaluated at the wrist for both the radial and ulnar arteries. The Allen maneuver should be performed if vascular injuries are suspected at the wrist. The brachial artery is easily palpated at the elbow, just medial to the lacertus fibrosus. Obliteration of the pulse implies a vascular problem proximally in the axillary or subclavian region. Venous tone and patterns should be observed. In axillary

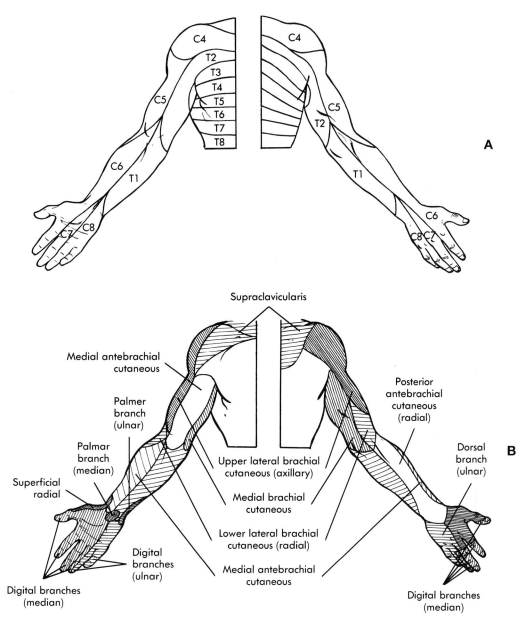

FIG. 4-53 Sensory distribution. **A,** Root dermatomes. **B,** Peripheral nerve distribution. *(From Nicholas JA, Hershman EB, editors:* The upper extremity in sports medicine, *St Louis, 1990, Mosby.)*

vein thrombosis, the venous pattern of the involved extremity is increased and the dorsal hand veins do not collapse when raised to the level of the heart (Fig. 4-54).

There are additional considerations that may affect these levels of compression. Movement of the head and neck; deep inspiration; and clavicular, scapular, and humeral movement, when performed in concert, can simultaneously alter structural relationships at one level or several levels and can cause impingement of nerves and vessels. Muscle hypertrophy resulting from occupational stress and obesity may compromise otherwise patent spaces. Loss of muscle tone and strength from a variety of causes, pain from unrelated but adjacent structures, chest deformity as a result of emphysema, postural portrayal of depressed mental status, poor working posture, and middle-age disuse atrophy (either singly or in combination) may alter potential spaces through sagging or displacement of the anatomic members.

Clavicular fractures with excessive callus or residual displacement of fragments and subacromial humeral luxation, blunt trauma to the upper thorax, postirradiation fibrosis, and the use of vibrating tools may either stretch part of the brachial plexus or damage vessel walls and result in thrombotic vessel wall complications. The following may contribute to compression symptoms: a cervical rib with or without a prefixed brachial plexus, a bifid clavicle, abnormal bony protuberances from the first thoracic rib, a fibrous remnant of the scalenus minimus muscle, abnormal scalene insertions on the first rib, and abnormal splitting of the scalenus medius by all or part of the brachial plexus. Either postural, dynamic, traumatic, or arteriosclerotic factors must be added to precipitate patient symptoms. Adson's test may be helpful in the diagnosis of thoracic outlet syndrome.

PROCEDURE

- The patient's elbow is flexed to 90 degrees (Fig. 4-55).
- The shoulder is abducted and externally rotated.
- As the examiner palpates the radial pulse, the patient rotates the head away from the involved extremity (Fig. 4-56).
- If the pulse disappears when the head is rotated, it is a positive test result for thoracic outlet syndrome.

Confirmation Procedures
Adson's test, costoclavicular maneuver, George's screening procedure, Halstead maneuver, reverse Bakody maneuver, Roos' test, shoulder compression test, and Wright's test

---

DIAGNOSTIC STATEMENT

Allen maneuver is positive on the right. This result indicates thoracic outlet syndrome.

CLINICAL PEARL

Altered relative position of the shoulder girdle to the neurovascular bundle, or vice versa, is a common element of thoracic outlet syndrome. However, a group of symptoms may be separated, in which there may be a static or gradual process under way that appears as a more general development without specific, separate, irritating incidents. Such a condition is labeled "postural" because of the alteration of the normal girdle relationship to the rest of the body.

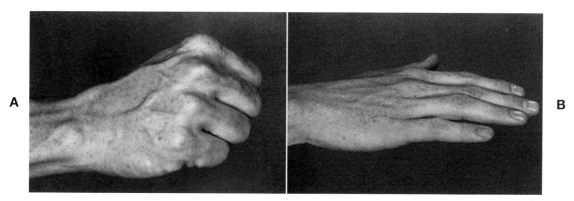

FIG. 4-54   Evaluation of axillary vein patency. **A,** Hand at side, normal prominent venous tone. **B,** Hand at heart level, veins collapse when axillary vein is patent. If the venous tone remains prominent in the elevated position, axillary vein thrombosis is suspected. *(From Nicholas JA, Hershman EB, editors:* The upper extremity in sports medicine, *St Louis, 1990, Mosby.)*

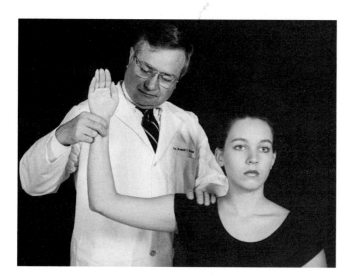

FIG. 4-55   The patient is seated. The examiner abducts the affected shoulder to 90 degrees. The patient's elbow is flexed to 90 degrees, and the shoulder is externally rotated. The radial pulse is located and recorded.

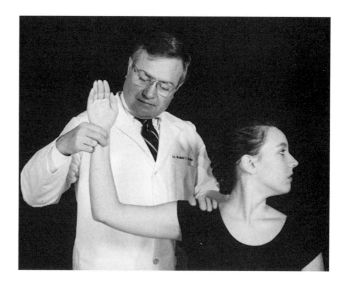

FIG. 4-56   The patient rotates the head to the opposite side. If the pulse disappears during this maneuver, the test is positive. The test is significant for thoracic outlet syndrome.

APLEY'S TEST

ALSO KNOWN AS APLEY'S SCRATCH TEST

Assessment for Degenerative Tendinitis of One of the Tendons of the Rotator Cuff, Usually the Supraspinatus Tendon

Comment

In healthy individuals, approximately 120-degree shoulder elevation is attributable to the glenohumeral joint. The remaining motion occurs at the scapulothoracic joint at a 2:1 ratio. There is considerable individual deviation from this 2:1 glenohumeral-scapulothoracic ratio among the general populace. Limitation at the glenohumeral joint leads to compensatory movement at the scapulothoracic joint during attempted elevation, which results in an altered or reverse scapulothoracic rhythm or ratio. This is observed as a shoulder-hike or girdle-hunching maneuver (Fig. 4-57).

Supraspinatus tendinitis is the most common type of tendinitis in the upper limb. This condition occurs most often in swimmers and tennis players or in other athletes who engage in sports that require repeated overhead movement of the arm.

The supraspinatus tendon passes beneath the acromion and inserts on the greater tubercle of the humerus, passing beneath the coracoacromial ligament that forms a fibrous arch over the tendon. Between the tendon and the overlying structures is the subacromial bursa.

Repeated abduction of the shoulder, unless it is maintained in external rotation, causes impingement of the tendon within the very narrow space between the humerus and the overlying acromion and ligament. This disorder is often called *impingement syndrome*. It has also been called *swimmer's shoulder.*

The microvasculature of the supraspinatus tendon is reduced where the tendon is wrung out by pressure during abduction. This site corresponds to that of tears in the supraspinatus tendon of geriatric patients. These tears may be the result of poor healing because of impaired circulation. Although tears are not as common in younger patients, the area affected is the same. Calcification sometimes occurs at this site.

The cause of this tendinitis is well defined and can be confirmed by horizontally adducting the patient's arm across the body. This move causes further impingement and reproduces the painful symptoms.

PROCEDURE

- The patient is seated and is instructed to place the affected hand behind the head and touch the opposite superior angle of the scapula (Fig. 4-58).
- The patient is then instructed to place the hand behind the back and attempt to touch the opposite inferior angle of the scapula (Fig. 4-59).
- Exacerbation of the patient's pain indicates degenerative tendinitis of one of the tendons of the rotator cuff, usually the supraspinatus tendon.

Confirmation Procedures

Impingement sign, subacromial push-button sign, and supraspinatus test

---

DIAGNOSTIC STATEMENT

Apley's scratch test (superior or inferior) is positive on the left. This result indicates tendinitis of the supraspinatus tendon.

CLINICAL PEARL

Apley's inferior is a useful test of internal rotation and extension. With severe restriction, the patient will not be able to get the hand behind the back at all. This movement is commonly affected in adhesive capsulitis.

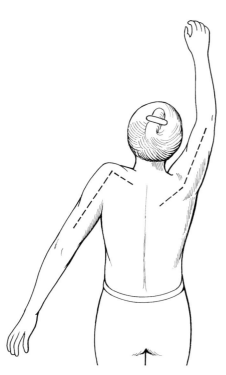

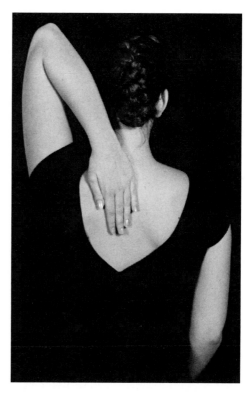

FIG. 4-57   Reverse scapulothoracic rhythm. *Broken lines* indicate the position of the scapular spine and humeral axis on each side, showing little or no movement of the left shoulder. This "shoulder hiking" attempt at abduction elevates rather than depresses the humeral head. *(From Saidoff DC, McDonough AL: Critical pathways in therapeutic intervention, St Louis, 1997, Mosby.)*

FIG. 4-58   The patient is seated and is instructed to place the hand of the affected arm behind the head and touch near the opposite scapula (Apley's scratch superior).

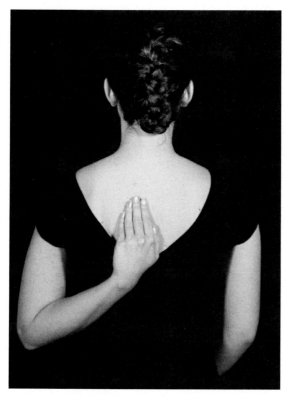

FIG. 4-59   The patient is then instructed to place the hand of the affected shoulder behind the back and attempt to touch near the opposite scapula (Apley's scratch inferior). If either position exacerbates the patient's pain, this indicates degenerative tendinitis of one of the tendons, usually the supraspinatus, of the rotator cuff.

Assessment for Anterior Shoulder Dislocation Trauma and Posterior Dislocation of the Humerus

Comment

Dislocation of the shoulder follows the loss of function of the restraining structures around the shoulder. This dislocation is a result of the same mechanism that causes subluxations. The most common type of dislocation of the shoulder in young patients is anteroinferior. This is pure dislocation, unaccompanied by fracture. As age advances, the ligaments become firmer and the bone less strong, so the dislocation may be accompanied by avulsion fracture, rather than a tear of the ligament. In the young patient, it is always the ligament or muscle that gives way. As the arm is forced into abduction and external rotation, the humeral head is thrust against the anterior portion of the glenohumeral joint. The coracoacromial ligament forces the humeral head downward, and it then emerges anteriorly and inferiorly into the redundant area of the capsule, which is protected by the glenohumeral ligaments. These ligaments give way when they are torn from the glenoid labrum because of avulsion of the labrum or actual disruption of the ligaments. The head of the humerus slips over the glenoid rim and immediately slides forward to lodge between the rim of the glenoid and coracoid process, and the arm drops toward the side but not against it. This is the classic dislocation of the shoulder in young patients. The damage to the ligament may be a transverse tear across the capsule; in addition, the capsular reinforcements known as the *glenohumeral ligaments* may split, with one passing above the humeral head and the other below it. In some instances, the ligaments actually grasp the humeral head to impede its reduction.

Posterior dislocation of the shoulder is uncommon. Such dislocation is caused by a direct driving force against the lower end of the humerus with the arm flexed forward. This force is transmitted up the arm, driving the head out posteriorly. No gross deformity of the shoulder is evident. The patient resists any motion of the shoulder, and on careful palpation, the examiner can feel less fullness of the humeral head in front and some increased fullness behind. There is also increased prominence of the coracoid. Such a dislocation is readily determined only if it is palpated very early, because within a short time, the swelling that is around the shoulder and that occurs from this extremely disabling injury will mask any physical findings.

Dislocations and subluxations (partial dislocation) of the glenohumeral joint often occur after indirect trauma with the arm abducted, extended, and externally rotated (anterior dislocation) and with the arm abducted, flexed, and internally rotated (posterior dislocation) (Fig. 4-60).

Two associated injuries may occur as a result of acute glenohumeral dislocation and instability. Because the shoulder is the most mobile joint in the body, bony restrictions do not provide substantial restraints. Rather, the fibrocartilaginous glenoid labrum deepens the articulation between the humeral head and the bony glenoid fossa (Fig. 4-61). When forces are great enough to dislocate the humerus from its confines within the glenoid, injury to the labrum occurs (Bankart lesion). A *Bankart lesion* is an avulsion of the capsule and glenoid labrum off of the anterior rim of the glenoid (Fig. 4-62).

The head of the humerus is subject to injury as a result of the anterior shoulder instability (Hill-Sachs lesion). The Hill-Sachs lesion is a compression or "impaction fracture" of the posterolateral aspect of the humeral head (Fig. 4-63).

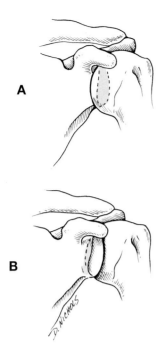

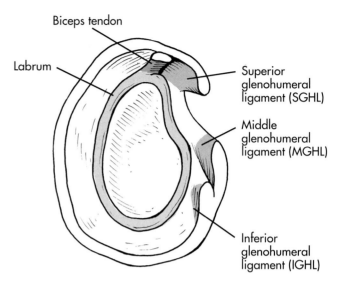

FIG. 4-60   Anterior and posterior glenohumeral dislocations. **A,** Anterior glenohumeral dislocation. **B,** Posterior glenohumeral dislocation. *(From Shankman GA: Fundamental orthopedic management for the physical therapist assistant, St Louis, 1997, Mosby.)*

FIG. 4-61   Anatomy of the glenoid labrum. *(From Shankman GA: Fundamental orthopedic management for the physical therapist assistant, St Louis, 1997, Mosby.)*

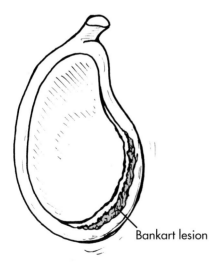

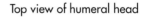
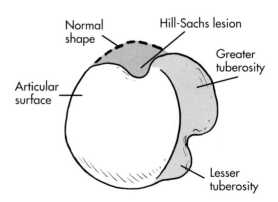

FIG. 4-62   Bankart lesion. *(From Shankman GA: Fundamental orthopedic management for the physical therapist assistant, St Louis, 1997, Mosby.)*

FIG. 4-63   Hill-Sachs lesion. *(From Shankman GA: Fundamental orthopedic management for the physical therapist assistant, St Louis, 1997, Mosby.)*

PROCEDURE

- The patient's shoulder is abducted and externally rotated (Fig. 4-64).
- If the patient shows apprehension or alarm and resists further motion, the test is positive (Fig. 4-65).
- This test may elicit a feeling that resembles the pain felt when the shoulder was previously dislocated.
- This test is performed slowly and cautiously; done too quickly, it is possible to dislocate the humerus.
- Anterior shoulder dislocation trauma is suggested by a positive test.
- To evaluate posterior shoulder dislocation, the shoulder is flexed and internally rotated (Fig. 4-66).
- A posterior force is applied on the patient's elbow.
- If the patient exhibits apprehension and resists further motion, the test is positive.
- A posterior dislocation of the humerus is suggested by a positive test.

Confirmation Procedures

Bryant's sign, Calloway's test, Dugas' test, Hamilton's test, Mazion's shoulder maneuver, and diagnostic imaging

DIAGNOSTIC STATEMENT

Apprehension test is positive for the right shoulder in the anterior portion. This result indicates shoulder dislocation trauma.

Apprehension test is positive for the right shoulder in the posterior portion. This result indicates shoulder dislocation trauma.

CLINICAL PEARL

These maneuvers are also known as the *drawer tests of Gerber and Ganz.* Any movements, clicks, or patient apprehension support the diagnosis of recurrent shoulder dislocation. Axial diagnostic images are made to confirm the diagnosis.

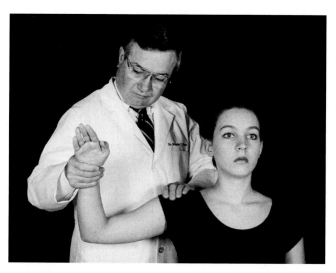

FIG. 4-64   The patient is seated comfortably with the arms at the sides. The shoulder is slowly abducted and externally rotated.

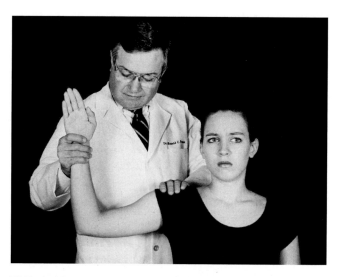

FIG. 4-65   A look or feeling of apprehension or alarm on the patient's face is the positive finding. The patient will resist further motion. This maneuver also may duplicate the feeling of an imminent dislocation. If performed too briskly, the humerus can dislocate. A positive test suggests anterior shoulder dislocation trauma.

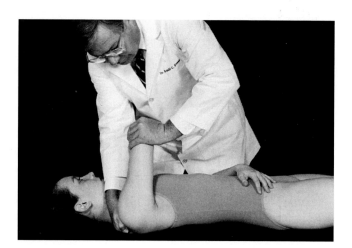

FIG. 4-66   For evaluating posterior shoulder dislocation, the patient should be supine. The shoulder is flexed and internally rotated. A posterior force is applied on the patient's elbow (forcing the humeral head posterior on the glenoid). A look of apprehension is a positive finding. The patient will resist further motion. A positive test suggests posterior dislocation of the humerus.

Assessment for Dislocation
of the Glenohumeral Articulation

Comment

The shoulder is the most commonly dislocated joint in the body. The typical mechanism of injury is abduction, extension, and external rotation, which results in an anterior dislocation. Axial loading of the internally rotated and extended arm, violent trauma, electrical shock, or convulsions can produce posterior dislocations. Severe trauma with hyperabduction forces on the upper extremity can produce an inferior dislocation. Because of the bony anatomy of the shallow glenoid and the round humeral head, initial dislocations can become locked by a wedge-shaped impression defect in the humeral head.

ORTHOPEDIC GAMUT 4-6

SHOULDER
DISLOCATIONS

Shoulder dislocations are classified in regard to the following:

1. The degree of instability (dislocation or subluxation)
2. The cause of the instability (traumatic or atraumatic)
3. The direction of the instability (anterior, posterior, or multidirectional)

The humerus is most commonly dislocated anteriorly (95%) or, in practice, anteriorly, medially, and inferiorly, coming to lie inferior to the coracoid process (Fig. 4-67). This may cause a cortical impaction of both the superior posterior aspect of the humerus (Hill-Sachs, or "hatchet," deformity) and the inferior aspect of the glenoid (Bankart lesion) or detachment of the anterior portion of the glenoid labrum.

Glenohumeral, AP, axillary lateral, and trans-scapular radiographs are necessary to document the direction and degree of instability. A Hill-Sachs lesion is best demonstrated by an AP view in internal rotation or the Stryker Notch view. An osseous Bankart or glenoid rim fracture is best demonstrated by the axillary West Point view.

Although posterior dislocations may be difficult to appreciate, they should not be missed. In general, they can be appreciated on the AP view by persistent internal rotation of the humerus and asymmetry of the glenohumeral joint (Fig. 4-68). An axillary view may be impossible to obtain, but a transthoracic ("swimmer's" view) or oblique (Y) view will confirm the diagnosis.

An unusual inferior dislocation, luxatio erecta, is caused by severe hyperabduction of the arm, whereby the humeral head impinges on the acromion. The acromion then acts as a fulcrum and thus causes an inferior displacement of the humeral head with the arm "locked" in abduction (Fig. 4-69).

Careful and early inspection in the acute dislocation injury reveals flattening and loss of the normal curvature of the shoulder, but swelling obliterates these findings later. Diagnostic imaging is needed to confirm the diagnosis. When shoulder dislocation is suspected, an axillary view is paramount to distinguish the exact position of the head of the humerus in relation to the glenoid process.

Dislocations of the shoulder are occasionally accompanied by injury to the axillary nerve with resulting loss of function of the deltoid muscle. With shoulder dislocations, the function of the deltoid and any sensory disturbance in the skin overlying the deltoid must be ascertained. The area over the deltoid is innervated by the axillary nerve, and assessment of the skin sensation will aid in predicting the

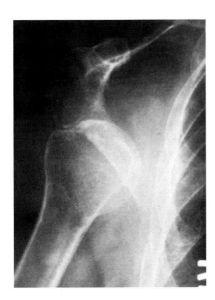

FIG. 4-67 Anterior dislocation of the right humerus. *(From Sutton D, Young JWR: A concise textbook of clinical imaging, ed 2, St Louis, 1995, Mosby.)*

A   **B**

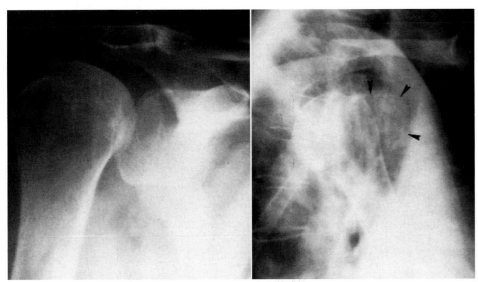

FIG. 4-68 **A,** Posterior dislocation of the humerus. **B,** A "swimmer's view." *(From Sutton D, Young JWR: A concise textbook of clinical imaging, ed 2, St Louis, 1995, Mosby.)*

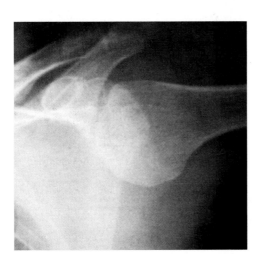

FIG. 4-69 Luxatio erecta. *(From Sutton D, Young JWR: A concise textbook of clinical imaging, ed 2, St Louis, 1995, Mosby.)*

recovery of the nerve. Dislocations of the shoulder rarely result in injury to other nerves and vessels of the upper extremity, but injuries of the posterior cord of the brachial plexus have been reported.

PROCEDURE

- The examiner views the characteristic lowering of the axillary fold (anterior and posterior pillars of the armpit) that is seen after trauma when dislocation of the glenohumeral articulation ensues (Figs. 4-70 and 4-71).

Confirmation Procedures

Apprehension test, Calloway's test, Dugas' test, Hamilton's test, Mazion's shoulder maneuver, and diagnostic imaging

DIAGNOSTIC STATEMENT

Bryant's sign is present in the right shoulder. This result indicates shoulder dislocation trauma.

CLINICAL PEARL

With dislocations of the shoulder, the axillary nerve may be injured. The patient is unable to contract the deltoid muscle, and there may be a small patch of anesthesia over the muscle. This anesthesia is usually a neurapraxia, which recovers spontaneously after a few weeks or months. The posterior cord of the brachial plexus occasionally is injured. This occurrence is somewhat alarming, but it usually recovers with time.

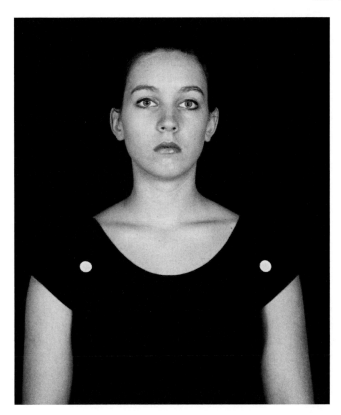

FIG. 4-70   The patient is seated with the arms comfortably at the sides.

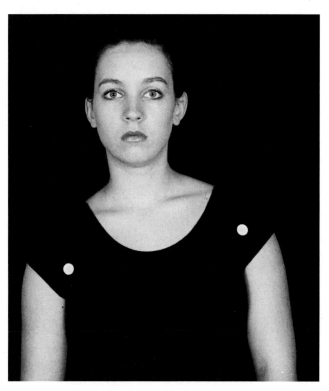

FIG. 4-71   If the sign is present, there is a characteristic lowering of the axillary fold (anterior and posterior pillars of the armpit) on the affected side. The sign is present when dislocation of the glenohumeral articulation has occurred.

CALLOWAY'S TEST

Assessment for Dislocation of the Humerus

Comment

Shoulder dislocation at the glenohumeral joint occurs anteriorly in 95% of the cases. The remaining 5% dislocate posteriorly. The incidence of anterior dislocation is attributed to the anatomic weakness of the anterior aspect of the joint.

The joint capsule is thin and loose. The capsule is reinforced by folds called *glenohumeral ligaments.* These ligaments attach from the humerus and fan out to attach to the superior anterior aspect of the glenoid fossa, partly to the glenoid labrum, and partly to a portion of the bone of the scapula. An opening in the capsule often exists between the superior and middle glenohumeral ligaments. This opening is called *Weitbrecht's foramen.* The opening may be a frank perforation or may be covered by a thin layer of the capsule. The articular cavity connects with the subscapular fossa through Weitbrecht's foramen. The humeral head dislocates through this opening, and dislocations may recur as a result of fraying or actual destruction of the middle glenohumeral ligament.

With dislocations, the glenoid labrum may be partially or completely detached and a tear may occur in the anteroinferior aspect. The glenoid labrum contains no fibrocartilage and is a redundant fibrous fold of the anterior capsule that disappears when the humerus is externally rotated. This pouch invites dislocation. The humeral head can protrude into this pouch, especially if an anatomic variant of the middle humeral ligament exists.

There are five types of dislocation, and the most common is the subcoracoid dislocation. The subclavicular and subglenoid types are less common and may be a progression of the subcoracoid type. All anterior types of dislocations can change into any of the other anterior types. The fifth type of dislocation, the posterior, or subspinous, is rare. The type of dislocation is determined by the location of the humeral head in relation to the glenoid seat when the diagnosis is made.

Primary anterior dislocations occur with equal frequency regardless of age, but recurrence of a dislocation is highest in the young and decreases after age 45. There is less recurrence in cases in which the primary dislocation was severe and resulted in greater hemorrhage and therefore greater scar formation in healing.

The sulcus sign is often present in shoulder instability. Grading of the sulcus sign is based on the distance between the inferior margin of the lateral acromion and the humeral head when a downward traction force is applied to the adducted arm (Fig. 4-72, *A*). Less than 1 cm of distance represents a 1+ sulcus, 1 to 2 cm indicates a 2+ sulcus, and more than 2 cm is a 3+ sulcus. A 3+ sulcus sign reflects laxity of the superior glenohumeral ligament and inferior glenohumeral ligament and is indicative of inferior instability. It is pathognomonic of multidirectional instability.

Apprehension tests are designed to induce anxiety and protect muscular contraction as the shoulder is brought to a position associated with instability. The anterior apprehension test is performed with the arm abducted and externally rotated. The examiner progressively increases the degree of external rotation and notes the development of patient apprehension. The posterior stress test (Fig. 4-72, *B*) is performed with the arm internally rotated and forward flexed to 90 degrees. Apprehension is unusual in this position, but pain or a palpable jump may be noted as the humerus is loaded in an AP direction and progressively adducted across the chest.

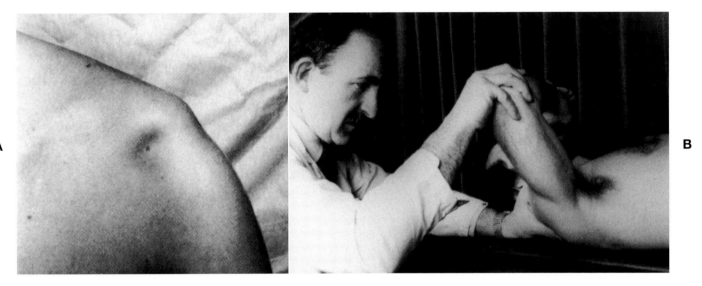

FIG. 4-72 Physical examination for shoulder instability. **A,** Sulcus sign. An extremely large sulcus is indicative of multidirectional instability. **B,** Posterior stress test. *(From Nicholas JA, Hershman EB, editors:* The upper extremity in sports medicine, *St Louis, 1990, Mosby.)*

Ligamentous laxity is commonly associated with shoulder instability and can be measured objectively on physical examination. The degree of thumb hyperabduction with the wrist volar flexed can be noted by the distance between the thumb and volar forearm. If the thumb reaches the forearm, the test is considered positive. An assessment is also made for index metacarpophalangeal hyperextension in excess of 90 degrees, elbow hyperextension, and knee hyperextension (Beighton Hypermobility Assessment) (Fig. 4-73).

PROCEDURE

- The test consists of measuring the girth of the shoulder joints bilaterally.
- This test is helpful in the examination of obese patients.
- The examiner loops a flexible tape measure through the axilla (Fig. 4-74).
- The girth is measured at the acromial tip.

- In a positive test, the girth of the affected joint is increased.
- The test is significant for dislocation of the humerus.

Confirmation Procedures
Apprehension test, Bryant's sign, Dugas' sign, Hamilton's test, Mazion's shoulder maneuver, and diagnostic imaging

---

DIAGNOSTIC STATEMENT

Calloway's test demonstrates an increased shoulder axillary circumference on the right. This increase is consistent with shoulder dislocation trauma.

CLINICAL PEARL

Shoulder dislocation results in severe pain. The patient supports the arm with the opposite hand and is hesitant to permit any kind of examination. The lateral outline of the shoulder may be flattened, and if the patient is not too muscular, a small bulge may be seen and felt just below the clavicle. The arm must always be examined for nerve and vessel injury.

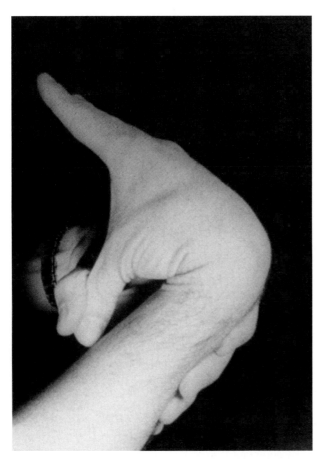

FIG. 4-73   Generalized ligamentous laxity is a patient with shoulder instability. *(From Nicholas JA, Hershman EB, editors: The upper extremity in sports medicine, St Louis, 1990, Mosby.)*

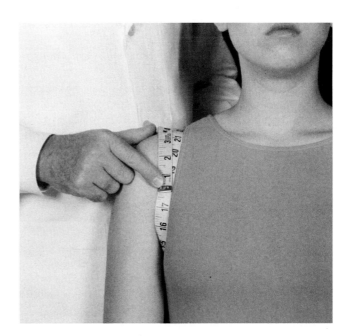

FIG. 4-74   The patient is seated comfortably with the arms at the sides. The examiner loops a flexible tape measure through the axilla and measures the girth of the affected shoulder at the acromial tip. The girth of the affected shoulder is compared with the girth of the unaffected shoulder. In a positive test, the girth of the affected joint is increased. The test is significant for dislocation of the humerus.

CODMAN'S SIGN

ALSO KNOWN AS DROP ARM TEST

Assessment for Tear in the Rotator Cuff Complex

Comment

Sudden tendon rupture in the shoulder results in immediate sharp pain. There is sometimes an audible pop in the shoulder. Mild swelling and ecchymosis of the upper anterior arm as well as a change of contour of the biceps muscle occur. Contraction of the musculature fibers takes the appearance of a firm ball of muscle that is more distal than normally expected and is palpable as a soft hump. This deformity will persist and is sometimes called the *Popeye sign* after the well-known cartoon character (Fig. 4-75).

One of the major functions of the rotator cuff is humeral head depression, although this function is progressively compromised during the evolution of the rotator cuff disorder. With progressive loss of this mechanism, the humeral head rises higher and higher as a result of the unrelenting upward pull of the deltoid. In the event of a major defect in the rotator cuff, the humeral head migrates even further proximally by protruding through the defect. A boutonniere deformity, just as in the finger, victimizes the buttonholed cuff by changing its line of pull so as to convert balancing forces into unbalancing forces (Fig. 4-76).

The thickness of the supraspinatus is approximately 6 mm. Diminution of the interval between the humeral head and the acromion, which is occupied by the supraspinatus and its surrounding soft tissues, suggests rupture of the rotator cuff. The interval diminishes with age in men only. A space of less than 6 mm is abnormal in a middle-age person (Fig. 4-77). Upward subluxation of the humeral head is almost always more pronounced on external than on internal rotation views (Fig. 4-78).

The acromiohumeral interval bears prognostic importance. Patients whose acromiohumeral distance is less than 7 mm often have larger tears and less strength and motion than others following cuff repair.

Complete tears of the tendinous cuff must be distinguished from incomplete tears. The clinical effects of the tears are different. An incomplete tear is one cause of the painful arc syndrome, and a complete tear seriously impairs the patient's ability to abduct the shoulder.

The tendon gives way under a sudden strain, usually caused by a fall or by overexertion. Age attrition of the tendon is a predisposing factor.

A tear of the tendinous cuff is mainly of the supraspinatus tendon, but it may extend into the adjacent subscapularis or infraspinatus tendons. Such a tear is close to the insertion of the tendons and usually involves the capsule of the joint, into which the tendons are blended. The edges of the rent retract, leaving a gaping hole that establishes a communication between the shoulder joint and the subacromial bursa.

With complete tears of the supraspinatus tendon, the patient is usually a male who is older than 60. After a strain or fall, the patient's complaints include pain at the tip of the shoulder and down the upper arm and an inability to raise the arm.

Examination reveals local tenderness below the margin of the acromion. When the patient attempts to abduct the arm, no movement occurs at the glenohumeral joint, but a range of 45 to 60 degrees of abduction can be achieved entirely by scapular movement. However, there is a full range of passive movement. If the arm is abducted with assistance beyond 90 degrees, the patient can sustain the abduction by deltoid action. The essential and characteristic feature in cases of torn supraspinatus tendon is the inability to initiate glenohumeral abduction. The usual explanation is that the early stages of abduction demand combining the action of the supraspinatus with the action of the deltoid muscle. This combined action supplies the main abduction force and the supraspinatus action that stabilizes the humeral head in the glenoid fossa.

A complete tear of the tendinous cuff must be distinguished from other causes of impaired glenohumeral abduction, especially the painful arc syndrome and paralysis of the abductor muscles (poliomyelitis or nerve injury). Inability to initiate glenohumeral abduction accompanied by enough power to sustain abduction once the limb has been raised passively is characteristic of a widely torn supraspinatus. With the painful arc syndrome, the power of abduction is retained, but the movement is painful. In a case of complete tear, arthrography will demonstrate communication between the joint and the subacromial bursa. The tear also may be visualized by ultrasound scanning.

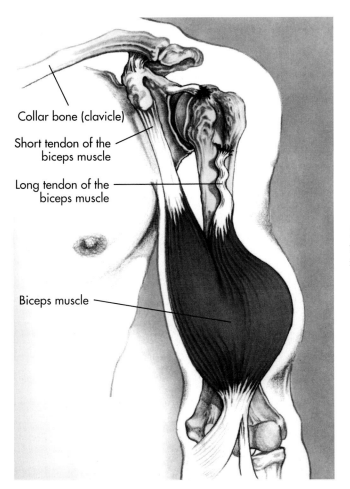

Collar bone (clavicle)

Short tendon of the
  biceps muscle

Long tendon of the
  biceps muscle

Biceps muscle

FIG. 4-75   Proximal long tendon biceps rupture with retraction of torn tendon ends.   *(From Saidoff DC, McDonough AL:* Critical pathways in therapeutic intervention, *St Louis, 1997, Mosby.)*

PROCEDURE

- The patient's arm is passively abducted (Figs. 4-79 and 4-80).
- The examiner suddenly removes support at some point above 90 degrees, which makes the deltoid contract suddenly (Fig. 4-81).
- If shoulder pain occurs and there is a hunching of the shoulder because rotator cuff function is absent, the sign is present for rotator cuff tear or, more specifically, rupture of the supraspinatus tendon.
- In a modification of Codman's sign, the patient's shoulder is abducted to 90 degrees passively.
- The patient tries to lower the arm slowly to the side in the same arc of movement.

- If the patient is unable to return the arm to the side slowly or has severe pain, the test is positive.
- A positive test suggests a tear in the rotator cuff complex.

Confirmation Procedures

Apley's scratch test, impingement sign, subacromial push-button sign, and supraspinatus test

---

DIAGNOSTIC STATEMENT

Codman's drop arm sign is present on the left. This result indicates a tear in the rotator cuff complex.

CLINICAL PEARL

The cardinal sign of cuff rupture is persistent weakness. The patient may be conscious of this weakness, but often the examiner must point it out. Sometimes the weakness is easily overlooked. The patient may be able to lift the arm into full abduction or beyond the point of a full-thickness cuff tear. However, if this action is resisted a little, sometimes by as little as the pressure of one finger, even a very strong patient may be unable to abduct or flex the shoulder well.

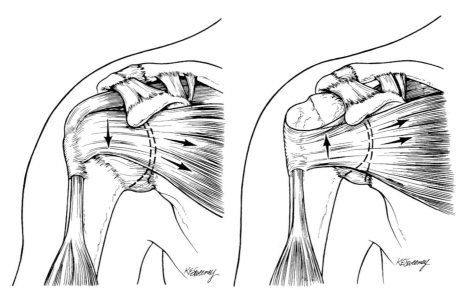

FIG. 4-76   Major cuff failure and retraction allow the humeral head to protrude upward through the cuff defect, creating a boutonniere lesion.   *(From Saidoff DC, McDonough AL:* Critical pathways in therapeutic intervention, *St Louis, 1997, Mosby.)*

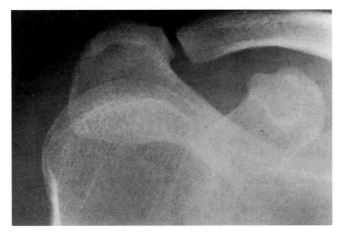

FIG. 4-77   Normal right acromioclavicular (AC) joint.   *(From Nicholas JA, Hershman EB, editors:* The upper extremity in sports medicine, *St Louis, 1990, Mosby.)*

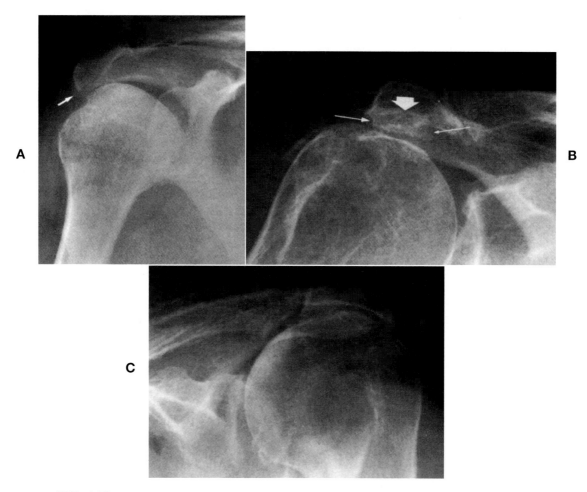

FIG. 4-78   Rotator cuff disease and impingement. **A,** Right shoulder; both the greater tuberosity and the acromion process are sclerotic. Hypertrophic changes of the peripheral margin of the acromion are also evident *(arrow)*. **B,** Right shoulder. There is bone formation *(long arrows)* along the undersurface of the acromion process *(large arrow)*. This occupies the subacromial space and is conformed to the humeral head contour. **C,** Left shoulder. Superior migration of the humeral head is evident.   *(From Nicholas JA, Hershman EB, editors: The upper extremity in sports medicine, St Louis, 1990, Mosby.)*

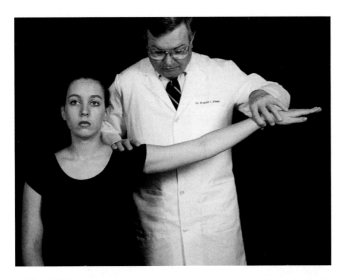

FIG. 4-79 The patient is seated. The examiner passively abducts the patient's affected arm.

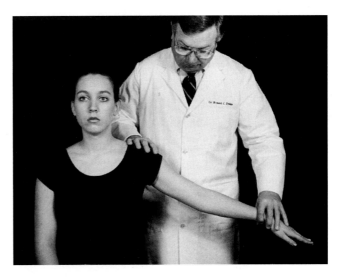

FIG. 4-80 The passive abduction is carried to a range slightly above 90 degrees.

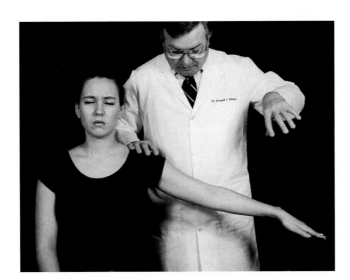

FIG. 4-81 The examiner suddenly removes support, making the deltoid contract suddenly. If the sign is present, shoulder pain and a hunching of the shoulder occur because rotator cuff function is absent. The sign is significant for rotator cuff tear (rupture of the supraspinatus tendon).

COSTOCLAVICULAR MANEUVER

Assessment for Thoracic Outlet Syndrome

Comment

Thoracic outlet compression syndrome refers to a common condition in which nerves or vessels or both are compressed between the root of the neck and axilla. Two clearly defined forms of this condition have been described. One is a neurologic syndrome that involves the lower trunk of the brachial plexus and is caused by abnormal nerve stretch or compression. The other is a vascular form that involves the subclavian artery and vein and is more common in men than in women.

ORTHOPEDIC GAMUT 4-7

THORACIC OUTLET SYNDROME

Depending on the mechanism and level of compression, several disorders are included under the title of thoracic outlet syndrome:

1. Cervical rib syndrome
2. Scalenus-anticus syndrome
3. Wright's hyperabduction syndrome
4. Pectoralis minor syndrome
5. Costoclavicular syndrome

The neurologic form of thoracic outlet syndrome often occurs in women of slim build and drooping shoulders. Presenting symptoms include aching pain in the side or back of the neck that extends across the shoulder and down along the inner aspect of the arm and paresthesias in the ulnar aspect of the hand. The sensory findings extend more proximally than an ulnar nerve lesion, whereas the motor findings include thenar and intrinsic muscle weakness and wasting.

An important sign reproduces the patient's symptoms by abducting and laterally rotating the arm at the shoulder with a flexed elbow while palpating the pulses at the wrist (Wright's maneuver).

The overhead exercise test may elicit symptoms of aching and fatigue in patients with thoracic outlet syndrome after 20 to 30 seconds of rapidly flexing and extending the fingers as the arm is held overhead (Roos' test).

As the neurovascular bundle enters the axillary canal, it runs through a narrow cleft beneath the clavicle and on top of the first rib. This cleft is a slitlike aperture over which the subclavius muscle arches, sometimes with a sharp, fusiform lower margin. Alterations and abnormalities in this cleft can compress the neurovascular bundle. Because the vein is the most medial structure running into the arm and lies in the narrowest part of the cleft, it suffers the most from any narrowing that develops. Abnormalities, fractures, and dislocations of the medial third of the clavicle or fractures of the first rib followed by excessive callus formation can constrict this space. The resulting symptoms are a sense of fullness in the hand and fingers and an aching, crampy pain in the forearm and hand. Vague shoulder or shoulder-arm discomfort may be mentioned, but the radiating pain is emphasized. The hand may be intermittently swollen, and sometimes superficial veins around the shoulder are engorged. Shoulder movement is not limited, which contrasts with shoulder-arm-hand syndrome, in which gross shoulder immobilization is prominent and hand symptoms are present. The radiating discomfort has the typically diffuse vascular pattern, which means the discomfort is not localized to nerve root or peripheral nerve distribution.

In addition to patients with obvious abnormality of the rib and clavicle, some patients develop this disturbance from a sagging shoulder girdle and atonic musculature. Normally, it is difficult to encroach upon the neurovascular bundle beneath the clavicle, but it is conceivable that some sagging occurs, and when tension in the bundle and enveloping sheath is added, the vessels may be compressed.

This costoclavicular disturbance can be separated from scalene and cervical rib disturbances by several findings.

There is no relation to cervical spine movements and no scalene or supraclavicular tenderness. The diagnostic images are different because no cervical rib is present. Arterial symptoms are occasionally prominent, but most of the disturbance is the result of venous obstruction. Costoclavicular compression can be differentiated from postural compression by the absence of any significant relation to body position either at work or while sleeping. Costoclavicular compression is also clearly differentiated from hyperabduction compression by the lack of significant correlation to shoulder movement.

PROCEDURE

- The radial pulse is palpated while the patient's shoulders are drawn down and in extension (Fig. 4-82).
- The cervical spine is flexed maximally (Figs. 4-83 and 4-84).
- If the pulses are lost, the test is positive.
- Thoracic outlet syndrome is suggested by a positive test.

Confirmation Procedures

Adson's test, Allen maneuver, George's screening procedure, Halstead maneuver, reverse Bakody maneuver, Roos' test, shoulder compression test, and Wright's test

---

DIAGNOSTIC STATEMENT

The costoclavicular maneuver is positive on the right. This result indicates costoclavicular thoracic outlet compression syndrome.

CLINICAL PEARL

Radiating discomfort from neurovascular compression can be associated with sleep or recumbency. This discomfort is a common disturbance that has many descriptive terms applied to it, including *Wartenberg's nocturnal dysesthesia, sleep tetany, waking numbness, nocturnal palsy,* and *morning numbness.*

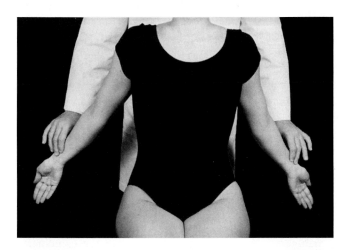

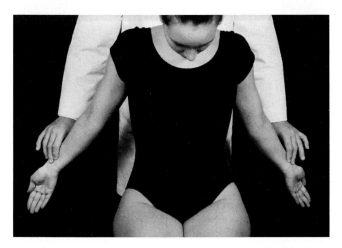

FIG. 4-82   The patient is seated comfortably with the arms at the sides. The examiner bilaterally palpates the radial pulse.

FIG. 4-83   The examiner extends the patient's shoulders as the patient flexes the cervical spine (chin to chest). The test is positive if the radial pulse of the affected arm disappears. A positive test indicates thoracic outlet syndrome.

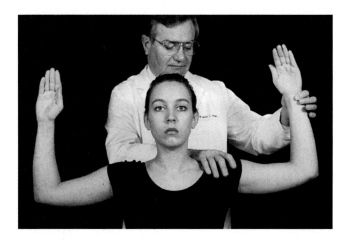

FIG. 4-84   An alternative is to have the patient actively abduct the shoulders and flex the elbows to 90 degrees. The examiner palpates the radial pulse of the affected arm and externally rotates the arm. The test is positive if the pulse disappears. A positive test indicates thoracic outlet syndrome. Before the arm is externally rotated in this position, a subtle sign of thoracic outlet syndrome may occur. This sign involves blanching of the hand of the affected arm. The examiner should use the unaffected side as a control.

DAWBARN'S SIGN

Assessment for Subacromial Bursitis

Comment

Like many other important joints, many of the major muscles surrounding the shoulder joint are "cushioned" by a bursal sac, which minimizes friction and subsequent irritation associated with movement. The most important bursae at the shoulder joint are the deltoid bursa and the subacromial bursa (Fig. 4-85).

A painful shoulder is a complaint that is common to all age groups and both sexes. To treat these patients effectively, the exact cause must be determined in each case. The use of *bursitis* as an all-inclusive term denoting the diagnosis and basis for therapy in the painful shoulder syndrome is irrational. Most of the body's bursae exist in or around the shoulder complex.

ORTHOPEDIC GAMUT 4-8

BURSAE LOCATIONS

The most commonly present bursae locations include the following (Fig. 4-86):

1. Subacromial and subdeltoid
2. Between the coracoid and the glenohumeral joint capsule
3. Summit of the acromion
4. Between the infraspinatus and the joint capsule
5. Between the teres major and the long head of the biceps
6. Between the subscapularis and the joint capsule
7. Anterior and posterior to the tendinous insertion of the latissimus dorsi
8. Behind the coracobrachialis muscle

Excluding traumatic causes, shoulder pain may radiate from a lesion of the cervical spine or may be the result of irritation from some other organ, such as the gallbladder or heart. However, shoulder pain most often originates as some derangement of the subacromial mechanism in the shoulder joint proper.

The subacromial mechanism of the shoulder joint is bounded above by the acromion and the coracoacromial ligament and below by the humeral head. The component structures of the shoulder include the subacromial, or subdeltoid, bursa; the musculotendinous, or rotator, cuff; the articular capsule of the shoulder joint; and the tendon sheath gliding mechanism of the long head of the biceps brachii muscle.

Most patients with shoulder pain will be found to have some lesion involving a component of this mechanism. The use of the blanket term *bursitis* to explain all of the derangements of the subacromial mechanism is the most important factor against successful management of the painful or stiff shoulder. All lesions of the subacromial mechanism may secondarily involve the subdeltoid bursa. It is rare that true primary subdeltoid bursitis is encountered. The most common derangements of the subacromial mechanism that cause shoulder pain are calcific deposits in the musculotendinous cuff, bicipital tendinitis, lesions of the acromioclavicular joint, and adhesive capsulitis of the shoulder joint.

PROCEDURE

- With the patient's arm comfortably at the side, deep palpation of the shoulder by the examiner elicits a well-localized, tender area (Fig. 4-87).
- With the examiner's finger still on the painful spot, the patient's arm is passively abducted by the examiner's other hand.
- The sign is present if the painful spot under the examiner's nonmoving finger disappears as the arm is abducted (Fig. 4-88).
- The sign is significant for subacromial bursitis.

Confirmation Procedure
Diagnostic imaging

DIAGNOSTIC STATEMENT

Dawbarn's sign is present in the left shoulder. This result indicates subacromial bursitis.

CLINICAL PEARL

Subacromial bursitis is not common as a primary condition. The condition may be caused by a direct blow over the shoulder. This blow causes an inflammatory reaction that is aggravated by further motion. Bursitis is usually a secondary reaction. The examiner should search for a primary lesion before beginning treatment.

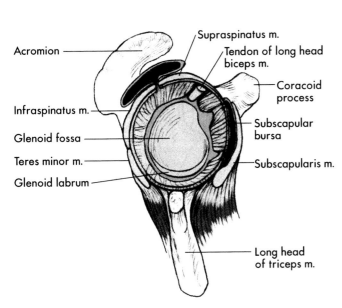

FIG. 4-85 Glenoid fossa and rotator cuff muscles. *(From Mathers LH, et al:* Clinical anatomy principles, *St Louis, 1996, Mosby.)*

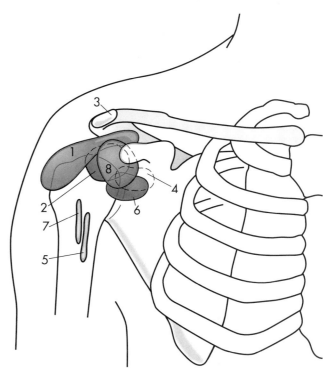

FIG. 4-86 Common shoulder bursae. See Orthopedic Gamut 4-8 for number key. *(From Saidoff DC, McDonough AL:* Critical pathways in therapeutic intervention, *St Louis, 1997, Mosby.)*

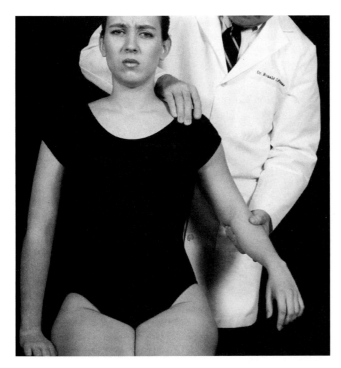

FIG. 4-87 The patient is seated with the arms comfortably at the side. The examiner palpates the affected shoulder deeply. A well-localized, tender area at the subacromial bursa is found.

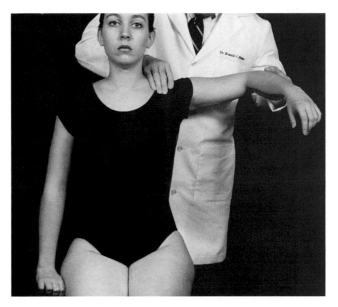

FIG. 4-88 While the examiner's finger is still on the painful spot, the patient's arm is passively abducted by the examiner's other hand. The sign is present when, as the arm is abducted, the painful spot disappears under the examiner's nonmoving finger. The sign is significant for subacromial bursitis.

Assessment for Shoulder Dislocation

Comment

Anterior dislocation is by far the most common pattern of shoulder dislocation. This type of dislocation occurs when the head of the humerus slips off and in front of the glenoid when the arm is abducted and extended.

ORTHOPEDIC GAMUT 4-9

ANTERIOR SHOULDER DISLOCATION

Radiographic appearances of anterior shoulder dislocation include the following:

1. Bankart lesion, which is an avulsion of a small fragment of the glenoid rim at the site of the triceps insertion (Fig. 4-89).
2. Flap fracture, an avulsion of the greater tuberosity (Fig. 4-90).
3. Hill-Sachs (hatchet) deformity, an impaction fracture of the posterosuperior surface of the humeral head produced by repetitive traumatization by the inferior glenoid rim after recurrent anterior glenohumeral joint dislocation

---

Once off the glenoid, the head slips medially when the arm is lowered. This slipping produces the characteristic profile of a dislocated shoulder. Because the head of the humerus is not lying in its normal position, the shoulder has a flatter appearance than usual and the elbow points outward. If the tip of the acromion and the lateral epicondyle can be joined by a straight line (Hamilton's test), the shoulder is dislocated.

This appearance and the observation that the patient supports the injured arm with the other hand makes it possible for the examiner to diagnose a dislocated shoulder from the other end of the examination room. A similarly flattened contour is also seen in patients with atrophied deltoid muscles and in displaced fractures of the surgical neck. However, in these patients, the humeral head is still in its normal position and the ruler test is negative.

Damage to the axillary nerve that occurs as it runs around the neck of the humerus causes partial or complete paralysis of the deltoid. The axillary nerve should be examined with an electromyogram (EMG) 3 and 6 weeks after the injury. If the examiner finds no change in pathologic findings between the two examinations, the nerve has been damaged and specific treatment may be necessary.

Brachial plexus injuries also occur if there has been a violent abduction strain. If dislocation occurs and causes neurologic damage, the results are often poor.

The axillary artery can be damaged by traction at the time of injury or by pressure from the humeral head. The radial pulse should be checked, and its presence should be recorded.

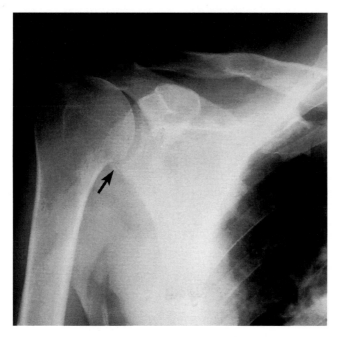

FIG. 4-89 Bankart lesion characterized by a small avulsion fragment of the inferior glenoid rim at the site of the triceps insertion *(arrow).* *(From Deltoff MN, Kogon PL: The portable skeletal x-ray library, St Louis, 1998, Mosby.)*

The humeral head occasionally buttonholes through the subscapularis. This action makes reduction impossible.

Chronic recurrent posterior subluxations are often demonstrable by the patient either by positioning the arm or by selected muscle contracture. It may be unilateral after trauma or bilateral with pain only on one side, with or without a precipitating traumatic event.

ORTHOPEDIC GAMUT 4-10

CHRONIC RECURRENT DISLOCATIONS

Four subsets of chronic recurrent dislocations are as follows:

1. Voluntary habitual (emotionally disturbed)
2. Voluntary
3. Not willful (muscular control)
4. Involuntary positional and involuntary unintentional (not demonstrable by patient)

The usual history is one of gradual onset in which subluxation of both shoulders can occur posteriorly either by contracture of the anterior deltoid and pectoralis (Fig. 4-91) or by arm position with the arm forward flexed (Fig. 4-92, *A*). Extension of the arm causes a sudden snap with a concomitant reduction (Fig. 4-92, *B*).

Although apprehension is common for anterior instability, it is not reliable for posterior instability.

PROCEDURE

- The patient places the hand of the affected shoulder on the opposite shoulder and attempts to touch the chest with the elbow (Fig. 4-93).
- The test is positive if the patient cannot touch the chest wall with the elbow (Fig. 4-94).
- The test is positive in shoulder dislocation.

Confirmation Procedures
Apprehension test, Bryant's sign, Calloway's test, Hamilton's test, Mazion's shoulder maneuver, and diagnostic imaging

---

DIAGNOSTIC STATEMENT

Dugas' test is positive on the left shoulder. This result indicates shoulder dislocation.

CLINICAL PEARL

In exceptional circumstances, the humeral head can become jammed below the glenoid with the arm pointing directly upward (luxatio erecta), presenting a spectacular appearance sometimes mistaken for hysteria. This condition is a true inferior dislocation. In contrast to anterior dislocation, the humeral head in this situation lies against the vessels and can cause ischemia. The rotator cuff is always damaged.

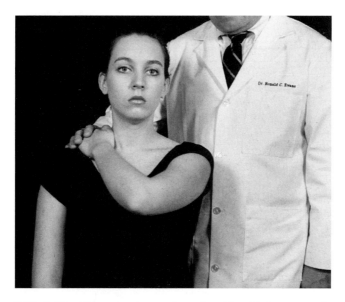

FIG. 4-93   The patient is seated comfortably with the arms at the sides. The patient places the hand of the affected shoulder on the opposite shoulder and attempts to touch the chest with the elbow.

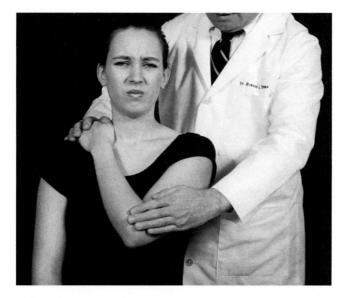

FIG. 4-94   If the patient cannot touch the chest wall with the elbow, the examiner confirms this by gently applying pressure to the elbow, attempting to approximate the elbow to the chest. Inability to move the elbow or increased pain is a positive sign. The presence of the sign indicates shoulder subluxation or dislocation.

Assessment for Subclavian Artery Stenosis or Occlusion

Comment

The vascular form of thoracic outlet syndrome is uncommon. It is characterized by a well-developed cervical rib producing stenosis and poststenotic dilation of the subclavian artery. The initial symptoms may vary from intermittent blanching of the hand and fingers as a result of embolization from a thrombus in the subclavian artery to a sudden catastrophic occlusion.

The Adson's test can be used to reproduce the symptoms by abducting and externally rotating the arm and raising the hand above the head. If the radial pulse disappears, a lesion of the subclavian artery should be suspected. It must be remembered that approximately 80% of healthy people demonstrate a positive Adson's test. Another provocative test is to have the patient raise both arms overhead and rapidly open and close the hand; this causes cramping very quickly if vascular thoracic outlet syndrome is present (Roos' test).

Effort thrombosis is a term used to describe a subclavian and axillary vein thrombosis caused by direct or indirect injury to the vein as a result of physical activity. This is a form of thoracic outlet syndrome that accounts for fewer than 2% of all reported incidents of deep vein thrombosis. Effort thrombosis has important short-term ramifications, such as severe disability and pulmonary embolism, that have been reported to occur in 12% of patients with subclavian vein thrombosis.

The symptoms and disability of effort thrombosis may persist for a prolonged period in 68% to 75% of patients. Although most cases result from trauma or use of cervical venous catheters, a small portion of the cases are related to various activities that require shoulder abduction.

The clinical presentation of effort thrombosis varies dramatically from intermittent, nonspecific symptoms that consist of a generalized aching of the arm, with a degree of fullness and swelling, to a dramatically swollen, painful arm with dependent rubor. Typically, this occurs in males 15 to 40 years of age, often after a particular physical activity. The symptoms may appear immediately or up to 2 weeks later. The most common symptom noted with time is increased swelling of the arm, which responds to elevation (venous tone assessment). Swelling may be accompanied by abnormal subcutaneous vein distension, which worsens if the arm is exercised.

In effort thrombosis, a venogram demonstrates occlusion of the axillary and subclavian veins, although the study itself may result in extension of the thrombosis. Doppler studies have been useful in distinguishing intermittent compression from thrombosis. Other noninvasive methods of evaluation include duplex scanning and impedance plethysmography.

Thoracic outlet syndrome describes the signs and symptoms resulting from proximal compression of the neurovascular structures supplying the upper limb.

The normal anatomy of the thoracic outlet, which extends from the intervertebral foramina and superior mediastinum to the axilla, must be considered not only in one plane but also in three dimensions to appreciate the potential mechanisms of compression.

The scalene muscles, which are the flexors and rotators of the neck, were formerly considered major causes of compression. This belief led not only to the term *scalenus anticus syndrome* but also to therapy directed solely at the release of these structures (scalenotomy). This method of therapy is a simple procedure with a high failure rate.

With many potential causes for compression, the three structures at risk—the subclavian artery, the vein, and the lower trunk of the brachial plexus—may be affected to significantly different degrees. The typical patient is likely to be a woman between the ages of 20 and 40. The ratio of women with thoracic outlet syndrome to men with the syndrome is 5:1. Complaints are often vague and hard to define.

PROCEDURE

- With the patient seated, the examiner assesses the patient's blood pressure bilaterally and records it (Fig. 4-95).
- The examiner also assesses the character of the patient's radial pulse bilaterally (Fig. 4-96).
- A difference of 10 mm Hg between the two systolic blood pressure readings and a feeble or absent radial pulse suggest possible subclavian artery stenosis or occlusion on the side of the feeble or absent pulse.
- If the test is negative, the examiner places a stethoscope over the supraclavicular fossa and auscultates the subclavian artery for bruits (Fig. 4-97).
- If bruits are present, subclavian artery stenosis or occlusion is suspected.

Confirmation Procedures

Adson's test, Allen maneuver, costoclavicular maneuver, Halstead maneuver, reverse Bakody maneuver, Roos' test, shoulder compression test, and Wright's test

---

DIAGNOSTIC STATEMENT

The results of George's screening procedure suggest subclavian artery stenosis or occlusion on the right.

CLINICAL PEARL

The shoulder joint can be linked with the hand in a symptom complex presenting the features of a reflex sympathetic disturbance. The shoulder symptoms may be due, in part, to the neurovascular upset that develops as a result of sympathetic stimulation. The shoulder complaint is usually secondary to some other factor, but the reflex dystrophy phenomenon has become so predominant that it is mislabeled as the cause when it is actually a result.

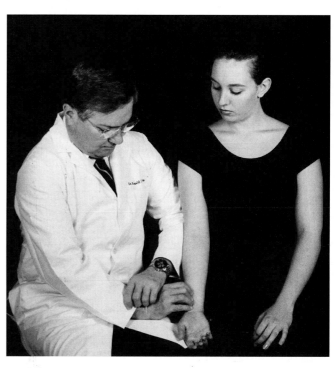

FIG. 4-96 The examiner bilaterally determines the character of the patient's radial pulse. A difference of 10 mm Hg between the two systolic blood pressures and a feeble or absent radial pulse suggests subclavian artery stenosis or occlusion on the side of the feeble or absent pulse.

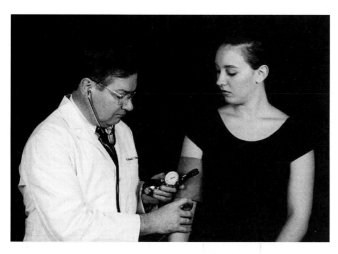

FIG. 4-95 The patient is seated. The examiner bilaterally assesses the patient's blood pressure and records the findings.

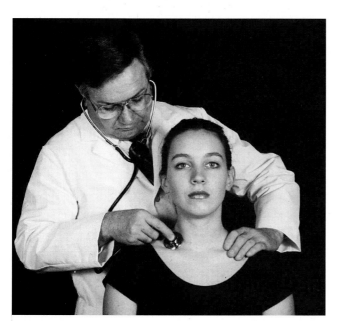

FIG. 4-97 If the first two procedures are negative, the examiner places a stethoscope over the supraclavicular fossa and auscultates the subclavian artery for bruits. If bruits are present, the screening procedure suggests a possible subclavian artery stenosis or occlusion.

HALSTEAD MANEUVER

Assessment for Thoracic Outlet Syndrome

Comment

Further out from the spinal cord, the nerve roots are grouped into trunks and cords that become intimately associated with the vascular bundle of the arm. The union takes place above the clavicle at a point where an additional cervical rib or tight scalenus anterior muscle may partially block the combined neurovascular bundle.

Compression of this bundle results in radiating discomfort and shoulder pain. However, the character of the pain changes from a well-defined neural pattern to a broad, more vague discomfort because of the vascular association. The general properties of both these pain conditions should be appreciated. Both conditions produce an aching neck, shoulder pain, a feeling of numbness, and tingling down the arm to the fingers. The inner aspect of the forearm and hand is the site usually involved, as opposed to the outer aspect of the thumb and index finger in the common cervical root lesions. The tingling that occurs often involves all of the fingers and produces a sense of fullness in the hand. If motor and sensory signs develop, they typically involve the ulnar supply because of pressure on the medial cord of the plexus. The small muscles of the hand may be involved, but either median or ulnar groups are singled out.

Entrapment neuropathy results from increased pressure on a nerve as it passes through an enclosed space. A nerve is most vulnerable to compression as it traverses a fibroosseous canal, where there is a disproportion of contents and capacity. Nerves that have previously been affected by a neuropathic process, as with diabetes or alcoholism, appear to be even more vulnerable to entrapment.

The signs and symptoms that accompany nerve entrapment may at times be subtle and easily confused with other orthopedic disorders.

Thoracic outlet syndrome is a term that encompasses a number of clinical entities. The syndrome results from compression of one or more of the neurovascular elements that pass through the superior thoracic aperture. In most cases, neurogenic entrapment accounts for the symptoms; rarely is there an isolated vascular lesion.

Patients usually experience sensory symptoms as the first manifestation of thoracic outlet syndrome. Paresthesias are common, which follow the ulnar nerve distribution along the medial aspect of the arm and forearm and then to the fourth and fifth fingers. Aching pain, radiating to the neck, shoulder, and arm, is common, often being more diffuse than the paresthesias. Carrying heavy objects, persistent abduction of the shoulder, and work that requires using the arms over the head may exacerbate these symptoms. Thoracic outlet syndrome is also more likely to occur in individuals with poor posture and drooping shoulders.

Signs of motor weakness, if they appear, usually follow the sensory complaints. Patients may describe a feeling of weakness or clumsiness in using the hand. Wasting of the thenar, hypothenar, and intrinsic muscles of the hand may be noted.

This distribution of atrophy, following a definite peripheral nerve pattern, is in contrast to progressive muscular atrophy, in which there is generalized involvement that does not follow a specific pattern.

Shoulder and arm movements are not particularly involved in either cervical rib or scalenus anticus disorders. Points of tenderness and soreness may be identified in the supraclavicular region away from the shoulder area proper and lying above the clavicle. When neck pain is present, it tends to be at the front, which is in contrast to the posterior discomfort of fibrositis and postural disorders.

PROCEDURE

- As the radial pulse of the affected arm is palpated, downward traction is applied on the extremity (Fig. 4-98).
- The neck is hyperextended (Fig. 4-99).
- Loss or diminution of the pulse suggests a positive test.
- If the test is negative, it is repeated with the patient rotating the head to the opposite side.
- Thoracic outlet syndrome is suggested by a positive test.

Confirmation Procedures

Adson's test, Allen maneuver, costoclavicular maneuver, George's screening procedure, reverse Bakody maneuver, Roos' test, shoulder compression test, and Wright's test

---

DIAGNOSTIC STATEMENT

Halstead maneuver is positive on the right shoulder. This result suggests the existence of thoracic outlet syndrome.

CLINICAL PEARL

Raynaud's disease, acroparesthesia, and thromboangiitis obliterans may be confused with thoracic outlet compression syndromes, but the former three conditions actually differ profoundly from outlet compression syndromes because Raynaud's disease, acroparesthesia, and thromboangiitis obliterans are not accompanied by shoulder discomfort, have no correlation to arm or shoulder movement, and are not affected by body posture.

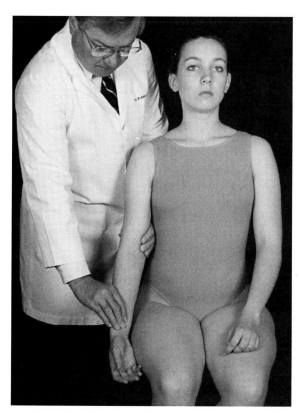

FIG. 4-98 The patient is seated comfortably with the arms at the sides. The examiner palpates the radial pulse of the affected arm.

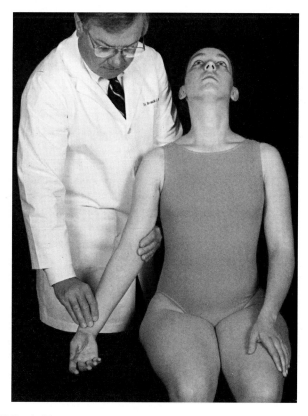

FIG. 4-99 The examiner applies downward traction on the affected extremity while the patient hyperextends the neck. Disappearance of the pulse is a positive test. A positive test indicates thoracic outlet syndrome. If the pulse does not disappear, the test is repeated with the patient's head rotated to the opposite side.

HAMILTON'S TEST

Assessment for Dislocation of the Shoulder

Comment

One of the consequences for superb mobility of the shoulder is frequent dislocation. A dislocated shoulder is an injury of the young, in whom it occurs more often than fracture of the neck of the humerus. Solid, healthy bone withstands abduction and twisting strain, but the weak capsule of the young gives way. Later in life, the bone becomes soft and the capsule contracts, so abduction and twisting result in shaft breaks while the joint remains intact. Young adults suffer this injury often. The most common accident that causes a dislocated shoulder is a fall with the arm outstretched for protection. The contribution of the elbow and body weight have been somewhat overlooked in explaining the mechanism of this injury. The essential episode is that the head of the humerus is forced against the weak anterior or anteroinferior capsule. In a fall, the outstretched hand absorbs the impact while the elbow is extended. As long as this extension is retained, a solid strut transmits the force to the superior or posterosuperior joint structures. The weight of the body alters this situation. As full weight is applied, momentary giving way or buckling of the elbow is inevitable. This breaks the solid strut, and the elbow must flex, which tilts the upper end of the humerus downward and forward. As the fall continues, the head slips off the glenoid rim easily. At this point, the extremity is in abduction and external rotation, exposing the posterosuperior part of the humeral head to the glenoid rim. The rim usually gets cut or creased. It is understandable that with repeated similar trauma, less and less force is needed to dislocate the humeral head. The humeral head commonly comes to lie at the front of the glenoid, resting on the rib. Occasionally, the humeral head lies higher, just below the clavicle.

In evaluating chronic laxity of the shoulder ligaments, the examiner first asks the patient to voluntarily reproduce subluxation of the shoulder to demonstrate laxity. Then provocative maneuvers to reproduce glenohumeral subluxations or dislocations can be done with the patient sitting, lying supine, or standing.

With the patient sitting, the examiner stabilizes the scapula by placing one finger on the coracoid and resting the body of the hand and forearm on the scapula. With the other hand, the index and middle fingers grasp the anterior humeral head and the thumb grasps the posterior head. A force is directed anteriorly and inferiorly (Fig. 4-100). Subluxation of the head over the anteroinferior glenoid rim is estimated as to degree. Pain may preclude this testing.

With the patient seated, abduction and external rotation of the involved arm and a force directed in an anteroinferior direction from behind may cause a palpable subluxation, labral crepitation, or frank dislocation (Fig. 4-101). The patient is most apprehensive and resists this maneuver when the arm is abducted to approximately 120 degrees and externally rotated. The patient's subjective apprehension that the shoulder may slip out of joint is considered a positive apprehension finding, whether or not there is actual joint subluxation.

Anterior (subcoracoid) glenohumeral joint dislocation (Fig. 4-102) is the most common (90%) of all four possible glenohumeral dislocations. The shoulder joint is the most commonly dislocated major body joint.

PROCEDURE

- If a straight edge (ruler or yardstick) can rest simultaneously on the acromial tip and the lateral epicondyle of the elbow, the test is positive (Fig. 4-103).
- The positive test is significant for dislocation of the shoulder.

Confirmation Procedures

Apprehension test, Bryant's sign, Calloway's test, Dugas' test, and Mazion's shoulder maneuver

---

DIAGNOSTIC STATEMENT

Hamilton's test is positive for the right shoulder. This result indicates dislocation trauma of the shoulder.

CLINICAL PEARL

Fractures of the humeral head that result in several fragments are usually accompanied by dislocation. Fracture dislocations of the humeral head present several problems: (1) the fragment may obstruct reduction and make open reduction necessary, (2) the reduction will be very unstable, (3) soft-tissue damage and hemorrhage into and around the shoulder lead to joint stiffness, and (4) avascular necrosis of the humeral head can follow fractures through the anatomic neck.

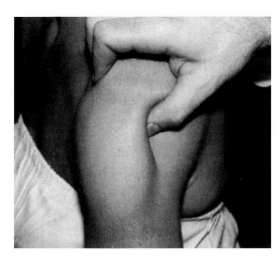

FIG. 4-100   Anteroinferior subluxation creates a void under the posterior acromion and a slight bulge below the coracoid. *(From Nicholas JA, Hershman EB, editors: The upper extremity in sports medicine, St Louis, 1990, Mosby.)*

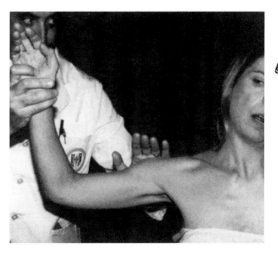

FIG. 4-101   Positive apprehension test. Attempts at anteroinferior subluxation of the abducted and externally rotated arm are exacerbated by forceful pressure on the proximal posterior humerus directed anteriorly. *(From Nicholas JA, Hershman EB, editors: The upper extremity in sports medicine, St Louis, 1990, Mosby.)*

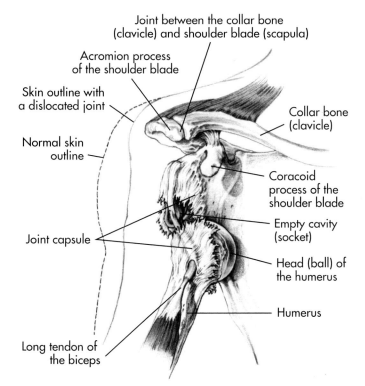

FIG. 4-102   Subcoracoid (anteroinferior) dislocation of the glenohumeral joint with tear of the glenoid labrum and joint capsule. *(From Saidoff DC, McDonough AL: Critical pathways in therapeutic intervention, St Louis, 1997, Mosby.)*

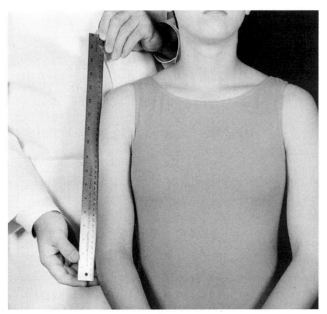

FIG. 4-103   The patient is seated comfortably with the arms at the sides. The examiner places a straight edge (ruler) at the lateral border of the affected shoulder from the acromion to the elbow. The test is positive if the straight edge can rest simultaneously on the acromial tip of the shoulder and the lateral epicondyle of the elbow. The test is significant for dislocation of the shoulder.

IMPINGEMENT SIGN

Assessment for Overuse Injury to the Supraspinatus or Biceps Tendons

Comment

The terminology for impingement lesions had led to confusion. Many names and causes for this condition have been cited, including *bursitis, tendinitis, acute trauma, overuse, instability, aging, tendon degeneration, vascular deficiencies,* and *mechanical impingement.* The rotator cuff is the only tendon situated between two bones.

ORTHOPEDIC GAMUT 4-11

IMPINGEMENT SYNDROME

The four stages of impingement syndrome are as follows:

Phase 1: edema and swelling (correlated with overuse tendinitis from activities requiring repetitive overhead arm action)

Phase 2: thickening and fibrosis (correlated with incomplete thickness rotator cuff tears)

Phase 3: comprises complete thickness tearing and bone changes (Fig. 4-104)

Phase 4: cuff tear arthropathy (occurs in a small percentage of neglected cuff tears) (Fig. 4-105)

The clinical presentations with impingement syndrome are recognized in young patients involved in activities using repetitive overhead arm motion. They become sore, and at times, a patient is unable to continue because of the pain that accompanies use of the arm at the level of the shoulder.

The differential diagnosis of rotator cuff impingement is adhesive capsulitis, nerve compression (C5-C6 disc) (Fig. 4-106), suprascapular neuropathy or other brachial plexus lesions, and shoulder instability.

The subacromial space is the most common site for impingement syndrome of symptoms in older active adults. This is usually associated with degenerative changes in the rotator cuff (Fig. 4-107, *A*).

Phase 2 impingement occurs more commonly in patients who are 35 to 50 years of age. Evidence of degeneration and fibrosis of the supraspinatus tendon and biceps tendon is noted (Fig. 4-107, *B*).

Phase 3 impingement involves a complete tear of the rotator cuff, most commonly the supraspinatus tendon (Fig. 4-107, *C*), less commonly the subscapularis tendon.

Tenosynovitis of the long head of the biceps is a common cause of shoulder pain in adults older than 40. This condition also may occur in young athletes from repeated strains, such as those caused by the throwing motion. The basic lesion is an inflammation of the tendon and its sheath in the bicipital groove. The disorder may be primary or secondary to disease of the overlying rotator cuff.

The biceps tendon may rupture as a result of advanced degeneration from chronic tendinitis. The rupture is usually complete and may follow a forceful contraction of the biceps muscle.

The biceps tendon may occasionally dislocate from the bicipital groove. The usual cause is a tear in the overlying subscapularis tendon as the result of degenerative changes. The condition also may result from a congenitally shallow groove. The disorder also may occur in the young patient after forceful external rotation and abduction of the shoulder. Recurrences are common and may be reproducible by the patient. Tenosynovitis often develops, leading to pain and stiffness.

PROCEDURE

- The patient's arm is slightly abducted and moved fully through flexion (Figs. 4-108 to 4-110).
- This move causes a jamming of the greater tuberosity into the anteroinferior acromial surface.
- A positive result is pain in the shoulder.
- A positive test suggests injury to the supraspinatus and sometimes to the biceps tendons.

Confirmation Procedures

Apley's test, subacromial push-button sign, supraspinatus press test, and Codman's sign

---

DIAGNOSTIC STATEMENT

Impingement sign is present in the right shoulder. This result indicates an overuse injury of the supraspinatus or biceps tendon.

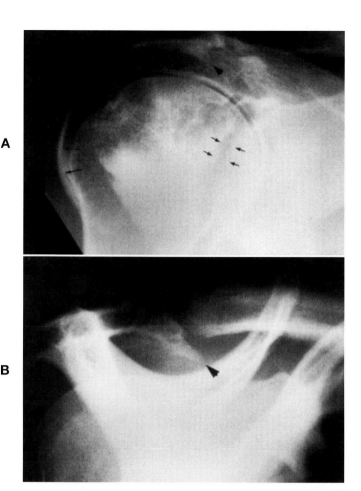

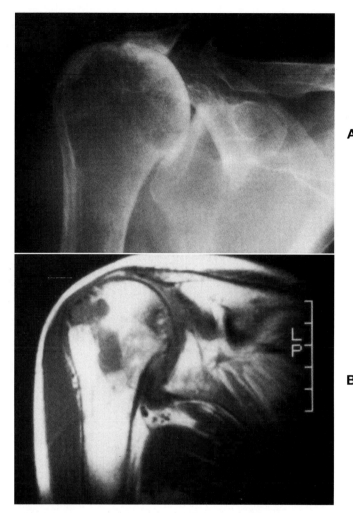

FIG. 4-104 Rotator cuff tear with stage III impingement. **A,** Calcification is seen extending into the superior portion of the coracoacromial ligament. **B,** This type III hooked acromion is the most common shape associated with tearing of the rotator cuff. *(From Nicholas JA, Hershman EB, editors:* The upper extremity in sports medicine, *St Louis, 1990, Mosby.)*

FIG. 4-105 Rotator cuff tear arthropathy with loss of the supraspinatus and superior migration of the humeral head. **A,** The humeral head thins out the acromion as a new facet is formed superiorly. The humeral head can no longer be fixed within the glenoid for adequate elevation or use of the intact deltoid. **B,** Magnetic resonance imaging demonstrates roughening and necrosis of the subchondral bone. *(From Nicholas JA, Hershman EB, editors:* The upper extremity in sports medicine, *St Louis, 1990, Mosby.)*

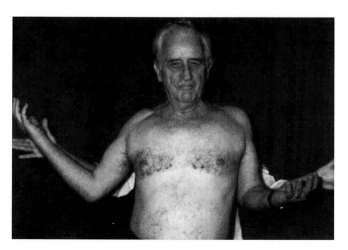

FIG. 4-106 Herniated C5-C6 disc resulting in external rotation weakness mimics rotator cuff tear of the left shoulder. Once the arms are released, the left arm falls in toward the stomach, demonstrating passive but not active external rotation. *(From Nicholas JA, Hershman EB, editors:* The upper extremity in sports medicine, *St Louis, 1990, Mosby.)*

CLINICAL PEARL

The archaic concept of the hunching girdle rhythm as the telltale mark of supraspinatus rupture needs to be discarded. Without resistance, a decrease in the range of motion may not be apparent. Motion must always be assessed against resistance. The presence of consistent weakness helps differentiate a tear from simple chronic tendinitis.

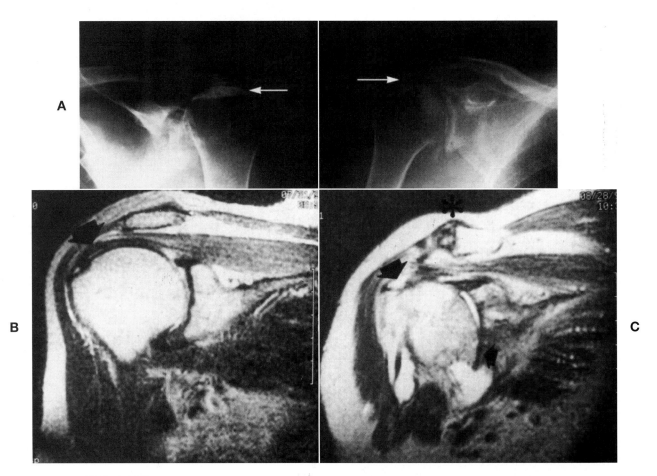

FIG. 4-107 **A,** Normal magnetic resonance imaging (MRI) scan of the shoulder. **B,** MRI of the shoulder showing a partial rotator cuff tear. **C,** MRI of the shoulder showing a complete tear of the rotator cuff. *(From Lewis CB, Knortz KA: Orthopedic assessment and treatment of the geriatric patient, St Louis, 1993, Mosby.)*

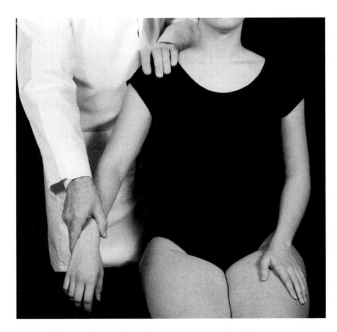

FIG. 4-108   The patient is seated comfortably with the arms at the sides. The examiner slightly abducts the patient's affected arm moving it through forward flexion.

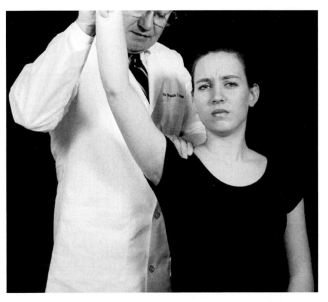

FIG. 4-109   Forward flexion causes jamming of the greater tuberosity against the anteroinferior acromial surface. Pain in the shoulder is a positive result. A positive test indicates an overuse injury to the supraspinatus and sometimes the biceps tendon.

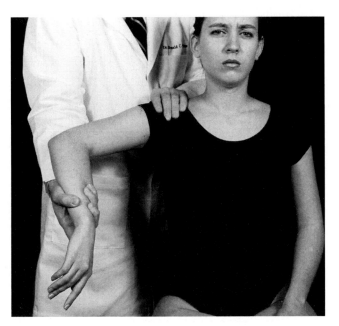

FIG. 4-110   As an alternative, the examiner can internally rotate the affected shoulder. This rotation occurs while the shoulder is abducted to 90 degrees and flexed at the elbow. The arm also can be moved into flexion, which will produce the same jamming effect.

LUDINGTON'S TEST

Assessment for Rupture of the Long Head of the Biceps Tendon

Comment

Although commonly diagnosed, bicipital tendinitis is not often seen in isolation and usually occurs in association with rotator cuff tendinitis or impingement or with glenohumeral instability. The bicipital tendon acts as a secondary stabilizer of the humeral head, and the translational movement seen with glenohumeral laxity can place increased stress on the tendon, leading to tendinitis.

Pain is usually felt over the anterior aspect of the shoulder, often radiating into the biceps muscle with well-localized tenderness over the tendon as it runs in the bicipital groove. Pain is felt with overhead activities and often with shoulder extension and elbow flexion. Examination may reveal features of impingement, rotator cuff tendinitis, and instability, all of which are important in determining the cause of bicipital tendinitis. Pain may be reproduced with resisted elbow flexion, supination, and shoulder flexion. Passive shoulder extension stretches the biceps and may be painful. Rupture of the tendon is evident when there is the characteristic deformity of the upper arm with bunching up of the lateral muscle belly of the biceps best seen with resisted elbow flexion and supination.

Acute rupture of the transverse humeral ligament can result in subluxation or dislocation of the tendon. This can present with symptoms similar to bicipital tendinitis, but often a more specific complaint is made of catching and a clicking sensation at the shoulder. Clinical examination may demonstrate subluxation of the tendon, which is felt as the arm is passively moved through internal and external rotation while in the 90-degree abducted position. Medial dislocation of the tendon is often found in association with tears of the subscapularis tendon.

The tendon of the long head of the biceps may be involved at several sites: its attachment to the superior glenoid labrum, which may be injured in a fall or throwing action (superior labrum anteroposterior [SLAP] lesion); as it runs across the glenohumeral joint (intraarticular); or as it runs in the bicipital groove (extraarticular). The transverse humeral ligament stabilizes the tendon in the bicipital groove, and if this mechanism is disrupted, subluxation or dislocation of the tendon can result. This tends to occur as the arm is rotated in the abducted position. The tendon can become inflamed, thickened, and fibrotic in chronic cases. Older patients may have attenuation and thinning of the tendon, and rupture may eventually ensue. This latter presentation is almost always indicative of underlying rotator cuff degeneration as the bicipital tendon appears to become stressed in its attempt to act as a humeral head depressor in cases of rotator cuff incompetence. Also, the presence of a complete rotator cuff tear exposes the intraarticular portion of the bicipital tendon to the overlying acromion and further impingement.

PROCEDURE

- The patient clasps both hands behind the head.
- The biceps tendons are in resting positions.
- The patient alternately contracts and relaxes the biceps muscles.
- As the patient contracts the muscles, the examiner palpates the biceps tendons (Fig. 4-111).
- The tendon will be felt to contract on the uninvolved side but not on the affected side.
- A positive test result is the loss of tendon contraction.
- A positive test suggests rupture of the long head of the biceps tendon.

Confirmation Procedures

Abbott-Saunders test, Speed's test, transverse humeral ligament test, and Yergason's test

---

DIAGNOSTIC STATEMENT

Ludington's test is positive on the right or left. This result indicates disruption of the biceps tendon.

CLINICAL PEARL

A double defect sometimes occurs, with the cuff giving way from the tuberosity on both sides of the tendon. Cuff laxity at this point seriously interferes with biceps function, and the tendon may slip medially over the lesser tuberosity and off the head.

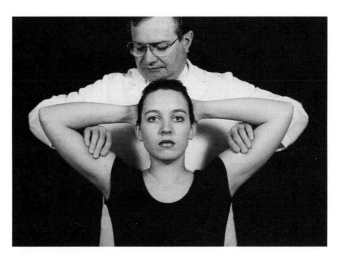

FIG. 4-111 Seated, the patient clasps both hands behind the head. The patient contracts and relaxes the biceps muscles. During this action, the examiner palpates the biceps tendons. The test is positive if tendon contraction is absent on the affected side. A positive test suggests a rupture of the long head of the biceps tendon.

MAZION'S SHOULDER MANEUVER

ALSO KNOWN AS SHOULDER ROCK TEST

Assessment for Significant Pathologic Process of the Shoulder

Comment

Pain felt in the cervicobrachial area may extend from the occiput to the arm or, at times, to the upper anterior chest and back.

Muscle strain and nerve root compression often follow this distribution. Tendinitis, arthritis, and trigger points usually cause a more localized discomfort that enables the patient to pinpoint the source of the pathologic process. One notable exception is the pain of acute subdeltoid bursitis. In this condition, the patient thinks that the discomfort can be located precisely in the musculature of the upper arm, but tenderness is always over the inflamed area, several centimeters higher, and beneath the acromion. Having the patient characterize the onset of the pain, including whether it was precipitated by acute or repeated trauma to the shoulder and neck, narrows the differential diagnosis. For example, continuous use of the arm above the head predisposes it to bursitis or tendinitis. Acute injury, of course, can result in obvious fractures or dislocations. Lacerations of the rotator cuff may be more elusive. Sudden lifting of a heavy object is all that is needed to tear the subacromial tendons.

Shoulder pain brought on by exertion, especially if the upper extremities are not being used, is more apt to be caused by coronary insufficiency than by a localized pathologic process.

The clinical history may be the key to diagnosis. For example, adhesive capsulitis follows immobilization of the joint, shoulder-arm-hand syndrome is a complication of myocardial infarction, and fibromyositis is associated with emotional tension. Shoulder pain of arthritis and polymyalgia rheumatica is insidious at the onset. The pain from both of the conditions is worse in the morning when the patient arises from sleep. Other disorders may be worse during the day. The temporal relationships of the pain are important to the diagnosis. Pain severity, constancy, and migratory nature are also important.

The most common complaint of patients with arthritis of the shoulder is pain. Typically, the pattern of pain is worsened with activities and somewhat relieved by rest. Patients often complain of night pain during recumbency. It is important to note a medication history with particular attention to oral steroids, which may cause osteonecrosis. Patients with rheumatoid arthritis are affected by mechanical changes from rotator cuff dysfunction as well as joint destruction in the glenohumeral joint. A general history combined with a physical examination should allow the examiner to limit the number of ancillary diagnostic tests to determine the cause of the arthritic condition. It is important that patients be examined in a relaxed atmosphere with full visualization of the entire upper trunk. Observation of range of motion with notation of scapulothoracic rhythm is helpful in determining what portion of the range is coming from the glenohumeral joint. Muscle examination includes strength measurement and examination for wasting or atrophy. Rotator cuff integrity, stability, and the patient's ability to perform activities such as combing hair, reaching the buttock, and dressing are assessed. Particular attention should be paid to loss of rotation.

PROCEDURE

- While standing or sitting, the patient places the palm of the affected upper limb over the top of the opposite clavicle (Fig. 4-112).
- From this position, the patient moves the elbow from the chest to the forehead, giving it an inferior to superior rocking motion (Figs. 4-113 and 4-114).
- The maneuver is positive if this action produces or aggravates shoulder or arm pain on the ipsilateral side.
- The pain of any significant pathologic process of the shoulder will be intensified and localized by this maneuver.

Confirmation Procedures

Apprehension test, Bryant's sign, Calloway's test, Dugas' test, Hamilton's test, and diagnostic imaging

---

DIAGNOSTIC STATEMENT

Mazion's shoulder maneuver is positive on the right. This result indicates a significant pathologic process of the shoulder.

CLINICAL PEARL

Adhesive capsulitis is a common but ill-understood affliction of the glenohumeral joint. Capsulitis is characterized by pain and uniform limitation of all movements but without radiographic change and with a tendency to a slow spontaneous recovery. There is no evidence of inflammatory or destructive change.

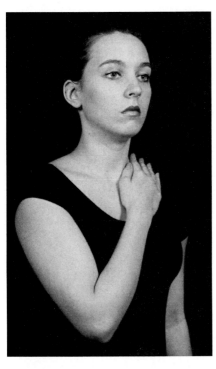

FIG. 4-112   While seated, the patient places the palm of the hand of the affected shoulder over the top of the opposite clavicle.

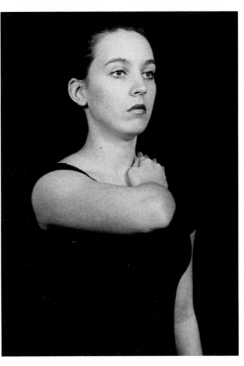

FIG. 4-113   The patient moves the elbow of the affected side from the chest toward the forehead.

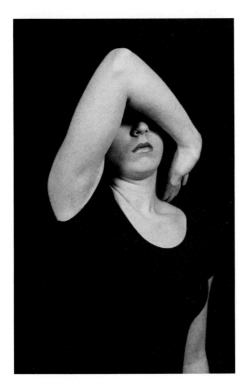

FIG. 4-114   This movement provides an inferior to superior rocking motion. The maneuver is positive if this action produces or aggravates shoulder or arm pain on the ipsilateral side. This maneuver will intensify and localize the pain of any significant shoulder pathology.

REVERSE BAKODY MANEUVER

Assessment for Cervical Foraminal Compression and Interscalene Compression

Comment

Thoracic outlet syndrome is a disorder characterized by compression of the subclavian artery, vein, or brachial plexus separately or, rarely, in combination. This compression results in a vascular or neurogenic syndrome, depending on which structure is involved. Neurogenic thoracic outlet syndrome is a neurologic syndrome caused by compression of the lower brachial plexus.

True, or classic, neurogenic thoracic outlet syndrome usually is caused by a congenital band that originates from the tip of the rudimentary cervical rib and inserts into the first rib. In this form, there is objective clinical and electrophysiologic evidence of peripheral nerve fiber injury that usually is limited to the lower trunk of the plexus. The typical patient is a young woman with weakness of the hand and wasting of the thenar more than the hypothenar eminence who experiences variable pain and paresthesia in the medial aspect of the upper extremity. Symptoms commonly are exacerbated by upper extremity activity. Multiple compression sites have been described, resulting in many "syndromes" (Fig. 4-115).

Electrodiagnostic examination is the most useful and objective diagnostic procedure in the diagnosis of neurogenic thoracic outlet syndrome. The compression results in a chronic, axon-loss, lower trunk brachial plexopathy (Fig. 4-116). Because all ulnar sensory fibers, all ulnar motor fibers, and the C8-T1 median fibers course the lower trunk, they are among the most obviously noted abnormalities on routine nerve conduction study (NCS).

A cervical rib is a congenital overdevelopment, bony or fibrous, of the costal process of the seventh cervical vertebra. A cervical rib often exists without causing symptoms, especially in the young. However, in adults, the tendency for gradual drooping of the shoulder girdle may lead to neurologic or vascular disturbance in the upper limb.

The overdeveloped costal process may be unilateral or bilateral, and it can range in size from a small bony protrusion, often with a fibrous extension, to a complete supernumerary rib. The subclavian artery and the lowest trunk of the brachial plexus arch over the rib. In some cases, the nerve trunk suffers damage at the site of pressure against the rib. This accounts for the neurologic manifestations. The vascular changes are accounted for by local damage to the subclavian artery, from which thrombotic emboli may be repeatedly discharged into the peripheral vessels of the upper limb.

A cervical rib is often symptomless. When symptoms occur, they usually begin during adult life. They may be neurologic, vascular, or combined.

The sensory symptoms are pain and paresthesia in the forearm and hand. These symptoms are most marked toward the medial (ulnar) side and are often relieved temporarily by changing the position of the arm. The motor symptoms include increasing weakness of the hand with difficulty carrying out the finer movements.

There is usually an area of sensory impairment and sometimes complete anesthesia in the forearm and hand. The affected area does not correspond in distribution to any of the peripheral nerves but may be related to the lowest trunk of the brachial plexus. There may be atrophy of the muscles of the thenar eminence or of the interosseous and hypothenar muscles.

The vascular changes that have been observed range from dusky cyanosis of the forearm and hand to gangrene of the fingers. The radial pulse may be weak or absent.

ORTHOPEDIC GAMUT 4-12

UPPER EXTREMITY NEUROGENIC SYNDROMES

The important alternative causes of upper extremity neurogenic syndromes include the following:

1. Central lesions (tumors involving the spinal cord or its roots)
2. Plexus lesions (tumors at the thoracic inlet Pancoast's tumor)
3. Distal nerve lesions (friction neuritis of the ulnar nerve at the elbow)
4. Pressure on the median nerve in the carpal tunnel

Occasionally, the neurologic manifestations characteristic of a cervical rib occur without a demonstrable skeletal deformity. The manifestations may have been ascribed to trapping of the nerves between the first rib and the clavicle (costoclavicular compression) or between the first rib and the scalenus anterior muscle, or to stretching of the lowest trunk of the brachial plexus over the normal first rib. More often, they are caused by a tough fibrous band in the scalenus medius muscle that may lead to kinking of the lowest trunk of the brachial plexus. The symptoms are easily

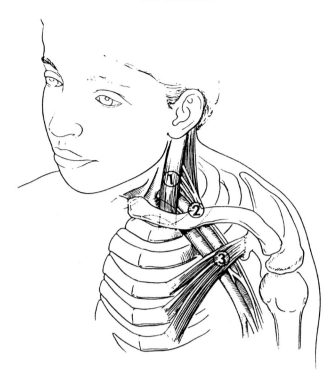

FIG. 4-115 The presumed sites of compression within the cervicoaxillary canal for the "scalenus anticus syndrome": *1,* Interscalene triangle, the costoclavicular syndrome; *2,* between the first rib and the clavicle; and *3,* the hyperabduction syndrome, beneath the pectoralis minor tendon. *(From Katirji B: Electromyography in clinical practice: a case study approach, St Louis, 1998, Mosby.)*

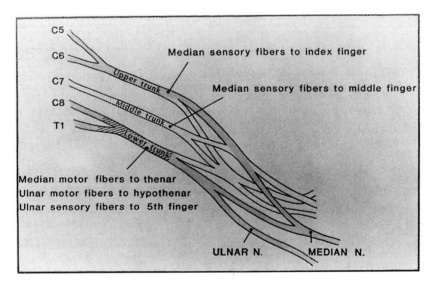

FIG. 4-116 Routine nerve conduction changes (median and ulnar) with neurogenic thoracic outlet syndrome. *(From Wilbourn AJ: Case report #7: true neurogenic thoracic outlet syndrome, Rochester, Minn, 1982, American Association of Electrodiagnostic Medicine.)*

confused with those from a prolapsed intervertebral disc between C7 and T1.

PROCEDURE

- While in the seated position, the patient actively places the palm of the affected extremity on top of the head, raising the elbow to a height approximately level with the head (Fig. 4-117).
- By elevating the arm, interscalene compression increases.
- The sign is present when the radiating pain appears or is worsened with this maneuver (Fig. 4-118).
- The sign helps differentiate between cervical foraminal compression and interscalene compression.

Confirmation Procedures

Adson's test, Allen maneuver, costoclavicular maneuver, George's screening procedure, Halstead maneuver, Roos' test, shoulder compression test, and Wright's test

DIAGNOSTIC STATEMENT

The presence of brachial plexus compression is indicated by the presence of a reverse Bakody sign on the right.

CLINICAL PEARL

Radiographs will show the abnormal rib. If it is small, it is clearly observed in the oblique projections. In cases of suspected vascular obstruction, arteriography is required.

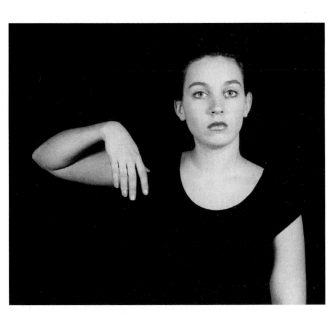

FIG. 4-117   While seated, the patient abducts and externally rotates the affected shoulder, moving the hand toward the top of the head.

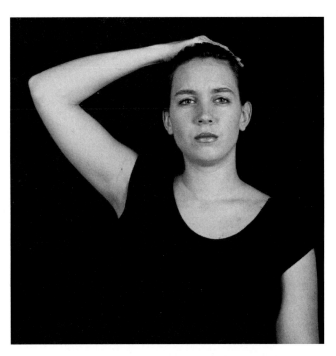

FIG. 4-118   The hand is placed on top of the head. The increase of pain in this position is a positive sign and indicates interscalene compression of the lower branches of the brachial plexus.

ROOS' TEST

Assessment for Thoracic Outlet Syndrome

Comment
The thoracic outlet syndrome complex refers to a series of neurovascular compression syndromes in the shoulder region. Thoracic outlet syndrome is recognized as an entrapment compression vasculopathy of the subclavian vessels. This more commonly involves the lower trunk or medial cord of the brachial plexus at any one of four sites (Fig. 4-119).

Costoclavicular syndrome occurs with compression of the subclavian artery, subclavian vein, and brachial plexus as they pass between the clavicle and the first rib. This syndrome is separate from the anterior scalene syndrome because of the vascular involvement.

The triangular costoclavicular space connects the cervical spine with the upper extremity and is called the *canalis cervicoaxillaris*. The boundaries of this space are as follows: anteriorly, the medial third of the clavicle and the subclavius muscle; posteriorly, the upper margin of the scapula; and posteromedially, the anterior third of the first rib and the insertions of the anterior and medial scalene muscles. The neurovascular bundle runs in the medial angle of this triangle. The subclavian vein lies medially in front of the anterior scalenus insertion on the first rib and deep to the costoclavicular ligament and thickening of the clavipectoral fascia, which extends from the coracoid process to the first rib (costocoracoid ligament). The subclavian artery briefly enters this space via the posterior scalene foramen to lie lateral to the subclavian vein. Passing between the anterior and medial scalene muscles, the brachial plexus joins the vascular bundle in the costoclavicular space.

When the costoclavicular space becomes narrowed by disease or dynamic compression, the neuromuscular structures are compromised. Although congenital anomalies are associated with thoracic outlet syndrome, functional or dynamic anatomy predominates as a cause for clinical disease.

ORTHOPEDIC GAMUT 4-13

COSTOCLAVICULAR NEUROVASCULAR SPACE

The following actions narrow the costoclavicular neurovascular space:

1. Raising the arm rotates the clavicle posteriorly into the space.
2. Displacing the shoulder posteriorly and interiorly rotates the clavicle posteriorly.
3. Inhaling deeply raises the first rib into the space because the clavicle does not rise with inspiration.

Patients with costoclavicular syndrome have subjective complaints similar to those of the anterior scalene syndrome (scalenus anticus syndrome). Although the neurologic complaints of pain, paresthesia, and hyperesthesia dominate in the anterior scalene syndrome, vascular symptoms dominate in the costoclavicular syndrome. Vein compression leads to temporary or permanent edema.

Clinical examination relies on the radial pulse evaluation, which occurs when the patient thrusts the chest forward and posteriorly and interiorly pulls the shoulders. Typically, the pulse weakens or disappears.

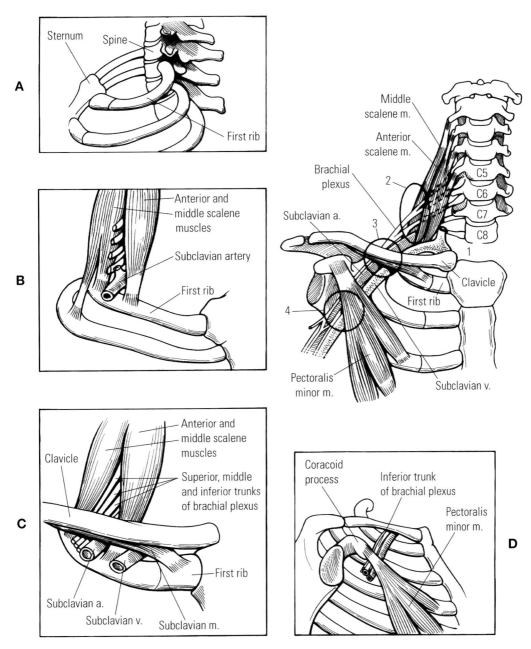

FIG. 4-119 The thoracic outlet has four sections. **A,** Sternocostovertebral space. **B,** The scalene triangle. **C,** The costoclavicular space. **D,** The coracopectoral space. *(From Saidoff DC, McDonough AL: Critical pathways in therapeutic intervention, St Louis, 1997, Mosby.)*

PROCEDURE

- While in the seated position, the patient positions both arms at 90 degrees and abducts and externally rotates them (Fig. 4-120).
- The patient repeatedly opens and closes the fists for up to 3 minutes (Fig. 4-121).
- If this maneuver reproduces the usual symptoms of discomfort, the patient probably has thoracic outlet syndrome (Fig. 4-122).

Confirmation Procedures

Adson's test, Allen maneuver, costoclavicular maneuver, George's screening procedure, Halstead maneuver, reverse Bakody maneuver, shoulder compression test, and Wright's test

---

DIAGNOSTIC STATEMENT

Roos' test is positive on the right. This result suggests thoracic outlet syndrome.

CLINICAL PEARL

Because all of the neurologic, arterial, and venous symptoms are consistently aggravated by both exercise and arm elevation, the most reliable test for the diagnosis of thoracic outlet syndrome is the 3-minute elevated-arm stress test (EAST).

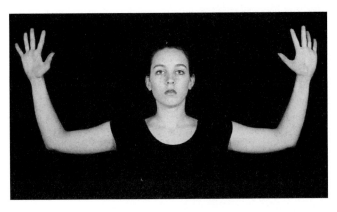

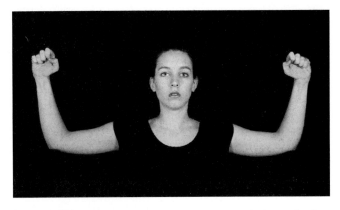

FIG. 4-120   While in the seated position, the patient places both arms in the 90-degree abducted and externally rotated position.

FIG. 4-121   The patient repeatedly opens and closes the fists slowly for 3 minutes.

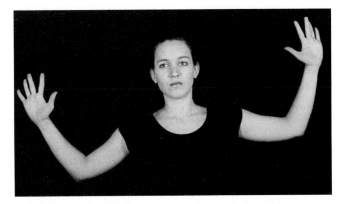

FIG. 4-122   If the test is positive, the usual symptoms are reproduced and the affected arm weakens. A positive test indicates thoracic outlet syndrome.

Assessment for Hyperabduction
Type of Thoracic Outlet Syndromes

Comment

The diagnosis of thoracic outlet syndrome is a clinical one that is largely reached by exclusion.

Ulnar nerve entrapment is suggested by nocturnal numbness, but patients never have sensory loss in the proximal or middle portions of the forearm. In addition, patients with ulnar nerve entrapment have no atrophy of the intrinsic muscles innervated by the median nerve in the thenar eminence. Carpal tunnel syndrome also can cause thenar atrophy, but the sensory loss, if present, manifests in the first two digits. Carpal tunnel syndrome is also differentiated from thoracic outlet syndrome by electrophysiologic studies indicating distal, not proximal, compression. In C8 cervical radiculopathy, there is compression with an almost identical pattern of T1 nerve fibers as in thoracic outlet syndrome. Neck pain, triceps weakness, reduced triceps reflex, and weakness of finger extensors provide a clue toward involvement of the C8 nerve root. Intramedullary or extramedullary spinal cord process such as syringomyelia, glioma of the spinal cord, extramedullary cervical tumor, infarction of the spinal cord, or meningioma in the foramen magnum may mimic thoracic outlet syndrome.

ORTHOPEDIC GAMUT 4-14

EXCLUDING THE THORACIC OUTLET

The following signs generally do not implicate the thoracic outlet:

1. Long tract signs such as brisk reflexes or extensor plantar response
2. Loss of tendon reflexes in the arms
3. Horner's syndrome
4. Weakness of the upper arm or shoulder

Pancoast's tumor, also known as *pulmonary superior sulcus tumor,* is accompanied by rapid and severe weakness of all of the small muscles of the hand and, in advanced cases, result in radiographically visible cancerous erosion of the first and second ribs, as well as possible hoarseness attributable to paralysis of one vocal cord.

Clavipectoral compression syndrome is a disorder that produces shoulder and other radiating symptoms but does not belong to the cervical root or scalenus or cervical rib classes. The syndrome resembles the latter because the findings suggest a vascular or neurovascular cause. Many forms of clavipectoral compression have been erroneously called *scalene* or *cervical rib* lesions. However, there are further distinguishing features that separate these conditions. The complete cause and pathology have not been firmly established, so clinical attributes are largely relied on for classification.

The symptom common to the group as a whole is paresthesia, or numbness and tingling, in the hand and fingers. Paresthesia develops after vague shoulder discomfort. The peripheral portion of the extremity, forearm, hand, and fingers quickly becomes the seat of the prominent discomfort, and the shoulder symptoms fade. The paresthesia follows no well-defined distribution, and the pattern is indistinct, particularly compared with the pain or numbness of peripheral nerve lesions. Often, both sides are involved. The vascular contribution is manifested by coldness, cyanotic hue, and crampy pain on effort. Writer's cramp is an example. Many of the symptoms and disorders have a striking relation to the position of the arm or the head. In many instances, the abducted position of the arm at work or rest is a potent irritant.

The fundamental pathologic process common to the group is stretching and compression of the neurovascular bundle at some point in the periclavicular, not clavicular, course. This possibility above the clavicle has been acknowledged in cervical rib and scalene lesions, but generally it has not been recognized that a similar disturbance may arise behind and below the clavicle as well. Pressure on the neurovascular bundle along the cervicoaxillary canal may develop directly behind the clavicle, below the clavicle, or behind the pectoralis minor. The bundle lies on a firm bed along its entire course, but the structures on top of it move in three separate zones. Superiorly, the clavicle rolls up and down and may pinch vessels on the first rib. Lower down, the costocoracoid membrane, as a remnant of the precoracoid primitive form, may tighten on the bundle through its connections with the enveloping fascia. Still more distally, the sharp edge of the pectoralis minor may become the compressing force or fulcrum. A soft bundle on a hard bed is easily crushed by these structures. Several special types of compression may be recognized: costoclavicular, postural, and hyperabduction. These conditions are to be differentiated from carpal tunnel syndrome, in which there is no shoulder involvement and the numbness and tingling are clearly confined to the median nerve distribution.

Patients with hyperabduction syndrome are usually young males of short, stocky stature who work long hours with the arms held above the shoulder level. Shoulder pain and finger paresthesia develop. In some instances, the discomfort appears without extreme abduction. Some patients are more prone than others to develop these symptoms. Patients prone to this condition are easily separated from the rest by their medical history, their youth, and the characteristically easy obliteration of the pulse during abduction.

PROCEDURE

- While the patient is seated upright, the examiner palpates the distal apex of the coracoid process and marks it with a flesh pencil (Fig. 4-123).
- With a hypothenar contact, the examiner applies downward pressure over the marked area (Fig. 4-124).
- Production of symptoms that are similar to neurovascular compression of the subclavian artery and brachial plexus constitutes a positive test.

- The test is significant for coracoid pressure syndrome, which is identical to the hyperabduction type of thoracic outlet syndromes.

Confirmation Procedures
Adson's test, Allen maneuver, costoclavicular test, George's screening procedure, Halstead maneuver, reverse Bakody maneuver, Roos' test, and Wright's test

DIAGNOSTIC STATEMENT

Shoulder compression test on the right is positive. This result indicates thoracic outlet compression caused by coracoid pressure.

CLINICAL PEARL

The neurovascular bundle may be compressed in the zone distal to the clavicle as the bundle passes beneath the costocoracoid membrane and pectoralis minor. The pectoralis minor has a particular contribution in this process and is a significant factor in creating the shoulder and radiating symptoms. A patient's degree of skeletal maturation has a great influence on the type of fracture that may result from trauma and the concern physicians have about the sequelae of such injuries. First, the relative softness of the bones of newborns and toddlers increases the likelihood of trauma producing a "greenstick fracture" rather than an ordinary fracture completely separating the two bone fragments. Another crucial consideration in the evaluation of fractures in children is the possible involvement of the epiphyseal plates of the bone in the fracture. If the line of a fracture crosses one of these areas of bone growth, the posthealing alignment of the bone on opposite sides of the plate is disturbed, and the subsequent growth and development of the bone will be asymmetric.

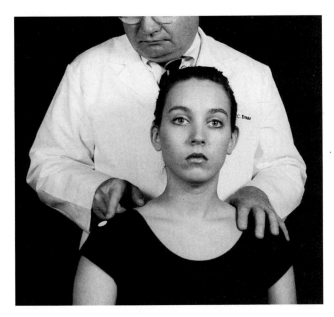

FIG. 4-123 The patient is seated comfortably with the arms at the sides. The examiner palpates the distal apex of the coracoid process and marks it.

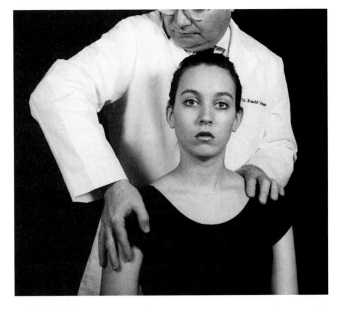

FIG. 4-124 With a hypothenar contact, the examiner applies downward pressure over the marked area. If the symptoms produced are similar to neurovascular compression of the subclavian artery and brachial plexus, this constitutes a positive test. The test is significant for coracoid pressure syndrome, which is identical to the hyperabduction type of thoracic outlet syndromes.

SPEED'S TEST

Assessment for Bicipital Tendinitis

Comment

The bicipital groove is between the greater and lesser tuberosities and lies along the anterior aspect of the surface of the humerus. The bicipital groove demonstrates varying configurations, depending on the height of the medial wall of the groove, formed by the lesser tuberosity (Fig. 4-125).

The long head of the biceps arises by a long, narrow tendon from the supraglenoid tubercle of the scapula. The long head passes through the shoulder joint and emerges from it to lie in the intertubercular sulcus (bicipital groove), where it is restrained by the transverse humeral ligament. The long head of the biceps is subject to the same type of impingement as the supraspinatus tendon, and it is initially difficult to differentiate the two. One distinguishing feature relates to internal and external rotation of the shoulder. In cases of bicipital tendinitis, rotation during abduction is usually painful, especially if the examiner applies slight pressure to the tendon in its groove while the patient's arm is passively maneuvered. In patients with supraspinatus tendinitis, the internally rotated position may be painful, but this pain will disappear when the humerus is rotated outward because the greater tubercle of the humerus no longer impinges on the acromion process.

The slight difference in the mechanics of these two types of tendinitis means that bicipital tendinitis occurs more often in patients who participate in activities involving throwing or paddling. Of course, bicipital tendinitis may occur in swimmers or other patients as well. Bicipital tendinitis is sometimes secondary to supraspinatus tendinitis because the latter may be accompanied by inflammation that involves the nearby biceps.

PROCEDURE

- Shoulder flexion by the patient is restricted (Fig. 4-126).
- The patient further resists forearm supinating and elbow extension.
- A positive test is indicated by increased tenderness in the bicipital groove (Fig. 4-127).
- A positive test suggests bicipital tendinitis.

Confirmation Procedures

Abbott-Saunders test, Ludington's test, transverse humeral ligament test, and Yergason's test

---

DIAGNOSTIC STATEMENT

Speed's test is positive on the right. This result indicates bicipital tendinitis.

CLINICAL PEARL

Tenosynovitis in the bicipital groove may develop into complete adherence of the tendon. This interdicts any extensive range of motion of the shoulder. The shoulder motion may remain restricted, or the biceps may rupture proximal to the groove.

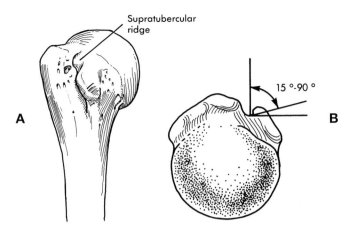

FIG. 4-125 **A,** Bicipital groove with supratubercular ridge. **B,** Angle of inclination of medial wall. *(From Nicholas JA, Hershman EB, editors:* The upper extremity in sports medicine, *St Louis, 1990, Mosby.)*

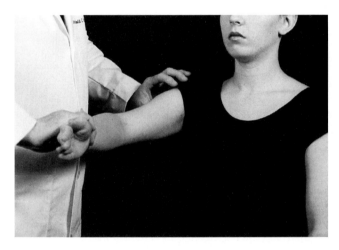

FIG. 4-126 While seated, the patient flexes the affected shoulder. The examiner then provides resistance.

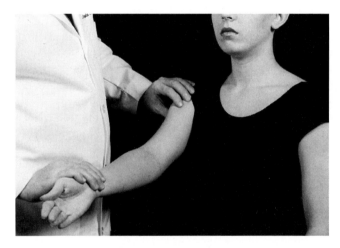

FIG. 4-127 While flexing the shoulder, the patient supinates the forearm and completely extends the elbow. A positive test elicits increased tenderness in the bicipital groove and indicates bicipital tendinitis.

SUBACROMIAL PUSH-BUTTON SIGN

ALSO KNOWN AS MAZION'S CUFF MANEUVER

Assessment for Rotator Cuff Tear of the Supraspinatus Tendon

Comment

Ruptures of the rotator cuff result from continued deterioration and degeneration. The tear may be partial or complete.

If the rupture is partial, the clinical findings are similar to those seen in chronic tendinitis. Even with complete rupture, the shoulder may have a full range of motion because of continued function of the other rotator muscles. Usually, however, with both partial and complete ruptures, there is some weakness in abduction or flexion. The weakness is usually most severe in abduction because the muscle most commonly torn is the supraspinatus. If the tear is more anterior into the subscapularis, forward flexion will be weak. It may be impossible to actively abduct the arm more than 45 or 50 degrees, after which further abduction is obtained by scapulothoracic motion. A painful "catch" may be noted on passive motion between 50 and 100 degrees, where compression of the swollen tissues between the tuberosity and the overlying arch occurs. Tenderness at the site of the tear is a common finding, and with complete ruptures, a defect in the cuff may be palpated through the deltoid muscle. Passive range of motion is often normal in the pain-free shoulder.

Atrophy of the cuff muscles is often present, and the "drop-arm" test may be positive.

Acute hemarthrosis and prominent ecchymosis down the arm may occasionally accompany longstanding rotator cuff tears, especially those with cuff-tear arthropathy. This is probably the result of further rupture with bleeding of remaining rotator cuff musculature. Chronic subdeltoid swelling usually means synovial fluid has escaped from the glenohumeral joint to the subacromial space and indicates a large rotator cuff rupture.

The rotator cuff is an almost complete tissue annulus that is attached to the humerus in the region of the anatomic neck and is formed by the fusion of the joint capsule with the musculotendinous insertions of the subscapularis in front, the supraspinatus above, and the teres minor and infraspinatus behind. The most important of these structures is the supraspinatus, which runs through a tunnel formed by the acromion and the coracoacromial ligament. The supraspinatus is separated from the acromion by part of the subdeltoid bursa.

The rotator cuff may suffer a large tear as a result of sudden traction to the arm. Such a tear occurs most readily in middle-age patients because of degenerative changes in the rotator cuff. Most commonly, the supraspinatus region is involved, and the patient has difficulty initiating abduction of the arm. In other cases, a torn or inflamed rotator cuff impinges the acromion during abduction, causing a painful arc of movement. Although the range of passive movement is not disturbed initially, limitation of rotation supersedes, so many of these cases become indistinguishable from adhesive capsulitis.

Any condition that decreases the functional space between the rotator cuff tendons and the rigid subacromial arch can cause impingement. Ultrasonography has some popularity in the evaluation of the rotator cuff. It is safe and noninvasive and is most accurate in large and moderately large tears. Magnetic resonance imaging (MRI) now plays a major role in diagnosing rotator cuff disease.

Most rotator cuff tears are associated with type 3 acromion.

ORTHOPEDIC GAMUT 4-15

ACROMION CHANGES

Three types of acromion changes observed in impingement syndrome are as follows:

Type 1: flat
Type 2: curved
Type 3: hooked

PROCEDURE

- The patient is seated with the upper extremities hanging limply at the sides.
- The examiner exerts strong finger or thumb pressure toward the midline at the clavicle, at a point even with the scapular spine (Fig. 4-128).
- The production or increase of shoulder pain indicates a positive test.

- The test is significant for rotator cuff tear of the supraspinatus tendon.

Confirmation Procedures

Apley's test, impingement sign, supraspinatus press test, and Codman's sign

---

DIAGNOSTIC STATEMENT

Subacromial push-button sign is positive on the right. This result indicates a rotator cuff tear of the supraspinatus tendon.

CLINICAL PEARL

Degenerative changes in the supraspinatus tendon may be accompanied by the local deposition of calcium salts. This process may continue without symptoms, although radiographic changes are obvious. However, the calcified material sometimes causes inflammatory changes in the subdeltoid area and results in sudden, severe, and incapacitating pain. When this occurs, the shoulder is acutely tender and is often swollen and warm to the touch.

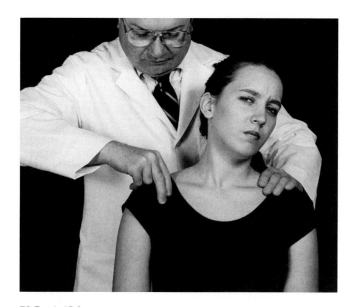

FIG. 4-128 The patient is seated with the upper extremities hanging limply at the sides. The examiner exerts strong finger or thumb pressure toward the midline of the clavicle, at a point even with the scapular spine. The production or increase of shoulder pain is a positive test. The test is significant for a rotator cuff tear, specifically a tear of the supraspinatus tendon.

SUPRASPINATUS PRESS TEST

Assessment for Tear of the Supraspinatus Tendon or Muscle

Comment

Supraspinatus syndrome (painful arc syndrome) is characterized by pain in the shoulder and upper arm during midrange abduction of the glenohumeral joint with freedom from pain at the extremes of the range. The syndrome is common to five distinct shoulder lesions: supraspinatus tendon tear, supraspinatus tendon inflammation, calcific deposits in the supraspinatus tendon, subacromial bursitis, and undisplaced fracture of the greater tuberosity.

The pain is produced mechanically by nipping of a tender structure between the tuberosity of the humerus and the acromion process and coracoacromial ligament.

Even in the normal shoulder, the clearance between the upper end of the humerus and the acromion process is small during abduction between 45 and 160 degrees. If a swollen and tender structure is present beneath the acromion, pain occurs during the arc of movement because the clearance is so small. In the neutral position and in full abduction, the clearance is greater and pain is less marked or absent.

The two classic views to rule out calcific tendinitis are AP views: with the arm in internal and external rotation.

In internal rotation, the Hill-Sachs posterior lateral humeral head impression fracture is seen as a straight line inside the most lateral portion of the head (Fig. 4-129). The Stryker notch view, a supplemental view, images the defect when the patient places a hand on top of his or her head.

If the greater tuberosity avulsed and is a fragment, it is not seen over the top of the humeral head. It is usually hidden in the AP view behind the humeral head and glenoid. The fragment is visualized either on the lateral scapular view or axillary view (Fig. 4-130).

A plain radiograph will identify and localize the calcific deposit to a particular tendon, usually the supraspinatus. In the formative phase of calcification, the deposit is well defined and homogeneously dense. In the resorptive phase, usually presenting as the acute condition, the deposit is less well defined, is irregular, and has a fluffy, less dense appearance (Fig. 4-131).

Whatever the primary cause, the clinical syndrome has the same general features, although they vary in degree.

ORTHOPEDIC GAMUT 4-16

SUPRASPINATUS SYNDROME

Variations of degeneration that lead to supraspinatus syndrome include the following:

1. In minor tearing of the supraspinatus tendon, tearing or strain of a few degenerate tendon fibers causes an inflammatory reaction with local swelling. Power is not as significantly impaired as it is after a complete tear of the rotator cuff.
2. With supraspinatus tendinitis, an inflammatory reaction is provoked by the degeneration of the tendon fibers.
3. Calcific deposits in the supraspinatus tendon occur when a white, chalky deposit forms within the degenerate tendon, and the lesion is surrounded by an inflammatory reaction. Pain occurs when the calcified material bursts into the surrounding tissue.
4. With subacromial bursitis, the bursal walls are inflamed and thickened by mechanical irritation.
5. With injury to the greater tuberosity, a contusion or undisplaced fracture of the greater tuberosity is a common cause.

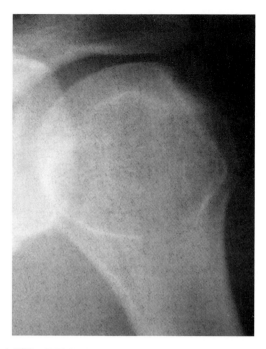

FIG. 4-129   Hill-Sachs posterolateral humeral head defect often is seen as a straight line on an internal rotation anteroposterior view. *(From Nicholas JA, Hershman EB, editors:* The upper extremity in sports medicine, *St Louis, 1990, Mosby.)*

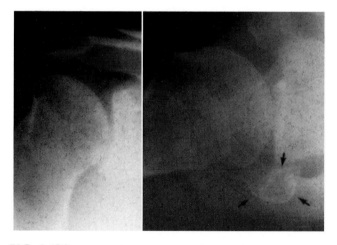

FIG. 4-130   External rotation and axillary view of a patient with a missed tuberosity avulsion. *(From Nicholas JA, Hershman EB, editors:* The upper extremity in sports medicine, *St Louis, 1990, Mosby.)*

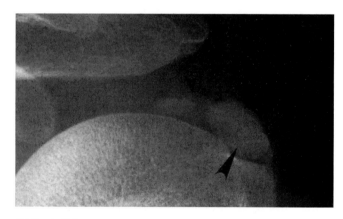

FIG. 4-131   Calcific tendinitis: formative stage *(large arrow)* and resorptive phase *(small arrow)*. *(From Klippel JH, Dieppe PA:* Rheumatology, *vol 1-2, ed 2, London, 1998, Mosby.)*

With the arm dependent, pain is absent or minimal. During abduction of the arm, pain begins at about 45 degrees and persists up to 160 degrees of movement. Above 160 degrees, the pain lessens or disappears. Pain is experienced again during descent from full elevation, in the middle arc of the range. The patient will often twist or circumduct the arm grotesquely to lower it as painlessly as possible. The severity of the pain varies from case to case. When the calcified deposit is in the supraspinatus tendon, the pain may be so intense that the patient is scarcely able to move the shoulder and is driven to seek emergency treatment.

PROCEDURE

- The patient abducts the shoulders to 90 degrees.
- The examiner resists the abduction (Fig. 4-132).
- The shoulders are medially rotated and angled 30 degrees forward (the patient's thumbs point to the floor) (Fig. 4-133).

- The examiner again resists abduction.
- If the patient exhibits weakness or experiences pain, the test is positive.
- Weakness and pain indicate a tear of the supraspinatus tendon or muscle.

Confirmation Procedures
Apley's test, Codman's sign, impingement sign, and subacromial push-button sign

DIAGNOSTIC STATEMENT

Supraspinatus test is positive on the right or left. This result indicates a tear of the supraspinatus tendon.

CLINICAL PEARL

Painful arc syndrome is sometimes confused with arthritis of the acromioclavicular joint, which also causes pain during a certain phase of the abduction arc. However, with acromioclavicular arthritis, the pain begins later in abduction (not below 90 degrees) and increases, rather than diminishes, as full elevation is achieved.

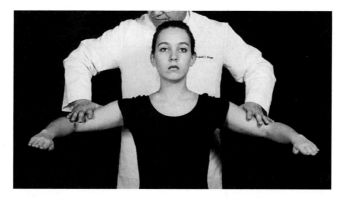

FIG. 4-132   While the patient is seated, the shoulders are abducted to 90 degrees with the arm in a neutral rotation. The examiner provides resistance to abduction.

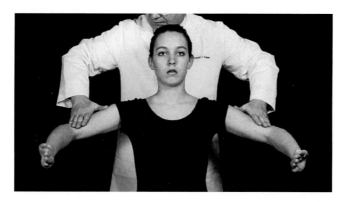

FIG. 4-133   The shoulders are internally rotated and angled 30 degrees forward so that the patient's thumbs point to the floor. The examiner again provides resistance to abduction. A positive test is indicated by pain or weakness in the affected shoulder, compared with the unaffected side. A positive test indicates a tear of the supraspinatus tendon or muscle.

TRANSVERSE HUMERAL LIGAMENT TEST

Assessment for Torn Transverse Humeral Ligament

Comment

Below and medial to the coracoacromial ligament, the long head of the biceps may be palpated beneath the capsule. The long head of the biceps is held in the groove by the transverse humeral ligament, a thickened prolongation of the capsule extending between the lesser and greater tuberosities.

ORTHOPEDIC GAMUT 4-17

BICEPS LONG HEAD STRUCTURE

The critical zones in the biceps long head structure are as follows:

1. The point at which the tendon arches over the humeral head
2. The point where the floor on which the tendon glides changes from bony cortex to articular cartilage

---

The bicipital retinaculum (Fig. 4-134) serves to hold the tendon of the long head of the biceps against the proximal humerus within the bicipital groove. The functional significance of this becomes apparent during shoulder elevation, which limits biceps contribution to either flexion or abduction by tethering of the long tendon within the bicipital groove. The retinaculum prevents the biceps from deflecting away from the humerus during contraction by keeping it straddled between the two tuberosities, thus limiting its leverage as a significant elevator.

Dimensions of the groove vary widely. Deep narrow apertures favor constriction of the tendon, and shallow flat grooves allow slipping and subluxation of the tendon. If the cuff zone at the top of the groove is torn, the tendon may slip out of the groove, particularly if the arm is abducted and externally rotated. Similarly, if strong force is applied while the arm is abducted and externally rotated, the tendon may be wrenched out of the groove.

PROCEDURE

- The patient's affected shoulder is passively abducted and internally rotated (Figs. 4-135 and 4-136).
- The examiner's fingers are placed on the bicipital groove.
- The patient's shoulder is passively externally rotated (Fig. 4-137).
- If a tendon snap in and out of the groove is felt as the external rotation occurs, the test is positive.
- A positive test suggests a torn transverse humeral ligament.

Confirmation Procedures

Abbott-Saunders test, Ludington's test, Speed's test, and Yergason's test

---

DIAGNOSTIC STATEMENT

Transverse humeral ligament test is positive on the left. This result indicates a torn transverse humeral ligament.

CLINICAL PEARL

Conditions involving the bicipital tendon and the bicipital groove are particularly pertinent to athletes because many sports involve the throwing motion of the arm. These athletes include baseball pitchers, football quarterbacks, batters, and tennis players. The throwing motion is especially inhibited by bicipital tendon problems. It is especially pertinent to recognize if the defect is an adhesive tenosynovitis, fraying of the tendon, or subluxation or dislocation of the tendon.

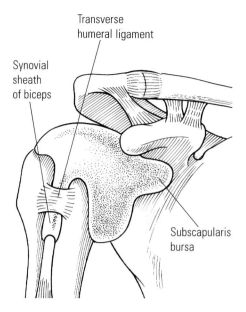

FIG. 4-134 Transverse humeral ligament. *(From Saidoff DC, McDonough AL:* Critical pathways in therapeutic intervention, *St Louis, 1997, Mosby.)*

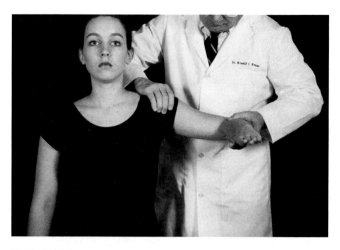

FIG. 4-135 The patient's shoulder is passively abducted with the elbow flexed to 90 degrees.

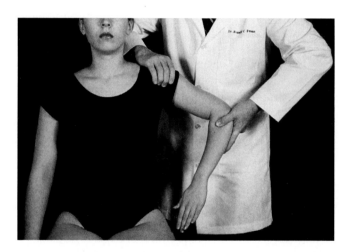

FIG. 4-136 The examiner's fingers are placed on the bicipital groove. The patient's shoulder is passively internally rotated.

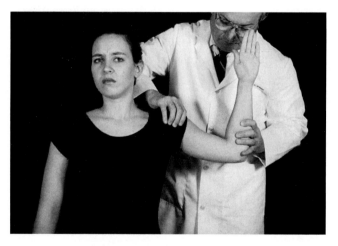

FIG. 4-137 While maintaining palpation of the bicipital groove, the shoulder is externally rotated passively. Tendon snap in and out of the groove as the external rotation occurs is a positive finding. A positive test suggests a torn transverse humeral ligament.

WRIGHT'S TEST

ALSO KNOWN AS HYPERABDUCTION MANEUVER

Assessment for Neurovascular Compromise of the Axillary Artery as Seen in the Hyperabduction Thoracic Outlet Syndromes

Comment

The Adson, hyperabduction, and costoclavicular maneuvers are provocative movements and postures that attempt to reproduce pain, paresthesias, a change in radial pulse, or a supraclavicular bruit.

The Hunter test is begun with the shoulder abducted to 90 degrees and the elbow flexed to 90 degrees. The arm is then straightened. A positive sign results in a painful shooting sensation down the arm in the distribution of the involved nerves, presumably from sudden traction of the tethered medial cord of the brachial plexus. Similar tension tests may be performed to stretch the ulnar and radial nerve tracts. The appropriate limb postures may be extrapolated when the various joints of the upper extremity are positioned to stretch each tract in relation to the axis of the joints it crosses (Fig. 4-138).

Elvey's upper extremity tension test (UETT) determines the mobility of the brachial plexus and nerve root, particularly the median nerve. Similar to the straight leg raising test in the lower extremities, this test may determine whether any restrictions of the nerve roots or plexus have occurred in those structures stretched by a sequence of upper extremity movements.

ORTHOPEDIC GAMUT 4-18

ELVEY'S TEST MOVEMENTS

The three superimposed component movements of Elvey's test are as follows:

1. Shoulder abduction and lateral rotation and extension behind the coronal plane
2. Forearm supination and elbow extension
3. Wrist and finger extension (Fig. 4-139)

With repetitive or prolonged hyperabduction of the arm, the neurovascular bundle in the axilla can be stretched under the pectoralis minor tendon and the coracoid process, resulting in symptoms of neurovascular compression.

When leaving the costoclavicular space, the three cords of the brachial plexus, the subclavian artery, and the subclavian vein pass under the insertion of the pectoralis minor muscle on the coracoid process. As this neurovascular bundle enters the axillary fossa, the artery and vein become known as the *axillary artery* and the *axillary vein*. As the upper extremity is abducted to 180 degrees, the neurovascular bundle is stretched around a fulcrum, which consists of the tendon of the pectoralis minor, the coracoid process, and the humeral head. The bundle almost reaches an angle of 90 degrees around the fulcrum. Unfortunately, the neurovascular bundle's course remains fixed, allowing no motion of the bundle. Compression at the fulcrum and tension along its components is the only way the bundle can compensate. Abduction of the arm produces a 30-degree elevation and a 35-degree posterior displacement of the clavicle, thereby narrowing the costoclavicular tunnel. The tunnel's anterior wall, consisting also of the pectoralis minor muscle, the subclavius muscle, and the costoclavicular ligament (the thickening of the clavipectoral fascia), is stretched and brought posteriorly further, pushing the neurovascular bundle against the fulcrum.

There are two critical anatomic points where compression of the neurovascular bundle may occur when the arm is hyperabducted. The first is where the bundle passes through the costoclavicular tunnel, or slit. The second is where the bundle passes under the pectoralis minor tendon at its insertion on the coracoid process. During abduction of the arm, the fixed neurovascular bundle can be compressed by the tendon of the pectoralis minor muscle as well as by the humeral head. The characteristic position that produces this compression is 180 degrees abducted and elbow flexion. This position commonly occurs during sleep or in certain occupations, such as that of electricians, painters, bricklayers, dry-wall hangers, or masons.

Pain, paresthesia, and numbness develop first in the fingers and later in the hand. In some patients, transitory ischemia and edema develop. These symptoms may resemble Raynaud's disease and are present in 38% of the patients

The most commonly encountered
causes of damage at the
various sites are indicated

C7 Root
By far the most common "acute cervical
disc lesion" occurs at this level. C6
and C5 less often. Other levels very rarely

C5 and C6 Roots
Most commonly involved roots
in cervical spondylosis.
C7 involved occasionally.
Others very rarely

Axillary nerve
Fracture of humeral neck
Dislocation of the humerus
Intramuscular injections

Radial nerve in spiral groove
Direct blow laterally. During
anesthesia medially. While drunk
medially ("Saturday night palsy").
Fractures of the humerus—
immediate or delayed

Lower trunk of the brachial plexus
Cervical rib syndrome. Altered anatomy
(outlet syndrome). Pancoast's tumor of
lung apex

Radial nerve in the axilla
Incorrect use of a crutch

Radial nerve (posterior
interosseus nerve)
Nerve enters forearm through
supinator muscle. Occupational
overuse of muscle may damage
nerve. Also occurs idiopathically.
Extensors of thumb and index
finger mainly affected

Ulnar nerve
Damage from repeated minor trauma
Prolonged bed rest
Delayed after fractures

Median nerve
At elbow. Rarely damaged by
direct trauma or fracture

(Anterior interosseus nerve)
Rarely damaged nerve lies very deep
Flexors of thumb and index finger are
affected by damage to nerve

Median nerve (carpal tunnel syndrome)
Nerve damaged by swelling or infiltration
of tunnel it transverses. Transiently seen
in pregnancy. Idiopathically in females.
Complicates rheumatoid arthritis.
Rarely seen in other systemic diseases

Ulnar nerve (deep branch)
Trauma to heel of the hand. Idiopathically
(often a ganglion found on exploration)
No sensory loss in typical cases

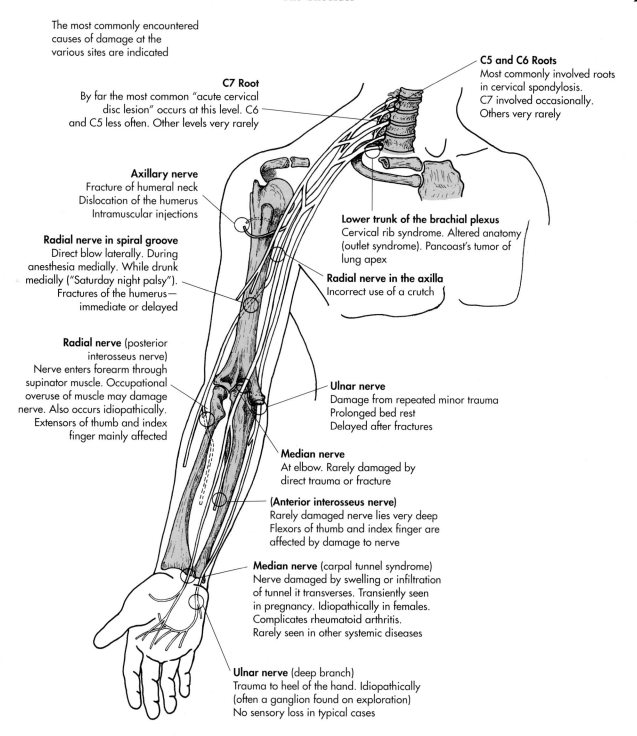

FIG. 4-138 Common sites of nerve injury in the upper extremity. *(From Saidoff DC, McDonough AL: Critical pathways in therapeutic intervention, St Louis, 1997, Mosby.)*

with hyperabduction syndrome. Neurologic symptoms are usually absent in hyperabduction syndrome because as paresthesia and pain develop, the patient corrects the arm position, so the nerve compression only lasts for a short time. If the arm is abducted to 180 degrees in patients with hyperabduction syndrome, symptoms can increase. The radial artery pulse may weaken or disappear. However, just as tests for the anterior scalene syndrome or costoclavicular syndrome can be positive in a normal position, the same results can be found when testing for hyperabduction syndrome.

PROCEDURE

- Before this test is started, the Allen maneuver at the wrist is performed to establish patency of the radial arteries.
- The patient is seated, with both arms hanging at the sides.
- The examiner palpates the patient's radial pulse (Fig. 4-140).
- Both arms, in turn, are passively abducted to 180 degrees (Fig. 4-141).
- The examiner notes the angle of abduction at which the radial pulse diminishes or disappears on the affected side (Fig. 4-142).

- The examiner compares the results with those on the unaffected side.
- The test is significant for neurovascular compromise of the axillary artery, as seen in hyperabduction thoracic outlet syndromes.
- Many patients have cessation of the radial pulse upon abduction without hyperabduction syndrome being present.
- If the nonaffected limb demonstrates radial pulse dampening or cessation at the same approximate degree of abduction as the affected side, the test is not positive for hyperabduction syndrome.

Confirmation Procedures
Adson's test, Allen maneuver, costoclavicular maneuver, George's screening procedure, Halstead maneuver, reverse Bakody maneuver, Roos' test, and shoulder compression test

DIAGNOSTIC STATEMENT

Wright's test is positive on the left. This result indicates hyperabduction thoracic outlet compression syndrome.

CLINICAL PEARL

In most instances of compression hyperabduction of the shoulder, the radial pulse is obliterated; however, obliteration of the radial pulse also may occur in the normal extremity. However, there is a difference. On the affected side, the marginal position is reached sooner than on the normal side. The marginal position is the level of abduction just below that which produces obliteration of the pulse. The patient is often aware of the exact level of abduction at which the symptoms occur.

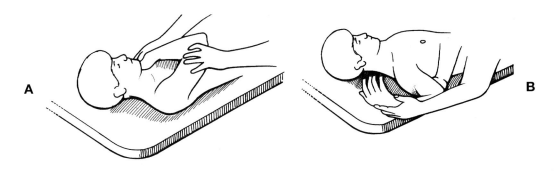

FIG. 4-139 Elvey's upper extremity tension test is a provocative sequence of motions that determines mobility (i.e., gliding) of the nerve tract, including the brachial plexus and nerve root. This particular test biases the median nerve and the anterior interosseous nerve for tension by way of mechanical stretch. **A,** First, the arm and scapula are place in a resting position. **B,** Next, the arm is placed in the position of 90 degrees shoulder abduction, lateral rotation, and elbow flexion with the forearm pronated. *(From Saidoff DC, McDonough AL: Critical pathways in therapeutic intervention, St Louis, 1997, Mosby.)*   *Continued*

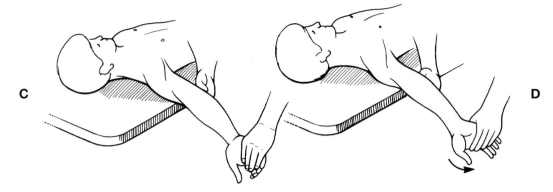

FIG. 4-139, cont'd **C,** The elbow and forearm are then extended and supinated. **D,** The wrist is then extended to reproduce symptoms. Cervical lateral flexion to the left or right may then be added. It is essential for the examiner to maintain each posture before superimposing the next position in this sequence. *(From Saidoff DC, McDonough AL:* Critical pathways in therapeutic intervention, *St Louis, 1997, Mosby.)*

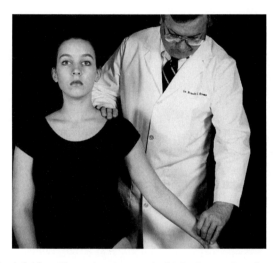

FIG. 4-140 The patient is seated with both arms hanging at the sides. The examiner palpates the radial pulse of the affected arm.

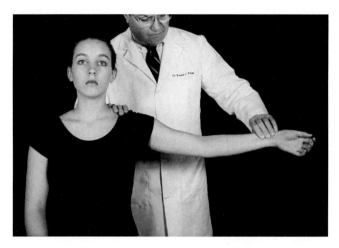

FIG. 4-141 The examiner abducts the affected arm to 180 degrees.

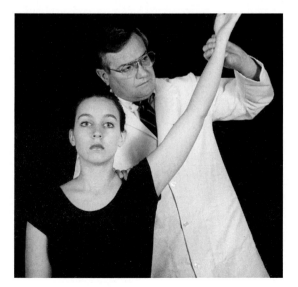

FIG. 4-142 The examiner notes the angle of abduction at which the radial pulse on the affected side diminishes or disappears. This angle is compared with the angle obtained on the unaffected side. The test is significant for neurovascular compromise of the axillary artery, as seen in hyperabduction thoracic outlet syndromes. If the nonaffected arm demonstrates radial pulse dampening or cessation at the same approximate angle of abduction, the test is not positive for hyperabduction syndrome.

YERGASON'S TEST

Assessment for Tenosynovitis or Involvement of the Transverse Humeral Ligament

Comment

The long head of the biceps follows a tortuous and hemmed-in course from its origin in the muscle belly to the supraglenoid tubercle. The type of trauma that usually produces tenosynovitis in the wrist, resulting in constrictive adhesions is not the mechanism commonly encountered at the long head of the biceps. The bicipital tendon area is not nearly so vulnerable to direct trauma, so tendinitis and tenosynovitis may develop gradually without definite acute episodes of injury.

The gliding of the long tendon of the biceps is guided by the coracohumeral ligament (Fig. 4-143). The ligament runs through the interval between the subscapularis and supraspinatus tendons, known as the *rotator interval,* and reinforces the glenohumeral joint capsule at that locale.

Following an activity such as the first game of the season for badminton or tennis or following a jerking strain after lifting with outstretched arms, discomfort is noted in the shoulder. Initially, the ache is indefinite and is not plainly related to motions that use the biceps tendon. Later, more acute pain develops, and the patient avoids lifting and keeps the arm at the side with the elbow flexed (this is the position of maximum comfort).

Examination reveals tenderness at the top and front of the shoulder. This tenderness is related to the tendon course across the upper end of the humerus. The tenderness follows into the bicipital groove and along the tendon into the arm. Deep palpation at the medial border of the deltoid delineates tenderness when pressure is applied along the tendon as the arm is rotated externally and internally. Flexion of the elbow and supination of the hand against resistance may produce pain that is referred to the front and inner aspects of the shoulder. In all shoulder lesions in which involvement of the biceps mechanism is suspected, diagnostic images that show the groove in profile should be acquired. With tendinitis or tenosynovitis, bony abnormalities are not unusual, but any abnormal contour of the groove may predispose the patient to development of the condition. If the groove is too flat or shallow, the tendon may slip out. If the groove is too deep, the tendon is roughened and squeezed. If there is spur formation, the tendon may become frayed.

PROCEDURE

- The patient flexes the elbow.
- The patient attempts to supinate the hand against resistance (Fig. 4-144).
- The patient then resists efforts to extend the elbow (Fig. 4-145).
- If pain over the intertubercular groove develops or is aggravated, the test is positive.
- A positive sign suggests tenosynovitis of the transverse humeral ligament.

Confirmation Procedures

Abbott-Saunders test, Ludington's test, Speed's test, and transverse humeral ligament test

---

DIAGNOSTIC STATEMENT

Yergason's test is positive on the right. This result indicates bicipital tenosynovitis or a torn transverse humeral ligament.

CLINICAL PEARL

The concept that the biceps tendon moves up and down the groove during motion at the glenohumeral joint is questionable. With the bicipital tendon and groove exposed under anesthesia, the biceps tendon remains fixed in the groove during motion. However, the head of the humerus glides up and down the tendon. Contraction of the biceps muscle, by supinating the forearm or flexing the elbow, makes the tendon taut but produces no motion of the tendon in the groove. All movements of the shoulder joint, regardless of the plane in which the arm is elevated, are accompanied by gliding motions of the humerus on the tendon.

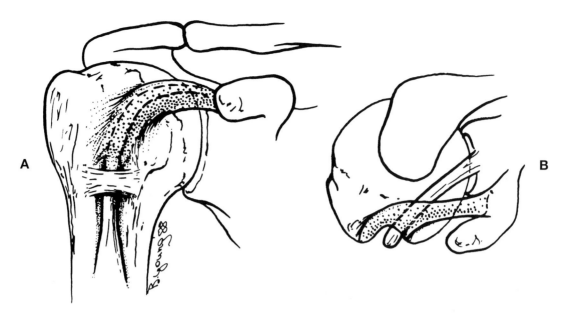

FIG. 4-143 The coracohumeral ligament thickens the rotator interval, inserts on either side of the bicipital groove, and is an important stabilizer of the biceps tendon. **A,** Anterior view. **B,** Superior view. *(From Saidoff DC, McDonough AL:* Critical pathways in therapeutic intervention, *St Louis, 1997, Mosby.)*

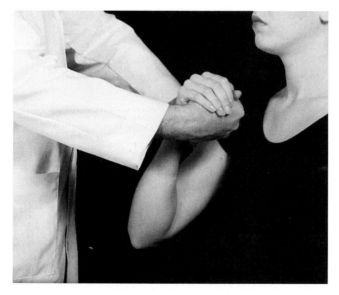

FIG. 4-144 The patient flexes the affected elbow. The patient resists efforts to extend the arm.

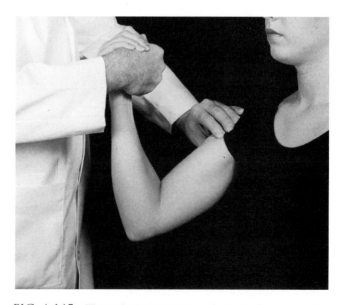

FIG. 4-145 The patient attempts to supinate the forearm against resistance. Pain over the intertubercular groove is a positive finding. A positive test suggests biceps tenosynovitis or involvement of the transverse humeral ligament.

CRITICAL THINKING

What is the cause of rotator cuff tears?

The process is secondary to repetitive microtrauma, degeneration, or impingement.

How is the strength of the supraspinatus and infraspinatus tested?

The supraspinatus is tested with the shoulder abducted to 90 degrees, flexed 30 degrees, and then maximally internally rotated. Downward pressure exerted by the examiner is resisted primarily by the supraspinatus. The infraspinatus is tested with the shoulder abducted at the side while the elbows are flexed 90 degrees. The examiner resists active external rotation.

What is the function of the long head of the biceps tendon?

The tendon has an important contribution as a humeral head depressor.

What are the most important capsule ligaments?

The inferior glenohumeral ligament complex is the most important because it resists anteroinferior shoulder translation when the arm is placed in abduction, external rotation, and extension.

What is a Bankart lesion?

The Bankart lesion is a detachment of the anteroinferior glenoid labrum from the bony glenoid rim.

What is a Hill-Sachs lesion?

A Hill-Sachs lesion is an osteochondral depression in the posterior humeral head.

What are the most common mechanisms for production of anterior and posterior shoulder dislocations?

Most dislocations occur through an indirect force applied to the arm. Anterior dislocations are produced by an external rotation and/or hyperextension force applied to the shoulder that is already in about 90 degrees of abduction. Posterior dislocations are caused by indirectly applied force to the arm when the shoulder is variably flexed, adducted, and internally rotated.

What physical findings are typical of an unreduced posterior dislocation?

External rotation and elevation are limited. The anterior shoulder is flattened and the coracoid process may be prominent.

Describe the basis and techniques for the sulcus tests.

The sulcus test demonstrates the degree of inferior laxity; it is thought to be a test of the superior glenohumeral ligament and the coracohumeral ligament.

What is the function of the rotator cuff muscles?

As a whole, the rotator cuff functions center the humeral head in the glenoid, thus adding stability and maximum leverage to shoulder motions.

What is the impingement syndrome?

Impingement is a general term used to describe pain originating from compression of inflamed tissue between the humeral head and the coracoacromial arch. Any condition that causes a narrowing of this "subacromial space" (structural abnormalities, physiologic abnormalities, or both) can lead to impingement.

How does a rotator cuff tear differ from impingement?

Rotator cuff tears are associated with impingement in 95% of cases. Impingement lesions have three progressive stages:

1. Edema and hemorrhage
2. Fibrosis and tendinitis
3. Rotator cuff tears, biceps tendon ruptures, and bony changes

Explain how bicipital tendinitis relates to impingement.

Inflammation of the tendon of the long head of the biceps occurs by the same mechanisms responsible for impingement. With elevation and rotation of the arm, the biceps tendon can be compressed between the head of the humerus, the acromion, and the coracoacromial ligament.

BIBLIOGRAPHY

Abrams WB, Berkow R: *The Merck manual of geriatrics,* Rahway, NJ, 1990, Merck Sharp & Dohme Research Laboratories.

Adams JC, Hamblen DL: *Outline of orthopaedics,* ed 11, Edinburgh, 1990, Churchill Livingstone.

Alario AJ: *Practical guide to the care of the pediatric patient,* St Louis, 1997, Mosby.

Allison D, Strickland N: *Acronyms & synonyms in medical imaging,* Oxford, 1996, ISIS Medical Media.

Altchek DW, et al: Arthroscopic acromioplasty: technique and results, *J Bone Joint Surg* 72A:1198, 1990.

American Medical Association: *Guides to the evaluation of permanent impairment,* ed 4, Chicago, 1993, American Medical Association.

American Medical Association: *How to use guides to the evaluation of permanent impairment,* ed 4, Falmouth, Colo, 1993, SEAK, Inc.

Anderson KN, Anderson LE: *Mosby's pocket dictionary of medicine, nursing, & allied health,* ed 2, St Louis, 1994, Mosby.

Apley AG, Solomon L: *Concise system of orthopaedics and fractures,* London, 1988, Butterworth-Heinemann.

Arntz CT, Jackins S, Matsen FA III. Prosthetic replacement of the shoulder for the treatment of defects in rotator cuff and the surface of the glenohumeral joint, *J Bone Joint Surg* 75A:485, 1993.

Ballinger PW: *Merrill's atlas of radiographic positions and radiologic procedures,* vol 1-3, ed 8, St Louis, 1995, Mosby.

Barabis J: Therapist's management of thoracic outlet syndrome. In Hunter JM, Schneider LH, Mackin EJ, Callahan AB, editors: *Rehabilitation of the hand: surgery and therapy,* ed 3, St Louis, 1990, Mosby.

Barkauskas VH, Stoltenberg-Allen K, Baumann LC, Darling-Fisher C: *Health & physical assessment,* ed 2, St Louis, 1998, Mosby.

Bateman JE: *Trauma to nerves in limbs,* Philadelphia, 1962, WB Saunders.

Bateman JE: The diagnosis and treatment of ruptures of the rotator cuff, *Surg Clin North Am* 43:1523, 1963.

Bateman JE: *The shoulder and neck,* ed 2, Philadelphia, 1978, WB Saunders.

Bergfeld JA: Acromioclavicular complex. In Nicholas JA, Hershman EB, editors: *The upper extremity in sports medicine,* St Louis, 1990, Mosby.

Berquist T: *MRI of the musculoskeletal system,* ed 3, Philadelphia, 1996, JB Lippincott.

Bland JH, Merrit JA, Boushey DR: The painful shoulder, *Semin Arthritis Rheum* 7:21, 1977.

Bloom RA: The active abduction view: a new maneuver in the diagnosis of rotator cuff tears, *Skeletal Radiol* 20:255, 1991.

Bozyk Z: Shoulder-hand syndrome in patients with antecedent myocardial infarctions, *Revmatologiia (mosk)* 6:103, 1968.

Brems JJ: Degenerative joints disease of the shoulder. In Nicholas J, Hershman E, editors: *The upper extremity in sports medicine,* St Louis, 1990, Mosby.

Brooks M, Evans R, Fairclough J: *Sports injuries,* ed 2, London, 1992, Gower Medical.

Brotzman SB: *Clinical orthopaedic rehabilitation,* St Louis, 1996, Mosby.

Brown DE, Neumann RD: *Orthopedic secrets,* Philadelphia, 1995, Hanley & Belfus.

Bucholz RW: *Orthopaedic decision making,* ed 2, St Louis, 1996, Mosby.

Bunker TD, Schranz PJ: *Clinical challenges in orthopaedics: the shoulder,* Oxford, 1998, ISIS Medical Media.

Burkhart SS: Arthroscopic treatment of massive rotator cuff tears, *Clin Orthop* 26:45, 1991.

Bush LH: The torn shoulder capsule, *J Bone Joint Surg* 57A:256, 1975.

Butler D: *Mobilisation of the nervous system,* Melbourne, 1991, Churchill Livingstone.

Cailliet R: *Shoulder pain,* Philadelphia, 1966, FA Davis.

Campbell JB, Campbell JM: *Mosby's survival guide to medical abbreviations & acronyms prefixes & suffixes symbols Greek alphabet,* St Louis, 1995, Mosby.

Canale ST: *Campbell's operative orthopaedics,* vol 1-4, ed 9, St Louis, 1998, Mosby.

Chandler TJ, et al: Shoulder strength, power and endurance in college tennis players, *Am J Sports Med* 20:455, 1992.

Chansky HA, Iannotti JP: The vascularity of the rotator cuff, *Clin Sports Med* 10:807, 1991.

Chappman S, Nakielny R: *Aids to radiological differential diagnosis,* ed 3, London, 1995, Bailliere Tindall.

Chard MD, et al: Shoulder disorders in the elderly: a community survey, *Arthritis Rheum* 34:766, 1991.

Cinquegranao D: Chronic cervical radiculitis and its relationship to "chronic bursitis," *Am J Phys Med Rehabil* 47:23, 1968.

Cipriano JJ: *Photographic manual of regional orthopaedic and neurological test,* ed 3, Baltimore, 1997, Williams & Wilkins.

Clark J, Sidles JA, Matsen FF: The repair of the glenohumeral joint capsule to the rotator cuff, *Clin Orthop* 254:29, 1990.

Codman EA: *The shoulder,* Boston, 1934, Author.

Cofield R: Degenerative and arthritic problems of the glenohumeral joint. In Rockwood C, Matsen F, editors: *The shoulder,* Philadelphia, 1990, WB Saunders.

Cohn RE: *Impairment rating examination and disability evaluation,* ed 3, Wilkesboro, NC, 1994, R Ernest Cohn.

Cooper DE, et al: Anatomy, histology and vascularity of the glenoid labrum, *J Bone Joint Surg* 74A:46, 1992.

Copeland SA, Gschwend N, Landi A, Saffar P: *Joint stiffness of the upper limb,* St Louis, 1997, Mosby.

Curwin S, Stanish WD: *Tendinitis: its etiology and treatment,* Lexington, 1984, The Collamore Press.

Dalton S, et al: Human shoulder tendon biopsy samples in organ culture produce procallagenase and tissue inhibitor of metalloproteinases, *Ann Rheum Dis* 54:571, 1995.

Dambro MR, Griffith JA: *Griffith's 5 minute clinical consult,* Baltimore, 1997, Williams & Wilkins.

D'Ambrogio KJ, Roth GB: *Positional release therapy assessment & treatment of musculoskeletal dysfunction,* St Louis, 1997, Mosby.

D'Ambrosia RD: *Musculoskeletal disorders: regional examination and differential diagnosis,* Philadelphia, 1977, JB Lippincott.

Dandy DJ: *Essential orthopaedics and trauma,* Edinburgh, 1989, Churchill Livingstone.

Dawson DM, Hallet M, Millender LH: *Entrapment neuropathies,* ed 2, Boston, 1990, Little, Brown.

Debeyre J, Patte D, Elmelik E: Repair of ruptures of the rotator cuff of the shoulder, *J Bone Joint Surg* 47B:36, 1965.

Deltoff MN, Kogon PL: *The portable skeletal x-ray library,* St Louis, 1998, Mosby.

Demeter SL, Andersson GBJ, Smith GM: *Disability evaluation,* St Louis, 1996, Mosby.

DePalma AF: *Surgery of the shoulder,* ed 2, Philadelphia, 1973, JB Lippincott.

Deshpande JK, Tobias JD: *The pediatric pain handbook,* St Louis, 1996, Mosby.

Dettenmeier PA: *Radiographic assessment for nurses,* St Louis, 1995, Mosby.

Doherty M: *Color atlas and text of osteoarthritis,* London, 1994, Wolfe.

Doherty M, Doherty J: *Clinical examination in rheumatology,* London, 1992, Wolfe.

Doherty M, George E: *Self-assessment picture tests in rheumatology,* London, 1995, Mosby-Wolfe.

Elster AD: *Questions and answers in magnetic resonance imaging,* St Louis, 1994, Mosby.

Engelman RM: Shoulder pain as a presenting complaint in upper lobe bronchogenic carcinoma: report of 21 cases, *Conn Med* 30:273, 1966.

Epstein O, Perkin GD, deBono DP, Cookson J: *Clinical examination,* ed 2, London, 1997, Mosby.

Farin PU, Jaroma H, Harju A, Soimakallio S: Shoulder impingement syndrome; sonographic evaluation, *Radiology* 176:845, 1990.

Feldmann E: *Current diagnosis in neurology,* St Louis, 1994, Mosby.

Ferezy JS: *The chiropractic neurological examination,* Gaithersburg, Md, 1992, Aspen.

Finke J: Neurologic differential diagnosis: the lower cervical region, *Dutsch Med Wochenschr* 90:1912, 1965.

Fornage B: *Musculoskeletal ultrasound,* New York, 1995, Churchill Livingstone.

Garn AN, Thorsen H, Lonnberg F: The effect of low-level laser therapy on musculoskeletal pain: a meta-analysis, *Pain* 52:63, 1993.

Garth W: Evaluating and treating brachial plexus injuries, *J Musculoskeletal Med* 55, 1994.

Gartsman GM: Arthroscopic acromioplasty for lesions of the rotator cuff, *J Bone Joint Surg* 72A:169, 1990.

Gascon J: A current problem: diagnosis of the shoulder pain syndrome, *Union Med Can* 94:463, 1965.

Gerard JA, Kleinfield SL: *Orthopaedic testing,* New York, 1993, Churchill Livingstone.

Gerber C, Krushell FJ: Isolated rupture of the tendon of the subscapularis muscle: clinical features in 16 cases, *J Bone Joint Surg* 73B:389, 1991.

Gilula LA, Yin Y: *Imaging of the wrist and hand,* Philadelphia, 1996, WB Saunders.

Gohlke F, Essigkrug B, Schmiz F: The pattern of the collagen fiber bundles of the capsule of the glenohumeral joint, *J Shoulder Elbow Surg* 3:111, 1994.

Goldie BS: *Orthopaedic diagnosis and management: a guide to the care of orthopaedic patients,* ed 2, Oxford, 1998, ISIS Medical Media.

Goldie I: Calcified deposits in the shoulder joint produced by calciphylaxis and their inhibition by triamcinolone: an experimental model, *Bull Soc Int Chir* 23:91, 1965.

Greenspan A: *Orthopedic radiology,* ed 2, Philadelphia, 1992, JB Lippincott.

Greenspan A, Montesano P: *Imaging of the spine in clinical practice,* London, 1993, Wolfe.

Greenstein GM: *Clinical assessment of neuromusculoskeletal disorders,* St Louis, 1997, Mosby.

Grossman ZD, et al: *Cost-effective diagnostic imaging the clinician's guide,* ed 3, St Louis, 1995, Mosby.

Halbach JW, Tank RT: The shoulder. In Gould JA, editor: *Orthopaedic and sports physical therapy,* ed 2, St Louis, 1990, Mosby.

Hale MS: *A practical approach to arm pain,* Springfield, Ill, 1971, Charles C Thomas.

Hammer WI: *Functional soft tissue examination and treatment by manual methods the extremities,* Gaithersburg, Md, 1991, Aspen.

Harryman DJ, et al: The role of the rotator interval capsule in passive motion and stability of the shoulder, *J Bone Joint Surg* 74A:53, 1992.

Harryman DT II, et al: Repairs of the rotator cuff, *J Bone Joint Surg* 73A:982, 1991.

Hartley A: *Practical joint assessment lower quadrant,* ed 2, St Louis, 1995, Mosby.

Hawkins RJ: *An organized approach to musculoskeletal examination and history taking,* St Louis, 1995, Mosby.

Hawkins RJ, Bokor D: Clinical evaluation of shoulder problems. In Rockwood C, Matshe F, editors: *The shoulder,* Philadelphia, 1990, WB Saunders.

Hawkins RJ, Kennedy JC: Impingement syndrome in athletics, *Am J Sports Med* 8:141, 1980.

Hawkins RJ, Mohtadi N: Rotator cuff problems in athletes. In DeLee JC, Drez D, editors: *Orthopaedic sports medicine: principals and practice,* vol 1, Philadelphia, 1994, WB Saunders.

Hijioka A, Suzuki K, Nakamura T, Hojo T: Degenerative change and rotator cuff tears: an anatomical study in 160 shoulders of 80 cadavers, *Arch Orthop Trauma Surg* 112:61, 1993.

Hinkle CZ: *Fundamentals of anatomy & movement a workbook and guide,* St Louis, 1997, Mosby.

Hornberger JP: *Exercise physiology therapeutic exercise,* Sarasota, Fla, 1991, Author.

Hsu HC, et al: Calcific tendinitis and rotator cuff tearing; a clinical and radiographic study, *J Shoulder Elbow Surg* 3:159, 1994.

Hurley J: Anatomy of the shoulder. In Nicholas J, Hershman E, editors: *The upper extremity in sports medicine,* St Louis, 1990, Mosby.

Iannotti JP, et al: Magnetic resonance imaging of the shoulder: sensitivity specificity and predictive value, *J Bone Joint Surg* 73A:17, 1991.

Itoi E, et al: Dynamic anterior stabilizers of the shoulder with the arm in abduction, *J Bone Joint Surg* 76B:834, 1994.

Jablonski S: *Dictionary of medical acronyms & abbreviations,* ed 3, Philadelphia, 1998, Hanley & Belfus.

Jehl J, Crummy P: *Essentials of radiologic surgery,* ed 6, Philadelphia, 1993, JB Lippincott.

Jobe C: Gross anatomy of the shoulder. In Rockwood C, Matsen F, editors: *The shoulder,* Philadelphia, 1990, WB Saunders.

Jobe FW, et al: The shoulder in sports. In Rockwood CA Jr, Matsen FA III, editors: *The shoulder,* Philadelphia, 1992, WB Saunders.

Kamkar A, Irrgang J, Whitney SL: Nonoperative management of secondary shoulder impingement syndrome, *J Orthop Sports Phys Ther* 17:21, 1993.

Kanner R: *Pain management secrets,* Philadelphia, 1997, Hanley & Belfus.

Kasdan ML: *Occupational hand & upper extremity injuries & diseases,* ed 2, Philadelphia, 1998, Hanley & Belfus.

Katirji B: *Electromyography in clinical practice: a case study approach,* St Louis, 1998, Mosby.

Katz WA: *Rheumatic diseases diagnosis and management,* Philadelphia, 1977, JB Lippincott.

Keats TH: *Atlas of normal roentgen variants,* ed 6, St Louis, 1996, Mosby.

Kendall HO, Kendall FP, Wadsworth GE: *Muscles testing and function,* ed 2, Baltimore, 1971, Williams & Wilkins.

Kessel L, Watson M: The painful arc syndrome: clinical classification as a guide to management, *J Bone Joint Surg* 59B:166, 1977.

Kircher MT, Cappuccino A, Torpey BM: Muscular violence as a cause of humeral fractures in pitchers, *Contemp Orthop* 26:475, 1993.

Kisner C, Colby LA: *Therapeutic exercise; foundations and techniques,* ed 2, Philadelphia, 1990, FA Davis.

Klippel JH, Dieppe PA: *Rheumatology,* vol 1-2, ed 2, London, 1998, Mosby.

Kronberg M, Nemeth G, Brostrom LA: Muscle activity and coordination in the normal shoulder: an electromyographic study, *Clin Orthop Rel Res* 257:76, 1990.

Kursuaogu-Brahme S, Gandry CR, Resnick D: Advanced imaging of the wrist, *Radiol Clin North Am* 228:307, 1990.

Lain TM: The military brace syndrome: a report of 16 cases of Erb's palsy occurring in military cadets, *J Bone Joint Surg* 51A:557, 1969.

Lavy CBD, Barrett DS: *Questions and answers on Apley's concise system of orthopaedics and fractures,* Oxford, 1991, Butterworth-Heinemann.

Leffert RD: Neurological problems. In Rockwood CA, Matsen FA, editors: *The shoulder,* vol 1, Philadelphia, 1990, WB Saunders.

Leffert RD, et al: Infra-clavicular brachial plexus injuries, *J Bone Joint Surg* 47B:9, 1965.

Legan JM, et al: Tears of the glenoid labrum: MR imaging of 88 arthroscopically confirmed cases, *Radiology* 179:241, 1991.

Lerner AJ: *The little black book of neurology,* ed 3, St Louis, 1995, Mosby.

Lewis CB, Knortz KA: *Orthopedic assessment and treatment of the geriatric patient,* St Louis, 1993, Mosby.

Lippitt S, Matsen F: Mechanisms of glenohumeral joint stability, *Clin Orthop* 291:20, 1993.

Litchfield R, et al: Rehabilitation of the overhead athlete, *J Orthop Sports Phys Ther* 18:433, 1993.

Loth TS: *Orthopedic boards review II: a case study approach,* St Louis, 1996, Mosby.

Lucas DB: Biomechanics of the shoulder joint, *Arch Surg* 107:425, 1973.

Magee DJ: *Orthopedic physical assessment,* ed 3, Philadelphia, 1997, WB Saunders.

Malen WJ, Bassett FH III, Goldner RD: Luxatio erecta: the inferior glenohumeral dislocation, *J Orthop Trauma* 4:19, 1990.

Malone TR, McPoil TG, Nitz AJ: *Orthopedic and sports physical therapy,* ed 3, St Louis, 1997, Mosby.

Marchiori DM: *Clinical imaging with skeletal, chest, and abdomen pattern differentials,* St Louis, 1999, Mosby.

Markey KL, DiBenedetto M, Curl WW: Upper trunk brachial plexopathy, *Am J Sports Med* 21:650, 1993.

Martin DR, Gaith WP: Results of orthoscopic debridement of glenoid labral tears, *Am J Sports Med* 23:4, 1995.

Martin JH: *Neuroanatomy text and atlas,* ed 2, Stamford, Conn, 1996, Appleton & Lange.

Mathers LH, et al: *Clinical anatomy principles,* St Louis, 1996, Mosby.

Matsen F, Arntz C: Rotator cuff failure. In Rockwood C, Matsen F, editors: *The shoulder,* Philadelphia, 1990, WB Saunders.

Matsen F, Arntz C: Subacromial impingement. In Rockwood C, Matsen F, editors: *The shoulder,* Philadelphia, 1990, WB Saunders.

Matsen FA III, Arntz CT: Rotator cuff tendon failure in the shoulder. In Matsen FA III, Rockwood CA Jr, editors: *The shoulder,* Philadelphia, 1990, WB Saunders.

Mazion JM: *Illustrated manual of neurological reflexes/signs/tests, part I; orthopedic signs/tests/maneuvers for office procedure, part II,* Orlando, 1980, Daniels Publishing.

McLaughlin HL: The "frozen" shoulder, *Clin Orthop* 20:126, 1961.

McRae R: *Clinical orthopaedic examination,* ed 3, Edinburgh, 1990, Churchill Livingstone.

McRae R: *Practical fracture treatment,* ed 3, New York, 1994, Churchill Livingstone.

Medical Economics Books: *Patient care flow chart manual,* ed 3, Oradell, NJ, 1982, Medical Economics Books.

Mellion MB: *Sports medicine secrets,* Philadelphia, 1994, Hanley & Belfus.

Mellion MB: *Office sports medicine,* ed 2, St Louis, 1996, Mosby.

Mendoza RX, Nicholas JA, Sands A: Principals of shoulder rehabilitation in the athlete. In Nicholas JA, Hershman EB, editor: *The upper extremity in sports medicine,* St Louis, 1990, Mosby.

Mengel MB, Schwiebert LP: *Ambulatory medicine the primary care of families,* ed 2, Stamford, Conn, 1996, Appleton & Lange.

Mennell JM: *The musculoskeletal system differential diagnosis from symptoms and physical signs,* Gaithersburg, Md, 1992, Aspen.

Mercier LR, Pettid FJ: *Practical orthopedics,* ed 4, St Louis, 1995, Mosby.

Merle D'Aubigne R: Nerve injuries in fractures and dislocations of the shoulder, *Surg Clin North Am* 43:1685, 1963.

Miller MD: *Review of orthopaedics,* Philadelphia, 1992, WB Saunders.

Mirvis SE, Young JWR: *Imaging in trauma and critical care,* Baltimore, 1991, Williams & Wilkins.

Misamore GW, Woodward C: Evaluation of degenerative lesions of the rotator cuff: a comparison of arthrography and ultrasonography, *J Bone Joint Surg* 73A:704, 1991.

Moore KL: *Clinically oriented anatomy,* ed 3, Baltimore, 1992, Williams & Wilkins.

Morrey BF, An K: *Biomechanics of the shoulder,* Philadelphia, 1990, WB Saunders.

Mosby-Year Book, Inc: *Expert 10-minute physical examination,* St Louis, 1997, Mosby-Year Book.

Moseley HF: *Shoulder lesions,* ed 3, Baltimore, 1969, Williams & Wilkins.

Moseley JB, et al: EMG analysis of the scapular muscles during a shoulder rehabilitation program, *Am J Sports Med* 10:128, 1992.

Murnaghan JP: Frozen shoulder. In Rockwood C, Matsen F, editors: *The shoulder,* Philadelphia, 1990, WB Saunders.

Neer CS: Anterior acromioplasty for the chronic impingement syndrome in the shoulder, *J Bone Joint Surg* 54A:41, 1972.

Neer CS II: *Shoulder reconstruction,* Philadelphia, 1990, WB Saunders.

Nettina SM: *The Lippincott manual of nursing practice,* ed 6, Philadelphia, 1996, Lippincott.

Neviaser JS: Musculoskeletal disorders of the shoulder region causing cervicobrachial pain: differential diagnosis and treatment, *Surg Clin North Am* 43:1703, 1963.

Newton RW: *Color atlas of pediatric neurology,* St Louis, 1995, Mosby-Wolfe.

Nielsen KD, Wester JU, Lorensten A: The shoulder impingement syndrome: the results of surgical decompression, *J Shoulder Elbow Surg* 3:12, 1994.

Nordin M, Andersson GBJ, Pope MH: *Musculoskeletal disorders in the workplace: principles and practice,* St Louis, 1997, Mosby.

Norris T: Treatment and physical examination of the shoulder. In Nicholas J, Hershman E, editors: *The upper extremity in sports medicine,* St Louis, 1990, Mosby.

O'Brien, SJ, et al: The anatomy and histology of the inferior glenohumeral ligament complex of the shoulder, *Am J Sport Med* 18:449, 1990.

O'Donoghue DH: *Treatment of injuries to athletes,* ed 3, Philadelphia, 1976, WB Saunders.

Olson WH, Brumback RA, Gascon G, Iyer V: *Handbook of symptom-oriented neurology,* ed 2, St Louis, 1994, Mosby.

Omer GE, Spinner M: *Management of peripheral nerve problems,* Philadelphia, 1980, WB Saunders.

O'Young B, Young MA, Stiens SA: *PM&R secrets,* Philadelphia, 1997, Hanley & Belfus.

Pagana KD, Pagana TJ: *Mosby's manual of diagnostic and laboratory tests,* St Louis, 1998, Mosby.

Pagnani MJ, Galinat BJ, Warren RF: Glenohumeral instability. In Nicholas JA, Hershman EB, editors: *The upper extremity in sports medicine,* St Louis, 1990, Mosby.

Parsons TA: The snapping scapula and subscapular exostosis, *J Bone Joint Surg* 55B:345, 1963.

Patten J: *Neurological differential diagnosis,* ed 2, London, 1996, Springer.

Pecina MM, Krmpotic-Nemanic J, Markiewitz AD: *Tunnel syndromes,* Boca Raton, Fla, 1991, CRC Press.

Pheasant S: *Ergonomics, work and health,* Gaithersburg, Md, 1991, Aspen.

Polley HF, Hunder GG: *Rheumatologic interviewing and physical examination of the joints,* ed 2, Philadelphia, 1978, WB Saunders.

Pollock RG, Duralde XA, Flatow EL, Bigliani LU: The use of arthroscopy in the treatment of resistant frozen shoulder, *Clin Orthop* 304:30, 1994.

Pronsati MP: Treatment of thoracic outlet syndrome comes under scrutiny, *Adv Physical Therapists* Sept:14, 1991.

Quigley TB: The nonoperative treatment of symptomatic calcareous deposits in the shoulder, *Surg Clin North Am* 43:1495, 1963.

Rachlin ES: *Myofascial pain and fibromyalgia trigger point management,* St Louis, 1994, Mosby.

Ravel R: *Clinical laboratory medicine clinical application of laboratory data,* ed 6, St Louis, 1995, Mosby.

Reilly PJ, Torg JS: Athletic injury to the cervical nerve roots and brachial plexus, *Op Tech Sports Med* 1:231, 1993.

Resnick D, Niwayama G: *Diagnosis of bone and joint disorders,* Philadelphia, 1995, WB Saunders.

Riley GP, et al: Glycosaminoglycans of human rotator cuff tendons: changes with age and in chronic rotator cuff tendinitis, *Ann Rheum Dis* 53:367, 1994.

Riley GP, et al: Tendon degeneration and chronic shoulder pain; changes in the collagen composition of the human rotator cuff tendons in rotator cuff tendinitis, *Ann Rheum Dis* 53:359, 1994.

Rizk TE, Pinals RS, Talaiver AS: Corticosteroid injections in adhesive capsulitis; investigation of their value and site, *Arch Phys Med Rehabil* 72:20, 1991.

Rockwood CA, Young DC: Disorders of the acromioclavicular joint. In Rockwood CA, Matsen FA, editors: *The shoulder,* vol 2, Philadelphia, 1990, WB Saunders.

Rodosky MW, Harner CD, Fu FH: The role of the long head of the biceps muscle and superior glenoid labrum in anterior stability of the shoulder, *Am J Sport Med* 22:121, 1994.

Rogers LR: *Radiology of skeletal trauma,* ed 2, London, 1992, Churchill Livingstone.

Rolak LA: *Neurology secrets,* ed 2, Philadelphia, 1998, Hanley & Belfus.

Roos DB, et al: Thoracic outlet syndrome, *Arch Surg* 93:71, 1966.

Rumack CM, Wilson SR, Charboneau JW: *Diagnostic ultrasound,* vol 1-2, ed 2, St Louis, 1998, Mosby.

Ruwe PA, et al: Can MR imaging effectively replace diagnostic arthroscopy? *Radiology* 183;335, 1992.

Saidoff DC, McDonough AL: *Critical pathways in therapeutic intervention,* St Louis, 1997, Mosby.

Schumacher HR, Bomalski JS: *Case studies in rheumatology for the house officer,* Baltimore, 1990, Williams & Wilkins.

Schumacher HR, Klippel JH, Koopman WJ: *Primer on the rheumatic diseases,* ed 10, Atlanta, 1993, Arthritis Foundation.

Selye H: The experimental production of calcified deposits in the rotator cuff, *Surg Clin North Am* 43:1483, 1963.

Shankman GA: *Fundamental orthopedic management for the physical therapist assistant,* St Louis, 1997, Mosby.

Silliman JF, Dean MT: Neurovascular injuries to the shoulder complex, *J Orthop Sports Phys Ther* 18:442, 1993.

Silliman JF, Hawkins RJ: Current concepts and recent advances in the athlete's shoulder, *Clin Sports Med* 10:693, 1991.

Silliman JF, Hawkins RJ: Classification and physical diagnosis of instability of the shoulder, *Clin Orthop* 291:7, 1993.

Skyhar MJ, Warren RF, Altchek DW: Instability of the shoulder. In Nicholas JA, Hershman EB, editors: *The upper extremity in sports medicine,* St Louis, 1990, Mosby.

Snyder SJ, Karzel RP, Del Pizzo W: SLAP lesions of the shoulder, *Arthroscopy* 6:274, 1990.

Snyder SJ, et al: Partial thickness rotator cuff tears: Results of arthroscopic treatment, *Arthroscopy* 7:1, 1991.

Sobel J, Pettrone F, Nirschl R: Prevention and treatment of upper extremity sports injuries. In Nicholas J, Hershman E, editors: *The extremity in sports medicine,* St Louis 1990, Mosby.

Soslowsky LJ, et al: Articular geometry of the glenohumeral joint, *Clin Orthop* 285:181, 1992.

Specht NT, Russo RD: *Practical guide to diagnostic imaging,* St Louis, 1998, Mosby.

Stedman TL: *Stedman's medical dictionary,* ed 25, Baltimore, 1990, Williams & Wilkins.

Steinbrocker O: The painful shoulder. In Hollander JL, McCarty DJ, editors: *Arthritis and allied conditions,* ed 8, Philadelphia, 1972, Lea & Febiger.

Stewart DL, Abeln SH: *Documenting functional outcomes in physical therapy,* St Louis, 1993, Mosby.

Stiles RG, Otte MT: Imaging of the shoulder, *Radiology* 188:603, 1993.

Stoller DW: *Magnetic resonance imaging in orthopaedics & sports medicine,* Philadelphia, 1993, JB Lippincott.

Strege D: Upper extremity. In Loth T, editor: *Orthopaedic boards review,* St Louis, 1993, Mosby.

Sutton D: *A textbook of radiology and imaging,* ed 5, London, 1993, Churchill Livingstone.

Sutton D, Young JWR: *A concise textbook of clinical imaging,* ed 2, St Louis, 1995, Mosby.

Tan JC, Horn SE: *Practical manual of physical medicine and rehabilitation,* St Louis, 1998, Mosby.

Taybi H, Lachman RS: *Radiology of syndromes, metabolic disorders, and skeletal dysplasias,* ed 4, St Louis, 1996, Mosby.

Thein LA: Rehabilitation of shoulder injuries. In Prentice WE, editor: *Rehabilitation techniques in sports medicine,* ed 2, St Louis, 1994, Mosby.

Thibodeau GA, Patton KT: *Anatomy & physiology,* ed 3, St Louis, 1996, Mosby.

Thibodeau GA, Patton KT: *Pocket reference to accompany anatomy & physiology,* ed 3, St Louis, 1996, Mosby.

Thompson JM: *Clinical outlines for health assessment,* St Louis, 1997, Mosby.

Toghill PJ: *Examining patients: an introduction to clinical medicine,* London, 1990, Edward Arnold.

Tollison CD, Satterthwaite JR, Tollison JW: *Handbook of pain management,* ed 2, Baltimore, 1994, Williams & Wilkins.

Torg JS, Shepard RJ: *Current therapy in sports medicine,* ed 3, St Louis, 1995, Mosby.

Townsend H, et al: Electromyographic analysis of the glenohumeral muscles during a baseball rehabilitation program, *Am J Sports Med* 19:264, 1991.

Turek SL: *Orthopaedics principles and their application,* ed 3, Philadelphia, 1977, JB Lippincott.

Uhthoff H, Sarkar K: Calcifying tendinitis. In Rockwood C, Matsen F, editors: *The shoulder,* Philadelphia, 1990, WB Saunders.

Van Holsbeeck M, Introcaso JH: *Musculoskeletal ultrasound,* St Louis, 1991, Mosby.

Wakefield TS, Frank RG: *The clinician's guide to neuro musculoskeletal practice,* Abbotsford, Wis, 1995, Allied Health of Wisconsin.

Wasilewski SA, Frankel U: Rotator cuff pathology, *Clin Orthop* 267:65, 1991.

Weineck J: *Functional anatomy in sports,* ed 2, St Louis, 1990, Mosby.

Weinstein SL, Buckwalter JA: *Turek's orthopaedics principles and their application,* ed 5, Philadelphia, 1994, JB Lippincott.

Whitenack SH, Hunter JM, Jaeger SH, Read RL: Thoracic outlet syndrome complex: diagnoses and treatment. In Hunter JM, Schneider LH, Mackin EJ, Callahan AD, editors: *Rehabilitation of the hand: surgery and therapy,* ed 3, St Louis, 1990, Mosby.

Williams GR, Rockwood CA: Fractures of the scapula. In DeLee JC, Drez D, editors: *Orthopaedic sports medicine: principals and practice,* vol 1, Philadelphia, 1994, WB Saunders.

Williams GR, Rockwood CA: Injuries to the acromioclavicular joint. In DeLee JC, Drez D, editors: *Orthopaedic sports medicine: principals and practice,* vol 1, St Louis, 1994, WB Saunders.

Williams MM, Snyder SJ, Buford D Jr: The Buford complex, the cord-like middle glenohumeral ligament and absent anterosuperior labrum complex; a normal anatomic capsulolabral variant, *Arthroscopy* 10:2417, 1994.

Windsor RE, Lox DM: *Soft tissue injuries: diagnosis and treatment,* Philadelphia, 1998, Hanley & Belfus.

Winter D: *Biomechanics and motor control of human movement,* ed 2, New York, 1990, Wiley-Interscience.

Wright IS: Neurovascular syndrome produced by hyperabduction of the arms, *Am Heart J* 29:1, 1945.

Wright IS: *Vascular diseases in clinical practice,* Chicago, 1948, Mosby.

Wright IS, et al: The subclavian steal and other shoulder girdle syndromes, *Trans Am Clin Climatol Assoc* 76:13, 1964.

Wright V: The shoulder-hand syndrome, *Rep Rheum Dis* 24:1, 1966.

Wuelker N, Plitz W, Roetman B: Biomechanical data concerning the shoulder impingement syndrome, *Clin Orthop* 303:242, 1994.

Yahara ML: Shoulder. In Richardson JK, Iglarsh ZA, editors: *Clinical orthopaedic physical therapy,* Philadelphia, 1994, WB Saunders.

Yergason RM: Supination sign, *J Bone Joint Surg* 12:160, 1931.

Yochum T, Rowe L: *Essentials of skeletal radiology,* ed 2, Baltimore, 1996, Williams & Wilkins.

Young DC, Rockwood CA: Fractures of the clavicle. In DeLee JC, Drez D, editors: *Orthopaedic sports medicine: principals and practice,* vol 1, Philadelphia, 1994, WB Saunders.

Young JWR, Mirvis SE, editors: *Imaging in trauma and critical care,* Baltimore, 1991, Williams & Wilkins.

Zitelli BJ, Davis HW: *Atlas of pediatric physical diagnosis,* ed 2, London, 1992, Wolfe.

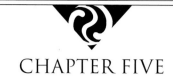

CHAPTER FIVE

THE ELBOW

AXIOMS IN ELBOW ASSESSMENT

- The elbow is a complex hinge joint.
- The elbow is essential to the positioning and full use of the hand.
- Soft-tissue lesions such as lateral epicondylitis and olecranon bursitis occur more often than joint disease.
- Diagnosis of elbow conditions is largely based on pain, location of swelling, presence of point tenderness, and the results of range-of-motion studies.

INTRODUCTION

Although the number of diseases that affect the elbow with any degree of frequency is small, examining the joint often provides clues to diagnosis of specific neuromuscular disease. Pain is the symptom that focuses attention on this joint and prompts the patient to visit the physician. Although it usually reflects a localized process at the elbow, the pain may be referred from the hand and wrist or from the shoulder and neck. Most actions of the elbow can be compensated for by the shoulder; therefore even moderate compromises of motion, provided they are painless, do not result in disability. Subtle flexion contractures may develop over years without the patient even being aware of them. In contrast, significant pain at the elbow can incapacitate the entire arm. Sleeves of clothing often cover the elbows, so swellings and deformities are cosmetically important only when they are exaggerated. It is important to note whether swelling is intracapsular or extracapsular, intramuscular or intermuscular. The earliest sign of joint effusion is induration of the capsule around the olecranon or epicondyles. In the flexed position, the hollows or the synovium may be totally filled.

TABLE 5-1

ELBOW JOINT CROSS-REFERENCE TABLE BY SYNDROME PROCEDURE

Elbow Test/Sign	Lateral Epicondylitis	Radiohumeral Bursitis	Cubital Tunnel Syndrome	Medial Epicondylitis	Neuropathy	Sprain
Cozen's test	•	•				
Elbow flexion test			•			
Golfer's elbow test				•		
Kaplan's sign	•					
Ligamentous instability test						•
Mills' test	•					
Tinel's sign at the elbow					•	

TABLE 5-2

ELBOW JOINT CROSS-REFERENCE TABLE BY SYNDROME

Cubital tunnel syndrome	Elbow flexion test
Lateral epicondylitis	Cozen's test
	Kaplan's sign
	Mills' test
Medial epicondylitis	Golfer's elbow test
Neuropathy	Tinel's sign at the elbow
Radiohumeral bursitis	Cozen's test
Sprain	Ligamentous instability test

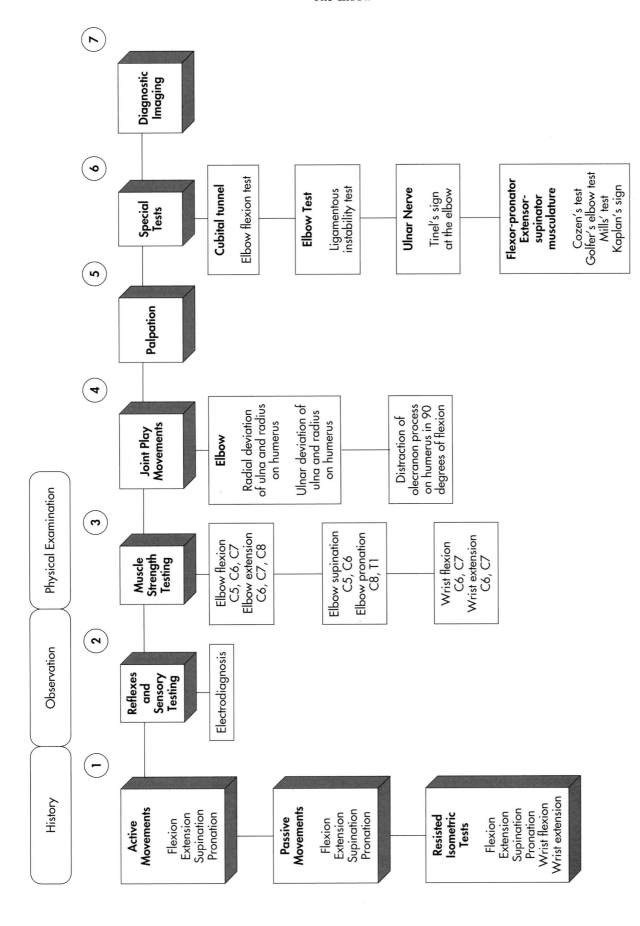

FIG. 5-1 Protocol of elbow joint assessment.

When the elbow is extended, the epicondyles and the tip of the olecranon should be at the same level. In normal elbow configuration, when a line is drawn between the epicondyles, the olecranon should be on the center of the line. When the elbow is flexed to an angle of 90 degrees, the tip of the olecranon lies directly distal to the line joining the epicondyles. If a line from the olecranon is drawn to each epicondyle, the three prominences and line should form an isosceles triangle.

If the triangle is normal, but abnormal in relation to the shaft of the humerus, there could be a supracondylar fracture in which the three bony landmarks are displaced posteriorly (Fig. 5-3).

ORTHOPEDIC GAMUT 5-1

ISOSCELES TRIANGLE OF THE ELBOW

If the triangle of the isosceles triangle of the elbow is abnormal, the following could exist:

1. Posterior elbow dislocation (Fig. 5-2)
2. Fracture of the epicondyle
3. Intracondylar fracture
4. Fracture of the olecranon

ORTHOPEDIC GAMUT 5-2

PRIMARY FUNCTIONS OF THE ELBOW

The elbow's primary functions are as follows:

1. Aid in positioning the hand in appropriate locations
2. Adjust height and length of the limb
3. Stabilize the upper extremity for power and fine motor work activities
4. Provide fulcrum for the arm in lifting

ORTHOPEDIC GAMUT 5-3

ELBOW JOINTS

The elbow consists of a complex set of joints that require careful assessment. The articulations of the joint are as follows:

1. Humeroulnar
2. Humeroradial
3. Proximal radioulnar

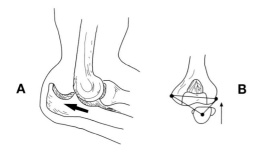

FIG. 5-2 **A,** Posterior elbow dislocation. **B,** Posterior view of elbow dislocation demonstrating the bony alignment. *(From Hartley A: Practical joint assessment upper quadrant, ed 2, St Louis, 1995, Mosby.)*

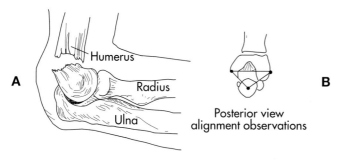

FIG. 5-3 **A,** Supracondylar fracture with olecranon impingement. **B,** Posterior view demonstrating the bony misalignment. *(From Hartley A: Practical joint assessment upper quadrant, ed 2, St Louis, 1995, Mosby.)*

The examination of the elbow must be preceded by a precise history to allow emphasis to be placed on particular areas. Complaints usually consist of pain, loss of movement, weakness, clicking, or locking. There may be sharply localized pain, typical of extraarticular pathology, deep joint pain, or the poorly localized pain of ulnar neuropathy with or without typical paresthesia extending to the hand (Fig. 5-4). The functional interplay between the elbow, shoulder, and wrist means that examination of all of these joints may be necessary (Table 5-3). Referred pain in the elbow, especially from the neck or shoulder, is usually diffuse. Examination must include comparison of right and left arms.

Pain of lateral elbow origin is usually diagnosed as radiohumeral bursitis, epicondylitis, or tennis elbow (Fig. 5-5). This problem involves either the origin of the wrist extensors (tendinitis) or, occasionally, radial nerve impingement by musculotendinous structures crossing the elbow joint (Fig. 5-6).

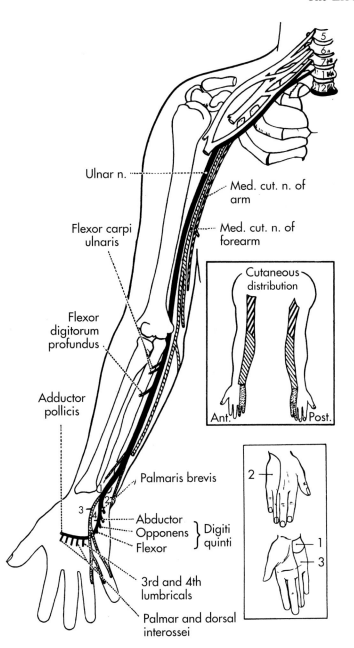

Ulnar n.

Med. cut. n. of arm

Med. cut. n. of forearm

Flexor carpi ulnaris

Flexor digitorum profundus

Adductor pollicis

Cutaneous distribution

Ant.   Post.

Palmaris brevis

Abductor
Opponens } Digiti
Flexor   quinti

3rd and 4th lumbricals

Palmar and dorsal interossei

FIG. 5-4   The course of the ulnar nerve.   *(From Katirji B:* Electromyography in clinical practice: a case study approach, *St Louis, 1998, Mosby.)*

TABLE 5-3

FUNCTIONAL ARC MEASUREMENTS FOR SELECTED ACTIVITIES OF DAILY LIVING

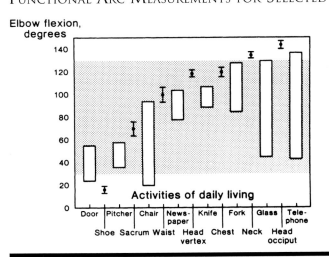

Elbow flexion, degrees

Activities of daily living

Door | Pitcher | Chair | News-paper | Knife | Fork | Glass | Tele-phone
Shoe   Sacrum   Waist   Head vertex   Chest   Neck   Head occiput

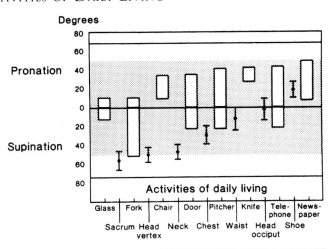

Degrees

Pronation

Supination

Activities of daily living

Glass | Fork | Chair | Door | Pitcher | Knife | Tele-phone | News-paper
Sacrum   Head vertex   Neck   Chest   Waist   Head occiput   Shoe

From Kelley WN, et al: *Textbook of rheumatology,* ed 5, Philadelphia, 1997, WB Saunders.

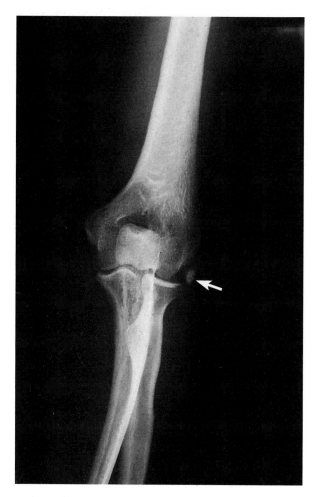

FIG. 5-5 Calcification of the common extensor tendon of the elbow *(arrow)*. *(From Deltoff MN, Kogon PL:* The portable skeletal x-ray library, *St Louis, 1998, Mosby.)*

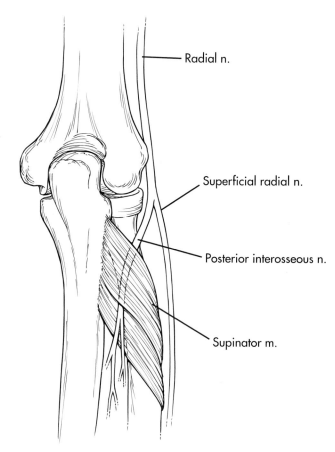

FIG. 5-6 In a posterior view, the radial nerve as it passes through the supinator musculature, travels around the head of the radius, and branches to the posterior interosseous nerves of the elbow. *(From Greenstein GM:* Clinical assessment of neuromusculoskeletal disorders, *St Louis, 1997, Mosby.)*

A similar problem may occur on the medial elbow epicondyle, because all of the wrist flexors and pronators originate from the medial epicondyle. Affected individuals use flexor-pronator muscle groups repetitively, isometrically or isokinetically. This is unusual, because forceful wrist flexor power is seldom used. Most powerful hand grasping is accomplished in the dorsiflexed wrist position.

Intraarticular abnormalities such as osteochondritis dissecans of the capitellum may result in lateral elbow pain (Fig. 5-7).

Osteochondritis dissecans of the elbow is an idiopathic disorder that affects the capitellum of the humerus, with ensuing avascular necrosis. It is usually seen in the dominant arm of adolescent boys, especially those involved in throwing sports (Fig. 5-8). Panner's disease is a condition of unclear origin in which there is osteochondrosis of the capitellum. It is seen most often in young boys who complain of tenderness and swelling over the lateral aspect

of the elbow with limited extension. Direct trauma or inadequate circulation through the elbow joint has been associated with osteochondritis of the capitellum (Fig. 5-9).

ORTHOPEDIC GAMUT 5-4

AVASCULAR NECROSIS OF THE CAPITELLUM

Possible causes of avascular necrosis of the capitellum of the elbow (Panner's disease) include the following:

1. Bacterial infection
2. Fracture
3. Heredity
4. Vascular insufficiency

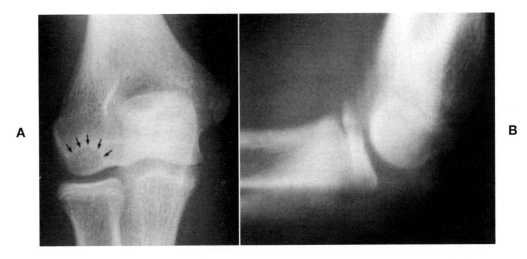

FIG. 5-7 **A,** Cyst outlined *(arrows)* in the capitellum compatible with either posttraumatic osteochondrosis or an osteochondral fracture. **B,** Traumatic osteochondrosis of the radial head. *(From Nicholas JA, Hershman EB: The upper extremity in sports medicine, ed 2, St Louis, 1995, Mosby.)*

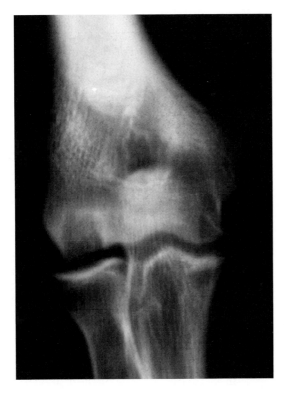

FIG. 5-8 Radiograph of osteochondritis dissecans of the capitellum. *(From Nicholas JA, Hershman EB: The upper extremity in sports medicine, ed 2, St Louis, 1995, Mosby.)*

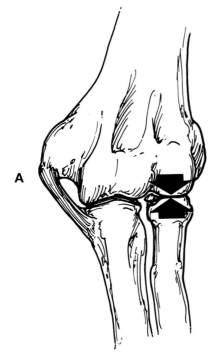

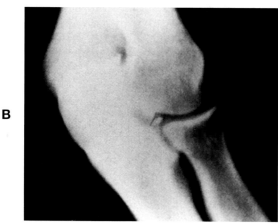

FIG. 5-9   **A** and **B,** Demonstration of radial head–capitellum compression and resultant loose bodies. *(From Nicholas JA, Hershman EB: The upper extremity in sports medicine, ed 2, St Louis, 1995, Mosby.)*

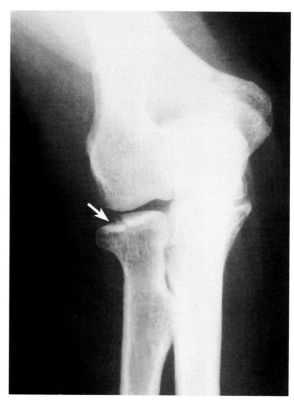

FIG. 5-10   Radial head fracture (chisel) of the lateral radial head *(arrow),* with inferior displacement of the fragment. *(From Deltoff MN, Kogon PL: The portable skeletal x-ray library, St Louis, 1998, Mosby.)*

ORTHOPEDIC GAMUT 5-5

HYPEREXTENSION INJURIES OF THE ELBOW

The structures of the elbow that can be injured with a hyperextension force include the following:

1. Biceps brachii, at its point of insertion on the neck of the radius
2. Brachialis, at its point of insertion on the ulna
3. Brachioradialis
4. Anterior portion of the medial (ulnar) and/or lateral (radial) collateral ligaments (the medial collateral ligament is injured more often because of the valgus position of the joint)
5. Elbow capsular and collateral ligament (they can avulse a piece of the condyle, most commonly the medial epicondyle)

An extremely minor fracture of the radial head (chisel fracture) might cause pain that could be confused with tennis elbow (Fig. 5-10). An injury occurring in children and adolescents in which the medial epicondyle is inflamed with partial separation of the apophysis is known as *little leaguer's elbow* (Fig. 5-11). Boxer's elbow (also called *hyperextension overload syndrome* or *olecranon impingement syndrome*) is caused by repetitive valgus extension of the elbow in the boxer's jab or in sports involving throwing (Fig. 5-12). Elbow joint hyperextension injuries usually result from falling on an outstretched arm. The elbow is extended and the forearm supinated (Fig. 5-13).

Pain in the elbow, particularly if it extends along the entire arm, without objective findings at the joint, suggests psychogenic rheumatism. Other diseases referring pain to the elbow include myocardial infarction, cervical root le-

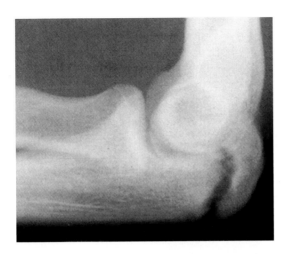

FIG. 5-11   Lateral elbow radiograph demonstrating the widened olecranon apophyseal plate. *(From Nicholas JA, Hershman EB:* The upper extremity in sports medicine, *ed 2, St Louis, 1995, Mosby.)*

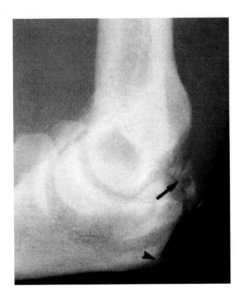

FIG. 5-12   Hypertrophic spurs at the posterior aspect of the olecranon process *(top arrow)*. *(From Nicholas JA, Hershman EB: The upper extremity in sports medicine, ed 2, St Louis, 1995, Mosby.)*

sions, thoracic outlet syndromes, or even subdeltoid bursitis. Psychogenic rheumatism is further suggested by a history of neurosis, strange behavior, or a bizarre and inconsistent history. Diagnostic imaging and laboratory tests are as unimpressive as the physical findings. Carpal tunnel syndrome may cause retrograde radiation of pain to the elbow.

Elbow joint complaints usually consist of pain, loss of movement, weakness, clicking, or locking. There may be sharply localized pain (typical of extraarticular pathology), deep joint pain, or poorly localized pain of ulnar neuropathy with or without typical paresthesias extending to the hand. The functional interplay between the elbow, shoulder, and wrist means that examination of all these joints may be necessary. Referred pain in the elbow, especially from the neck or shoulder, is usually diffuse (Table 5-4).

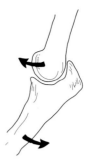

FIG. 5-13   Elbow hyperextension injury mechanism, with olecranon impingement. *(From Hartley A:* Practical joint assessment upper quadrant, *ed 2, St Louis, 1995, Mosby.)*

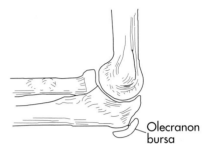

FIG. 5-14   The olecranon bursa. *(From Hartley A:* Practical joint assessment upper quadrant, *ed 2, St Louis, 1995, Mosby.)*

TABLE 5-4

UPPER EXTREMITY PERIARTICULAR SYNDROME DIFFERENTIAL DIAGNOSTIC LIST

Region	Periarticular Syndrome	Monarticular Syndrome
Shoulder	Subacromial bursitis	Pancoast tumor
	Long-head bicipital tendinitis	Brachial plexopathy
	Rotator cuff tear	Cervical nerve root injury
Elbow	**Olecranon bursitis**	**Ulnar nerve**
	Epicondylitis	**entrapment**
Wrist	Extensor tendinitis (including de Quervain's tenosynovitis)	Carpal tunnel syndrome
	Gonococcal tenosynovitis	
Hand	Palmar fasciitis (Dupuytren's contracture)	
	Ligamentous or capsular injury	

Modified from Kelley WN, et al: *Textbook of rheumatology,* ed 5, Philadelphia, 1997, WB Saunders.

True elbow pain can be related to joint disease; however, it is more commonly caused by lesions of the periarticular tissues. Inflammation of the olecranon bursa (draftsman's elbow) may be secondary to a number of conditions, including repetitive or acute trauma, rheumatoid arthritis, gout, and pseudogout (Fig. 5-14). It is also known as *student's elbow* and *miner's elbow.*

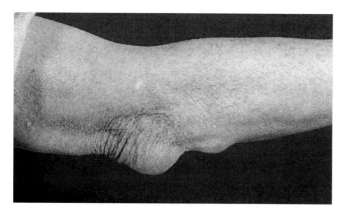

FIG. 5-15   Olecranon bursitis as seen with rheumatoid arthritis; note also the rheumatoid nodule distal to the joint. *(From Klippel JH, Dieppe PA:* Rheumatology, *vol 1-2, ed 2, London, 1998, Mosby.)*

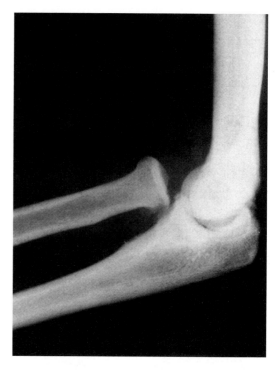

FIG. 5-16   Anterior dislocation of the radial head. *(From Nicholas JA, Hershman EB:* The upper extremity in sports medicine, *ed 2, St Louis, 1995, Mosby.)*

The olecranon bursa is prone to injury by friction or a blow. In addition, because of its position, swelling occurs easily and is readily visible. It may also be involved in crystal arthropathies (gout or rarely calcium pyrophosphate arthritis) or in generalized inflammatory arthritis, especially rheumatoid arthritis in which swelling of the olecranon bursa may be seen in association with rheumatoid nodules on the ulnar border of the forearm (Fig. 5-15).

A traumatic or overuse form of osteochondritis of the radial head occurs in some sports that involve throwing. This is especially evident in the teenage athletes. The radioulnar joint may be affected by loose bodies and synovial osteochondromatosis. Traumatic partial subluxation of the radial head through the annular ligament occurs in children younger than 8 years of age (Fig. 5-16). A "pushed elbow" describes subluxation of the radial head in a proximal direction, which is often seen after a person falls on an outstretched hand. A "pulled elbow" is subluxation of the radial head in a distal direction, which may follow a forceful traction to the forearm.

ESSENTIAL ANATOMY

The elbow acts as a lever system that, along with the other joints, changes the direction of the upper extremity to put the hand in the most effective functional position. The elbow consists of three bones: the distal end of the humerus and the proximal ends of the radius and the ulna (Figs. 5-17 to 5-19). The three articulating surfaces are enclosed in a single synovial cavity. The olecranon bursa is the largest bursa of the elbow, although several smaller bursae are present (Fig. 5-20).

The three major deep nerves of the forearm are the radial, medial, and ulnar nerves. The radial nerve lies anterior to the lateral epicondyle in the arm in its anterior compartment (Fig. 5-21).

The median nerve enters the forearm by passing between the two heads of pronator teres and descends in the anterior compartment of the forearm, traveling between the flexor digitorum superficialis and flexor digitorum profundus muscles (Fig. 5-22).

At the elbow, the ulnar nerve lies in a groove on the posterior surface of the medial epicondyle of the humerus and travels between the two heads of the flexor carpi ulnaris to enter the forearm (see Fig. 5-22).

Arterial supply to the forearm depends entirely on branches of the brachial artery (Fig. 5-23). The radial artery courses to the lateral side of the forearm and aligns itself with the radius. The ulnar artery is the larger of the two branches of the brachial artery (Fig. 5-24).

ESSENTIAL MOTION ASSESSMENT

Tissue approximation limits elbow flexion to 140 to 150 degrees. Retained flexion motion of 130 degrees or less is an impairment in the activities of daily living (Fig. 5-25).

Elbow extension is 0 degrees. Up to 10 degrees of hyperextension is still within normal limits if the patient has no history of trauma to the joint. The inability to return the elbow to within 10 degrees of the neutral position is an impairment in the activities of daily living (Fig. 5-26).

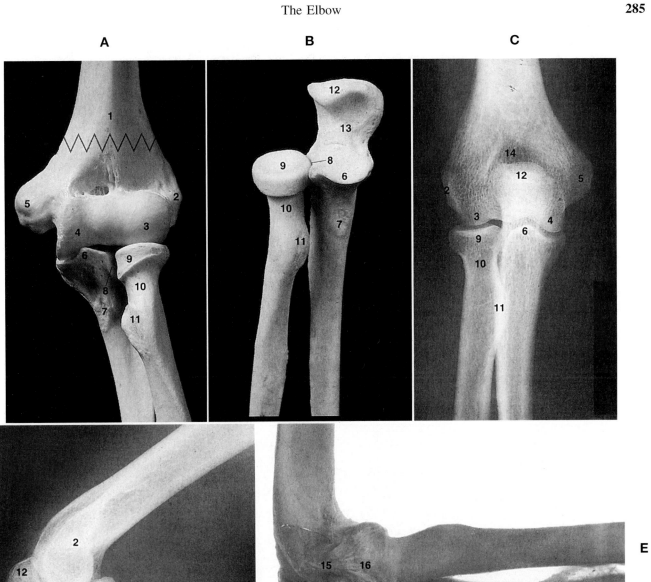

FIG. 5-17   Radiographic anatomy of the elbow. **A-C,** Anteroposterior views. **D-E,** Lateral views.
(From Greenstein GM: Clinical assessment of neuromusculoskeletal disorders, *St Louis, 1997, Mosby.)*

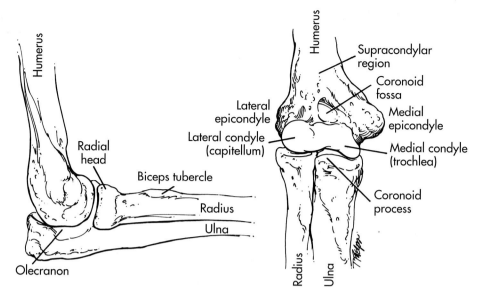

FIG. 5-18   Osseous anatomy of the elbow. *(From Nicholas JA, Hershman EB: The upper extremity in sports medicine, ed 2, St Louis, 1995, Mosby.)*

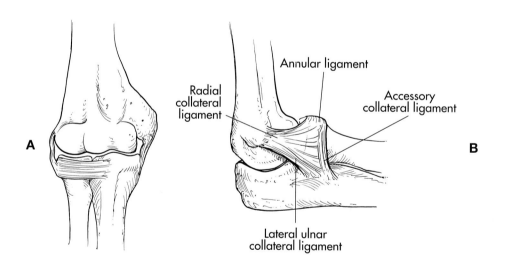

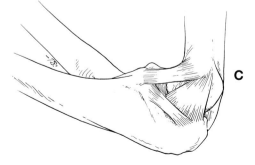

FIG. 5-19   Ligament anatomy of the elbow joint. **A,** Annular ligament. **B,** Lateral collateral ligament complex. **C,** Medial collateral ligament complex. *(From Nicholas JA, Hershman EB: The upper extremity in sports medicine, ed 2, St Louis, 1995, Mosby.)*

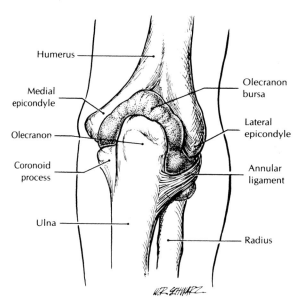

FIG. 5-20   Elbow joint (posterior view). *(From Barkauskas VH, Stoltenberg-Allen K, Baumann LC, Darling-Fisher C:* Health & physical assessment, *ed 2, St Louis, 1998, Mosby.)*

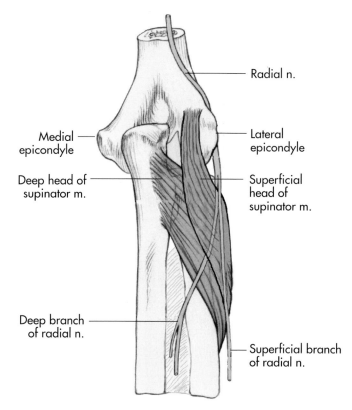

FIG. 5-21   Radial nerve at the elbow. *(From Mathers LH, et al:* Clinical anatomy principles, *St Louis, 1996, Mosby.)*

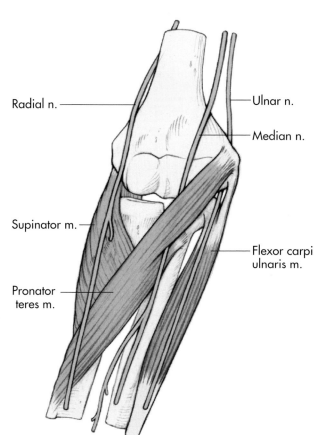

FIG. 5-22   Potential sites for compression of nerves in the proximal forearm (anterior view, right elbow). *(From Mathers LH, et al:* Clinical anatomy principles, *St Louis, 1996, Mosby.)*

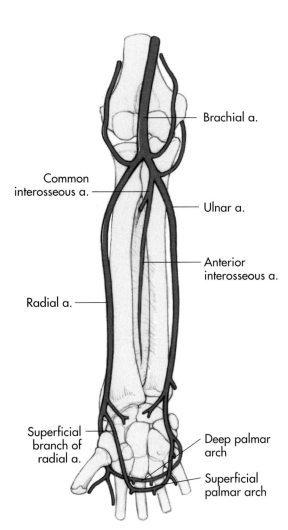

FIG. 5-23 Arterial supply to the forearm (anterior view). *(From Mathers LH, et al:* Clinical anatomy principles, *St Louis, 1996, Mosby.)*

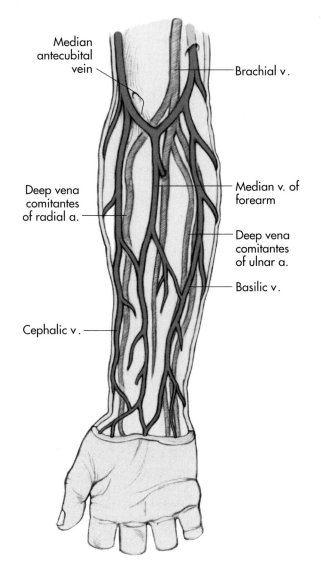

FIG. 5-24 Superficial and deep veins of the forearm (anterior view). *(From Mathers LH, et al:* Clinical anatomy principles, *St Louis, 1996, Mosby.)*

The valgus angle of the elbow ranges from 0 to 15 degrees. This allows the forearm to extend beyond the width of the pelvis. The carrying angle enables the forearm to sustain high tensile stresses. Variations in the carrying angle are cubitus valgus (forearm farther than the arm) and cubitus varus (forearm carried more medial) (Fig. 5-27). A gunstock deformity is a cubitus varus deformity of the elbow. Gunstock deformities are usually secondary to fractures or epiphyseal injury to the distal humerus. The carrying angle is a normal finding and is not indicative of an elbow occult pathology.

Supination of the elbow is limited by tissue stretch to 90 degrees. Retained supination motion of 60 degrees or less is an impairment in the activities of daily living (Fig. 5-28).

Elbow pronation is the same as supination, 80 to 90 degrees. Retained pronation motion of 70 degrees or less is an impairment in the activities of daily living (Fig. 5-29).

ESSENTIAL MUSCLE FUNCTION ASSESSMENT

The arm is divided by fascial septa into anterior and posterior compartments. The lateral and medial intermuscular septa (Figs. 5-31 and 5-32) attach to the humerus

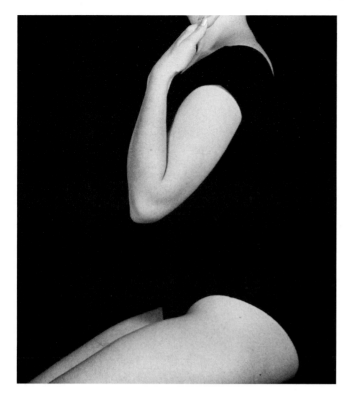

FIG. 5-25   Tissue approximation limits elbow flexion to 140 to 150 degrees. Retained flexion motion of 130 degrees or less is an impairment in the activities of daily living.

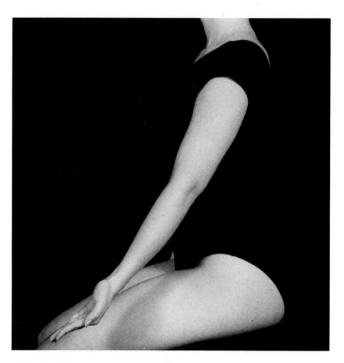

FIG. 5-26   Elbow extension is 0 degrees. Ten degrees of hyperextension is within normal limits if equal bilaterally and in the absence of injury. The inability to return the elbow to within 10 degrees of the neutral position is an impairment in the activities of daily living.

and radiate medially and laterally to the skin, dividing the arm.

The prime movers in flexion of the elbow are the biceps brachii (musculocutaneous nerve, C5, C6), brachialis (musculocutaneous nerve, C5, C6), and brachioradialis (radial nerve, C5, C6) muscles. The flexor muscles of the forearm arising from the medial epicondyle of the humerus are the accessory muscles (Fig. 5-33).

The prime mover in extension of the elbow is the triceps brachii muscle (radial nerve, C7, C8); the anconeus muscle is an accessory. When the arm is horizontally abducted, the long head of the triceps is shortened over the shoulder joint. When the shoulder is flexed, the long head of the triceps is shortened over the elbow joint and elongated over the shoulder joint (Fig. 5-34).

Although the triceps and anconeus act together in extending the elbow joint, the two muscles can be differentiated. The belly of the anconeus muscle is below the elbow joint and is easily distinguished from the triceps by palpation. Paralysis of the anconeus materially reduces the strength of elbow extension (Fig. 5-35).

The primary supinators are the biceps brachii and the supinator. The accessory muscle in this movement is the brachioradialis. In addition to its role in supination, the biceps also functions as an elbow flexor. Its total biceps

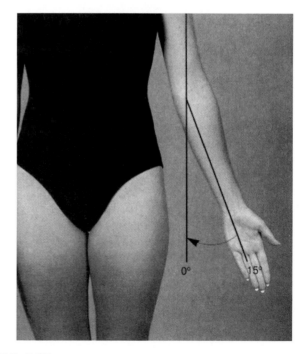

FIG. 5-27   The expected carrying angle of the arm is between 0 and 15 degrees in the adult. (*From Barkauskas VH, Stoltenberg-Allen K, Baumann LC, Darling-Fisher C:* Health & physical assessment, *ed 2, St Louis, 1998, Mosby.*)

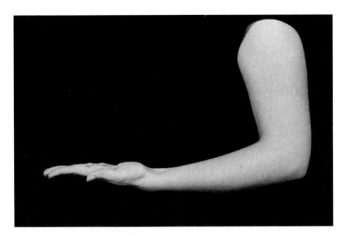

FIG. 5-28   Supination of the elbow is limited, by tissue stretch, to 90 degrees. Retained supination motion of 60 degrees or less is an impairment in the activities of daily living.

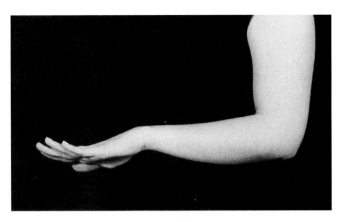

FIG. 5-29   Elbow pronation, 80 to 90 degrees, is the same as supination. Retained pronation motion of 70 degrees or less is an impairment in the activities of daily living.

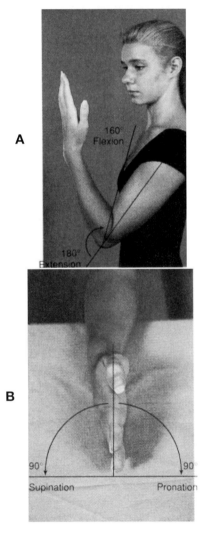

FIG. 5-30   Range of motion of the elbow. **A,** Flexion and extension. **B,** Pronation and supination. *(From Barkauskas VH, Stoltenberg-Allen K, Baumann LC, Darling-Fisher C:* Health & physical assessment, *ed 2, St Louis, 1998, Mosby.)*

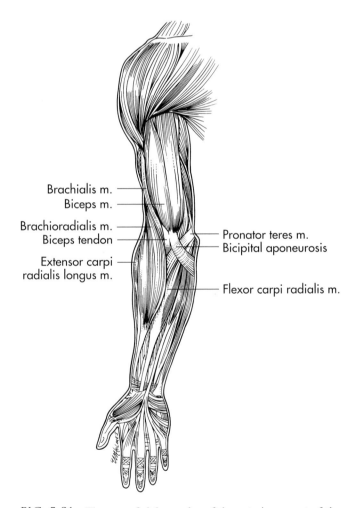

FIG. 5-31   The superficial muscles of the anterior aspect of the elbow. *(From Nicholas JA, Hershman EB:* The upper extremity in sports medicine, *ed 2, St Louis, 1995, Mosby.)*

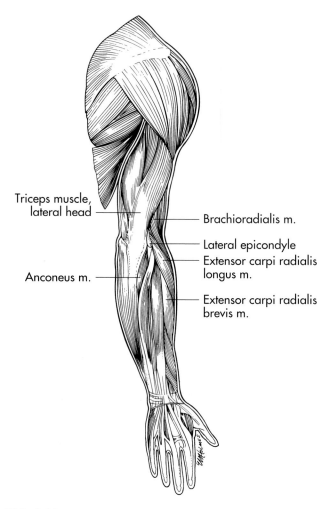

Triceps muscle,
lateral head

Anconeus m.

Brachioradialis m.

Lateral epicondyle

Extensor carpi radialis
longus m.

Extensor carpi radialis
brevis m.

FIG. 5-32   The superficial muscles of the posterior aspect of the elbow.   *(From Nicholas JA, Hershman EB:* The upper extremity in sports medicine, *ed 2, St Louis, 1995, Mosby.)*

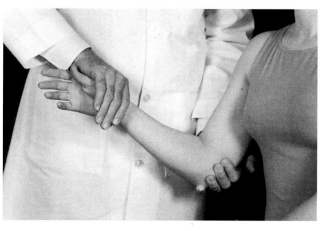

FIG. 5-33   The prime movers in flexion of the elbow are the biceps brachii (musculocutaneous nerve, C5, and C6), brachialis (musculocutaneous nerve, C5, and C6), and brachioradialis (radial nerve, C5, and C6) muscles. The flexor muscles of the forearm that arise from the medial epicondyle of the humerus are the accessory muscles. For testing flexion of the elbow, the patient sits with the arm at the side, the elbow slightly flexed, and the forearm supinated. The examiner stabilizes the patient's arm by grasping it with one hand. The patient is instructed to flex the elbow through its range of motion against graded resistance applied by the examiner. The examiner's other hand is just proximal to the patient's wrist. If the biceps and brachialis are weak, as in a musculocutaneous lesion, the patient will pronate the forearm before flexing the elbow. With this type of lesion, the patient is using the brachioradialis, extensor carpi radialis longus, pronator teres, and wrist flexors.

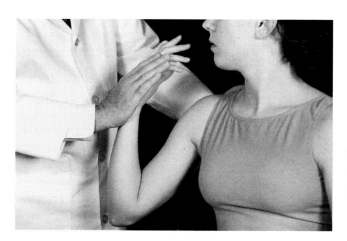

FIG. 5-34   The prime mover in extension of the elbow is the triceps brachii muscle (radial nerve, C7, and C8), and the anconeus muscle is an accessory. The patient is seated. To test extension of the elbow, the examiner fixes the patient's arm as described for flexion and instructs the patient to move the elbow through the range of extension motion while providing graded resistance with the other hand just proximal to the patient's wrist. When the arm is horizontally abducted, the long head of the triceps is shortened over the shoulder joint. When the shoulder is flexed, the long head of the triceps is shortened over the elbow joint and elongated over the shoulder joint.

FIG. 5-35 Although the triceps and anconeus act together in extending the elbow joint, the two muscles can be differentiated. The belly of the anconeus muscle is below the elbow joint and is easily distinguished from the triceps by palpation. The branch of the radial nerve that innervates the anconeus arises near the midhumeral level and is long. It is possible for a lesion to involve only this branch, leaving the triceps unaffected. Paralysis of the anconeus materially reduces the strength of elbow extension. The muscle grade of good in-elbow extension strength is actually the result of a normal triceps and a zero anconeus function.

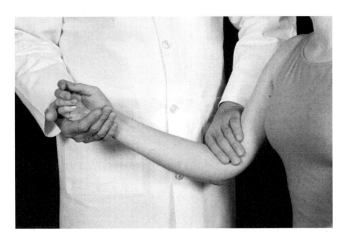

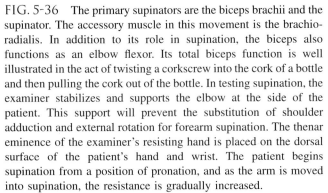

FIG. 5-36 The primary supinators are the biceps brachii and the supinator. The accessory muscle in this movement is the brachioradialis. In addition to its role in supination, the biceps also functions as an elbow flexor. Its total biceps function is well illustrated in the act of twisting a corkscrew into the cork of a bottle and then pulling the cork out of the bottle. In testing supination, the examiner stabilizes and supports the elbow at the side of the patient. This support will prevent the substitution of shoulder adduction and external rotation for forearm supination. The thenar eminence of the examiner's resisting hand is placed on the dorsal surface of the patient's hand and wrist. The patient begins supination from a position of pronation, and as the arm is moved into supination, the resistance is gradually increased.

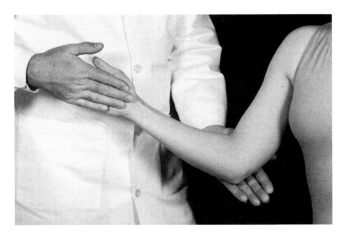

FIG. 5-37 The primary pronators are the pronator teres and the pronator quadratus. The accessory muscle in this movement is the flexor carpi radialis. The examiner stabilizes the patient's elbow just proximal to the joint. This stabilization prevents the substitution of shoulder abduction and internal rotation for pure forearm pronation. The resisting hand is adjusted so that the thenar eminence presses against the volar surface of the hand. This adjustment requires only that the examiner turn the resisting hand from the dorsal to the volar surface of the patient's hand. The patient begins forearm pronation from a position of supination. As the patient moves into pronation, the resistance is increased.

function is well illustrated in the act of twisting a corkscrew into the cork of a bottle and then pulling the cork out of the bottle (Fig. 5-36).

The primary pronators are the pronator teres and the pronator quadratus. The accessory muscle in this movement is the flexor carpi radialis. Pronation and supination are complex movements (Fig. 5-37) that occur simultaneously around an axis best described as an imaginary line between the head of the radius proximally and the medial end of the triangular articular disc distally. In the proximal radioulnar joint, the head of the radius can rotate within the perimeter created by the annular ligament (Fig. 5-38).

Essential Imaging

The elbow position of function is 90 degrees of flexion with the forearm midway between supination and pronation. In this position, the olecranon process of the ulna and the medial and lateral epicondyles of the humerus normally form an isosceles triangle when viewed posteriorly; this is known as the *triangle sign*. If there is a fracture, dislocation, or degeneration leading to loss of bone and/or cartilage, the distance between the apex and base decreases, and the isosceles triangle no longer exists (Fig. 5-39).

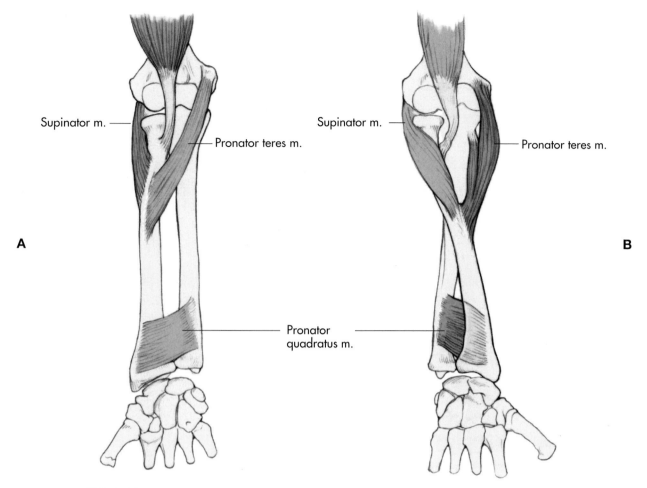

Supinator m. —

— Pronator teres m.

Supinator m. —

— Pronator teres m.

A

B

Pronator
quadratus m.

FIG. 5-38   Muscles mediating supination (**A**) and pronation (**B**). *(From Mathers LH, et al:* Clinical anatomy principles, *St Louis, 1996, Mosby.)*

ORTHOPEDIC GAMUT 5-6

THE ELBOW JOINT

Plain radiographic films demonstrate that the elbow is a compound joint consisting of the following:

1. The articulation of the trochlea of the humerus with the trochlear notch of the ulna
2. The articulation of the capitulum of the humerus with the superior surface of the radial head

Extension of the elbow is limited by the olecranon of the ulna as it contacts the olecranon fossa of the humerus (Figs. 5-40 and 5-41); flexion of the elbow is limited only by the apposition of the muscle masses of the arm and forearm and the bones themselves (Figs. 5-42 and 5-43). Lateral shift of the olecranon process during elbow flexion can result in a medial incongruity of the olecranon-trochlear joint space. A medial incongruity of more than 5 mm is a potential cause of ulnar nerve compression (Figs. 5-44 to 5-47).

Computed tomography (CT) is a successful adjunct to plain film radiography in demonstrating subtle elbow injury. CT studies are particularly helpful in demonstrating occult fractures and osteochondral injuries, as well as in localizing loose bodies and osteophytes located out of the plane of conventional radiographs (Fig. 5-48).

Muscles in the forearm have a variety of attachments. They are found in two large groupings: the anterior and posterior forearm muscles (Fig. 5-49). Magnetic resonance imaging (MRI) of patients is useful in identifying recalcitrant lateral epicondylitis (Fig. 5-50).

Arthrography of the elbow can be carried out using either single- or double-contrast techniques (Fig. 5-51).

As it crosses the cubital fossa at the elbow, the brachial artery remains superficial, covered only by the bicipital aponeurosis and the median cubital vein (Fig. 5-52).

Text continued on p. 300

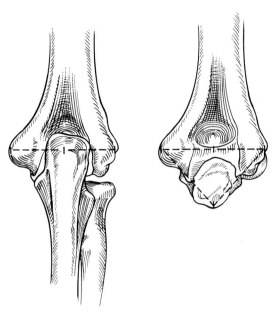

FIG. 5-39   Relationship of the palpable landmarks of the medial and lateral epicondyles of the humerus and the olecranon tip of the ulna.   *(From Nicholas JA, Hershman EB: The upper extremity in sports medicine, ed 2, St Louis, 1995, Mosby.)*

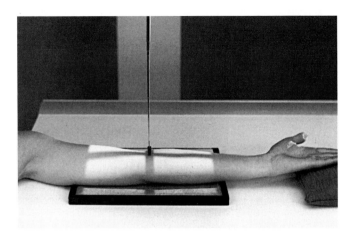

FIG. 5-40   Anteroposterior positioning of the elbow.   *(From Ballinger PW: Merrill's atlas of radiographic positions and radiologic procedures, vol 1-3, ed 8, St Louis, 1995, Mosby.)*

FIG. 5-41   Anteroposterior radiograph of the elbow.   *(From Ballinger PW: Merrill's atlas of radiographic positions and radiologic procedures, vol 1-3, ed 8, St Louis, 1995, Mosby.)*

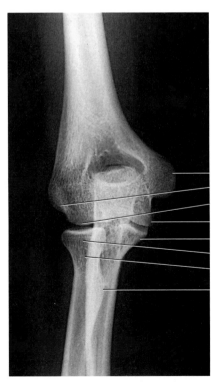

Medial epicondyle
Lateral epicondyle
Capitulum (capitellum)
Trochlea
Proximal ulna
Radial head
Radial neck
Radial tuberosity

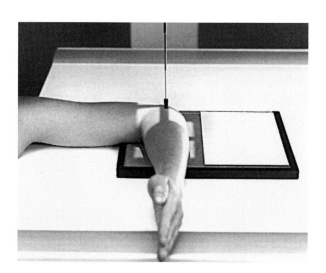

FIG. 5-42 Lateral positioning of the elbow. *(From Ballinger PW: Merrill's atlas of radiographic positions and radiologic procedures, vol 1-3, ed 8, St Louis, 1995, Mosby.)*

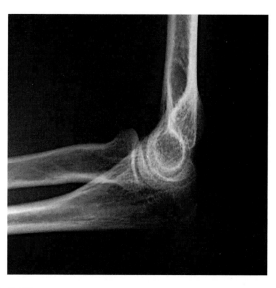

FIG. 5-43 Lateral radiograph of the elbow. *(From Ballinger PW: Merrill's atlas of radiographic positions and radiologic procedures, vol 1-3, ed 8, St Louis, 1995, Mosby.)*

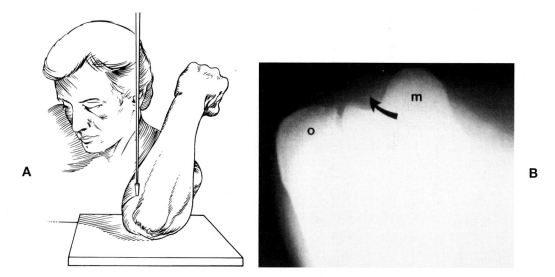

FIG. 5-44 **A,** Cubital tunnel view. **B,** Cubital tunnel radiograph of normal elbow. *Curved arrow,* Cubital tunnel; *m,* medial epicondyle; *o,* olecranon process. *(From Nicholas JA, Hershman EB: The upper extremity in sports medicine, ed 2, St Louis, 1995, Mosby.)*

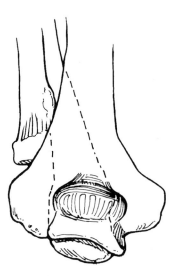

FIG. 5-45 Posteroanterior axial olecranon process. *(From Ballinger PW:* Merrill's atlas of radiographic positions and radiologic procedures, *vol 1-3, ed 8, St Louis, 1995, Mosby.)*

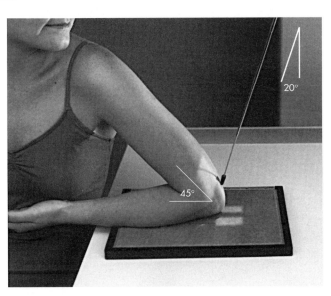

FIG. 5-46 Posteroanterior axial positioning of olecranon process with central ray angled at 20 degrees. *(From Ballinger PW:* Merrill's atlas of radiographic positions and radiologic procedures, *ed 8, St Louis, 1995, Mosby.)*

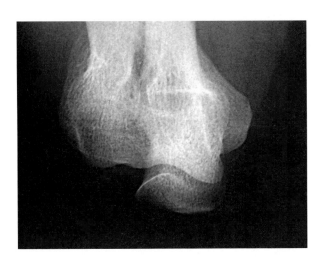

FIG. 5-47 Posteroanterior radiograph of axial olecranon process with central ray angulation at 20 degrees. *(From Ballinger PW:* Merrill's atlas of radiographic positions and radiologic procedures, *vol 1-3, ed 8, St Louis, 1995, Mosby.)*

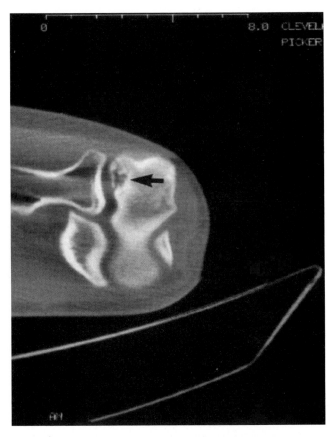

FIG. 5-48 Computed tomography scan made through the joint line of the elbow demonstrates osteochondritis dissecans in the subchondral bone of the capitellum. *(From Nicholas JA, Hershman EB:* The upper extremity in sports medicine, *ed 2, St Louis, 1995, Mosby.)*

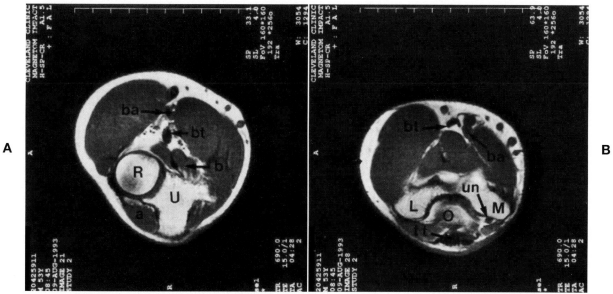

FIG. 5-49   These T$_1$-weighted spin-echo images of a normal elbow demonstrate the signal intensities of normal tissues. **A,** Level of radioulnar articulation. **B,** Level of intercondylar region. *(From Nicholas JA, Hershman EB: The upper extremity in sports medicine, ed 2, St Louis, 1995, Mosby.)*

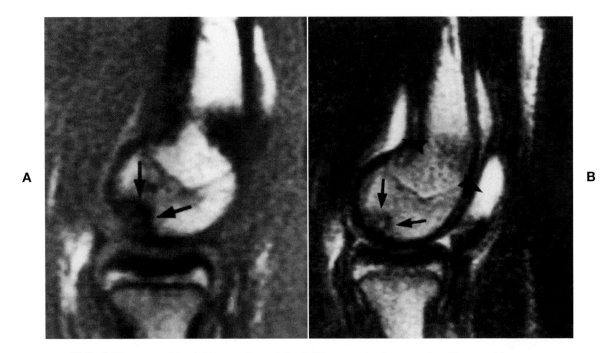

FIG. 5-50   T₁-weighted **(A)** and T₂-weighted **(B)** spin-echo images of a 12-year-old gymnast documenting the clinically suspected diagnosis of osteochondritis dissecans. *(From Nicholas JA, Hershman EB: The upper extremity in sports medicine, ed 2, St Louis, 1995, Mosby.)*

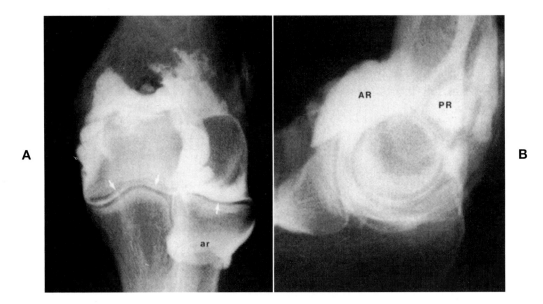

FIG. 5-51   Anteroposterior **(A)** and lateral **(B)** radiographs of the elbow made during a single-contrast elbow arthrogram demonstrate the articular cartilage *(arrows)* with normal filling of the anterior recess *(AR)*, the posterior recess *(PR)*, and the annular recess *(ar)*.   *(From Nicholas JA, Hershman EB: The upper extremity in sports medicine, ed 2, St Louis, 1995, Mosby.)*

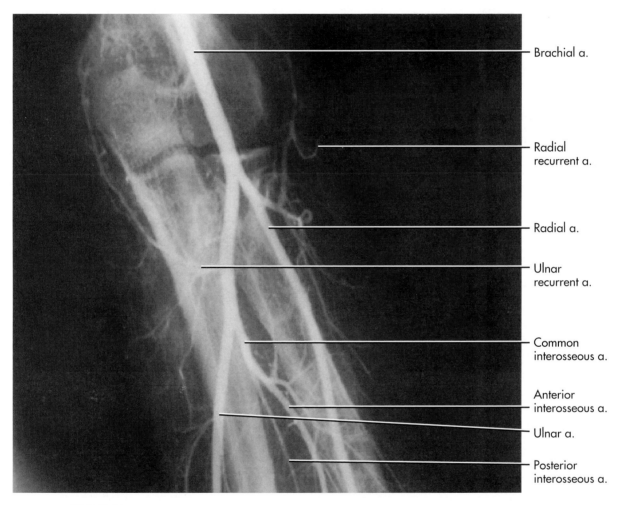

FIG. 5-52   Brachial artery arteriogram.   *(From Mathers LH, et al:* Clinical anatomy principles, *St Louis, 1996, Mosby.)*

COZEN'S TEST

Assessment for Lateral Epicondylitis and Radiohumeral Bursitis

Comment

The syndrome of chronic and disabling pain in the elbow, particularly near the radiohumeral articulation, is commonly and mistakenly designated tennis elbow rather than epicondylitis or radiohumeral bursitis. There is often a lack of specificity regarding the origin of this type of pain. Tennis elbow diagnosis is similar to shin splints or belly ache, having no relation to the type of injury.

The understanding of the pathoanatomy of tennis elbow has been aided significantly by surgical experience over the past decade. Many concepts advanced by investigators of prior decades have proven flawed including the terminology.

The histologic evaluation of tennis elbow tendinosis identifies a noninflammatory response in tendon. This histopathology has been named *angiofibroblastic tendinosis* (Fig. 5-53) and is likely the result of a degenerative and avascular process.

The location of tendinosis is classically in the extensor carpi radialis brevis (ECRB) tendon (100%) and the extensor communis (EC) tendon (35%) laterally and in the pronator teres (PT) and the flexor carpi radialis (FCR) (95%) medially.

Because of the proximity of the epicondyle, the radiohumeral joint, and the supinator aponeurosis, diagnosis of exact tissue involvement can be confusing (Fig. 5-54). Often, the conditions are caused by the same mechanisms, overuse of the elbow joint.

Lateral epicondylitis generally results from repetitive overuse of the wrist and forearm in patients older than 35 years of age who have a high activity level or demanding activity technique and who sometimes have an inadequate fitness level. Although tenderness and swelling occur near the lateral epicondyle, histopathologic studies confirm that the lateral epicondyle of the humerus itself is not injured and that acute inflammation is not the primary problem. Rather, a granulation tissue identified as angiofibroblastic hyperplasia occurs in the ECRB tendon origin as a result of eccentric overload in an area of poor vascularity. Hence, the term *tendinosis* is perhaps more appropriate that *tendinitis*.

An objective measurement is infrared thermography of the affected elbow, which shows a discrete localized area of increased heat near the lateral epicondyle in 98% of affected elbows (Fig. 5-55). Analysis of the gradient across the abnormal area reveals a correlation with clinical severity.

PROCEDURE

- The patient clenches a fist tightly, dorsiflexes it, and maintains a pronated position.
- The examiner, while grasping the patient's lower forearm, applies a flexing force to the dorsiflexion posture of the patient's wrist (Fig. 5-56).
- The test is positive if it reproduces acute lancinating pain in the region of the lateral epicondyle.
- The test is significant for epicondylitis or radiohumeral bursitis.

Confirmation Procedures
Golfer's elbow test, Mills' test, and Kaplan's sign

ORTHOPEDIC GAMUT 5-7

EXTENSOR-SUPINATOR APONEUROTIC ATTACHMENT

The various conditions on the lateral side of the elbow of the extensor-supinator aponeurotic attachment to the lateral epicondyle are as follows:

1. Radioulnar synovitis, marked by development of a pannus of synovium between the radius and ulna
2. Strain in the aponeurosis itself, often directly over the radial head
3. Radiohumeral bursitis

DIAGNOSTIC STATEMENT

Cozen's test is positive for the right elbow. This result suggests lateral epicondylitis or radiohumeral bursitis.

CLINICAL PEARL

Cozen's is the easiest test to perform for lateral epicondylitis. The patient often has already discovered the pain that accompanies resisted dorsiflexion of the wrist, such as when lifting a gallon of milk. Although the pain of epicondylitis is sometimes exquisite and sharply localized, the condition does not truly differentiate itself from tendinitis or bursitis.

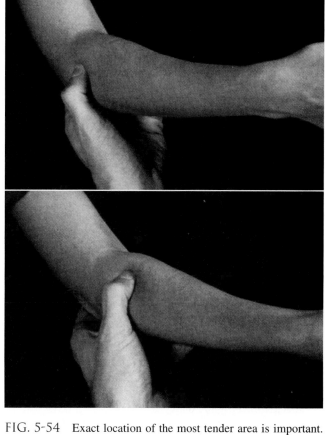

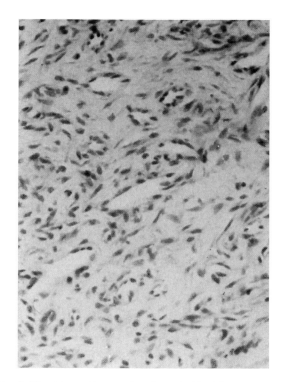

FIG. 5-53   Photomicrograph of angiofibroblastic tendinosis. *(From Torg JS, Shepard RJ: Current therapy in sports medicine, ed 3, St Louis, 1995, Mosby.)*

FIG. 5-54   Exact location of the most tender area is important. **A,** Thumb is over the common extensor tendon and radial head. **B,** Thumb is over the supinator and radial nerve. *(From Nicholas JA, Hershman EB: The upper extremity in sports medicine, ed 2, St Louis, 1995, Mosby.)*

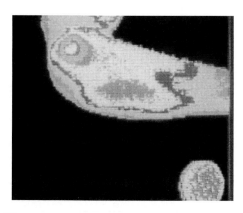

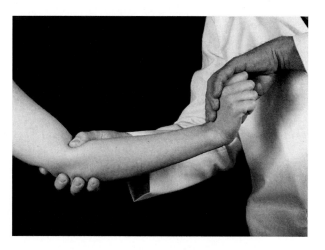

FIG. 5-55   An infrared thermographic pattern in lateral epicondylitis showing localized "hot spot." *(From Klippel JH, Dieppe PA: Rheumatology, vol 1-2, ed 2, London, 1998, Mosby.)*

FIG. 5-56   With the patient seated and the affected elbow slightly flexed and pronated, the patient makes a fist. The patient actively dorsiflexes the hand and wrist. The examiner applies steady pressure against the dorsum of the patient's hand in an attempt to flex it. The patient resists this movement. Pain elicited at or near the lateral epicondyle suggests epicondylitis.

ELBOW FLEXION TEST

Assessment for Cubital Tunnel Syndrome and Ulnar Nerve Palsy at the Elbow

Comment

The ulnar nerve may be compressed at a point just distal to the medial epicondyle through the two heads of the flexor carpi ulnaris. The ulnar nerve is given off from the brachial plexus in the axilla. While medial to the brachial artery, the nerve passes down the extremity until it reaches the distal third of the arm. At this point, the nerve and the brachial artery diverge, and the nerve enters the groove between the medial epicondyle of the humerus and the olecranon. The ulnar nerve passes between the humeral and ulnar heads of the flexor carpi ulnaris muscle and descends to the wrist and hand. This path is along the ulnar aspect of the forearm.

Within the bony groove at the elbow, the nerve is susceptible to compression. The compression can result from direct trauma or changes that occur within the groove and cause gradual impingement. Sometimes, a slow and progressive ulnar palsy is the delayed result of a fracture or soft-tissue injury at the elbow that has produced scarring. Changes in configuration of the groove that are caused by osteoarthritis are occasionally seen with ulnar damage. In addition to severe, direct trauma that affects the elbow joint and may produce immediate or delayed ulnar palsy, repeated, mild trauma may be an overlooked factor. Habitual leaning on the elbow on a desk or constant use of the elbow as a support at work may cause tardy ulnar palsy.

The restrictive opening that the nerve passes through at the elbow is formed by an aponeurotic arch between the olecranon and the medial epicondyle. The floor of this arch is the medial ligament of the elbow joint. This unyielding passageway is somewhat snug. Tissue edema in this region may produce nerve compression.

If the ulnar nerve lesion is at or below the midforearm, clawing of the two fingers that are innervated by the ulnar nerve can occur. Clawing occurs because the extrinsic muscles producing interphalangeal joint flexion are neurologically spared (Fig. 5-57).

Compression neuropathy of the ulnar nerve as it traverses the elbow is often a complication of local trauma, particularly as a result of fractures of the humerus. Constriction of the nerve in a fibroosseous tunnel is possible.

The osseous portion of the cubital tunnel is formed anteriorly by the medial epicondyle, the fibrous portion by the ulnohumeral ligaments laterally, and the aponeurosis of the two heads of the flexor carpi ulnaris posteromedially (Fig. 5-58). The size of the tunnel is reduced when the elbow is placed in flexion.

Without a history of trauma, it may be difficult to give a precise cause for cubital tunnel syndrome. However, chronic pressure over the ulnar groove, which may be exerted by occupational stress or from unusual elbow positioning, is an etiologic source. Arthritic conditions that result in synovitis at the elbow, or osteophyte production, can also cause compression of the nerve.

Paresthesias are noted in the distribution of the ulnar nerve. The neuropathy often is bilateral. Symptoms are aggravated by prolonged use of the elbow in flexed position. Most patients will demonstrate atrophy of intrinsic muscles and weakness in pinch and grasp (Figs. 5-59 and 5-60). There may be wasting of the hypothenar muscles and slight clawing of the fourth and fifth fingers. A positive Wartenberg's sign indicates weakness in adduction of the fifth finger.

Differentially, compression of the ulnar nerve can occur at the other locations, including the cervical spine, thoracic outlet, and Guyon's canal. Cubital ulnar tunnel syndrome must be differentiated from tardy ulnar palsy. In ulnar palsy, neuropathy develops years after an injury (Fig. 5-61).

Other sites in the forearm for potential compression include the dense fibrous arcade of Struthers and the roof of the cubital tunnel formed by the cubital tunnel retinaculum (Fig. 5-62).

ORTHOPEDIC GAMUT 5-8

SITES OF COMPRESSION

The following are potential sites of compression along the course of the ulnar nerve:

1. The arcade of Struthers
2. The proximal edge of the cubital tunnel retinaculum
3. The cubital tunnel
4. The deep flexor pronator aponeurosis

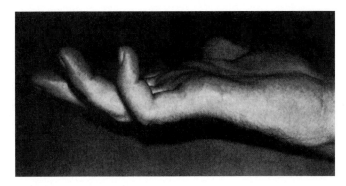

FIG. 5-57   Ulnar claw hand.   *(From Katirji B:* Electromyography in clinical practice: a case study approach, *St Louis, 1998, Mosby.)*

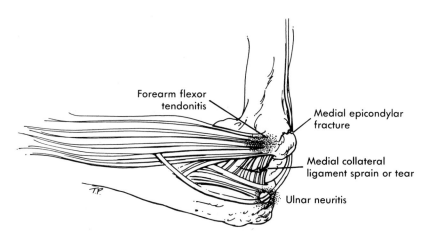

FIG. 5-58   Causes of medial elbow pain.   *(From Nicholas JA, Hershman EB:* The upper extremity in sports medicine, *ed 2, St Louis, 1995, Mosby.)*

PROCEDURE

- The patient completely flexes the elbow.
- The elbow is held in the flexed position for up to 5 minutes (Fig. 5-63).
- If tingling or paresthesia occurs in the ulnar distribution of the forearm and hand, the test is positive.
- A positive finding suggests the presence of cubital tunnel syndrome.

Confirmation Procedures

Tinel's sign at the elbow and electrodiagnosis

DIAGNOSTIC STATEMENT

The elbow flexion test is positive on the right. This result indicates cubital tunnel syndrome.

The elbow flexion test is positive on the right. This result suggests compression of the ulnar nerve in the cubital tunnel.

CLINICAL PEARL

This test is not only useful for cubital tunnel syndrome; it may also reveal the mechanism that resulted in injury to the ulnar nerve. The fully flexed elbow is a common posture for the arm during sleep, naturally or chemically induced. Patients may wake up with ulnar palsy symptoms that stem from prolonged neural compression and anoxia.

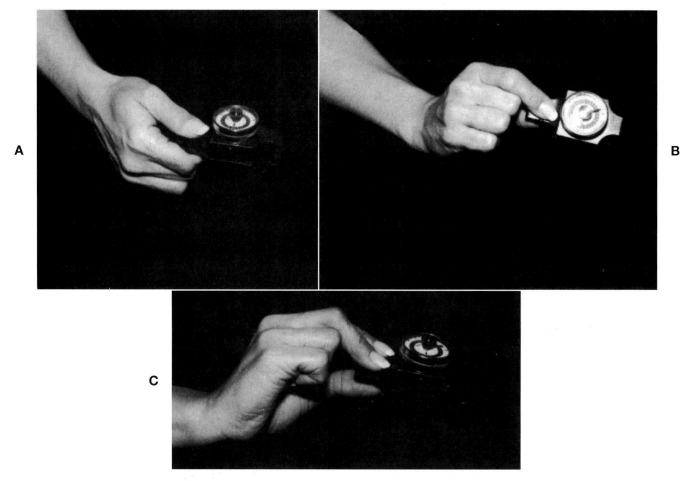

FIG. 5-59   Evaluation of pinch grip. **A,** Assessment of lateral or "key" pinch. **B,** Tip-to-tip pinch. **C,** Chuck pinch.   *(From Lewis CB, Knortz KA: Orthopedic assessment and treatment of the geriatric patient, St Louis, 1993, Mosby.)*

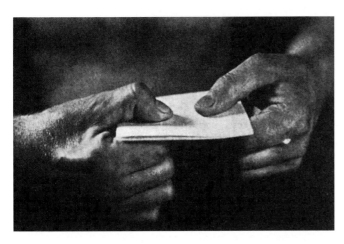

FIG. 5-60   Froment's sign in an ulnar nerve lesion. The patient is directed to pull a piece of paper apart using both hands. The affected hand flexes the thumb by using the flexor pollicis longus to prevent the paper from slipping out of the hand. This masks the weakness of the adductor pollicis. *(From Katirji B:* Electromyography in clinical practice: a case study approach, *St Louis, 1998, Mosby.)*

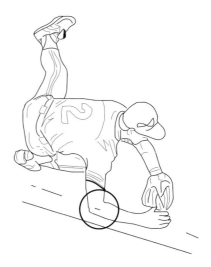

FIG. 5-61   Fall onto the elbow. *(From Hartley A:* Practical joint assessment upper quadrant, *ed 2, St Louis, 1995, Mosby.)*

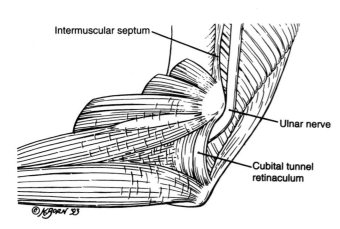

FIG. 5-62   The ulnar nerve passes behind the intermuscular septum and medial condyle. It enters the cubital tunnel beneath the cubital tunnel retinaculum. *(From Torg JS, Shepard RJ:* Current therapy in sports medicine, *ed 3, St Louis, 1995, Mosby.)*

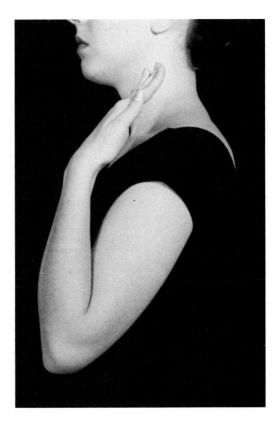

FIG. 5-63   The seated patient maintains a fully flexed elbow for as long as possible. The norm is 5 minutes or longer with no symptoms produced. Ulnar paresthesia developing in less than 5 minutes suggests cubital tunnel syndrome.

GOLFER'S ELBOW TEST

Assessment for Medial Epicondylitis

Comment

Epicondylitis is a type of involvement that is peculiar to the elbow and develops along the medial and lateral epicondyles. The extensor-supinator muscles arise along the lateral epicondyle, and the flexor-pronator muscles arise along the medial epicondyle, where they have an aponeurotic attachment.

Epicondylitis occurs either by contusion of the area or, more commonly, by strain (Fig. 5-64). Characteristic irritation develops at the attachment of the aponeurosis to the bone. Pain, which is aggravated by gripping, occurs along the involved epicondyle. When the patient clenches the fist, one of the first phases of action is strong contraction of carpal extensors to fix the wrist. If this contraction did not occur, the wrist would go into flexion, and an ineffective fist would result.

Although epicondylitis may follow an acute strain, it more often results from chronic degenerative changes. These changes are caused by attrition of the aponeurotic fibers at the elbow. If there is degenerative change, there may be calcification or even spur formation over the epicondyle.

In medial epicondylitis, valgus stress is applied to the elbow while palpating over the medial joint line beneath the ulnar collateral ligament (Fig. 5-65). Occasionally, some patients will have asymptomatic ulnar collateral ligament attenuation and valgus laxity, while others with a significant ligament injury will have no palpable laxity at all (Fig. 5-66).

Valgus stress radiographs, obtained using manual stress or a graded pressure device, document excessive medial joint opening and confirm ligament laxity (Figs. 5-67 and 5-68).

The medial collateral ligament of the elbow is the most important ligament for stability of the elbow joint. It is divided into three bundles according to anatomic location: anterior, posterior, and transverse (Fig. 5-69).

PROCEDURE

- The patient is seated, the patient's elbow is flexed slightly, and the hand is supinated (Fig. 5-70).
- The patient flexes the wrist against resistance (Fig. 5-71).
- Medial epicondyle pain suggests epicondylitis.
- In more severe medial epicondylitis, the flexor muscle groups are weakened and the elbow-wrist mechanism can be extended by the examiner (Fig. 5-72).
- Full extension of the elbow-wrist joint localizes the lesion more sharply in medial aponeurosis contractures.

Confirmation Procedures

Cozen's test, Kaplan's sign, and Mills' test

DIAGNOSTIC STATEMENT

The golfer's elbow test is positive on the left. This result suggests epicondylitis at the medial epicondyle.

The golfer's elbow test is positive on the left. This result suggests flexor-pronator aponeurosis tendinitis at the medial epicondyle.

CLINICAL PEARL

This test is a reverse procedure of Cozen's test. Cozen's test relies on resisted wrist dorsiflexion, but the golfer's elbow test relies on resisted elbow-wrist flexion. The pain associated with medial epicondylitis spreads down the forearm and is often confused with carpal tunnel syndrome symptoms.

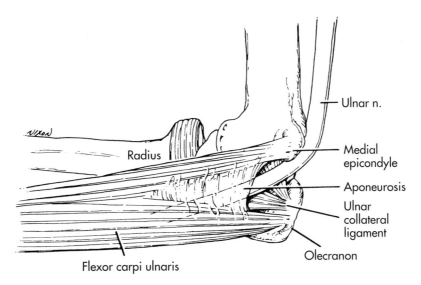

Ulnar n.

Radius

Medial epicondyle

Aponeurosis

Ulnar collateral ligament

Olecranon

Flexor carpi ulnaris

FIG. 5-64   The medial surface of the elbow demonstrating the course of the ulnar nerve through the ulnar groove and cubital tunnel.   *(From Kincaid JC: The electrodiagnosis of ulnar neurotherapy at the elbow,* Muscle Nerve *11:1005, 1988, Wiley Publishing.)*

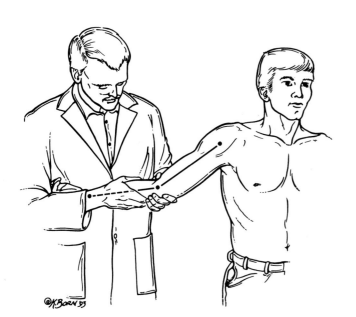

FIG. 5-65   Examination for evaluating medial instability of the elbow.   *(From Torg JS, Shepard RJ:* Current therapy in sports medicine, *ed 3, St Louis, 1995, Mosby.)*

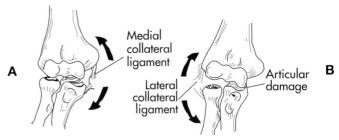

A

Medial collateral ligament

Lateral collateral ligament

Articular damage

B

FIG. 5-66   **A,** Valgus overstretch damage to the elbow. **B,** Varus overstretch damage to the elbow.   *(From Hartley A:* Practical joint assessment upper quadrant, *ed 2, St Louis, 1995, Mosby.)*

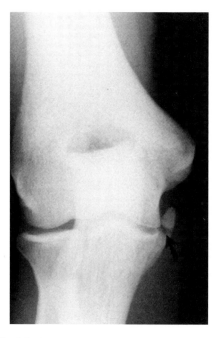

FIG. 5-67   Medial traction spur. *(From Nicholas JA, Hershman EB: The upper extremity in sports medicine, ed 2, St Louis, 1995, Mosby.)*

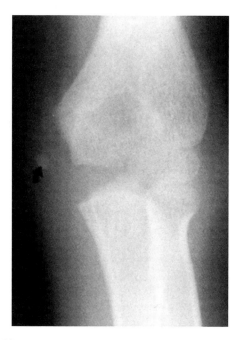

FIG. 5-68   Complete avulsion of the medial epicondylar apophysis *(arrow)* can occur in an acute injury from throwing sports rather than chronic degradation. *(From Nicholas JA, Hershman EB: The upper extremity in sports medicine, ed 2, St Louis, 1995, Mosby.)*

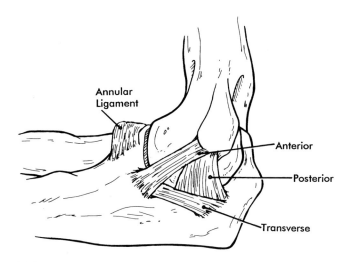

FIG. 5-69   Medial ligaments of the elbow. *(From Bucholz RW: Orthopaedic decision making, ed 2, St Louis, 1996, Mosby.)*

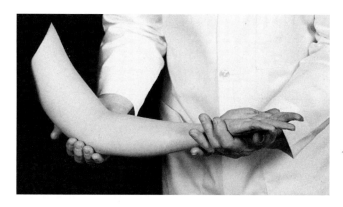

FIG. 5-70   The seated patient slightly flexes the elbow. The hand and wrist are in supination.

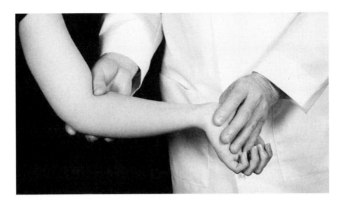

FIG. 5-71 The examiner applies steady pressure to the supinated hand in an attempt to extend the elbow and wrist. The patient resists this movement with active flexion. Pain elicited at the medial epicondyle suggests epicondylitis.

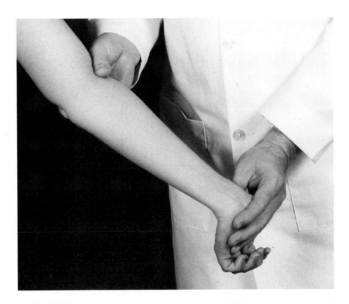

FIG. 5-72 With severe medial epicondylitis, the examiner is able to overcome the flexor muscle groups and extend the elbow and wrist fully. With aponeurosis contractures present, the full extension of the elbow and wrist localizes the lesion more sharply.

KAPLAN'S SIGN

Assessment for Lateral Epicondylitis

Comment

Lateral epicondylitis is a symptom complex that presents with pain at the elbow, especially during extension of the wrist or fingers against resistance. It is usually caused by a tear in the conjoined tendons of the extensor muscles. It is often associated with an osseous avulsion or spur on the lateral epicondyle of the humerus. Direct compression of the dorsal interosseous nerve at or distal to the level of the supinator also presents the same symptoms.

On palpation, there is pain in the area of the lateral epicondyle. This continues down the dorsal aspect of the forearm over the wrist extensors and the extensor digitorum communis.

Etiologic factors include direct trauma to the elbow joint in the area of the lateral epicondyle or, more commonly, a muscle strain secondary to athletic activities. If direct trauma is the underlying cause, tangential diagnostic images of the lateral epicondyle should be obtained. The images may demonstrate the presence of small osteophytes within the substance of the conjoined tendon.

osteophyte at the tip of the olecranon. The axial view demonstrates the articulation of the olecranon and postero-medial osteophytes with the trochlea (Fig. 5-73).

Although patients do not usually recall a specific traumatic episode, they do admit that symptoms of low-grade pain and morning stiffness were brought on or aggravated by certain repetitive activities, such as tennis, golf, and pipe fitting. A grasping motion that stretches the epicondylar muscle attachments will accentuate the pain.

Other pathologic conditions include arthritis of the radiohumeral joint, radiohumeral bursitis, traumatic synovitis of the radiohumeral joint through forced extension and supination, and periostitis or osteitis of the epicondyle (Fig. 5-74).

The presence of immunoglobin M-rheumatoid factor (IgM-RF) enzymes and HLA-B27 antigen in cases of epicondylitis suggests that the recurring tenosynovitis (epicondylitis) represents an incomplete form of rheumatoid disease (Fig. 5-75).

Although the radial nerve may be compressed under the brachioradialis muscle, this is a rare event and is painful more distally than tennis elbow.

ORTHOPEDIC GAMUT 5-9

IMAGING OF THE ELBOW

Standard plain film imaging of the elbow involves five views:

1. Anteroposterior (AP)
2. Lateral
3. Medial
4. Lateral obliques
5. Axial

The lateral and oblique views, taken at 45 degrees oblique to the AP, may reveal characteristic formation of an

---

ORTHOPEDIC GAMUT 5-10

ELBOW SWELLING

The following are common local swelling locations of the elbow:

1. Olecranon bursa and the radiohumeral bursa
2. Muscle strains or contusions to the tendon, belly, or tenoperiosteal junction
3. Intracapsular effusion

Marked posterior joint swelling usually is olecranon bursitis, whereas anterior and posterior swelling often is caused by intracapsular effusion (Fig. 5-76).

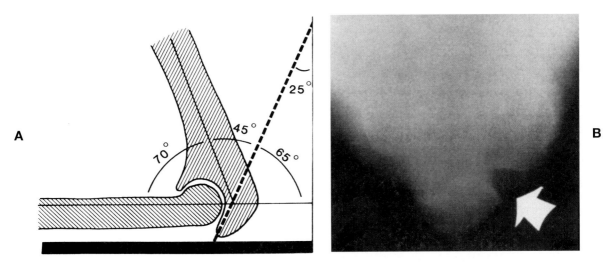

FIG. 5-73   **A,** A diagram demonstrating the radiographic position for the axial (tangential) view of the elbow. **B,** Axial view revealing the posteromedial osteophyte and profile of the trochlear articulation.   *(From Torg JS, Shepard RJ: Current therapy in sports medicine, ed 3, St Louis, 1995, Mosby.)*

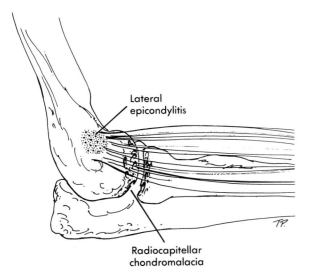

FIG. 5-74   Causes of lateral elbow pain.   *(From Nicholas JA, Hershman EB: The upper extremity in sports medicine, ed 2, St Louis, 1995, Mosby.)*

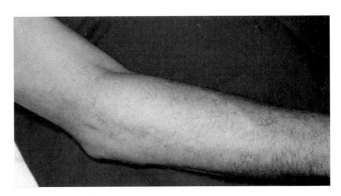

FIG. 5-75   Rheumatoid nodules.   *(From Epstein O, Perkin GD, deBono DP, Cookson J: Clinical examination, ed 2, London, 1997, Mosby.)*

The use of fluoroquinolone antibiotics (ciprofloxacin, ofloxacin, norfloxacin, enoxacin, lomefloxacin) has been implicated in epicondylitis. The intense pain at the epicondyle appears very shortly after administration of the first dose of the drug and is not relieved by conservative treatment. Ultrasonography reveals extensive inflammatory pannus with pseudonecrotic areas. MRI confirms the lesions and demonstrates subclinical abnormality of the adjoining tendons.

PROCEDURE

- While the patient is seated, the affected upper limb is held straight out with the wrist in slight dorsiflexion.
- Grip strength is assessed with a dynamometer (Fig. 5-77).
- This maneuver is repeated as the examiner firmly encircles the patient's forearm with both hands or with a strap placed approximately 1 to 2 inches below the elbow joint line (Fig. 5-78).
- The sign is present if initial grip strength improves and lateral elbow pain diminishes.

Confirmation Procedures
Cozen's test, golfer's elbow test, and Mills' test

DIAGNOSTIC STATEMENT

Kaplan's sign is present on the left. This result suggests lateral epicondylitis.

CLINICAL PEARL

Kaplan's sign is a good test for discerning the efficacy of tennis-elbow support in the management of a patient's condition. Obviously, if the grip does not improve while the brace is in place, the musculature and epicondylar tissues are not being supported adequately. The condition may be so severe that the use of a brace is not helpful.

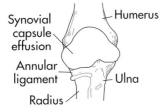

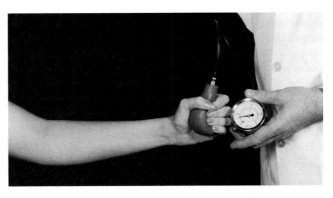

FIG. 5-76   Intracapsular effusion from an anterior view.   *(From Hartley A: Practical joint assessment upper quadrant, ed 2, St Louis, 1995, Mosby.)*

FIG. 5-77   With the elbow flexed slightly and the hand in a position of function, the seated patient grips a dynamometer. The examiner records the findings.

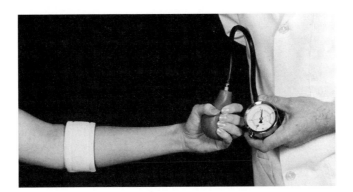

FIG. 5-78   The grip strength is tested again with the elbow supported by either a tennis elbow strap or the examiner's hands. Increased grip strength and decreased elbow pain indicate lateral epicondylitis.

Assessment for Medial or Lateral Collateral Ligament Instability at the Elbow

Comment

Because the elbow is a stable joint, ligament injury is uncommon. It is impossible to sprain the elbow by excessive flexion. In excessive extension, the olecranon impinges against the back of the humerus, and the continuing force parts the coronoid from the trochlea of the humerus. This also results in an injury to the anterior portion of the collateral ligament, particularly on the medial side. This injury may vary from a partial tear to complete rupture of the ligaments and capsule. As the force stops short of complete rupture, the elbow flexes, the tension releases, and no feeling of instability occurs at the elbow joint. This lack of instability is seen because of the inherent, bony structure of the elbow and because the elbow does not require the same degree of stability for bearing weight that is necessary in the knee.

The patient with an injury of excessive elbow extension will have a history of elbow hyperextension and of severe pain on the medial and sometimes the lateral side of the elbow. This pain is relieved by flexion. The symptoms at the time of examination vary according to the severity of the injury. Pain is ordinarily not a prominent factor, but there will be localized tenderness at the site of the tear, either along the ulna on the medial side or along the epicondyle. There may also be pain along the lateral collateral ligament at the site of the tear. Any attempt to extend the arm causes pain, and motion is stopped, short of complete extension, by a muscle spasm.

The collateral ligaments also may be sprained by lateral motion. Forced abduction of the extended arm will damage the medial ligaments (Fig. 5-79). Forced adduction will damage the lateral ligaments (Fig. 5-80). Instability is extremely uncommon. It is difficult to determine whether the rupture of the ligaments is complete unless there has been complete dislocation of the elbow. A sprain-fracture caused by an avulsion of the ligament with a bony fragment may be revealed by diagnostic imaging. Symptoms of lateral stresses will be localized to the one side and accompanied by the same findings as for hyperextension. These findings include tenderness along the site of the tear, local swelling, and pain during attempts to reproduce the causative force.

PROCEDURE

- The examiner stabilizes the patient's arm with one hand at the elbow, and the other hand is placed at the wrist.
- The patient's elbow is slightly flexed (20 to 30 degrees), and an adduction (varus) force is applied to test the lateral collateral ligament (Fig. 5-81).
- An abduction (valgus) force is then applied to test the medial collateral ligament (Fig. 5-82).

Confirmation Procedure

Diagnostic imaging

DIAGNOSTIC STATEMENT

Abduction stress is positive on the right for sprain of the lateral collateral ligaments of the elbow.

Abduction stress is positive on the right for sprain of the medial collateral ligaments of the elbow.

CLINICAL PEARL

It is not uncommon in elbow ligamentous testing for osseous reductions to be felt or heard. During this procedure, the radial head may be reduced because of a minor subluxation, or simple adhesion releases may occur. The testing may become the treatment.

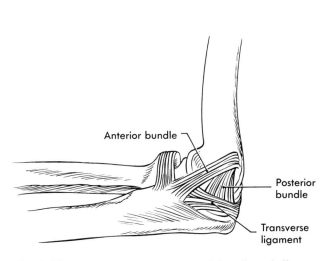

FIG. 5-79 Medial view of the medial collateral ligament bundles. *(From Nicholas JA, Hershman EB: The upper extremity in sports medicine, ed 2, St Louis, 1995, Mosby.)*

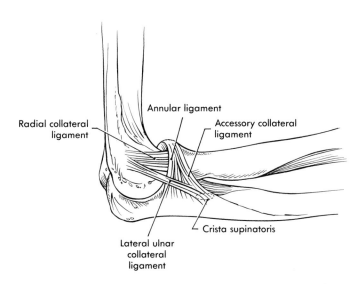

FIG. 5-80 Lateral view of the lateral collateral and annular ligaments. *(From Nicholas JA, Hershman EB: The upper extremity in sports medicine, ed 2, St Louis, 1995, Mosby.)*

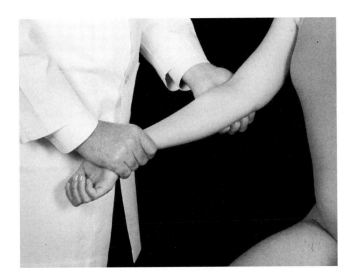

FIG. 5-81 The patient is seated comfortably with the elbow slightly flexed (20 to 30 degrees) and the hand and arm in supination. The examiner stabilizes the elbow while applying an abduction (valgus) force to the distal forearm. This tests the medial collateral ligaments. Pain indicates sprain.

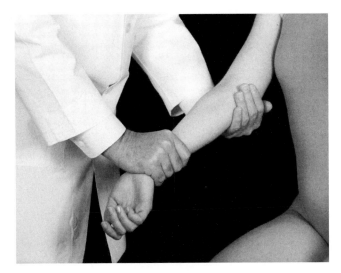

FIG. 5-82 The procedure described in Fig. 5-81 is repeated with an adduction force applied to the distal forearm while the examiner stabilizes the elbow. This procedure assesses the lateral collateral ligaments. Pain indicates sprain.

MILLS' TEST

ALSO KNOWN AS MILLS' MANEUVER

Assessment for Lateral Epicondylitis

Comment

Used synonymously with the term *tennis elbow,* lateral epicondylitis is one of the most common lesions of the arm. Approximately 1% to 3% of the population is affected by it, mostly those between 40 and 60 years of age, the dominant arm being affected most frequently. Some 40% to 50% of tennis players suffer with it, mainly older players. It is found most often in nonathletes, and the majority are not manual workers. Many cannot describe any specific precipitating factors.

There have been more than 25 suggested causes of the condition, and this reflects the use of the diagnosis nonspecifically for lateral elbow pain. It is believed that most cases result from a musculotendinous lesion of the common extensor tendon at the attachment to the lateral epicondyle or nearby, especially that portion derived from extensor carpi radialis brevis.

Age is an important factor because lateral epicondylitis rarely occurs before the age of 30. Adult maturity is associated with alterations in the enthesis, including changes in collagen content, reduction in cells and ground substance, and increases in lipids, which then probably predispose it to injury.

Lateral epicondylitis usually arises slowly and apparently spontaneously; a blow or acute traumatic strains are relatively rarely remembered. Pain is localized to the lateral epicondyle but may spread up and down the upper limb. Grip is impaired because of the pain, and this may result in restricted daily activities. Tenderness over the epicondyle is usual, although maximum tenderness is sometimes found at

nearby sites. The other cardinal sign is increased pain on resisting wrist dorsiflexion with the elbow in extension.

It is important to exclude other conditions that produce elbow pain, especially that referred from the cervical spine or shoulder, as well as arthritis of the elbow, although this is usually obvious.

A nerve entrapment around the elbow may produce diagnostic confusion. Radial tunnel syndrome or compression of the posterior interosseous nerve can produce lateral elbow and upper foramen pain. Compression of the posterior interosseous nerve may occur where it passes through supinator muscle just below the elbow joint. A well-defined arcade of Frohse is present in 30% of patients and makes a compression neuropathy more likely. Diffuse pain, symptoms distal to the lateral epicondyle, and the presence of muscle weakness may be useful distinguishing features.

PROCEDURE

- The patient's forearm, fingers, and wrist are passively flexed (Figs. 5-83 to 5-85).
- The forearm is pronated and extended (Figs. 5-86 and 5-87).
- The test is positive if elbow pain increases.
- A positive test indicates lateral epicondylitis (tennis elbow).

Confirmation Procedures

Cozen's test, golfer's elbow test, Kaplan's sign, and diagnostic imaging

---

DIAGNOSTIC STATEMENT

Mills' test is positive on the right. This result indicates lateral epicondylitis of the elbow.

CLINICAL PEARL

Mills' test is also a treatment maneuver. One of the principles of management for lateral epicondylitis is the sectioning of the aponeurosis from the epicondyle. In the final maneuvers of Mills' test, this separation is accomplished.

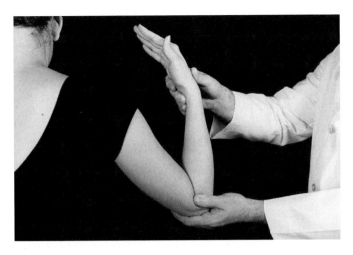

FIG. 5-83   The patient is seated. The examiner passively and fully flexes the elbow.

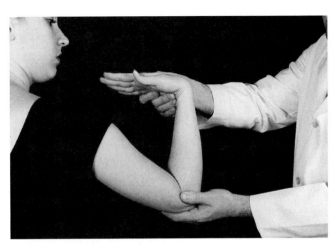

FIG. 5-84   After passively and fully flexing the patient's elbow, the examiner flexes the patient's wrist.

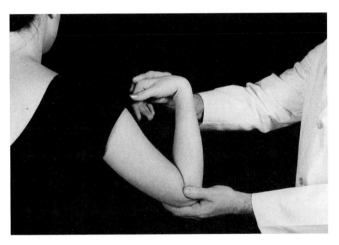

FIG. 5-85   After attaining the position described in Fig. 5-84, the patient's fingers are fully flexed. The forearm, wrist, and hand are all fully flexed in supination.

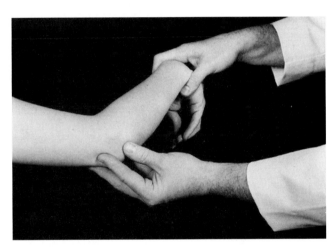

FIG. 5-86   The examiner maintains wrist and finger flexion while extending the patient's elbow.

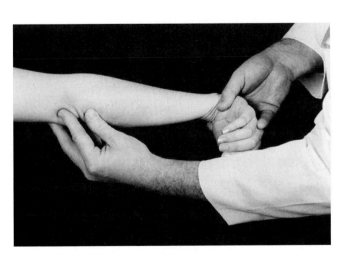

FIG. 5-87   At maximum elbow extension, with the wrist and fingers still flexed, the forearm is pronated. Pain at the lateral epicondyle indicates epicondylitis. All of the movements associated with this procedure should be accomplished in a smooth continuous manner.

TINEL'S SIGN AT THE ELBOW

ALSO KNOWN AS FORMICATION SIGN, DISTAL TINGLING ON PERCUSSION (DTP) SIGN, AND HOFFMAN-TINEL'S SIGN

Assessment for Ulnar or Radial (Posterior Interosseous) Neuropathy at the Elbow

Comment

Nerve roots and peripheral nerves may be injured by a blunt object that causes a contusion or by a sharp object that produces a partial or complete laceration. The nerve also can be injured by a severe stretch, resulting from a traction injury. In addition, nerves are particularly vulnerable to prolonged ischemia, which can lead to necrosis.

In neuropraxia, there is only slight damage to the nerve with transient loss of conductivity, particularly in its motor fibers. In neuropraxia, wallerian degeneration, which is the breakdown of the myelin sheaths into lipid material and fragmentation of the neurofibrils, does not occur. Complete recovery from neuropraxia may be expected within a few days or weeks.

In axonotmesis, the injury damages axons, which are prolongations of the cells in the spinal cord, but does not damage the structural framework of the nerve. The axons distal to the injury undergo wallerian degeneration. Peripheral regeneration of the axons occurs along the intact neural tubes to the appropriate end organs. This regeneration occurs very slowly, approximately 1 mm each day, or 3 cm each month. If axonotmesis in a nerve occurred 9 cm proximal to its site of entrance into a muscle, it would take approximately 3 months for the regenerating axons to reinnervate that muscle.

In the injury of neurotmesis, the internal neural structural framework and the enclosed axons are divided, torn, and destroyed. Wallerian degeneration occurs in the distal segment. Because the axons in the proximal segment have lost their neural tubes, natural regeneration is improbable. The neurofibrils and fibrous elements grow out of the divided end of the nerve to produce a bulbous neuroma. The only hope of recovery lies in excision of the damaged section of the nerve and accurate approximation of the freshened ends. Even under ideal circumstances, recovery is less than complete.

Immediately after nerve injury, there is a loss of conductivity in motor, sensory, and autonomic fibers. The muscles supplied by the nerve root or peripheral nerve exhibit a flaccid paralysis and later undergo atrophy. A loss of cutaneous sensations, deep sensation, and position sense can be detected. The autonomic deficit is characterized by a lack of sweating (anhidrosis) in the cutaneous distribution of the nerve. There is a temporary vasodilation and resultant warm skin, followed by vasoconstriction and cold skin.

The precise diagnosis concerning both the type of injury and its location can be helped by the appropriate electrical tests, which include nerve conduction, strength curve, and electromyography (Fig. 5-88).

The prognosis depends on the type of injury (neuropraxia, axonotmesis, or neurotmesis). If recovery does take place, it is evidenced first by return of muscle power in the most proximally supplied muscle. Return of sensation follows a definite pattern. Deep sensation returns first, followed by pain and position sense. As regeneration of axons proceeds along the nerve, the regenerated portion becomes hypersensitive. Tapping over the injured area causes a tingling sensation. Assessing the distal limit of this phenomenon at intervals makes it possible to determine the progress of regeneration (Fig. 5-89).

PROCEDURE

- While the patient is seated, the examiner taps the groove between the olecranon process and the lateral epicondyle with a neurologic reflex hammer (Fig. 5-90).
- The same is repeated for the groove between the olecranon process and the medial epicondyle.
- Hypersensitivity indicates neuritis or neuroma of the respective nerve.

Confirmation Procedure
Electrodiagnosis

DIAGNOSTIC STATEMENT

Tinel's sign is present in the medial epicondylar groove of the right elbow. This sign suggests ulnar neuropathy.

Tinel's sign is present in the lateral epicondylar groove of the right elbow. This sign suggests involvement of the superficial radial nerve.

CLINICAL PEARL

It must be remembered that the tingling elicited by the Tinel's sign represents regeneration. Pain and tingling represent injury and degeneration. The more distally the tingling is felt from the site of percussion, the more distally the axons have regenerated.

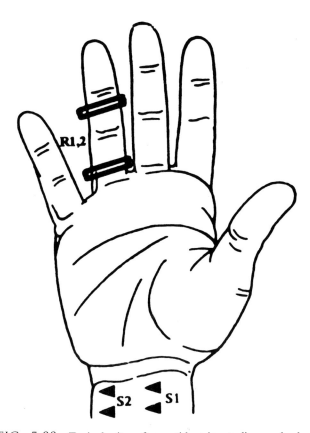

FIG. 5-88 Typical sites for antidromic median and ulnar sensory latencies stimulation while recording the ring finger. *S1* is the median stimulation site; *S2* is the ulnar stimulation site. *R1,2* is the recording site for both responses. *(From Preston DC, et al: The median-ulnar latency difference studies are comparable in mild carpal tunnel syndrome,* Muscle Nerve *17:1419, 1994, Wiley Publishing.)*

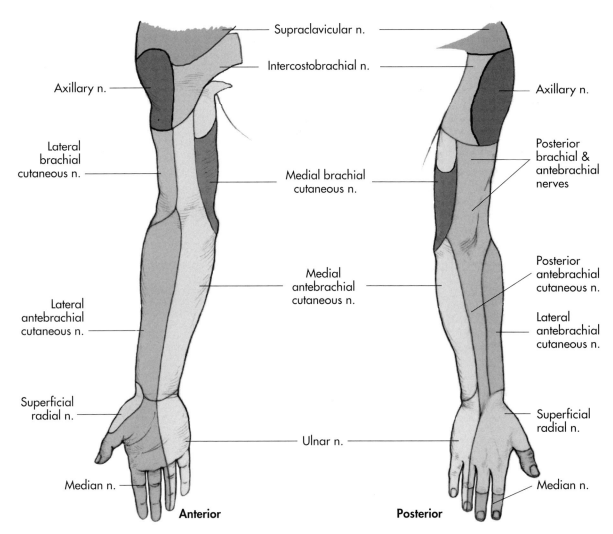

FIG. 5-89 Cutaneous innervation of the upper extremity. *(From Mathers LH, et al:* Clinical anatomy principles, *St Louis, 1996, Mosby.)*

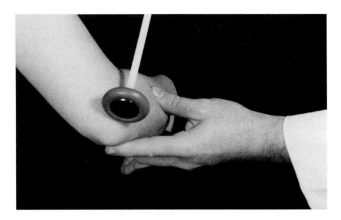

FIG. 5-90 The patient is seated comfortably with the elbow flexed to 90 degrees. The examiner percusses the superficial radial nerve at the lateral epicondylar groove. Tingling that radiates down the lateral forearm indicates regeneration associated with superficial radial nerve palsy. Pain radiating down the lateral forearm is associated with injury and superficial radial nerve degeneration. The same procedure is repeated for the medial epicondylar groove and the ulnar nerve.

CRITICAL THINKING

What articulations make up the elbow joint?
Humeroulnar joint, humeroradial joint, and proximal radioulnar joint

List the functions of the elbow.
The elbow positions the hand in space, effectively lengthens and shortens the upper extremity, stabilizes the upper extremity for power and detailed work activities, and provides power to the arm for lifting.

Describe the carrying angle of the elbow.
The carrying angle of the elbow is the normal anatomic valgus angulation between the upper arm and forearm when the elbow is fully extended. The normal angle is 5 to 10 degrees in males and 10 to 15 degrees in females.

What is a gunstock deformity of the arm?
A gunstock deformity refers to a cubitus varus deformity of the elbow.

What muscles originate from the medial epicondyle?
Flexor carpi radialis, flexor carpi ulnaris, palmaris longus, flexor digitorum superficialis, flexor digitorum profundus, and pronator teres

What muscles originate from the lateral epicondyle?
Extensor carpi radialis, extensor carpi radialis longus, palmaris longus, extensor digitorum communis, supinator, and anconeus

List the ligaments of the elbow.
Medially, the ulnar collateral ligament; laterally, the radial collateral ligament and annular ligament

What is the normal position of function of the elbow?
90 degrees flexion with the forearm midway between supination and pronation

What is the most common congenital anomaly of the elbow?
Radial head dislocation

What is Panner disease?
Panner disease is osteochondrosis of the capitellum. It is seen most often in young males.

What is osteochondritis dissecans of the elbow?
Osteochondritis dissecans is an idiopathic disorder affecting the capitellum of the humerus, with avascular necrosis.

Describe tennis elbow.
This term has traditionally been used to describe numerous symptoms of the elbow. It most commonly refers to lateral epicondylitis, in which the extensor carpi radialis brevis is affected by repetitive strain injury.

Describe Cozen's test.
The examiner stabilizes the elbow. The patient makes a fist, pronates the forearm, and extends the wrist against resistance. This can cause pain in the lateral epicondyle.

What is usually responsible for medial epicondylitis, or golfer's elbow?
Repetitive strain injury of the flexor-pronator musculature at or near its insertion on the medial epicondyle.

How is medial epicondylitis tested?
The examiner resists wrist flexion and forearm pronation, causing medial epicondyle pain.

Describe boxer's elbow.
Boxer's elbow is a hyperextension overload syndrome or olecranon impingement syndrome caused by repetitive valgus extension of the elbow.

Describe little leaguer's elbow.
Little leaguer's elbow is an injury occurring in children and adolescents in which the medial epicondyle is inflamed and there is partial separation of the apophysis.

Where does ulnar nerve entrapment at the elbow typically occur?
The cubital tunnel, which is a passageway formed by the two heads of the ulnar collateral ligament and the tendon of the flexor carpi ulnaris

Describe draftsman's elbow.
Draftsman's elbow is inflammation of the olecranon bursa. It is also known as *student's elbow* and *miner's elbow*.

What are "pushed elbow" and "pulled elbow"?
Pushed elbow is subluxation of the radial head in proximal direction, which is often seen after a person falls on an outstretched hand. Pulled elbow is subluxation of the radial head in a distal direction, which may follow a forceful traction to the forearm.

BIBLIOGRAPHY

Adams JC, Hamblen DL: *Outline of orthopaedics,* ed 11, Edinburgh, 1990, Churchill Livingstone.

American Medical Association: *Guides to the evaluation of permanent impairment,* ed 4, Chicago, 1993, American Medical Association.

American Medical Association: *How to use guides to the evaluation of permanent impairment,* ed 4, Falmouth, 1993, SEAK.

American Orthopaedic Association: *Manual of orthopaedic surgery,* Chicago, 1972, The Association.

Anderson KN, Anderson LE: *Mosby's pocket dictionary of medicine, nursing, & allied health,* ed 2, St Louis, 1994, Mosby.

Angelo RL, Soffer SR: Elbow anatomy relative to arthroscopy. In Andrews Jr, Soffer SR, editors: *Elbow arthroscopy,* St Louis, 1994, Mosby.

Apfelberg DB, Larson SJ: Dynamic anatomy of the ulnar nerve at the elbow, *Plast Reconstr Surg* 51:76, 1973.

Apley AG, Solomon L: *Concise system of orthopaedics and fractures,* London, 1988, Butterworth-Heinemann.

Ballinger PW: *Merrill's atlas of radiographic positions and radiologic procedures,* vol 1-3, ed 8, St Louis, 1995, Mosby.

Barkauskas VH, Stoltenberg-Allen K, Baumann LC, Darling-Fisher C: *Health & physical assessment,* ed 2, St Louis, 1998, Mosby.

Bateman JE: *Trauma to nerves in limbs,* Philadelphia, 1962, WB Saunders.

Beals RK: The normal carrying angle of the elbow, *Clin Orthop* 119:194, 1976.

Beetham WP, Polley HF, Slocumb CH, Weaver WF: *Physical examination of the joints,* Philadelphia, 1965, WB Saunders.

Bennett JB, Tullos HS: Acute injuries to the elbow. In Nicholas JA, Hershman EB, editors: *The upper extremity in sports medicine,* St Louis, 1990, Mosby.

Berquist T: *MRI of the musculoskeletal system,* ed 3, Philadelphia, 1996, JB Lippincott.

Blackwell JR, Cole KJ: Wrist kinematics in expert and novice tennis players performing the backhand stoke: implications for tennis elbow, *J Biomech* 27:509, 1994.

Boyd HB, McLeod AC: Tennis elbow, *J Bone Joint Surg* 55A:1183, 1973.

Bradley WG: *Disorders of peripheral nerves,* Oxford, 1974, Blackwell Scientific.

Brooks M, Evans R, Fairclough J: *Sports injuries,* ed 2, London, 1992, Gower Medical.

Brotzman SB: *Clinical orthopaedic rehabilitation,* St Louis, 1996, Mosby.

Brown DE, Neumann RD: *Orthopedic secrets,* Philadelphia, 1995, Hanley & Belfus.

Bucholz RW: *Orthopaedic decision making,* ed 2, St Louis, 1996, Mosby.

Canale ST: *Campbell's operative orthopaedics,* vol 1-4, ed 9, St Louis, 1998, Mosby.

Carson WG, Meyer JF: Diagnostic arthroscopy of the elbow: surgical techniques and arthroscopic portal anatomy. In McGinty JB, editor: *Operative arthroscopy,* New York, 1991, Raven.

Chapman S, Nakielny R: *Aids to radiological differential diagnosis,* ed 3, London, 1995, Bailliere Tindall.

Cipriano JJ: *Photographic manual of regional orthopaedic and neurological tests,* ed 3, Baltimore, 1997, Williams & Wilkins.

Cohn RE: *Impairment rating examination and disability evaluation,* ed 3, Wilkesboro, NC, 1994, R Ernest Cohn.

Conway JE, Jobe FW, Glousman RE, Pink M: Medial instability of the elbow in throwing athletes: treatment by repair or reconstruction of the ulnar collateral ligament, *J Bone Joint Surg* 74A:67, 1992.

Copeland SA, Gschwend N, Landi A, Saffar P: *Joint stiffness of the upper limb,* St Louis, 1997, Mosby.

Daffner RH: *Clinical radiology, the essentials,* Baltimore, 1993, Williams & Wilkins.

Dambro MR, Griffith JA: *Griffith's 5 minute clinical consult,* Baltimore, 1997, Williams & Wilkins.

D'Ambrosia RD: *Musculoskeletal disorders, regional examination and differential diagnosis,* Philadelphia, 1977, JB Lippincott.

Dandy DJ: *Essential orthopaedics and trauma,* Edinburgh, 1989, Churchill Livingstone.

Dawson DM, Hallett M, Millender LH: Pathology of nerve entrapment. In Dawson DM, Hallett M, Wilbourn A, editors: *Entrapment neuropathies,* ed 2, Boston, 1990, Little & Brown.

Delagi E, Perrotto L, Iazzetti J, Morrison D: *An anatomic guide for the electromyographer,* Springfield, Ill, 1975, Charles C Thomas.

Dellon AL, Hament W, Gittelshon A: Nonoperative management of cubital tunnel syndrome: an 8 year prospective study, *Neurology* 43:1673, 1993.

Deltoff MN, Kogon PL: *The portable skeletal x-ray library,* St Louis, 1998, Mosby.

Demeter SL, Andersson GBJ, Smith GM: *Disability evaluation,* St Louis, 1996, Mosby.

Dimitru D: *Electrodiagnostic medicine,* Philadelphia, 1995, Hanley & Belfus.

Doherty M: *Color atlas and text of osteoarthritis,* London, 1994, Wolfe.

Doherty M, Doherty J: *Clinical examination in rheumatology,* London, 1992, Wolfe.

Doherty M, George E: *Self-assessment picture tests in rheumatology,* London, 1995, Mosby-Wolfe.

Edeiken J: *Roentgen diagnosis of diseases of bone,* ed 4, Baltimore, 1990, Williams & Wilkins.

Elster AD: *Questions and answers in magnetic resonance imaging,* St Louis, 1994, Mosby.

Epstein O, Perkin GD, deBono DP, Cookson J: *Clinical examination,* ed 2, London, 1997, Mosby.

Feldmann E: *Current diagnosis in neurology,* St Louis, 1994, Mosby.

Folberg CR, Weiss AP, Akelman E: Cubital tunnel syndrome, part 1: presentation and diagnosis, *Orthop Rev* 23:136, 1994.

Fornage B: *Musculoskeletal ultrasound,* New York, 1995, Churchill Livingstone.

Fritz RC, Brody GA: MR imaging of the wrist and elbow, *Clin Sports Med* 14:315, 1995.

Garden RS: Tennis elbow, *J Bone Joint Surg* 43B:100, 1961.

Gardner E: *Fundamentals of neurology,* ed 4, Philadelphia, 1963, WB Saunders.

Gerard JA, Kleinfield SL: *Orthopedic testing,* New York, 1993, Churchill Livingstone.

Gilula LA, editor: *The traumatized wrist and hand: radiographic and anatomic correlation,* Philadelphia, 1992, Saunders.

Gilula LA, Yin Y: *Imaging of the wrist and hand,* Philadelphia, 1996, WB Saunders.

Grant JCB, Basmajian JV: *Grant's method of anatomy,* ed 7, Baltimore, 1965, Williams & Wilkins.

Greenspan A: *Orthopedic radiology,* ed 2, Philadelphia, 1992, JB Lippincott.

Greenstein GM: *Clinical assessment of neuromusculoskeletal disorders,* St Louis, 1997, Mosby.

Grossman ZD, et al: *Cost-effective diagnostic imaging: the clinician's guide,* ed 3, St Louis, 1995, Mosby.

Hale MS: *A practical approach to arm pain,* Springfield, Ill, 1971, Charles C Thomas.

Hammer WI: *Functional soft tissue examination and treatment by manual methods the extremities,* Gaithersburg, Md, 1991, Aspen.

Hartley A: *Practical joint assessment upper quadrant,* ed 2, St Louis, 1995, Mosby.

Hawkins RJ: *An organized approach to musculoskeletal examination and history taking,* St Louis, 1995, Mosby.

Hinkle CZ: *Fundamentals of anatomy & movement: a workbook and guide,* St Louis, 1997, Mosby.

Ho CP, Sartoris DJ: Magnetic resonance imaging of the elbow, *Rheum Dis Clin North Am* 17:705, 1991.

Hollinshead WH: *Anatomy for surgeons,* vol 3, *The back and limbs,* ed 2, New York, 1969, Harper & Row.

Hoppenfeld S: *Physical examination of the spine and extremities,* New York, 1976, Appleton-Century-Crofts.

Jablonski S: *Dictionary of medical acronyms & abbreviations,* ed 3, Philadelphia, 1998, Hanley & Belfus.

Jehl J, Crummy P: *Essentials of radiologic surgery,* ed 6, Philadelphia, 1993, JB Lippincott.

Kaplan EB: Treatment of tennis elbow (epicondylitis) by denervation, *J Bone Joint Surg* 41A:147, 1959.

Kasch MC: Acute hand injuries. In Pedretti LW, Zolton B, editors: *Occupational therapy: practice skills for physical dysfunction,* ed 3, St Louis, 1990, Mosby.

Kasdan ML: *Occupational hand & upper extremity injuries & diseases,* ed 2, Philadelphia, 1998, Hanley & Belfus.

Katirji B: *Electromyography in clinical practice: a case study approach,* St Louis, 1998, Mosby.

Katz WA: *Rheumatic diseases diagnosis and management,* Philadelphia, 1977, JB Lippincott.

Kendall HO, Kendall FP, Wadsworth GE: *Muscles: testing and function,* ed 3, Baltimore, 1992, Williams & Wilkins.

Klippel JH, Dieppe PA: *Rheumatology,* vol 1-2, ed 2, London, 1998, Mosby.

Lavy CBD, Barrett DS: *Questions and answers on Apley's concise system of orthopaedics and fractures,* Oxford, 1991, Butterworth-Heinemann.

LeHuec JC, et al: Epicondylitis after treatment with fluoroquinolone antibiotics, *J Bone Joint Surg* 77B:293, 1995.

Lerner AJ: *The little black book of neurology,* ed 3, St Louis, 1995, Mosby.

Lewis CB, Knortz KA: *Orthopedic assessment and treatment of the geriatric patient,* St Louis, 1993, Mosby.

Loth TS: *Orthopedic boards review II: a case study approach,* St Louis, 1996, Mosby.

Magee DJ: *Orthopedic physical assessment,* ed 3, Philadelphia, 1997, WB Saunders.

Malmivaara A, et al: Rheumatoid factor and HLA antigens in wrist tenosynovitis and humeral epicondylitis, *Scand J Rheumatol* 24:154, 1995.

Malone TR, McPoil TG, Nitz AJ: *Orthopedic and sports physical therapy,* ed 3, St Louis, 1997, Mosby.

Martin JH: *Neuroanatomy text and atlas,* ed 2, Stamford, Conn, 1996, Appleton & Lange.

Mathers LH, et al: *Clinical anatomy principles,* St Louis, 1996, Mosby.

Mazion JM: *Illustrated manual of neurological reflexes/signs/tests, part 1, orthopedic signs/tests/maneuvers for office procedure, part II,* Orlando, 1980, Daniels Publishing.

McRae R: *Clinical orthopaedic examination,* ed 3, Edinburgh, 1990, Churchill Livingstone.

Medical Economics Books: *Patient care flow chart manual,* ed 3, Oradell NJ, 1982, Medical Economics Books.

Mellion MB: *Sports medicine secrets,* Philadelphia, 1994, Hanley & Belfus.

Mellion MB: *Office sports medicine,* ed 2, St Louis, 1996, Mosby.

Mennell JM: *The musculoskeletal system differential diagnosis from symptoms and physical signs,* Gaithersburg, Md, 1992, Aspen.

Mercier LR, Pettid FJ: *Practical orthopedics,* ed 4, St Louis, 1995, Mosby.

Meyers JF: Elbow arthroscopy. In Shahriaree H, editor: *O'Connor's textbook of arthroscopic surgery,* Philadelphia, 1992, JB Lippincott.

Mills GP: The treatment of tennis elbow, *Dr Med J* 1:12, 1928.

Mitchell SW: *Injuries of nerves and their consequences,* Philadelphia, 1972, JB Lippincott.

Moore KL: *Clinically oriented anatomy,* ed 3, Baltimore, 1992, Williams & Wilkins.

Mosby-Year Book, Inc: *Expert 10-minute physical examination,* St Louis, 1997, Mosby.

Murphy BJ: MR imaging of the elbow, *Radiology* 184:525, 1992.

Newman JS, et al: Detection of soft-tissue hyperemia: value of power Doppler sonography, *AJR Am J Roentgenol* 163:385, 1994.

Nicholas JA, Hershman EB: *The upper extremity in sports medicine,* ed 2, St Louis, 1995, Mosby.

Nirschi RP: Patterns of failed healing in tendon injury. In Buckwalter J, Leadbetter W, Goodwin P, editors: *Sports induced soft tissue inflammation,* Chicago, 1991, American Academy of Orthopedic Surgeons.

Nirschi RP: Elbow tendinosis/tennis elbow, *Clin Sports Med* 4:851, 1992.

Nirschi RP: Muscle and tendon trauma. In Morrey BF, editor: *The elbow and its disorders,* Philadelphia, 1993, Saunders.

Nordin M, Andersson GBJ, Pope MH: *Musculoskeletal disorders in the workplace: principles and practice,* St Louis, 1997, Mosby.

Nordin M, Frankel VH: *Basic biomechanics of the musculoskeletal system,* ed 2, Philadelphia, 1989, Lea & Febiger.

O'Donoghue DH: *Treatment of injuries to athletes,* ed 3, Philadelphia, 1976, WB Saunders.

O'Drsicoll SW, Ball DF, Morrey BF: Posterolateral rotary instability of the elbow, *J Bone Joint Surg* 73A:440, 1991.

O'Drsicoll SW, et al: The anatomy of the lateral ulnar collateral ligament, *Clin Anat* 5:296, 1992.

O'Dwyer KJ, Howie CR: Medial epicondylitis of the elbow, *Int Orthop* 19:69, 1995.

Omer GE, Spinner M: *Management of peripheral nerve problems,* Philadelphia, 1980, WB Saunders.

Osborne G: Compression neuritis of the ulnar nerve at the elbow, *Hand Clin* 2:10, 1970.

Parkes JC: Overuse injuries of the elbow. In Nicholas JA, Hershman EB, editors: *The upper extremity in sports medicine,* St Louis, 1990, Mosby.

Pecina MM, Krmpotic-Nemanic J, Markiewitz AD: *Tunnel syndromes,* Boca Raton, Fla, 1991, CRC Press.

Peterson AR, et al: Variations in dorsomedial hand innervation, electrodiagnostic implications, *Arch Neurol* 49:870, 1992.

Pheasant S: *Ergonomics, work and health,* Gaithersburg, Md, 1991, Aspen.

Polley HF, Hunder GG: *Rheumatologic interviewing and physical examination of the joints,* ed 2, Philadelphia, 1978, WB Saunders.

Potter HG, et al: Lateral epicondylitis: correlation of MR imaging, surgical, and histophysiologic findings, *Radiology* 196:43, 1995.

Preston DC, et al: The median-ulnar latency difference studies are comparable in mild carpal tunnel syndrome, *Muscle Nerve* 17:1469, 1994.

Regan W, Korinek S, Morrey B, An K-N: Biomechanical study of ligaments around the elbow joint, *Clin Orthop* 271:170, 1991.

Regan W, Lester E, Coorac R, Morrey BF: Microscopic histopathology of chronic refractory lateral epicondylitis, *Am J Sports Med* 20:746, 1992.

Regan WD, Morrey BF: Physical examination of the elbow. In Morrey BF, editor: *The elbow and its disorders,* Philadelphia, 1993, WB Saunders.

Reid DC: *Sports injury assessment and rehabilitation,* New York, 1992, Churchill Livingstone.

Resnick D, Niwayama G: *Diagnosis of bone and joint disorders,* Philadelphia, 1995, WB Saunders.

Roetert EP, et al: The biomechanics of tennis elbow, an integrated approach, *Clin Sports Med* 14:47, 1995.

Rosenbaum RB, Ochoa JL: *Carpal tunnel syndrome and other disorders of the median nerve,* Boston, 1993, Butterworth-Heinemann.

Rosenberg ZS, et al: The elbow: MR features of nerve disorders, *Radiology* 188:235, 1993.

Saidoff DC, McDonough AL: *Critical pathways in therapeutic intervention,* St Louis, 1997, Mosby.

Salter RB: *Textbook of disorders and injuries of the musculoskeletal system,* Baltimore, 1970, Williams & Wilkins.

Sandifer PH: *Neurology in orthopaedics,* London, 1967, Butterworths.

Sauser DD, Thodorson SH, Fahr LM: Imaging of the elbow, *Radiol Clin North Am* 28:923, 1990.

Schumacher HR, Klippel JH, Koopman WJ: *Primer on the rheumatic diseases,* ed 10, Atlanta, 1993, Arthritis Foundation.

Seddon H: *Surgical disorders of the peripheral nerves,* Baltimore, 1968, Williams & Wilkins.

Smith FM: *Surgery of the elbow,* ed 2, Philadelphia, 1972, WB Saunders.

Spinner M, Spencer PS: Nerve compression lesions of the upper extremity: a clinical and experimental review, *Clin Orthop* 104:46, 1974.

Stedman TL: *Stedman's medical dictionary,* ed 25, Baltimore, 1990, Williams & Wilkins.

Stoller DW: *Magnetic resonance imaging in orthopaedics & sports medicine,* Philadelphia, 1993, JB Lippincott.

Storen G: The radiocapitellar relationship, *Acta Chir Scand* 116:144, 1995.

Sunderland S: *Nerves and nerve injuries,* Baltimore, 1968, Williams & Wilkins.

Tan JC, Horn SE: *Practical manual of physical medicine and rehabilitation,* St Louis, 1998, Mosby.

Timmerman LA, Andrews JR: Undersurface tear of the ulnar collateral ligament in baseball players, *Am J Sports Med* 22:33, 1994.

Toghill PJ: *Examining patients: an introduction to clinical medicine,* London, 1990, Edward Arnold.

Torg JS, Shepard RJ: *Current therapy in sports medicine,* ed 3, St Louis, 1995, Mosby.

Tullos HS, King JW: Lesions of the pitching arm in adolescents, *JAMA* 220:264, 1972.

Turek SL: *Orthopaedics principles and their application,* ed 3, Philadelphia, 1977, JB Lippincott.

Vanderpool DW, Chalmers J, Lamb DW, Whiston TR: Peripheral compression lesions of the ulnar nerve, *J Bone Joint Surg* 50B:792, 1968.

Wadsworth TG: *The elbow,* New York, 1982, Churchill Livingstone.

Ward WL, Belhobek GH, Anderson TE: Arthroscopic elbow findings: correlation with preoperative radiographic studies, *Arthroscopy* 8:498, 1992.

Warwick R, Williams PL: *Gray's anatomy,* ed 35, Philadelphia, 1973, WB Saunders.

Watchmaker GP, Lee G, Mackinnon SE: Intraneural topography of the ulnar nerve in the cubital tunnel facilitates anterior transposition, *J Hand Surg Am* 19:915, 1994.

Watt: Magnetic resonance imaging in orthopaedics, *J Bone Joint Surg* 73:534, 1991.

Weinstein SL, Buckwalter JA: *Turek's orthopaedics principles and their application,* ed 5, Philadelphia, 1994, JB Lippincott.

Wiens E, Lane S: The anterior interosseous nerve syndrome, *Can J Surg* 21:354, 1978.

Wilson FC: *The musculoskeletal system,* Philadelphia, 1975, JB Lippincott.

Windsor RE, Lox DM: *Soft tissue injuries: diagnosis and treatment,* Philadelphia, 1998, Hanley & Belfus.

Winter D: *Biomechanics and motor control of human movement,* ed 2, New York, 1990, Wiley-Interscience.

Yochum T, Rowe L: *Essentials of skeletal radiology,* ed 2, Baltimore, 1996, Williams & Wilkins.

THE FOREARM, WRIST, AND HAND

AXIOMS IN FOREARM, WRIST, AND HAND ASSESSMENT

- Pain in the wrist and hand may have origin in the bones and joints, periarticular soft tissues, nerve roots, peripheral nerves, and vascular structures.

- Pain in the wrist and hand may also be referred from the cervical spine, thoracic outlet, shoulder, or elbow.

INTRODUCTION

Chronic wrist pain has often been called the *lower back pain of hand conditions.* Both areas offer the clinician significant diagnostic and therapeutic challenges. As in the examination of the lower back, a precise evaluation based on thorough knowledge of regional anatomy is essential to successful management.

The wrist joint is probably the most complicated joint in the body because of its unique arrangement and articulation of the radiocarpal and intercarpal joints. Ligamentous injuries to the carpus can lead to significant and possibly permanent disability. Diagnosis may be difficult with persistent degrees of carpal instability. Definitive treatment modalities have not been perfected. As with most joint injuries, a more thorough understanding of the anatomy and pathogenesis of these injuries is useful.

Carpal injuries represent a spectrum of bony and ligamentous damage. The names given to the various injuries describe the resultant damage apparent only on radiographs, for example, *lunate dislocation, perilunate dislocation, scaphoid fracture, transscaphoid perilunate fracture-dislocation,* or *transscaphoid transtriquetral perilunate fracture-dislocation.* Each injury is not an entity but part of a continuum.

TABLE 6-1

FOREARM, WRIST, AND HAND CROSS-REFERENCE TABLE BY ASSESSMENT PROCEDURE

Forearm, Wrist, and Hand

Test/Sign	Arterial Stenosis	Rheumatoid Arthritis	Digit Contractures	Carpal Fracture	Sprain	Denervation	Tenosynovitis	Aseptic Necrosis	Ulnar Neuropathy	Neuroma	Colles' Fracture	Carpal Tunnel Syndrome	Anterior Interosseous Syndrome
Allen's test	•												
Bracelet test		•											
Bunnell-Littler test			•										
Carpal lift sign				•	•								
Cascade sign		•		•									
Dellon's moving two-point discrimination test						•			•				
Finkelstein's test							•						
Finsterer's sign				•				•					
Froment's paper sign									•				
Interphalangeal neuroma test										•			
Maisonneuve's sign											•		
Phalen's sign												•	
Pinch grip test													•
Shrivel test						•							
Test for tight retinacular ligaments			•										
Tinel's sign at the wrist									•			•	
Tourniquet test	•								•			•	
Wartenberg's sign									•				
Weber's two-point discrimination test						•			•				
Wringing test												•	

TABLE 6-2

FOREARM, WRIST, AND HAND CROSS-REFERENCE TABLE BY SYNDROME OR TISSUE

Syndrome	Test/Sign	Syndrome	Test/Sign
Anterior interosseous syndrome	Pinch grip test	Denervation	Dellon's moving two-point discrimination test
			Shrivel test
Arterial stenosis	Allen's test		Weber's two-point discrimination test
	Tourniquet test	Digit contractures	Bunnell-Littler test
Aseptic necrosis	Finsterer's sign		Test for tight retinacular ligaments
Carpal fracture	Carpal lift sign	Neuroma	Interphalangeal neuroma test
	Cascade sign	Rheumatoid arthritis	Bracelet test
	Finsterer's sign		Cascade sign
Carpal tunnel syndrome	Phalen's sign	Sprain	Carpal lift sign
	Tinel's sign at the wrist	Tenosynovitis	Finkelstein's test
		Ulnar neuropathy	Dellon's moving two-point discrimination test
	Tourniquet test		Froment's paper sign
	Wringing test		Tinel's sign at the wrist
Colles' fracture	Maisonneuve's sign		Tourniquet test
			Wartenberg's sign
			Weber's two-point discrimination test

ORTHOPEDIC GAMUT 6-1

WRIST CARPAL SYSTEM

Injury of the wrist carpal system is determined by the following:

1. The type of three-dimensional loading
2. The magnitude and direction of the forces involved
3. The position of the hand at the time of impact
4. The biomechanical properties of the bones and ligaments

A stable and pain-free wrist is a prerequisite for normal hand function. In contrast, a painful, unstable, or deformed wrist impairs function. The wrist, a common target of rheumatoid arthritis, is adversely affected by the reaction of synovial tissue on capsuloligamentous structures, articular cartilage, and subchondral bone. The mechanical forces of the different muscle groups acting across the wrist also contribute to deformities.

The initial evaluation of a patient with an injured wrist must be thorough and methodical. In recent years, increased understanding of carpal mechanics and instability patterns, with and without fractures, has increased the importance of accurate examination of the wrist. The diagnosis of "sprained wrist" is not adequate in establishing a proper treatment regimen. By taking a careful history, performing an exact examination, and using appropriate diagnostic aids such as motion views, tomography, bone scans, and arthrog-

raphy, the clinician can establish an accurate diagnosis of wrist injury. It is only after an accurate diagnosis is established that a rational, therapeutic regimen can be prepared.

As with any other orthopedic problem, assessment of wrist and hand disorders begins with a complete history (Box 6-1). Painful disorders of the forearm, wrist, and hand can be classified based on the tissue of origin of pain and its distribution.

ESSENTIAL ANATOMY

The bones of the hand can be divided into four units: a central fixed unit for stability and three mobile units for dexterity and power. The fixed unit comprises the eight carpal bones tightly bound to the second and third metacarpals (Fig. 6-2).

ORTHOPEDIC GAMUT 6-2

MOBILE UNITS OF THE WRIST

The three mobile units projecting from the fixed unit of the wrist are as follows:

1. The thumb, for powerful pinch and grasp and fine manipulations
2. The index finger, for precise movements alone or with the thumb
3. The middle, ring, and little fingers for power grip

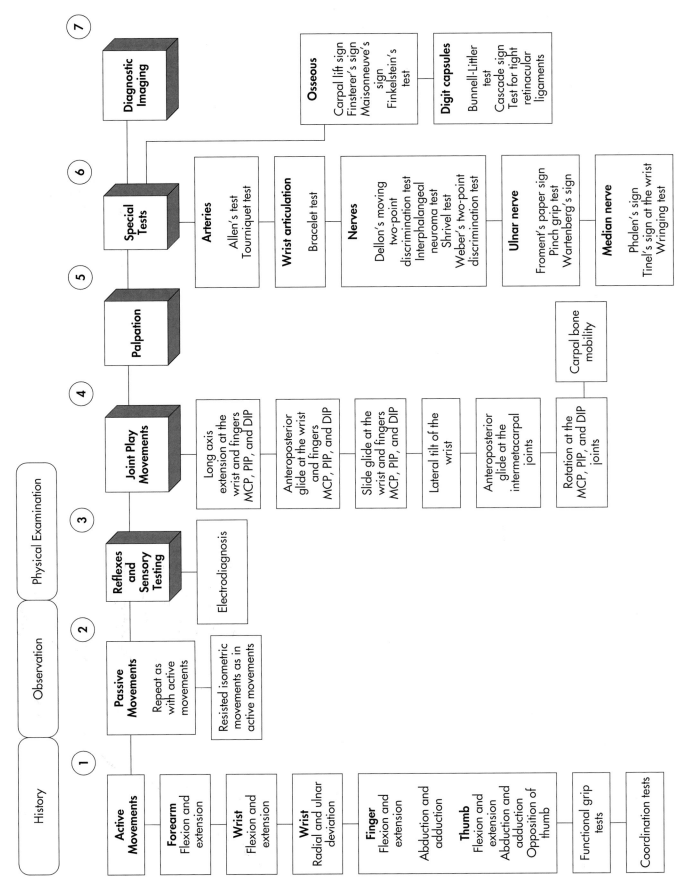

FIG. 6-1 Forearm, wrist, and hand assessment. *DIP,* Distal interphalangeal; *MCP,* metacarpophalangeal; *PIP,* proximal interphalangeal.

Précis of Forearm Wrist and Hand Diagnostic Consideration

SKIN AND SUBCUTANEOUS TISSUE
Forearm
Dorsal hand
Palmar hand
Digits

BONES AND JOINTS
Forearm
Wrist
Hand
Digits
　Metacarpophalangeal joints
　Interphalangeal joints
　Thumb articulations

FLEXOR MUSCLE SYSTEM
Forearm
Carpal tunnel
Palm and digits

EXTENSOR MUSCLE SYSTEM
Forearm
Extensor retinaculum
Dorsal hand
Extensor hood mechanism

NERVES
Superficial nerves
Deep nerves
　Radial nerve
　Ulnar nerve
　Median nerve

VESSELS
Arteries
Veins
Lymphatics

The carpal bones form a volar concave arch or carpal tunnel. The four bony prominences are joined by the flexor retinaculum (transverse carpal ligament), which forms the roof of the carpal tunnel. The flexor retinaculum straps down the flexor tendons as they cross at the wrist. The ulnar nerve, artery, and vein cross over the retinaculum but are sometimes covered by a fibrous band—the superficial part of the transverse carpal ligament—to form the ulnar tunnel, or Guyon's canal. The eight carpals (Fig. 6-3) are arranged in two roughly parallel rows, each row extending from lateral to medial. Each of the carpal bones articulates with adjacent carpal bones by small synovial joints, and small individual ligaments unite adjacent bones (Fig. 6-4).

The wrist transmits force between the hand and forearm. Force (Fig. 6-5) passes through the capitate bone of the distal carpal row, the scaphoid and lunate bones of the proximal carpal row, and onward proximally to the distal end of the radius. These are the bones most likely to be fractured or dislocated in injury of the hand-wrist mechanism. Of the two long bones of the forearm, only the radius has true articulation with the carpal bones (Fig. 6-6).

ORTHOPEDIC GAMUT 6-3

RADIOCARPAL JOINT

The radiocarpal joint consists of the following:

1. The distal surface of the radius
2. The scaphoid and lunate bones
3. The triangular fibrocartilage connecting the medial side of the distal radius with the ulnar styloid process
4. The triquetrum

As described earlier, the flexor retinaculum (Fig. 6-7) is a strong fibrous ligament extending across the anterior surface of the wrist, connecting the tubercles of scaphoid and trapezium laterally with the pisiform and hamulus of the carpal tunnel. On the posterolateral side of the wrists is a triangular region bounded by several tendons, known as the *anatomic snuff box* (Fig. 6-8). The tendons of extensor carpi radialis longus and brevis lie in the floor of the snuff box, as do the scaphoid bone and the radial artery.

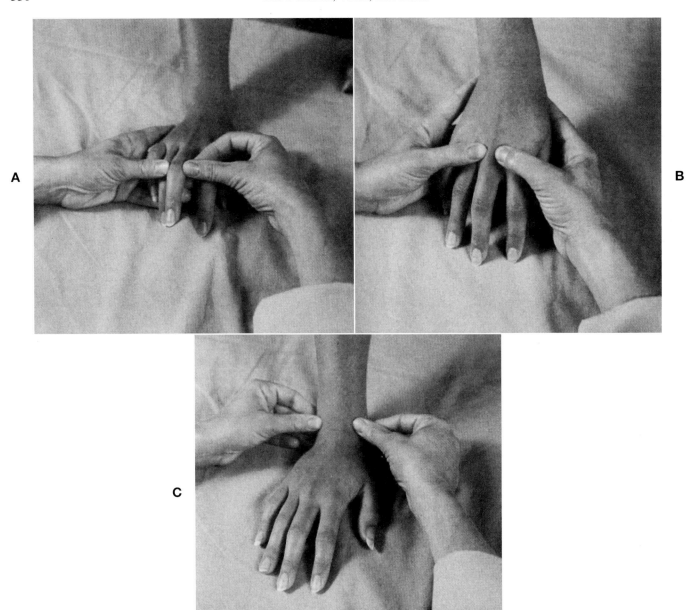

FIG. 6-2 Palpation of joints of the hand and wrist. **A,** Interphalangeal joints. **B,** Metacarpophalangeal joints. **C,** Radiocarpal groove and wrist. *(From Barkauskas VH, et al:* Health & physical
assessment, *ed 2, St Louis, 1998, Mosby.)*

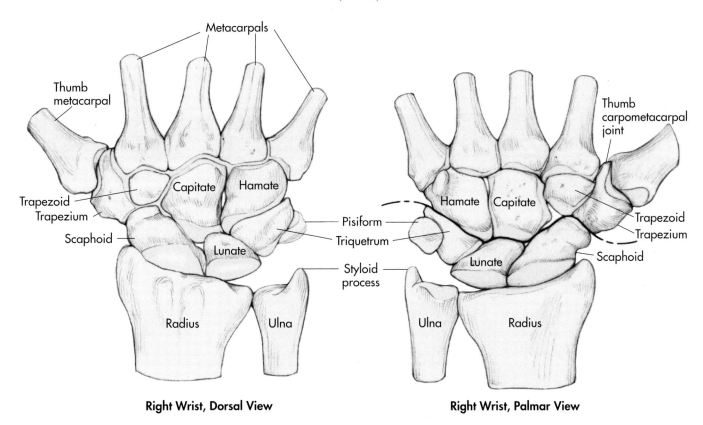

Right Wrist, Dorsal View   **Right Wrist, Palmar View**

FIG. 6-3   Carpal bones, dorsal and palmar views. *(From Mathers LH, et al:* Clinical anatomy principles, *St Louis, 1996, Mosby.)*

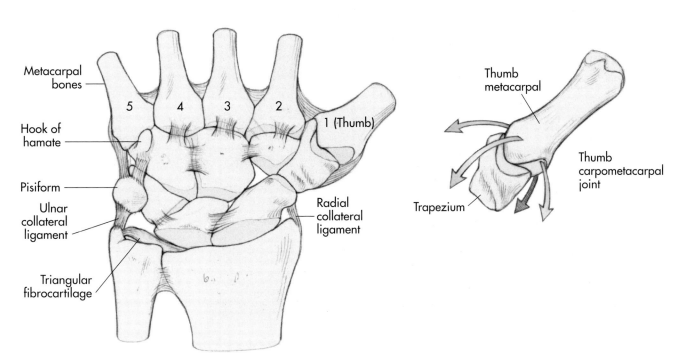

FIG. 6-4   Wrist ligaments and the carpometacarpal joint of the thumb. *(From Mathers LH, et al:* Clinical anatomy principles, *St Louis, 1996, Mosby.)*

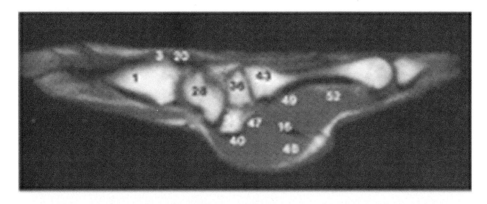

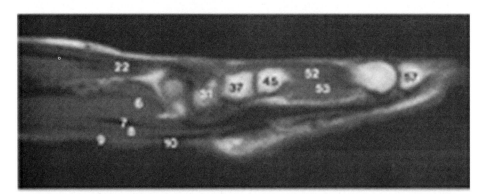

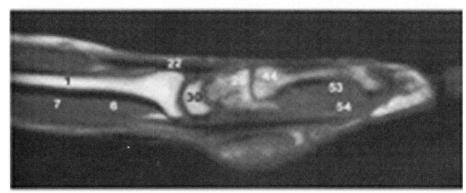

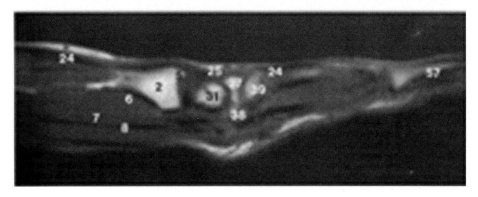

1	Radius
2	Ulna
3	Dorsal tubercle of radius
5	Styloid process of ulna
6	Pronator quadratus muscle
7	Flexor digitorum profundus muscle
8	Tendon of flexor digitorum profundus muscle
9	Flexor digitorum superficialis muscle
10	Tendon of flexor digitorum superficialis muscle
16	Tendon of flexor pollicis longus muscle
20	Tendon of extensor carpi radialis brevis muscle
22	Tendon of extensor digitorum muscle
24	Tendon of extensor digiti minimi muscle
25	Tendon of extensor carpi ulnaris muscle
28	Scaphoid
29	Capitate
30	Lunate
31	Triquetral
35	Trapezium
36	Trapezoid
37	Hamate
38	Hook of hamate
39	Base of fifth metacarpal
40	Abductor pollicis brevis muscle
43	Base of second ⎫
44	Base of third ⎬ metacarpal
45	Base of fourth ⎭
47	Opponens pollicis muscle
48	Flexor pollicis brevis muscle
49	Adductor pollicis muscle
52	Dorsal interossei muscles
53	Ventral interossei muscles
54	Lumbrical muscle
57	Shaft of proximal phalanx

FIG. 6-5   Magnetic resonance imaging through the wrist. Sagittal sections. *(From Mathers LH, et al: Clinical anatomy principles, St Louis, 1996, Mosby.)*

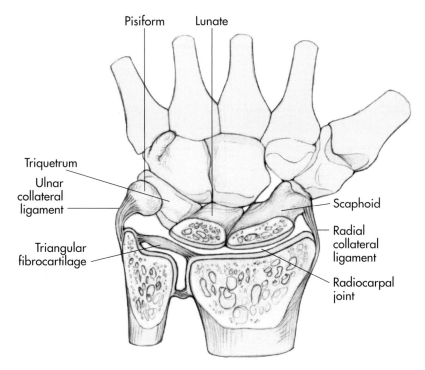

Pisiform   Lunate

Triquetrum

Ulnar collateral ligament

Triangular fibrocartilage

Scaphoid

Radial collateral ligament

Radiocarpal joint

FIG. 6-6   Interior of the radiocarpal joint, anterior view, right wrist. *(From Mathers LH, et al: Clinical anatomy principles, St Louis, 1996, Mosby.)*

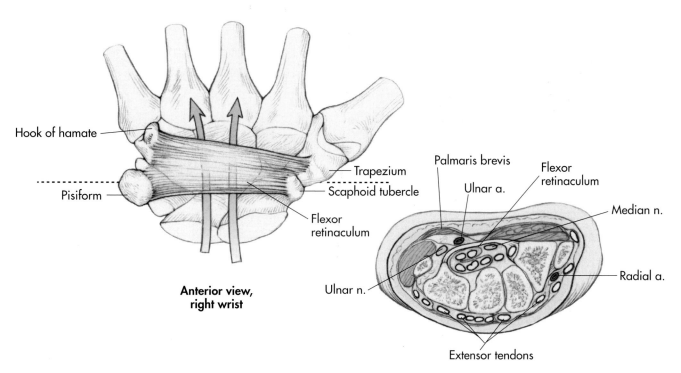

Hook of hamate

Pisiform

Trapezium

Scaphoid tubercle

Flexor retinaculum

Anterior view, right wrist

Palmaris brevis

Ulnar a.

Flexor retinaculum

Median n.

Radial a.

Ulnar n.

Extensor tendons

FIG. 6-7   Flexor retinaculum and wrist in cross-section. *(From Mathers LH, et al: Clinical anatomy principles, St Louis, 1996, Mosby.)*

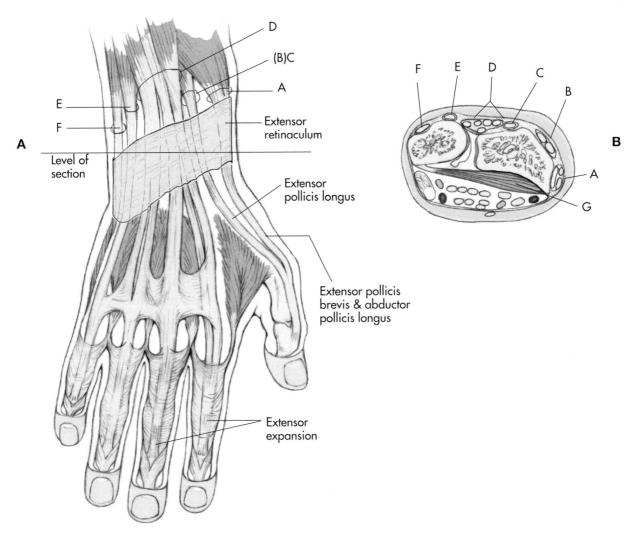

FIG. 6-8   Dorsum of the hand and wrist (**A**) and cross section through distal ulna and radius (**B**).
(From Mathers LH, et al: Clinical anatomy principles, *St Louis, 1996, Mosby.)*

ESSENTIAL MOTION ASSESSMENT

Movements of the wrist comprise flexion, extension, and ulnar and radial deviation. Flexion-extension movements of the fingers occur at both the metacarpophalangeal (MCP) and the interphalangeal joints (Fig. 6-9).

Movements of the thumb are described in terms different from those applied to the other digits because the thumb is positioned in a way that is different from the way the fingers are positioned, and the thumb is capable of unique movements not possible in the other digits.

Opposition is a unique capability, possessed only by the thumb. The goal of opposition is to cause the "pulp" surface (i.e., the rounded eminence directly opposite the nail) of the distal phalanx to face the pulp surfaces of the other digits.

This capability is essential to realizing the full range of capabilities for grasping and manipulating objects with the hand.

Creating a cup-shaped recess in the palm of the hand requires movement of the other four digits. This recess allows an object to be cradled in the palm before the fingers are closed over it.

For examination of the wrist/hand range of motion, the middle finger is considered midline (Fig. 6-10). Wrist flexion decreases as the fingers are flexed. Movements of flexion and extension are ultimately limited by muscles and ligaments (Figs. 6-11 and 6-12).

Finger abduction is 20 to 30 degrees at the MCP joints. Finger adduction is 0 degrees at the same joint. The loss of finger abduction or adduction has minimal effect on the

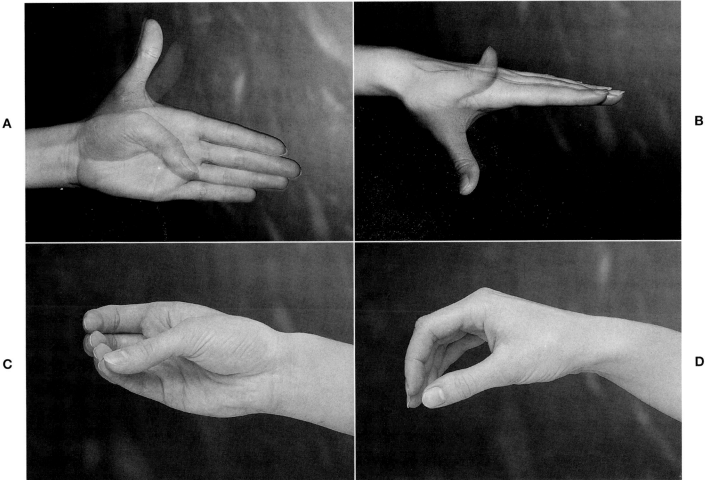

FIG. 6-9   Examples of thumb movements. **A,** Flexion-extension. **B,** Abduction-adduction. **C,** Opposition. **D,** Hand in neutral position. *(From Mathers LH, et al:* Clinical anatomy principles, *St Louis, 1996, Mosby.)*

activities of daily living. Thumb flexion at the carpometacarpal joint is in a range of 45 to 50 degrees. At the MCP joint, the range is 50 to 55 degrees. At the interphalangeal joint, thumb flexion is in a range of 80 to 90 degrees. Extension of the thumb at the interphalangeal joint is 0 to 5 degrees. Thumb abduction is 60 to 70 degrees. Thumb adduction is 30 degrees. Seventy degrees or less of retained flexion of the thumb at the interphalangeal joint and 50 degrees or less retained flexion at the MCP joint are considered impairments of the thumb in the activities of daily living. Zero degrees of extension at the interphalangeal joint is considered the sole impairment of extension for the thumb. Forty degrees or less of radial abduction and 25 degrees or less of adduction are considered impairments of the thumb in the activities of daily living (Fig. 6-13).

ESSENTIAL MUSCLE FUNCTION ASSESSMENT

ORTHOPEDIC GAMUT 6-4

MUSCLES OF THE HAND

The muscles controlling the movements of the hand are divided into the following two groups:

1. Extrinsic muscles that originate within the arm and forearm
2. Intrinsic muscles whose origins and insertions are entirely within the hand (Figs. 6-14 to 6-18)

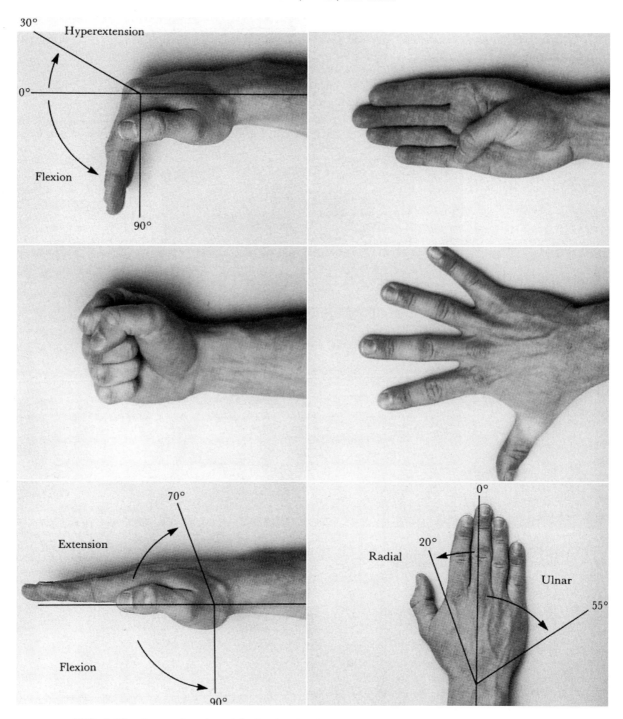

FIG. 6-10   Range of motion of the hand and wrist.   *(From Barkauskas VH, et al: Health & physical assessment, ed 2, St Louis, 1998, Mosby.)*

ESSENTIAL IMAGING

The importance of routine posteroanterior (PA) and lateral radiographs in neutral position of the wrist cannot be overemphasized.

With PA wrist radiographs, the scaphoid and the distance between the carpal bones can be assessed

(Figs. 6-19 and 6-20). A gap of 3 mm or more between the scaphoid and the lunate is abnormal and indicates a tear in the scapholunate interosseous ligament. A supinated, clenched-fist anteroposterior (AP) radiograph accentuates this gap.

On the lateral radiograph, an angle between the long axis of the scaphoid and the lunate greater than 70 degrees

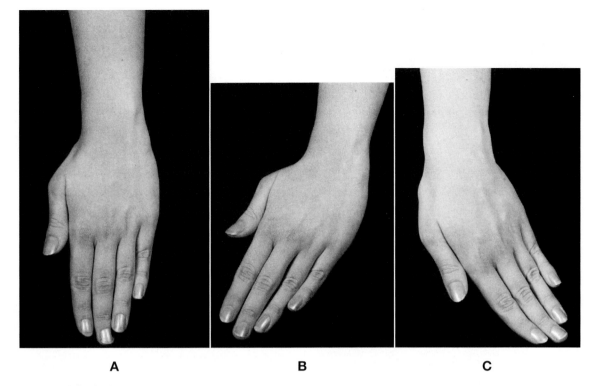

A   **B**   **C**

FIG. 6-11   The wrist in a neutral position **(A).** Radial deviation **(B).** Ulnar deviation **(C).** Radial deviation of 15 degrees or less and ulnar deviation of 30 degrees or less are impairments of the forearm in the activities of daily living.

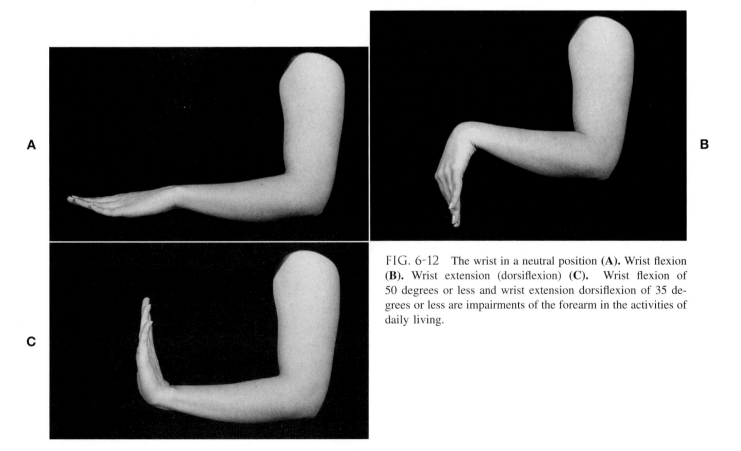

FIG. 6-12   The wrist in a neutral position **(A).** Wrist flexion **(B).** Wrist extension (dorsiflexion) **(C).** Wrist flexion of 50 degrees or less and wrist extension dorsiflexion of 35 degrees or less are impairments of the forearm in the activities of daily living.

A

B

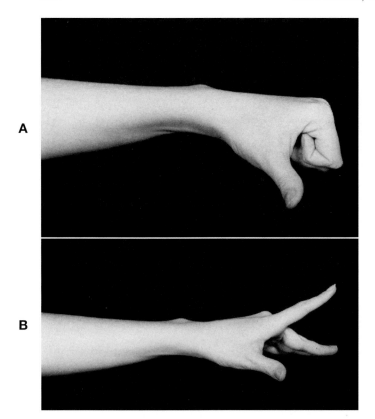

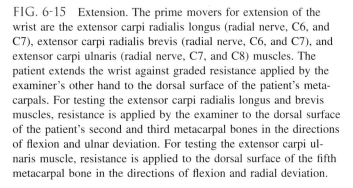

FIG. 6-13   Finger flexion (**A**) at the metacarpophalangeal joints. Extension (**B**) at the metacarpophalangeal joints. Extension of the proximal interphalangeal joints. Retained active finger flexion of 80 degrees or less at the metacarpophalangeal joint, 90 degrees or less at the proximal interphalangeal joint, and 60 degrees or less at the distal interphalangeal joint serve as an impairment of the fingers in the activities of daily living. Retained active extension of 10 degrees or less at the metacarpophalangeal joint serves as the sole impairment of the fingers in the activities of daily living.

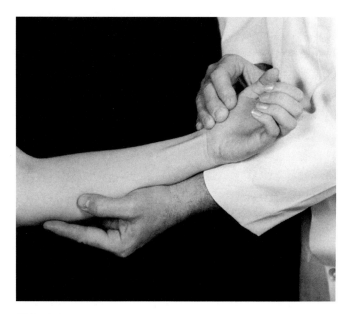

FIG. 6-14   Flexion. The prime movers for flexion of the wrist are the flexor carpi radialis (median nerve, C6, and C7) and the flexor carpi ulnaris (ulnar nerve, C8, and T1) muscles. The palmaris longus muscle is an accessory muscle used for this motion. The patient flexes the wrist against graded resistance provided by the fingertips of the examiner's other hand placed in the patient's palm. The flexor carpi radialis muscle is tested when the examiner provides resistance on the palmar side of the base of the second metacarpal bone in the directions of extension and ulnar deviation. The flexor carpi ulnaris is tested when the examiner applies resistance on the palmar side of the base of the fifth metacarpal bone in the directions of extension and radial deviation.

FIG. 6-15   Extension. The prime movers for extension of the wrist are the extensor carpi radialis longus (radial nerve, C6, and C7), extensor carpi radialis brevis (radial nerve, C6, and C7), and extensor carpi ulnaris (radial nerve, C7, and C8) muscles. The patient extends the wrist against graded resistance applied by the examiner's other hand to the dorsal surface of the patient's meta-carpals. For testing the extensor carpi radialis longus and brevis muscles, resistance is applied by the examiner to the dorsal surface of the patient's second and third metacarpal bones in the directions of flexion and ulnar deviation. For testing the extensor carpi ul-naris muscle, resistance is applied to the dorsal surface of the fifth metacarpal bone in the directions of flexion and radial deviation.

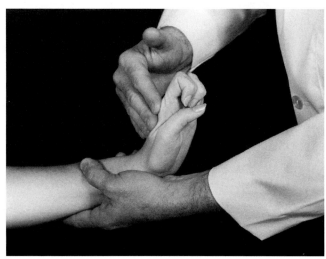

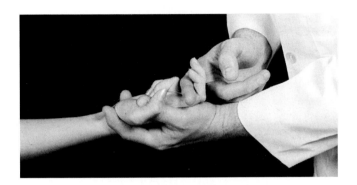

FIG. 6-16   Flexion of the interphalangeal joints of the fingers is accomplished by the long flexor tendons. Of the two long flexor tendons, the flexor digitorum sublimis has its main action on the middle finger joint. To test for sublimis action, the profundus tendon to the finger in question must be put completely out of action by passively flexing the metacarpophalangeal joint and by hyperextending the adjacent fingers. In tests for profundus action, the finger must be held passively and extended at both the proximal and middle finger joints.

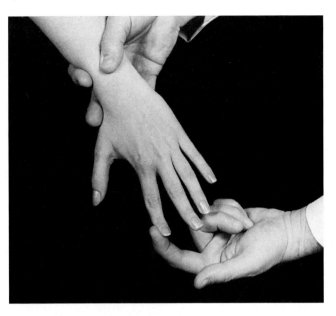

FIG. 6-17   The intrinsic muscles of the hand consist of a central group containing the interossei and lumbricales and the two lateral groups of hypothenar and thenar eminences. Many actions have been attributed to the lumbricales, but they have no powerful individual action of their own and can operate only with the stronger interossei.

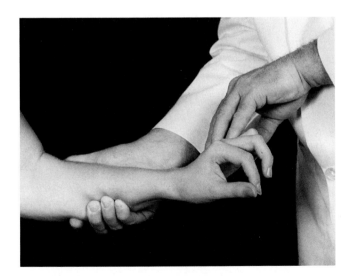

FIG. 6-18   The interosseous and lumbrical muscles are of fundamental importance in the extension of the fingers.

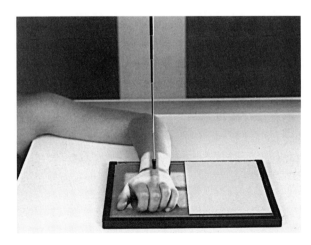

FIG. 6-19   Posteroanterior positioning of the wrist. (*From Ballinger PW:* Merrill's atlas of radiographic positions and radiologic procedures, *vol 1-3, ed 8, St Louis, 1995, Mosby.*)

is abnormal and is consistent with scapholunate dissociation (Figs. 6-21 and 6-22). An angle of 30 degrees or less is also abnormal and could signify ulnocarpal instability.

Special plain radiographs can further identify pathologic conditions. A carpal tunnel view, which is a radiograph with the wrist in full extension, fingers extended, and the beam in front of the third metacarpal, helps the examiner visualize fractures of the hook of the hamate (Figs. 6-23 and 6-24). The pisotriquetral area can be better seen with lateral radiographs of the hand and forearm in 10 to 15 degrees of supination.

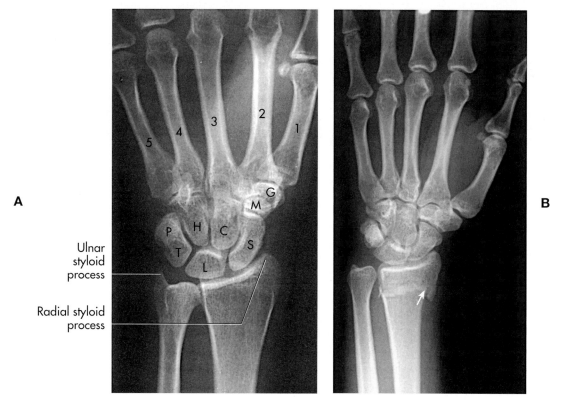

FIG. 6-20 **A,** Posteroanterior radiograph of the wrist. *C,* Capitate; *G,* trapezium; *H,* hamate; *L,* lunate; *M,* trapezoid; *P,* pisiform; *S,* scaphoid; *T,* triquetrum. **B,** Posteroanterior radiograph showing fracture *(arrow).* *(From Ballinger PW:* Merrill's atlas of radiographic positions and radiologic procedures, *vol 1-3, ed 8, St Louis, 1995, Mosby.)*

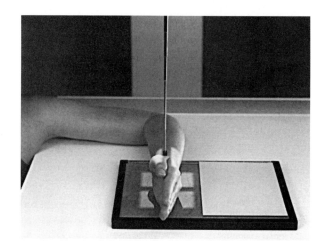

FIG. 6-21 Lateral positioning of wrist with ulnar surfaces to the film. *(From Ballinger PW:* Merrill's atlas of radiographic positions and radiologic procedures, *vol 1-3, ed 8, St Louis, 1995, Mosby.)*

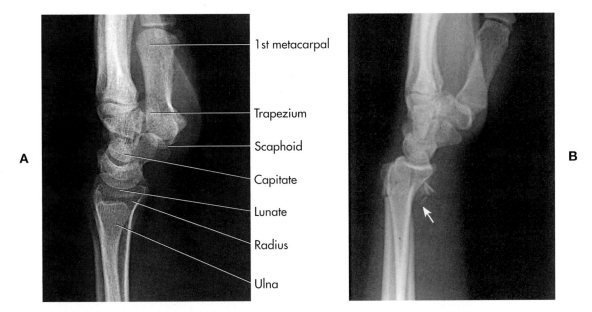

FIG. 6-22 **A,** Lateral wrist radiograph (ulnar surface to film). **B,** Lateral with fracture *(arrow).*
(From Ballinger PW: Merrill's atlas of radiographic positions and radiologic procedures, *vol 1-3, ed 8, St Louis, 1995, Mosby.)*

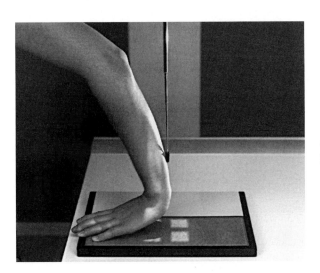

FIG. 6-23   Tangential (superoinferior) carpal canal. *(From Ballinger PW:* Merrill's atlas of radiographic positions and radiologic procedures, *vol 1-3, ed 8, St Louis, 1995, Mosby.)*

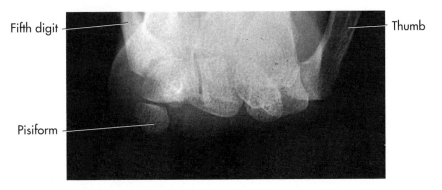

FIG. 6-24   Tangential radiograph of carpal canal (superoinferior). *(From Ballinger PW:* Merrill's atlas of radiographic positions and radiologic procedures, *vol 1-3, ed 8, St Louis, 1995, Mosby.)*

ALLEN'S TEST

Assessment for Peripheral Vascular Obstruction at the Wrist

Comment

The blood supply of the hand is largely anterior or palmar in position. All of the arterial supply enters on the front of the wrist, and at least half of the venous drainage leaves by the same route. Both arterial and venous systems are subject to many variations. Age has some influence on the state of the system. Arteriovenous anastomoses are poorly developed in children. In elderly persons, both the arteries and the veins become elongated, large, and tortuous. In the absence of local vascular trauma, sympathetic dystrophy influence of vascular homeostasis must be considered.

Sympathetic dystrophy and sympathetic-mediated pain dysfunction are the most serious of the complications that can occur after injuries to the wrist.

Sympathetic pain is a diffuse, disabling hypersensitivity in one or more peripheral nerve autonomous zones. The pain initiates with burning pain, cold sensitivity, hyperhidrosis, and painful motion. Reflex sympathetic dystrophy (RSD) presents an exaggerated response of the tissue to injury, producing intense and prolonged pain, vasomotor disturbance, and associated trophic changes. The pain and discomfort of RSD crosses several dermatome distributions. Clinical characteristics include protecting and guarding the extremity; holding or carrying the hand and wrist; and limiting use of the limb in pinch, grasp, and daily activities (Fig. 6-25).

Diagnosis of RSD is initially based on clinical symptoms and signs for the upper extremity. This includes painful disuse of the hand and wrist with a high degree of awareness. Supportive laboratory testing includes positive bone scans (Fig. 6-26), hypervascularity (thermography), and positive sweat test with autonomic dysfunction and quantitative sudomotor axon reflex test (QSART). Later, osteoporosis can help confirm the diagnosis. The sympathetic dystrophy scale is effective in confirming and rating the severity of this syndrome (Box 6-2).

The superficial and deep palmar arterial arches are so named because of their relationship to the flexor tendons. These arches are connected to the dorsal carpal arterial arch (which lies deep in the extensor tendons) by a proximal and distal row of perforating arteries that pass between the metacarpal shafts.

The extensive anastomoses between the various vessels allow occlusion of an arch within its length without serious risk to the distal blood supply. Even when both the radial and ulnar arteries are occluded at the wrist, the blood supply usually can be maintained through collateral circulation that, in such cases, will pass mainly through the perforating arteries. The digital arteries of a finger are of sufficient caliber to allow survival of the fingertip.

ORTHOPEDIC GAMUT 6-5

RSD LIMB PROTECTION

The following are three stages of RSD limb protection by the patient:

1. Not allowing palpation or percussion or even light touch of the affected tissue
2. Loss of use, stiffness of soft tissues, loss of joint motion, development of contracture, and atrophy of skin; warmth of hypervascularity turns to coldness; strength and function diminish further
3. Shiny, dry skin; degeneration of muscle tone; further joint stiffness; and both joint and muscle contracture

---

BOX 6-2

Putative Diagnostic Criteria for Reflex Sympathetic Dystrophy (RSD)

CLINICAL SYMPTOMS AND SIGNS
1. Burning pain
2. Hyperpathia or allodynia
3. Temperature or color changes
4. Edema
5. Hair or nail growth changes

LABORATORY RESULTS
6. Thermometry or thermography
7. Bone radiograph
8. Three-phase bone scan
9. Quantitative sweat test
10. Response to sympathetic block

INTERPRETATION: IF TOTAL OF POSITIVE FINDINGS IS
>6 Probable RSD
3-5 Possible RSD
<3 Unlikely RSD

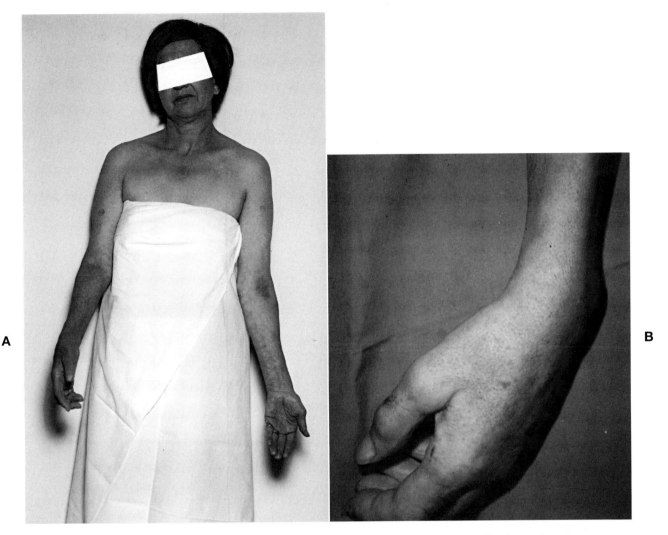

FIG. 6-25   Sympathetic dysfunction, typically with limb disuse, can be observed on inspection of the patient as a whole **(A)** or the hand and wrist in particular **(B).**   *(From Cooney WP, Linscheid RL, Dobyns JH: The wrist diagnosis and operative treatment, vol 1-2, St Louis, 1998, Mosby.)*

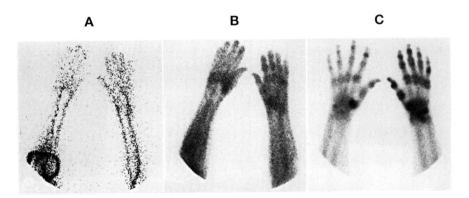

FIG. 6-26   Triphasic bone scan in sympathetic dystrophy. **A,** Injection phase. **B,** Early phase. **C,** Late phase.   *(From Cooney WP, Linscheid RL, Dobyns JH: The wrist diagnosis and operative treatment, vol 1-2, St Louis, 1998, Mosby.)*

The veins that drain blood from the hand are either superficial or deep systems. The superficial veins start on the dorsum of the fingers and collect their blood from the plexuses on the palmar and lateral sides of the fingers. The superficial veins run in several trunks parallel to the long axis of the fingers and drain into the cephalic and basilic veins via the dorsal venous network. There is no consistent pattern for this dorsal network, but in general, the cross communications are scanty. The deep veins of the hand and forearm are small and do not drain as much blood as the superficial system.

ORTHOPEDIC GAMUT 6-6

PULSES IN THE WRIST

Pulses can be palpated at the wrist in the following three places:

1. The radial artery lying just medial to the radial styloid process, which passes toward the hand
2. The ulnar artery, which passes just lateral (in the anatomic position) to the pisiform bone
3. The deep radial artery, which crosses the floor of the anatomic snuff box

---

Occlusion of the ulnar artery at the wrist may produce symptoms similar to those seen with ulnar tunnel syndrome. This disorder usually is secondary to some repetitive trauma to the ulnar aspect of the hand, such as when the hand is used as a mallet (hypothenar hammer syndrome). This disorder produces a thrombosis of the ulnar artery and results in ischemic manifestations such as pain, pallor, paresthesias, and decreased temperature of the affected digits. Local tenderness may be present, and Allen's test is often positive.

PROCEDURE

- The patient is seated and instructed to make a tight fist to express blood from the palm. The examiner uses finger pressure to occlude the radial and ulnar arteries (Figs. 6-27 and 6-28).
- The patient opens and closes the fist to express any remaining blood (Fig. 6-29). The examiner releases the arteries one at a time (Fig. 6-30).
- The sign is negative if the pale skin of the palm flushes immediately after an artery is released.
- The sign is positive if the skin of the palm remains blanched for more than 5 seconds. This test, which should be performed before Wright's test, Eden's test, and the shoulder hyperabduction maneuver, is significant for revealing vascular occlusion of the artery tested.

Confirmation Procedures

Tourniquet test and vascular assessment

DIAGNOSTIC STATEMENT

Allen's test is positive for the left wrist. This result suggests ulnar arterial occlusion.

Allen's test is positive after performing left wrist radial artery occlusion. This result suggests radial arterial occlusions.

CLINICAL PEARL

This test will often elicit paresthesia when an underlying distal peripheral nerve entrapment syndrome exists (carpal tunnel syndrome [CTS]). The test is used as an early indicator of other general pathologic conditions only when paresthesia is elicited.

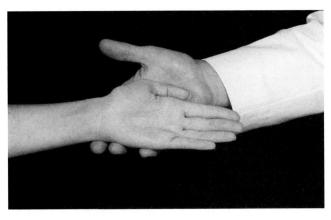

FIG. 6-27   The patient is seated with the elbow of the affected arm flexed and the forearm supinated.

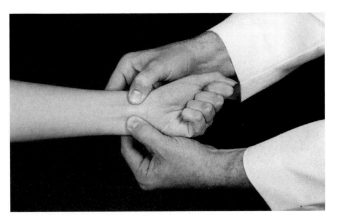

FIG. 6-28   With the patient's arm in the position of that described in Fig. 6-27, the radial and ulnar arteries are occluded by the examiner. The examiner will use both hands to occlude the arteries.

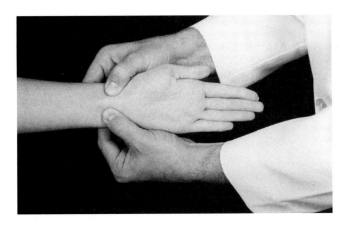

FIG. 6-29   While the radial and ulnar arteries are occluded, the patient opens and closes the hand repeatedly to express the blood from the tissue. Arterial occlusion is maintained.

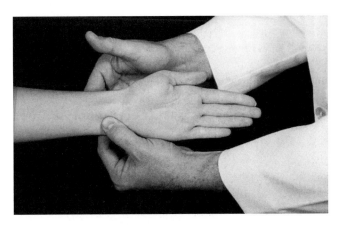

FIG. 6-30   The patient opens the hand, which should be blanched by ischemia. The examiner opens one artery, radial or ulnar. The filling time of the hand is recorded. If circulation fails to return within 5 seconds or less, this represents vascular compromise. The test is repeated for the remaining artery.

Assessment for Degenerative Changes of the Wrist Articulations (Rheumatoid Arthritis)

Comment

The hands and wrists are extremely important in the differential diagnosis of orthopedic diseases. Many of these disorders, which number more than 100, affect only the hands, and most of them strike at one time or another. In the two hands and wrists, an examiner may witness more than 60 articulations activated by dozens of muscles, tendons, ligaments, and bones. In a single glance, an examiner may witness the manifestations not only of one joint complex but also of an entire clinical syndrome.

The hands are in constant motion during the waking hours and even during sleeping hours. The hands are used in most activities of daily living, such as working, eating, and playing; the slightest compromise of function will be quickly bothersome to the patient. Such a disease has an effect psychosocially, too, because the hands are often noticed by others and they cannot be concealed for long. Handshaking, dining, and touching have cardinal roles in interpersonal relationships. No orthopedic examination is complete without a thorough assessment of symptoms, physical findings, and functions of the hands.

Osteoarthritis is a degenerative joint disease characterized by a progressive loss of articular cartilage and formation of new bone at the joint surfaces and subchondral area (Fig. 6-31). When located in the distal interphalangeal (DIP) joints, they are Heberden's nodes. When located in the proximal interphalangeal joints, they are Bouchard's nodes.

Visible evidence of rheumatoid arthritis and clues at the wrist level include the following: early swelling in one or more of the extensor tendon sheaths (Fig. 6-32) dorsally; swelling and tenderness just proximal to the transverse carpal ligament palmarly; or diffuse swelling of the entire wrist joint area, visible medially (Fig. 6-33), dorsally (Fig. 6-34), and laterally (Fig. 6-35); or a combination of these. Inflammation may or may not be visible (Figs. 6-36 to 6-38).

Rheumatoid arthritis usually begins in the proximal interphalangeal (PIP) joints, with development of typical fusiform swelling. At a later stage, the MCP and carpal joints may be affected.

There is a gradual loss of articular cartilage, as evidenced by narrowing of the joint spaces, and decalcification of bone occurs, particularly at a point adjacent to the affected joint. Along with these joint changes, there may be a weakness of grip as a result of atrophy of the intrinsic muscles. As the disease progresses, there is increasing deformity with flexion contractures of the MCP joints, ulnar deviation of the fingers, and adduction of the thumb.

The characteristic changes of adult rheumatoid arthritis are found most commonly in the hands. Although arthritis may present as a monarticular process, multiple joints are usually symmetrically affected. The onset of arthritis is usually gradual, and some of the early signs may be morning stiffness, weakness, paresthesia, and relative disability. Uncapping jars and holding a coffee cup may be difficult, and fastening buttons may be frustrating.

Examination of someone with arthritis reveals that the palms are moist and red while the fingers are tremulous. Fist formation, grip strength, and pinching are impaired, especially after prolonged disuse of the hands. The following findings suggest, but are not pathognomonic of, rheumatoid

---

ORTHOPEDIC GAMUT 6-7

RHEUMATOID DEFORMITY

Rheumatoid deformity of the wrist usually presents as the following:

1. Dorsal, distal, and then ulnar displacement of the distal ulna ("caput ulnae syndrome")
2. Subluxation of the carpus, usually palmarly with supination and radial deviation leading to a zigzag collapse of the wrist and secondary increased ulnar drift

3. Foreshortening and widening of the carpus
4. End-point deformities in which the patient presents with subluxation, dislocation, or ankylosis of the wrist
5. Digit stance deformities, particularly extension or flexion stance alterations during cascade testing
6. Signs of neurovascular alterations

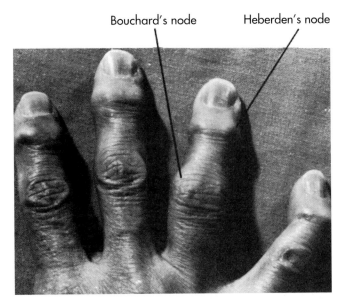

FIG. 6-31   Nodules of the hand associated with osteoarthritis.
(From Barkauskas VH, et al: Health & physical assessment, *ed 2, St Louis, 1998, Mosby.)*

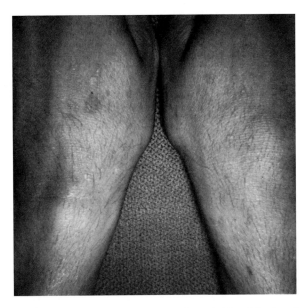

FIG. 6-32   Bilateral early rheumatoid arthritis of both wrists.
(From Cooney WP, Linscheid RL, Dobyns JH: The wrist diagnosis and operative treatment, *vol 1-2, St Louis, 1998, Mosby.)*

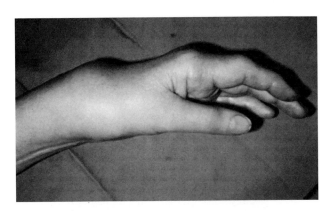

FIG. 6-33   Radial-lateral view of rheumatoid arthritis of the left wrist and hand with a moderate amount of arthritis involving the wrist, metacarpophalangeales, and interphalangeales. *(From Cooney WP, Linscheid RL, Dobyns JH:* The wrist diagnosis and operative treatment, *vol 1-2, St Louis, 1998, Mosby.)*

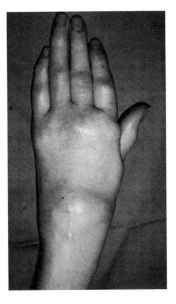

FIG. 6-34   Dorsal view of the same wrist in Fig. 6-33. *(From Cooney WP, Linscheid RL, Dobyns JH:* The wrist diagnosis and operative treatment, *vols 1-2, St Louis, 1998, Mosby.)*

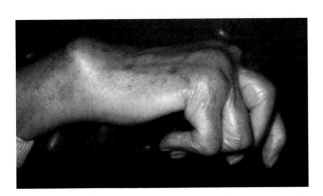

FIG. 6-35   Lateral view of a rheumatoid arthritis wrist with "caput distal ulnae." *(From Cooney WP, Linscheid RL, Dobyns JH:* The wrist diagnosis and operative treatment, *vol 1-2, St Louis, 1998, Mosby.)*

arthritis: symmetric swelling of the PIP joints, boutonniere or swan-neck deformities of several PIP joints, swelling or tenderness of the MCP joints, ulnar deviation or subluxation of these MCP and PIP joints, synovitis of the wrist (especially at the distal ulna), tenderness of the distal ulna, and swelling of the extensor carpi ulnaris tendon. More than one of these makes rheumatoid arthritis a likely diagnosis. The symptom complex of MCP joint swelling with ulnar deviation of the fingers, dorsal interosseous muscle atrophy, and extensor swelling at the wrist is virtually pathognomonic of rheumatoid arthritis. Caput ulnae syndrome also has a high degree of specificity. Subcutaneous nodules in the elbow and forearm may point to early diagnosis of this syndrome. The skin is moist, warm, lightly mottled, and thin and may be transparent (Fig. 6-39).

The erythrocyte sedimentation rate is elevated, but a normal value does not rule out the disease. Early in the disease, the latex fixation test is most often negative, and only soft-tissue swelling is found when using diagnostic imaging. The test for rheumatoid factor eventually becomes positive in 70% of patients. Subchondral osteoporosis, erosive changes, and joint-space narrowing later appear on the diagnostic images.

PROCEDURE

- The examiner gives mild to moderate lateral compression of the lower ends of the radius and ulna (Fig. 6-40).
- This compression causes acute forearm, wrist, and hand pain (Fig. 6-41).
- The test is significant for rheumatoid arthritis.

Confirmation Procedures
Clinical laboratory and diagnostic imaging

DIAGNOSTIC STATEMENT

Bracelet test is positive on the right. This result indicates rheumatoid involvement of the wrist.

CLINICAL PEARL

The bracelet test can be similar to a manual tourniquet test. The examiner must carefully compress osseous structures and not occlude arterial structures.

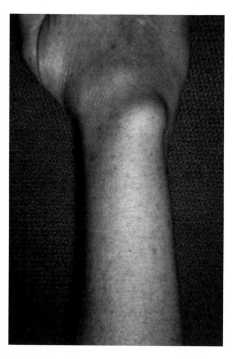

FIG. 6-36   The "caput ulnae" deformity in rheumatoid arthritis. *(From Cooney WP, Linscheid RL, Dobyns JH: The wrist diagnosis and operative treatment, vol 1-2, St Louis, 1998, Mosby.)*

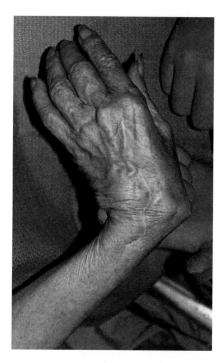

FIG. 6-37   Dorsal view of a rheumatoid arthritis wrist that has dislocated ulnarward.   *(From Cooney WP, Linscheid RL, Dobyns JH: The wrist diagnosis and operative treatment, vol 1-2, St Louis, 1998, Mosby.)*

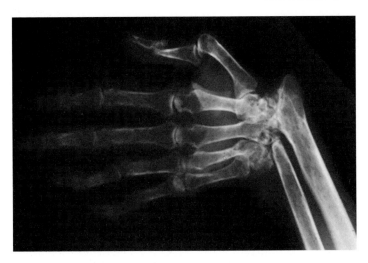

FIG. 6-38   Rheumatoid arthritis with the severe ulnar translation and angulation of the wrist. *(From Cooney WP, Linscheid RL, Dobyns JH: The wrist diagnosis and operative treatment, vol 1-2, St Louis, 1998, Mosby.)*

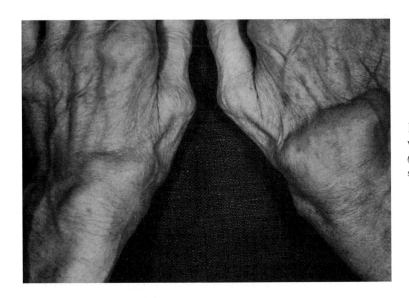

FIG. 6-39   Dorsal view of paired rheumatoid arthritis wrists shows diffuse extensor tenosynovitis on the right. *(From Cooney WP, Linscheid RL, Dobyns JH: The wrist diagnosis and operative treatment, vol 1-2, St Louis, 1998, Mosby.)*

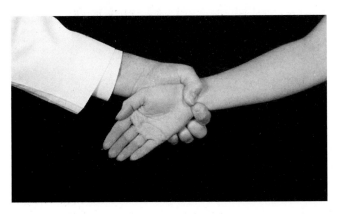

FIG. 6-40   The patient is seated with the elbow flexed. The examiner grasps the affected wrist, applying lateral compression to the distal radius and ulna. This may cause acute pain that indicates rheumatoid arthritis of the wrist.

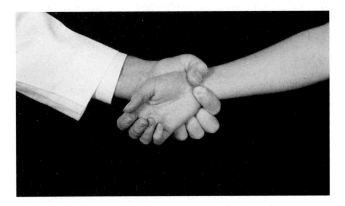

FIG. 6-41   While the examiner applies the lateral compression, the patient attempts to make a fist. This action, which will intensify the pain, will detect and localize the structures more involved in the arthritic degeneration.

Assessment for Interphalangeal Capsular Contractures

Comment

Osteoarthritis is a common abnormality that affects the hands. This type of arthritis attacks the DIP joints, where bony enlargement occurs. Sometimes, acute Heberden's nodes, characterized by erythematous periarticular inflammation, occur. Osseous hypertrophy of the PIP joints is characteristic of Bouchard's nodes. Heberden's and Bouchard's nodes may affect one or all of the fingers, but the effects are usually symmetric. Except for the thumb, the MCP joints are not involved. Rheumatoid arthritis usually involves the ulnar aspect of the hand, and osteoarthritis typically involves the radial aspect. The first carpometacarpal (CMC) joint is one of the joints most commonly involved. The wrists are usually spared, except for some volar swelling that occurs when there is an associated CTS. Contrary to what is widely believed, the erythrocyte sedimentation rate is sometimes slightly elevated. Other than that, systemic manifestations are lacking. Deformities such as ankylosis of the DIP joints, flexion contractures of the PIP joints, and unstable subluxation of the first MCP or CMC joints are common (Fig. 6-42). Lateral deviations at both the DIP and PIP joints, particularly when radiad at one digit and ulnad at another, are more suggestive of osteoarthritis than they are of rheumatoid arthritis. Although extensive deformations may occur, disability is usually not great. Diagnostic images will show characteristic subchondral sclerosis, marginal spur formation, joint space narrowing, and cystic changes at the involved joint.

With a pathologic condition such as arthritis, there is usually an inflammatory lesion in the muscles, the cell elements of which include lymphocytes, plasma cells, epithelioid cells, and occasionally mononuclear, eosinophile, and polymorphonuclear cells. These cells usually have a nodular arrangement in the tissue but occasionally are scattered. Muscles demonstrate degeneration as evidenced by enlargement, increase in number, and vacuolization of the nuclei. Muscle fibers shrink and break into small elements. Many of the fibers are replaced by fatty and fibrous connective tissue. The blood vessels thicken with collagen and periadventitial or paraadventitial round-cell infiltration. These changes involve the extensor mechanism, subcutaneous tissue, joint capsule, connective tissue septa, and the intrinsic muscles. The PIP joints usually demonstrate limitation of motion, so the patient cannot oppose the fingertip to the thumb tip. When the patient tries to grasp an object with the fingers, the thumb opposes the PIP joint. This pressure will eventually lead to a thumb that pushes the fingers in an ulnar direction (Fig. 6-43).

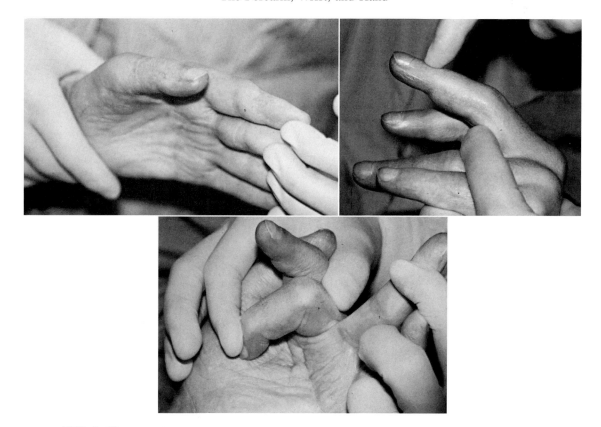

FIG. 6-42   Intrinsic contracture and Volkmann's contracture of the forearm secondary to axillary artery disruption.   *(From Cooney WP, Linscheid RL, Dobyns JH:* The wrist diagnosis and operative treatment, *vol 1-2, St Louis, 1998, Mosby.)*

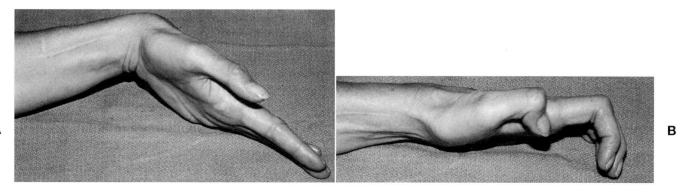

FIG. 6-43   **A,** Active digital extension in Volkmann's contracture. **B,** Wrist extension causes tight flexor tenodesis of the fingers and thumb at all joints.   *(From Cooney WP, Linscheid RL, Dobyns JH:* The wrist diagnosis and operative treatment, *vol 1-2, St Louis, 1998, Mosby.)*

PROCEDURE

- The examiner slightly extends the MCP joint while moving the PIP joint into flexion (Figs. 6-44 and 6-45).
- A PIP joint that cannot be flexed indicates a tight intrinsic muscle or contracture of the joint capsule. This is a positive finding (Fig. 6-46).
- This joint will not flex fully if the capsule is tight (Fig. 6-47).

Confirmation Procedures

Cascade sign, test for tight retinacular ligaments, clinical laboratory tests, and diagnostic imaging

DIAGNOSTIC STATEMENT
Bunnel-Littler test is positive for the right hand at the index finger. This result suggests capsular contracture consistent with osteoarthritis.

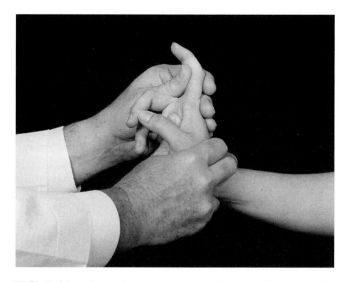

FIG. 6-44   The patient is seated with the elbow flexed and the forearm pronated. The examiner slightly extends the metacarpophalangeal joint of the digit under examination.

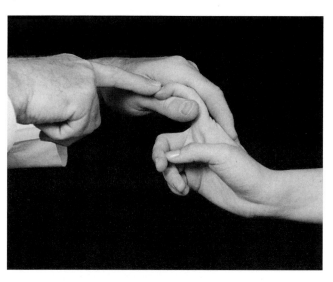

FIG. 6-45   After extending the metacarpophalangeal joint, the examiner tries to move the proximal interphalangeal joint into flexion. The test is positive if the proximal interphalangeal joint cannot be flexed. This result indicates tight intrinsic musculature or contracture of the joint capsule.

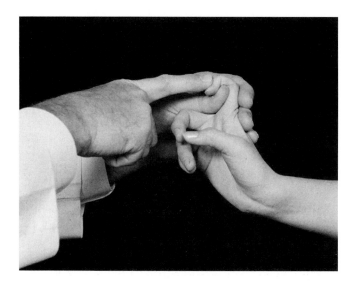

FIG. 6-46   From the position attained in Fig. 6-45, the examiner then slightly extends the proximal interphalangeal joint of the digit and tries to move the distal interphalangeal joint into flexion.

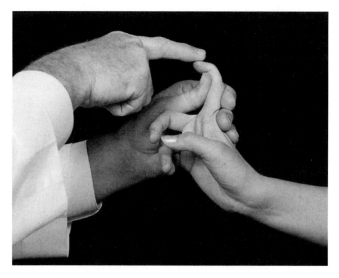

FIG. 6-47   The test is positive if the distal interphalangeal joint cannot be flexed. This indicates tight intrinsic musculature or contracture of the joint capsule.

CARPAL LIFT SIGN

Assessment for Carpal Fracture or Sprain

Comment

Because a sprain is a ligament injury, by definition, it is uncommon in the wrist. Most of the so-called sprains that are commonly diagnosed are not sprains at all but rather are strains of tendon attachments or injuries to the bone. The ligaments of the wrist permit a large amount of motion in the radiocarpal joint but very little motion in the intercarpal joints. The massive ligaments on the volar aspect of the wrist are so strong that a hyperextension injury is more likely to produce an incomplete fracture of the carpal bones, a contusion of the articular surfaces, or possibly a chondral fracture rather than a tearing of the ligaments. With hyperextension, there may actually be slipping of one row of carpals on the other. It is this slipping that permits damage to the dorsal carpal ligaments, but it is rather difficult to demonstrate. Suffice it to say that with the common dorsiflexion injury of the wrist, the damage is usually on the dorsal aspect. Therefore the examiner should be wary of the diagnosis of sprain of the wrist with a common dorsiflexion injury. During dorsiflexion of the wrist, pain is more common over the back of the wrist and forearm than over the front. However, stress on the ligament would appear to have been on the volar side. If there is tenderness over the carpus, careful x-ray study should be made, and the carpal bones should be studied closely regarding their position and condition.

Fractures of the scaphoid are the most common fractures occurring in the wrist joint. These injuries are also prone to complications, most notably nonunion, malunion, and late degenerative changes. Although scaphoid fracture is still predominately a fracture seen in men, it is not uncommon in active women (Fig. 6-48). The most common fracture line is through the scaphoid midpoint. The scaphoid takes a good deal of stress at the wrist, whether it is in dorsiflexion or palmar flexion, because of its position bridging the two rows of carpals.

Subluxation and dislocation may accompany ligament injury and may have peculiar characteristics when they occur in the wrist. Dislocation of the radiocarpal joint is extremely uncommon even though it occurs as the result of violent action. A complete carpal dislocation is also uncommon and is obviously a serious injury. Both conditions are accompanied by deformity and disability, are readily diagnosed, and usually receive good treatment. Diagnosing the exact dislocation through the carpus is difficult, but careful x-ray examination of both the normal and injured wrist in several positions will reduce the margin of error. It is particularly important for these conditions to be diagnosed early because, as with most dislocations, the longer the dislocation remains unreduced, the greater the likelihood that it will recur and permanent residual impairment will result.

The outer layer of the deep fascia of the dorsum of the hand is continuous with the antebrachial fascia. The deep fascia is modified over the wrist to form the dorsal carpal ligament. On either side of the hand, the deep fascia becomes fused with the second and fifth metacarpals, with the inner layer forming a compartment through which the extensor tendons can move freely. Distally, the deep fascia fuses with the capsules of the MCP joints and adjacent periosteum. The inner layers invest the underlying carpal and metacarpal bones and interosseous muscles.

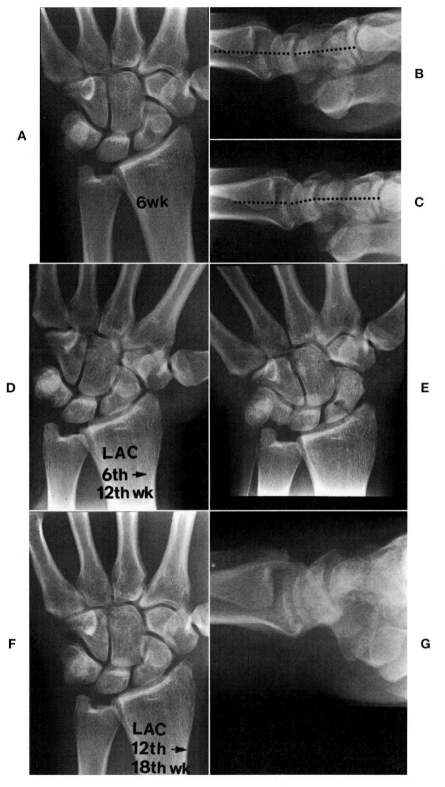

FIG. 6-48   Sprain of wrist. Initial radiograph was negative. **A-G,** Course of healing over 18 weeks.   *(From Cooney WP, Linscheid RL, Dobyns JH: The wrist diagnosis and operative treatment, vol 1-2, St Louis, 1998, Mosby.)*

PROCEDURE

- While fixing the other fingers to the examination table, the examiner applies pressure to the dorsum of the digit being examined.
- The patient attempts to lift or extend the finger off the table (Fig. 6-49).
- The sign is present if this action causes pain at the dorsum of the wrist.
- The presence of this sign indicates carpal fracture or sprain.

Confirmation Procedures

Finsterer's sign, Maisonneuve's sign, Finkelstein's test, and diagnostic imaging

---

DIAGNOSTIC STATEMENT

Carpal lift sign is present for the left wrist. This result suggests fracture in the proximal or distal row of carpals or in the base of a metacarpal.

CLINICAL PEARL

Carpal lift is accomplished when the finger is extended against resistance. The earliest sign of carpal fracture or degeneration, before using imaging, is the pain elicited with this test. With a carpal fracture, the carpal lift shifts the bony fragments and produces the corresponding discomfort.

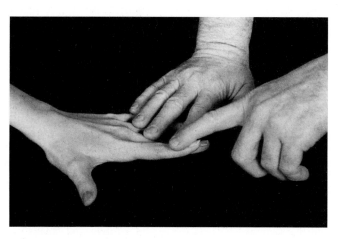

FIG. 6-49   The patient is seated with the elbow flexed. The arm is pronated, and the affected hand and wrist are resting flat on the examining table. While fixing the other fingers to the examination table, the examiner applies pressure to the dorsum of the digit under examination. The patient attempts to lift or extend the finger from the table. The sign is present if this action causes pain at the dorsum of the wrist. Such pain indicates carpal fracture or sprain. The pain may be emanating from the proximal or distal row of carpals or from the base of a metacarpal. The examiner should test each digit.

Assessment for Internal Derangement of Carpometacarpal Articulations and Internal Derangement of Phalanges

Comment

In the normal wrist and hand, the digits are medially deviated slightly in relation to the carpal bones. In addition, the metacarpals are at an angle to each other. These positions increase the dexterity of the hand and oblique flexion of the medial four digits and contribute to deformities seen in conditions such as rheumatoid arthritis and phalangeal fractures.

Treatment of fractures of the proximal phalanx is difficult because of the necessity of restoring alignment (Fig. 6-50). Fractures of the base are often angulated volarly because of the pull of the intrinsic muscles. The degree of angulation is difficult to visualize by lateral radiograph because the proximal phalanges of the uninjured fingers are superimposed on the film. An oblique radiograph is helpful, but it may fail to show the true severity of the angulation.

Volar angulation of the fracture is often noticed by a depression on the dorsal aspect of the bone, which can be palpated as the examiner's finger moves across the MCP joint and along the dorsal aspect of the phalanx.

Rheumatoid arthritis is a connective-tissue disease characterized by chronic inflammatory changes in the synovial membranes and other structures and by migratory swelling and stiffness of the joints in the early stage. Rheumatoid arthritis is also characterized by a variable degree of deformity, ankylosis, and invalidism in its late stage.

The cause of rheumatoid arthritis has not been determined, but a slight familial tendency has been demonstrated. Hypotheses of the etiologic factors have included infection, abnormality of peripheral circulation, endocrine imbalance, metabolic disturbance, allergic phenomenon, faulty adaptation to physical or psychic stress, and many other concepts. Evidence suggests that infection by slow viruses or organisms of the *Mycoplasma* species may play a role, but proof is lacking. The autoimmune mechanisms may be the underlying cause, and proteolytic enzymes released from disrupted lysosomes within the joint may play a part in the chronic synovial inflammation and the destruction of articular cartilage.

Rheumatoid arthritis currently is regarded as one of a group of connective-tissue diseases that exhibit somewhat similar clinical and pathologic changes. Other members of the group include systemic lupus erythematosus, polyarteritis nodosa, dermatomyositis, progressive systemic sclerosis, and rheumatic fever.

In the hand and wrist, the lesions of rheumatoid arthritis are characteristic and progressively disabling. The thumb is often drawn into adduction, the fingers deviate toward the ulnar side, and individual digits may develop grotesque deformities and severe restriction of function (Fig. 6-51). Arthritic destruction at the wrist may result in dorsal subluxation of the distal end of the ulna, medial subluxation of the carpus on the radius, and radial deviation of the hand. The inflammatory synovial reaction damages the joints and involves the tendon sheaths and tendon in producing a variety of deformities.

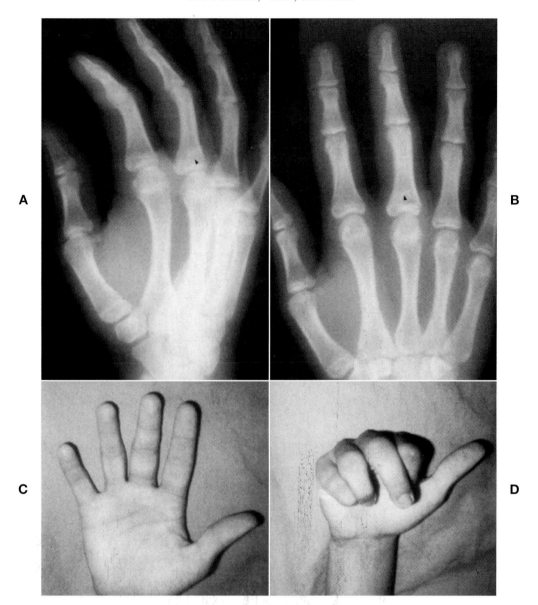

FIG. 6-50   The oblique fracture at the base of the proximal phalanx of the middle finger. **A** and **B,** Anteroposterior and oblique radiographs. **C** and **D,** Clinical examination.   *(From Nicholas JA, Hershman EB:* The upper extremity in sports medicine, *ed 2, St Louis, 1995, Mosby.)*

PROCEDURE

- The patient is seated, elbow flexed and forearm supinated. The patient flexes the fingers at the MCP and PIP joints, as if the hand is gripping a golf club. A complete fist should not be made (Fig. 6-52).
- In the normal hand, the longitudinal axis of the four fingers converges over or near the scaphoid tubercle (Fig. 6-53).
- The sign is present if any of the fingers are askew, which indicates internal derangement of the metacarpals, carpals, or both (Fig. 6-54).

Confirmation Procedures

Bunnel-Littler test, test for tight retinacular ligaments, clinical laboratory, and diagnostic imaging

DIAGNOSTIC STATEMENT

Cascade sign is present. This result suggests rheumatoid arthritis in the carpals of the left wrist.

Cascade sign is present in the left hand. This result suggests internal derangement of the wrist and hand.

CLINICAL PEARL

A faulty cascade of the fingers, indicating internal derangement of the wrist and hand, is an impediment of the hand grasp in daily activities. Patients usually have adopted accommodating grips. Pain or grip weakness is what precipitates the need for professional care.

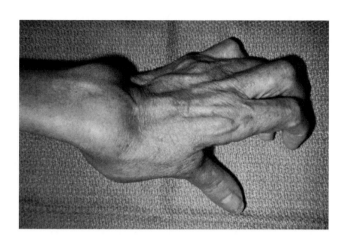

FIG. 6-51 Rheumatoid arthritis wrist that has translated palmarward. *(From Cooney WP, Linscheid RL, Dobyns JH: The wrist diagnosis and operative treatment, vol 1-2, St Louis, 1998, Mosby.)*

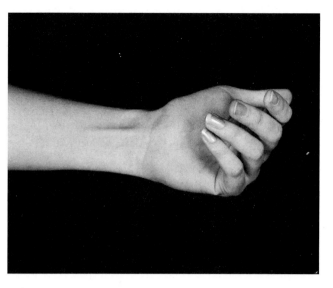

FIG. 6-52 The patient is seated with the elbow flexed and the forearm supinated. The patient flexes the fingers at the metacarpophalangeal and proximal interphalangeal joints, as if the hand is gripping a golf club. A complete fist should not be made.

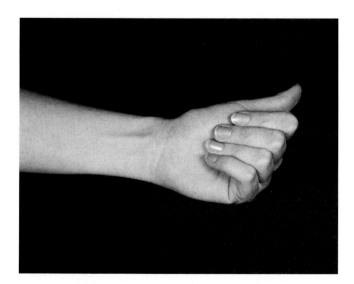

FIG. 6-53 In the normal hand, the longitudinal axis of the four fingers converges over or near the scaphoid tubercle.

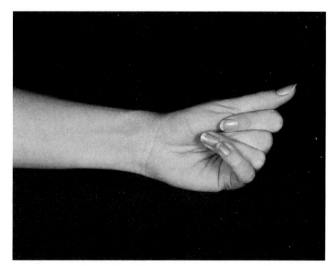

FIG. 6-54 The sign is present if any of the fingers are askew, which indicates internal derangement of the metacarpals or carpals or both.

DELLON'S MOVING TWO-POINT DISCRIMINATION TEST

Assessment for Dermatome Sensory Disturbances

Comment

Sensation is the acceptance and activation of impulses in the afferents of the nervous system. There are four primary modes of sensation that are determined by the peripheral terminal endings of the sensory axons. These modes are the mechanoreceptors (touch-pressure), nociceptors (pain), and thermoreceptors (cold and warmth). Determination of the electrical conduction velocity of sensory nerves is the only objective way to measure sensation.

Sensibility is the cutaneous appreciation and precise interpretation of sensation. For example, two-point discrimination is a judgment, not a primary sensation. There is no correlation between sensory nerve conduction velocity and two-point discrimination values after repair of peripheral nerves.

Atrophy of the opponens muscle is a finding in advanced carpal tunnel syndrome (CTS) (Fig. 6-55, *A*). Opponens muscle weakness alone can be an earlier finding in CTS but is difficult to identify. To test for motor weakness associated with CTS, the clinician should examine only the opponens muscle. To do this, the patient is asked to place the back of the hands on a table and point the thumb tip at the ceiling (Fig. 6-55, *B*). The examiner then attempts to flatten the thumb on the table with two fingers. Most people with normal opponens power are able to prevent the force of the examiner's two fingers from flattening the thumb to the table.

Normal cutaneous sensation provides normal-quality sensibility that has been termed *tactile gnosia.* All current testing to examine the degree of loss of sensibility is related to cutaneous touch-pressure sensation. The sensation of touch is mediated through myelinated axons that are termed *quickly adapting* and *slowly adapting* in relation to their peripheral receptors. Touch-pressure can be divided into moving touch and constant (static) pressure, in relation to the receptors that are stimulated. Moving touch can be demonstrated with a 30 cycles per second (cps) tuning fork for flutter, which will affect the Meissner corpuscles, or a 256 cps tuning fork for vibration, which will affect the Pacini corpuscles. Static pressure, which will affect the Merkel discs, is evaluated by the Weber two-point discrimination test (Merkel discs) and the von Frey test. Moving touch is evaluated by the moving two-point discrimination test or using the ridge sensimeter. Functional tests, such as a picking-up test or coin test, evaluate both receptor populations. The tests are subjective and related to factors other than sensation, such as comprehension, motor strength, and coordination or concentration.

ORTHOPEDIC GAMUT 6-8

TWO-POINT DISCRIMINATION

The normal threshold for two-point discrimination distance for the volar surface of the hand varies according to the zone being tested:

1. Between the fingertip and the DIP joint, two-point discrimination is normal from 3 to 5 mm, diminished if 6 to 10 mm, and absent if greater than 10 mm.
2. Between the DIP joint and the PIP joint, normal is 3 to 6 mm, diminished is 7 to 10 mm, and absent is greater than 10 mm.
3. Between the PIP joint and the finger web, normal is 4 to 7 mm, diminished is 9 to 10 mm, and absent is greater than 10 mm.
4. Between the web and the distal palmar crease, normal is 5 to 8 mm, diminished is 9 to 20 mm, and absent is greater than 20 mm.
5. Between the distal crease and the central palm, normal is 6 to 9 mm, diminished is 10 to 20 mm, and absent is greater than 20 mm.
6. At the base of the palm and wrist, normal is 7 to 10 mm, diminished is 11 to 20 mm, and absent is greater than 20 mm.
7. The threshold for the dorsal surface is higher in all zones: normal is 7 to 12 mm, diminished is 13 to 20 mm, and absent is greater than 20 mm.
8. Below the elbow but above the wrist, normal is 40 to 50 mm, diminished is between 55 and 80 mm, and absent is greater than 80 mm.
9. Above the elbow, normal is 65 to 75 mm, diminished is between 80 and 100 mm, and absent is greater than 100 mm.

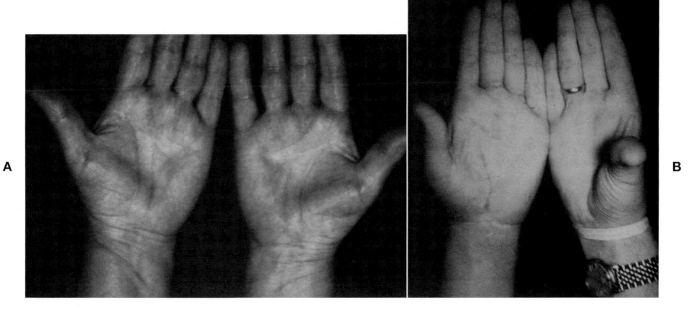

FIG. 6-55 **A,** Marked opponens muscle atrophy on the right compared with normal thenar muscle size and strength on the left. **B,** Examination for opponens pollicis muscle function. *(From Cooney WP, Linscheid RL, Dobyns JH: The wrist diagnosis and operative treatment, vol 1-2, St Louis, 1998, Mosby.)*

PROCEDURE

- Two blunt points are moved proximally and distally in the long axis of the digit (Fig. 6-56).
- One or two points of the Boley gauge are randomly used.
- The distance between the two points is decreased until the two points can no longer be distinguished (Fig. 6-57).
- The object is to determine whether the patient can discriminate between being touched with one or two points and the minimum distance at which two points touching the skin are recognized.
- Several areas on the uninvolved hand should be checked because some patients have congenitally abnormal two-point discrimination.

The testing instrument can be a Boley gauge, a blunt-eye caliper, or a paper clip. Testing is begun distally and proceeds proximally. The points of the caliper are set at 10 mm and are brought progressively closer together after each accurate response is obtained. The pressure from the testing instrument should not produce an ischemic area on the skin. When the two points are applied, they make contact simultaneously, and the line between the points is in the longitudinal axis of the finger. The patient closes the eyes for this test and indicates immediately if one or two points are felt. From 3 to 5 seconds should be allowed between application of the points. A series of one or two points is applied with varied sequence in each finger zone, and the procedure is performed three times. If the patient does not report two of the three correctly, the result is considered a failure at that distance. If the patient correctly identifies the number of points applied, the testing distance is decreased by 5 mm. There are 10 applications of two points and 10 applications of one point, both of which occur randomly. The total incorrect one-point applications are subtracted from the total of correct two-point applications. A score of 5 or more is considered passing.

Abnormal skin texture, such as heavy scales or calluses, has a marked influence on the test results. Testing can be done in the presence of edema or infection, but the results demonstrate the sensibilities present, which may not reflect the true status of the nerve.

Confirmation Procedures
Interphalangeal neuroma testing, shrivel test, Weber's two-point discrimination test, and electrodiagnosis

---

DIAGNOSTIC STATEMENT

Dellon's moving two-point discrimination test is positive in the index finger on the left hand. This result suggests a pathologic condition of the median nerve.

CLINICAL PEARL

A Janet's test can be performed simultaneously with Dellon's test. If the patient's responses are bizarre and do not follow anatomic distributions, psychogenic anesthesia is suspected. The patient is instructed to say "yes" when the stimulus is felt and "no" when the stimulus is not felt. The patient will say "no" if functional anesthesia exists.

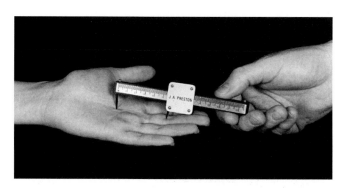

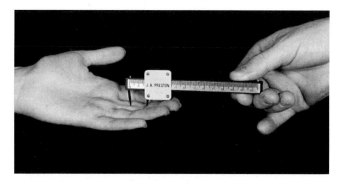

FIG. 6-56 The patient is seated with the elbow flexed. The hand is supinated and is resting on the examining table. The Boley gauge is set at 10 mm of distance or greater. The gauge is applied to the proximal axis of the digit under investigation. The two points must make contact simultaneously and with equal pressure. The patient's eyes should be closed.

FIG. 6-57 The gauge is moved distally, keeping in the long axis of the finger. The gauge distance is decreased in increments of 5 mm. The test is positive for loss of sensibility if the gauge cannot be perceived as two points at the expected threshold distances for the area tested.

FINKELSTEIN'S TEST

Assessment for de Quervain's Disease (Hoffman's Disease, Tenosynovitis of the Thumb)

Comment

Stenosing tenosynovitis of the tendon sheath of the abductor pollicis longus and the extensor pollicis brevis was first clearly recognized by de Quervain (1895). In this process, an additional etiologic agent may be the presence of accessory tendons in the sheath.

As the tendons to the thumb cross over the lower end of the radius on its radial aspect, they pass through tunnels of grooves on the lower end of the radius (Fig. 6-58). A fibrous retinaculum forms the roof of these tunnels. In particular, the long abductor and short extensor of the thumb pass directly over the styloid process of the radius. Multiple tendons of the abductor may pass through the same sheath, which is subcutaneous. Tenosynovitis in this area is common, usually as a result of overuse of the wrist and thumb. These tendons slide through the tunnel not only during movements of the thumb but also during movements of the wrist while the thumb is fixed. As the condition progresses, the tendons swell, the sheath thickens, and a situation arises that is analogous to trigger finger. While one tendon slides through the groove, another one hangs and doubles up. In the early stages, the tendon may then slip through the constriction with a palpable click.

de Quervain's disease (Hoffman's disease) usually affects women between the ages of 30 and 60 years. This disease is usually the result of repetitive thumb abduction or extension or of ulnar wrist deviation. It is more common in repetitive activities such as keyboarding, filing, carpentry, assembly-line work, and golfing. Pain, tenderness, and swelling over the first dorsal compartment, increased with thumb motion, dominate the physical findings. Palpable crepitus is occasionally present over the compartment. Affected individuals develop bilateral involvement 30% of the time. Differential diagnosis includes entrapment of the superficial branch of the radial nerve, arthrosis of the thumb axis and surrounding joints, and intersection syndrome.

During the early stage of de Quervain's disease, use of the wrist is increasingly painful. Swelling appears over the styloid of the radius. This tissue feels very firm and tender when palpated. The tendon sheath is tender and often swollen (Fig. 6-59).

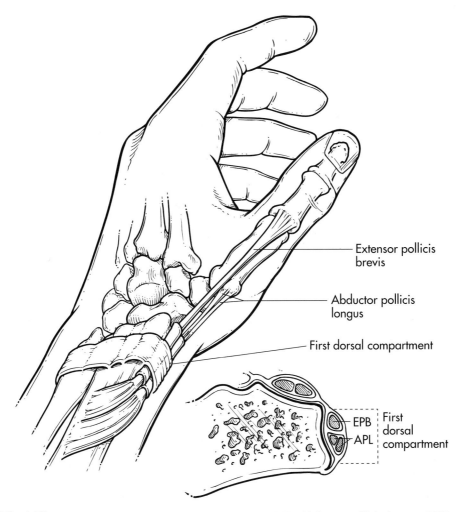

FIG. 6-58   Anatomy of the first dorsal compartment. *APL,* Abductor pollicis longus; *EPB,* extensor pollicis brevis. *(From Cooney WP, Linscheid RL, Dobyns JH:* The wrist diagnosis and operative treatment, *vol 1-2, St Louis, 1998, Mosby.)*

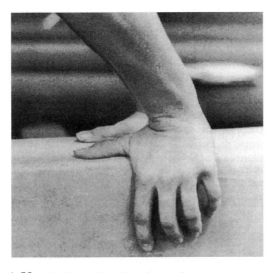

FIG. 6-59   Position of hand on beam that causes symptoms of both ulnar sprains and radial tendonitis (de Quervain's tenosynovitis). *(From Nicholas JA, Hershman EB:* The upper extremity in sports medicine, *ed 2, St Louis, 1995, Mosby.)*

PROCEDURE

- The patient makes a fist with the thumb inside the fingers. The examiner deviates the wrist in an ulnar direction (Figs. 6-60 and 6-61).
- If it produces pain over the abductor pollicis longus and the extensor pollicis brevis tendons at the wrist, the test is positive (Fig. 6-62).
- Pain indicates tenosynovitis in these two tendons.

Confirmation Procedures

Carpal lift sign, Finsterer's sign, Maisonneuve's sign, clinical laboratory testing, and diagnostic imaging

DIAGNOSTIC STATEMENT

Finkelstein's test is positive for the left wrist. This result indicates stenosing tenosynovitis of the extensor pollicis longus.

CLINICAL PEARL

Finkelstein's test produces an exquisitely painful response when stenosing tenosynovitis is present. Initially, it is somewhat easier to determine the severity of the condition when the patient actively tucks the thumb in and then deviates the hand and wrist in an ulnar direction. Depending on the response this produces, the passive test can then be performed. The pain elicited by this test is discrete and can be long lasting once excited.

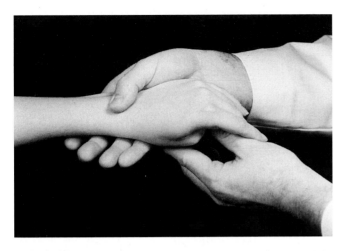

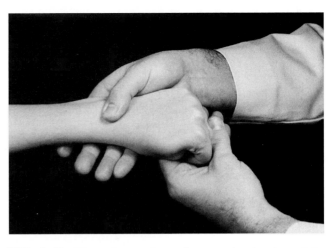

FIG. 6-60   The patient is seated with the elbow flexed and the forearm pronated. The examiner tucks the affected thumb into the palm of the patient's hand.

FIG. 6-61   The patient makes a fist over the thumb, and the examiner helps maintain the fist.

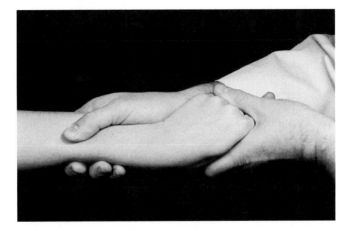

FIG. 6-62   The examiner moves the hand and wrist into sharp ulnar deviation. Pain elicited at the abductor pollicis longus and the extensor pollicis brevis tendons indicates stenosing tenosynovitis.

Assessment for Lunate Carpal Septic Necrosis

Comment

Following trauma, whether severe or trivial, the carpal bones may undergo aseptic necrosis. However, often no history of trauma is obtainable. Most commonly, the semilunar bone is affected (Kienbock's disease), less often the scaphoid bone is affected (Preiser's disease), and rarely are the other hand bones affected (Fig. 6-63). The amount of aseptic necrosis varies in degree. Regardless, the necrotic trabeculae are slowly resorbed and replaced by creeping substitution. Resorption often is incomplete, and cystlike areas form that are filled with fibrous tissue or amorphous debris. The articular cartilage degenerates and is replaced by fibrocartilage. The carpal bones become irregular, and the inevitable result is degenerative arthritis of the entire wrist joint.

Radiographic evaluation of the carpus is accomplished with a wrist series, which includes a neutral PA and neutral lateral. The series is completed with pronated PA views of the wrist in radial and ulnar deviation, along with an AP grip or clenched fist view.

The cause of Kienbock's disease is unknown but thought to be related to antecedent trauma, with microfracture perhaps disrupting the vascular supply to the lunate.

ORTHOPEDIC GAMUT 6-9

KIENBOCK'S DISEASE

Kienbock's disease staging follows:

I. Normal x-ray examination; abnormal bone scan or magnetic resonance imaging (MRI) scan
II. Linear or compression fracture
III. Increased bony density
IV. Collapse
V. Arthritis

The scaphoid articulates with five bones, is predominately covered by articular cartilage, and is the most commonly fractured carpal bone. Blood supply to the proximal pole may be tenuous, with approximately one third of scaphoids having one or no vascular foramina proximal to the scaphoid waist (midportion). As a result, proximal fractures require longer periods of immobilization for union, with avascular necrosis of the proximal pole seen in 30% of mid-third fractures and almost 100% of proximal pole fractures.

Symptoms that occur even before roentgenographic evidence appears include wrist pain that radiates up the forearm, tenderness over the affected bone, swelling of the wrist, and limitation of motion, usually dorsiflexion. By passively dorsiflexing either the long finger, if the semilunar bone is involved, or the thumb and index finger, if the scaphoid bone is involved, pain is reproduced.

A prominent feature of Kienbock's disease is its insidious onset, which often occurs without known prior injury. There has been a considerable difference of opinion about the events leading up to this initial complex of findings. Of the possibilities, the occurrence of a simple transverse fracture, resulting from a single episode of trauma; numerous compression fractures, resulting from repeated compression strains; and lunate or perilunate dislocation, leading to avascular necrosis in anatomically at-risk individuals, are the most popular. These theories have not been supported by well-conceived studies. On the other hand, it is clear that once the process of lunate necrosis has begun, a consistent and progressive sequence of events follows.

PROCEDURE

- The sign is present when grasping an object hard, clenching the hand, or making a fist fails to show the normal prominence of the third metacarpal on the dorsal surface and when percussion of the third metacarpal elicits tenderness just distal to the center of the wrist joint (Figs. 6-64 and 6-65).
- The test is significant for Kienbock's disease (aseptic necrosis of the lunate).

Confirmation Procedures

Carpal lift sign, Maisonneuve's sign, Finkelstein's test, and diagnostic imaging

---

DIAGNOSTIC STATEMENT

Finsterer's sign is present in the right wrist. This result suggests lunate carpal aseptic necrosis.

CLINICAL PEARL

For this sign, all the metacarpal heads are percussed. This gross, low-frequency vibration will localize any cortical defect.

A 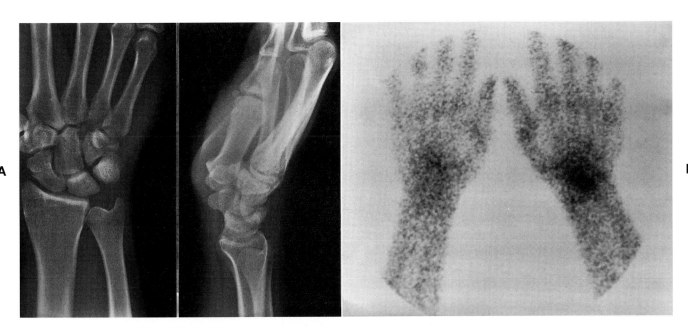 B

FIG. 6-63   Stage 1 Kienbock's disease. **A,** Normal appearance of radiographs of the wrist. **B,** Increased uptake at the lunate level on the bone scan.   *(Modified from Cooney WP, Linscheid RL, Dobyns JH: The wrist diagnosis and operative treatment, vol 1-2, St Louis, 1998, Mosby.)*

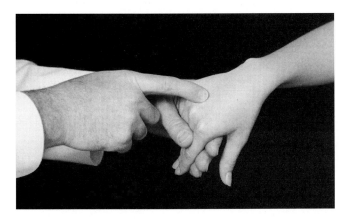

FIG. 6-64   The patient is seated with the elbow flexed and the arm pronated. The examiner locates the proximal head of the third metacarpal. This may be a site of discomfort and abnormal bony contour.

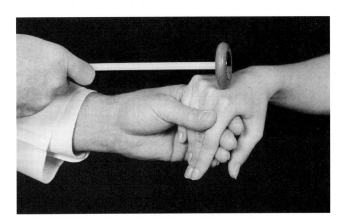

FIG. 6-65   The examiner percusses the proximal head of the third metacarpal with a reflex hammer or tuning fork. Pain elicited distal to the center of the wrist indicates Kienbock's disease (aseptic necrosis of the carpal lunate).

FROMENT'S PAPER SIGN

ALSO KNOWN AS FROMENT'S SIGN

Assessment for Ulnar Nerve Palsy

Comment

Testing the function of the median and ulnar nerves is the important first step in the evaluation of injuries of the volar aspect of the wrist.

Neuralgic amyotrophy, a disorder with many synonyms, is believed to be an inflammatory disease that afflicts the brachial plexus or one or more peripheral nerves in the shoulder girdle or upper extremity. It is a rare disorder with an estimated annual incidence of 1.64 cases per 100,000 population. It most often affects adults, peaking during their 20s. Males are affected twice as often as females. It usually is unilateral, but it sometimes is bilateral and asymmetric; it rarely is recurrent. Most cases have no specific precipitating factors, but some follow upper respiratory tract infection, vaccination, childbirth, and surgical procedures.

As the name implies, neuralgic amyotrophy is characterized by painful weakness of the upper limb. There is an abrupt onset of deep, boring shoulder pain, which is severe, worse during the night, and maximal during the first few days of illness. Many patients visit the emergency room for pain control. Typically, the patient notices upper limb weakness during the first week, as the pain starts to subside. Sensory loss usually is mild but may be more prominent in severe cases. Deep tendon reflexes are depressed or absent if the appropriate muscles are weakened significantly.

The anterior interosseous nerve is a purely motor branch of the median nerve. Entrapment may result from compression by aberrant or accessory muscles, fibrous bands beneath the pronator teres, or by pressure from an enlarged bicipital muscle.

Because there are no sensory fibers in the anterior interosseus nerve, the patient has no sensory complaints and experiences only motor weakness. The typical pattern is loss of distal flexion of the thumb and index finger, giving a characteristic pinch sign (Fig. 6-66). The pronator quadratus is tested with the elbow fully flexed.

Severance of the median nerve at the wrist results in the inability to oppose the thumb and anesthesia of the volar surface of the thumb; the index finger; and the long, radial half of the ring finger. When this severance occurs, sensation is the most important function lost. In adults, the recovery of sensation is rarely complete after repair of the median nerve. Although a casual examination may show that the patient appreciates pinprick and light touch in a normal manner, a careful examination reveals loss or diminution of two-point discrimination. The patient thereby loses a measure of tactile gnosia, which is essential for rapid and precise manipulation of small objects and for the tactile differentiation of objects.

Severance of the ulnar nerve at the wrist results in the loss of function of the dorsal and volar interossei, the adductor pollicis, the hypothenar muscles, and the lumbricales to the ring and little fingers. The patient exhibits anesthesia over the volar surface of the little finger and over the ulnar half of the volar surface of the ring finger. The key function lost is the use of the adductor pollicis and the first dorsal interosseous. The adductor is essential for strong pinching by the thumb. The first dorsal interosseous stabilizes the index finger against the thumb during pinching. The strength of the ulnar-innervated intrinsic muscles fails to return to functional levels in 75% of all ulnar nerve injuries in adults.

PROCEDURE

- The patient grasps a piece of paper between any two fingers (Fig. 6-67).
- Failure to maintain the grip when the paper is pulled away indicates ulnar nerve paralysis (Fig. 6-68).
- This result indicates a positive test.
- The test indicates ulnar nerve paralysis.

Confirmation Procedures

Pinch grip test, Wartenberg's sign, and electrodiagnosis

DIAGNOSTIC STATEMENT

Froment's test is positive for the left hand, which indicates ulnar nerve palsy.

CLINICAL PEARL

A change from a tip-to-tip pinch grip position to a pulp-to-pulp position is the earliest sign of ulnar entrapment (anterior interosseous nerve lesions must be differentiated). An electromyogram (EMG) requires more gross muscle deficiency for conclusive findings, and the nerve conduction velocity (NCV) may be equivocal in the early stages of nerve degeneration.

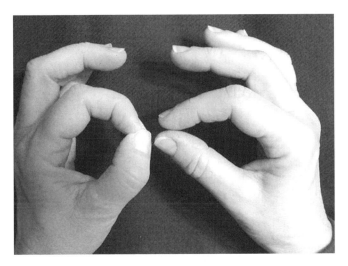

FIG. 6-66   Anterior interosseous nerve paralysis.

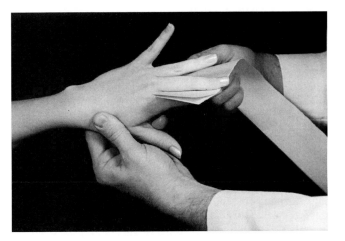

FIG. 6-67   The patient's elbow is flexed, and the forearm is pronated. The patient abducts the fingers from each other. The examiner places a sheet of paper between any two fingers, and the patient adducts the fingers, gripping the paper. Failure to maintain this grip as the examiner tugs on the paper suggests ulnar nerve paralysis.

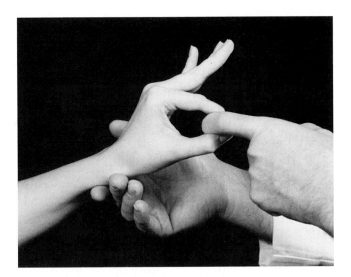

FIG. 6-68   In a modification of the Froment's paper test, the patient adducts and flexes the tip of the finger to the tip of the thumb. The examiner tries to pull the digits apart. Failure of the fingers to maintain sufficient strength to resist this motion suggests ulnar nerve paralysis (anterior interosseous nerve lesions must be differentiated by electromyogram).

INTERPHALANGEAL NEUROMA TEST

Assessment for Interdigital Neuroma

Comment

Neuromas can form at the cut end of an injured nerve. A neuroma incontinuity may develop along the pathway of an injured nerve. Neurofibroma is a nerve tumor arising from the Schwann cells and fibrocytes. This tumor is usually intertwined with the nerve fascicles, and complete removal requires a segmental resection of the nerve and reconstruction with a nerve graft (Fig. 6-69). Neurofibrolipoma is a benign nerve tumor with elements of fibrous and lipomatous hyperplasia. Like the neurofibroma, it tends to be intimately associated with nerve, and removal requires segmental nerve resection.

When stimulated, the neuromas may cause exquisite discomfort in the extremity. This usually consists of a pins-and-needles sensation or a shooting pain that radiates from a localized area. Sometimes, the pain may become so severe and diffuse that it spreads up the entire extremity. This spread of pain from a neuroma to the point where it involves the entire extremity may be due to the fiber interaction in injured nerves. Alternatively, painful nerve impulses stimulate or excite the internuncial pool of the spinal cord so much that normal impulses reaching this area from the periphery are interpreted as painful.

Such painful neuromas often are confused with the phantom limb syndrome. This does not imply that the phantom limb syndrome is caused by a painful neuroma. The point is that the painful neuroma so excites and stimulates certain areas of the central nervous system that the phantom sensation becomes painful.

Painful neuromas should not be confused with causalgia. Pain produced by neuromas should not be called *minor causalgia* because this only adds to the confusion.

PROCEDURE

- Neuromas should be carefully sought out by examination of the area using a slender instrument for palpating, such as the blunt end of a reflex hammer (Fig. 6-70).
- A localized spot in a scar will cause severe pain and is associated with paresthesia.
- The neuroma itself may be felt as a discrete mass.

Confirmation Procedures

Dellon's moving two-point discrimination test, shrivel test, Weber's two-point discrimination test, and electrodiagnosis

---

DIAGNOSTIC STATEMENT

Interdigital probing reveals the presence of a neuroma in continuity in the median nerve at the base of the first phalanx of the left hand.

CLINICAL PEARL

Although neuromas in continuity develop more frequently in the lower extremity and near amputations, they do develop elsewhere. Neuromas in continuity are observed at the bifurcation of nerve branches near the base of digits. This may result from the chronic mechanical irritation caused by malalignment of the digit structures.

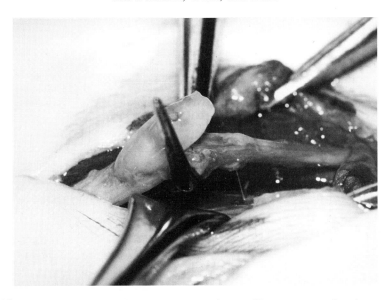

FIG. 6-69 Myxomatous neurofibroma. Intraneural neurofibroma appeared to be carpal tunnel syndrome at presentation. The encapsulated lesion is dissected from the median nerve. *(From Cooney WP, Linscheid RL, Dobyns JH: The wrist diagnosis and operative treatment, vol 1-2, St Louis, 1998, Mosby.)*

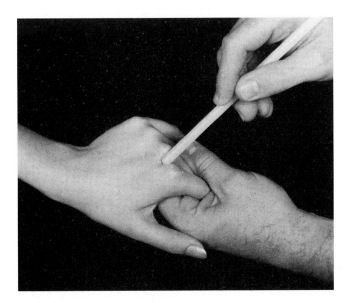

FIG. 6-70 The patient's forearm is pronated. The metacarpophalangeal interdigital tissues are probed with the blunt end of a reflex hammer. If a neuroma is present, severe pain and paresthesia will be elicited. The neuroma may be palpated as a discrete mass.

Assessment for Colles' Fracture

Comment

A fracture through the flared distal metaphysis of the radius, also known as *Colles' fracture,* is a common fracture in adults older than age 50. This type of fracture occurs more often in women than in men and has the same age and sex incidence as fractures of the neck of the femur. Both fractures occur through bone that has become markedly weakened by a combination of senile and postmenopausal osteoporosis.

The incidence of Colles' fracture is particularly high when walking conditions are slippery because the typical mechanism of injury is as follows: the patient either slips or trips, and in an attempt to break the fall, the patient lands on the open hand with the forearm pronated. This pressure breaks the wrist. Therefore the forces that fracture the distal end of the radius involve not only dorsiflexion and radial deviation but also supination, all of which account for the typical fracture deformity.

The fracture pattern is constant, the main fracture line being transverse within the distal 2 cm of the radius. Radiographs in traction following closed reduction are helpful in determining the severity of injury and potential for instability.

ORTHOPEDIC GAMUT 6-10

COLLES' FRACTURE

Poor results from Colles' fracture are caused by the following:

1. Residual dorsal tilt more than 20 degrees (normal, 11 to 12 degrees of volar tilt)
2. Radial inclination more than 10 degrees (normal, 22 to 23 degrees)
3. Articular incongruity more than 2 mm
4. Radial translation more than 2 mm

Unstable injuries are often the result of cortical comminution (dorsal with Colles', volar in Smith's) (Fig. 6-71). Impact forces at the time of injury may compress trabecular bone, especially in older individuals with osteopenia.

There may be only two major fragments, but comminution of the thin cortex is common, especially in the osteoporotic bone of the elderly. The ulnar styloid is often avulsed. The distal end of an intact radius extends beyond

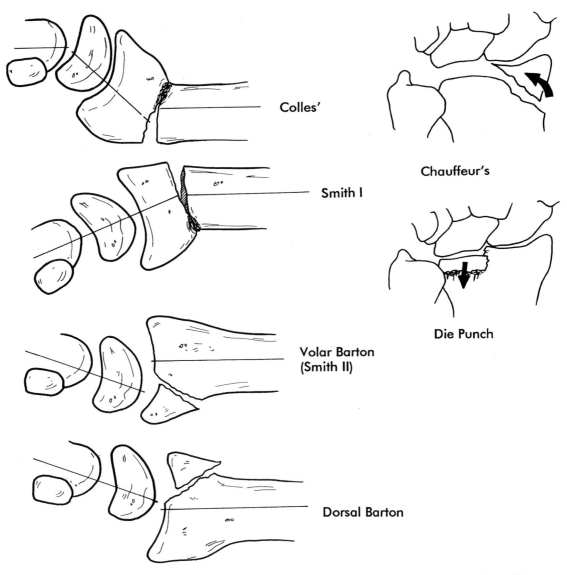

FIG. 6-71 Distal radius fracture classification. *(From Bucholz RW: Orthopaedic decision making, ed 2, St Louis, 1996, Mosby.)*

the distal end of the ulna. The joint surface is angulated 15 degrees toward the anterior (palmar) aspect of the wrist. After a Colles' fracture, these relationships are reversed, and there is always some degree of subluxation of the distal radioulnar joint.

The clinical deformity, often called a *dinner fork* deformity, is typical. In addition to the swelling, there is an obvious jog just proximal to the wrist resulting from the posterior displacement and posterior tilt of the distal radial fragment. The hand is radially deviated, and although it is often less obvious clinically, the wrist appears supinated in relation to the forearm.

Two main types of Colles' fractures can be identified. With the stable type of fracture, there is one main transverse fracture line with little cortical comminution. In the unstable type, there is gross comminution, particularly of the dorsal cortex, and marked crushing of the cancellous bone (Fig. 6-72). The intact periosteal hinge is on the dorsal aspect of the fracture in both types.

Median nerve injury occurring coincident with a Colles' fracture (laceration or contusion) is rare but should be considered when the fracture is compound. Most early-median nerve problems are related to the progressive edema and hematoma that follow injury and to the reduction of the fracture. During the healing phase, exuberant fracture callus, especially in the presence of persistent bony deformity, can result in median nerve symptoms. The residual scarring and thickening that follow healing can eventually result in CTS or tardy median nerve palsy at a much later date.

PROCEDURE

- A positive Maisonneuve's sign is characterized by marked hyperextensibility (dorsiflexion) of the hand (Fig. 6-73).
- The sign is present in Colles' fracture.

Confirmation Procedures
Carpal lift sign, Finsterer's sign, Finkelstein's test, and diagnostic imaging

---

DIAGNOSTIC STATEMENT

Maisonneuve's sign is present in the left wrist. This sign indicates a Colles' fracture of the radius.

CLINICAL PEARL

Maisonneuve's sign remains a finding long after the fracture healing process is completed. A marked hyperextension of the wrist, with or without complaint, warrants imaging.

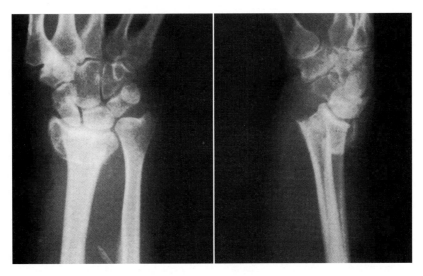

FIG. 6-72   Typical Colles' fracture with dorsal and radial displacement.   *(Modified from Mercier LR, Pettid FJ:* Practical orthopedics, *ed 4, St Louis, 1995, Mosby.)*

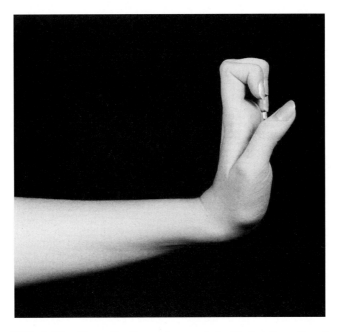

FIG. 6-73   The patient's arm is pronated with the elbow flexed. The hand and wrist are actively dorsiflexed. The sign is present if marked hyperextension of the wrist is apparent. The sign is present in Colles' fracture.

PHALEN'S SIGN

ALSO KNOWN AS PHALEN'S SIGN AND PRAYER SIGN

Assessment for Carpal Tunnel Syndrome (Median Nerve Palsy)

Comment

In the distal forearm, the median and ulnar nerves are surrounded by soft tissues and untethered by bone or dense ligamentous tissues. Distal to the sublimis muscle belly, the median nerve lies just beneath the fascia and is protected only by the palmaris longus tendon. Within the carpal tunnel, the median nerve is in the most volar layer of structures and is easily compressed by the volar carpal ligament. The four unyielding walls of the carpal tunnel fix the volume of the tunnel and guarantee compression of the contained structures if edema or bone fragments occupy part of the available space.

The median nerve may be compressed in the carpal tunnel, producing CTS. Usually, there is pain over the median nerve distribution. As the disease progresses, a definite pattern of hypesthesia or anesthesia will appear over this area. Opposition of the thumb may disappear before there are definite sensory changes in the hand (Fig. 6-74). The large fibers (motor) in the nerves are damaged more than the smaller fibers (sensory) in such types of indirect trauma. Percussion of the median nerve at the flexor crease of the wrist may produce paresthesia along the median nerve. As the disease further progresses, the pain may reach the forearm and even the shoulder. The symptoms may be more prominent at night.

The symptoms are aggravated by temporarily occluding the circulation of the arm above the elbow. A partially injured nerve is more susceptible to ischemia than is a normal one. Therefore paresthesia and numbness will appear first along the median nerve distribution rather than in the ulnar nerve.

Several provocative signs for CTS have been discovered and are extremely useful in diagnosing the condition. The nerve is located just ulnar to the palmaris longus tendon. Tinel's sign demonstrates irritability of a nerve, as evidenced by direct tapping with a reflex hammer or finger directly on the median nerve. If struck vigorously, any peripheral nerve responds by sending electric shock sensations in the distribution of the nerve. In CTS, tapping the median nerve at the wrist causes tingling or paresthesias (or both) in part or all of the distribution in the hand.

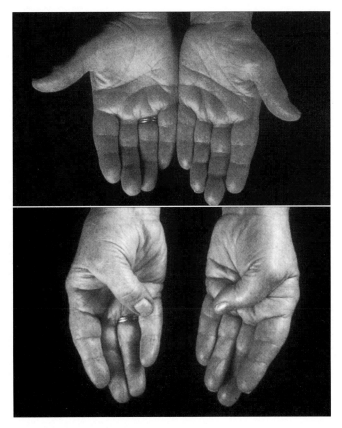

FIG. 6-74 Carpal tunnel syndrome. *(From Epstein O et al: Clinical examination, ed 2, London, 1997, Mosby.)*

Occasionally, an electric shock sensation also is transmitted proximally toward the elbow or shoulder.

Phalen's test (Fig. 6-75, *A*) is performed by asking the patient to maximally palmar flex the wrist for 60 seconds. The test is considered positive if paresthesias occur in the median nerve distribution of the hand. Modifications of this test include placing the hand in maximum dorsiflexion with the fingers extended (reverse Phalen's) (Fig. 6-75, *B*) or holding the fingers flexed (Berger's test), which may crowd the lumbrical muscles into the tunnel of Guyon.

The carpal compression test is preferred as the most accurate provocative sign in CTS. The patient opposes the thumb to the small finger and flexes the wrist (Fig. 6-75, *C*). The examiner's thumb firmly compresses the area between the two tendons, indenting the skin 4 to 5 mm. In CTS, paresthesias in the median nerve distribution occur within 60 seconds. Paresthesias within 15 seconds or less indicate more advanced disease.

PROCEDURE

- The patient's wrists are flexed maximally. The position is held for up to 1 minute as the dorsums are pushed together (Fig. 6-76).
- Tingling sensations that radiate into the thumb, the index finger, and the middle and lateral half of the ring finger are a positive sign.
- A positive sign indicates CTS caused by median nerve compression (Fig. 6-77).

Confirmation Procedures

Tinel's sign at the wrist, wringing test, electrodiagnosis, and diagnostic imaging (MRI)

DIAGNOSTIC STATEMENT

Phalen's sign is present in the right (or left) wrist. This sign indicates CTS and median nerve palsy.

CLINICAL PEARL

Phalen's sign duplicates the wrist flexion/extension maneuvers that irritate the median nerve. The presence of Phalen's sign is a good indicator that wrist splints will be useful in the management of the CTS. As a screening test, a reverse Phalen's maneuver can be performed. The patient is asked to press the hands together in the vertical plane and raise the elbows until they are horizontal. Loss of any dorsiflexion should be obvious. The most common cause of lost dorsiflexion is stiffness after a Colles' fracture.

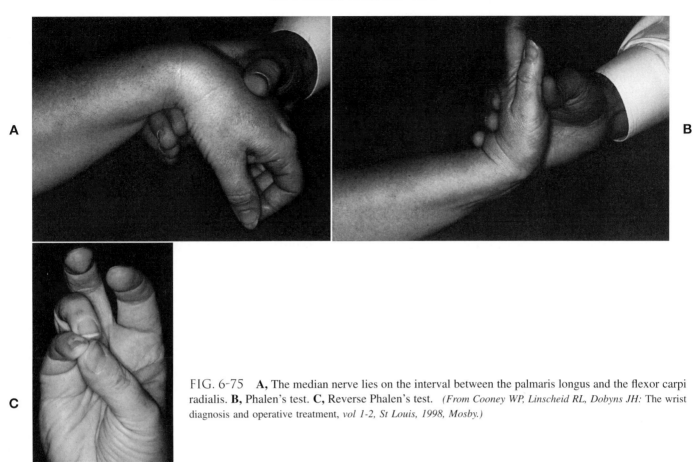

FIG. 6-75 **A,** The median nerve lies on the interval between the palmaris longus and the flexor carpi radialis. **B,** Phalen's test. **C,** Reverse Phalen's test. *(From Cooney WP, Linscheid RL, Dobyns JH: The wrist diagnosis and operative treatment, vol 1-2, St Louis, 1998, Mosby.)*

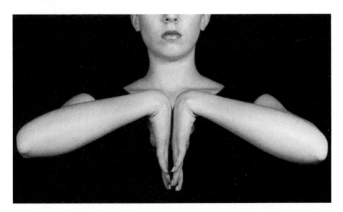

FIG. 6-76 The patient is seated with both elbows flexed and the arms pronated. The wrists are flexed, and the dorsal surfaces of the hands are approximated to each other. The position is maintained for at least 60 seconds. In addition, the elbows can be dropped slightly to increase the wrist flexion angle. Median nerve paresthesia indicates carpal tunnel syndrome. In the flexed wrist position, the syndrome is caused by neural ischemia.

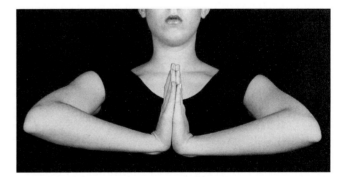

FIG. 6-77 A reversed position for this test is with the patient's wrists extended and the palms of the hands approximated to each other. The patient maintains this position for at least 60 seconds. Median nerve paresthesia indicates carpal tunnel syndrome that is caused by neural stretch and compression by surrounding tissues.

PINCH GRIP TEST

Assessment for Anterior Interosseous Nerve Syndrome

Comment

In anterior interosseous nerve syndrome, the pronator quadratus is nonfunctioning. Pronation is accomplished entirely by the pronator teres, and selective pronation tests are positive in varying degrees. The pronator teres muscle is strongest while the elbow joint is in extension and weaker while the elbow is flexed to 145 degrees. The patient pronates the arm against resistance if the pronator quadratus is nonfunctioning. The patient will have more pronation power while the arm is extended, when the pronator teres is at its maximum advantage, than while the elbow is flexed, when the pronator quadratus contributes its force in pronation (Fig. 6-78).

After supplying the pronator teres, flexor carpi radialis, palmaris longus, and flexor digitorum sublimis muscles, the median nerve divides into two branches. The main trunk continues into the hand, and the anterior interosseous branch supplies the flexor pollicis longus, the flexor digitorum profundus to the index and middle fingers, and the pronator quadratus. Compression of the anterior interosseous branch of the median nerve in the forearm, usually secondary to anomalous muscle and tendon origins, produces the anterior interosseous syndrome. The characteristic physical finding of this compression is paralysis of the muscles that this section of the nerve supplies. The Jamar hydraulic dynamometer provides an accurate and reliable method of measuring grip strength (Fig. 6-79). The adjustable handle allows an accurate evaluation of overall hand strength. Grip strength is altered by the size of the objects being grasped; therefore readings should be taken in all five grip spans. Measuring grip strength requires that the arm be held at the side. The elbow should be flexed at 90 degrees with the wrist held in a neutral position. The patient is instructed to apply a grip force smoothly without rapid wrenching or jerking motions. The examiner should ensure that substitute patterns are not used. Initially, the right and left hand should be tested alternately. The noninvolved extremity may be used for comparison.

During physical examination, there is weakness of grip and a characteristic pinch grip in which the index finger is extended at the DIP joint with hyperflexion of the PIP joint. The MCP joint of the thumb has increased flexion, and the interphalangeal (IP) joint is hyperextended. Thenar muscle function and sensory function in the median nerve distribution are normal.

Various injuries to the hand and wrist can interfere with the worker's ability to perform activities requiring grip.

Grip depends on skeletal mobility, joint integrity, and a combination of contraction and relaxation of the intrinsic and the extrinsic muscle groups.

ORTHOPEDIC GAMUT 6-11

STAGES OF HAND GRASP

Hand grasp consists of three stages:

1. Opening of the hand
2. Closing of the digits to grasp an object
3. Regulating the force of pressure

ORTHOPEDIC GAMUT 6-12

DIVISIONS OF HAND GRASP

Hand grasp is divided into two types:

1. Power
2. Precision

The intrinsic muscles play an important role in required finger motion. Precision grip is required in grasping a smaller object or a ball (Figs. 6-80 to 6-82).

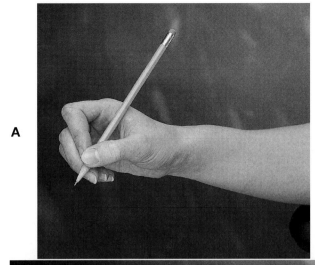

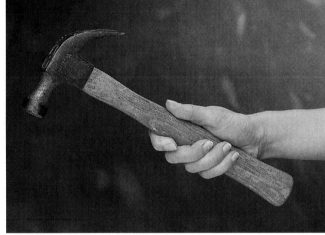

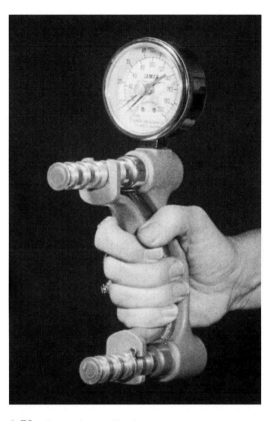

FIG. 6-78 Precision and power grips. **A,** In the precision grip, the wrist and fingers are flexed by the larger muscles and the intrinsic hand muscles make small incremental movements of the fingers. **B,** The power grip involves the long flexor tendons and the palmar muscles, and the object is to create a rigid grip on the object being held. *(From Mathers LH, et al: Clinical anatomy principles, St Louis, 1996, Mosby.)*

FIG. 6-79 Jamar hydraulic dynamometer. *(From Nicholas JA, Hershman EB: The upper extremity in sports medicine, ed 2, St Louis, 1995, Mosby.)*

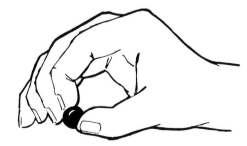

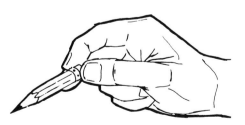

FIG. 6-80 Opposition occurs between the thumb and index finger and is used for picking up small objects. *(From Malick MH: Manual on static hand splinting, Pittsburgh, 1972, Harmarville Rehabilitation Center.)*

FIG. 6-81 Three-point prehension is used to grasp and stabilize large objects most commonly during functional activity. *(From Malick MH: Manual on static hand splinting, Pittsburgh, 1972, Harmarville Rehabilitation Center.)*

PROCEDURE

- The patient pinches the tips of the index finger and thumb together in tip-to-tip pinch (Fig. 6-83).
- If the patient is unable to pinch tip to tip and has a pulp-to-pulp pinch of the index finger and thumb, this is a positive sign for anterior interosseous nerve syndrome (Fig. 6-84).
- This sign may indicate entrapment of the anterior interosseous nerve (Figs. 6-85 and 6-86).

Confirmation Procedures

Froment's paper sign, Wartenberg's sign, and electrodiagnosis

---

DIAGNOSTIC STATEMENT

Pinch-grip testing on the left is positive. This result indicates anterior interosseous nerve syndrome in the forearm.

CLINICAL PEARL

Even minor irritation of the anterior interosseous nerve produces this sign. The inability to pinch grip tip to tip influences the patient's ability to pick up small objects, which is the dysfunction that usually causes the patient to seek professional care.

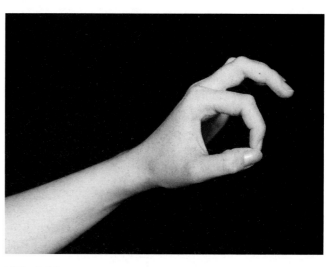

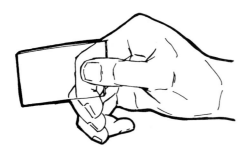

FIG. 6-82   Lateral or key pinch. The most powerful form of pinch. *(From Malick MH: Manual on static hand splinting, Pittsburgh, 1972, Harmarville Rehabilitation Center.)*

FIG. 6-83   The patient pinches the tip of the index finger to the tip of the thumb in tip-to-tip pinch.

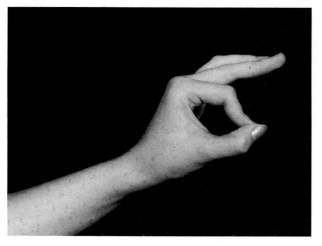

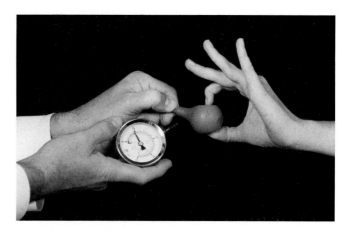

FIG. 6-84   If the grip is tip to pulp or pulp to pulp, the test is positive. A positive test indicates involvement of the anterior interosseous nerve.

FIG. 6-85   The pinch grip also can be determined with pinch dynamometers. Again, the normal grip is tip to tip. The grip strength of each digit is recorded.

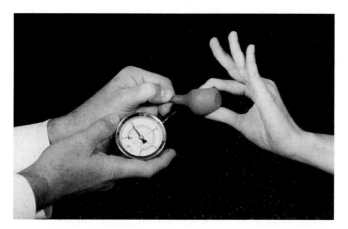

FIG. 6-86   The abnormal grip is tip to pulp or pulp to pulp, both of which produce a corresponding loss of pinch-grip strength.

SHRIVEL TEST

Also Known as O'Riain's Sign

Assessment for Peripheral Nerve Denervation

Comment
O'Riain has recorded a common but unappreciated observation: The skin of denervated fingers does not wrinkle or shrivel as normal skin does when immersed in warm water. This objective test can be performed without the patient's concentration or cooperation and is particularly indicated for use with small children. Shriveling of the skin returns progressively with recovery of nerve function. O'Riain recommends immersion in water at approximately 40° C for 30 minutes. Smooth skin indicates a loss of sensibility. The patient may have already noticed this phenomenon with routine bathing.

PROCEDURE
- The affected fingers are placed in warm (40° C) water for approximately 30 minutes (Fig. 6-87).
- The fingers are removed from the water and skin wrinkling is observed, especially over the finger pulp (Fig. 6-88).

- Normal fingers wrinkle; denervated fingers do not.
- O'Riain's sign is valid only in the first 90 to 120 days after injury, consistent with reactions of degeneration.

Confirmation Procedures
Dellon's moving two-point discrimination test, interphalangeal neuroma test, Weber's two-point discrimination test, and electrodiagnosis

---

DIAGNOSTIC STATEMENT

O'Riain's sign is present on the second and third digits of the right hand. The presence of this sign indicates denervation.

CLINICAL PEARL

Muscle wasting in CTS is a good illustration of the trophic relationship that exists between striated muscle and the nerves that innervate them. When the nerve input to such a muscle is interrupted, the muscle wastes away, loses its strength, and in time, becomes much reduced in size. Even when the nerve-muscle relationship remains intact, if physiologic transmission of impulses is blocked, the muscle similarly wastes away. Smooth muscle is innervated by autonomic nerves, but no such trophic relationship exists in the case of smooth muscle.

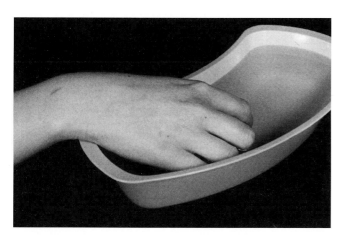

FIG. 6-87   The patient's fingers are immersed in warm (40° C) water for approximately 30 minutes.

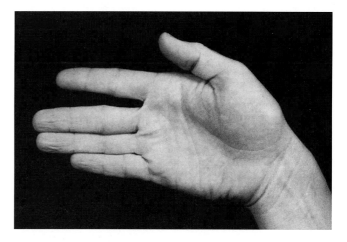

FIG. 6-88   After the patient removes the digits from the water, skin wrinkling is noted. If the skin of the pulp of a finger is not wrinkled, the test is positive. A positive shrivel test indicates denervation of that area. This sign usually is not elicited after 90 to 120 days following injury.

TEST FOR TIGHT RETINACULAR LIGAMENTS

Assessment for Fixation of Phalangeal Retinacular Ligaments

Comment

A study of the structure and function of the dorsal aponeurosis is essential for understanding the forces that are active during flexion and extension of the finger. The dorsal aponeurosis is the main structural basis for the integration and coordination of the extensor and intrinsic muscles.

An important portion of the terminal tendon is the retinacular ligament. This ligament consists of two parts: a transverse layer that is spread over both lateral tendons and a very slender but strong band that merges with the most lateral fibers of the terminal tendon. The first or broad thin ligament passes proximally across the PIP joint. Some of the ligament's fibers reach as far as the flexor tendon sheath over the first phalanx, to which they adhere. The fibers of the second or oblique ligament pass underneath the transverse part of the retinacular ligament and insert into the lateral border of the first phalanx. Therefore the lateral aspect of the PIP joint is crossed by two structures: the lateral tendon and the retinacular ligament. At the level of the PIP joint, the dorsal aponeurosis forms a hood that is drawn over the joint, further reinforcing the joint at its sides.

The position of the lateral tendon and the retinacular ligament is important, especially the oblique part of the ligament in relation to the axis of motion of the PIP joint. In the fully extended joint, the lateral tendon passes dorsally, and the oblique band passes ventrally to the axis. This relation changes as the joint is flexed, until both structures become displaced ventrally. Disruption of the terminal extensor mechanism at the DIP joint produces an extensor lag at that joint. This lesion, the mallet finger, which has also been referred to as a *baseball finger,* is incurred when an object, often a ball, strikes the tip of the extended finger, forcing it suddenly into flexion. This activity tears the extensor mechanism from the base of the distal phalanx. The tendon may be just stretched or attenuated, or it may be torn completely from the bone, resulting in a soft-tissue mallet finger. If the deformity is associated with a fracture in which a fragment of bone comes off from the dorsum of the distal phalanx with the tendon, a mallet fracture is present.

There may be erythema over the dorsum of the joint and some pain with the injury, but there can be remarkably few symptoms. Inability to actively extend the distal phalanx is present to a varying degree. The exact amount of extension loss can be better estimated when the distal phalanx is compared with an adjacent normal finger because many patients normally hyperextend at the DIP joint (Fig. 6-89).

On the dorsal side of the second phalanx, a triangular lamina of connective tissue that joins the two lateral tendons with each other prevents both tendons from sliding off the base of the second phalanx. According to Bunnell, a fascial sheet extending from the lateral band to the collateral ligament and to the base of the second phalanx causes the volar shift of the lateral bands during flexion.

ORTHOPEDIC GAMUT 6-13

PIP DISLOCATIONS

Acute dorsal PIP dislocations are categorized as follows:

I. Hyperextension: joint surfaces in contact
II. Dorsal dislocation: with dorsal dislocation of the middle phalanx on the proximal phalanx (bayonet)
III. Proximal dislocation: fracture of the volar base of the middle phalanx

---

PROCEDURE

- The PIP joint is placed in a neutral position as the DIP joint is flexed passively (Fig. 6-90).
- If the DIP joint does not flex, the ligaments or capsule are tight or contracted.
- If the PIP joint flexes easily, the retinacular ligaments are tight but the capsule is normal.

Confirmation Procedures

Bunnel-Littler test, Cascade sign, clinical laboratory testing, and diagnostic imaging

---

DIAGNOSTIC STATEMENT

The test for tight retinacular ligaments is positive at the DIP joint of the index finger of the right hand. This result indicates fixation of the ligaments.

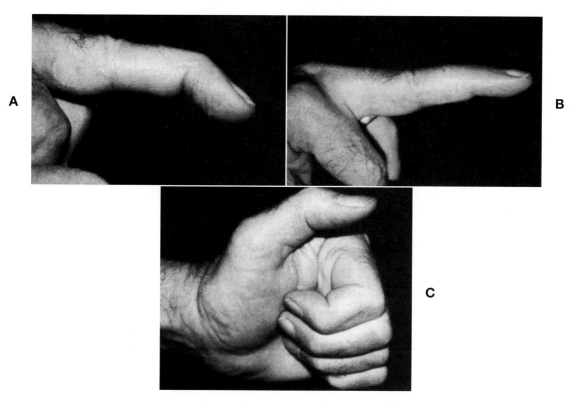

FIG. 6-89   Mallet finger. **A,** Forty-five-degree extensor lag at the distal joint. **B** and **C,** Range of motion achieved at 4 months.   *(From Nicholas JA, Hershman EB:* The upper extremity in sports medicine, *ed 2, St Louis, 1995, Mosby.)*

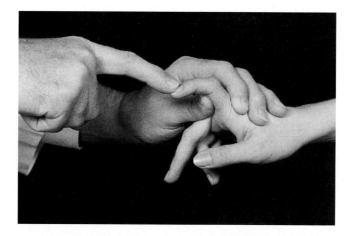

FIG. 6-90   The patient's elbow is flexed, and the forearm is pronated. The examiner fixes the proximal interphalangeal joint in the neutral position. The examiner tries to flex the distal interphalangeal joint. If the joint does not flex, the collateral ligaments and the joint capsule are tight. If the joint flexes freely, the collateral ligaments are tight, and the joint capsule is normal.

TINEL'S SIGN AT THE WRIST

Assessment for Peripheral Neuropathy in Median or Ulnar Nerve Distribution

Comment

Pressure applied to an injured nerve trunk often produces a tingling sensation that is transmitted to the periphery of the nerve and localized to a precise cutaneous region. Pain is a sign of nerve irritation; tingling is a sign of regeneration. More precisely, tingling reveals the presence of regenerating axons.

The point of nerve irritation is present as a localized pain that is felt at the point where pressure is applied. If this pain extends along the nerve trunk, it is most intense at the point of pressure. This type of pain is associated with pain produced by pressure of the muscles, and the muscular pain is most often more pronounced than the pain along the nerve trunk.

Although the tingling of regeneration is not a painful sensation, it is a vaguely disagreeable feeling. The patient may compare the sensation with that of an electric shock. This sensation may be felt at the point of compression but is most commonly felt in the skin along the corresponding nerve distribution. The patient does not experience pain in the muscles adjacent to the nerve where tingling is found.

The two types of sensation, pain and tingling, produced by pressure on the nerve are easily differentiated in all cases. The two sensations rarely exist simultaneously in the same nerve or, more exactly, at the same point during examination of a nerve. The sensations may follow one another along the same nerve trunk. The two different signs produced by pressure applied to the nerve are similar to the symptoms that are revealed by examination of the skin sensation. Regeneration of the nerve is manifested by paresthesia of a more constant type such as that associated with hypoesthesia produced by touch, by puncture, and especially by slight friction of the skin.

However, in all cases, pain indicates irritation of the axons and tingling indicates their regeneration. These are much easier to differentiate than the signs of cutaneous sensibility. The symptoms of neural compression also are more constant and appear much earlier. They furnish more precise, more localized, and more important information.

In total nerve interruption along the course of the nerve trunk, a definite zone can be found where pressure produces tingling in the cutaneous distribution of the nerve. This zone of tingling is not extended. It does not exceed 2 or 3 cm. This zone indicates that, at this precise point, the suddenly interrupted axons have undergone local degeneration.

With complete interruptions of the nerve produced by very tight entrapment, the same characteristics of fixation, prominence, and precise limitation are found, but the zone of tingling is more extended.

It is possible in certain instances to find along the course of the same nerve two different sites of tingling corresponding to two different lesion levels.

Incomplete interruption of a nerve or, more exactly, lesions permitting the passage of regenerating axons are characterized by progressive extension of the tingling. The same progressive extension of the tingling zone is found in incomplete interruption with nerve irritability.

Tingling induced by pressure of the nerve does not appear before the fourth or even the sixth week after trauma. The tingling disappears as soon as the nerve returns to its normal structure and the newly formed axons become mature. After 8 or 10 months, the tingling stops. Tingling may be absent in certain, rare cases.

The first clinical manifestation of regeneration of a nerve is that paresthesia occurs while the nerve is being percussed. As this is done, beginning distally and proceeding proximally, a point will be reached at which the patient feels a tingling or buzzing sensation accompanied by radiation of sensation down to the involved area. The advancing edge of this sensitive area in the nerve is measured at monthly intervals using some bony prominence as a guide. The steady progress of this sensation down the nerve is a rough test of recovery.

A sign of CTS, called the *volar hot dog,* is a firm hot dog–type swelling at the wrist. This sausage-shaped structure (1 cm wide and 2.5 cm long) is located on the ulnar side of the palmaris longus tendon (Fig. 6-91) and extends proximally from the wrist crease.

Although CTS is diagnosed on the basis of the patient's history and clinical examination, imaging and electrodiagnostic studies may be useful in confirming the diagnostic impression.

The most important electrodiagnostic study is the measurement of sensory nerve conduction velocity across the carpal tunnel. A slowed conduction velocity, along with prolongation of distal motor latency, lends support to the diagnosis of CTS.

PROCEDURE

- The carpal tunnel is percussed at the wrist (Fig. 6-92).
- Tingling in the thumb, index finger, forefinger, and the middle and lateral half of the ring finger is a positive finding.
- Tingling and paresthesia must be felt distal to the point of percussion for a positive finding.
- The test can demonstrate the rate of regeneration of the sensory fibers.
- The most distal point of the abnormal sensation represents the distal limit of nerve regeneration.

Confirmation Procedures

Phalen's sign, Wartenberg's sign, electrodiagnosis, and diagnostic imaging (MRI)

DIAGNOSTIC STATEMENT

Tinel's sign is present at the left wrist, producing paresthesia along the median nerve distribution. This suggests media nerve neuropathy.

CLINICAL PEARL

Tinel's sign is extremely useful in identifying (1) the most proximal point of nerve regeneration or (2) the most distal point of nerve degeneration. These points are one and the same. Tinel's is most evidenced at the Valleix points (tender points) along the course of the peripheral nerve (as in a neuralgia/neuritis). The examiner also may slide the tip of the index finger across the palm, noting frictional resistance and temperature. Increased thenar resistance from lack of sweating and temperature rise (vasodilation) may occur with median involvement.

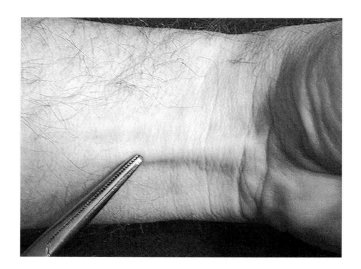

FIG. 6-91 Palmaris longus tendon. The hemostat tip identifies the tissue of the palmaris longus tendon, a major landmark in carpal canal compression syndromes.

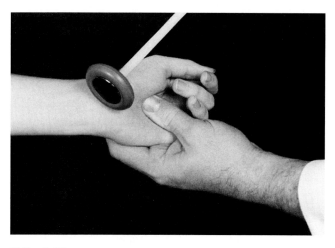

FIG. 6-92 The patient's elbow is flexed and the forearm supinated. The wrist and hand are slightly dorsiflexed by the examiner. The examiner percusses the volar surface of the wrist over the carpal tunnel with a reflex hammer or tuning fork. Tingling that is along the median nerve distribution and distal to the point of percussion indicates regeneration of the nerve. Pain following the same distribution, above and below the point of percussion, indicates neural inflammation and degeneration. Percussion at the tunnel of Guyon reveals the condition of the ulnar nerve as it passes into the hand.

TOURNIQUET TEST

Assessment for Neural Irritability as a Result of Posterior Interosseous or Median Nerve Compression

Comment

Significant diminution of blood flow to individual digits or to an entire hand results in pale nail beds, slow capillary recovery after skin compression, diminished bleeding after skin puncture, lowering of the skin temperature, and pain of varying intensity. Symptoms and signs of pain, pulselessness, pallor, paresthesia, and paralysis indicate arterial insufficiency or inadequate capillary perfusion. The coexistence of pallor with cyanosis and rubor is consistent with vasoconstriction and subsequent vasodilation.

Pallor and a significant drop in skin temperature will cause pain that is moderately severe and described as a deep, dull, aching sensation. As the ischemia state persists, pain becomes more intense.

The term *Raynaud's disease* is used to describe vasospasm without an underlying primary disease. If vasospasm is associated with a known connective-tissue disease, Raynaud's phenomenon is implied. Recognition of Raynaud's syndrome and the patient's response to this condition is important in explaining pain and cold tolerance associated with a known pathologic condition. When the symptoms of pain occur in a digit of the hand or on the entire extremity, the existence of adequate blood flow in the large and small vessels must be determined.

In patients known to have a nerve lesion, such as ulnar nerve compression at the elbow, posterior interosseous nerve compression in the supinator muscle, or median nerve compression at the wrist, diminished blood flow will cause abnormal sensory changes to occur earlier than would happen in the normal patient. Motor weakness occurs more quickly when partial or complete ischemia occurs.

Various conditions, such as atherosclerotic stenosis, thromboembolism, or compression of major arteries in the thoracic outlet, cause pain, claudication, paresthesia, and intermittent episodes of pallor. The lesions may be partial or complete, and the clinical symptoms vary according to the degree of ischemia (Figs. 6-93 and 6-94).

Acute occlusion of the ulnar artery is associated with unrelenting pain, pallor, and later, rubor and cyanosis. Cold tolerance is diminished, and intrinsic muscle weakness occurs.

Obliteration of the brachial artery because of trauma causes the occurrence of an anterior compartment compression of the forearm muscles, vessels, and nerve and causes pallor of the hand, diminished pulse volume, and severe pain. The effect of diminished arterial inflow and lessened venous outflow on pain has been calibrated by analyzing the effects of traumatic lesions at various levels of the extremity. Decompression of a tight compartment anterior to the elbow and in the forearm will diminish pain almost immediately. Elimination of nerve compression syndromes at the wrist and elbow will provide measurable relief of pain.

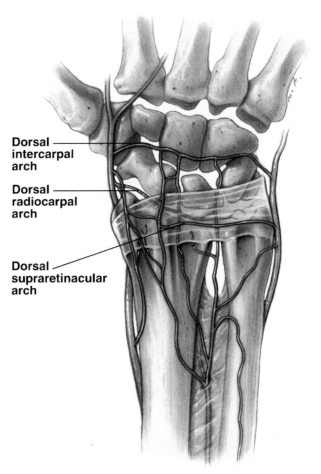

Dorsal intercarpal arch

Dorsal radiocarpal arch

Dorsal supraretinacular arch

FIG. 6-93   Intercarpal arches and anastomoses on the dorsal side of the wrist.   *(From Cooney WP, Linscheid RL, Dobyns JH:* The wrist diagnosis and operative treatment, *vol 1-2, St Louis, 1998, Mosby.)*

Causalgia is a mixed nerve lesion with accompanying or secondary vascular insufficiency. Sympathetic dystrophy is a part of the spectrum that may occur, although no particular nerve injury is demonstrated. Median nerve distributions are commonly present, but the ulnar nerve is rarely involved. There is, however, a vasospastic element that occurs secondary to a major or minor insult of the extremity or an adjacent organ.

PROCEDURE

- Application of a pneumatic tourniquet to a normal extremity with pressure elevated to 20 mm of mercury above the patient's resting diastolic blood pressure will obliterate arterial inflow and venous outflow, slow motor nerve conduction, decrease sensory conduction, and cause severe pain in the hand and forearm, all of which occur at the site of tourniquet compression (Fig. 6-95).
- Anoxia and nerve compression occur simultaneously, and muscle weakness is evident within 3 to 5 minutes.
- Digital paresthesia occurs, and sensation diminishes gradually to anesthesia in about 30 minutes.

- These painful sensations are a combination of muscle and nerve ischemia and nerve compression.
- The appearance of symptoms at less than 300 mm of pressure or sooner than 3 to 5 minutes is a positive test result.
- A positive test indicates neural instability as a result of posterior interosseous nerve or median nerve compression syndromes (Fig. 6-96).

Confirmation Procedures
Allen's test and vascular assessment

DIAGNOSTIC STATEMENT

The tourniquet test is positive in the left forearm. This result indicates neural irritability as a result of posterior interosseous or median nerve compression.

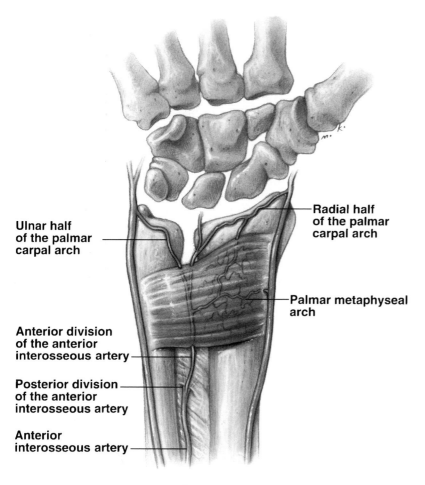

**Ulnar half
of the palmar
carpal arch**

**Radial half
of the palmar
carpal arch**

**Palmar metaphyseal
arch**

**Anterior division
of the anterior
interosseous artery**

**Posterior division
of the anterior
interosseous artery**

**Anterior
interosseous artery**

FIG. 6-94   The palmar extrinsic vascular supply of the wrist. *(From Cooney WP, Linscheid RL, Dobyns JH: The wrist diagnosis and operative treatment, vol 1-2, St Louis, 1998, Mosby.)*

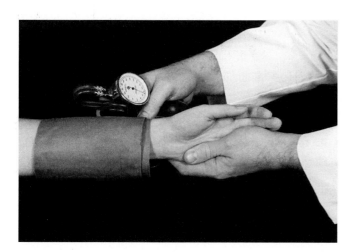

FIG. 6-95   The patient's elbow is flexed, and the arm is supinated and resting on the examination table. A blood pressure cuff is applied to the forearm at a spot above the area of complaint. The cuff is inflated to 20 mm Hg above the patient's resting diastolic blood pressure. Pressure may be increased to reach blanching of the distal extremity. Arm and hand pain, paresthesia, and muscle weakness appearing in less than 5 minutes indicate arterial insufficiency.

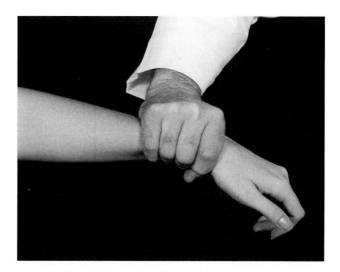

FIG. 6-96   A modified tourniquet test is performed with the examiner occluding the circulation of the extremity manually instead of using a blood pressure cuff. The same principles apply, but this modification does not rely on the accuracy of the pressure to establish occlusion of the arteries.

WARTENBERG'S SIGN

Assessment for Ulnar Palsy

Comment

The ulnar nerve descends from the medial cord of the brachial plexus on the medial side of the arm and pierces the medial intramuscular septum. The nerve continues in a groove behind the medial humeral epicondyle into the forearm. A branch to the flexor carpi ulnaris is given off in the region of the elbow and, distal to this, a branch to the medial half of the flexor digitorum profundus. The nerve trunk enters the forearm posteriorly between the two heads of the flexor carpi ulnaris. The nerve is constricted by a fibrous band between the muscle and the ulna, and it is here that the nerve trunk is vulnerable to compression. The nerve, which lies to the medial side of the ulnar artery in the distal half of the forearm and proximal to the wrist, emerges from under the flexor carpi ulnaris to enter the canal of Guyon, the roof of which is the volar carpal ligament. From here, the nerve passes between the pisiform and hamate bones, and at this point, the nerve divides into a deep motor branch to the ulnar innervated intrinsic muscles and a superficial sensory branch. The latter supplies both the dorsal and volar aspects of the ulnar side of the hand, all of the small fingers, and the ulnar half of the ring finger. The deep motor branch swings across the midpalm, dorsal to the flexor tendons, as it gives off branches to the palmaris brevis and the three hypothenar muscles: the abductor, opponens, and flexor digiti quinti. The nerve then supplies the four dorsal and three volar interossei, the lumbricales of the small and ring fingers, the adductor pollicis, and the deep head of the flexor pollicis brevis. Proximal to the wrist, the palmar and dorsal cutaneous nerves of the hand are given off.

The ulnar nerve is the most commonly injured nerve of the upper extremity. Open wounds, especially at the wrist, are the most common cause of injury, but compression or irritation of the nerve at either the wrist or the elbow can occur. The major functional loss in low median nerve palsy is a sensory loss. Loss of ulnar nerve function, as with radial nerve function, is a motor loss. Anesthesia in the ulnar distribution of the hand, at its worst, is an inconvenience, but loss of all the interossei and the adductor pollicis interferes seriously with the strength and effectiveness of the patient's grasp.

Ulnar clawhand (main en griffe) is primarily caused by loss of the interossei, the major function of which is to flex the MCP joints. With the loss of the interossei, the action of the extrinsic finger extensors is unopposed, and a hyperextension deformity of the MCP joints begins. As the volar capsule of these joints stretches, the deformity, which may be barely present in the recently injured extremity, progresses. Lumbricales one and two are most commonly median innervated. Therefore the index and middle fingers usually do not develop the deformity. The interossei and lumbricales also act as IP joint extensors, and with their paralysis, these joints are held in flexion by the now-unopposed flexor digitorum profundi and flexor digitorum sublimis. These flexors are overactive in their attempt to compensate for the lack of the interossei as MCP flexors. Thus a vicious cycle is started. The more the patient attempts to correct the deformity actively, the more exaggerated it will become. The degree of clawing is usually less apparent in the high ulnar palsy than when the ulnar half of the flexor digitorum profundus is spared.

Workers involved in activities that require repetitive forearm rotation along with ulnar deviation of the wrist can develop a branch of the radial nerve that was originally described in nonathletes by Wartenberg. This condition is also seen in workers who wear equipment that encompasses the wrist. Anatomically, the radial sensory nerve is located in a subcutaneous position between the extensor carpi radialis longus and the brachioradialis at the junction of the mid and distal thirds of the forearm. The fascia at this point of transition sends fibers from the musculotendinous area of the brachioradialis to the extensor carpi radialis longus. These fibers create a relatively unyielding bridge under the nerve, which is the most common location of entrapment.

The patient experiences pain and numbness over the dorsoradial aspect of the hand and thumb. Pertinent physical findings include Tinel's sign over the nerve and exacerbation of symptoms with wrist flexion and ulnar deviation. Most obvious in the ulnar clawhand is the apparent deformity of clawing, which is a loss of the transverse arch of the hand, and visible atrophy of the interossei, particularly the first dorsal interosseous muscle mass (Fig. 6-97). Hypothenar atrophy also occurs. The next most apparent condition is the clumsy grip and the marked weakness of grasp. Normal grip strength in the adult male is approximately 90 pounds and is 53 pounds for females. In the ulnar-palsied hand, the grip strength will be only one fourth to one third of that. It is this weakness that is most responsible for gross dysfunction of the hand, such as the loss of the ability to grasp a shovel or a suitcase handle.

More disabling for fine sophisticated use of the hand is the interference with normal pinch or prehension. The average strength of pinch in the adult male is 20 to 25 pounds, but with ulnar palsy, the strength is only 10% to 20% of that. This loss in strength is due to paralysis of the adductor pollicis, half of the flexor pollicis brevis, and the first dorsal interosseous muscles. The paralysis of these muscles leads not only to weakness but also to gross deformity of pinch, manifested by hyperextension of the thumb MCP joint and hyperflexion of the thumb IP joint. A good test of adductor pollicis and first dorsal interosseous function is to observe the position of the fingers for pinch and test the muscle strength of each digit. Palpation of the first dorsal interosseous muscle on the radial side of the second metacarpal and the adductor pollicis is deep in the thumb web. This can be done while the patient attempts maximum strength of pinch.

The ulnar pinch deformity represents a reversal of the normal longitudinal arch of the first metacarpal and thumb, the integrity of which depends on the presence of the adductor pollicis and normal MCP flexion. Many variations of classic ulnar-palsied pinch are possible and are caused by variations in median and ulnar innervation of the intrinsics, whether the patient has loose or tight joints.

Ulnar palsy is usually caused by trauma of the ulnar nerve as it passes behind the medial humeral epicondyle. The most common causes are old fractures of the elbow and arthritis. Paresthesia or hypesthesia develop in the ulnar nerve distribution with increasing weakness of the intrinsic muscles. Percussion of the nerve in the epicondylar groove will produce paresthesia along its course.

PROCEDURE

- The patient performs a hard grasp strength test with a dynamometer.
- The examiner observes the position and function of the digits in the action.
- If the position of abduction is assumed by the little finger, the sign is present (Fig. 6-98).
- The sign is present in ulnar palsy.

Confirmation Procedures

Froment's paper sign, pinch grip test, and electrodiagnosis

DIAGNOSTIC STATEMENT

Wartenberg's sign is present in the left hand. The presence of this sign suggests ulnar palsy.

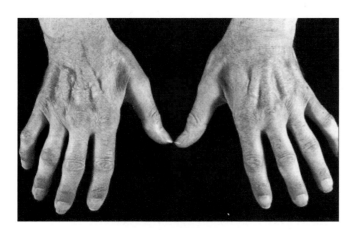

FIG. 6-97   Bilateral ulnar nerve lesions.   *(From Epstein O, et al: Clinical examination, ed 2, London, 1997, Mosby.)*

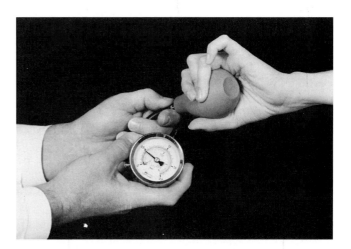

FIG. 6-98   The patient grasps a dynamometer for grip-strength testing. The sign is present if the fifth digit remains abducted and does not contribute to the grip strength. The presence of the sign indicates ulnar nerve paralysis.

WEBER'S TWO-POINT DISCRIMINATION TEST

Assessment for Diminished Peripheral Nerve Sensibility

Comment

The human nervous system is bombarded simultaneously by a multitude of stimuli. The afferent input is limited by the inconstant threshold of the peripheral nerve endings and the specialized receptor organs associated with them. Sensation is the acceptance and activation of impulses in the afferent nerve fibers of the nervous system.

The brain receives and elaborates a continuously changing flood of sensations. Varied sensations are synthesized into three-dimensional experiences. Central neural mechanisms, such as memory storage and introspection, influence the conscious perception of the external and internal environment. Sensibility is the conscious appreciation and interpretation of the stimulus that produced sensation.

Tactile discrimination requires interpretation by the cerebral cortex.

ORTHOPEDIC GAMUT 6-14

TACTILE DISCRIMINATION

Four types of tactile discrimination are the following:

1. Stereognosis
2. Graphesthesia
3. Extinction
4. Two-point discrimination

Stereognosis is the ability to recognize objects by touching and manipulating them. Stereognosis should be tested with universally familiar objects, such as a key, safety pin, or coin (Fig. 6-99).

In graphesthesia, the patient identifies letters or numbers written on the palm with a blunt point. The patient who does not have graphesthesia can correctly identify the letters or numbers inscribed (Fig. 6-100).

To test for extinction, the examiner should touch the same areas on both sides of the body simultaneously. Failure of the patient to perceive touch on one side is called the *extinction phenomenon*. Normally, sensation is perceived on both sides.

Position sense (kinesthetic sensation) is facilitated by proprioceptive receptors in the muscles, tendons, and joints. Perception of the position, orientation, and motion of limbs and body parts is obtained from kinesthetic sensations.

A sensory unit is a single first-order afferent neuron, including all peripheral and central branches.

ORTHOPEDIC GAMUT 6-15

QUALITIES OF SENSIBILITY

Five elementary qualities of sensibility can be evoked by stimulation via the following:

1. Touch-pressure
2. Warmth
3. Coldness
4. Pain
5. Movement and position

ORTHOPEDIC GAMUT 6-16

NEURAL SENSORY UNIT

The following factors influence the neural sensory unit:

1. The diameter of the first-order afferent neuron
2. The properties of the sensory receptors
3. The size and population of the receptive field
4. The threshold for the entire sensory unit

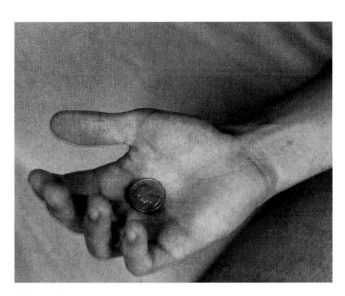

FIG. 6-99   Testing for stereognosis.   *(From Barkauskas VH et al:* Health & physical assessment, *ed 2, St Louis, 1998, Mosby.)*

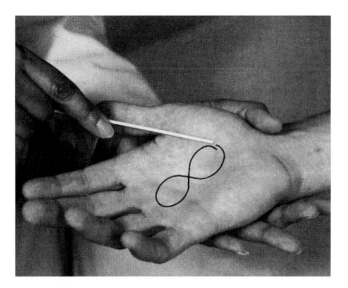

FIG. 6-100   Testing for graphesthesia.   *(From Barkauskas VH, et al:* Health & physical assessment, *ed. 2, St Louis, 1998, Mosby.)*

- The test should be demonstrated while the patient is watching the procedure. The patient then closes the eyes.
- Several areas on the uninvolved hand should be checked because some patients have congenitally abnormal two-point discrimination.
- The testing instrument can be a Boley gauge, a blunt-eye caliper, or an ordinary paper clip. Testing is begun distally and proceeds proximally (Fig. 6-101).
- The points of the caliper are set at 10 mm and are brought together progressively as accurate responses are obtained (Fig. 6-102).
- The pressure from the testing instrument should not produce an ischemic area on the skin.
- When two points are applied, they make contact simultaneously.
- The patient indicates immediately if one or two points are felt.
- An interval of 3 to 5 seconds should be allowed between application of the points.
- A series of one or two points is applied with varied sequence in each finger zone.
- The procedure is done three times; if the patient does not record two of the three correctly, the result is considered a failure at that test distance.
- If the patient correctly identifies the number of points applied, the testing distance is decreased in varying increments.

- There are 10 applications of two points and 10 applications of one point at random.
- The total incorrect one-point applications are subtracted from the total of correct two-point applications.
- A score of 5 or more is considered passing.

Abnormal skin texture, such as heavy scales or calluses, has a marked influence on the test results. Testing can be done in the presence of edema or infection, but the results demonstrate the sensibilities present, which may not reflect the true status of the nerve.

Confirmation Procedures
Dellon's moving two-point discrimination test, interphalangeal neuroma test, shrivel test, and electrodiagnosis

---

DIAGNOSTIC STATEMENT

Weber's two-point discrimination testing demonstrates diminished sensibility (13 to 20 mm) at the dorsal surface of the base of the thumb. This result suggests nerve receptor or impulse transmission deficits.

CLINICAL PEARL

As with Dellon's moving two-point discrimination test, bizarre responses are reason for suspicion as to the origin of the symptoms. Janet's test can help identify psychogenic anesthesia.

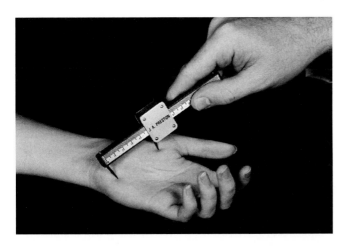

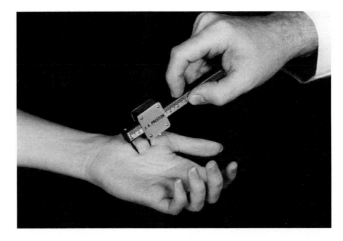

FIG. 6-101   The patient is seated with the elbow flexed. The arm is supinated and resting on the examination table. The hand is relaxed. The Boley gauge is set for 10 mm or more distance. The contact points are made randomly, beginning at the distal portions of the hand. The contacts must touch simultaneously and with equal pressure. The patient's eyes are closed.

FIG. 6-102   As the testing progresses, the gauge contacts are reset closer together in 5-mm increments. If the patient cannot detect the points in two out of three attempts, the test is positive. A positive test indicates diminished sensibility for the area tested, according to established norms.

WRINGING TEST

Assessment for Elbow, Wrist, or Hand Derangement

Comment

The median nerve enters the hand through the carpal tunnel, a bony trough covered with a stout fibrous roof called the *flexor retinaculum,* which it shares with nine tendons, each covered with two layers of synovium. The carpal tunnel is a defined space with rigid and semirigid circumferential boundaries. The tube of space making up the carpal tunnel provides a channel for passage of all the flexor tendons of the thumb and digits from the forearm to the hand. The median nerve also passes through this space, completing the contents of the carpal canal. In addition to providing a protected passageway for these vital structures into the hand, the transverse carpal ligament functions as a pulley to increase the power of the flexor tendons. The underlying bones form the floor of the carpal canal and are somewhat more distal (Fig. 6-103).

There is no room for the tissues to expand, and any swelling of the tendons or the synovium around them compresses the median nerve.

The most common overall cause of CTS is fluid retention, of which the most common cause is pregnancy. However, overuse of the tendons from repeated forceful movements of the wrist, either at work or recreation, is probably the most common cause of CTS referred to orthopedic and neurosurgical clinics. Any condition that causes synovial thickening, including rheumatoid arthritis and Colles' fracture, can also be responsible.

Median nerve compression causes paresthesia in the median nerve distribution, which is the front of the thumb, index finger, middle finger, and the radial half of the ring finger. The palm is not involved because the palmar branch of the median nerve arises above the wrist.

The symptoms are worse at night, and the patient will wake and fling the hand up and down to try and relieve the symptoms. In time, the paresthesia is replaced by pain, which can be felt as far up as the elbow, and eventually by numbness in the median distribution.

Most patients notice the little finger is not affected, and those who report that all the fingers are involved should be treated with suspicion.

The differential diagnosis includes peripheral neuropathy, mononeuritis, cervical spondylosis, and tumors of the thoracic outlet that involve the brachial plexus, but these are often forgotten because CTS is such a common condition. If there is any doubt, the diagnosis can be confirmed by nerve conduction studies.

PROCEDURE

- The patient, using both hands, wrings a towel (Fig. 6-104).
- Paresthesia in the hand indicates CTS.
- Pain elicited at the elbow indicates epicondylitis.
- Wrist discomfort indicates arthropathy or carpal derangement.

Confirmation Procedures

Phalen's sign, electrodiagnosis, diagnostic imaging, and further testing based on the area of localized complaint

---

DIAGNOSTIC STATEMENT

Wringing test is positive for the right (or left) wrist and hand and elicits paresthesia of the right (or left) hand. This result indicates CTS.

CLINICAL PEARL

The wringing test is useful to determine the area for primary investigation. The patient also may be asked to hold both wrists in a fully flexed position for 1 to 2 minutes. The appearance or exacerbation of paresthesia suggests CTS. This test is the most sensitive clinical test for CTS. Advanced CTS can produce thenar atrophy and distal phalangeal acroasphyxia. The wringing test is particularly useful in eliciting responses in more subtle afflictions of the median nerve.

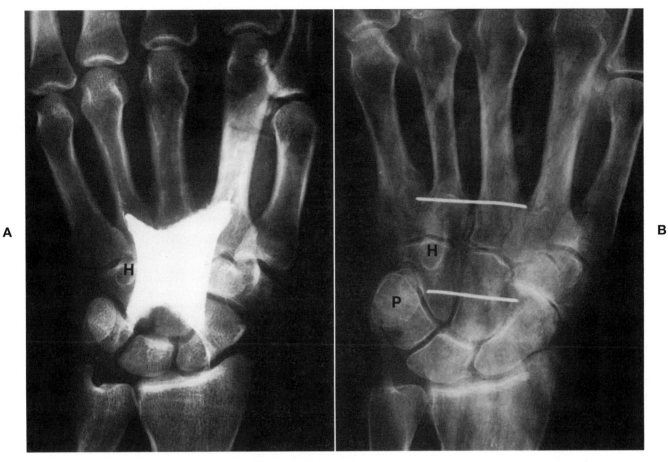

FIG. 6-103 **A,** Radiographic contrast material outlining the borders of the carpal tunnel. **B,** Lines representing border of carpal tunnel superimposed on radiograph. *(From Cooney WP, Linscheid RL, Dobyns JH: The wrist diagnosis and operative treatment, vol 1-2, St Louis, 1998, Mosby.)*

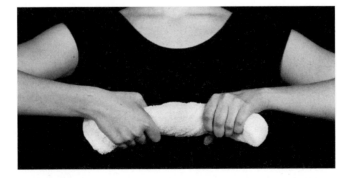

FIG. 6-104 The patient, using both hands, wrings a towel. Maximum effort is applied. The test will localize the discomfort to the primary site of origin. If the test elicits pain at the elbow, epicondylitis is suspected. If the discomfort is felt at the wrist, arthropathy or carpal derangement is suspected. Paresthesia in the hand suggests carpal tunnel syndrome.

BIBLIOGRAPHY

Abrams WB, Berkow R: *The Merck manual of geriatrics,* Rahway, 1990, Merck Sharp & Dohme Research Laboratories.

Adams JC, Hamblen DL: *Outline of orthopaedics,* ed 11, Edinburgh, 1990, Churchill Livingstone.

Agee JM, et al: Endoscopic release of the carpal tunnel: a randomized prospective multicenter study, *J Hand Surg* 17A:987, 1992.

Alario AJ: *Practical guide to the care of the pediatric patient,* St Louis, 1997, Mosby.

Amadio PC: The Mayo Clinic and carpal tunnel syndrome, *Mayo Clin Proc* 67:42, 1992.

American Board of Chiropractic Orthopedists: *Proceedings 1997,* New Orleans, 1997, American Board of Chiropractic Orthopedists.

American Medical Association: *Guides to the evaluation of permanent impairment,* ed 4, Chicago, 1993, The Association.

American Medical Association: *How to use guides to the evaluation of permanent impairment,* ed 4, Falmouth, Conn, 1993, SEAK.

American Society for Surgery of the Hand: *The hand examination and diagnosis,* Aurora, Colo, 1978.

Anderson B, Kayes S. Treatment of flexor tenosynovitis of the hand trigger finger with corticosteroids: a prospective study of the response to local injection, *Arch Intern Med* 151:153, 1991.

Apley AG, Solomon L: *Concise system of orthopaedics and fractures,* London, 1988, Butterworth-Heinemann.

Aulicino P: Neurovascular injuries in the hands of athletes, *Hand Clin* 6:455, 1990.

Baird KS, Crossan JF, Ralston SH: Abnormal growth factor and cytokine expression in Dupuytren's contracture, *J Clin Pathol* 46:425, 1993.

Baird KS, et al: T-cell-mediated response in Dupuytren's disease, *Lancet* 341:1622, 1993.

Ballinger PW: *Merrill's atlas of radiographic positions and radiologic procedures,* vol 1-3, ed 8, St Louis, 1995, Mosby.

Barkauskas VH, et al: *Health & physical assessment,* ed 2, St Louis, 1998, Mosby.

Beckenbaugh RD, et al: Kienbock's disease: the natural history of Kienbock's disease and consideration of lunate fractures, *Clin Orthop* 149:98, 1980.

Bell JA: Sensibility evaluation. In Hunter JM, et al, editors: *Rehabilitation of the hand,* St Louis, 1978, Mosby.

Belsole RJ, et al: Computed analyses of the pathomechanics of scaphoid waist nonunions, *J Hand Surg* 16A:899, 1991.

Berger RA: Endoscopic carpal tunnel release, a current perspective, *Hand Clin* 10:625, 1994.

Birchard D, Pichora D: Experimental corrective scaphoid osteotomy for scaphoid malunion with abnormal wrist mechanics, *J Hand Surg* 15A:863, 1990.

Bourne G: *The structure and function of nervous tissue,* New York, 1968, Academic Press.

Braithwaite IJ, Jones WA: Scapho-lunate dissociation occurring with scaphoid fracture, *J Hand Surg* 17B:286, 1992.

Brashear HR Jr, Raney RB: *Shands' handbook of orthopaedic surgery,* St Louis, 1978, Mosby.

Brondum V, Larsen CF, Skov O: Fracture of carpal scaphoid: frequency and distribution in a well-defined population, *Eur J Radiol* 15:118, 1992.

Brooks M, Evans R, Fairclough J: *Sports injuries,* ed 2, London, 1992, Gower Medical.

Brotzman SB: *Clinical orthopaedic rehabilitation,* St Louis, 1996, Mosby.

Brown DE, Neumann RD: *Orthopedic secrets,* Philadelphia, 1995, Hanley & Belfus.

Brown M: The well elderly. In Guccione A, editor: *Geriatric physical therapy,* St Louis, 1993, Mosby.

Brown MG, Keyser B, Roghtnberg ES: Endoscopic carpal tunnel release, *J Hand Surg* 17A:1009, 1992.

Brown RA, et al: Carpal tunnel release: a prospective, randomized assessment of open and endoscopic methods, *J Bone Joint Surg* 75A:1265, 1993.

Buchler U: *Wrist instability,* St Louis, 1996, Mosby.

Bucholz RW: *Orthopaedic decision making,* ed 2, St Louis, 1996, Mosby.

Bunnell S: Surgery of the rheumatic hand, *J Bone Joint Surg* 27:759, 1955.

Burton RI: Extensor tendons-late reconstruction. In Green DP, editor: *Operative hand surgery,* ed 3, New York, 1993, Churchill Livingstone.

Cahalan T, et al: Biomechanics of the golf swing in players with pathologic conditions of the forearm, wrist, and hand, *Am J Sports Med* 19:288, 1991.

Cailliet R: *Hand pain and impairment,* ed 2, Philadelphia, 1975, FA Davis.

Cambridge CA: Range of motion measurements of the hand. In Hunter JM, et al, editors: *Rehabilitation of the hand,* ed 3, St Louis, 1990, Mosby.

Canale ST: *Campbell's operative orthopaedics,* vol 1-4, ed 9, St Louis, 1998, Mosby.

Canoso JJ: Bursitis, tenosynovitis, ganglions, and painful lesions of the wrist, elbow and hand, *Curr Opin Rheumatol* 2:276, 1990.

Christiansen TG, et al: Diagnostic value of ultrasound in scaphoid fractures, *Injury* 22:397, 1991.

Chusid JG, McDonald JJ: *Correlative neuroanatomy and functional neurology,* Los Altos, Calif, 1962, Lange Medical.

Cipriano JJ: *Photographic manual of regional orthopaedic and neurological test,* ed 3, Baltimore, 1997, Williams & Wilkins.

Cobb TK, et al: Anatomy of the flexor retinaculum, *J Hand Surg* 18A:91, 1993.

Cohn RE: *Impairment rating examination and disability evaluation,* ed 3, Wilkesboro, NC, 1994, R Ernest Cohn.

Collo MC, et al: Evaluating arthritic complaints, *Nurse Pract* 15:9, 1991.

Compson JP, Waterman JK, Spencer JD: Dorsal avulsion fractures of the scaphoid: diagnostic implications and applied anatomy, *J Hand Surg* 18B:58, 1993.

Cooney WP III, Dobyns JH, Linscheid RL: Complications of Colles' fracture, *J Bone Joint Surg* 62A:613, 1980.

Cooney WP III, Linscheid RL, Dobyns JH: External pin fixation for unstable Colles' fracture, *J Bone Joint Surg* 61A:840, 1979.

Cooney WP III, Linscheid RL, Dobyns JH: *The wrist diagnosis and operative treatment,* vol 1-2, St Louis, 1998, Mosby.

Copeland SA, et al: *Joint stiffness of the upper limb,* St Louis, 1997, Mosby.

Dambro MR, Griffith JA: *Griffith's 5 minute clinical consult,* Baltimore, 1997, Williams & Wilkins.

D'Ambrogio KJ, Roth GB: *Positional release therapy assessment & treatment of musculoskeletal dysfunction,* St Louis, 1997, Mosby.

D'Ambrosia RD: *Musculoskeletal disorders regional examination and differential diagnosis,* Philadelphia, 1977, JB Lippincott.

Dandy DJ: *Essential orthopaedics and trauma,* Edinburgh, 1989, Churchill Livingstone.

Dellon AL, Curtis RM, Edgerton MT: Evaluating recovery of sensation in the hand following nerve injury, *Johns Hopkins Med J* 130:235, 1972.

Dellon AL, Curtis RM, Edgerton MT: Reeducation of sensation in the hand after nerve injury and repair, *Plast Reconstr Surg* 53:297, 1974.

Deltoff MN, Kogon PL: *The portable skeletal x-ray library,* St Louis, 1998, Mosby.

Demeter SL, Anderson GBJ, Smith GM: *Disability evaluation,* St Louis, 1996, Mosby.

Deshpande JK, Tobias JD: *The pediatric pain handbook,* St Louis, 1996, Mosby.

Dettenmeier PA: *Radiographic assessment for nurses,* St Louis, 1995, Mosby.

Dias JJ, et al: Suspected scaphoid fractures, the value of radiographs, *J Bone Joint Surg* 72B:98, 1990.

Dilley DF, Tonkin MA: Acute calcific tendinitis in the hand and wrist, *J Hand Surg* 16B:215, 1991.

Doherty M: *Color atlas and text of osteoarthritis,* London, 1994, Wolfe.

Doherty M, Doherty J: *Clinical examination in rheumatology,* London, 1992, Wolfe.

Doherty M, George E: *Self-assessment picture tests in rheumatology,* London, 1995, Mosby-Wolfe.

Doyle JR: Extensor tendons-acute injuries. In Green DP, editor: *Operative hand surgery,* ed 3, New York, 1993, Churchill Livingstone.

Dray GJ, Eaton RG: Dislocation and ligament injuries in the digits. In Green DP, editor: *Operative hand surgery,* ed 3, New York, 1993, Churchill-Livingstone.

Duchenne GB: *Physiology of motion* (translated by Emanuel B. Kaplan), Philadelphia, 1975, WB Saunders.

Elster AD: *Questions and answers in magnetic resonance imaging,* St Louis, 1994, Mosby.

Epstein O, et al: *Clinical examination,* ed 2, London, 1997, Mosby.

Evangelisti S, Realve VF: Fibroma of tendon sheath as a cause of carpal tunnel syndrome, *J Hand Surg* 17A:1026, 1992.

Feldmann E: *Current diagnosis in neurology,* St Louis, 1994, Mosby.

Ferezy JS: *The chiropractic neurological examination,* Gaithersburg, Md, 1992, Aspen.

Finkelstein H: Stenosing tendovaginitis at the radial styloid process, *J Bone Joint Surg* 12:509, 1930.

Finneson BE: *Diagnosis and management of pain syndromes,* Philadelphia, 1969, WB Saunders.

Flatt AE: *The care of minor hand injuries,* St Louis, 1972, Mosby.

Frykman G: Fracture of the distal radius including sequelae-shoulder-hand-finger syndrome, disturbance in the distal radioulnar joint and impairment of nerve function: a clinical and experimental study, *Acta Orthop Scand Suppl* 108:1, 1967.

Frykman GK: *The orthopedic clinics of North America,* vol 12(2), Philadelphia, April 1981 and April 1984, WB Saunders.

Gabel G, Bishop AT, Wood MB: Flexor carpi radialis tendinitis. part II: results of operative treatment, *J Bone Joint Surg* 76A:1015, 1994.

Garcia JH: *Neuropathology the diagnostic approach,* St Louis, 1997, Mosby.

Gelberman RH, et al: The vascularity of the lunate bone and Kienbock's disease, *J Hand Surg* 5A:272, 1980.

Goldie BS: *Orthopaedic diagnosis and management: a guide to the care of orthopaedic patients,* ed 2, Oxford, 1998, ISIS Medical Media.

Goldner JL: Volkmann's ischemic contracture. In Flynn JE, editor: *Hand surgery,* ed 2, Baltimore, 1975, Williams & Wilkins.

Goldner JL, et al: Metacarpophalangeal joint arthroplasty with silicone-Dacron prosthesis, Niebauer type, six and a half years experience, *J Bone Joint Surg* 2:200, 1977.

Gordon M: *Nursing diagnosis: process and application,* ed 3, St Louis, 1994, Mosby.

Green DP: Carpal dislocations and instabilities. In Green DP, editor: *Operative hand surgery,* ed 3, New York, 1993, Churchill-Livingstone.

Greenstein GM: *Clinical assessment of neuromusculoskeletal disorders,* St Louis, 1997, Mosby.

Grossman ZD, et al: *Cost-effective diagnostic imaging the clinicians guide,* ed 3, St Louis, 1995, Mosby.

Guimberteau JC, Panconi B: Recalcitrant non-union of the scaphoid treated with a vascularized bone graft based on the ulnar artery, *J Bone Joint Surg* 72A:88, 1990.

Hammer WI: *Functional soft tissue examination and treatment by manual methods: the extremities,* Gaithersburg, Md, 1991, Aspen.

Hartley A: *Practical joint assessment upper quadrant,* ed 2, St Louis, 1995, Mosby.

Harvey FJ, Harvey PM, Horsely MW: De Quervain's disease: surgical or nonsurgical treatment, *J Hand Surg* 15A:83, 1990.

Hawkins RJ: *An organized approach to musculoskeletal examination and history taking,* St Louis, 1995, Mosby.

Hinkle CZ: *Fundamentals of anatomy & movement a workbook and guide,* St Louis, 1997, Mosby.

Hoppenfeld S: *Physical examination of the spine and extremities,* New York, 1976, Appleton-Century-Crofts.

Hornberger JP: *Exercise physiology therapeutic exercise,* Sarasota, Fla, 1991, Joseph P Hornberger.

Hunter JM: Recurrent carpal tunnel syndrome, epineural fibrous fixation, and traction neuropathy, *Hand Clin* 7:491, 1991.

Imaeda T, et al: Magnetic resonance imaging in scaphoid fractures, *J Hand Surg* 17B:20, 1992.

Johnson MK: *The hand book,* Springfield, Ill, 1973, Charles C Thomas.

Jonsson K: Nonunion of a fractured scaphoid tubercle, *J Hand Surg* 15A:283, 1990.

Jupiter JB: Current concepts review: fractures of the distal end of the radius, *J Bone Joint Surg* 73A:461, 1991.

Kanner R: *Pain management secrets,* Philadelphia, 1997, Hanley & Belfus.

Kasdan ML: *Occupational hand & upper extremity injuries & diseases,* ed 2, Philadelphia, 1998, Hanley & Belfus.

Katirji B: *Electromyography in clinical practice: a case study approach,* St Louis, 1998, Mosby.

Katz WA: *Rheumatic diseases diagnosis and management,* Philadelphia, 1977, JB Lippincott.

Keats TE: *Atlas of roentgenographic measurement,* ed 6, St Louis, 1990, Mosby.

Kendall HO, Kendall FP, Wadsworth GE: *Muscle testing and function,* ed 2, Baltimore, 1971, Williams & Wilkins.

Kerluke L, McCabe SJ: Nonunion of the scaphoid: a critical analysis of recent natural history studies, *J Hand Surg* 18A:1, 1993.

Kerr CD, Sybert DR, Albarracin NS: An analysis of flexor synovium in idiopathic carpal tunnel syndrome: report of 625 cases, *J Hand Surg* 17A:1028, 1992.

Kiebhaber TR, Stern P: Upper extremity tendinitis and overuse syndrome in the athlete, *Clin Sports Med* 11:39, 1992.

Klippel JH, Dieppe PA: *Rheumatology,* vol 1-2, ed 2, London, 1998, Mosby.

Kloth LC, McCulloch JM, Feedar JA: *Wound healing: alternatives in management,* Philadelphia, 1990, FA Davis.

Koenigsberg R: *Churchill's illustrated medical dictionary,* New York, 1989, Churchill Livingstone.

Kraemer BA, Young BL, Arfken S: Stenosing flexor tenosynovitis, *South Med J* 83:806, 1990.

Landsmeer JMF: *Atlas of anatomy of the hand,* Edinburgh, 1976, Churchill Livingstone.

Larsen CF, Brondum V, Skov O: Epidemiology of scaphoid fractures in Odense, Denmark, *Acta Orthop Scand* 63:216, 1992.

Lavy CBD, Barrett DS: *Questions and answers on Apley's concise system of orthopaedics and fractures,* Oxford, 1991, Butterworth-Heinemann.

Lee MLH: The intraosseous arterial pattern of the carpal lunate bone and its relation to avascular necrosis, *Acta Orthop Scand* 33:43, 1963.

Lerner AJ: *The little black book of neurology,* ed 3, St Louis, 1995, Mosby.

Leslie BM, Ericson WB Jr, Morehead JR: Incidence of a septum within the first dorsal compartment of the wrist, *J Hand Surg* 15A:88, 1990.

Lewis CB, Knortz KA: *Orthopedic assessment and treatment of the geriatric patient,* St Louis, 1993, Mosby.

Lewis MH: Median nerve decompression after Colles' fracture, *J Bone Joint Surg* 60B:195, 1978.

Lindstrom G, Nystrom A: Incidence of post-traumatic arthrosis after primary healing of scaphoid fractures: a clinical and radiological study, *J Hand Surg* 15B:11, 1990.

Lindstrom G, Nystrom A: Natural history of scaphoid non-union, with special reference to "asymptomatic" cases, *J Hand Surg* 17B:697, 1992.

Linscheid RL, Dobyns JH: Rheumatoid arthritis of the wrist, *Ortho Clin North Am* 2:649, 1971.

Linscheid RL, et al: Traumatic instability of the wrist, *J Bone Joint Surg* 54A:1612, 1972.

Linscheid RL, et al: Instability patterns of the wrist, *J Hand Surg* 8A:682, 1983.

Lister G: *The hand: diagnosis and indications,* Edinburgh, 1977, Churchill Livingstone.

Lluch AL: Thickening of the synovium of the digital flexor tendons: cause or consequence of the carpal tunnel syndrome? *J Hand Surg* 17B:209, 1992.

Lynch AC, Lipscomb PR: The carpal-tunnel syndrome and Colles' fractures, *JAMA* 185:363, 1963.

Magee DJ: *Orthopedic physical assessment,* ed 3, Philadelphia, 1997, WB Saunders.

Malone TR, McPoil TG, Nitz AJ: *Orthopedic and sports physical therapy,* ed 3, St Louis, 1997, Mosby.

Mannerfelt L, et al: Rupture of the extensor pollicis longus tendon after Colles' fracture and by rheumatoid arthritis, *J Hand Surg* 15B:49, 1990.

Marchiori DM: *Clinical imaging with skeletal, chest, and abdomen pattern differentials,* St Louis, 1999, Mosby.

Martin JH: *Neuroanatomy text and atlas,* ed 2, Stamford, Conn, 1996, Appleton & Lange.

Mathers LH, et al: *Clinical anatomy principles,* St Louis, 1996, Mosby.

Mayfield JK: Mechanism of carpal injuries, *Clin Orthop* 149:45, 1980.

Mayfield JK, Johnson RP, Kilcoyne RF: Carpal dislocations: pathomechanics and progressive perilunar instability, *J Hand Surg* 5:226, 1980.

Mayfield JK, et al: Biomechanical properties of human carpal ligaments, *Orthop Trans* 3:143, 1979.

Mayo Clinic: *Clinical examinations in neurology,* ed 3, Philadelphia, 1971, WB Saunders.

Mazion JM: *Illustrated manual of neurological reflexes/signs/tests, part I, Orthopedic signs/tests/maneuvers for office procedure, part II,* Orlando, 1980, Daniels Publishing.

McCarty DJ, Koopman WJ, editors: *Arthritis and allied conditions,* ed 12, Philadelphia, 1993, Lea & Febiger.

McLain RF, Steyer CM: Tendon ruptures with scaphoid nonunion, a case report, *Clin Orthop* 255:117, 1990.

McNurty RY, et al: Kinematics of the wrist, II, clinical applications, *J Bone Joint Surg* 600:955, 1978.

McRae R: *Clinical orthopaedic examination,* ed 3, Edinburgh, 1990, Churchill Livingstone.

Medical Economics Books: *Patient care flow chart manual,* ed 3, Oradell, NJ, 1982, Medical Economics Books.

Mellion MB: *Sports medicine secrets,* Philadelphia, 1994, Hanley & Belfus.

Mellion MB: *Office sports medicine,* ed 2, St Louis, 1996, Mosby.

Mennell JM: *The musculoskeletal system differential diagnosis from symptoms and physical signs,* Gaithersburg, Md, 1992, Aspen.

Mercier LR, Pettid FJ: *Practical orthopedics,* ed 4, St Louis, 1995, Mosby.

Millender LH, Nalebuff EA, Feldon PG: Rheumatoid arthritis, In Green D, editor: *Operative hand surgery,* New York, 1982, Churchill Livingstone.

Minamikawa Y, et al: de Quervain's syndrome: surgical and anatomical studies of the fibroosseous canal, *Orthopedics* 14:545, 1991.

Mino DE, Palmer AK, Levinsohn EM: The role of radiography and computerized tomography in the diagnosis of subluxation and dislocation of the distal radioulnar joint, *J Hand Surg* 8A:23, 1983.

Moberg E: Criticism and study of methods for examining sensibility of the hand, *Neurology* 12:8, 1962.

Moberg E: Relation of touch and deep sensation to hand reconstruction, *Am J Surg* 109:353, 1965.

Mody BS, et al: Nonunion of fractures of the scaphoid tuberosity, *J Bone Joint Surg* 75B:423, 1993.

Moldaver J: Tinel's signits characteristics and significance, *J Bone Joint Surg* 60A:412, 1978.

Mosby-Year Book, Inc.: *Expert 10-minute physical examination,* St Louis, 1997, Mosby-Year Book.

Mourad LA: *Orthopedic disorders,* St Louis, 1991, Mosby.

Mulliken JB: Cutaneous vascular anomalies. In McCarthy JG, editor: *Plastic surgery, vol 5, tumors of the head and neck and skin,* Philadelphia, 1990, WB Saunders.

Naidu SH, Heppenstall RB: Compartment syndrome of the forearm and hand, *Hand Clin* 10:13, 1994.

Nakamura P, Imaeda T, Miura T: Scaphoid malunion, *J Bone Joint Surg* 73B:134, 1991.

Nakamura R, et al: Analysis of scaphoid fracture displacement by three-dimensional computed tomography, *J Hand Surg* 16A:485, 1991.

Nakamura R, et al: Scaphoid non-union with D.I.S.I. deformity, a survey of clinical cases with special reference to ligamentous injury, *J Hand Surg* 16B:156, 1991.

Nettina SM: *The Lippincott manual of nursing practice,* ed 6, Philadelphia, 1996, Lippincott.

Newton RW: *Color atlas of pediatric neurology,* St Louis, 1995, Mosby-Wolfe.

Nicholas JA, Hershman EB: *The upper extremity in sports medicine,* ed 2, St Louis, 1995, Mosby.

Nolan WV III, et al: Results of treatment of severe carpal tunnel syndrome, *J Hand Surg* 17A:1020, 1992.

Nordin M, Anderson GBJ, Pope MH: *Musculoskeletal disorders in the workplace: principles and practice,* St Louis, 1997, Mosby.

O'Donoghue DH: *Treatment of injuries to athletes,* ed 3, Philadelphia, 1976, WB Saunders.

Olson WH, et al: *Handbook of symptom-oriented neurology,* ed 2, St Louis, 1994, Mosby.

Omer GE, Spinner M: *Management of peripheral nerve problems,* Philadelphia, 1980, WB Saunders.

Omer GE Jr: Evaluation and reconstruction of the forearm and hand after acute traumatic peripheral nerve injuries, *J Bone Joint Surg* 50A:1454, 1968.

Omer GE Jr: Sensation and sensibility in the upper extremity, *Clin Orthop* 104:30, 1974.

Omer GE Jr, Vogel JA: Determination of physiological length of a reconstructed muscle tendon unit through muscle stimulation, *J Bone Joint Surg* 47A:304, 1965.

Omer GE Jr, et al: The neurovascular cutaneous island pedicles for deficient median nerve sensibility: new technique and results of serial functional tests, *J Bone Joint Surg* 52A:1181, 1970.

O'Riain S: Shrivel test: a new and simple test of nerve function in the hand, *BMJ* 3:615, 1973.

O'Young B, Young MA, Stiens SA: *PM&R secrets,* Philadelphia, 1997, Hanley & Belfus.

Pagnanelli DM, Barrer SJ: Bilateral carpal tunnel release at one operation: report of 228 patients, *Neurosurgery* 31:1030, 1992.

Pahle JA, Raunio P: The influence of wrist position on finger deviation in the rheumatoid hand: a clinical and radiological study, *J Bone Joint Surg* 51B:664, 1969.

Palmer AK: Fractures of the distal radius. In Green DP, editor: *Operative hand surgery,* ed 2, New York, 1993, Churchill Livingstone.

Palmer AK, Glisson RR, Werner FW: Ulnar variance determination, *J Hand Surg* 7:376, 1982.

Palmer AK, Livensohn EM, Kuzma GR: Arthrography of the wrist, *J Hand Surg* 8:15, 1983.

Palmer DH, et al: Endoscopic carpal tunnel release, *Arthroscopy* 9:498, 1993.

Patten J: *Neurological differential diagnosis,* ed 2, London, 1996, Springer.

Pecina MM, Krmpotic-Nemanic J, Markiewitz AD: *Tunnel syndromes,* Boca Raton, Fla, 1991, CRC Press.

Perleik PC, Guilford WB: Magnetic resonance imaging to assess vascularity of scaphoid nonunions, *J Hand Surg* 16A:479, 1991.

Phalen GS: The carpal-tunnel syndrome: seventeen years' experience in diagnosis and treatment of six hundred fifty-four hands, *J Bone Joint Surg* 48A:211, 1966.

Pheasant S: *Ergonomics, work and health,* Gaithersburg, Md, 1991, Aspen.

Pitner MA: Pathophysiology of overuse injuries in the hand and wrist, *Hand Clin* 6:355, 1990.

Porter JN: Raynaud's syndrome. In Sabiston DC Jr, editor: *Davis Christopher textbook of surgery,* Philadelphia, 1977, WB Saunders.

Protas JM, Jackson WT: Evaluating carpal instabilities with fluoroscopy, *AJR Am J Roentgenol* 135:137, 1980.

Resnick D, Niwayama G: *Diagnosis of bone and joint disorders,* Philadelphia, 1981, WB Saunders.

Royle SG: Compartment syndrome following forearm fracture in children, *Injury* 21:73, 1990.

Saidoff DC, McDonough AL: *Critical pathways in therapeutic intervention,* St Louis, 1997, Mosby.

Sampson SP, Wisch D, Badalamente MA: Complications of conservative and surgical treatment of de Quervain's disease and trigger fingers, *Hand Clin* 10:73, 1994.

Scheck M: Long-term follow up of treatment of comminuted fractures of the distal end of the radius by transfixation with Kirschner wires and cast, *J Bone Joint Surg* 44A:337, 1962.

Schumacher HR, Klippel JH, Koopman WJ: *Primer on the rheumatic diseases,* ed 10, Atlanta, 1993, Arthritis Foundation.

Sennwald G: *The wrist,* New York, 1990, Springer-Verlag.

Shankman GA: *Fundamental orthopedic management for the physical therapist assistant,* St Louis, 1997, Mosby.

Silver D: Circulatory problems of the upper extremity. In Sabiston DC Jr, editor: *Davis Christopher textbook of surgery,* Philadelphia, 1985, WB Saunders.

Smith KL, Harvey FJ, Stalley PD: Nonunion of a pathologic juvenile scaphoid fracture after osteomyelitis, *J Hand Surg* 16A:493, 1991.

Southmayd WW, Millender LH, Nalebuff EA: Rupture of the flexor tendons in the index finger after Colles' fracture case report, *J Bone Joint Surg* 57A:562, 1975.

Specht NT, Russo RD: *Practical guide to diagnostic imaging,* St Louis, 1998, Mosby.

Spencer PS: The traumatic neuroma and proximal stump, *Bull Hosp Jt Dis Orthop Inst* 35:85, 1974.

Spinner M: *Injuries of the major branches of peripheral nerves of the forearm,* Philadelphia, 1972, WB Saunders.

Stern PJ: Tendinitis, overuse syndromes, and tendon injuries, *Hand Clin* 6:467, 1990.

Stewart DL, Abeln SH: *Documenting functional outcomes in physical therapy,* St Louis, 1993, Mosby.

Stoller DW: *Magnetic resonance imaging in orthopaedics & sports medicine,* Philadelphia, 1993, JB Lippincott.

Sugden P, et al: Dermal dendrocytes in Dupuytren's disease: a link between the skin and pathogenesis? *J Hand Surg* 18B:662, 1993.

Sunderland S: *Nerves and nerve injuries,* Baltimore, 1968, Williams & Wilkins.

Sutton D, Young JWR: *A concise textbook of clinical imaging,* ed 2, St Louis, 1995, Mosby.

Swanson AB, et al: Pathogenesis of rheumatoid deformities in the hand. In Cruess RL, Mitchell NS, editors: *Surgery of rheumatoid arthritis,* Philadelphia, 1971, JB Lippincott.

Taleisnik J: The ligaments of the wrist, *J Hand Surg* 1A:110, 1976.

Taleisnik J: Rheumatoid arthritis of the wrist. In Strickland JW, Steichen JB, editors: *Difficult problems in hand surgery,* St Louis, 1982, Mosby.

Tan JC, Horn SE: *Practical manual of physical medicine and rehabilitation,* St Louis, 1998, Mosby.

Taybi H, Lachman RS: *Radiology of syndromes, metabolic disorders, and skeletal dysplasias,* ed 4, St Louis, 1996, Mosby.

Thibodeau GA, Patton KT: *Anatomy & physiology,* ed 3, St Louis, 1996, Mosby.

Thibodeau GA, Patton KT: *Pocket reference to accompany anatomy & physiology,* ed 3, St Louis, 1996, Mosby.

Thompson JM: *Clinical outlines for health assessment,* St Louis, 1997, Mosby.

Thompson JS, Phelph TH: Repetitive strain injuries, how to deal with the epidemic of the 1990's, *Postgrad Med* 88:143, 1990.

Thorson E, Szabo RM: Common tendinitis problems in the hand and forearm, *Orthop Clin North Am* 23:65, 1992.

Tiel-van Buul MM, et al: Radiography of the carpal scaphoid, experimental evaluation of "the carpal box" and first clinical results, *Invest Radiol* 27:954, 1992.

Tiel-van Buul MM, et al: Radiography and scintigraphy of suspected scaphoid fracture, a long-term study in 160 patients, *J Bone Joint Surg* 75B:61, 1993.

Tinel J: *Nerve wounds: Symptomatology of peripheral nerve lesions caused by war wounds* (translated by F Rothwell; edited by CA Joll), New York, 1918, William Wood.

Toghill PJ: *Examining patients: an introduction to clinical medicine,* London, 1990, Edward Arnold.

Tollison CD, Satterthwaite JR, Tollison JW: *Handbook of pain management,* ed 2, Baltimore, 1994, Williams & Wilkins.

Torg JS, Shepard RJ: *Current therapy in sports medicine,* ed 3, St Louis, 1995, Mosby.

Trumble TE, Benirschke SK, Vedder NB: Ipsilateral fractures of the scaphoid and radius, *J Hand Surg* 18A:8, 1993.

Tubiana R: *The hand,* Philadelphia, 1981, WB Saunders.

Turek SL: *Orthopaedics principles and their application,* ed 3, Philadelphia, 1977, JB Lippincott.

Urbaniak JR: Complication of treatment of carpal tunnel syndrome. In Gelberman RH, editor: *Operative nerve repair and reconstruction,* vol 2, Philadelphia, 1991, JB Lippincott.

US Preventative Services Task Force: *Guide to clinical preventive services,* ed 2, Alexandria, 1996, International Medical Publishing.

Vance RM, Gelberman RH: Acute ulnar neuropathy with fractures at the wrist, *J Bone Joint Surg* 60A:962, 1978.

Van Holsbeeck M, Introcaso JH: *Musculoskeletal ultrasound,* St Louis, 1991, Mosby.

Vidal MA, et al: Preiser's disease, *Ann Chir Main Memb Super* 10:227, 1991.

von Prince K: Occupational therapy's interest in function following peripheral nerve injury, *Med Bull US Army, Europe* 23:143, 1966.

von Prince K, Butler B: Measuring sensory function of the hand in peripheral nerve injuries, *Am J Occup Ther* 21:385, 1967.

Wakefield TS, Frank RG: *The clinicians guide to neuro musculoskeletal practice,* Abbotsford, Wisc, 1995, Allied Health of Wisconsin, S.C.

Warwick R, Williams PL: *Gray's anatomy,* Philadelphia, 1973, WB Saunders.

Weineck J: *Functional anatomy in sports,* ed 2, St Louis, 1990, Mosby.

Weinstein S: Tactile sensitivity of the phalanges, *Percept Mot Skills* 14:351, 1962.

Weinstein SL, Buckwalter JA: *Turek's orthopaedics principles and their application,* ed 5, Philadelphia, 1994, JB Lippincott.

Weiss A-PC, Akelman E, Tabatabai M: Treatment of de Quervain's disease, *J Hand Surg* 19A:595, 1994.

Weiss AP, Steichen JB: Synovial sarcoma causing carpal tunnel syndrome, *J Hand Surg* 17A:1024, 1992.

Werner JL, Omer GE Jr: Evaluating cutaneous pressure sensation of the hand, *Am J Occup Ther* 24:247, 1970.

Williams TM, et al: Verification of the pressure provocative test in carpal tunnel syndrome, *Ann Plast Surg* 19:8, 1992.

Windsor RE, Lox DM: *Soft tissue injuries: diagnosis and treatment,* Philadelphia, 1998, Hanley & Belfus.

Witczak JW, Masear VR, Meyer RD: Triggering of the thumb with de Quervain's stenosing tendovaginitis, *J Hand Surg* 15A:265, 1990.

Witt J, Pess G, Gelberman RH: Treatment of de Quervain's tenosynovitis: a prospect study of the results of injection of steroids and immobilization in a splint, *J Bone Joint Surg* 73A:219, 1991.

Wynn-Parry CB: *Rehabilitation of the hand,* ed 3, London, 1973, Butterworths.

Yacoe ME, et al: Dupuytren's contracture: MR imaging findings and correlation between MR signal intensity and cellularity of lesions, *AJR Am J Roentgenol* 160:813, 1993.

Yosipovitch G, et al: Trigger finger in young patients with insulin dependent diabetes, *J Rheumatol* 17:951, 1990.

Younger CP, DeFiore JC: Rupture of the flexor tendons to the fingers after a Colles' fracture: a case report, *J Bone Joint Surg* 59A:828, 1977.

Zoega H: Fracture of the lower end of the radius with ulnar nerve palsy, *J Bone Joint Surg* 48V:514, 1966.

THE THORACIC SPINE

AXIOMS IN THORACIC SPINE ASSESSMENT

- The thoracic spine requires evaluation in isolation and together with the cervical and lumbar spine.
- Thoracic pain can be perplexing and difficult to diagnose.
- The most commonly involved area is the thoracolumbar junction.

INTRODUCTION

Thoracic spinal pain and dysfunction present a particularly challenging clinical dilemma. Thoracic spinal pain may arise from somatic as well as visceral origins. Pain felt along the thoracic spine may arise from the ribs, the abdomen, or the vertebral column.

The thoracic spine is the part of the vertebral column that is most rigid because of the rib cage. The rib cage, in turn, provides protection for the heart and lungs.

Thoracic pain occurs as a referred visceral symptom. This pain can be from the chest and abdomen. The pain may also appear as a symptom of a problem of musculoskeletal origin. Sudden pain in the thoracic region occurs less often than in the more mobile cervical and lumbar spines.

The structure of the thorax as a whole is such that overall motion of this portion of the spine is limited.

ORTHOPEDIC GAMUT 7-1

THORACIC AREA PAIN

The following are diagnostic keys for thoracic area pain:

1. Identify postural strain syndromes.
2. Identify radicular syndromes.
3. Always check for myelopathy.

ORTHOPEDIC GAMUT 7-2

THORACIC SPINE

The stabilizing influences for the thoracic spine include the following:

1. The first element is the vertebral articular process. The interlocking arrangement of the thoracic facets prevents anterior displacement of the vertebra and forms the imbrication of the thoracic spine.
2. The second primary stabilizing influence of the thoracic spine is the vertebral body. At the posterior of the vertebral bodies, the height of the body is greater than in the anterior. This contributes to the thoracic spine kyphosis.
3. The third stabilizing influence is the structure of the ribs and their attachments to the spine. The ribs help stiffen the thoracic spine.
4. The fourth primary stabilizing influence for the thoracic spine is the structure of the intervertebral disc. The thoracic spine intervertebral discs are more narrow and thin than in the cervical or lumbar spines. They are also less elastic than all the other disc tissues of the spine.

TABLE 7-1

THORACIC SPINE CROSS-REFERENCE TABLE BY ASSESSMENT PROCEDURE

Disease Assessed

Thoracic Spine Test/Sign	Scoliosis	Ankylosing Spondylitis	Intervertebral Disc Syndrome	Sprain	Tuberculosis	Myelopathy	T1-T2 Nerve Root	Rib Injury	Intercostal Syndrome	Fracture	Strain	Fibrositis
Adam's positions	●											
Amoss's sign		●	●	●								
Anghelescu's sign					●							
Beevor's sign						●						
Chest expansion test		●										
First thoracic nerve root test							●					
Forestier's bowstring sign		●										
Passive scapular approximation test							●					
Rib motion test		●						●	●			
Schepelmann's sign								●	●			
Spinal percussion test			●	●						●	●	
Sponge test												●
Sternal compression test								●				

TABLE 7-2

THORACIC SPINE CROSS-REFERENCE TABLE BY SYNDROME OR TISSUE

Syndrome	Test/Sign	Syndrome	Test/Sign
Ankylosing spondylitis	Amoss's sign	Myelopathy	Beevor's sign
	Chest expansion test	Rib injury	Rib motion test
	Forestier's bowstring sign		Schepelmann's sign
	Rib motion test		Sternal compression test
Fibrositis	Sponge test	Scoliosis	Adam's positions
Fracture	Spinal percussion test	Sprain	Amoss's sign
Intercostal syndrome	Rib motion test		Spinal percussion test
	Schepelmann's sign	Strain	Spinal percussion test
Intervertebral disc syndrome	Amoss's sign	T1-T2 nerve root	First thoracic nerve root test
	Spinal percussion test		Passive scapular approximation test
		Tuberculosis	Anghelescu's sign

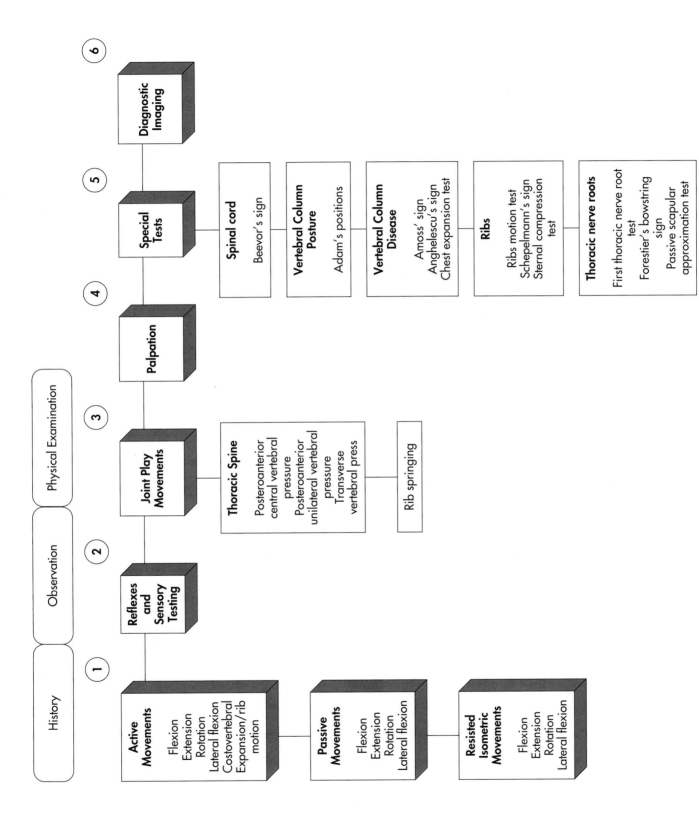

FIG. 7-1 Thoracic spine assessment.

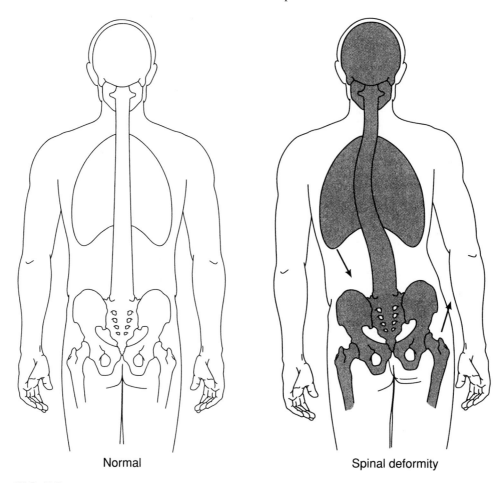

Normal   Spinal deformity

FIG. 7-2   Deformity of the spine. *(From Barkauskas VH, et al:* Health & physical assessment, *ed 2, St Louis, 1998, Mosby.)*

Added to the bony and discal stabilizing influences of the thoracic spine are the muscles supporting the spinal column. The thoracic spinal column serves as the attachment for many of the muscles of the trunk, shoulder, and arm.

Among these muscles are the trapezius and latissimus dorsi. The deeper muscles of the trunk include the levator scapulae, rhomboid major, and rhomboid minor. Still deeper are the sacrospinalis muscle groups, which include the spinalis dorsi, longissimus dorsi, and the iliocostalis lumborum.

During an examination of the thorax and thoracic spine, the assessment is primarily of the thoracic spine. The examination is extensive. Without a history of specific trauma or injury to the thoracic spine, the examiner must be prepared to assess the other implicated tissues. For problems superior to the thoracic spine, a thorough examination of the cervical spine and upper limb is a part of the examination scheme. If a problem exists inferior to the thoracic spine, the examination of the lumbar spine and lower limb is completed.

The shape of the spine and its structural relationship to the shoulder girdle, thorax, and pelvis should be assessed.

The normal spinal curvatures are concave at the cervical area, convex at the thoracic area, and concave at the lumbar area. Any differences in heights of the shoulders and the iliac crests should be noted. Unusual heights of the iliac crests suggest uneven leg lengths. Variations in spinal curvature may indicate a structural problem. Scoliosis is a deformity of the spine that appears as a lateral deviation (Fig. 7-2). The normal anteroposterior curve needs to be assessed as well (Fig. 7-3, *A*). Kyphosis is a flexion deformity (Fig. 7-3, *B*). When the angle of the defect is sharp, the apex is called a *gibbus.* Lordosis (swayback) is an extension deviation of the spine, commonly in the lumbar area (Fig. 7-3, *C*).

ESSENTIAL ANATOMY

There are 12 thoracic vertebrae. They are characterized by downswept spines, prominent transverse processes, and heart-shaped bodies, and they are unique in articulating with the normal 12 pairs of ribs. Ribs 1 to 10 articulate both with the vertebral body and its transverse process. Ribs 11 and

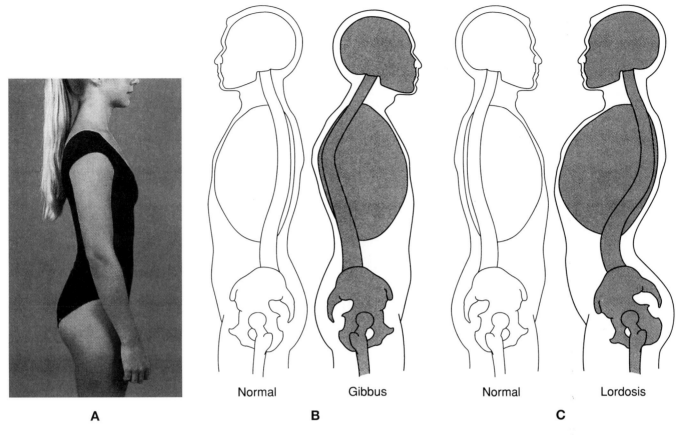

Normal | Gibbus | Normal | Lordosis

A | B | C

FIG. 7-3 **A,** Normal curvature of the spine. **B,** Kyphosis. **C,** Lordosis and extension deformity of the spine. *(From Barkauskas VH, et al:* Health & physical assessment, *ed 2, St Louis, 1998, Mosby.)*

12 articulate only with the vertebral body and are not jointed to the transverse processes on these vertebrae. The thoracic spine and the ribs are intimately related to many neural, vascular, and visceral structures (Figs. 7-4 and 7-5). Each intercostal nerve (and the subcostal and upper two lumbar nerves) sends a white ramus communicans to the sympathetic ganglion of the same level. Each intercostal nerve provides sensory, motor (somatic motor), and sympathetic (visceral motor to blood vessels and sweat glands) innervation to the thoracic or abdominal wall.

ESSENTIAL MOTION ASSESSMENT

The facets of the thoracic vertebrae are oriented 60 degrees to the horizontal plane. These facets are more vertically oriented than the articular processes of the cervical region. This vertical orientation dramatically limits forward flexion. Extension is limited by the inferior articular processes contacting the laminae of the vertebrae below and by contact between adjacent spinous processes.

Rotation is the dominant movement in the thoracic region (Fig. 7-6).

ORTHOPEDIC GAMUT 7-3

THORACOLUMBAR SPINE

To assess range of motion of the thoracolumbar spine, the patient is directed to do the following:

1. Slowly bend forward at the waist and try to touch the toes (while observed for scoliosis) (Figs. 7-7 and 7-8).
2. Bend back as far as possible (hyperextend the spine) (Fig. 7-9).
3. Bend to the right and left side as far as possible (lateral bending with the pelvis stabilized) (Fig. 7-10).
4. Turn to the right and left in a circular motion (with the pelvis stabilized) (Figs. 7-11 and 7-12).

Text continued on p. 420

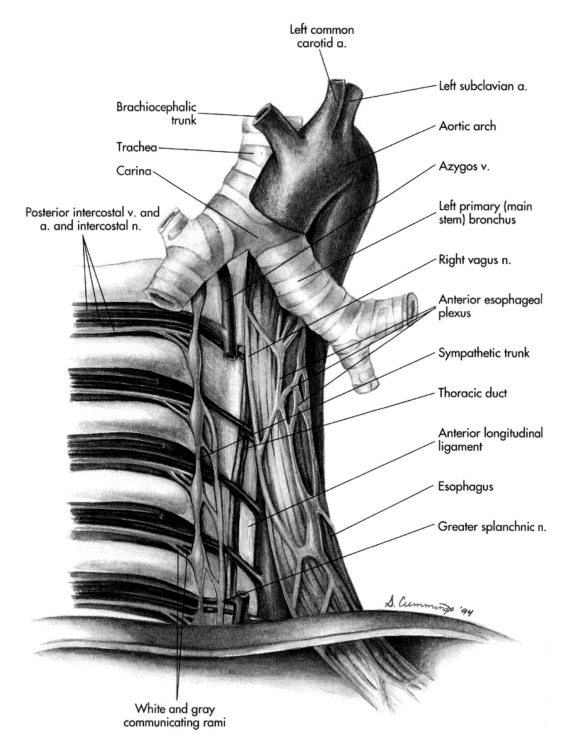

FIG. 7-4   Relationship of the vertebrae and the ribs to the vessels and nerves of the thorax. *(From Cramer GD, Darby SA: Basic and clinical anatomy of the spine, spinal cord, and ANS, St Louis, 1995, Mosby.)*

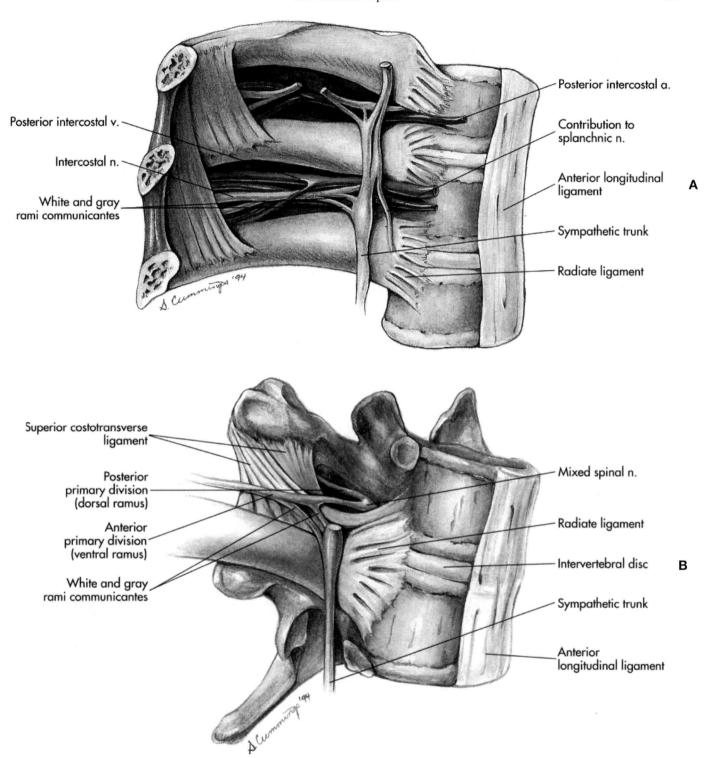

Posterior intercostal v.

Intercostal n.

White and gray rami communicantes

Posterior intercostal a.

Contribution to splanchnic n.

Anterior longitudinal ligament

Sympathetic trunk

Radiate ligament

A

Superior costotransverse ligament

Posterior primary division (dorsal ramus)

Anterior primary division (ventral ramus)

White and gray rami communicantes

Mixed spinal n.

Radiate ligament

Intervertebral disc

Sympathetic trunk

Anterior longitudinal ligament

B

FIG. 7-5   **A,** Nerves and vessels related to three adjacent vertebrae and the ribs that articulate with them. **B,** Close-up of the nerves associated with a single thoracic motion segment.   *(From Cramer GD, Darby SA: Basic and clinical anatomy of the spine, spinal cord, and ANS, St Louis, 1995, Mosby.)*

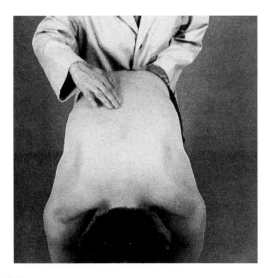

FIG. 7-6   Palpation of the spinal processes as the patient bends forward. *(From Barkauskas VH, et al:* Health & physical assessment, *ed 2, St Louis, 1998, Mosby.)*

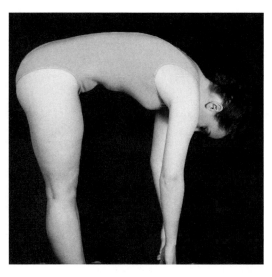

FIG. 7-7   Flexion range of motion in the thoracic spine is 20 to 45 degrees. In an indirect measurement of the thoracic range of motion, the length of the spine from the C7 spinous process to the T12 spinous process is measured. The patient bends forward, and the spine is again measured. A minimum of a 2.7-cm difference is considered normal. A measurement from the C7 spinous process to S1 can also be made. The spine is measured a second time with the patient bending. A minimum of a 10-cm difference is normal. Alternatively, the patient bends forward attempting to touch the toes. The patient tries to keep the knees straight. The distance from the patient's fingertips to the floor is assessed.

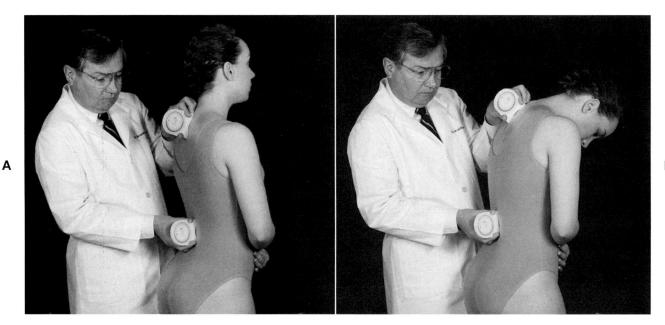

A   B

FIG. 7-8   For testing flexion with an inclinometer, the patient is seated or standing. One inclinometer is placed in the sagittal plane at the T1 level and the other at the T12 level, also in the sagittal plane **(A).** Both instruments are zeroed. If seated, the patient places the hands on the hips, and if standing, the patient crosses the arms in front of the chest. The thoracic spine is flexed forward so as not to involve lumbar spine motion **(B).** Both instrument readings are recorded. The T12 value is subtracted from the T1 value to arrive at the thoracic flexion angle. Retained flexion of the thoracic spine of 30 degrees or less is an impairment of the thoracic spine in the activities of daily living.

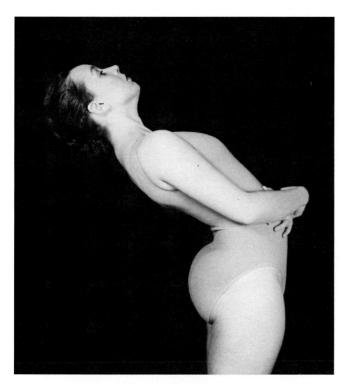

FIG. 7-9   Extension in the thoracic spine is normally 25 to 35 degrees. The distance between C7 and T12 spinous processes is determined with a tape measure. A minimum of a 2.5-cm difference in tape measure length between standing and extension is normal.

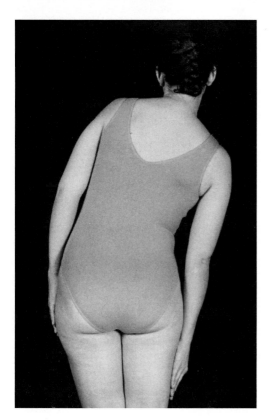

FIG. 7-10   Lateral flexion is approximately 20 to 40 degrees to the right and left. For accuracy of movement, the patient runs a hand down the side of the leg, without bending forward or backward. The distance from the fingertips to the floor is measured. The measurements are compared bilaterally. The distances should be equal.

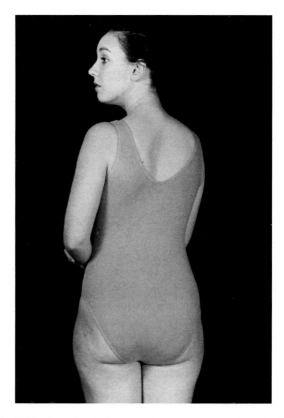

FIG. 7-11   Rotation in the thoracic spine is approximately 35 to 50 degrees. The patient rotates to the right or left. The examiner assesses the amount of rotation, comparing both ways.

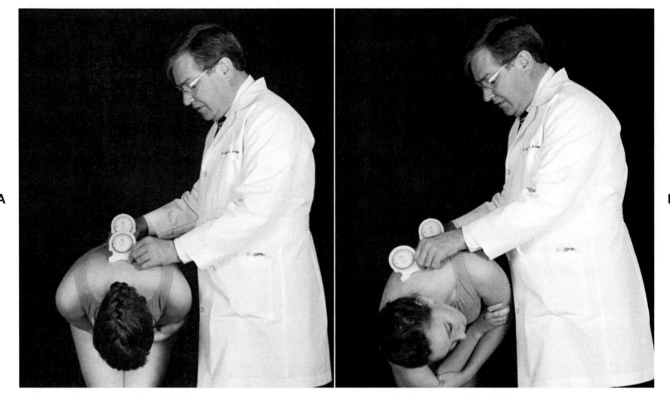

FIG. 7-12   When an inclinometer is used to assess thoracic spinal rotation, the patient is standing. The patient is flexed forward. The patient may brace the position with the arms. One inclinometer is placed at the T1 level in the coronal plane and the other at the T12 level also in the coronal plane (**A**). Both instruments are zeroed. The patient rotates to one side and the angles indicated on both instruments are recorded (**B**). The T12 measurement is subtracted from the T1 measurement to arrive at the thoracic rotation angle. The measurements are repeated for rotation to the opposite side. Retained active rotation of the thoracic spine of 20 degrees or less is an impairment of the function of the thoracic spine in the activities of daily living.

ESSENTIAL MUSCLE FUNCTION ASSESSMENT

In addition to the bony and discal stabilizing influences of the thoracic spine, there are also muscles supporting the spinal column. The thoracic spinal column serves as the attachment for many of the muscles of the trunk, shoulder, and arm.

Among these muscles are the trapezius and latissimus dorsi. The deeper muscles of the trunk include the levator scapulae, rhomboid major, and rhomboid minor. Still deeper are the sacrospinalis muscle groups. These include the spinalis dorsi, longissimus dorsi, and iliocostalis lumborum.

The trapezius muscle attaches to the spinous processes from the upper cervicals to the lower thoracic spine. In the lower part, the muscle overlaps the long attachment of the latissimus dorsi muscle.

The latissimus dorsi muscle attaches to the spinous processes, beginning in the midthoracic region, and extends to the pelvis. The trapezius and latissimus dorsi are the two most superficial muscles of the back. In addition to movement, these muscles also serve to enclose the deeper muscle layers.

The deeper muscles are broad and flat and are not as frequently subjected to injury. These muscles are the levator scapulae, rhomboid major, and rhomboid minor. They lie under the trapezius, in the upper portion of the dorsal spine. The muscles extend down toward the level of the upper limit of the latissimus dorsi.

Still deeper are the muscles that run from the spine to the pelvis and form the sacrospinalis group. This group is a combination of many muscles, whose course parallels the spinal column. The sacrospinalis group of muscles includes the spinalis dorsi, longissimus dorsi, and iliocostalis lumborum.

The sacrospinalis group fills the sulcus between the spinous processes, the bodies of the vertebrae, and the arc of the ribs. This group of muscles interdigitates in such a manner that each muscle supports the others. These muscles make up the lumbar mass of muscles

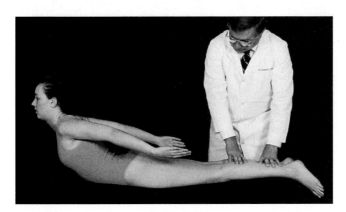

FIG. 7-13   The patient is prone. The hip extensors must be given fixation of the pelvis to the thighs, and the examiner must stabilize the legs firmly on the examining table. The patient then attempts trunk extension. The ability to complete spine extension and hold against strong pressure with hands clasped behind the head is normal. The ability to perform this only with the hands behind the back is good. If performed only with the hands clasped behind the back, the ability to lift the thorax so that the xiphoid process of the sternum is raised slightly from the table is fair. When marked weakness is present, usually such weakness extends throughout the back. If cervical extensors can lift the head, a head-raising movement can furnish slight resistance against other back extensors. When the lower back is strong and the upper back is weak, an attempt to raise the thorax will result in the back extensors extending the lower back by anteriorly tilting the pelvis, but the thorax will not be lifted from the table.

that extends from the occiput to the sacrum and laterally to the spinous processes.

These muscles have multiple actions depending on the relationship between them. One muscle may serve to stabilize the spine while another muscle member moves.

The back extensors are the most important of all the trunk muscles. There are several reasons why abdominal muscles are discussed in detail in literature and back extensors have little emphasis. Weakness of the lower back musculature is seldom encountered except in paralytic cases. The incidence among nonparalytic, or so-called normal individuals is probably less than 1%.

On the other hand, abdominal muscle weakness is commonly encountered. Parts of the abdominal muscles can be tested separately, but the back extensors can be tested only as a group.

During the trunk extension test, the latissimus dorsi, quadratus lumborum, and trapezius assist back extensors.

The head and neck extensor muscles and the hip extensors should be tested before the back extensors are tested (Fig. 7-13).

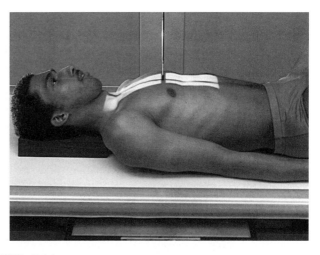

FIG. 7-14   Anteroposterior thoracic vertebrae. *(From Ballinger PW: Merrill's atlas of radiographic positions and radiologic procedures, vol 1-3, ed 8, St Louis, 1995, Mosby.)*

ESSENTIAL IMAGING

A number of radiographic views have been frequently described to evaluate the osseous and soft-tissue anatomy of the thoracic spine. Frontal (anteroposterior [AP]) (Figs. 7-14 and 7-15), lateral (left) (Figs. 7-16 to 7-18), and "swimmer's" views (Figs. 7-19 to 7-24) are the standard evaluation projections (Fig. 7-25).

Although plain x-ray films are generally unreliable in the early detection and assessment of osteoporosis, plain film findings of osteoporosis can be a helpful adjunct to the diagnosis. The trabecular bone becomes sparse, resulting in overall reduction in bone density.

Nontraumatic compression deformities are a sure sign that bone density is compromised.

ORTHOPEDIC GAMUT 7-4

COMPRESSION DEFORMITIES

Compression deformities may take several shapes:

1. An isolated central end-plate impression may be present.
2. Biconcave end-plate deformities may be present.
3. The segment may lose anterior vertebral body height with maintenance of the end-plate integrity.
4. The segment may demonstrate loss of anterior and posterior vertebral body height.
5. Fractures of the ribs are quite common.

Text continued on p. 426

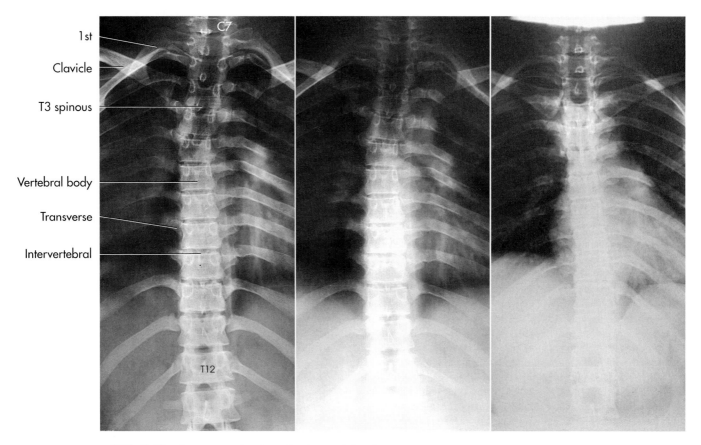

1st

Clavicle

T3 spinous

Vertebral body

Transverse

Intervertebral

C7

T12

FIG. 7-15   Anteroposterior thoracic views of the thorax.   *(From Ballinger PW:* Merrill's atlas of radiographic positions and radiologic procedures, *vol 1-3, ed 8, St Louis, 1995, Mosby.)*

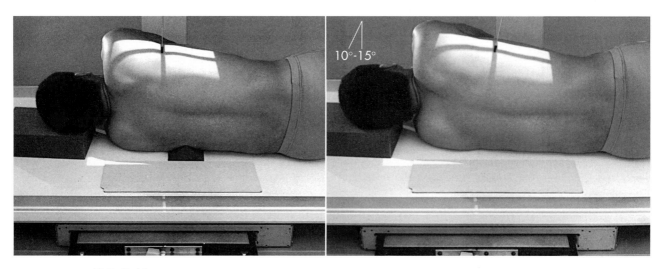

10°-15°

FIG. 7-16   Recumbent lateral thoracic spine.   *(From Ballinger PW:* Merrill's atlas of radiographic positions and radiologic procedures, *vol 1-3, ed 8, St Louis, 1995, Mosby.)*

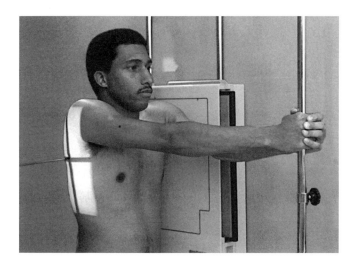

FIG. 7-17   Upright lateral thoracic spine.   *(From Ballinger PW:* Merrill's atlas of radiographic positions and radiologic procedures, *vol 1-3, ed 8, St Louis, 1995, Mosby.)*

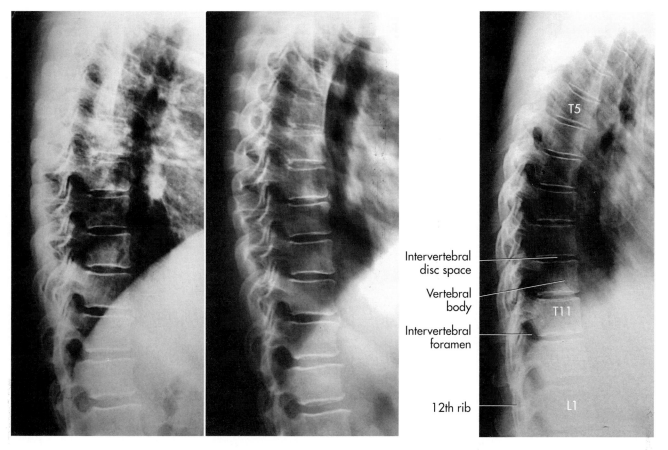

FIG. 7-18   Lateral thoracic spine.   *(From Ballinger PW:* Merrill's atlas of radiographic positions and radiologic procedures, *vol 1-3, ed 8, St Louis, 1995, Mosby.)*

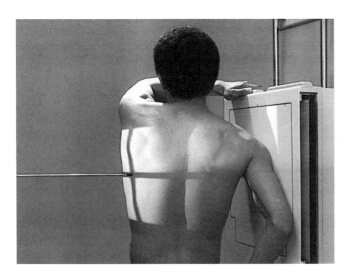

FIG. 7-19 Posteroanterior oblique zygapophyseal joints. *(From Ballinger PW:* Merrill's atlas of radiographic positions and radiologic procedures, *vol 1-3, ed 8, St Louis, 1995, Mosby.)*

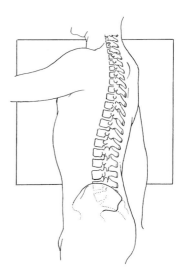

FIG. 7-20 Posteroanterior oblique Z-joints, right anterior oblique for joints closest to film. *(From Ballinger PW:* Merrill's atlas of radiographic positions and radiologic procedures, *vol 1-3, ed 8, St Louis, 1995, Mosby.)*

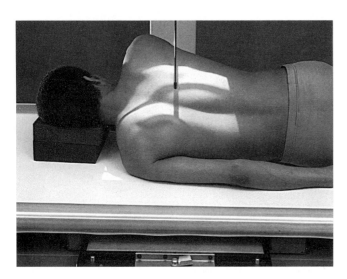

FIG. 7-21 Posteroanterior oblique Z-joints, left anterior oblique for joints closest to film. *(From Ballinger PW:* Merrill's atlas of radiographic positions and radiologic procedures, *vol 1-3, ed 8, St Louis, 1995, Mosby.)*

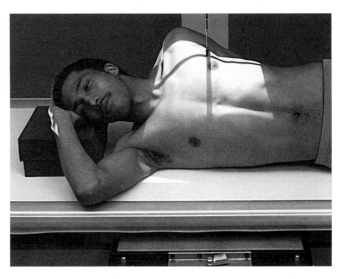

FIG. 7-22 Anteroposterior oblique Z-joints, right posterior oblique for joints farthest from film. *(From Ballinger PW:* Merrill's atlas of radiographic positions and radiologic procedures, *vol 1-3, ed 8, St Louis, 1995, Mosby.)*

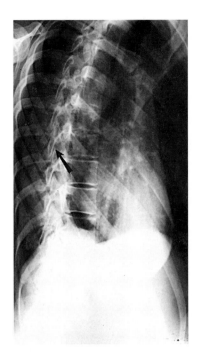

FIG. 7-23   Upright posteroanterior oblique Z-joints. *(From Ballinger PW:* Merrill's atlas of radiographic positions and radiologic procedures, *vol 1-3, ed 8, St Louis, 1995, Mosby.)*

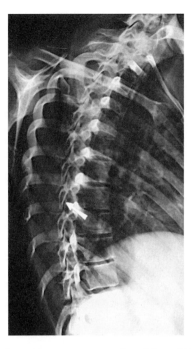

FIG. 7-24   Recumbent anteroposterior oblique Z-joints. *(From Ballinger PW:* Merrill's atlas of radiographic positions and radiologic procedures, *vol 1-3, ed 8, St Louis, 1995, Mosby.)*

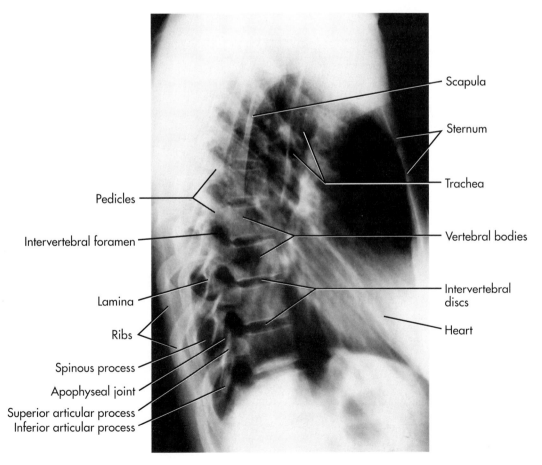

FIG. 7-25   Lateral radiographic view of the thoracic spine and ribs.   *(From Greenstein GM:* Clinical assessment of neuromusculoskeletal disorders, *St Louis, 1997, Mosby.)*

ADAM'S POSITIONS

Assessment for Pathologic or Structural Scoliosis

Comment

The spinal column centers the mass of the torso and head in a line along the vertical axis that falls through the pelvis. Disturbances of the spine, such as the curvatures associated with scoliosis, may significantly alter the normal balance and coordination of the spine (Table 7-3).

Scoliosis, or lateral curvature of the spine, may be idiopathic, congenital, or neuromuscular in origin. Idiopathic scoliosis is responsible for 85% to 95% of all cases of scoliosis. Infantile idiopathic scoliosis spans the ages of 0 to 3 years. Juvenile idiopathic scoliosis occurs in patients aged 4 to 10 years, and adolescent idiopathic scoliosis occurs in patients older than 10 years of age (Fig. 7-26).

A slight lateral curve with the convexity on the same side as handedness (i.e., convexity to the left in left-handed individuals) is normally found in the upper thoracic region (Fig. 7-27). The diagnosis usually is made on routine physical examination. Attention should be focused on the problem in all children, but especially in those between the ages of 10 and 14 years, when spinal growth is most rapid (Fig. 7-28). The diagnosis is confirmed by a standing plain film study of the spine (Fig. 7-29). Pathologic anomalies at birth are responsible for scoliosis in some individuals. Usually, the problem results from a "failure of formation" (Fig. 7-30).

Scoliosis is also classified as either structural or nonstructural. Structural curves are fixed and nonflexible and fail to correct with side bending. Nonstructural curves, on the other hand, are flexible and readily correct with side bending.

TABLE 7-3

THORACIC SPINE SYNDROMES

	Sprain or Strain	Vertebral Subluxation	Scoliosis	Scheuermann's Disease
Physical examination findings	Palpable tenderness over intervertebral joint Supraspinous ligament tenderness Pain on twisting, cervical flexion, or extreme extension Paraspinal myospasm or hypertonicity	Pain over spinous process or supraspinous ligament Flexion or extension fixation; malposition Loss of normal springy end-feel Alteration of normal muscle or joint physiology	Structural deformity, such as hip or pelvis unleveling, leg length discrepancy, posterior scapula, high shoulder Muscular asymmetry and unilateral hypertonicity Lateral curvature of spine Chronologic age versus skeletal maturity	Kyphotic deformity of dorsal spine Rigid musculature of thoracic spine Discomfort of back in growing children and adolescents Tight anterior shoulder girdle and thorax
X-ray findings	Usually unremarkable	Normal Need to rule out concomitant mechanical factors that can delay recovery	Lateral deviation of spine (D1 to S1 view)	End-plate irregularity, abnormal vertebral ossification patterns, anterior plate or body deformity, involvement of three or more vertebral bodies More than 40°-45° of kyphosis

Modified from Brier SR: *Primary care orthopedics,* St Louis, 1999, Mosby.

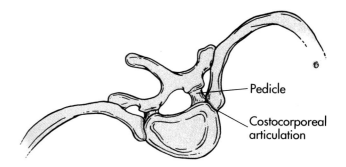

Pedicle

Costocorporeal articulation

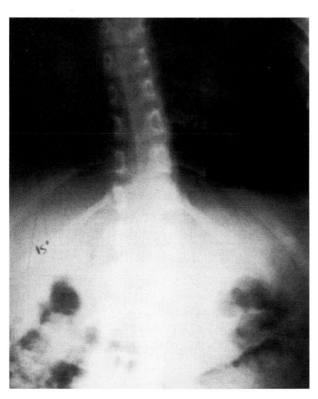

FIG. 7-26 Scoliosis. *(From Brier SR: Primary care orthopedics, St Louis, Mosby, 1999.)*

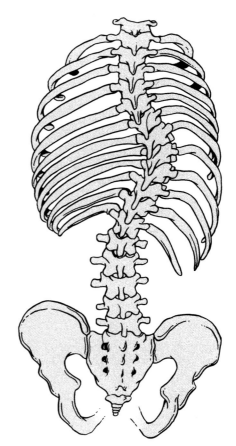

FIG. 7-27 Posterior view of a scoliotic spine. *(From Cramer GD, Darby SA: Basic and clinical anatomy of the spine, spinal cord, and ANS, St Louis, 1995, Mosby.)*

Curvature of the spine in the AP direction in which the convexity is directed posteriorly is termed *kyphosis.* This curvature exists in the normal spine at the thoracic and sacral regions. Disease of the discs and vertebral bodies is the most common cause. Congenital kyphosis is rare and usually is secondary to a localized malformation of the spine.

Senile kyphosis is relatively common in the elderly patient and may be symptomatic (Fig. 7-31).

Scheuermann's kyphosis is a fixed kyphosis that develops near the time of puberty. The cause is unknown, but the deformity is caused by typical wedging abnormalities in the dorsal and dorsolumbar spine that result in a decrease in the anterior height of the vertebrae. Mild forms may clinically resemble postural round back. Wedging of the vertebrae, irregularity of the end plates, and typical Schmorl's nodules are seen on the lateral view, usually between T2 and T12 (Fig. 7-32). Synostoses and osteophyte formation are not uncommon in adults. *Gibbus* refers to a focal flexion deformity (Fig. 7-33).

Few conditions produce decreased kyphosis. The lordotic interscapular thoracic spine (Pottenger's saucering) involves the T2 to T6 vertebrae. This type of flattened thoracic spine may have its beginning in the juvenile years, ages 2 through 5. The cause of this flattened spine may be a congenital fixation of the thoracic spine.

The examiner should also be aware that if a thoracolumbar kyphosis exists, the kyphosis is caused by a postural deficit, resulting from poor postural habits. This cause of kyphosis is most prevalent in adolescents. A patient with this condition is not round-shouldered, rather round-backed. The classification for thoracolumbar kyphosis is round back type I or type II. Type I results from postural habitus and type II from structural abnormalities. Among causes for thoracolumbar kyphosis are juvenile osteochondrosis (Scheuermann's disease) and vertebra plana (Calvé's disease).

The lower the thoracolumbar kyphosis occurs in the thoracic spine, the more it is a fixed and unyielding kyphosis. The patient may have normal and supple flexion in the areas of the spine above the thoracolumbar kyphosis.

Concerning the thoracic kyphosis, the examiner must observe for gibbus deformity. The gibbus deformity is associated with spinal tuberculosis and involves only two or three vertebral elements. The gibbus is a short, sharply angled, and acute kyphosis. This may also be observed in significant compression fracture of one or more thoracic vertebrae.

Often, with the dramatic and adverse changes of thoracic kyphosis, there is a parallel development of lateral curvature (scoliosis).

The presence of scoliosis needs to be determined. Nonstructural scoliosis is associated with poor postural habits. When the patient with nonstructural or postural scoliosis assumes proper standing or seated attitudes, the scoliosis disappears. Poor posture, hysteria, nerve root irritation, inflammation in the spine area, leg length discrepancy, or hip contracture can cause nonstructural scoliosis.

An idiopathic structural scoliosis does not have any specific cause. Structural changes may result from a congenital problem, such as wedge vertebrae, hemivertebrae, or failure of segmentation. The increase or decrease of kyphosis in a juvenile will alert the examiner to other postural deficits that may indicate the onset of scoliosis.

Senile scoliosis is the result of spinal column changes associated with aging of the adult thoracic spine. A scoliotic curve develops but does not have all the characteristics demonstrable in adolescent scoliosis. Upon a more thorough examination, senile scoliosis might actually be mild or moderate adolescent structural scoliosis that was previously undetected. Changes or increases in curvature usually result from the effects of gravity or injury to the thoracic spine. These patients often are experiencing thoracic pain and are surprised to learn that scoliosis exists.

Once scoliosis is identified, the degree of curvature has to be determined. Accurate techniques of measurement must be used. Once a particular method of curvature measurement is established, all further studies must be measured in the same way.

PROCEDURE

- If the patient has an S or C scoliosis, the curvature may straighten when the spine flexes forward.
- If it does, it is a negative sign and evidence of functional scoliosis.
- A positive sign occurs when the scoliosis does not improve after flexing forward.

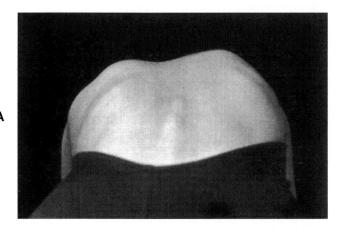

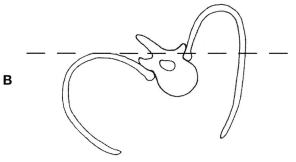

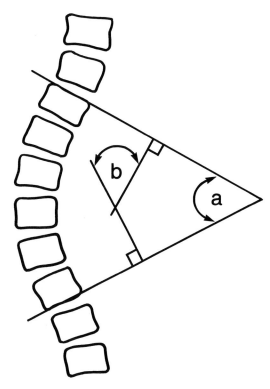

FIG. 7-28 **A,** Scoliosis with rib prominence from vertebral rotation is best exhibited on forward bending. **B,** Cross section of the chest showing rib distortion from vertebral rotation. *(From Mercier LR, Pettid FJ:* Practical orthopedics, *ed 4, St Louis, 1995, Mosby.)*

FIG. 7-29 Cobb method of measuring the severity of a curve. *(From Mercier LR, Pettid FJ:* Practical orthopedics, *ed 4, St Louis, 1995, Mosby.)*

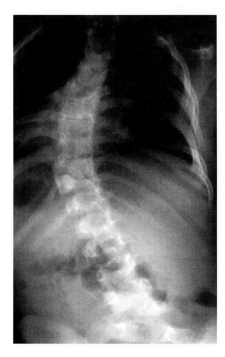

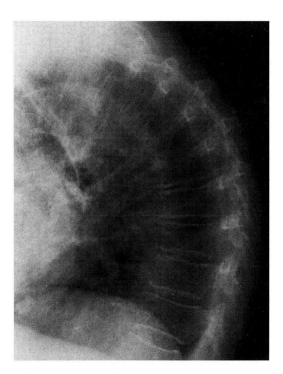

FIG. 7-30 Thoracolumbar curve with hemivertebra. *(From Brier SR:* Primary care orthopedics, *St Louis, Mosby, 1999.)*

FIG. 7-31 Senile kyphosis. *(From Mercier LR, Pettid FJ:* Practical orthopedics, *ed 4, St Louis, 1995, Mosby.)*

- A positive sign is evidence of pathologic or structural scoliosis, and it indicates altered morphology, pathology, trauma, and subluxation.
- A posterior Adam's position requires the examiner to be behind the patient (Figs. 7-34 and 7-35).
- An anterior Adam's position requires the examiner to be in front of the patient (Fig. 7-36).

Confirmation Procedures
Postural assessment and diagnostic imaging

DIAGNOSTIC STATEMENT

An anterior Adam's position reveals mild left convex cervicothoracic scoliosis, without the rib humping sign.

A posterior Adam's position reveals a moderate right convex thoracolumbar scoliosis, with a marked rib humping sign.

CLINICAL PEARL

When the scoliotic curvature disappears in the Adam's position, the curves are mild to moderate, or less than 25 degrees. These curves have more of a functional component than a structural component and are amenable to conservative management.

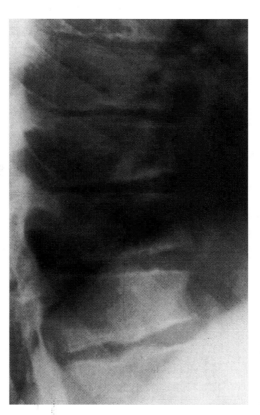

FIG. 7-32   Scheuermann's disease.   *(From Mercier LR, Pettid FJ: Practical orthopedics, ed 4, St Louis, 1995, Mosby.)*

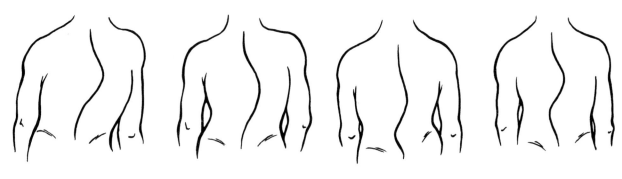

Right thoracic curve

Right thoracic lumbar curve

Left lumbar curve

Right thoracic and left lumbar curve (double major curve)

FIG. 7-33 Examples of scoliosis curve patterns. *(From Barkauskas VH, et al:* Health and physical assessment, *ed 2, St Louis, 1998, Mosby.)*

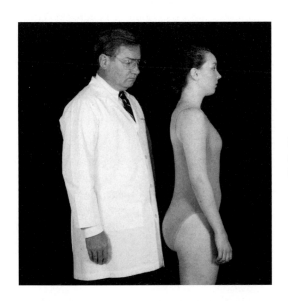

FIG. 7-34 The patient is standing. The examiner notes any spinal asymmetry, scapular winging, chest rotational deformity, and so forth.

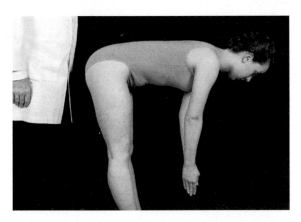

FIG. 7-35 For posterior Adam's position, the patient flexes forward at the waist. The arms are allowed to hang toward the floor, and the hands are placed together in a prayer position. The examiner, who is posterior to the patient, observes the thoracolumbar spine for deformity, which includes persistent scoliotic curvature, rib humping, and muscular atrophy.

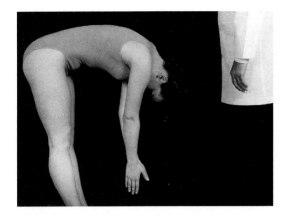

FIG. 7-36 In anterior Adam's position, the patient assumes the Adam's position by flexing the spine at the waist and also flexing the cervical spine. The examiner, who is anterior to the patient, observes for upper thoracic scoliosis defects.

AMOSS'S SIGN

Assessment for Ankylosing Spondylitis, Severe Sprain, or Intervertebral Disc Syndrome

Comment

The early erosive sclerotic changes of bone adjacent to the sacroiliac joints in ankylosing spondylitis are well recognized. Less well recognized is the fact that similar erosive sclerotic changes may on occasion involve the intervertebral disc and adjacent bone, producing a lesion termed *spondylodiscitis.*

The radiographic appearance of spondylodiscitis is fairly typical (Fig. 7-37). Erosion of the subchondral bony plates widens the disc space. The surrounding bone becomes sclerotic and radiodense. Either erosion or sclerosis may be more prominent. The reported incidence of spondylodiscitis is 5% to 6%. It occurs most frequently in the lower thoracic spine.

Ankylosing spondylitis, an ascending disease, affects the thoracic region after the lumbar. Patients with this condition experience back pain, but the anterolateral chest pain and the limited chest expansion are what bother them the most. In some, these symptoms may occur rather early in the life of the disease, but they usually become bothersome after 6 years of illness. Chest pain, which usually occurs during inspiration, and limited chest expansion are primarily caused by involvement of costovertebral and manubriosternal joints, as well as the costochondral junctions and the clavicular joints. The girdlelike restriction may cause a sense of anxiety and dyspnea, particularly upon exertion. However, respiratory problems are surprisingly uncommon, although restricted ventilatory volumes are detected by pulmonary function studies. Of course, should concomitant disease result in impaired diaphragmatic breathing, then a problem is likely to develop.

Tenderness is elicited over the manubriosternal joint, the costochondral junctions, and the entire dorsal spine. With more advanced disease, a dorsal kyphosis is evident, and the thoracic cage remains in the expiratory position. Chest expansion, normally no less than 1 inch in females and 1.5 inches in males, may be diminished by 50% or more. A football abdomen, a spherical protrusion, may result from abdominal breathing.

The posture of the hang-dog cervical spine, dorsal kyphosis with the chest cage fixed in expiration, straightening of the lumbar spine, marked flexion contractures of the hips and knees, and a gaze that is fixed on the floor are highly characteristic of the terminal stage of ankylosing spondylitis and should offer no problems with diagnosis.

Ankylosing spondylitis may be primarily or secondarily associated with a variety of conditions. Most of these disorders follow manifestation of spondylitis, but some may precede the actual onset of musculoskeletal symptoms by several months and occasionally by years. In some instances, these allied conditions may overlap one another. Aortitis may be found both in idiopathic ankylosing spondylitis and in Reiter's syndrome. Heel pain is common to psoriatic arthritis, Reiter's syndrome, and enteropathic arthropathy, whether or not there is associated inflammation of the spine. The detection of HLA-B27 antigen, not only in ankylosing spondylitis but also in Reiter's disease and psoriatic arthritis, creates an even closer relationship between these conditions.

PROCEDURE

- The recumbent patient places the hands far behind the body and tries to arise from the supine position to the seated position.
- The patient can also be in a side-lying position (Fig. 7-38).
- The examiner should note the patient's position of comfort and any spinal complaints that the patient presents.
- The patient arises from the side-lying position to a sitting position (Fig. 7-39).
- The sign is present when either action elicits a localized thoracic or thoracolumbar spinal pain.
- The sign suggests ankylosing spondylitis, severe sprain, or intervertebral disc syndrome.

Confirmation Procedures

Chest expansion test, Forestier's bowstring sign, clinical laboratory testing, and diagnostic imaging

---

DIAGNOSTIC STATEMENT

Amoss's sign is present and suggests the presence of ankylosing spondylitis. Further laboratory testing is warranted.

CLINICAL PEARL

It is occasionally observed that the patient defers to a side-lying posture when trying to stand after lying supine. This is Amoss's sign. Amoss's sign may not produce pain, but it reveals stiffness and lack of mobility and is still useful for detecting chronic spondylitis, which, at the least, requires imaging of the thoracolumbar spine.

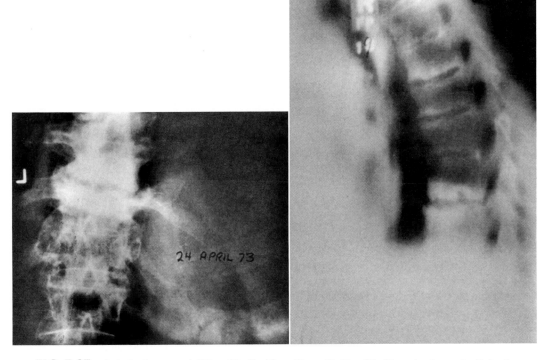

FIG. 7-37   Ankylosing spondylitis with discitis.   *(From Watkins RG:* The spine in sports, *St Louis, 1996, Mosby.)*

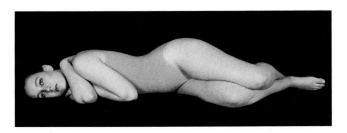

FIG. 7-38   The patient is in a side-lying position on the examining table. The examiner notes the position of comfort and any spinal complaints that the patient expresses.

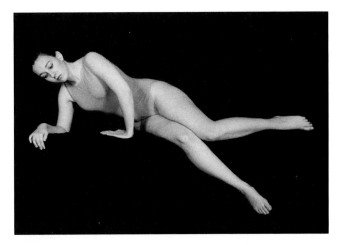

FIG. 7-39   The patient arises from the side-lying position to a seated position. The sign is present when this action elicits a localized thoracic or thoracolumbar spinal pain. The sign suggests ankylosing spondylitis, severe sprain, or intervertebral disc syndrome.

ANGHELESCU'S SIGN

Assessment for Tuberculosis of the Vertebrae or Other Destructive Processes of the Spine

Comment

Spinal infections are rare, constituting only 2% to 4% of all cases of osteomyelitis. Often, patients with vertebral osteomyelitis have few systemic symptoms, such as fever or sepsis, and may have normal white blood cell counts; therefore delay in diagnosis is not uncommon. A high index of suspicion is necessary to accurately diagnose spinal infections in the early stages.

With tuberculous spondylitis, any single vertebra or several vertebrae may be involved. The disease most often involves the lower thoracic and the lumbar spine. The infection starts in the cancellous bone area of the vertebral body. Most commonly, an exudative reaction with marked hyperemia produces severe generalized osteoporosis. The body softens and easily yields to compression forces. In the thoracic spine, normal kyphotic curve increases the pressure on the vertebrae anteriorly, and anterior wedging is severe. An angular kyphosis results if the vertebral body is crushed.

The infection advances and destroys the epiphyseal cortex, the intervertebral disc, and the adjacent vertebrae. The infective exudate may spread anteriorly beneath the anterior longitudinal ligament to reach the neighboring vertebrae.

Infection of the posterior bony arch and the transverse processes is unusual. More commonly, granulation tissue develops and compresses the spinal cord and the nerve roots. Pressure on nerve structures is more likely in the thoracic spine, where the caliber of the spinal canal is small. Sequestra and bone fragments do not often extrude into the canal, limited by the strong posterior longitudinal ligament.

The most common vertebral infection is an exudative type that constitutes a severe hypergic reaction. This causes an extreme degree of osteoporosis that spreads rapidly. Abscess formation is common, and constitutional symptoms are pronounced.

PROCEDURE

- Anghelescu's sign is for identifying tuberculosis of the vertebrae or other destructive processes of the spine.
- In the supine position, the patient places weight on the head and heels while lifting the body upward (Fig. 7-40).
- Inability to hyperextend the spine indicates a disease process (Fig. 7-41).

Confirmation Procedures

Chest expansion test, Forestier's bowstring sign, clinical laboratory testing, and diagnostic imaging

---

DIAGNOSTIC STATEMENT

Anghelescu's sign is present and strongly suggests tuberculous spondylitis. Further laboratory testing and diagnostic images are warranted.

CLINICAL PEARL

When testing for Anghelescu's sign, the loss of the ability to achieve a near opisthotonos posture is significant. Although the true opisthotonos posture involves the cervical spine, very few patients normally have enough strength in the neck to accomplish this.

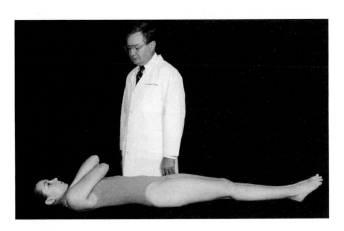

FIG. 7-40 The patient is supine on the examining table. The examiner observes for postural symmetry and notes any positions of antalgia.

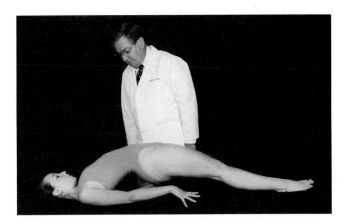

FIG. 7-41 From the supine position, the patient attempts to extend the thoracic spine sufficiently to raise it from the table. Without thoracic spinal pathology, the patient will be able to rest the weight of the body on the heels and the shoulders (a near opisthotonos posture). This position cannot be achieved in tuberculous spondylitis.

BEEVOR'S SIGN

Assessment for Myelopathy Associated with the T10 Spinal Level

Comment

Probably the most important diagnosis to make in thoracic and thoracic-radiating pain is that of a thoracic disc herniation. The incidence of thoracic disc herniation is 1 in 1 million. Pressure on the exiting thoracic nerve at that level produces pain in the chest and back. Pressure on or damage to the spinal cord carries the grave risk of permanent cord injury. A thoracic disc herniation can result in paraplegia, with weakness and numbness in the legs and complete loss of bowel, bladder, sexual, and leg function. Up to 50% of patients with thoracic disc herniation can have significant spinal cord injury.

Thoracic disc herniation may present with a great variety of symptoms. In the lower thoracic spine, a flaccid neurologic loss may occur rather than the spastic presentation of an upper thoracic disc herniation, and it often mimics lumbar spine disease. Lower herniated thoracic disc may present with the signs and symptoms of neurogenic claudication or sciatica. Upper thoracic disc herniations at T1-T2 or T2-T3 may present as a cervical spine problem, with pain radiating to the medial aspect of the arm, hand, and shoulder, with possible intrinsic hand weakness and/or Horner's syndrome.

Within the thoracic spine, there is overlap of dermatomes. The dermatomes follow the ribs, and the absence of only one dermatome may lead to no loss in sensation at all.

Absence of the abdominal reflexes may be an early sign of corticospinal disease, which is a common sign of multiple sclerosis but is by no means pathognomonic of this disease. When the abdominal reflexes are absent, hyperreflexia of the lower extremities and the Babinski sign are present.

The fifth thoracic (T5) segment is at the level of the nipple, T10 at the umbilicus, and T12 at the groin.

The motor and sensory roots become progressively longer as they proceed from their respective cord segments to their points of exit.

Acute postinfectious polyneuropathy (Guillain-Barré syndrome), an acute idiopathic polyneuritis, is a disease of unknown origin characterized by rapid onset of ascending weakness with associated sensory disturbance. All races, all age groups, and both sexes are susceptible to this disease. Peripheral nerve demyelination and often a mononuclear inflammatory reaction characterize the pathologic picture. There are numerous theories as to causation of this disease. One theory is that the disease results from an autoimmune reaction against a peripheral nerve antigen, specifically myelin. Other theories postulate that the disease is secondary to a bacterial, viral, or neurotoxic substance. About half of the cases of acute postinfectious polyneuropathy will occur after an upper respiratory or gastrointestinal infection.

The typical medical history includes an acute upper respiratory illness followed by a few days of pins-and-needles paresthesia, followed by lower extremity weakness, which is characteristically a symmetrically ascending motor weakness accompanied by minimal sensory changes and intact sphincter control. Aching or tenderness may be present, but neither is a prominent feature. A minority of patients exhibits profound sensory losses. Temporary bowel or bladder paralysis may occur but occurs in a lesser degree than the lower extremity paralysis. The disease may ascend to involve the bulbar muscles, resulting in respiratory paralysis and death. The course of the disease ranges from several days to a week. If the patient survives the first 2 weeks, the prognosis is good. Motor power returns gradually over the course of a year.

PROCEDURE

- Beevor's sign, although not an abdominal reflex, is seen during an examination.
- In this test, the recumbent patient lifts his or her head off the examining table (Figs. 7-42 and 7-43).
- Normally, the upper and lower abdominal muscles contract equally and the umbilicus does not move or drift.
- When the lower abdominal muscles alone are weakened, the umbilicus will be drawn upward by the contraction of the intact upper musculature (Figs. 7-44 and 7-45).
- This effect is associated with a spinal cord lesion at the T10 level.

Confirmation Procedures

Sensory assessment, reflex testing, electrodiagnosis, and diagnostic imaging (magnetic resonance imaging [MRI])

DIAGNOSTIC STATEMENT

Beevor's sign is present, as demonstrated by cephalad-umbilical drift. This sign reveals lower abdominal muscular weakness and suggests myelopathy associated with the T10 spinal level.

CLINICAL PEARL

In the presence of prolonged illness followed by lower extremity paresthesia (regardless of how minor), this test needs to be performed. Beevor's sign affords an early, noninvasive indicator of the existence of thoracic spinal cord myelopathy.

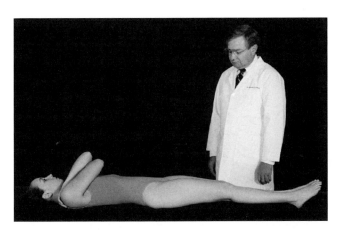

FIG. 7-42   The patient is supine on the examining table. The abdominal muscles are palpated, and the position of the umbilicus established.

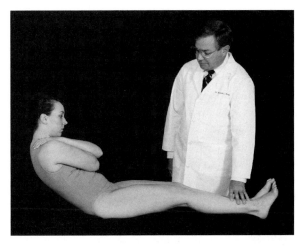

FIG. 7-43   The examiner fixes the patient's legs to the table with mild downward pressure. The patient performs a partial sit-up, with the arms folded across the chest. The examiner notes any drift of the umbilicus. During a sit-up, the uppermost fibers of the abdominal musculature are primarily the ones tested. Drift occurs toward the stronger or uninvolved musculature. Cephalad drift implicates lower thoracic spine involvement. Caudad drift implicates upper thoracic spine involvement, but not above T7.

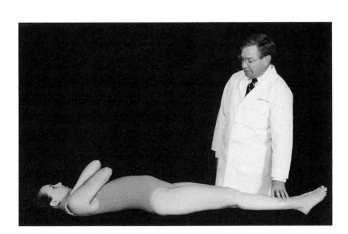

FIG. 7-44   If extensive abdominal muscle weakness or paresis exists, the back will arch from the table as the patient attempts the partial sit-up. The thorax may pull away from the pelvis until it is firmly fixed by extension of the thoracic spine. The arching of the back stretches the abdominal muscles, and they may appear firm under tension. The examiner needs to be careful not to mistake this tautness for firmness resulting from actual contraction of the muscles.

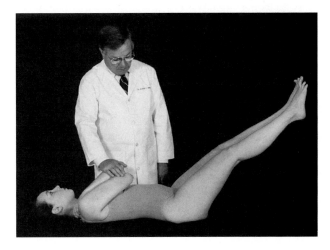

FIG. 7-45   As an alternative, the patient can perform a partial bilateral leg lift to test the abdominal musculature. In this procedure, the examiner can apply a mild downward pressure to the patient's thorax, fixing it to the examining table for stability. Umbilical drift is noted. Leg-lifting primarily tests the lowermost fibers of the abdominal musculature.

CHEST EXPANSION TEST

Assessment for Spinal Ankylosis

Comment

Children breathe abdominally. Women perform upper thoracic breathing. Men are upper and lower thoracic breathers. In the aged, the breathing is in the lower thoracic and abdominal regions. Chest wall movement that occurs during breathing displaces the pleural surfaces, thorax musculature, nerves, and ribs. Breathing and coughing accentuate pain if any of these structures are injured.

In pectus carinatum (pigeon chest), the sternum projects more anterior and inferior. This deformity increases the AP dimension of the chest and can impair ventilation volume.

In pectus excavatum (funnel chest), the sternum is displaced posteriorly by an overgrowth of the ribs. The AP dimension of the chest is decreased. The heart is displaced or compressed.

In barrel chest, often associated with emphysema, the sternum projects anterior and superior and the AP chest diameter is increased.

Ankylosing spondylitis is a disease of the spine. It occurs in late adolescence or early adulthood and is characterized pathologically by progressive inflammation of the spine, sacroiliac joints, and the larger joints of the extremities—particularly the hips, knees, and shoulders—leading to fibrous or bony ankylosis and deformity.

Ankylosing spondylitis starts insidiously in a young adult. Symptoms at first are vague and poorly localized. Aching and stiffness around both sacroiliac joints occur as a morning backache that subsides with activity but returns after sitting in one position for prolonged periods. The pain and stiffness become progressively worse and spread slowly, within 6 months to a year, to the rest of the spine. Limitation of motion appears first in the lower spine but is finally notable throughout the spine. Chest expansion is restricted because of disease of the costovertebral joints.

The early roentgenographic features usually are those of bilateral sacroiliitis. Eventually, there may be complete fusion of the sacroiliac and hip joints as healing takes place following the inflammation. As the disease progresses, calcifications of the anulus fibrosis and paravertebral ligaments develop, which give rise to the so-called bamboo-spine appearance characteristic of ankylosing spondylitis (Fig. 7-46). The HLA-B27 antigen is important in the diagnosis of ankylosing spondylitis. This antigen occurs in nearly 100% of Caucasian patients with ankylosing spondylitis.

PROCEDURE

- The chest diameter is measured at the level of the fourth intercostal space.
- The measurement is taken as the patient exhales maximally (Fig. 7-47).
- A second measurement is made as the patient inhales deeply (Fig. 7-48).
- The normal difference between inspiration and expiration is 5.75 to 7.62 cm (1.5 to 3 inches).

Confirmation Procedures

Amoss's sign, Forestier's bowstring sign, clinical laboratory testing, range-of-motion testing, spirometer testing, and diagnostic imaging of the pelvis and sacroiliac joints

---

DIAGNOSTIC STATEMENT

Chest expansion in this female patient is 1.91 cm (0.75 inches), which suggests thoracic involvement by ankylosing spondylitis.

Chest expansion in this male patient is 2.54 cm (1 inch), which suggests the existence of ankylosing spondylitis that affects the thoracic spine.

CLINICAL PEARL

Chest expansion measurements are sensitive indicators of early involvement of the costovertebral joints in ankylosing spondylitis. The chest expansion test is often positive before the patient realizes a change in chest comfort.

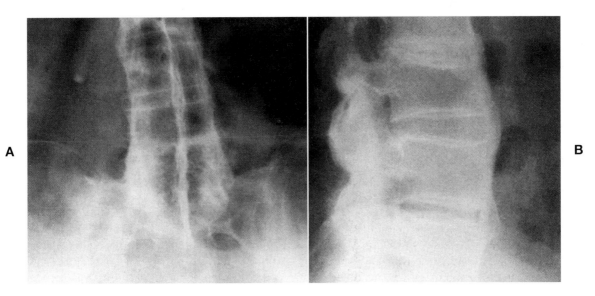

FIG. 7-46   Ankylosing spondylitis. **A,** Anteroposterior view. **B,** Lateral view.   *(From Mercier LR, Pettid FJ: Practical orthopedics, ed 4, St Louis, 1995, Mosby.)*

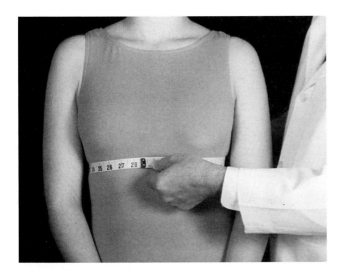

FIG. 7-47   The patient is standing with the arms at the sides. The examiner places a tape measure around the patient's chest at any of the following points: (1) at the fourth intercostal space, (2) at the axillary level, (3) at the level of the nipples, or (4) at the T10 rib level. The patient exhales maximally, and the chest diameter is measured.

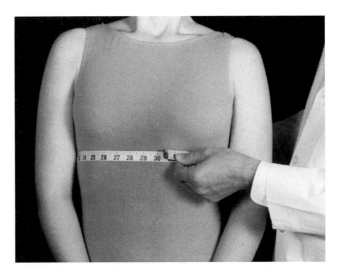

FIG. 7-48   The patient inhales deeply, and a second measurement is made. The normal difference between inspiration and expiration is 5.75 to 7.62 cm (1.5 to 3 inches). Decreases, in the absence of trauma, suggest ankylosing spondylitis.

Assessment for First or Second Thoracic Nerve Root Involvement

Comment

Thoracic disc herniations are rare, seen in less than 0.3% of the population, and affect both men and women equally from the fourth through the sixth decades of life. The most common segments affected are between the ninth and twelfth thoracic vertebrae.

Central disc prolapse generally produces symptoms of spastic paraparesis, increased deep tendon reflexes, and a positive Babinski response. However, lateral thoracic disc protrusions produce signs more consistent with nerve root compression.

ORTHOPEDIC GAMUT 7-6

NERVOUS SYSTEM

The four components of the nervous system that refer pain or discomfort follow:

1. The spinal cord
2. The dural sleeve of a nerve root
3. The nerve trunk
4. A peripheral or cutaneous nerve

Compression of the spinal cord usually results in paresthesias (pins and needles) that are bilateral and disregard segmentation of the body. Other associated neural structures, compressed simultaneously, cause pain that follows dermatome patterns.

At the point of emergence from the dura, a dural sleeve invests the nerve root. Pressure on the dural sleeve produces discomfort. Pain occurs in all or any part of the dermatome. Paresthesia, a compression phenomenon, occurs at the distal end of the dermatome. Paresthesia often conspicuously occupies an area supplied by multiple nerve roots. The paresthesia has no edge or depth, and numbness displaces paresthesia. Pressure on a nerve root causes analgesia. Minimal pressure evokes paresthesia.

Weakness results from compression of the nerve root within the parenchyma. Weakness is discernible during resisted movements.

In compression of a nerve root, pressure on the surrounding dural sleeve, at the transverse process, will hurt. Impaired conduction along a nerve leads to muscle weakness, manifested during resisted movements. Paresthesia

rather than numbness represents a release phenomenon. The lesion always lies proximal to the upper edge of the paresthetic area.

In compression of a peripheral nerve or cutaneous nerve, numbness, rather than paresthesia, occupies the cutaneous area supplied by the nerve. The edge is well defined, and toward the center of the area, full anesthesia is often demonstrable.

The dura mater does not conform to the rules of segmental reference. The dura mater descends from the foramen magnum of the skull to the inferior edge of the first or second sacral vertebra. The dura mater keeps the spinal cord buffered in cerebrospinal fluid. From the dura mater protrude 30 pairs of nerve roots covered by the dural sheath.

Compression or stretching of the dura mater causes extrasegmentally referred pain. The dura mater is adjacent to the intervertebral discs and vulnerable to posterior pressure exerted by the posterior longitudinal ligament.

Dura mater pain often pervades many dermatomes simultaneously. This pain is a common cause of scapular pain, and the symptoms are usually central or unilateral. Pressure on the dura mater at thoracic levels may radiate pain to the base of the neck, and this pain also may radiate to the posterior or anterior aspect of the trunk. The pain will spread over many dermatomes simultaneously. The symptoms usually are central or unilateral.

Pressure on the dura mater at lumbar levels may cause pain that reaches the lower thorax in the posterior, the lower abdomen, the upper buttocks, the sacrum, and the coccyx. Again, many dermatomes may be occupied simultaneously.

Pain perceived elsewhere in places other than its true site is referred pain. Nearly all pain is referred. The examiner's task is to determine the origin of the pain.

The sensory cortex determines the site where symptoms are referred. The sensory cortex attributes the impulses it receives to the appropriate areas of the body. With stimuli to the skin, the sensory cortex achieves a high degree of accuracy. Over time, a stimulus reaching certain cells in the cortex is interpreted as damage in a specific area of the skin.

The same cortical cells receive a painful stimulus arising from a deep-seated structure. The sensory cortex interprets this new impulse based on experience. Pain is referred to the area of skin served by those particular cortical cells.

The area of skin associated with sensory cells is the dermatome. The dermatome corresponds to the embryologic neural segment from which the structure was derived. Thus the sensory cortex will refer a pain in tissue of T5 segmental origin to the T5 dermatome and from the T8 structure to the T8 dermatome.

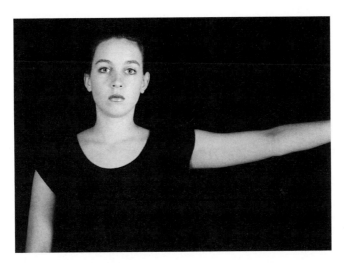

FIG. 7-49   The patient is seated and abducts the shoulder to 90 degrees. The arm is pronated.

The 40 dermatome segments of a 1-month-old fetus are distributed horizontally. At this stage, the dermatomes are superimposed directly over the segments from which they are derived. The growth of the four limbs draws the dermatomes down the arms and the legs. However, in the trunk, the original arrangement of circular dermatome bands remains intact.

PROCEDURE

- Pain from stretching the first thoracic nerve root via the ulnar nerve identifies the T1 or T2 roots.
- Disc lesions at either level are rarities and are not accompanied by easily identifiable neurologic signs.
- If weakness is present, the possibility of serious disease should be considered.
- The affected arm is abducted to 90 degrees. The elbow is flexed with the pronated forearm to 90 degrees (Figs. 7-49 to 7-51).

- The patient places the hand behind the neck (Fig. 7-52).
- The ulnar nerve and the T1 nerve root are stretched.
- A positive test is indicated by scapular pain on the ipsilateral side.

Confirmation Procedures
Cervical range of motion, thoracic spinal range of motion, reflex testing, sensory assessment, electrodiagnosis, Roos' test, and diagnostic imaging

---

DIAGNOSTIC STATEMENT

Stretch of the first thoracic nerve root is positive on the left because scapular pain is produced. This result indicates nerve root compression at T1.

ORTHOPEDIC GAMUT 7-7

PAIN REFERRAL

Pain referral rules are as follows:

1. Pain refers segmentally. A T5 tissue refers pain to the T5 dermatome. Pain can occupy all or any part of the dermatome. If the patient describes symptoms straddling more than one dermatome or if the pain migrates from one dermatome to another, four possibilities arise: (a) The patient is describing a nonorganic pain; (b) the lesion itself is shifting, which often happens with vertebral element displacements; (c) the lesion is spreading, as in metastasis; or (d) the pain stems from a tissue that cannot refer pain segmentally. An exception of importance is the dura mater, which refers pain extrasegmentally.
2. Pain refers distally. The source of symptoms is sought locally or proximally.
3. Referred pain does not cross the midline. A T5 left rib will not cause discomfort on the right side of the body. A pain felt centrally must originate from a

central structure. Pain that cannot be accounted for by a unilateral structure must be sought centrally. A pain alternating from one side of the body to the other must have a central source. That central source must be able to shift from one side to the other, such as during an intervertebral disc displacement.
4. The extent of pain reference is controlled. The referred pain is controlled by the size of the dermatome and the position in the dermatome of the tissue lesion. A large dermatome permits greater reference than a small one. A lesion in the proximal part of the dermatome refers pain farther than a lesion in the distal part.
5. The more intense the pain the greater the number of cortical cells excited. The spread to adjacent cells in the sensory cortex is interpreted as an enlargement of the painful area.
6. The deeper a soft-tissue lesion lies, the larger the reference to be expected. However, bone lesions produce minimal pain radiation.

CLINICAL PEARL

The first thoracic nerve root stretch indicates nerve root compression. This stretch can also indicate the existence of an inflammation of the lower two branches of the brachial plexus, a nonvascular thoracic outlet syndrome. This diagnosis is further confirmed by Roos' test.

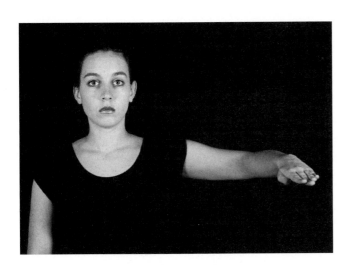

FIG. 7-50 The elbow is flexed to 90 degrees.

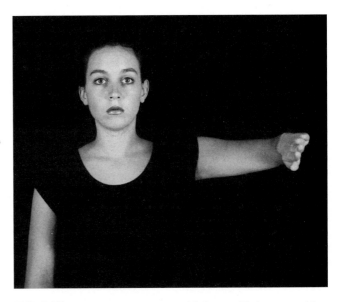

FIG. 7-51 The forearm is pronated fully to a 90-degree position, which should not be uncomfortable at this point.

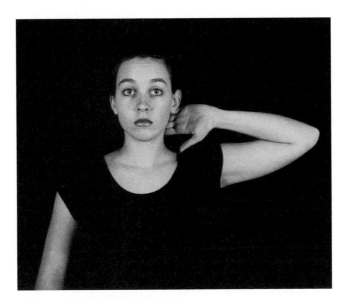

FIG. 7-52 The elbow is fully flexed, and the pronated hand is placed behind the head. Pain elicited in the scapular region suggests T1 nerve root involvement.

FORESTIER'S BOWSTRING SIGN

Assessment for Ankylosing Spondylitis

Comment
It is well recognized that severe flexion deformities of the spine may occur in patients with ankylosing spondylitis.

ORTHOPEDIC GAMUT 7-8

THORACIC KYPHOSIS

Patients with thoracic kyphosis are classified into the following two groups:

1. In the first group, there is a major increase in thoracic kyphosis, with an associated loss of lumbar lordosis and a rigid spine. With sufficient extension of the lumbar spine, compensation can be achieved for the thoracic kyphosis, allowing a horizontal gaze and erect posture (Fig. 7-53).
2. Patients in the second group have thoracic kyphotic deformity but maintain a normal or even increased (compensatory) cervical and lumbar lordosis.

Ankylosing spondylitis is an inflammation of the joints of the spine that often results in bony ankylosis. The process is chronic, usually low grade, and begins mainly in young men. Early symptoms include pain and stiffness of the back; later, there is disability because of the so-called poker spine.

On one hand, ankylosing spondylitis is a disease of the cartilaginous and fibrocartilaginous joints of the spine. On the other hand, the disease affects the diarthrodial articulations, such as the sacroiliac joint, the hips, and the shoulders. Ankylosing spondylitis is primarily an axial disease. However, in approximately 35% of the patients, peripheral involvement of the hands, knees, ankles, and other joints does occur and is sometimes the first manifestation of the disease. However, it is rare that peripheral arthritis results in significant deformity. All axial joints, including the manubriosternal, costovertebral, and symphysis pubis, may be affected.

Although ankylosing spondylitis is an entity distinct from rheumatoid arthritis, the early pathologic changes are similar. Like rheumatoid arthritis, ankylosing spondylitis is a synovial disease characterized grossly by proliferative granulation tissue, adhesions of the joint, and probably a greater tendency for fibrous and bony ankylosis. The earliest findings of the disease are found in the sacroiliac joint and typify those also seen in the apophyseal joints of the lumbar, dorsal, and cervical spine as well as the shoulders, hips, costovertebral, manubriosternal, and symphysis pubis articulations. Joint spaces are initially widened because of proliferative synovitis that gives way to erosive changes of the articular margins, narrowing, and then fusion.

There may be no semblance of a joint. The histologic counterpart of these findings is synovial membrane thickening with plasma cell and lymphocyte infiltration that are arranged in nests surrounding the smaller synovial blood vessels. Foci of chronic inflammation also may be found in adjacent bone, usually independent of the synovial process.

Most of the patient's discomfort and disability are caused by involvement of the dorsolumbar spine, albeit the sacroiliacs are concomitantly affected. Muscle pains, initially diffuse, may become increasingly concentrated in the dorsolumbar region. Stiffness is profound at times. Bending, lifting, and turning become formidable chores. Examination usually shows mild to severe direct tenderness of the dorsolumbar apophyseal joints, marked paravertebral muscle spasm, straightening of the lumbar spine, and sometimes an ironed-out appearance caused by muscle atrophy. Limitation of motion can be marked even if symptoms are minimal or absent.

The normal arching of the spine during flexion is lost, but this may not be fully appreciated because of the compensatory flexion at the hips. Lateral flexion of the dorsolumbar spine cannot be disguised so well. It is sometimes lost. Minor limitations of motion can be confirmed by marking a point 10 cm above the fifth lumbar process and measuring the linear distance between the fifth lumbar spinous process and this point during flexion and extension. The distance should normally increase by 5 cm (2 inches) or more (Schober test). Spondylitis of the dorsolumbar area, even if a fixed ankylosis ensues, usually does not pose a serious threat of disability.

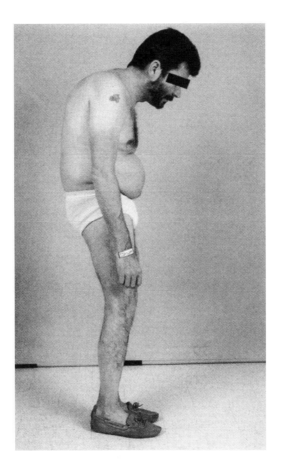

FIG. 7-53 Ankylosing spondylitis. *(From Watkins RG:* The spine
in sports, *St Louis, 1996, Mosby.)*

Patients who seek help because of the apparent spinal deformity may have their main deformity in the hip joints, the lumbar spine, or the thoracic spine, or it may be primarily cervical in situation (Fig. 7-54). The most reliable measure of trunk deformity is the chin-brow to vertical angle. This is a measure of the angle formed by a line from the brow to the chin through the vertical, when the patient stands with the hips and knees extended, and the neck in its neutral or fixed position (Fig. 7-55).

PROCEDURE

- The standing patient performs side bending and reveals ipsilateral tightening and contracture of the paraspinal musculature (Figs. 7-56 and 7-57).

- Normally, the contralateral musculature demonstrates tightening (Fig. 7-58).
- The test is significant for ankylosing spondylitis.

Confirmation Procedures

Amoss's sign, Anghelescu's sign, chest expansion test, clinical laboratory testing, and diagnostic imaging

DIAGNOSTIC STATEMENT

Forestier's bowstring sign is present on the left. This sign suggests the presence of ankylosing spondylitis in the thoracolumbar spine.

CLINICAL PEARL

Although the presence of Forestier's bowstring sign suggests spondylitis, this test also indicates strain and intervertebral disc involvement. Any loss of symmetric motion must be examined further.

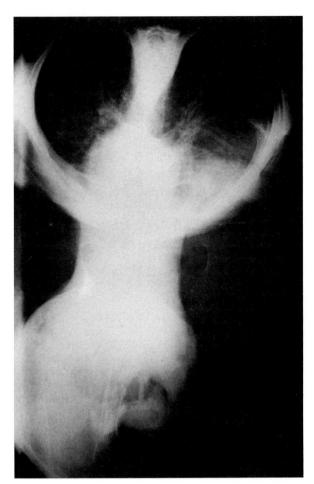

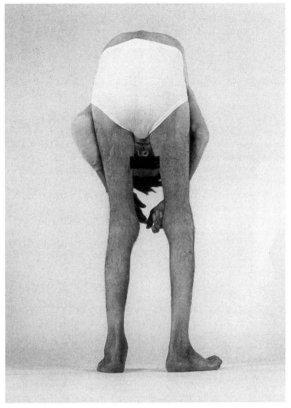

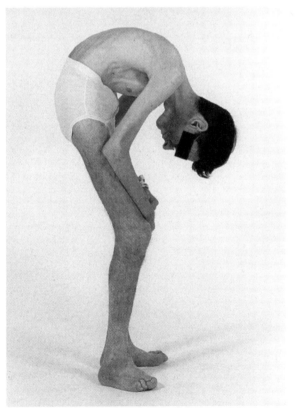

FIG. 7-54   Ankylosing spondylitis demonstrating complexity of spinal deformity.   *(From Watkins RG: The spine in sports, St Louis, 1996, Mosby.)*

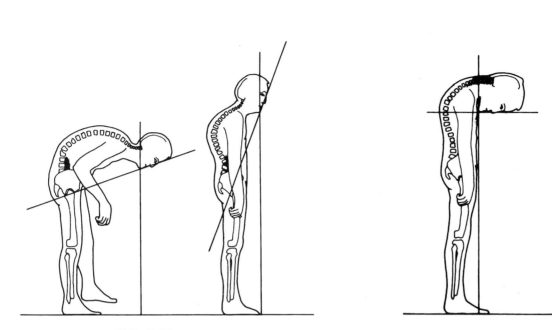

FIG. 7-55 Measurement of the degree of kyphotic deformity of the spine in ankylosing spondylitis using the chin-to-vertical angle. *(From Watkins RG:* The spine in sports, *St Louis, 1996, Mosby.)*

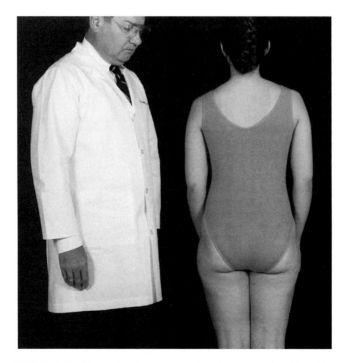

FIG. 7-56 The patient is standing with the arms at the sides. The examiner notes any loss of symmetry of the spinal musculature and notes the posture.

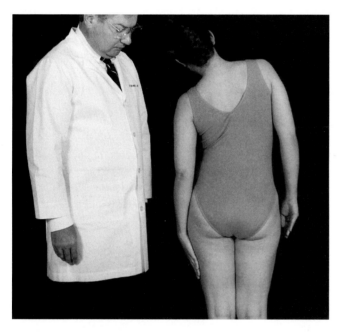

FIG. 7-57 The patient flexes the thoracic spine laterally. The sign is present when there is tightening or contracture of the musculature on the same side as flexion. This suggests ankylosing spondylitis.

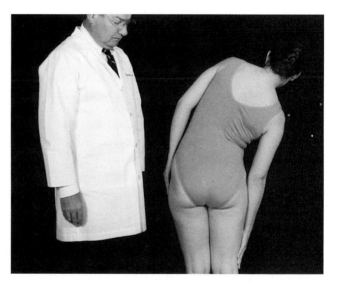

FIG. 7-58 The lateral flexion is compared bilaterally. Motion toward the opposite side is expected to produce normal tightening on the contralateral side. Overall, this tightening represents asymmetric motion of the thoracic spine.

PASSIVE SCAPULAR APPROXIMATION TEST

Assessment for T1 or T2 Nerve Root Problem

Comment
The scapular reflex is a contraction of the scapular muscles upon stimulation of the interscapular region. This reflex demonstrates the integrity of the cord between the upper two or three dorsal and lower two or three cervical nerves. However, only a third of the patients exhibit a good reflex response. The examiner should observe the quality of the skin's vascular response following the reflex stimulus. Each side should be equally hyperemic.

The dorsal (erector spinae) reflex is a local contraction of the erector spinae musculature that follows stimulation of the skin along the border of the muscle. This reflex demonstrates integrity of the dorsal region of cord.

These reflexes are carried out by stimulating the respective area with a Wartenberg pinwheel or a reflex hammer. Reflexes are examined bilaterally.

In acute intervertebral disc herniation, sequestered disc fragments are forced into the spinal canal. Although compression of the theca may be slight, impingement of the anterior median longitudinal artery, an end artery, produces ischemia of the spinal cord over several segments.

The critical zone of the spinal cord is that portion of the cord that lies within the area of the spinal canal extending from the vertebral segments T4 to T9. This portion of the spinal canal is the narrowest zone of the canal and corresponds to that part of the cord possessing the least amount of vascular supply. Therefore the spinal cord may be compromised by two factors: compression and interruption of the vascular supply. Ischemia produces edema and central necrosis of the cord.

Injury to the long thoracic nerve often occurs along with sprain or other injury at the base of the neck. The long thoracic nerve comes directly off the nerve roots and does not participate in the brachial plexus. The nerve passes down and supplies the various striations of the serratus anterior. Bruising or damage to this nerve may occur and pass unrecognized until distressing winging of the scapula is noted. The cause of this winging may be a sharp blow at the base of the neck that laterally impinges the nerve against the lower cervical vertebrae. Because the long thoracic nerve is primarily a motor nerve, there is usually little pain or discomfort to guide the examiner. There may be weakness or complete paralysis of the nerve, resulting in loss of fixation of the scapula to the chest wall.

PROCEDURE
- The examiner passively approximates the patient's scapulae (Fig. 7-59).
- Ipsilateral T1 or T2 nerve root problem is indicated by scapular pain (Fig. 7-60).

Confirmation Procedures
First thoracic nerve root test, Roos' test, electrodiagnosis, and diagnostic imaging

---

DIAGNOSTIC STATEMENT

Passive scapular approximation test is positive on the right (or left). This result suggests a compression syndrome at the T1 or T2 nerve root.

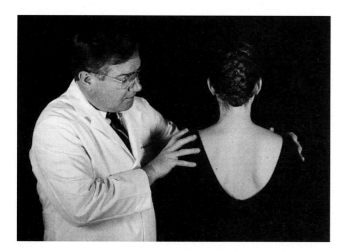

FIG. 7-59 The patient is standing, with the arms at the sides. The examiner observes for thoracic spinal symmetry and posture.

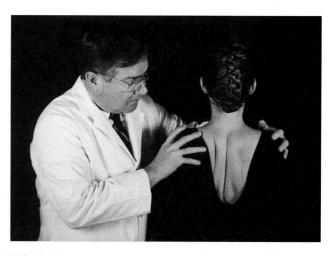

FIG. 7-60 The examiner approximates the scapulae by pulling the shoulder tips backward. Pain in the scapular area indicates a T1 or T2 nerve root involvement.

RIB MOTION TEST

Assessment for Hypermobile or Hypomobile Costal Structures

Comment

The costocorporeal articulation is a joint between the head of a rib and the adjoining typical thoracic vertebrae.

The ligaments of the costotransverse articulation include the articular capsule, costotransverse ligament (both described previously), superior costotransverse ligament, and lateral costotransverse ligament.

The costovertebral joints are synovial joints that are found between the ribs and the vertebral body (Fig. 7-61). There are 24 of these joints, and they are divided into two parts. Ribs 1, 10, 11, and 12 form joints with a single vertebra. Ribs 2 through 9 have an intraarticular ligament. The intraarticular ligament divides the joint into two parts, so each rib forms a joint with two adjacent vertebrae. Ribs 2 through 9 also articulate with the intervening intervertebral disc.

The costotransverse joints are synovial joints found between the ribs and the transverse processes of the vertebrae for ribs 1 through 10. Ribs 11 and 12 do not form a joint with the transverse processes. Therefore this joint does not exist at these two levels.

The costochondral joints are formed between the ribs and the costal cartilage. The sternocostal joints are found between the costal cartilage and the sternum. The costochondral joints of ribs 2 through 6 are synovial. The first rib costal cartilage is united with the sternum by a synchondrosis and is not synovial. Ribs form joints with an adjacent rib or costal cartilage. At each of these articulations, a synovial interchondral joint exists.

The ribs help stiffen the thoracic spine. The ribs articulate with the demifacets on vertebrae T2 to T9. For T1 and T10 vertebrae, there is a complete facet for ribs 1 and 10, respectively. The first rib forms a joint with T1 only, the second rib with T1 and T2, and so on.

Ribs 1 through 7 articulate with the sternum directly and are classified as true ribs. Ribs 8, 9, and 10 join with the costocartilage of the rib above and are classified as false ribs. Ribs 11 and 12 are classified as floating ribs because they do not attach to the sternum or costal cartilages at their distal ends.

Ribs 11 and 12 form joints only with the bodies of T11 and T12 vertebrae. These ribs do not have a joint with the transverse processes of the vertebrae or with the costocartilage of the rib above. The ribs are held by ligaments to the body of the vertebrae and to the transverse processes of the same vertebrae. Some of these ligaments also bind the ribs to the vertebrae above.

At the top of the rib cage, the ribs are horizontal. As the rib cage descends, the ribs become more and more oblique. Rib 12 is more vertical than horizontal. During inspiration, the ribs are pulled up and forward. The first six ribs increase the AP dimension of the chest, mainly by rotating around their long axes. Downward rotation of the rib neck is associated with depression of the chest. Upward rotation of the same portion of the ribs is associated with chest elevation. Collectively, these motions are known as the *pump handle action.* These movements are accompanied by elevation of the manubrium and sternum, superior and anterior.

Ribs 7 through 10 mainly increase lateral, or transverse, dimension. The ribs move superiorly, posteriorly, and medially to increase the infrasternal angle, or inferiorly, anteriorly, and laterally to decrease the angle. These movements are known as the *bucket handle action.*

Ribs 8 through 12 move laterally in a caliper action that increases the lateral dimension.

The ribs are elastic in children but become increasingly brittle with age. In the anterior half of the chest, the ribs are subcutaneous. In the posterior half, the ribs are covered by muscles.

PROCEDURE

- As the supine patient inhales and exhales, the AP movement of the ribs is palpated (Fig. 7-62).
- Restriction in motion is noted.
- Rib abnormalities during exhalation suggest an elevated rib (lowest rib).
- Rib abnormalities during inhalation suggest a depressed rib (uppermost rib).

Confirmation Procedures

Chest expansion test, sternal compression test, and diagnostic imaging

---

DIAGNOSTIC STATEMENT

Rib motion for ribs 5 to 7 on the right is inhibited during inhalation. This result suggests a depressed fifth rib.

Rib motion for ribs 5 to 7 on the right is inhibited during exhalation. This inhibition of movement suggests an elevated seventh rib.

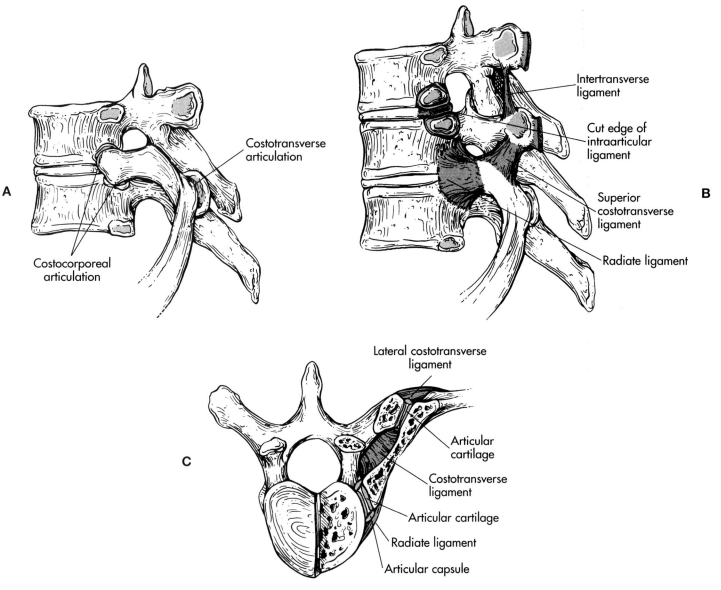

FIG. 7-61 Costovertebral articulations. **A,** Bony costocorporeal and costotransverse articulations. **B,** Ligamentous attachments of these joints. **C,** Superior view.   *(From Cramer GD, Darby SA: Basic and clinical anatomy of the spine, spinal cord, and ANS, St Louis, 1995, Mosby.)*

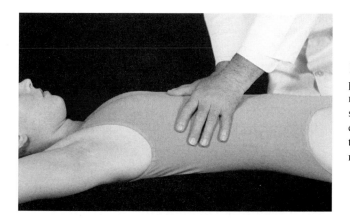

FIG. 7-62   With the patient supine, the examiner's hands are placed over the chest. The examiner feels for the anteroposterior movement of the ribs as the patient inhales and exhales. Any restriction or difference in motion is noted. Rib abnormalities during exhalation suggest an elevated rib. Rib abnormalities during inhalation suggest a depressed rib. A depressed rib is usually the uppermost rib. An elevated rib is usually the lowest rib.

SCHEPELMANN'S SIGN

Assessment for Costal and Intercostal Tissue Integrity

Comment

Any fixation or aberrant movement of the costovertebral articulations, or ribs, can have an impact on the synovial joints of the dorsal spine. It is not uncommon to find concomitant loss of joint play at the rib angle and corresponding vertebral motor unit. It is suggested that the rib cage may act as a splint to the thoracic spine. This splinting effect may prevent stresses placed directly on the midspine. In addition, it may be one of the reasons that thoracic disc herniations are less common. The fully developed ribs protect the underlying thoracic viscera, while simultaneously providing attachment sites for a wide variety of muscles (Table 7-4).

Because a multitude of muscles attach to the chest, almost any manifestation of strain may occur. Strain may be caused by violent exertion or by overstretching of the muscles. The symptoms depend entirely on the area involved. In the long muscles of the back of the thorax, this condition may be indistinguishable from or may be a part of a lumbar strain. In the front of the chest, the strain may involve the muscles of the abdominal wall, where the muscles attach to the lower ribs. Strain also may involve the intercostal muscles, although this is uncommon because the muscles are well protected by other muscle structures. These muscles do not act forcibly enough to rupture their fibers. A strain is much more likely to involve an area connecting to the chest than the chest itself. This is particularly true of the scapular muscles. Strain of the rhomboids will occur either at the scapular attachment or along the spine much more often than at the costal attachment. Similarly, the serrati may be more likely to get injured in their substance than in their costal origins. Careful analysis of the active motion that causes pain will usually determine the proper muscle group.

Strain of the muscle at its attachment to the rib is likely to be more painful than it is disabling. However, there may be considerable attendant muscle spasms that will splint the chest and interfere with deep breathing. These spasms may actually prevent certain types of activity. A strain of the abdominal recti attached to the lower ribs may interdict undertaking of certain sports, such as rowing or wrestling, in which forcible use of the abdominal muscles is required. Similarly, a spasm of the shoulder muscles may interdict throwing.

PROCEDURE

- Schepelmann's sign identifies rib integrity (Fig. 7-63).
- The patient raises the arms while in the seated position and then bends laterally.
- If pain is created on the concave side, it is caused by intercostal neuritis (Fig. 7-64).
- If pain is created on the convex side, the diagnosis is intercostal myofascitis (Fig. 7-65).
- Intercostal myofascitis must be differentiated from the fibrous inflammation of pleurisy.

Confirmation Procedures

Rib motion testing, chest expansion test, Amoss's sign, Forestier's bowstring sign, sternal compression test, and diagnostic imaging

---

TABLE 7-4

THORACIC CAGE ARCHITECTURE

Region	Tissues
Superiorly	Sternocleidomastoid, sternohyoid, sternothyroid, and anterior, middle, and posterior scalene muscles
Anteriorly	Pectoralis major and minor muscles, mammary glands
Posteriorly	Serratus posterior superior and inferior, and deep back muscles; trapezius, rhomboid minor and major, scapula and all muscles related to it reset against the thoracic cage
Laterally	Serratus anterior muscles
Inferiorly	Abdominal muscles attaching to thoracic cage (i.e., rectus abdominis, external and internal abdominal oblique, and transverses abdominis)

Adapted from Cramer GD, Darby SA: *Basic and clinical anatomy of the spine, spinal cord, and ANS*, St Louis, 1995, Mosby.

DIAGNOSTIC STATEMENT

Schepelmann's sign is present on the left, concave side. The presence of this sign suggests intercostal neuritis.

Schepelmann's sign is present on the left, convex side. The presence of this sign suggests intercostal myofascitis.

CLINICAL PEARL

Schepelmann's test provides an efficient method for localizing rib injury. The patient moves actively and can limit the motion according to the pain.

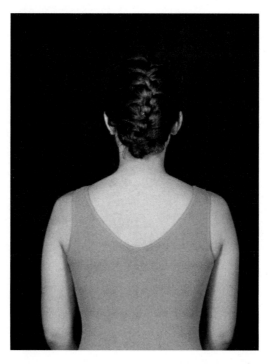

FIG. 7-63 The patient is seated comfortably, and the spinal contours are noted.

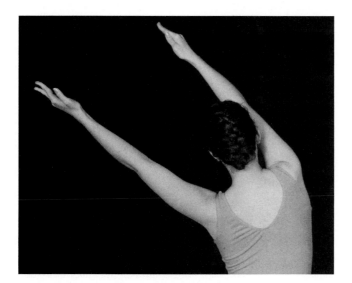

FIG. 7-64 The patient fully abducts the shoulders, bringing the hands overhead. The patient flexes the thoracic spine laterally. Pain elicited on the side of flexion (concave) indicates intercostal neuritis. Pain elicited on the convex side indicates intercostal myofascitis.

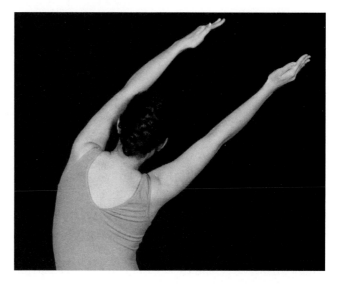

FIG. 7-65 The test is performed bilaterally.

SPINAL PERCUSSION TEST

Assessment for Spinal Osseous and Paraspinal Soft-Tissue Integrity

Comment

Several mechanisms of injury to the thoracic spine can lead to a sprain or strain disability. Flexion and extension loading in a ballistic fashion can damage the joints and paravertebral soft tissues of the thoracic spine. Lifting can also injure the midspine if the weight is too heavy or the mechanics are incorrect. Excessive contraction and rotation can place undue strain on the facet joints and erector muscles of the spine.

Multiple-level spinal fractures, which may be contiguous or separated, are estimated to occur in 3% to 5% of patients with spinal fractures (Fig. 7-66). Multiple noncontiguous spinal fractures rarely occur without injury to the spinal cord. There are three patterns of injury (Fig. 7-67).

ORTHOPEDIC GAMUT 7-9

MULTIPLE-LEVEL SPINAL FRACTURES

The three patterns of injury in multiple-level spinal fractures are as follows:

Pattern A: The primary lesion occurs between C5 and C7, with secondary injuries at T12 or the lumbar spine.

Pattern B: The primary injury occurs at T2 and T4, with secondary injuries in the cervical spine.

Pattern C: The primary injury occurs between T12 and L2, with secondary injuries from L4 to L5.

Patients with multiple-level, noncontiguous fractures usually have a disproportionate number of primary vertebral injuries in the middle and upper thoracic spine.

In thoracolumbar spine injuries, a three-column concept of spinal injury exists (Fig. 7-68). The anterior column contains the anterior longitudinal ligament, the anterior half of the vertebral body, and the anterior portion of the annulus fibrosus. The middle column consists of the posterior longitudinal ligament, the posterior half of the vertebral body, and the posterior aspect of the annulus fibrosus. The posterior column includes the neural arch, the ligamentum flavum, the facet capsules, and the interspinous ligaments.

ORTHOPEDIC GAMUT 7-10

THORACOLUMBAR FRACTURES

The thoracolumbar fracture classifications (based on three-column concepts) follow:

1. Wedge compression fractures cause isolated failure of the anterior column and result from forward flexion.
2. In stable burst fractures, the anterior and middle columns fail because of a compressive load.
3. In unstable burst fractures, the anterior and middle columns fail in compression, and the posterior column is disrupted.
4. Chance fractures are horizontal avulsion injuries of the vertebral bodies caused by flexion about an axis anterior to the anterior longitudinal ligament.
5. In flexion distraction injuries, the flexion axis is posterior to the anterior longitudinal ligament. The anterior column fails in compression, and the middle and posterior columns fail in tension.
6. Translational injuries are characterized by malalignment of the neural canal, which has been totally disrupted. Usually, all three columns have failed in shear.

There is a significantly increased incidence of fractures of the spine because of osteoporosis in the later years of life. Even after relatively minor trauma, compression fractures with vertebral collapse are common in older people. After age 70 in the asymptomatic population, the incidence of such fractures is 20%. In the aging spine, the cause of such fractures may be spontaneous and obscure without a major traumatic event. The fractures may occur because of sneezing, raising windows, or lifting weights. The patient can experience severe pain in the spine, although absence of discomfort is common. Minor falls may also produce such fractures. In addition to having back pain, these patients may have local tenderness and may be reluctant to move while in bed to avoid further pain. Some patients have root pain, and a very small minority have injury to the spinal cord. Approximately 15% of such patients may develop paralytic ileus, particularly in association with fractures of T12 and L1. It is generally considered that retroperitoneal hemorrhage is the underlying factor in the production of the ileus

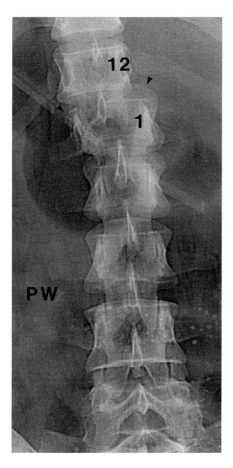

FIG. 7-66 Anteroposterior view of the thoracolumbar spine shows noncontiguous translation injury at T12-L1 level. *(From Canale ST: Campbell's operative orthopaedics, vol 1-4, ed 9, St Louis, 1998, Mosby.)*

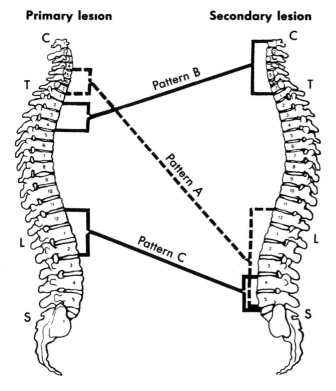

FIG. 7-67 Three patterns of multiple level injury. *(From Canale ST: Campbell's operative orthopaedics, vol 1-4, ed 9, St Louis, 1998, Mosby.)*

either by the size of the hemorrhage or by irritation of the celiac plexus.

Osteoporosis is the most commonly seen metabolic disease in the United States. It is almost universally found in the elderly and, like atherosclerosis, develops slowly over many years. The two most common types of osteoporosis are postmenopausal and "age associated" (sometimes called *senile*). The age-associated form is seen equally in males and females. The postmenopausal type is the most common symptomatic form of osteoporosis. This disorder becomes increasingly more common with age, usually developing within 15 to 20 years after menopause. It is estimated that 1.5 million fractures occur yearly because of osteoporosis. The disorder is less common in African Americans and more common in Caucasians and Asians. Spontaneous fractures, vertebral collapse, and osteoporosis are often discovered as incidental findings on roentgenograms (Fig. 7-69).

PROCEDURE

- While the patient is seated or standing and the thoracic spine is slightly flexed, the examiner percusses the spinous processes and the associated musculature of each of the thoracic vertebrae with a neurologic reflex hammer.

- Evidence of localized pain indicates a possible fractured vertebra.
- Evidence of radicular pain indicates a possible disc lesion.
- Because of the nonspecific nature of this test, other conditions also will elicit a positive pain response.
- If a ligamentous sprain exists, percussion of the spinous processes will elicit pain (Fig. 7-70).
- Percussion of the paraspinal musculature will elicit a positive sign for strain (Fig. 7-71).

Confirmation Procedures
Soto-Hall sign, Dejerine sign, Valsalva maneuver, Lhermitte's sign, and diagnostic imaging

---

DIAGNOSTIC STATEMENT

Spinal percussion elicits pain on the spinous process of T4. This pain suggests osseous injury at that level.

Spinal percussion elicits pain at the paraspinals on the left of T5. This pain suggests soft-tissue injury at that level.

CLINICAL PEARL

When soft-tissue percussion reproduces the complaint, the examiner may expect the same phenomenon from applications of ultrasound to the tissue. The uses of such therapies may be delayed until the soft tissue is no longer reactive to percussion.

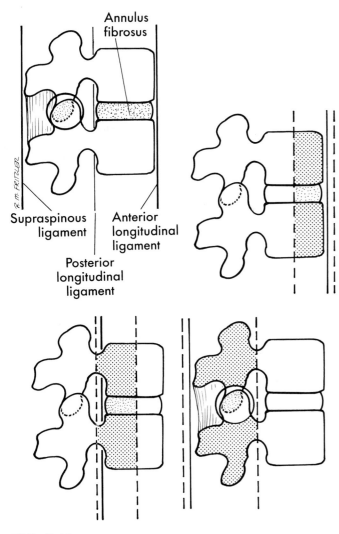

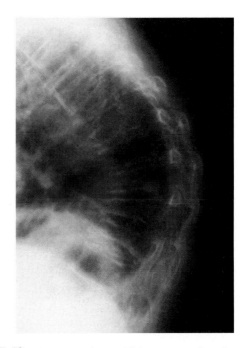

FIG. 7-68 Three-column classification of spinal instability. *(From Canale ST:* Campbell's operative orthopaedics, *vol 1-4, ed 9, St Louis, 1998, Mosby.)*

FIG. 7-69 Osteoporosis. Multiple compression fractures are present. *(From Mercier LR, Pettid FJ:* Practical orthopedics, *ed 4, St Louis, 1995, Mosby.)*

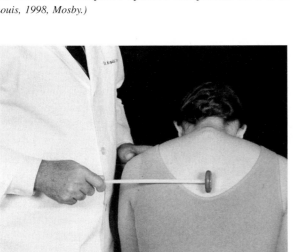

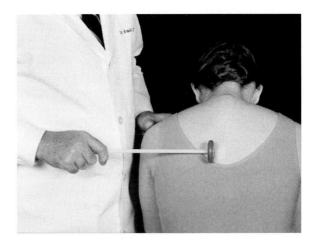

FIG. 7-70 In the seated or standing position, the patient flexes the thoracic spine, exposing the spinous processes as much as possible. The examiner percusses the spinous processes of each vertebra. Localized pain is evidence of a fracture or severe sprain. Radiating pain suggests intervertebral disc syndrome.

FIG. 7-71 The paravertebral tissues are percussed. Pain elicited in the soft tissues suggests muscular strain and highly sensitive myofascial trigger points.

SPONGE TEST

Assessment for Acute Inflammatory Lesions of the Spine

Comment

Minor injuries of the soft tissue result from mild overuse or overstretching. Severe thoracic soft-tissue injuries are characterized by traumatic effusion, pain, and loss of function. Traumatic effusion consists of four types of physiologic tissue reactions.

Tissue tearing or crushing with rupture of the blood vessels causes bleeding into the tissue. The capillaries are constricted in the injury area or site. Resultant clotting seals the damaged vessels. Fibroblasts begin the repair process, and lymphatic drainage takes place.

Local inflammation causes the undamaged capillaries to dilate and become more permeable, allowing inflammatory exudates to form. The exudates stimulate fibroblast repair and white blood cell activity with resultant local heat, redness, swelling, and pain.

There is formation of tissue thickening or tissue adhesions from the blood and exudates, especially if any of the lymphatics are damaged or if the circulation is impaired.

If a thoracic spinal joint is involved in the soft-tissue injury, synovial effusion may result. With muscle strain, the interstitial exudates and fluids gel when the muscle is at rest. The patient experiences a stiffening of the muscle upon resting the injured part. This stiffening is followed by the onset of a cramp or spasm of the injured muscle, and associated pain and ache occur in the part. This pain is completely relieved by movement. As the exudates are forced out of the tissue, through mechanical action of muscle contraction, the part is no longer stiff or sore. However, after excessive movement, the strained muscle fibers are once again aggravated and become uncomfortable. The patient is forced to rest the part, and the cycle begins again.

Myofascial fibrositis, an inflammatory nonsuppurative condition affecting the interstitial tissues of the body, is an established clinical syndrome. Previous terms applied to this condition often caused confusion. These terms are *nonarticular rheumatism, fibromyositis, myositis,* and *muscular rheumatism.* Other commonly used terms include *wry neck* and *lumbago.*

Primary myofascial fibrositis occurs independent of pathologic causes elsewhere in the body. Secondary myofascial fibrositis is myofascial inflammation that is secondary to the development of another pathologic condition and is associated with conditions such as rheumatoid arthritis, osteoarthritis, hypertrophic or degenerative arthritis, spondylosis, septic foci, rheumatic fever, diabetes, and influenza. Secondary myofascial fibrositis may also be the residual effect of traumatic injuries.

When the tissues involved fail to heal completely after injury, the condition of myofascial inflammation is called a *residual* complication.

Older patients who develop clinical cases of myofascial fibrositis experience a gradual onset of their symptoms (senile myofascial fibrositis). The etiology of this type of myofascial fibrositis is one that is mixed and complex and is probably associated with a combination of factors that include endocrine imbalances, dietary deficiencies, and degenerative tissue changes.

Normal fibrous tissue is made up of bands of collagen, fibroblasts, elastic tissue fibrils, fluid spaces, reticuloendothelial cells, capillaries, and nerves.

The inflammatory reaction of these tissues includes the swelling and fragmentation of the bands of collagen and the proliferation of fibroblasts. If the fibroblasts proliferate, the proliferation causes contractures and blocks the free flow of tissue fluids. This blockage results in difficulty moving the joints and produces pressure on the vessels and nerves in the immediate vicinity. Although small nodules form, they are often too small to be palpated. The nodules are discovered because of tenderness produced by pressure or other means.

The onset of the clinical symptoms may be sudden or insidious. The limitation of joint movement in acute cases is caused by muscle spasm. In chronic cases, the spasm may be mixed with contractures. Postinertial dyskinesia, which is the "gelling" stiffness that results from movement of a part that has been rested, is a consistent complaint.

Swelling of the tissues is sometimes found by the examiner. However, the swelling sensation often is subjective. The nodules that have been described are located by palpation, especially when the nodules form over a firm undersurface, such as bone. By carefully searching the area, the examiner can discern acutely tender areas of myofascial fibrositis, which are called *trigger points.*

Sensitive areas in the soft tissues throughout the body have been described for years. Pressure on these areas causes local and referred pain into distal areas of the body. These tender areas are often identified as symptoms of the following conditions: myofascial pain syndrome, myalgia, myositis, fibrositis, fibromyositis, fibromyalgia fascitis, myofascitis, muscular rheumatism, strain, and sprain.

The small hypersensitive area that makes up a trigger site may be stimulated by pressure, goading, needling, excessive heat, local icing, and motion.

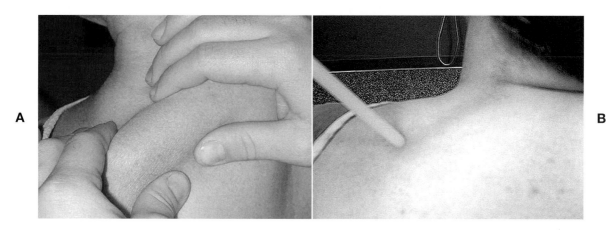

FIG. 7-72   Skin-rolling tenderness **(A)** and reactive hyperemia **(B)**.

Trigger points are characterized as hard nodules of fibrous connective tissue that surrounds sparse muscle fibers. There also are infiltrations of lymphocytes. Trigger points may be worsened by stress, infection, or metabolic upset.

Myofascial fibrositis is classified as acute, subacute, or chronic, depending on the pain, pressure sensitivity, reflex spasm, swelling, impaired mobility, and increased temperature in the area.

Diagnostic criteria for myofascial fibrositis include exquisite pain and tenderness, circumscribed painful tissue hardening, and pressure on the trigger point, which causes pain referral.

Predisposing factors for myofascial fibrositis include chronic muscular strain, repeated excessive muscular activity, direct trauma, chilling of fatigued muscles, arthritis, nerve root injury, and psychogenic anxiety.

The cardinal symptom of fibromyalgia is diffuse, chronic pain. The pain often begins in one location, particularly the neck and shoulders, but then becomes more generalized. Generally, patients state that "it hurts all over" and have difficulty locating the site of pain arising from articular or nonarticular tissues. Patients often describe the muscle pain as burning, radiating, or gnawing and the intensity of the pain as modest or severe, but varying greatly. Most patients also report profound fatigue. Headaches, either tension or more typical migraine headaches, and symptoms suggestive of irritable bowel syndrome are present in more than 50% of patients. True Raynaud's phenomenon or a Raynaud's-like excess sensitivity to cold have also been commonly reported.

Patients invariably complain of muscle weakness; however, formal muscle testing does not reveal significant weakness, provided the pain does not prevent the patient from achieving maximal effort. The only reliable finding on examination is the presence of multiple tender points. Nine pairs of tender points should be examined routinely. Patients with fewer than 11 tender points certainly can be diagnosed with fibromyalgia provided other symptoms and signs are present. Other common findings on examination include muscle "spasm" or taut bands of muscle, sometimes referred to by patients as nodules; skin sensitivity, in the form of skin roll tenderness of dermatographism (Fig. 7-72); or purplish mottling of the skin, especially of the legs following exposure to the cold. Myofascial pain syndromes also overlap with fibromyalgia (Table 7-5). The relationship

TABLE 7-5

MISDIAGNOSES THAT MAY BE GIVEN TO PATIENTS WHO EVENTUALLY ARE FOUND TO HAVE THE FIBROMYALGIA SYNDROME

Systemic lupus erythematosus/ rheumatoid arthritis	Inflammatory bowel disease
Early spondyloarthropathy	Sciatica
Multiple sclerosis	Neuropathy
Depression	Interstitial cystitis
Hypochondriasis	Metabolic myopathy
Somatoform pain disorder	Inflammatory myopathy
Malingering	Alzheimer's disease
Hypothyroidism	Meniérè's disease
	Polymyalgia rheumatica

From Kelley WN, et al: *Textbook of rheumatology*, ed 5, Philadelphia, 1997, WB Saunders.

of trigger points and tender points is not clear. The location of the trigger point is deep within the muscle belly. Trigger points result in decreased muscle stretch and pain with contraction. A "twitch response" (or jump sign), pathognomonic of an active trigger point, is a visible or palpable contraction of the muscle produced by a rapid snap of the examining finger on the taut band of muscle. There is a characteristic referred pain pattern (Fig. 7-73).

PROCEDURE

- A hot moist sponge is passed up and down the spine several times (Figs. 7-74 and 7-75).
- If any lesion of the spine is present, pain is felt as the sponge passes over the lesion.
- The test is positive for acute inflammatory lesions of the spine.

Confirmation Procedures
Palpation, thoracic spinal range of motion, and thoracic spinal muscle testing

DIAGNOSTIC STATEMENT

The sponge test is positive at the midthoracic spine and reveals focal areas of tenderness. This result suggests local tissue inflammation.

CLINICAL PEARL

As with spinal percussion, the focal areas of tenderness found with the sponge test may be hypersensitive to mechanical stimulation. This sensitivity represents spasmophilia and must be absent before aggressive physical therapy can begin.

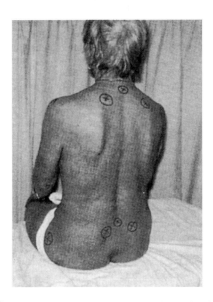

FIG. 7-73   Trigger points in the cervical and lumbar regions.
(From Mosby's medical, nursing, & allied health dictionary, *St Louis, 1998, Mosby.)*

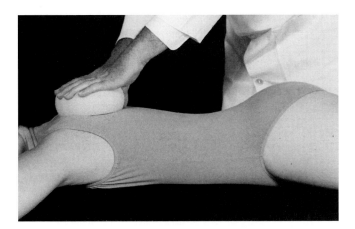

FIG. 7-74   The patient is prone. The examiner notes spinal symmetry and any muscular induration. A hot sponge is placed at the superior aspect of the thoracic spine.

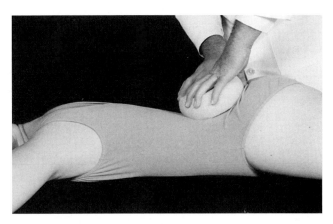

FIG. 7-75   The sponge is passed down the spinal column to the lumbosacral area. This is repeated several times. Pain is felt in locally inflamed areas as the sponge passes over them. This pain indicates local acute inflammation.

STERNAL COMPRESSION TEST

Assessment for Costal Structure Fracture

Comment

Also known as *Tietze's syndrome*, costochondritis is an inflammation of the rib cartilage at the costosternal junction. The differential diagnosis includes angina pectoris, intercostal strain and neuralgia, rib subluxation, and in cases of substantial trauma, rib fracture. The patient with costochondritis complains of point tenderness over one or two rib heads or costal junctions lateral to the sternum (Table 7-6). Symptoms are most commonly localized to the second, third, or fourth costochondral junctions. Abduction of the arm reproduces the patient's pain, which may radiate down the arm. Acute inflammation causes discomfort or pain on deep inspiration as the rib cage expands. Bogginess or swelling over the costal cartilage is possible but does not always occur.

Fractures of the ribs are common, and they usually are caused by a direct blow from a blunt object. In this instance, there is likely to be a fracture of one or, at most, two ribs. Forceful compression of the chest in one of its diameters may produce single or multiple fractures. In the first instance, the patient will relate a history of a blow to the chest that may have been forceful enough to knock the wind out of the person and cause severe localized pain. As the patient tries to breathe deeply, there is severe pain. Muscle spasm splints the chest and prevents deep breathing. The result is rapid, shallow respiration caused by the combination of air hunger and pain during inspiration. In the second instance, the patient may relate a history of being crushed in a pileup or of falling forcibly onto a side with an object between the chest and the ground. Here again, the patient will experience labored breathing accompanied by severe pain. Careful examination at the time

TABLE 7-6

THORAX AND RIB SYNDROMES

	Costochondritis (Tietze's Syndrome)	Intercostal Strain	Intercostal Neuralgia	Costovertebral Syndrome	Pectoralis Strain
Physical examination findings	Painful arm abduction Palpable tenderness at costosternal junction Commonly at 2nd to 4th rib cartilage Normal results on cardiac examination Exacerbation of pain on stretching of pectoralis muscle	Palpable tenderness at rib interspace Splinting or spasm of affected intercostal muscle Reproduction of pain at deep inspiration with arms overhead	Painful rib interspace Possible strain of intercostal muscle Referral of pain from anterior to posterior or vice versa Exacerbation of pain with deep inspiration or spinal rotation Need to rule out infection (e.g., herpes zoster) and organic disease	Tenderness over rib angle or head Fixation of costovertebral articulation Inferoanterior subluxation of corresponding dorsal vertebral level Muscle guarding, spasm over affected rib cage Palpable spinal rotation or cervicodorsal fixation Referral to anterior thorax possible	Pain on examination at pectoralis muscle, either proximally or distally Swelling or bogginess of muscle belly Discomfort on abduction of arm Ecchymosis at injury site possible Pain reproduced by adduction against resistance Need to rule out costochondral injury, avulsion of pectoralis tendon at proximal humerus
X-ray findings	Usually normal Need to rule out rib fracture in cases of blunt trauma	Not applicable	Only needed for suspected organic disease or rib trauma	Not applicable	Not applicable unless rupture or avulsion is suspected

Adapted from Brier SR: *Primary care orthopedics,* St Louis, 1999, Mosby.

of injury will elicit tenderness directly over the rib or ribs, and pain occurs in this same area during deep breathing. Although direct pressure on the involved rib is avoided, compression of the chest will cause pain. If the sixth rib is broken at the anterior axillary line, pressure made directly backward on the sternum will cause pain in the area of the fracture, and deep inspiration will be painful. Any attempt at coughing or sneezing is disastrous. A patient who tries to do so will grab the chest and attempt to restrict the motion manually.

There may be a palpable defect in the rib if the fracture is complete, and it is possible to elicit crepitus. Manipulation to elicit such an effect is not justifiable. Fracture can be differentiated from a simple contusion because contusion does not usually cause pain during motion of the rib.

PROCEDURE

- While the patient is in the supine position, the examiner exerts downward pressure on the sternum (Fig. 7-76).
- Localized pain at the lateral border of the ribs indicates a rib fracture.

Confirmation Procedures

Chest expansion test, Schepelmann's test, and diagnostic imaging

DIAGNOSTIC STATEMENT

The sternal compression test is positive and elicits pain at the lateral border of the sixth rib on the right. This result suggests rib fracture.

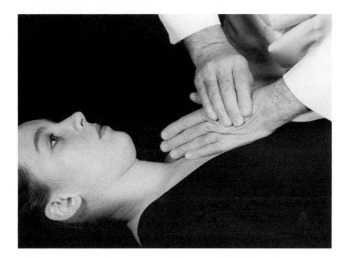

FIG. 7-76 The patient is supine, with the arms at the sides or crossed low over the abdomen. The examiner places the ulnar aspect of one hand in the vertical axis of the sternum. The other hand is placed on top of it. The examiner exerts a downward pressure on the sternum. Localized pain in the ribs indicates fracture.

CRITICAL THINKING

List the seronegative spondyloarthropathies.
(1) Ankylosing spondylitis, (2) psoriatic arthritis, (3) reactive arthritis (Reiter's syndrome), and (4) juvenile ankylosing spondylitis

List the common features of the seronegative spondyloarthropathies.
1. Predilection for inflammatory lesions of axial skeleton
2. Oligoarticular peripheral joint arthritis
3. Enthesitis-inflammation at bony insertion of tendons, ligaments, and articular capsules
4. Frequent extraarticular inflammation of eye (uveitis), heart (aortitis), skin, and mucous membranes
5. Tendency to afflict young adults (mostly men)
6. Strong association with HLA-B27
7. Negative rheumatoid factor

List the three basic types of spinal deformity.
Scoliosis, kyphosis, and lordosis

List the common classifications of scoliosis.
- Congenital scoliosis
- Adolescent idiopathic scoliosis
- Infantile and juvenile idiopathic scoliosis
- Neuromuscular scoliosis

List other disease processes in which scoliosis and kyphosis are also seen.
- Neurofibromatosis
- Spinal cord injuries
- Metabolic disorders
- Marfan's syndrome
- Infections
- Tumors
- Dwarfism

What is the prevalence of adolescent idiopathic scoliosis?
Curves of more than 10 degrees occur in approximately 3% of the population in North America, whereas curves greater than 20 degrees occur in 0.2% to 0.3% of the population. Curves greater than 20 degrees have a female:male ratio of 9:1.

Describe the physical examination for a patient with scoliosis.
Asymmetries in the shoulder, scapula, waistline, or pelvic regions are identified. The Adam's position is performed.

What is Adam's position?
The patient stands with feet together and knees straight and bends forward at the waist. The arms are held dependent with the hands together, palms and fingers opposed. The examiner compares the sides of the back for asymmetry. Prominence of the scapula or rib (called *rib hump*) is observed.

What is infantile and juvenile idiopathic scoliosis?
Infantile scoliosis occurs from 0 through 3 years of age. Juvenile scoliosis occurs between ages 4 and 10 years.

What is kyphosis?
Kyphosis is a change in the alignment of a segment of the spine in the sagittal plane that increases the posterior convex angulation.

What is the prevalence of Scheuermann's disease?
Scheuermann's disease is found in approximately 1% of the general population, with a slight female dominance (female:male ratio is 1.4:1).

What are the three columns of the spine?
The *anterior* column includes the anterior longitudinal ligament, the anterior portion of the annulus, and the anterior half of the vertebral body. The *middle* column consists of the posterior longitudinal ligament, the posterior portion of the annulus, and the posterior portion of the vertebral body. The *posterior* column is made up of the pedicles, facets, lamina, and posterior ligamentous complex, including the interspinal ligaments, ligamentum flavum, and facet joint capsule.

Describe a compression fracture.
A compression fracture results in a typical anterior wedging of the vertebral body in the anterior column. The middle and posterior columns generally are not involved.

What is a burst fracture?
A burst fracture is a fracture of the anterior and middle columns; varying degrees of the fracture fragments are displaced into the neural canal.

What is a flexion-distraction injury?
A flexion-distraction injury, also known as a *Chance fracture,* is common in motor vehicle accidents when the victim is wearing only a lap seatbelt. The fracture involves the anterior, middle, and posterior columns or the posterior ligaments.

BIBLIOGRAPHY

Abrams WB, Berkow R: *The Merck manual of geriatrics,* Rahway NJ, 1990, Merck Sharp & Dohme Research Laboratories.

Adams JC, Hamblen DL: *Outline of orthopaedics,* ed 11, Edinburgh, 1990, Churchill Livingstone.

Adams RD, Victor M: *Principles of neurology,* ed 3, New York, 1985, McGraw-Hill.

Alario AJ: *Practical guide to the care of the pediatric patient,* St Louis, 1997, Mosby.

American Medical Association: *Guides to the evaluation of permanent impairment,* ed 4, Chicago, 1993, The Association.

American Medical Association: *How to use guides to the evaluation of permanent impairment,* ed 4, Falmouth, Conn, 1993, SEAK.

American Orthopaedic Association: *Manual of orthopaedic surgery,* Chicago, 1972, The Association.

Aminoff MJ: *Electrodiagnosis in clinical neurology,* ed 2, New York, 1986, Churchill Livingstone.

Anderson PA, et al: Flexion distraction and chance injuries to the thoracolumbar spine, *J Orthop Trauma* 5:153, 1991.

Ansel BM: Rheumatic disorders in childhood, *Clin Rheum Dis* 2:303, 1976.

Apley AG, Solomon L: *Concise system of orthopaedics and fractures* London, 1988, Butterworth-Heinemann.

Appelrouth D, Gottlieb NL: Pulmonary manifestations of ankylosing spondylitis, *J Rheumatol* 2:446, 1975.

Asbury AK, McKhann GM, McDonald WI: *Disease of the nervous system,* Philadelphia, 1986, WB Saunders.

Avioli LV: Senile and post-menopausal osteoporosis, *Adv Intern Med* 21:391, 1976.

Avioli LV: Osteoporosis, pathogenesis and therapy. In Avioli LV, Vrane SM, editors: *Metabolic bone disease,* New York, 1977, Academic Press.

Avioli LV: Significance of osteoporosis: a growing national health care problem, *Orthop Rev* 21:1126, 1992.

Baker AB, Joynt RJ: *Clinical neurology,* New York, 1985, Harper & Row.

Ballinger PW: *Merrill's atlas of radiographic positions and radiologic procedures,* vol 1-3, ed 8, St Louis, 1995, Mosby.

Barkauskas VH, et al: *Health & physical assessment,* ed 2, St Louis, 1998, Mosby.

Bauer DC, et al: Factors associated with appendicular bone mass in older women, *Ann Intern Med* 118:657, 1993.

Beetham WP, et al: *Physical examination of the joints,* Philadelphia, 1965, WB Saunders.

Bennett RM, et al: A multidisciplinary approach to fibromyalgia treatment, *J Musculoskel Med* 8:21, 1991.

Benson MKD, Byrnes DP: The clinical syndromes and surgical treatment of thoracic intervertebral disc prolapse, *J Bone Joint Surg* 57B:471, 1975.

Berg EE: The sternal-rib complex: a possible fourth column in thoracic spine fractures, *Spine* 18:1916, 1993.

Bernat JL: A dangerous backache, *Hosp Pract (Off)* 12:36, 1977.

Blount WP, Moe JH: *The Milwaukee brace,* Baltimore, 1973, Williams & Wilkins.

Boden SD, et al: *The aging spine: essentials of pathophysiology, diagnosis and treatment,* Philadelphia, 1991, WB Saunders.

Bogduk N, Twomey LT: *Clinical anatomy of the lumbar spine,* ed 2, Melbourne, 1991, Churchill Livingstone.

Bogduk N, Valencia F: Innervation and pain patterns of the thoracic spine. In Grant R, editor: *Physical therapy of the cervical and thoracic spine,* ed 2, New York, 1994, Churchill Livingstone.

Bondilla KK: Back pain: osteoarthritis, *J Am Geriatr Soc* 25:62, 1977.

Bordurant FJ, et al: Acute spinal cord injury: a study using physical examination and magnetic resonance imaging, *Spine* 15:161, 1990.

Bourdillon JR: *Spinal manipulation,* ed 3, New York, 1982, Appleton-Century-Crofts.

Bradford DS: Juvenile kyphosis, *Clin Orthop* 128:45, 1977.

Bradford DS, et al: Scheuermann's kyphosis and roundback deformity: results of Milwaukee brace treatment, *J Bone Joint Surg* 56A:740, 1974.

Bradford DS, et al: Scheuermann's kyphosis: results of surgical treatment by posterior spine arthrodesis in 22 patients, *J Bone Joint Surg* 57A:439, 1975.

Brashear HR, Raney RB: *Shand's handbook of orthopaedic surgery,* St Louis, 1978, Mosby.

Brier SR: *Primary care orthopedics,* St Louis, 1999, Mosby.

Brooks M, Evans R, Fairclough J: *Sports injuries,* ed 2, London, 1992, Gower Medical.

Brotzman SB: *Clinical orthopaedic rehabilitation,* St Louis, 1996, Mosby.

Brown CW, et al: The natural history of thoracic disc herniation, *Spine* 17:597, 1992.

Brown DE, Neumann RD: *Orthopedic secrets,* Philadelphia, 1995, Hanley & Belfus.

Brown MD: Diagnosis of pain syndromes of the spine, *Orthop Clin North Am* 6:233, 1975.

Bucholz RW: *Orthopaedic decision making,* ed 2, St Louis, 1996, Mosby.

Buckwalter J: Spine update: aging and degeneration of the human intervertebral disc, *Spine* 20:1307, 1995.

Bunnell WP: Treatment of idiopathic scoliosis, *Orthop Clin North Am* 10:813, 1979.

Cailliet R: *Scoliosis: diagnosis and management,* Philadelphia, 1975, FA Davis.

Canale ST: *Campbell's operative orthopaedics,* vol 1-4, ed 9, St Louis, 1998, Mosby.

Carman DL, et al: Measurement of scoliosis and kyphosis radiographs, intraobserver and interobserver variation, *J Bone Joint Surg* 72A:328, 1990.

Cipriano JJ: *Photographic manual of regional orthopaedic and neurological test,* ed 3, Baltimore, 1997, Williams & Wilkins.

Cohn RE: *Impairment rating examination and disability evaluation,* ed 3, Wilkesboro, NC, 1994, R Ernest Cohn.

Cramer GD, Darby SA: *Basic and clinical anatomy of the spine, spinal cord, and ANS,* St Louis, 1995, Mosby.

Croft P, Schollum J, Silman A: Population study of tender point counts and pain as evidence of fibromyalgia, *Br Med J* 309:696, 1994.

Crosby EC, Humphrey T, Lauer EW: *Correlative anatomy of the nervous system,* New York, 1962, Macmillan.

Cyriax J: *Textbook of orthopaedic medicine, vol 1: diagnosis of soft tissue lesions,* London, 1982, Bailliere Tindall.

Cyriax JH, Cyriax PJ: *Illustrated manual of orthopaedic medicine,* London, 1983, CM Publications.

Daffner RH, et al: The radiology assessment of post-traumatic vertebral stability, *Skeletal Radiol* 19:103, 1990.

Dambro MR, Griffith JA: *Griffith's 5 minute clinical consult,* Baltimore, 1997, Williams & Wilkins.

D'Ambrogio KJ, Roth GB: *Positional release therapy assessment & treatment of musculoskeletal dysfunction,* St Louis, 1997, Mosby.

D'Ambrosia RD: *Musculoskeletal disorders: regional examination and differential diagnosis,* Philadelphia, 1977, JB Lippincott.

Dandy DJ: *Essential orthopaedics and trauma,* Edinburgh, 1989, Churchill Livingstone.

Dawson DM, Hallett M, Millender LH: *Entrapment neuropathies,* Boston, 1983, Little, Brown.

DeJong RN: *The neurologic examination,* ed 4, New York, 1978, Harper & Row.

Deltoff MN, Kogon PL: *The portable skeletal x-ray library,* St Louis, 1998, Mosby.

Demeter SL, Andersson GBJ, Smith GM: *Disability evaluation,* St Louis, 1996, Mosby.

Deshpande JK, Tobias JD: *The pediatric pain handbook,* St Louis, 1996, Mosby.

Dettenmeier PA: *Radiographic assessment for nurses,* St Louis, 1995, Mosby.

Dickson RA: Conservative treatment for idiopathic scoliosis, *J Bone Joint Surg* 67B:176, 1985.

Doherty M: *Color atlas and text of osteoarthritis,* London, 1994, Wolfe.

Doherty M, Doherty J: *Clinical examination in rheumatology,* London, 1992, Wolfe.

Doherty M, George E: *Self-assessment picture tests in rheumatology,* London, 1995, Mosby-Wolfe.

Elattrache N, Fadale PD, Fu F: Thoracic spine fracture in a football player, *Am J Sports Med* 21:157, 1984.

Elster AD: *Questions and answers in magnetic resonance imaging,* St Louis, 1994, Mosby.

Engelman EG, Engleman EP: Ankylosing spondylitis: recent advances in diagnosis and treatment, *Med Clin North Am* 61:347, 1977.

Epstein O et al: *Clinical examination,* ed 2, London, 1997, Mosby.

Feldmann E: *Current diagnosis in neurology,* St Louis, 1994, Mosby.

Ferezy JS: *The chiropractic neurological examination,* Gaithersburg, Md, 1992, Aspen.

Ferris B, Edgar M, Leyshon A: Screening for scoliosis, *Acta Orthop Scand* 59:417, 1988.

Garcia F, Florez MT, Conejero JA: A butterfly vertebra or a wedge fracture? *Int Orthop* 17:7, 1993.

Garcia JH: *Neuropathology: the diagnostic approach,* St Louis, 1997, Mosby.

Gartland JJ: *Fundamentals of orthopaedics,* London, 1968, E & S Livingstone.

Gavin TM, Shurr DG, Patwardhan AG: Orthotic treatment for spinal disorders. In Weinstein SL, editor: *The pediatric spine,* New York, 1993, Raven.

Gertzbein SD: Spine update: classification of thoracic and lumbar fractures, *Spine* 19:626, 1994.

Goldenberg DL: Fatigue in rheumatic disease, *Bull Rheum Dis* 44:4, 1995.

Goldie BS: *Orthopaedic diagnosis and management: a guide to the care of orthopaedic patients,* ed 2, Oxford, 1998, ISIS Medical Media.

Goldstein LA, Waugh TR: Classification and terminology of scoliosis, *Clin Orthop* 93:10, 1973.

Greenspan A, Montesano P: *Imaging of the spine in clinical practice,* London, 1993, Wolfe.

Greenstein GM: *Clinical assessment of neuromusculoskeletal disorders,* St Louis, 1997, Mosby.

Gregersen GG, Lucas DB: An in vivo study of the axial rotation of the human thoracolumbar spine, *J Bone Joint Surg* 49A:247, 1967.

Grieve GP: *Common vertebral joint problems,* New York, 1981, Churchill Livingstone.

Grootboom MJ, Govender S: Acute injuries of the upper dorsal spine, *Injury* 24:389, 1993.

Grossman ZD, et al: *Cost-effective diagnostic imaging: the clinician's guide,* ed 3, St Louis, 1995, Mosby.

Hamilton MG, Thomas HG: Intradural herniation of a thoracic disc presenting as flaccid paraplegic: case report, *Neurosurgery* 27:482, 1990.

Harvey J, Tanner S: Low back pain in young athletes: a practical approach, *Sports Med* 12:394, 1991.

Harvey MA, James B: *Differential diagnosis,* Philadelphia, 1972, WB Saunders.

Hawkins RJ: *An organized approach to musculoskeletal examination and history taking,* St Louis, 1995, Mosby.

Heim HA: Scoliosis, *Clin Symp* 25:1, 1973.

Hinkle CZ: *Fundamentals of anatomy & movement: a workbook and guide,* St Louis, 1997, Mosby.

Hollingshead WH, Jenkins DR: *Functional anatomy of the limbs and back,* Philadelphia, 1981, WB Saunders.

Hornberger JP: *Exercise physiology: therapeutic exercise,* Sarasota, Fla, 1991, Joseph P Hornberger.

James JP: The etiology of scoliosis, *J Bone Joint Surg* 52B:410, 1970.

Judge RD, Zuidema GD, Fitzgerald FT: *Clinical diagnosis: a physiologic approach,* Boston, 1982, Little, Brown.

Kanner R: *Pain management secrets,* Philadelphia, 1997, Hanley & Belfus.

Kapandji IA: *The physiology of the joints: the trunk and vertebral column,* vol 3, New York, 1974, Churchill Livingstone.

Katirji B: *Electromyography in clinical practice: a case study approach,* St Louis, 1998, Mosby.

Katz WA: *Rheumatic diseases: diagnosis and management,* Philadelphia, 1977, JB Lippincott.

Keats TE, Lusted LB: *Atlas of roentgenographic measurements,* ed 6, St Louis, 1990, Mosby.

Keim HA: *The adolescent spine,* New York, 1982, Springer-Verlag.

Kelley WN, et al: *Textbook of rheumatology,* vol 1, ed 4, Philadelphia, 1993, Saunders.

Kendall HO, Kendall FP, Wadsworth GE: *Muscle testing and function,* ed 2, Baltimore, 1971, Williams & Wilkins.

Kimura J: *Electrodiagnosis in disease of nerve and muscle: principles and practice,* Philadelphia, 1983, FA Davis.

Klippel JH, Dieppe PA: *Rheumatology,* vol 1-2, ed 2, London, 1998, Mosby.

Koenigsberg R: *Churchill's illustrated medical dictionary,* New York, 1989, Churchill Livingstone.

Korovessis P, Sidiropoulos P, Dimas A: Complete fracture-dislocation of the thoracic spine without neurologic deficit: case report, *J Trauma* 36:122, 1994.

Kostuik JP: Adult scoliosis. In Weinstein J, Wiesel SW, editors: *The lumbar spine,* Philadelphia, 1990, WB Saunders.

Krupp MA, Chatton MJ: *Current diagnosis and treatment,* Los Altos, Calif, 1972, Lange Medical.

Lavy CBD, Barrett DS: *Questions and answers on Apley's concise system of orthopaedics and fractures,* Oxford, 1991, Butterworth-Heinemann.

Lerner AJ: *The little black book of neurology,* ed 3, St Louis, 1995, Mosby.

Levene DL: *Chest pain: an integrated diagnostic approach,* Philadelphia, 1977, Lea & Febiger.

Lewis CB, Knortz KA: *Orthopedic assessment and treatment of the geriatric patient,* St Louis, 1993, Mosby.

Lonstein JE, Winter RB: Milwaukee brace treatment of adolescent idiopathic scoliosis—review of 1020 patients, *J Bone Joint Surg* 76A:1207, 1994.

MacConaill MA, Basmajian JV: *Muscles and movements: a basis for human kinesiology,* Baltimore, 1969, Williams & Wilkins.

Macnab I: *Backache,* Baltimore, 1977, Williams & Wilkins.

Magee DJ: *Orthopedic physical assessment,* ed 3, Philadelphia, 1997, WB Saunders.

Maigne JY, Maigne R, Guerin-Surville H: Upper thoracic dorsal rami: anatomic study of their medial cutaneous branches, *Surg Radiol Anat* 13:190, 1991.

Maigne R: *Orthopaedic medicine: a new approach to vertebral manipulation,* Springfield, Ill, 1972, Charles C Thomas.

Maitland GD: *Vertebral manipulation,* London, 1973, Butterworths.

Malone TR, McPoil TG, Nitz AJ: *Orthopedic and sports physical therapy,* ed 3, St Louis, 1997, Mosby.

Manniche C, et al: Clinical trial of intensive muscle training for chronic low back pain, *Lancet* 24:1473, 1988.

Marchiori DM: *Clinical imaging with skeletal, chest, and abdomen pattern differentials,* St Louis, 1999, Mosby.

Marrero GH: Juvenile kyphosis, *Spine State Art Rev* 4:173, 1990.

Martin JH: *Neuroanatomy text and atlas,* ed 2, Stamford, Conn, 1996, Appleton & Lange.

Mathers LH, et al: *Clinical anatomy principles,* St Louis, 1996, Mosby.

Mazion JM: *Illustrated manual of neurological reflexes/signs/tests, part I, orthopedic signs/tests/maneuvers for office procedure, part II,* Orlando, 1980, Daniels Publishing.

McGoey BV, et al: Effect of weight loss on musculoskeletal pain in the morbidly obese, *J Bone Joint Surg* 72B:322, 1990.

McKenzie RA: *The lumbar spine: mechanical diagnosis and therapy,* Wikanae, New Zealand, 1981, Spinal Publications.

McRae R: *Clinical orthopaedic examination,* ed 3, Edinburgh, 1990, Churchill Livingstone.

Medical Economics Books: *Patient care flow chart manual,* ed 3, Oradell, NJ, 1982, Medical Economics Books.

Mellion MB: *Sports medicine secrets,* Philadelphia, 1994, Hanley & Belfus.

Mellion MB: *Office sports medicine,* ed 2, St Louis, 1996, Mosby.

Mengel MB, Schwiebert LP: *Ambulatory medicine: the primary care of families,* ed 2, Stamford, Conn, 1996, Appleton & Lange.

Mennell JM: *The musculoskeletal system differential diagnosis from symptoms and physical signs,* Gaithersburg, Md, 1992, Aspen.

Mercier LR, Pettid FJ: *Practical orthopedics,* ed 4, St Louis, 1995, Mosby.

Modic MT, Masaryk TJ, Ross JS: *Magnetic resonance imaging of the spine,* ed 2, St Louis, 1994, Mosby.

Moe JH, Kettleson DN: Idiopathic scoliosis, *J Bone Joint Surg* 52A:1509, 1970.

Moe JH, Winter RB, Bradford DS, Lonstein JF: *Scoliosis and other spinal deformities,* Philadelphia, 1978, WB Saunders.

Moldofsky H: Chronobiological influences on fibromyalgia syndrome: theoretical and therapeutic implications, *Baillieres Clin Rheumatol* 8:801, 1994.

Moll JH, Wright V: Measurement of spinal movement. In Jayson M, editor: *Lumbar spine and back pain,* New York, 1976, Grune & Stratton.

Moll JMH, Wright V: An objective clinical study of chest expansion, *Ann Rheum Dis* 31:1, 1972.

Montgomery SP, Erwin WE: Scheuermann's kyphosis: long-term results of Milwaukee brace treatment, *Spine* 6:5, 1981.

Moore KL: *Clinically oriented anatomy,* ed 3, Baltimore, 1992, Williams & Wilkins.

Morrisey RT, et al: Measurement of Cobb angle on radiographs of patients who have scoliosis, evaluation of intrinsic error, *J Bone Joint Surg* 72A:320, 1990.

Mosby-Year Book, Inc: *Expert 10-minute physical examination,* St Louis, 1997, Mosby-Year Book.

Nash CL: Scoliosis bracing, *J Bone Joint Surg* 62A:848, 1980.

Nash CL, Moe JH: A study of vertebral rotation, *J Bone Joint Surg* 52A:223, 1969.

Netter F: *The Ciba collection of medical illustration, vol 8: The musculoskeletal system,* Summitt, NJ, 1990, Ciba Geigy.

Nettina SM: *The Lippincott manual of nursing practice,* ed 6, Philadelphia, 1996, Lippincott.

Newton RW: *Color atlas of pediatric neurology,* St Louis, 1995, Mosby-Wolfe.

Noonan KJ, et al: Use of the Milwaukee brace for progressive idiopathic scoliosis, *J Bone Joint Surg* 78A:557, 1996.

Nordin M, Andersson GBJ, Pope MH: *Musculoskeletal disorders in the workplace: principles and practice,* St Louis, 1997, Mosby.

O'Connor MI, Carrier BI: Metastatic disease of the spine, *Orthopedics* 15:611, 1992.

O'Donoghue DH: *Treatment of injuries to athletes,* ed 4, Philadelphia, 1984, WB Saunders.

Olson WH, et al: *Handbook of symptom-oriented neurology,* ed 2, St Louis, 1994, Mosby.

Omer GE, Spinner M: *Management of peripheral nerve problems,* Philadelphia, 1980, WB Saunders.

O'Young B, Young MA, Stiens SA: *PM&R secrets,* Philadelphia, 1997, Hanley & Belfus.

Panjabi MM: The stabilizing system of the spine, part II, neutral zone and instability hypothesis, *J Spinal Disord* 5:390, 1992.

Panjabi MM, White AA: *Clinical biomechanics of the spine,* ed 2, Philadelphia, 1990, JB Lippincott.

Panjabi MM, et al: Thoracolumbar burst fracture: a biomechanical investigation of its multidirectional flexibility, *Spine* 19:578, 1994.

Papaioannu T, Stokes I, Kenwright J: Scoliosis associated with limb length inequality, *J Bone Joint Surg* 64A:59, 1982.

Patten J: *Neurological differential diagnosis,* ed 2, London, 1996, Springer.

Pheasant S: *Ergonomics, work and health,* Gaithersburg, Md, 1991, Aspen.

Pope MH, Frymoyer JW, Krag MH: Diagnosing instability, *Clin Orthop* 279:60, 1992.

Prescott E, et al: Fibromyalgia in the adult Danish population: I. a prevalence study, *Scand J Rheumatol* 22:233, 1993.

Rachlin ES: *Myofascial pain and fibromyalgia trigger point management,* St Louis, 1994, Mosby.

Ramsey RG: *Neuroradiology,* Philadelphia, 1987, WB Saunders.

Resnick NW, Greenspan SL: Senile osteoporosis reconsidered, *JAMA* 261:1025, 1989.

Riggs BL, Melton LJ III: *Osteoporosis: etiology, diagnosis and management,* New York, 1988, Raven.

Rodnitzky RL: *Van Allen's pictorial manual of neurologic tests,* St Louis, 1988, Mosby.

Rolak LA: *Neurology secrets,* ed 2, Philadelphia, 1998, Hanley & Belfus.

Rothman RH, Simeone FA: *The spine,* Philadelphia, 1982, WB Saunders.

Rowland LP: *Merritt's textbook of neurology,* ed 7, Philadelphia, 1984, Lea & Febiger.

Ruge D, Wiltse LL: *Spinal disorders: diagnosis and treatment,* Philadelphia, 1977, Lea & Febiger.

Rumball K, Jarvis J: Seat-belt injuries of the spine in young children, *J Bone Joint Surg* 74B:572, 1992.

Sacsh BL, et al: Primary osseous neoplasms of the thoracic and lumbar spine, *Orthop Trans* 8:422, 1984.

Saidoff DC, McDonough AL: *Critical pathways in therapeutic intervention,* St Louis, 1997, Mosby.

Schumacher HR, Klippel JH, Koopman WJ: *Primer on the rheumatic diseases,* ed 10, Atlanta, 1993, Arthritis Foundation.

Shankman GA: *Fundamental orthopedic management for the physical therapist assistant,* St Louis, 1997, Mosby.

Simmons EH: Kyphotic deformity of the spine in ankylosing spondylitis, *Clin Orthop* 128:65, 1977.

Simmons EH, Bernstein AJ: Fractures of the spine in ankylosing spondylitis. In Floman Y, Farcy JP, Argenson C, editors: *Thoracolumbar spine fractures,* New York, 1993, Raven.

Simmons EH, Graziano GP, Heffner R Jr: Muscle disease as a cause of kyphotic deformity in ankylosing spondylitis, *Spine* 16:5351, 1991.

Simons GW, Sty JR, Storkshak RJ: Retroperitoneal and retrofascial abscesses, *J Bone Joint Surg* 65A:1041, 1983.

Sledge CB, Poss R: *The year book of orthopedics 1997,* St Louis, 1997, Mosby.

Spapen HD, et al: The straight back syndrome, *Neth J Med* 36:29, 1990.

Specht NT, Russo RD: *Practical guide to diagnostic imaging,* St Louis, 1998, Mosby.

Spivak JM, Vaccaro AR, Cotler JM: Thoracolumbar spine trauma, I, evaluation and classification, *J Am Acad Orthop Surg* 3:345, 1995.

Starlanyl D, Copeland ME: *Fibromyalgia & chronic myofascial pain syndrome: a survival manual,* Oakland, Calif, 1996, New Harbinger.

Stewart DL, Abeln SH: *Documenting functional outcomes in physical therapy,* St Louis, 1993, Mosby.

Stillerman C, Weiss M: Management of thoracic disc disease, *Clin Neurosurg* 38:325, 1992.

Stoller DW: *Magnetic resonance imaging in orthopaedics & sports medicine,* Philadelphia, 1993, JB Lippincott.

Sunderland S: *Nerves and nerve injuries,* ed 2, New York, 1979, Churchill Livingstone.

Sutton D, Young JWR: *A concise textbook of clinical imaging,* ed 2, St Louis, 1995, Mosby.

Tan JC, Horn SE: *Practical manual of physical medicine and rehabilitation,* St Louis, 1998, Mosby.

Taybi H, Lachman RS: *Radiology of syndromes, metabolic disorders, and skeletal dysplasias,* ed 4, St Louis, 1996, Mosby.

Thibodeau GA, Patton KT: *Anatomy & physiology,* ed 3, St Louis, 1996, Mosby.

Thibodeau GA, Patton KT: *Pocket reference to accompany anatomy & physiology,* ed 3, St Louis, 1996, Mosby.

Thompson JM: *Clinical outlines for health assessment,* St Louis, 1997, Mosby.

Toghill PJ: *Examining patients: an introduction to clinical medicine,* London, 1990, Edward Arnold.

Tollison CD, Satterthwaite JR, Tollison JW: *Handbook of pain management,* ed 2, Baltimore, 1994, Williams & Wilkins.

Torg JS, Shepard RJ: *Current therapy in sports medicine,* ed 3, St Louis, 1995, Mosby.

Tsou PM: Embryology of congenital kyphosis, *Clin Orthop* 128:18, 1977.

Tsou PM, Yau A, Hodgson AR: Embryogenesis and prenatal development of congenital vertebral anomalies and their classification, *Clin Orthop* 152:211, 1980.

Turek SL: *Orthopaedics principles and their application,* ed 3, Philadelphia, 1977, JB Lippincott.

Turner PG, Green JH, Galasko CS: Back pain in childhood, *Spine* 14:812, 1989.

Van Holsbeeck M, Introcaso JH: *Musculoskeletal ultrasound,* St Louis, 1991, Mosby.

Veeming A, et al: The posterior layer of the thoracolumbar fascia, its function in load transfer from spine to legs, *Spine* 20:753, 1995.

Vernon L, Dooley J, Acusta A: Upper lumbar and thoracic disc pathology: a magnetic resonance imaging analysis, *J Neuromusculoskeletal System I* 59:63, 1993.

Wakefield TS, Frank RG: *The clinician's guide to neuro musculoskeletal practice,* Abbotsford, Wisc, 1995, Allied Health of Wisconsin, S.C.

Watkins RG: *The spine in sports,* St Louis, 1996, Mosby.

Wedgewood RJ, Schaller JG: The pediatric arthritides, *Hosp Pract (Off Ed)* 12:83, 1977.

Weineck J: *Functional anatomy in sports,* ed 2, St Louis, 1990, Mosby.

Weinerman SA, Bockman RS: Medical therapy of osteoporosis, *Orthop Clin North Am* 21:109, 1990.

Weinstein SL: Adolescent idiopathic scoliosis: prevalence and natural history, *Am Acad Orthop Surg Lect* 38:115, 1989.

Weinstein SL, Buckwalter JA: *Turek's orthopaedics principles and their application,* ed 5, Philadelphia, 1994, JB Lippincott.

White AA: Kinematics of the normal spine as related to scoliosis, *J Biomech* 4:405, 1971.

White AH, Schofferman JA: *Spine care,* vol 1-2, St Louis, 1995, Mosby.

White AW, Panjabi MM: *Clinical biomechanics of the spine,* Philadelphia, 1990, JB Lippincott.

White KP, Nielson WR: Cognitive behavioral treatment of fibromyalgia syndrome: a follow-up assessment, *J Rheumatol* 22:717, 1995.

White KP, et al: Fibromyalgia in rheumatology practice: a survey of Canadian rheumatologists, *J Rheumatol* 22:722, 1995.

Whiteside TE: Traumatic kyphosis of the thoracolumbar spine, *Clin Orthop* 128:78, 1977.

Whitmore I, Willan PLT: *Multiple choice questions in human anatomy,* London, 1995, Mosby.

Wiles P, Sweetnam R: *Essentials of orthopaedics,* London, 1965, JA Churchill.

Williams P, Warwick R: *Gray's anatomy,* ed 36, Philadelphia, 1980, WB Saunders.

Windsor RE, Lox DM: *Soft tissue injuries: diagnosis and treatment,* Philadelphia, 1998, Hanley & Belfus.

Wolfe F, et al: The prevalence and characteristics of fibromyalgia in the general population, *Arthritis Rheum* 38:19, 1995.

Wyke B: Morphological and functional features of the innervation of the costovertebral joints, *Folia Morphol* 23:296, 1975.

Zatouroff M: *Diagnosis in color: physical signs in general medicine,* ed 2, London, 1996, Mosby-Wolfe.

Zitelli BJ, Davis HW: *Atlas of pediatric physical diagnosis,* ed 2, London, 1992, Wolfe.

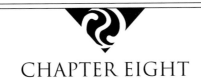

CHAPTER EIGHT

THE LUMBAR SPINE

AXIOMS OF LUMBAR SPINE ASSESSMENT

- Back pain is common from the second decade of life on.
- Intervertebral disc disease and disc herniation are most prominent in the third and fourth decades of life.
- Back and posterior thigh pain arises from many areas of the spine, including the facet joints, longitudinal ligaments, and the periosteum of the vertebrae.
- Radicular pain often extends below the knee in the affected dermatome.

INTRODUCTION

As many as 90% of patients with back pain have a mechanical reason for their pain. Mechanical low back pain may be defined as pain secondary to overuse of a normal anatomic structure or pain secondary to trauma or deformity of an anatomic structure. The age of a patient is helpful in determining the potential cause of back pain. In considering spondyloarthropathies, clinical characteristics help in differentiating the diseases belonging in this group (Fig. 8-2). The sex of the patient may also help select potential causes of low back pain. Certain disorders occur more often in males, whereas others are associated more commonly with females. Others occur equally in both sexes (Table 8-3).

Other than the common cold, back pain is the most prevalent human affliction. As stated earlier, most patients have a mechanical cause (muscle strain or annular tear) for their back pain and do not have an underlying, serious, systemic medical illness.

Even if treatment involves only a localized part of the lumbar spine, in each case, the lumbar spine has to be considered as a functional unit consisting of bones, ligaments, intervertebral discs, muscles, and all other soft tissues. Because of their central location, spinal elements represent the focal point for the equilibrium of the body. Because of the many connections and relations, spinal changes influence some organs directly, and the functional equilibrium of the spine depends on the efficient performance of other organs.

The spine contributes to many mutual relationships within the total body. With its equilibrium (statics), the spine exerts, influences, and receives forces (dynamics), all of which are interwoven with the far-reaching chain of motion (kinetics). In addition, the spine is able to exercise considerable influence on neighboring structures as well as on remote organs. This is its action on nerves and blood vessels. To a considerable degree, this complicated system depends on the metabolism, the mineral metabolism of the bones, and the nutrition of the bradytrophic ligamentous and

TABLE 8-1

LUMBAR SPINE CROSS-REFERENCE TABLE BY ASSESSMENT PROCEDURE

Disease Assessed

Lumbar Spine Test/Sign	Intervertebral Disc Syndrome	Sciatica	Intervertebral Foramen Encroachment	Dural Adhesions	Subluxation	Mechanical Lower Back	Cord Tumor	Spinal Neuropathy	Sprain	Hip Lesion	Femoral Nerve	L2-L3-L4	Meningitis	Sacroiliac Lesion	Hamstring Spasm	Myofascitis	Denervation	Fracture	Lower Extremity Joints
Antalgia sign	•																		
Bechterew's sitting test	•	•	•	•	•														
Bilateral leg-lowering test	•		•			•													
Bowstring sign								•											
Bragard's sign	•	•					•	•											
Cox sign	•																		
Demianoff's sign						•													
Deyerle's sign		•																	
Double leg-raise test	•					•			•										
Ely's sign								•			•	•							
Fajersztajn's test	•	•		•															
Femoral nerve traction test								•			•	•							
Heel/toe walk test	•	•						•											
Hyperextension test											•	•							
Kemp's test	•					•		•											
Kernig/Brudzinski sign													•						
Lasègue differential sign								•											
Lasègue rebound test	•																		
Lasègue sitting test		•						•											
Lasègue test	•	•	•	•		•	•							•					
Lewin punch test	•																		
Lewin snuff test	•	•																	
Lewin standing test		•													•				
Lewin supine test	•	•												•		•			
Linder's sign																			
Matchstick test	•																•		
Mennell's sign														•					
Milgram's test	•						•												
Minor's sign	•													•				•	
Nachlas test					•	•								•					
Neri's sign	•					•								•					
Prone knee-bending test											•	•							
Quick test																			•
Schober's test						•													
Sicard's sign		•						•											
Sign of the buttock						•				•									
Skin pinch test	•					•										•	•		
Spinal percussion test	•					•			•									•	
Straight-leg-raising test	•			•			•												
Turyn's sign		•																	
Vanzetti's sign		•																	

TABLE 8-2

Lumbar Spine Cross-Reference Table By Syndrome or Tissue

Cord tumor	Bragard's sign	Lower extremity joints	Quick test
	Lasègue test	Mechanical lower back	Bilateral leg-lowering test
	Milgram's test		Demianoff's sign
	Straight-leg-raising test		Double leg-raise test
Denervation	Matchstick test		Kemp's test
	Skin pinch test		Lasègue test
Dural adhesions	Bechterew's sitting test		Nachlas test
	Fajersztajn's test		Neri's sign
	Lasègue test		Schober's test
	Straight-leg-raising test		Sign of the buttock
Femoral nerve	Ely's sign		Skin pinch test
	Femoral nerve traction test		Spinal percussion test
	Hyperextension test	Meningitis	Kernig/Brudzinski sign
	Prone knee-bending test	Myofascitis	Lewin supine test
Fracture	Minor's sign		Skin pinch test
	Spinal percussion test	Sacroiliac lesion	Lasègue test
Hamstring spasm	Lewin standing test		Lewin supine test
Hip lesion	Ely's sign		Mennell's sign
	Sign of the buttock		Minor's sign
Intervertebral disc syndrome	Antalgia sign		Nachlas test
	Bechterew's sitting test		Neri's sign
	Bilateral leg-lowering test	Sciatica	Bechterew's sitting test
	Bragard's sign		Bragard's sign
	Cox sign		Deyerle's sign
	Double leg-raise test		Fajersztajn's test
	Fajersztajn's test		Heel/toe walk test
	Heel/toe walk test		Lasègue sitting test
	Kemp's test		Lasègue test
	Lasègue rebound test		Lewin snuff test
	Lasègue test		Lewin standing test
	Lewin punch test		Lewin supine test
	Lewin snuff test		Sicard's sign
	Lewin supine test		Turyn's sign
	Matchstick test		Vanzetti's sign
	Milgram's test	Spinal neuropathy	Bowstring sign
	Minor's sign		Bragard's sign
	Neri's sign		Ely's sign
	Skin pinch test		Femoral nerve traction test
	Spinal percussion test		Heel/toe walk test
	Straight-leg-raising test		Kemp's test
Intervertebral foramen encroachment	Bechterew's sitting test		Lasègue differential sign
	Bilateral leg-lowering test		Lasègue sitting test
	Lasègue test		Sicard's sign
L2-L3-L4	Femoral nerve traction test	Sprain	Double leg-raise test
	Hyperextension test		Spinal percussion test
	Prone knee-bending test	Subluxation	Bechterew's sitting test
			Nachlas test

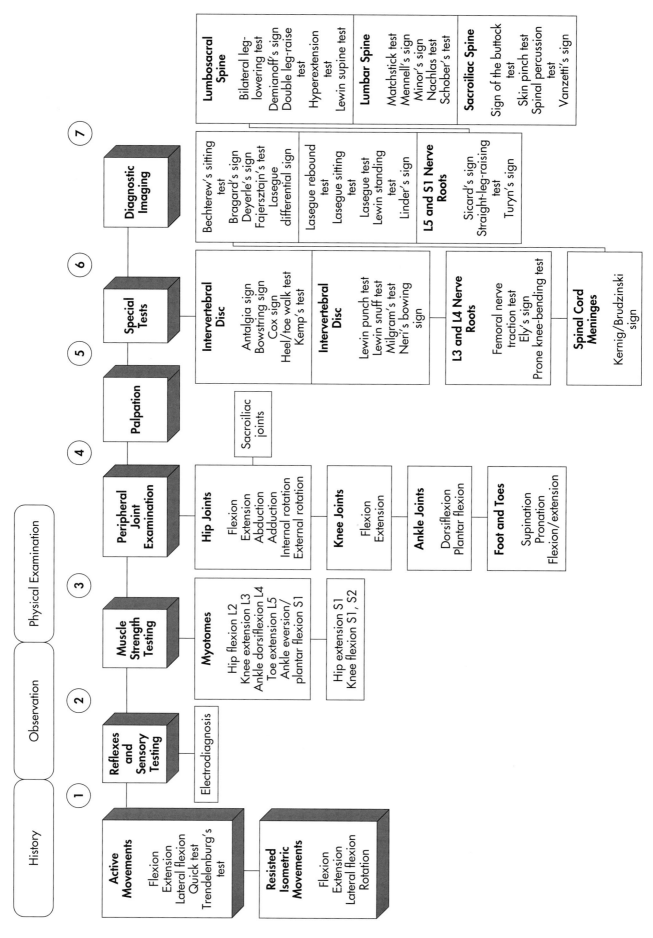

FIG. 8-1 Lumbar spine assessment.

A

Typical pattern of peripheral arthritis: predominantly of
  lower limb, asymmetric
Tendency to radiographic sacroiliitis
Absence of rheumatoid factor
Absence of subcutaneous nodules and other
  extra-articular features of rheumatoid arthritis
Overlapping extra-articular features characteristic of the
  group (such as anterior uveitis)
Significant familial aggregation
Association with HLA-B27

B

Ankylosing spondylitis
Reiter's syndrome/reactive arthritis
Arthropathy of inflammatory bowel disease (Crohn's
  disease, ulcerative colitis)
Psoriatic arthritis
Undifferentiated spondyloarthropathies
Juvenile chronic arthritis: juvenile onset ankylosing
  spondylitis

FIG. 8-2   **A,** Clinical characteristics of spondyloarthropathies.
B, Diseases belonging to the spondyloarthropathies. *(From Kelley
WN, et al:* Textbook of rheumatology, *ed 5, Philadelphia, 1997,
WB Saunders.)*

TABLE 8-3

GENDER PREVALENCE IN LOW BACK PAIN

Male predominance	Female predominance
Spondyloarthropathies	Polymyalgia rheumatica
Vertebral osteomyelitis	Fibromyalgia
Benign and malignant neoplasms	Osteoporosis
Paget's disease	Parathyroid disease
Retroperitoneal fibrosis	
Peptic ulcer disease	
Work-related mechanical	
disorders	

Data from Klippel JH, Dieppe PA: *Rheumatology,* vol 1-2, ed 2, London,
1998, Mosby.

disc tissues. Improper function of the endocrine glands also
affects the spine.

During fetal development, the spine may be exposed to
many influences, such as drug-induced malformations, lack
of oxygen, or radiation.

Occupational and daily-living stresses, as well as
traumatic influences, may combine to have an unfavorable
effect when coupled with the aging process, which has a
marked effect on the disc apparatus and the bony substance.
More resources for the diagnosis and treatment of spinal
diseases are available today than previously.

Degeneration of posture during early years, lack of
exercise, physical weakness, and degenerative changes in
later life have taken on a serious social significance for the
cultures of industrialized nations.

The spine is an intricate and interesting mechanical
structure. The spine's functions are mechanical, and it is
well suited for serving its basic mechanical roles. The
materials used to execute the design are appropriate for
enhancing these functions. The spine must transfer loads
from the trunk to the pelvis, must allow for physiologic
motion, and must protect the spinal cord from damage.
When a proper appreciation of normal anatomy and
mechanics has been gained, the pathophysiology of the
diseased or deformed spine becomes clear.

The lumbar spine is designed to withstand loading and
to provide truncal mobility. The primary plane of motion is

during flexion-extension, although there is significant axial
rotation at the L5 level. This rotation in the lower lumbar
spine is particularly important, considering that the annulus
fails and tears with torsional forces. Coupling in the lumbar
spine is the opposite of cervical and thoracic spine coupling.
The spinous processes move toward the concavity of the
curve in physiologic lateral flexion.

Optimal spinal mobility in relation to age is difficult to
pin down. The only generalization it is possible to make is
that spinal mobility is probably greatest during adolescence
and early adulthood. This tendency is significant when
planning treatment and in determining prognoses.

The anatomic structures of the lumbosacral spine
receive specific types of sensory innervation that are
associated with distinct qualities of pain (Table 8-4).

ESSENTIAL ANATOMY

There are five lumbar vertebrae, numbered L1 to L5,
followed by five fused sacral bodies that form the sacrum
and the coccyx. The alignment of the lumbar spine generally
has a lordotic contour. The normal lordosis is 30 to 50
degrees (apex L3) in a standing person.

Lumbar vertebrae are specialized for weight bearing
and strength. They have strong, thick bodies (Fig. 8-3) and
stout spines and transverse processes to which attach several
large paravertebral muscles (Fig. 8-4). The anterior longitudinal ligament extends from the sacrum to the inferior
surface of the occipital bone.

The intrinsic musculature of the back is innervated
by the posterior primary rami of segmental spinal nerves
(Fig. 8-5). These nerves also innervate the skin and subcutaneous tissues overlying the intrinsic muscles of the back,
the vertebral column, and the meninges.

Within the intervertebral foramina, the ventral and
dorsal roots of each segment unite to form a true spinal

TABLE 8-4

SUMMARY OF THE CHARACTERISTICS OF LOW BACK PAIN OF VARIOUS ORIGINS

Source of Pain	Distribution	Nature	Aggravating Factors	Neurologic Changes
Spinal pain	Sclerotomal Local	Sharp Dull	Motion	None
Discogenic pain	Sclerotomal	Deep, aching	Increased intradiscal pressure (e.g., bending, sitting, Valsalva maneuver)	None
Nerve root pain	Radicular	Paresthesias Numbness	Root stretching	Present
Multiple lumbar spinal stenosis pain	Radicular Sclerotomal	Paresthesias Spinal claudication pattern	Lumbar extension Walking	Present
Referred visceral pain	Dermatomal	Deep, aching	Related to affected organ	None

From Kelley WN, et al: *Textbook of rheumatology,* ed 5, Philadelphia, 1997, WB Saunders.

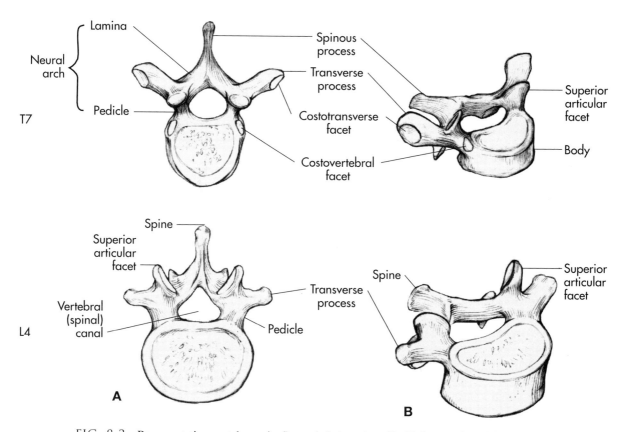

FIG. 8-3   Representative vertebrae. **A,** Superoinferior view. **B,** Right anterior oblique views. *(From Mathers LH, et al: Clinical anatomy principles, St Louis, 1996, Mosby.)*

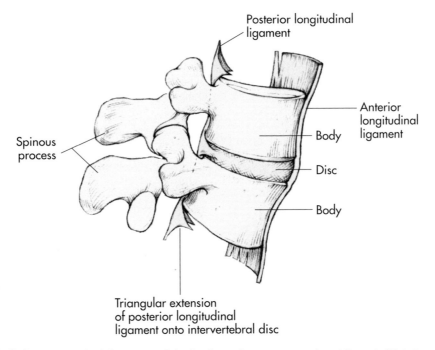

FIG. 8-4   Longitudinal ligaments of the lumbar spine.   *(From Mathers LH, et al:* Clinical anatomy principles, *St Louis, 1996, Mosby.)*

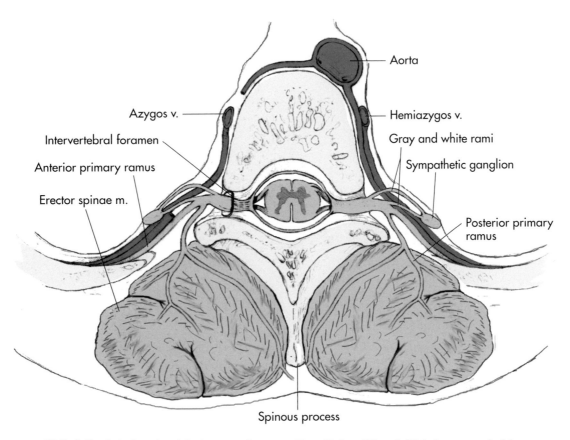

FIG. 8-5   Spinal cord and the intercostal space.   *(From Mathers LH, et al:* Clinical anatomy principles, *St Louis, 1996, Mosby.)*

nerve (Fig. 8-6). Spinal nerves represent all of the axons leaving and entering the spinal cord at that level (Fig. 8-7).

Below L2, the vertebral canal contains the many nerve roots that make up the cauda equina (so named because it resembles the many hairs in a horse's tail)

(Fig. 8-8). The systematic dermatome pattern is evident as consecutive segments in order from proximal to distal along the cephalic border of the limb and then from distal to proximal along the caudal border of the limb (Fig. 8-9). The posterior margin of the annulus and the posterior longitudinal ligament are supplied by the sinuvertebral

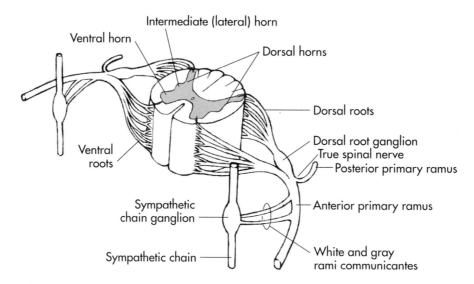

FIG. 8-6 Spinal cord and sympathetic chain. (*From Mathers LH, et al:* Clinical anatomy principles, *St Louis, 1996, Mosby.*)

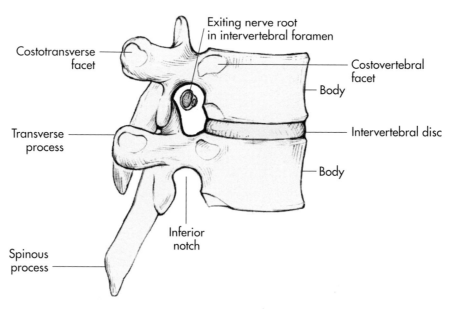

FIG. 8-7 Intervertebral foramen. (*From Mathers LH, et al:* Clinical anatomy principles, *St Louis, 1996, Mosby.*)

nerve, which is formed by a branch of the ventral rami (somatic) and a branch of the gray ramus communicans (autonomic) (Fig. 8-10).

ESSENTIAL MOTION ASSESSMENT

Range-of-motion findings are most helpful in pinpointing a vertebral structure that may be compromised in the lumbar spine. Pain at an early point in the extension of the lumbar spine suggests an inflamed posterior joint or pars pathology. Painful lumbar flexion in the early-to-middle range connotes a faulty disc mechanism or muscular stain. Because the terminal range of flexion causes the facet joint capsule to stretch, a pain response at this point may indicate a posterior joint sprain.

Patients with acute spasm or significant trauma often have multidirectional complaints and severe limitation of motion in all planes. Therefore range-of-motion testing may be initially inconclusive as to the severity of the injury.

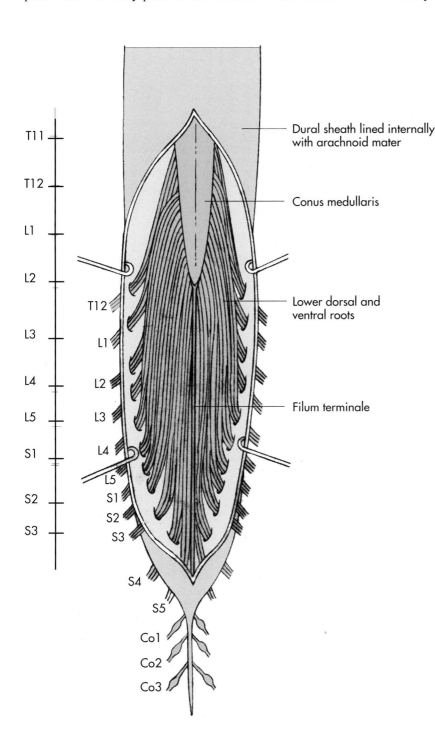

T11
T12
L1
L2
L3
L4
L5
S1
S2
S3

T12
L1
L2
L3
L4
L5
S1
S2
S3
S4
S5
Co1
Co2
Co3

Dural sheath lined internally with arachnoid mater

Conus medullaris

Lower dorsal and ventral roots

Filum terminale

FIG. 8-8   Cauda equina.   *(From Mathers LH, et al:* Clinical anatomy principles, *St Louis, 1996, Mosby.)*

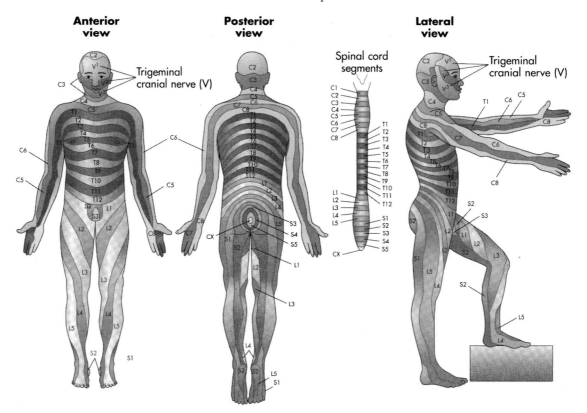

FIG. 8-9 Dermatomes. Segmental dermatome distribution of spinal nerves to the front, back, and side of the body. *C,* Cervical segments; *CX,* coccygeal segment; *L,* lumbar segments; *S,* sacral segments; *T,* thoracic segments. *(From Thibodeau GA, Patton KT:* Structure and function of the body, *St Louis, 1997, Mosby.)*

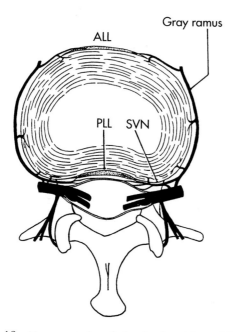

FIG. 8-10 Nerve supply of the lumbar intervertebral disc. *ALL,* Anterior longitudinal ligaments; *PLL,* posterior longitudinal ligaments; *SVN,* sinuvertebral nerves. *(From Nicholas JA, Hershman EB:* The lower extremity & spine in sports medicine, *vol 1-2, ed 2, St Louis, 1995, Mosby.)*

To assess the contribution made to flexion by the lumbar spine, the examiner should mark the spine at the lumbosacral junction, and then 10 cm above and 5 cm below this point. On forward flexion, the distance between the two upper marks should increase by approximately 4 cm, the distance between the lower two remaining unaltered (Figs. 8-11 to 8-14).

ESSENTIAL MUSCLE FUNCTION ASSESSMENT

The erector spinae consist of a minor portion, spinalis, and two major portions, longissimus and iliocostalis. The spinalis connects spinous processes, and the longissimus and iliocostalis connect homologous portions of the costal and transverse elements of the lumbar, thoracic, and cervical vertebrae and skull (Fig. 8-15).

Useful in screening is muscle testing of the legs, which measures strength on a 5-point scale for extension and flexion (knee), abduction and adduction (hip), and eversion and inversion, and dorsiflexion and plantar flexion (foot) (Table 8-5).

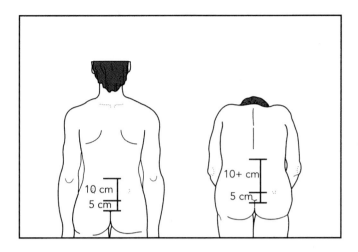

FIG. 8-11 Measuring lumbar flexion. *(From Epstein O, Perkin GD, deBono DP, Cookson J:* Clinical examination, *ed 2, London, 1997, Mosby.)*

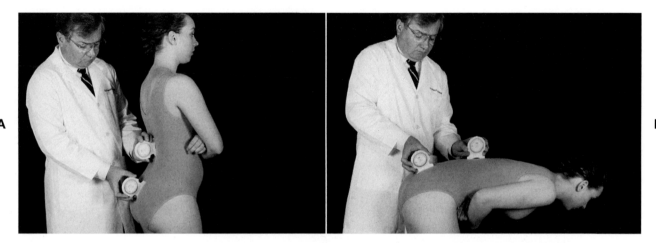

A

B

FIG. 8-12 For flexion, 80 degrees of movement is normal. Movement must occur from the lumbar spine and not the hips or thoracic spine. How far forward the patient is able to bend is compared with the straight-leg-raising tests. When using an inclinometer to measure the lumbar flexion range of motion, the patient is standing. One inclinometer is placed over the T12 spinous process in the sagittal plane. The second inclinometer is placed at the level of the sacrum, also in the sagittal plane **(A).** Both inclinometers are zeroed at these positions. The patient flexes forward and the angle of both inclinometers is recorded **(B).** The sacral inclination is subtracted from the T12 inclination to obtain the lumbar flexion angle. Flexion movement of 60 degrees or less is an impairment to the lumbar spine in the activities of daily living.

ORTHOPEDIC GAMUT 8-1

LOWER EXTREMITY MUSCULATURE

The innervation lower extremity musculature is sequential:

1. L2 and L3 supply hip flexion
2. L4 and L5 hip extension
3. L3 and L4 supply knee extension
4. L5 and S1 knee flexion
5. L4 and L5 supply ankle dorsiflexion
6. S1 and S2 ankle plantar flexion
7. L4 supplies ankle inversion
8. L5 and S1 supply ankle eversion

FIG. 8-13 Extension is limited to 35 degrees in the lumbar spine. Extension, as measured with an inclinometer, is performed with the patient standing. One inclinometer is placed over the T12 spinous process in the sagittal plane. The second inclinometer is placed at the sacrum, also in the sagittal plane. Both instruments are zeroed in this position. The patient extends the lumbar spine, and the angles of both instruments are recorded. The sacral inclination angle is subtracted from the T12 inclination angle to obtain the lumbar extension angle. Lumbar extension range of motion that is 20 degrees or less is an impairment to the lumbar spine in the activities of daily living.

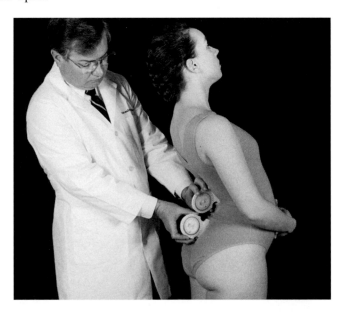

A
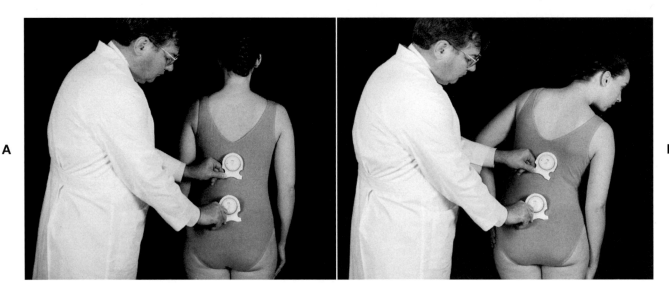
B

FIG. 8-14 Lateral flexion is approximately 25 degrees in the lumbar spine. The patient slides a hand down the side of the leg. The patient cannot bend forward or backward during the movement. The movement is compared to the opposite side. To use an inclinometer to measure the lateral lumbar flexion, the patient is standing and the lumbar spine is in neutral position. One inclinometer is placed at the T12 spinous process, in the coronal plane. The second inclinometer is placed at the superior aspect of the sacrum, in the coronal plane. Both instruments are zeroed to this position (**A**). The patient laterally flexes the lumbar spine to one side, and the inclinations of both instruments are recorded (**B**). The sacral angle is subtracted from the T12 angle to obtain the lumbar lateral flexion angle. The procedure is repeated for the range of motion to the opposite side. Lateral flexion of 20 degrees or less to either side is an impairment of the lumbar spine in the activities of daily living.

For patients in which the objective findings do not match the subjective complaints, close observation helps identify the inconsistencies (Table 8-6). A finding of three or more of the five signs of the Waddell Index is clinically significant. Isolated positive signs are ignored.

The most superficial layer of tissue, below the subcutaneous layer, contains the thoracolumbar fascia. This tissue attaches medially to the thoracic spinous processes and inferiorly to the iliac crest and lateral crest of the sacrum. Laterally, the tissue serves as the origin of the latissimus dorsi and transversus abdominis muscles. Superiorly, the tissue attaches to the angles of the ribs in the thoracic region. Below the fascia lie the superficial multisegmental muscles, collectively named the *erector spinae muscles*. Their origin is a

TABLE 8-5

Lᴜᴍʙᴀʀ Rᴀᴅɪᴄᴜʟᴀʀ Sʏɴᴅʀᴏᴍᴇs

Disc Level	Any Central Disc Herniation	L5/S1	L4/L5	L3/L4
Nerve root involved	Cauda equina (L4/L5 > L5/S1)	S1	L5	L4
Pain referral pattern	Perineum	Unilateral	Unilateral	Unilateral
	Low back	Low back	Low back	Low back
	Buttocks	Buttocks	Buttocks	Buttocks
	Either or both legs	Posterior leg	Lateral leg and thigh	Posterolateral leg
Motor deficit	Unilateral or bilateral leg weakness	Unilateral weakness; plantar flexion of foot; difficulty with toe walking	Unilateral weakness; dorsiflexion of foot; difficulty with heel walking	Unilateral quadriceps weakness
Sensory deficit	Perineum/buttocks, low back, thighs, legs, feet	Lateral foot, posterolateral calf	Lateral calf; between 1st and 2nd toes	Knee distal, anterior thigh
Reflexes compromised	Ankle jerk	Ankle jerk	0	Knee jerk

From Demeter SL, Andersson GBJ, Smith GM: *Disability evaluation,* St Louis, 1996, Mosby.

thick tendon attached to the posterior aspect of the sacrum, iliac crest, lumbar spinous processes, and supraspinous ligament. The muscle fibers split into three columns at the level of the lumbar spine: the lateral iliocostalis, the intermediate longissimus, and the more medial spinalis. The action of this group of muscle is to extend the spine. With unilateral action, the muscle group flexes the spine to one side.

Deep to the erector spinae lie the transversospinal muscles, including the multifidus and rotators. The multifidus originates at the posterior surface of the sacrum, the aponeurosis of the sacrospinalis, the posterior superior iliac spine, and the posterior sacroiliac ligament. The multifidus inserts two to four segments above its origin, into the spinous processes. The multifidus extends the spine and rotates it toward the opposite side. The rotators have similar attachments and action, but they ascend only one or two segments. Additional deep muscles include the interspinalis, which connects pairs of adjacent lumbar spinous processes, and the intertransversarii (medial, dorsal lateral, and ventral lateral groups), which connect pairs of adjacent transverse process. These muscles extend and bend the column to the same side, respectively.

The forward and lateral flexor muscles of the lumbar spine are located anterior and lateral to the vertebral bodies and transverse processes. The iliopsoas consists of two separate muscular heads: the iliacus and psoas major. The origins of the psoas major arise from the intervertebral disc by five slips, each of which starts from adjacent upper and lower margins of two vertebrae, and membranous arches that emanate from the bodies of the four upper lumbar vertebrae. These arches permit the lumbar arteries and veins and the sympathetic rami communicates to pass beneath them. The iliacus arises from the iliac fossa and joins the

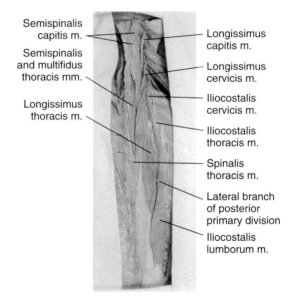

FIG. 8-15   Fifth layer of back muscles of the right side.   *(From Cramer GD, Darby SA: Basic and clinical anatomy of the spine, spinal cord, and ANS, St Louis, 1995, Mosby.)*

psoas under the inguinal ligament. The iliacus then crosses the hip joint capsule and inserts into the lesser trochanter of the femur. These muscles flex the lumbar spine and bend it toward the same side. The quadratus lumborum, which lies lateral to the vertebral column, arises from the posterior part of the iliac crest and iliolumbar ligament and inserts into the twelfth rib and the tips of the transverse processes of the upper four lumbar vertebrae. This muscle fixes the diaphragm during inspiration and bends the trunk toward the same side when it acts alone (Figs. 8-16 to 8-18).

TABLE 8-6

NONORGANIC PHYSICAL SIGNS INDICATING ILLNESS BEHAVIOR

	Physical Disease/Normal Illness Behavior	Abnormal Illness Behavior
Symptoms		
Pain	Anatomic distribution	Whole leg pain
		Tailbone pain
Numbness	Dermatomal	Whole leg numbness
Weakness	Myotomal	Whole leg giving away
Time pattern	Varies with time and activity	Never free of pain
Response to treatment	Variable benefit	Intolerance of treatments
		Emergency admissions to hospital
Signs		
Tenderness	Anatomic distribution	Superficial
		Widespread nonanatomic
Axial loading	No lumbar pain	Lumbar pain
Simulated rotation	No lumbar pain	Lumbar pain
Straight leg raising	Limited on distraction	Improves with distraction
Sensory	Dermatomal	Regional
Motor	Myotomal	Regional, jerky, giving way

From Demeter SL, Andersson GBJ, Smith GM: *Disability evaluation,* St Louis, 1996, Mosby.

FIG. 8-16   During trunk extension, back extensors are assisted by the latissimus dorsi, quadratus lumborum, and trapezius. The patient is lying prone on the examination table. Hip extensors must give fixation of the pelvis to the thighs, and the examiner must stabilize the legs firmly on the table. The patient then extends the trunk.

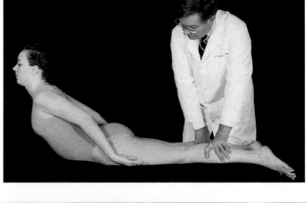

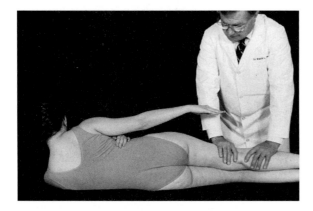

FIG. 8-17   Lateral flexion of the trunk requires a combination of lateral flexion and hip abduction. The patient is side-lying, with the head, upper trunk, pelvis, and lower extremities in a straight line. The top arm is extended down along the side. The patient is not allowed to hold on to the pelvis and attempt to pull up with the hand. The under arm is forward, across the chest. This rules out assistance by pushing up with the elbow. The legs must be held down by the examiner to counterbalance the weight of the trunk. During the test, the patient laterally flexes the trunk away from the examination table.

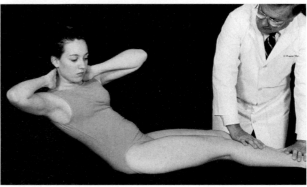

FIG. 8-18   Raising the trunk obliquely forward combines trunk flexion and rotation. It is accomplished by the combined actions of the external oblique on one side, the internal oblique on the opposite side, and the rectus abdominis. The patient is supine on the examination table, and the legs are supported by the examiner. The patient clasps the hands behind the head. The patient flexes, rotates the trunk, and holds the position.

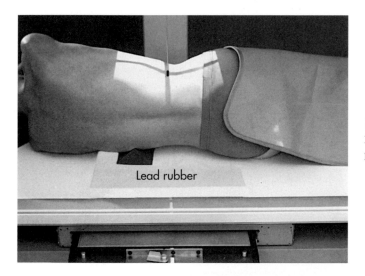

Lead rubber

FIG. 8-19   Lateral lumbar spine.   *(From Ballinger PW, editor:* Merrill's atlas of roentgenographic positions and standard radiologic procedures, *ed 8, St Louis, 1995, Mosby.)*

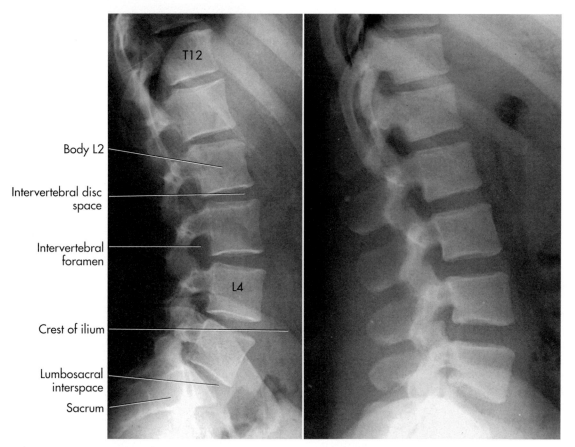

T12

Body L2

Intervertebral disc space

Intervertebral foramen

L4

Crest of ilium

Lumbosacral interspace

Sacrum

FIG. 8-20   Lateral lumbar spine.   *(From Ballinger PW, editor:* Merrill's atlas of roentgenographic positions and standard radiologic procedures, *ed 8, St Louis, 1995, Mosby.)*

ESSENTIAL IMAGING

A variety of radiographic views can be taken when the lumbosacral region is evaluated. The standard views consist of the anteroposterior (AP), lateral (Figs. 8-19 and 8-20), oblique (Figs. 8-21 to 8-23), and either a frontal or a lateral lumbosacral spot (Figs. 8-24 and 8-25).

The AP projection has generally been used for recumbent examinations. This places the lumbar spine fully arched by extension of the lower limbs. The extended limb position accentuates the lordotic curve, which increases the angle between the vertebral bodies and the divergent rays, with resultant distortion of the bodies as well as poor delineation of the intervertebral disc spaces (Figs. 8-26 and 8-27). The lordotic curve can be reduced and the intervertebral disc

FIG. 8-21   Anteroposterior oblique lumbar spine. *(From Ballinger PW, editor:* Merrill's atlas of roentgenographic positions and standard radiologic procedures, *ed 8, St Louis, 1995, Mosby.)*

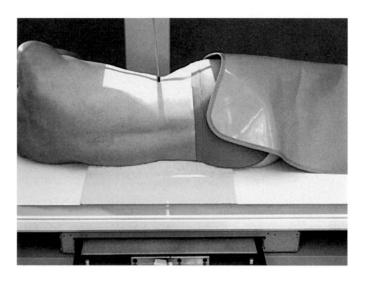

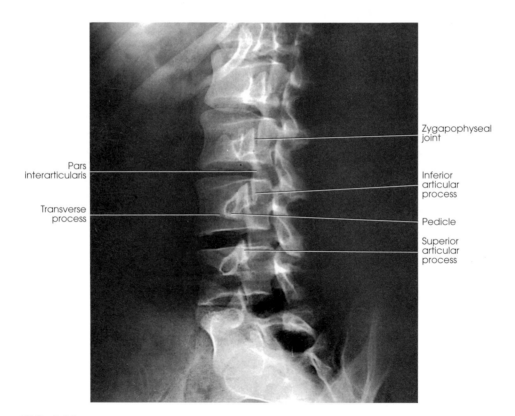

Zygapophyseal joint

Pars interarticularis

Inferior articular process

Transverse process

Pedicle

Superior articular process

FIG. 8-22   Anteroposterior oblique lumbar spine right posterior oblique. *(From Ballinger PW, editor:* Merrill's atlas of roentgenographic positions and standard radiologic procedures, *ed 8, St Louis, 1995, Mosby.)*

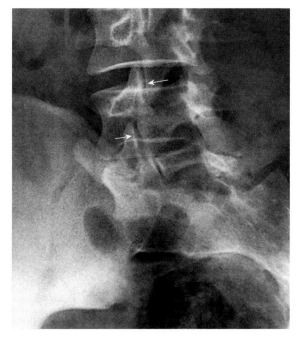

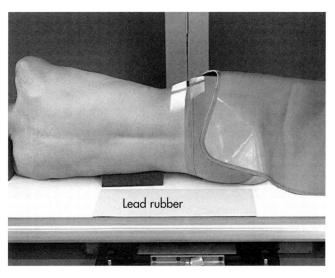

FIG. 8-23   Anteroposterior oblique lumbar spine right posterior oblique.   *(From Ballinger PW, editor:* Merrill's atlas of roentgenographic positions and standard radiologic procedures, *ed 8, St Louis, 1995, Mosby.)*

FIG. 8-24   Lateral L5-S1.   *(From Ballinger PW, editor:* Merrill's atlas of roentgenographic positions and standard radiologic procedures, *ed 8, St Louis, 1995, Mosby.)*

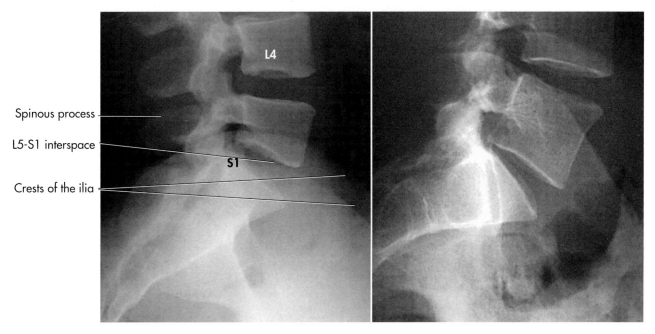

FIG. 8-25   Lateral L5-S1.   *(From Ballinger PW, editor:* Merrill's atlas of roentgenographic positions and standard radiologic procedures, *ed 8, St Louis, 1995, Mosby.)*

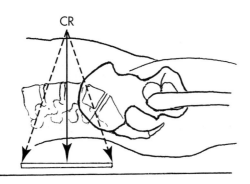

FIG. 8-26 Lumbar spine demonstrating intervertebral disc spaces and diverging central ray are not parallel. *(From Ballinger PW, editor: Merrill's atlas of roentgenographic positions and standard radiologic procedures, ed 8, St Louis, 1995, Mosby.)*

spaces clearly delineated in the AP projection simply by flexing the hips and knees enough to place the back in firm contact with the table (Figs. 8-28 to 8-30).

Bone scintigraphy is of limited utility in patients with low back pain (Fig. 8-31).

Computed tomography (CT) is useful for evaluating abnormalities of the lumbosacral spine, where the spatial anatomy is complex (Fig. 8-32). CT can visualize cortical bone destruction, calcified tumor matrix, and soft-tissue extension of tumors affecting the spine and is superior to magnetic resonance imaging (MRI) in this regard (Fig. 8-33). MRI is an excellent technique to view the spinal cord. MRI identifies syringomyelia, atrophy, cord infarction, cord injury, multiple sclerosis, and intramedullary tumors (Fig. 8-34). MRI can identify the vertebral bodies in which bone marrow has been replaced with tumor (Fig. 8-35).

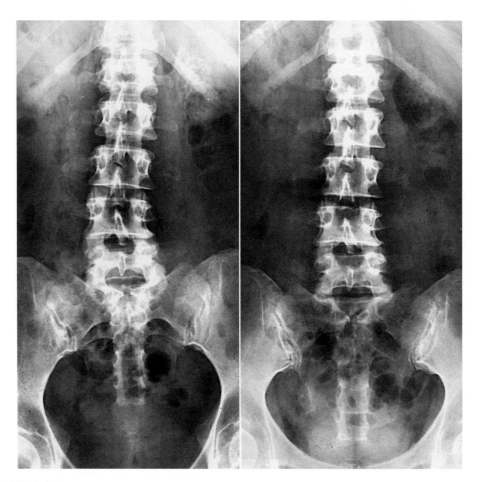

FIG. 8-27 Anteroposterior lumbar spine. *(From Ballinger PW, editor: Merrill's atlas of roentgenographic positions and standard radiologic procedures, ed 8, St Louis, 1995, Mosby.)*

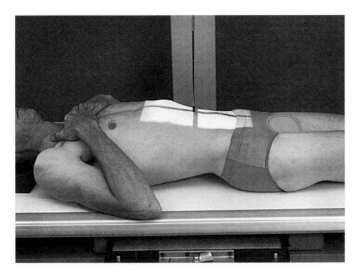

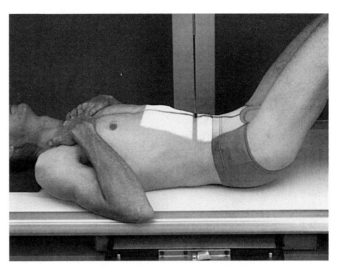

FIG. 8-28   Anteroposterior lumbar spine with the limbs extended, creating increased lordotic curve. *(From Ballinger PW, editor: Merrill's atlas of roentgenographic positions and standard radiologic procedures, ed 8, St Louis, 1995, Mosby.)*

FIG. 8-29   Anteroposterior lumbar spine with limbs flexed, decreasing lordotic curve. *(From Ballinger PW, editor: Merrill's atlas of roentgenographic positions and standard radiologic procedures, ed 8, St Louis, 1995, Mosby.)*

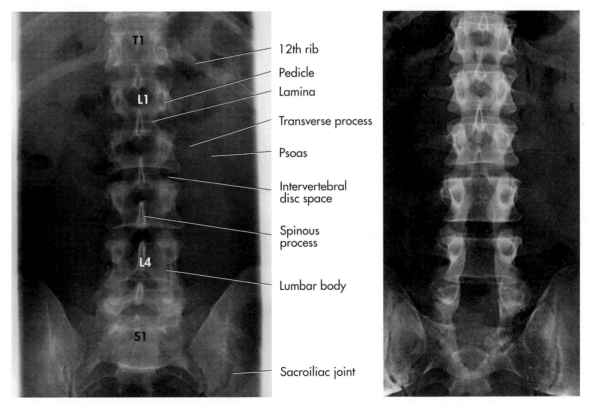

FIG. 8-30   Anteroposterior lumbar spine. *(From Ballinger PW, editor: Merrill's atlas of roentgenographic positions and standard radiologic procedures, ed 8, St Louis, 1995, Mosby.)*

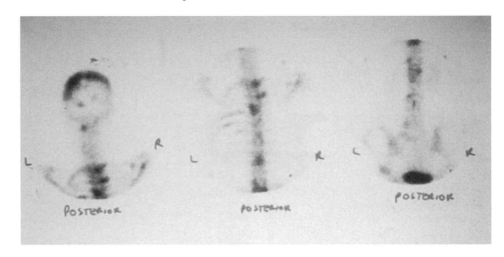

FIG. 8-31 A bone scan demonstrating the random uptake of radioisotope. Note the absence of uptake symmetry and variation of sizes of the foci throughout the skeleton. *(From Deltoff MN, Kogon PL: The portable skeletal x-ray library, St Louis, 1998, Mosby.)*

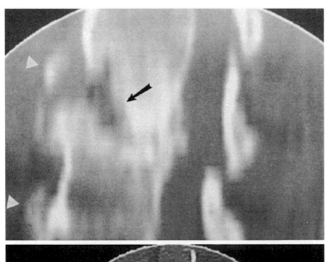

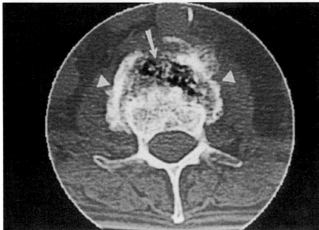

FIG. 8-32 CT with sagittal reformation reveals ligamentous ossification *(arrowheads)* with a vacuum phenomenon within the fracture cleft *(arrows)*. Fracture through a bamboo spine is more common in ankylosing spondylitis than in this case. *(From Sartoris DJ: Musculoskeletal imaging: the requisites, St Louis, 1996, Mosby.)*

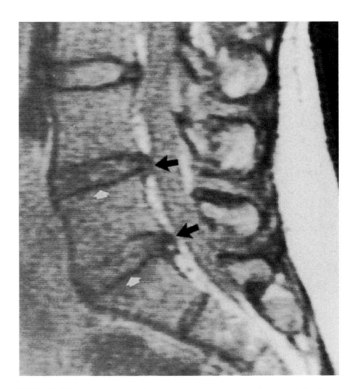

FIG. 8-33 On a T_1-weighted sagittal image, abnormal findings include posterior disc protrusion *(black arrows)* and decreased signal intensity in the nucleus pulposus *(white arrows)* at L4-L5 and L5-S1. *(From Sartoris DJ: Musculoskeletal imaging: the requisites, St Louis, 1996, Mosby.)*

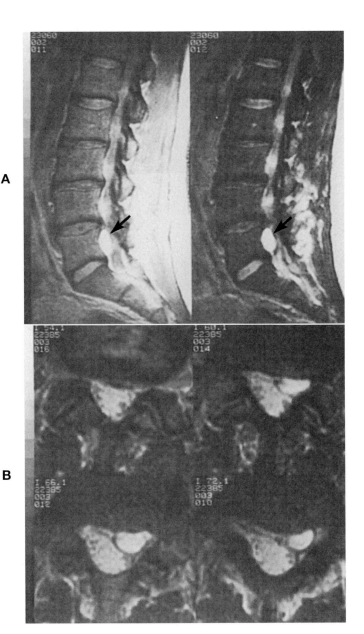

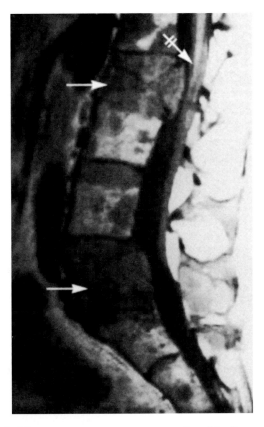

FIG. 8-34 Epidural hematoma. **A,** Sagittal proton density and double echo T$_2$-weighted images (TR/TE 2500/30, 70 ms) demonstrate a large ventral extradural soft-tissue mass, which is of relatively high signal intensity on both proton density and double echo T$_2$-weighted sequences *(arrows)*. **B,** Axial T$_2$-weighted images (TR/TE 3000/70 ms) in this patient with acute epidural hematoma demonstrate the relatively large ventrolateral extradural soft-tissue mass with high signal intensity, resulting in left-sided subarticular impingement of the traversing left L5 nerve root. *(From Kirkaldy WH: Managing low back pain, ed 4, Philadelphia, 1999, Churchill Livingstone.)*

FIG. 8-35 T$_1$-weighted MRI scan reveals mild effacement of the thecal sac *(crossed arrow)* and multiple hypointense regions where normal hyperintense marrow has been replaced by tumor tissue *(arrows)*. This is particularly the case at L5, which appears homogeneously hypointense. *(From Marchiori DM: Clinical imaging with skeletal, chest, and abdomen pattern differentials, St Louis, 1999, Mosby.)*

Assessment for Posterolateral, Posteromedial, and Posterocentral Intervertebral Disc Protrusion

Comment

Small disc lesions can cause significant spinal impairment. Central lesions may cause thecal sac displacement or lumbar spinal canal compromise (Fig. 8-36).

Two major types of low back abnormalities center around the intervertebral disc: acute impairment from herniated discs and chronic impairment from degenerative disc disease (Table 8-7).

The usual pressure in the nucleus pulposus is 30 pounds per square inch (psi). This pressure is 30% to 40% less in the standing position than in the seated position and is 50% less in the reclining position than in the seated position. Cerebrospinal fluid pressure is 100 to 200 mm H_2O in the recumbent position and 400 mm H_2O in the seated posture.

ORTHOPEDIC GAMUT 8-2

DISC INJURIES

Definitions of disc injuries follow:

1. *Disc protrusion* is present when nuclear material does not extend beyond the annulus in a contained HNP.
2. *Disc extrusion* is a focal herniation contained by the posterior longitudinal ligament that extends into the spinal canal.
3. *Sequestered disc* is a free fragment that has broken off or through the annular peripheral fibers in the vertebral canal (prolapsed).

TABLE 8-7

LUMBAR DISC SYNDROMES

	Lumbar Herniated Nucleus Pulposus	Degenerative Disc Disease
Physical examination findings	Back or leg pain	Morning stiffness
	Sciatic nerve tension signs:	Lumbopelvic hypomobility
	Positive straight leg raise <60°	Pain in lumbar flexion
	Positive Bragard's sign	History consistent with spinal degeneration
	Positive bowstring test	
	Positive Bechterew's test	
	Painful arc of lumbar flexion, extension, or both	
	True nerve root signs:	
	Radiculopathy	
	Motor or sensory deficit	
	Paresthesias	
	Diminished or absent deep tendon reflexes	
	Possible antalgia, muscle spasm, instability	
X-ray findings	Need to rule out organic pathology	Radiologic signs in acute exacerbation
	Hypolordosis secondary to muscle spasm	Spur formation
	Possible loss of intervertebral disc height	Loss of intervertebral disc height
	Possible diagnosis of degenerative arthritis	Discogenic spondylosis
		Compatible findings on CT or MRI scans

Adapted from Brier SR: *Primary care orthopedics,* St Louis, 1999, Mosby.
CT, Computed tomography; *MRI,* magnetic resonance imaging.

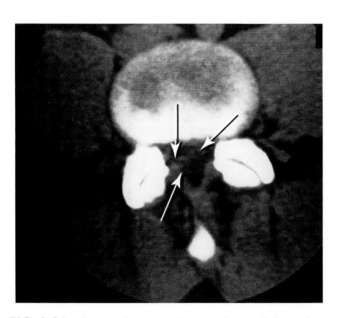

FIG. 8-36   Computed tomography scan demonstrating a large right paracentral herniated disc at the L4-L5 level.   *(From Brier SR: Primary care orthopedics, St Louis, 1999, Mosby.)*

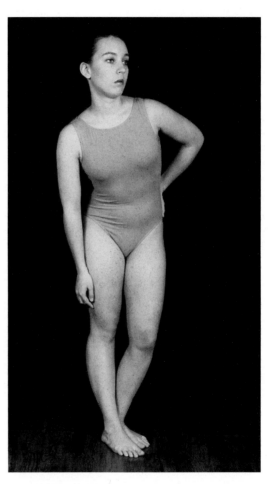

FIG. 8-37   When the disc protrudes lateral to the nerve root, the patient assumes an antalgic lean away from the side of the disc lesion or pain. In this illustration, the patient is experiencing left leg sciatica.

A disc may protrude either lateral to a nerve root, medial to a nerve root, under a nerve root, or central to the nerve root.

Approximately 90% or more of the lumbar lesions occur at either the L4-L5 or L5-S1 disc level. The L4-L5 disc usually compresses the fifth lumbar nerve root, resulting in pain sensations down the lower extremity in the L5 dermatome. The L5-S1 disc usually compresses the first sacral nerve root, resulting in pain distribution down the S1 dermatome. Of these patients, 60% will have an antalgic lean. Two factors are important: the side of sciatic pain distribution and the side of antalgic inclination. By evaluating the antalgic posture, the examiner may determine whether the problem is a medial, central, or lateral disc protrusion.

PROCEDURE

- When the disc protrudes lateral to the nerve root, the patient assumes an antalgic lean away from the side of the disc lesion or pain (Fig. 8-37).
- When the disc protrudes medial to the nerve root, the patient assumes an antalgic lean into the side of the disc lesion or pain (Fig. 8-38).
- With a central disc lesion, the patient assumes a flexed posture of the lumbar spine, with or without leaning to either side (Fig. 8-39).

- With protrusion under the nerve root, the patient may not lean at all.

Confirmation Procedures
Bowstring sign, Cox sign, heel/toe walk test, Kemp's test, Lewin punch test, Lewin snuff test, Milgram's test, and Neri's sign

DIAGNOSTIC STATEMENT

The patient demonstrates antalgic positioning toward the right, away from the left side sciatica. This result suggests a left side lateral disc protrusion.

The patient demonstrates a left side antalgic posturing toward the side of pain. This posture suggests a left side medial disc protrusion.

The patient demonstrates a fixed and slightly flexed antalgic posture with no lateral flexion component. This posture suggests a central disc protrusion.

CLINICAL PEARL

If the antalgia is not readily apparent in a static posture, it will appear with forward flexion of the trunk. If a disc protrusion exists, even in the mildest degree, trunk flexion exerts enough pressure to irritate the inflamed muscle or to stretch neural structures over the bulging disc. The antalgia is manifested at this point.

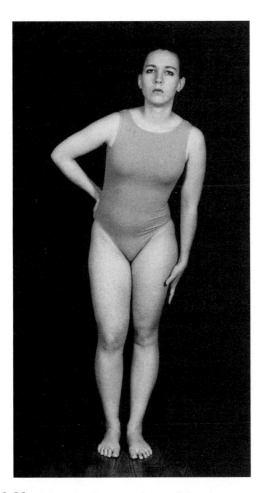

FIG. 8-38   When the disc protrudes medial to the nerve root, the patient assumes an antalgic lean into the side of the disc lesion or pain. In this illustration, the patient is experiencing left leg sciatica.

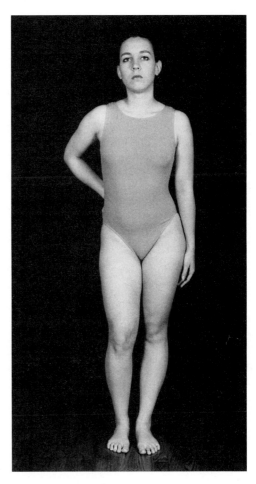

FIG. 8-39   With a central disc lesion, the patient assumes a flexed posture of the lumbar spine, with or without leaning to either side.

BECHTEREW'S SITTING TEST

Assessment for Sciatica, Intervertebral Disc Lesion, Vertebral Exostoses, Dural Sleeve Adhesions, Muscular Spasm, or Vertebral Subluxation

Comment

The dura mater of the lumbar spine has a series of attachments to neighboring vertebrae and ligaments. These attachments are found at each segmental level and are usually found in the region of the intervertebral disc. They have been referred to as the *dural attachment complex* or *Hoffmann ligaments*.

The neural elements pass over an intervertebral disc before exiting through an intervertebral foramen (IVF) (Fig. 8-40).

A typical lumbar IVF (Fig. 8-41) is sometimes described as being shaped like an inverted teardrop or an inverted pear.

Compression, or entrapment, of neural elements as they pass through the nerve root canal or the IVF can occur. Causes of such compression include degenerative changes of the superior articular facets and posterior vertebral bodies, intervertebral disc protrusion, and pressure from the superior pedicle of the IVF.

Lumbar disc protrusions are a common cause of lower back pain with sciatica. This protrusion usually occurs against a background of degenerative joint disease. The disc protrusion of a young adult is likely to be traumatic and should not be classified as osteoarthritis.

The precipitating trauma of an intervertebral disc syndrome is usually slight. The annulus fibrosus ruptures posteriorly, and a fragment of the nucleus is extruded into the vertebral canal. In other instances, there may be a frank prolapse of the nucleus pulposus through the tear. If there is concomitant rupture of the posterior longitudinal ligament, the protrusion may be in the midline posteriorly. This is instead of a usual posterolateral position. The fibrocartilage or nucleus pulposus may impinge on the related nerve root and compress it against the lamina and ligamentum flavum. Because the rupture is usually to one side of the midline, only one nerve root is affected in its extrathecal course. Because the roots of the cauda equina run vertically within the theca, one or more of these passing caudal nerves also may be compressed. If the rupture is in the midline, roots on both sides may be involved. If it is large enough, the protrusion also may compress the cauda equina. Most disc lesions are at the L4-L5 or L5-S1 level. It is only here that a disc lesion produces the syndrome of lower backache with sciatica. Unlike the situation in the cervical spine, cord compression is not a feature of lumbar disc lesions because the spinal cord ends opposite the lower border of L1. However, cauda equina compression can occur at these levels.

The apophyseal joints are usually involved pari passu with disc degeneration. They are also part of the pattern of joint involvement in multiple osteoarthritis and are likely to contribute to the patient's symptoms.

Pain is aggravated by movement of the spine, such as rolling over in bed, and by any maneuver that causes elevation of the cerebrospinal fluid pressure within the theca. Pain is more constantly aggravated by maneuvers that stretch the sciatic nerve. Forward flexion of the lumbar spine or straight leg raising with the patient supine produces pain.

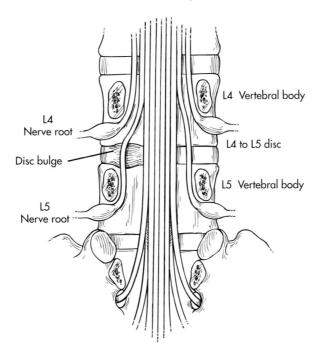

FIG. 8-40   Lumbar intervertebral discs and the exiting nerve roots.   *(From Greenstein GM:* Clinical assessment of neuromusculoskeletal disorders, *St Louis, 1997, Mosby.)*

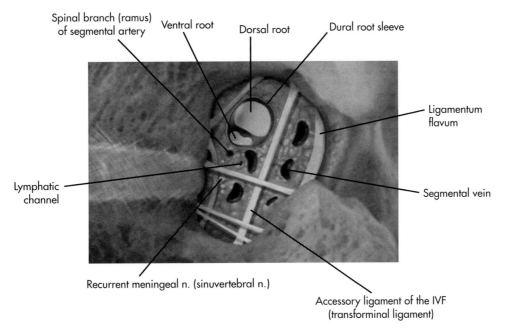

FIG. 8-41   The lumbar intervertebral foramen. *IVF,* Intervertebral foramen.   *(From Greenstein GM:* Clinical assessment of neuromusculoskeletal disorders, *St Louis, 1997, Mosby.)*

The back usually is held rigid, and movements are limited by muscle spasm, which results in antalgia to one side or the other and flattening of the lumbar lordosis. Forward flexion is more limited than lateral flexion.

PROCEDURE

- While in a seated position, the patient attempts to extend each leg, one at a time (Figs. 8-42 and 8-43).
- The examiner resists the patient's attempts at hip flexion with downward pressure on the thigh (Fig. 8-44).
- This extension is followed by an attempt to extend both legs.
- The test is positive if backache or sciatic pain is increased or the maneuver is impossible.
- In disc involvement, extending both legs will usually increase the spinal and sciatic discomfort.
- A positive test indicates sciatica, a disc lesion, exostoses, adhesions, spasm, or subluxation.

Confirmation Procedures

Bragard's sign, Deyerle's sign, Fajersztajn's test, Lasègue differential sign, Lasègue rebound test, Lasègue sitting test, Lasègue test, Lewin standing test, Lindner's sign, Sicard's sign, straight-leg-raising test, and Turyn's sign

DIAGNOSTIC STATEMENT

Bechterew's sitting test is positive on the left and elicits pain that begins in the lumbar spine and radiates down the left leg. This result suggests a disc lesion in the lumbar spine and nerve root irritation on the left.

CLINICAL PEARL

Simple flattening or even reversal of the lumbar curve often is not associated with radicular pain. The pain is localized in the lower lumbar spine, and any movement of the spine accentuates the pain. In these instances, the prime pathologic feature is sprain of an intervertebral joint rather than root irritation.

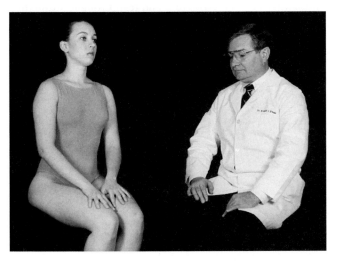

FIG. 8-42   The patient is in the seated position.

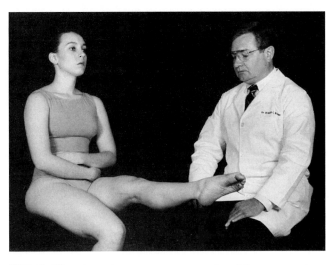

FIG. 8-43   The patient attempts to extend each leg one at a time.

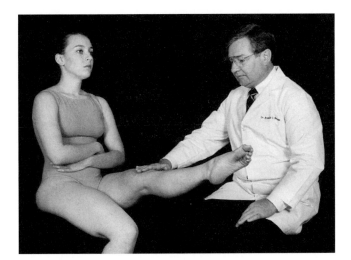

FIG. 8-44   The examiner resists the patient's attempts at hip flexion with downward pressure on the thigh. The test is positive if the maneuver increases backache or sciatic pain or if the maneuver is impossible. Unilateral leg testing is followed by the patient's attempt to extend both legs simultaneously. With disc involvement, extending both legs will usually increase the spinal and sciatic discomfort. A positive test indicates sciatica, disc lesion, exostoses, adhesions, spasm, or subluxation.

Assessment for Mechanical Lumbosacral Lesion, Intervertebral Disc Lesion, or Vertebral Exostoses

Comment

The lumbar Z joints are complex synovial joints that are oriented in the vertical plane (Fig. 8-45).

During rotation of the lumbar region, distraction, or gapping, occurs between adjacent lumbar articular facets on the side of rotation. An articular capsule covers the posterior aspect of each lumbar Z joint. Effusion within the Z joint may enter the superior recess and as little as 0.5 ml of effusion may cause the superior recess of the capsule to enter the anteriorly located IVF. Such a protrusion of the Z joint is known as a *synovial cyst*.

Degenerative changes of the Z joints often accompany aging. Such changes include an inflammatory reaction at the synovial lining of the Z joint, changes of the articular cartilage, loose bodies in the Z joint, and laxity of the joint capsule.

Degeneration of the disc leads to increased rotational instability of the Z joints, resulting in further degeneration of these structures.

Osteophytes (bony spurs) often develop with age on the superior and inferior articular processes. Often, this occurs on the periphery of the Z joint along the attachment sites of the ligamentum flavum or the articular capsule.

As the legs are raised or lowered, they exert a strong, downward pull on the pelvis. This pull is in opposition to the upward pull of the abdominal muscles. If the patient can tilt the pelvis posteriorly to flex the spine and hold the low back flat on an examining table as the legs are raised or lowered, the abdominal muscles must act to hold that position.

If the abdominal muscles are weak and the hip flexor muscles are strong, the back cannot be held flat while the legs are raised or lowered. The lower back will appear hyperextended as the legs are raised, and the abdominal muscles will be put on stretch.

The actions of various segments of the abdominal muscles are so closely allied with and interdependent on other parts that no specific functions can be ascribed to any single segment.

From a mechanical standpoint, the pelvis can be tilted toward the posterior rib cage by an upward pull on the pubis, by a downward pull on the ischium, and by an oblique pull from the anterior iliac crest. The muscle or muscle fibers that lie in these lines of pull are the rectus abdominis, the hip extensors, and the lateral fibers of the external oblique. These muscles act to tilt the pelvis posteriorly, whether the subject is standing or lying supine. During double leg raising from a supine position, the hip extensors cease to actively assist in tilting the pelvis posteriorly. The rectus abdominis and the external oblique muscles assume the major roles if an effort is made to flex the lumbar spine and keep the lower back flat on the examination table, while the thoracic spine remains extended. Without the resistance of the lower extremities, the pelvis can be tilted posteriorly by the external oblique without assistance from the rectus abdominis. Against resistance, as occurs during double leg raising, the rectus abdominis must come into strong action.

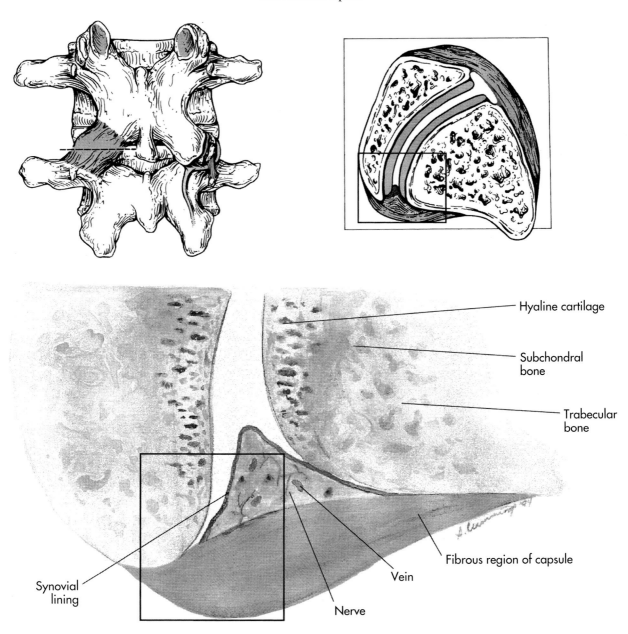

FIG. 8-45 The zygapophyseal joint (Z joint). *(From Greenstein GM:* Clinical assessment of neuromusculoskeletal disorders, *St Louis, 1997, Mosby.)*

The abdominal muscles elongate, and the back starts to arch if the patient's strength is not sufficient to maintain the pelvis in posterior tilt.

At the initiation of double leg raising or leg lowering, the thorax will show a tendency for the ribs to pull inward, decreasing the infrasternal angle. This movement is compatible with the line of pull and the action of the external oblique.

PROCEDURE

- The patient lowers the straightened legs from a 90-degree angle to a 45-degree angle (Figs. 8-46 and 8-47).
- The test is positive if the legs drop or if the move produces pain.
- A positive test indicates lumbosacral involvement, disc lesions, or exostoses.

Confirmation Procedures

Demianoff's sign, double leg-raise test, hyperflexion test, Lewin supine test, matchstick test, Mennell's sign, Minor's sign, Nachlas test, Quick test, Schober's test, sign of the buttock, skin pinch test, spinal percussion test, and Vanzetti's sign

---

DIAGNOSTIC STATEMENT

The bilateral leg-lowering test is positive and elicits lower back pain. This result indicates mechanical lumbosacral involvement.

CLINICAL PEARL

Because of the presence of the nociceptive nerve ending within the annulus fibrosus of the disc, annular tears can cause pain in the lower back, buttocks, sacroiliac region, and lower extremity. This pain can occur without nerve compression by a disc protrusion. Disc protrusion that does not compress the nerve root can cause an inflammatory response and secondary radiculitis by chemically induced inflammatory neural pain.

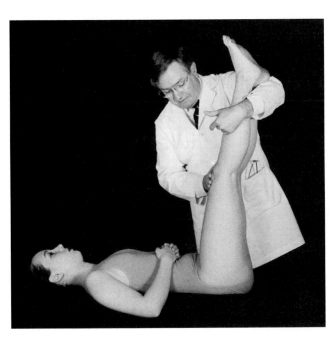

FIG. 8-46 The patient is supine with both legs fully extended. The examiner lifts both legs, simultaneously, to a near 90-degree, hip-flexion angle.

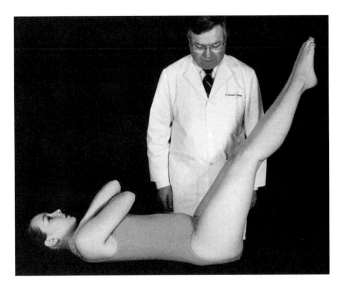

FIG. 8-47 From this elevated leg position, the patient is instructed to lower the legs from a 90-degree angle to a 45-degree angle. The test is positive if the legs drop or if lower back pain is produced. A positive test indicates lumbosacral involvement, disc lesions, or exostoses.

Assessment for Lumbar Nerve Root Compression

Comment

Lower back pain often is associated with sciatica and can be elicited in the posterior part of a degenerated disc because the posterior longitudinal ligament in this region contains sensory nerve fibers. However, lower back pain is not the direct result of nerve root compression. Disc degeneration does not elicit a referred radiating pain that can be confused with the pain of lumbosacral nerve root compression. Lower back pain is present in most cases of sciatica and often appears earlier than does the radiating pain. In some cases, the pain has its onset with the onset of the radiating pain. The lower back pain is not as important in the diagnosis as the levels and sites of nerve root compression.

In adults, the cord ends near the caudal end of the first lumbar vertebra. In its caudal extension, the dural sac encloses the lumbosacral nerve roots. At each segment, a pair of nerve roots, symmetrically enclosed by dural nerve root sleeves, leaves the dural sac and departs from the spinal canal through the intervertebral foramina at that level. In the lower lumbar region, the point of departure of the nerve roots from the dural sac is more cranial than the point at which the nerve roots depart from the spinal canal through their respective intervertebral foramina. The difference in height amounts to about one segment.

All of the lower sacral nerve roots depart from the tapering end cone of the dural sac, which is caudal to the level of the L5 disc. This end cone varies in how far it reaches into the sacral canal. The levels at which the lower sacral nerve roots depart from the dural sac are different in individual cases.

The neurologic symptoms caused by disc protrusions bulging from different lumbar discs depend on the nerve root that is closest to the site of the disc protrusion, making it the first one compressed. At their point of departure from the dural sac, the nerve roots are firmly fixed to the dural sac and cannot, at this point, be easily pushed aside by disc protrusions. This firmness contributes to the occurrence of typical nerve root syndromes caused by disc protrusions located near the point from which the nerve roots depart.

ORTHOPEDIC GAMUT 8-3

LUMBOSACRAL NERVE ROOTS

After leaving the dural sac, the lumbosacral nerve roots run caudally and laterally in the direction that they depart from the spinal canal:

1. The fourth lumbar root (L4) leaves the dural sac slightly caudal of the intervertebral disc between the third and fourth lumbar vertebrae (third lumbar disc).
2. The fifth lumbar root (L5) leaves the dural sac near the level of the fourth lumbar disc.
3. The first sacral root (S1) leaves the dural sac medial of S1 and slightly below the level of the L5 disc.

PROCEDURE

- With the patient in the supine position, the examiner moves the patient's leg until it is above the examiner's shoulder.
- At this point, firm pressure should be exerted on the hamstring muscles (Fig. 8-48).
- If pain is not elicited, pressure is applied to the popliteal fossa.
- Pain in the lumbar region or radiculopathy is a positive sign for nerve root compression.

Confirmation Procedures

Antalgia sign, Cox sign, heel/toe walk test, Kemp's test, Lewin punch test, Lewin snuff test, Milgram's test, and Neri's sign

---

DIAGNOSTIC STATEMENT

Bowstring sign is present on the left. The presence of this sign indicates lumbosacral nerve root compression.

CLINICAL PEARL

Nerve roots must change their lengths depending on the degree of flexion, extension, lateral flexion, and rotation of the lumbar spine. Lumbar nerve roots that are limited in motion by fibrosis of either intraspinal or extraspinal origin will create traction on the nerve root complex, causing ischemia and secondary neural dysfunction.

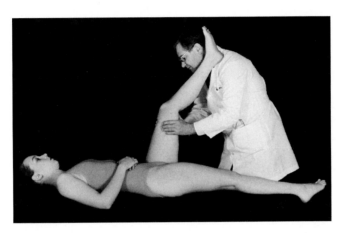

FIG. 8-48   The patient is in the supine position with both legs fully extended. The examiner places the patient's affected leg atop a shoulder. The examiner exerts firm pressure near the insertion of the hamstring muscles. If this maneuver is painful, firm pressure is applied to the popliteal fossa. Pain in the lumbar region or radiculopathy is a positive sign for nerve root compression.

BRAGARD'S SIGN

Assessment for Sciatic Neuritis, Spinal Cord Tumor, Intervertebral Disc Lesions, and Spinal Nerve Irritation

Comment

An intervertebral disc typically consists of a nucleus pulposus surrounded by an anulus fibrosus, both sandwiched between superior and inferior vertebral end-plates (Fig. 8-49). The nucleus pulposus of a lumbar intervertebral disc consists of a central core of a well-hydrated proteoglycan matrix surrounded by fibrocartilage. The anulus fibrosus consists of 10 to 12 concentric lamellae of collagen fibers. In any given lamella, the collagen fibers run in parallel at an angle of about 65 degrees to the vertical, but the direction of this angle alternates in successive layers.

Pain in the segmental distribution of a root is the hallmark of root compression syndrome. Pain in the spine and restriction of spinal movement are common and are the result of local involvement of the sensitive tissues and the root. Herniated disc, metastatic malignancy, a primary neoplasm, recent trauma, or inflammation may be responsible.

Pain that radiates down the leg follows the primary anterior division of the nerve and may be localized by the patient anywhere in the distribution of the root. This root pain is aggravated by spinal movement, local pressure over the nerve, or straining of the nerve. Pressure over the muscle in the area of pain usually produces discomfort.

Paresthesia in root distribution is common and usually is experienced distally, in the foot. This paresthesia may be aggravated or relieved by the same factors that influence the pain, but the paresthesia is constant.

Weakness and atrophy in the corresponding myotonic distribution result from prolonged or severe root compression, and stretch reflexes, with arcs that are largely or entirely incorporated in the involved root, will be diminished or lost.

Suspicion of a single nerve root compression syndrome should be prompted by the combination of a history of pain and the presence of paresthesia in the appropriate distribution of one nerve root only. Findings necessary to confirm the diagnosis are those that relate spinal movement to the radiating pain, those that demonstrate muscular weakness and tenderness in the myotome, and those that localize sensory and reflex deficits to the dermatome and myotome.

A herniated intervertebral disc produces a persistent, unilateral, isolated syndrome. Bilateral and multiple nerve root involvement can be caused by extensive degenerative joint disease. When nerve root involvement is progressive and acute or subacute, metastatic malignancy or inflammation is suggested.

Nerve root compression may herald an intraspinal mass that later will impinge on the spinal cord or cauda equina. The examiner must always look closely for motor, sensory, and reflex changes below the affected root because these changes may indicate involvement of the cord or cauda equina.

A herniated intervertebral disc is the most common cause of frank root compression syndromes affecting the extremities.

PROCEDURE

- If the Lasègue or straight-leg-raising tests are positive, the leg is lowered below the point of discomfort, and the foot is sharply dorsiflexed (Fig. 8-50).
- The sign is present if pain is increased.
- The presence of the sign is a finding associated with sciatic neuritis, spinal cord tumors, intervertebral disc lesions, and spinal nerve irritations.

Confirmation Procedures

Bechterew's sitting test, Deyerle's sign, Fajersztajn's test, Lasègue differential sign, Lasègue rebound test, Lasègue sitting test, Lasègue test, Lewin standing test, Lindner's sign, Sicard's sign, straight-leg-raising test, and Turyn's sign

---

DIAGNOSTIC STATEMENT

Bragard's sign is present. This result indicates sciatic neuritis on the left.

CLINICAL PEARL

Either the Bragard's sign or Hyndman's sign (for neck flexion movement) must be accomplished as a finishing maneuver in any positive straight-leg-raising test. Pain that increases during neck flexion, ankle dorsiflexion, or both indicates an inflamed nerve root. Pain that does not increase with these maneuvers may indicate a problem in the hamstring area or in the lumbosacral or sacroiliac joints.

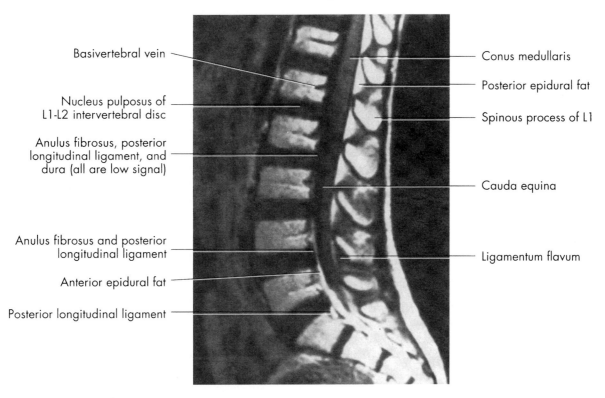

Basivertebral vein

Nucleus pulposus of
L1-L2 intervertebral disc

Anulus fibrosus, posterior
longitudinal ligament, and
dura (all are low signal)

Anulus fibrosus and posterior
longitudinal ligament

Anterior epidural fat

Posterior longitudinal ligament

Conus medullaris

Posterior epidural fat

Spinous process of L1

Cauda equina

Ligamentum flavum

FIG. 8-49   T₁-weighted (SE 800/20) midline sagittal image of the lumbar spine.   *(From Enzmann DR, DeLaPaz RL, Rubin JB:* Magnetic resonance of the spine, *St Louis, 1990, Mosby.)*

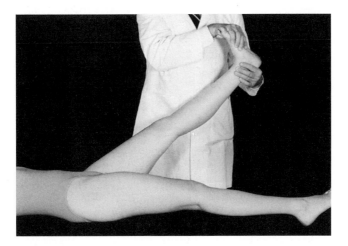

FIG. 8-50   If a straight-leg-raising test is positive, the affected leg is lowered just below the angle of pain production and is held by the examiner. The examiner sharply dorsiflexes the foot. The sign is present if the pain is duplicated or increased. The presence of the sign indicates sciatic neuritis, spinal cord tumors, intervertebral disc lesions, and spinal nerve irritations.

COX SIGN

Assessment for Prolapse of Intervertebral Disc Nucleus

Comment

In general, the intervertebral discs of the lumbar region are the thickest of the spine (Fig. 8-51).

The lumbar discs become shorter during the day because they carry the load of the torso relaxation. They usually regain their shape within 5 hours of sleep (creep). During the active hours, the discs require movement to maintain proper hydration. In fact, decreased movement and decreased axial loading have been strongly associated with disc degeneration.

Several maneuvers tighten the sciatic nerve and compress an inflamed nerve root against a herniated lumbar disc. With the straight-leg-raising tests, the L5 and S1 nerve roots move several millimeters at the level of the foramen. The L4 nerve root moves a smaller distance, and the proximal roots show little motion. The straight-leg-raising tests are most important and valuable for detecting lesions of the L5 and S1 nerve roots. Young patients with herniated discs have marked propensities for positive straight-leg-raising tests. Although the test itself is not pathognomonic, a negative test rules out the possibility of a herniated disc. After age 30, a negative straight-leg-raising test no longer precludes this diagnosis.

The straight-leg-raising tests are performed while the patient is supine. The examiner raises the affected leg slowly. Only when leg pain or radicular symptoms are reproduced is the straight-leg-raising test considered positive. Back pain alone is not a positive finding for straight leg raising.

Many variations of the straight-leg-raising test have been developed. Contralateral straight leg raising is performed in a way similar to the straight-leg-raising test except that, with the former test, the examiner raises the unaffected leg. If this movement reproduces the patient's sciatica in the affected extremity, the test is positive. This result suggests a herniated disc and is an indication that the prolapse, although it may be large, is medial to the nerve root in the axilla.

When the roots of the femoral nerve are involved, they are tensed, not by the straight-leg-raising test but by the reverse of straight leg raising, such as hip extension and knee flexion.

PROCEDURE

- Cox sign occurs during straight leg raising when the pelvis rises from the table instead of the hip flexing (Figs. 8-52 and 8-53).
- Cox sign is present when patients have a prolapse of the nucleus into the intervertebral foramen.

Confirmation Procedures

Antalgia sign, bowstring sign, heel/toe walk test, Kemp's test, Lewin punch test, Lewin snuff test, Milgram's test, and Neri's sign

---

DIAGNOSTIC STATEMENT

Cox sign is present during straight leg raising on the left. This sign indicates a prolapse of nuclear material into the neural foramen.

CLINICAL PEARL

Cox sign is a consistent finding associated with disc prolapse. The sign often is overlooked in the patient's pain presentation. A false-negative test result may occur if the examiner does not observe the movements of the buttocks on the affected side. The sign is present the moment hip flexion motion is locked and the buttock rises from the examination table.

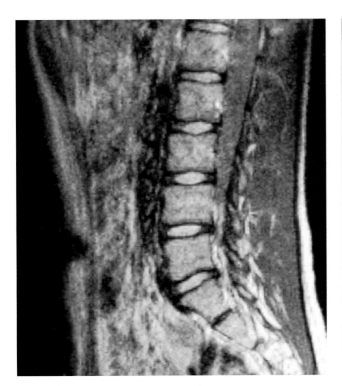 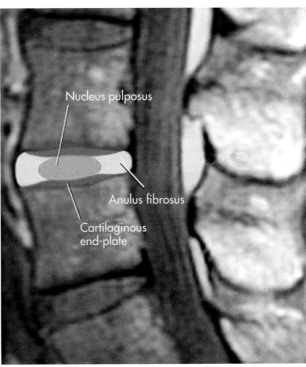

FIG. 8-51 Midsagittal magnetic resonance imaging scan of the lumbar spine. *(From Greenstein GM: Clinical assessment of neuromusculoskeletal disorders, St Louis, 1997, Mosby.)*

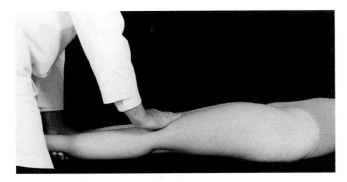

FIG. 8-52 The patient is supine with the legs fully extended. The examiner places one hand under the ankle of the affected leg and the other hand on the knee.

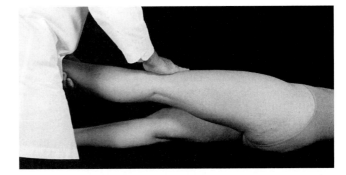

FIG. 8-53 The examiner performs a straight-leg-raising test on the affected leg. Cox sign is present if, during the straight leg raising, the pelvis rises from the table rather than the hip flexing. The sign is present in patients with prolapse of the nucleus into the intervertebral foramen.

DEMIANOFF'S SIGN

Assessment for Spasm of the Sacrolumbalis (Iliocostalis Lumborum) Musculature

Comment

Back strain can be defined as nonradiating lower back pain associated with mechanical stress to the lumbosacral spine. The exact number of patients with back strain is difficult to determine. Most patients with back pain (90%) have it for a mechanical reason. Of patients with mechanical lower back pain, back strain may account for 60% to 70%.

The cause of back strain is not always clear, but it may be related to muscular strain secondary to either a specific traumatic episode or continuous mechanical stress. The lumbosacral spine has two major biomechanical functions. The first function is to support the upper body in a balanced, upright position while allowing the second function—locomotion. In a static, upright position, maintenance of erect posture is achieved through a balance among the expansile pressure of the intervertebral discs, the stretch placed on the anterior and posterior longitudinal and facet joint ligaments, and the sustained involuntary tone of the surrounding lumbosacral and abdominal muscles. The balance of the spine is also related to the reciprocal physiologic curves in the cervical, thoracic, and lumbosacral areas of the vertebral column. The balance in curvature results in an individual's posture. Proper alignment is also influenced by structures in the pelvis and lower extremities, including the hip joint capsule and the hamstring and gluteus maximus muscles.

Movement of the lumbar spine is associated with a lumbar pelvic rhythm that results in the simultaneous reversal of the lumbar lordosis and rotation of the hips. During flexion and extension of the lumbar spine, tension is produced in the paraspinous, hamstring, and gluteal muscles; the fascia that surrounds the muscles; and the ligaments that support the vertebral bodies and discs. In addition to the normal stresses placed on these structures during lowering and raising of the torso, the stresses on these anatomic structures are increased to an even greater degree when an individual must lift a heavy object. During lateral flexion, paraspinous muscle activity increases on both sides of the spine, but it primarily increases on the side toward the lateral flexion. During axial rotation of the spine, the erector spinae muscles on the ipsilateral side and the rotator and multifidus muscles on the contralateral side are active. Lateral flexion is accomplished by contraction of the abdominal wall oblique muscles with the ipsilateral quadratus lumborum and psoas major muscles.

Spinal infections involving the vertebrae and the intervertebral discs, usually referred to as *disc space infections* because of the characteristic radiographic appearance, are rare causes of low back pain. When present and in the early stages, spinal infection may be confused with back strain.

Although a number of serious conditions, including benign and malignant tumors, Paget's disease, vascular disease, infections, and fractures, cause discomfort in the lower back, most patients who experience low back pain do not have underlying medical disease. The history of a previous infection, and in particular a urinary tract infection with abdominal symptoms, suggests the possibility of disc space infection. Pyogenic infections of the lower spine usually present with persistent increasing pain. Pyrexia, local tenderness, muscle spasm, constitutional symptoms, and neurologic deficits may or may not be present. Pain radiating to the abdomen or both legs and the presence of abdominal discomfort and symptoms may confuse the diagnosis.

ORTHOPEDIC GAMUT 8-4

DISC SPACE INFECTION

The radiographic evidence of established disc space infection includes the following:

1. Symmetric destruction of adjacent end-plate surfaces of two vertebrae
2. Loss of disc height
3. Reactive new bone formation
4. Sclerosis of bone end-plates, with or without evidence of bone destruction or bone formation
5. Soft-tissue abscesses
6. Kyphosis or subluxation after there has been significant bone destruction

---

The early diagnosis of a disc space infection requires a high level of clinical suspicion. Any patient in whom this possibility is considered should have blood cultures, urine cultures, a complete blood count, erythrocyte sedimentation rate (ESR), and AP and lateral radiographs of the spine. The radiographs may show evidence of soft-tissue expansion around the disc height. A bone scan may be helpful, showing a localized hot spot before radiographic change, and spinal MRI may show the abscess and disc space changes in the early stage of evolution. In addition, CT scans, as carried out in the case, may help delineate the anatomic changes.

PROCEDURE

- While the patient is in a supine position, the examiner performs a straight-leg-raising test with either leg.
- The sign is present when this action produces a pain in the lumbar region.
- This pain prevents the patient from raising the leg high enough to form an angle, between the examination table and the leg, of 15 degrees or more (Fig. 8-54).
- The sign differentiates pain that originates in the sacrolumbalis muscles from lumbar pain of any other origin.

- When the test is positive, it demonstrates that the pain is caused by the stretching of the sacrolumbalis (iliocostalis lumborum).

Confirmation Procedures
Bilateral leg-lowering test, double leg-raising test, hyperextension test, Lewin supine test, matchstick test, Mennell's sign, Minor's sign, Nachlas test, Quick test, Schober's test, sign of the buttock, skin pinch test, spinal percussion test, and Vanzetti's sign

---

DIAGNOSTIC STATEMENT

Demianoff's sign is present. This sign indicates strain of the sacrolumbalis musculature.

CLINICAL PEARL

Demianoff's sign is clearly separate from Cox sign. Demianoff's sign involves production of lower back pain, which prevents further raising of the leg. Sciatica is absent. Cox sign is present when the pelvis is locked, which prevents further elevation of the leg because of increasing sciatica.

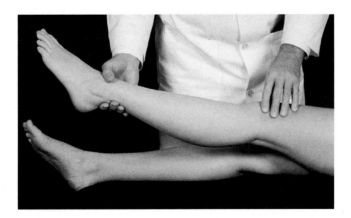

FIG. 8-54 The patient is in a supine position. The examiner performs a straight-leg-raising test on the affected leg. The sign is present when this action produces a pain in the lumbar region. The pain prevents the examiner from raising the leg high enough to form an angle of 15 degrees or more with the examination table. When the sign is present, it demonstrates that pain occurs because of the stretching of the sacrolumbalis (iliocostalis lumborum) musculature.

DEYERLE'S SIGN

Assessment for Sciatic Nerve Irritation

Comment

Patients with acute low back pain often complain of pain that radiates from the low back into the posterior thigh.

Patients with lesions compressing the L2 and L3 nerve roots may experience pain on the medial and lateral portions of the posterior thigh. Occasionally, L4 lesions may also cause similar symptoms and signs. The phase of degeneration or spondylosis often determines the level of intervention (Table 8-8).

The pain pattern that is associated with nerve root irritation resulting from a movable lamina arch or neural arch (spondylolisthesis) resembles the pain caused by compression of the nerve root by an intervertebral disc or by compression of the nerve root by other mechanical means. Pain usually occurs when the spine is extended or when the spinous process is compressed or manipulated, causing secondary irritation of the dura. Pain may radiate along the course of the femoral or sciatic nerve, depending on the site of the bone abnormality.

Degenerative arthritis in the hip or alteration of the hip joint capsule or of the surrounding osseous structures may cause pain anteriorly, laterally, and posteriorly in the groin. Pain radiation may be associated with this through the lateral femoral cutaneous nerve, through the obturator nerve along the medial aspect of the thigh, or through branches of the sciatic nerve along the posterior thigh.

Destructive lesions of the sacrum, pelvis, pubis, or ischium cause pain along the femoral, obturator, or sciatic nerves. The onset of this pain may be vague and gradual, and the distribution of the pain may be deep, with few cutaneous changes. The radiculopathy may resemble a primary nerve root irritation.

PROCEDURE

- While the patient is seated, the affected leg is passively extended at the knee until pain is reproduced (Fig. 8-55).
- The knee is then slightly flexed while strong pressure is applied by the examiner into the popliteal fossa (Fig. 8-56).
- The sign is present if this pressure increases radicular symptoms.
- The sign demonstrates irritation of the sciatic nerve above the knee.
- This irritation is caused by stretching the nerve over an abnormal mechanical obstruction.

Confirmation Procedures

Bechterew's sitting test, Bragard's sign, Fajersztajn's test, Lasègue differential sign, Lasègue rebound test, Lasègue sitting test, Lasègue test, Lewin standing test, Lindner's sign, Sicard's sign, straight-leg-raising test, and Turyn's sign

---

DIAGNOSTIC STATEMENT

Deyerle's sign is present on the left. This sign indicates irritation of the sciatic nerve above the knee.

CLINICAL PEARL

Deyerle's sign is a variation of the Lasègue sitting test. The sign demonstrates the effects of inflammation or partial denervation (neural compression) in the sciatic distribution. The pain response may be caused by myalgic hyperalgesia as a response to denervation hypersensitivity.

TABLE 8-8

OVERVIEW OF SCHEME OF TREATMENT RELATIVE TO THE PHASE OF SPONDYLOSIS

Phase	Lesion	Treatment
Dysfunction	Facet joint	Mobilization, manipulation, injection
	Sacroiliac joint	Mobilization, manipulation, injection
	Myofascial syndromes	Contract stretching, injection
	Disc herniation	Epidural injection, discectomy
Unstable	Disc herniation	Epidural injection, discectomy
	Segmental instability	Injection, fusion
	Lateral stenosis	Nerve root block, decompression, fusion
	Central stenosis	Epidural injection, decompression, fusion
	Degenerative olisthesis	Epidural injection, decompression, fusion
	Isthmic olisthesis	Epidural injection, decompression, fusion
Stabilization	Disc herniation	Epidural injection, discectomy
	Lateral stenosis	Nerve root block, decompression
	Central stenosis	Epidural injection, decompression
	Degenerative olisthesis	Epidural injection, decompression, rarely fusion
	Isthmic olisthesis	Epidural injection, decompression, rarely fusion

From Kirkaldy WH: *Managing low back pain,* ed 4, Philadelphia 1999, Churchill Livingstone.

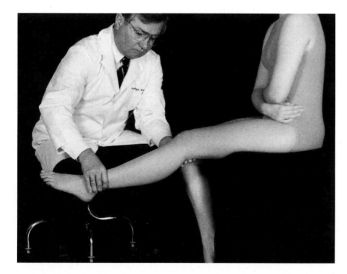

FIG. 8-55 The patient is seated. The examiner extends the patient's affected leg to the point at which pain is reproduced.

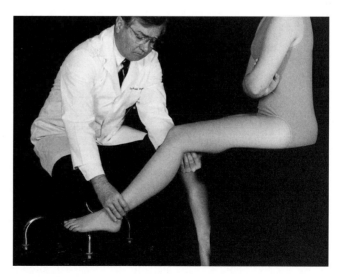

FIG. 8-56 The knee is slightly flexed while strong pressure into the popliteal fossa is applied by the examiner. The sign is present if radicular symptoms are increased.

DOUBLE LEG-RAISE TEST

ALSO KNOWN AS BILATERAL STRAIGHT LEG-RAISING TEST

Assessment for Lumbosacral Joint Involvement

Comment

Sprain is common in the mobile lumbar spine, which has many ligaments giving support to the various joints. The supraspinous ligament, which extends along the tips of the spinous processes, is particularly susceptible. A sprain involving this ligament can be diagnosed by tenderness over the ligament or over the tip of the spinous process, where the ligament attaches. Active contraction of the muscles to pull the spine into hyperextension is pain free, as is passive extension. Active flexion of the back, which occurs during an attempt to sit up from the supine position, is pain free until tension is put on the spinous process by forcing the head toward the knees. Passive hyperflexion of the spine will cause pain.

Injury to other ligaments of the back is much more difficult to diagnose. The interspinous ligament is rarely damaged because it has elastic fibers and is not readily overstretched. However, the articular ligaments around the apophyseal joints are commonly damaged, as are the anterior spinal and the lateral spinal ligaments. Whether or not the ligamentum flavum is damaged by hyperflexion is problematic because it is also an elastic structure and probably will allow as much motion without damage as the range of flexion of the back will permit. Diagnosis of these sprains depends on whether tests that bring stress upon certain areas are used. With a sprain, passive movements that put stress on the involved ligament will cause pain. For example, sprain of the capsule on the left will cause pain during lateral flexion to the right or during flexion of the trunk.

Persistent low back pain without nerve root tension signs should signal the possibility of a stress reaction or fracture of the pars interarticularis.

Spondylolysis appearing between ages 6 and 7 is caused by a fatigue fracture of the pars interarticularis and is seldom caused by one acute, traumatic event.

Patients with an impending or existing pars fractures complain of low back pain. Young patients often report that they have been playing a sport, even though they had a backache and some spasm, and that they noted a sudden worsening of symptoms after a specific traumatic episode.

Affected patients often complain of chronic, dull, aching, or cramping pain in the low back. The pain may be unilateral or bilateral, usually "along the belt line." The ache is usually constant and worsens with rotation or hyperextension of the low back. There are usually no radicular findings or true sciatic tension signs present. The range of motion, although painful, is usually full. There may be palpable, paraspinal spasms and hamstring tightness. Commonly, having the patient stand on one leg and bend backward (Jackson's test) reproduces and accentuates the pain if a fatigue fracture is present (Fig. 8-57). In the presence of a unilateral defect, hyperextension while standing on the ipsilateral leg will worsen the pain on the side of the defect.

PROCEDURE

- While the patient is supine, the examiner performs a straight-leg-raising test on each of the lower extremities, noting the angle at which the pain is produced.
- Next, both lower limbs are raised together (Fig. 8-58).
- If pain is produced at an earlier angle by raising both legs together, the test is positive (Fig. 8-59).
- In the presence of disc disease with resulting vertebral instability, the double leg-raising movement will cause pain in the lumbar area.
- The test is specific and highly accurate for lumbosacral joint involvement.

Confirmation Procedures

Bilateral leg-lowering test, Demianoff's sign, hyperextension test, Lewin supine test, matchstick test, Mennell's sign, Minor's sign, Nachlas test, Quick test, Schober's test, sign of the buttock, skin pinch test, spinal percussion test, and Vanzetti's sign

---

DIAGNOSTIC STATEMENT

The double leg-raise test is positive and elicits pain in the lumbosacral spine. This result indicates lumbosacral joint involvement and implies a ligamentous sprain.

CLINICAL PEARL

Atypical cases of disc prolapse are common. A definite history of injury or strain is often lacking. The pain may begin gradually rather than suddenly, and the symptoms may be confined to the back and never radiate down the leg. On the other hand, the pain is sometimes felt predominantly in the limb and is scarcely perceptible in the back.

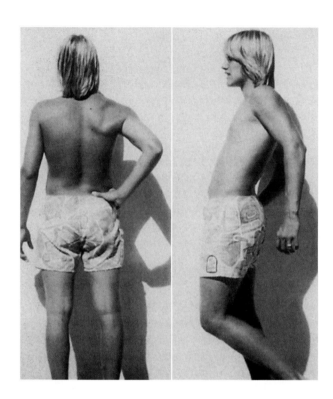

FIG. 8-57   Jackson's one-legged hyperextension test. The patient stands on one leg and hyperextends the back. Back pain will be reproduced on the symptomatic side if there is an impending pars fracture.

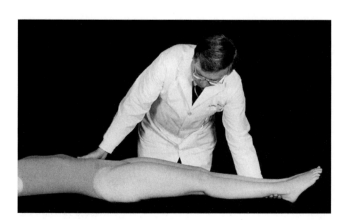

FIG. 8-58   The patient is supine with both legs fully extended. The examiner performs a straight-leg-raising test on each of the lower extremities and notes the angle at which the pain is produced. The examiner then raises both lower limbs together.

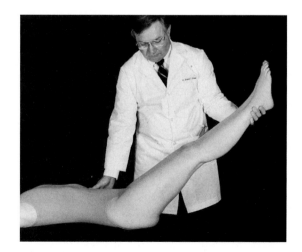

FIG. 8-59   If raising both legs together produces pain at an earlier angle than raising each leg singly, then the sign is positive. The test is specific and highly accurate for lumbosacral joint involvement.

ELY'S SIGN

ELY'S HEEL-TO-BUTTOCK TEST

Assessment for Lumbar Radicular or Femoral Nerve Inflammation

Comment

The size of the lumbar vertebral canal ranges from 12 to 20 mm in its AP dimension at the midsagittal plane and 18 to 27 mm in its transverse diameter. Stenosis has been defined as a narrowing below the lowest value of the range of normal (Table 8-9).

The dura mater of the lumbar spine has a series of attachments to neighboring vertebrae and ligaments. They have been referred to as the *dural attachment complex* or *Hoffmann ligaments* (Fig. 8-60). Narrowing of the vertebral canal (spinal canal) is most often known as *spinal canal stenosis.* Lumbar spinal canal stenosis affects the nerves of the cauda equina or the dorsal and ventral roots as they leave the vertebral canal and enter IVFs. The exiting nerve roots travel through the more narrow, lateral aspect of the vertebral canal, known as the *lateral recess,* before entering

---

TABLE 8-9

DIMENSIONS OF THE LUMBAR VERTEBRAL FORAMINA (VERTEBRAL CANAL)*

Dimension	Size (Range)†
Anteroposterior (in midsagittal plane)	12-20 mm
Transverse (interpedicular distance)	18-27 mm

From Cramer GD, Darby SA: *Basic and clinical anatomy of the spine, spinal cord, and ANS,* St Louis, 1995, Mosby.

*Dimensions below the lowest value indicate spinal (vertebral) canal stenosis (Dommisse & Louw, 1990). A typical vertebral foramen is rather triangular (trefoil) in shape. However, the upper lumbar vertebral foramina are more rounded than the lower lumbar foramina. L1 is the most rounded, and each succeeding lumbar vertebra becomes increasingly triangular, with L5 the most dramatically trefoil of all.

†Dimensions of lumbar vertebral foramina are usually smaller than those of the cervical region but larger than those of the thoracic region.

---

the IVF. As the roots pass through this region of the vertebral canal, pressure may be placed on them. This is known as *lateral recess stenosis.*

In sequestration of nuclear tissue adjacent to or under a nerve, adhesions may form within and without the nerve root sheath, binding the root firmly to the floor of the spinal canal. During movements of the trunk and legs, the nerve roots are no longer freely movable or capable of moving in and out of the intervertebral foramina without tension. When fixed to the floor of the spinal canal or within the foramina, the nerve roots are subjected to abnormal tension during movement of the trunk and legs, particularly movements that require the extended leg to flex at the hip. Tension on the nerve roots causes radicular pain.

The condition is characterized by the localization of the pain in the dermatome supplied by the affected nerve root. The pain, although often widely distributed throughout the dermatome, occasionally is limited to a small area within it. Although dermatomal in distribution, nerve root pain in the leg seldom extends beyond the ankle. However, any associated dermatomal paresthesia or dysesthesia is usually most prominent distally and may be described in the foot.

Pain is present in the spinal column and is temporarily associated with pain in the leg, with paresthesia, or both.

Root pain often is produced or aggravated by coughing, sneezing, and straining (e.g., during defecation) or by any other measures that suddenly increase intrathoracic and intraabdominal pressure. Such increases in pressure block venous flow from the epidural space through the intervertebral veins. Because the intervertebral veins do not contain valves, such increases in pressure may also permit a return of blood with consequent distension of the veins in the epidural space. This condition in turn forces the dura, which envelops the nerve roots, toward the spinal cord. Because the nerve roots are affixed to the spinal cord proximally and peripherally at the intervertebral foramen, the displacement of the dura results in stretching of the involved nerve root. This stretching results in pain if the root is diseased. In addition, distension of the intervertebral vein may result in direct compression of the nerve root.

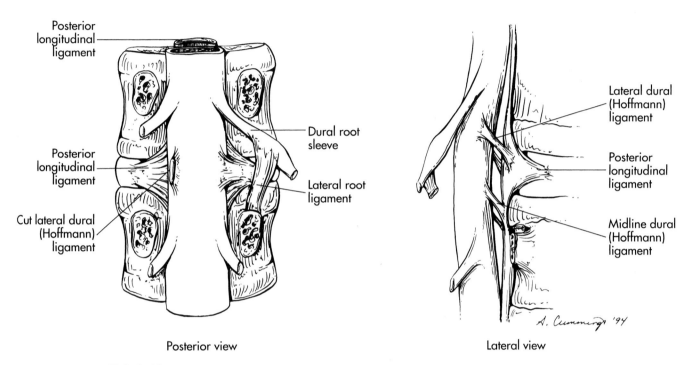

Posterior longitudinal ligament

Posterior longitudinal ligament

Cut lateral dural (Hoffmann) ligament

Dural root sleeve

Lateral root ligament

Lateral dural (Hoffmann) ligament

Posterior longitudinal ligament

Midline dural (Hoffmann) ligament

Posterior view

Lateral view

FIG. 8-60   Attachments of the dura mater to surrounding structures.   *(From Cramer GD, Darby SA: Basic and clinical anatomy of the spine, spinal cord, and ANS, St Louis, 1995, Mosby.)*

Root pain may awaken the patient at night after several hours of sleep and may be relieved 15 to 30 minutes after the patient assumes an upright position. The patient may learn to prevent the pain by sleeping in a chair. However, in contrast to peripheral neuritis, the position is the important determining factor. If the patient lies down in a similar position during the day, the pain occurs as it does at night. This feature of root pain has its basis in the lengthening of the spinal column that takes place when the horizontal position is assumed and the shortening that takes place when the patient is in the upright position. Because the length of the spinal cord remains the same regardless of the position assumed by the patient, the lengthening of the spinal column results in a tensing of, or traction on, the nerve roots that emerge from the lumbar and sacral segments of the cord. From these segments, the roots course downward and outward to emerge from their respective intervertebral foramina.

PROCEDURE

- The patient is prone, with the toes hanging over the edge of the table and legs relaxed.
- One or the other heel is approximated to the opposite buttock (Figs. 8-61 and 8-62).

- After flexion of the knee, the thigh is hyperextended.
- With any significant hip lesion, it will be impossible to do this test normally.
- With irritation of the iliopsoas muscle or its sheath, it will be impossible to extend the thigh to any normal degree.
- This test will aggravate inflammation of the lumbar nerve roots and will be accompanied by production of femoral radicular pain.
- The test will also stretch lumbar nerve root adhesions, which will be accompanied by upper lumbar discomfort.

Confirmation Procedures
Femoral nerve traction test and prone knee-bending test

DIAGNOSTIC STATEMENT

Ely's sign is present on the left. This sign indicates femoral nerve or radicular inflammation.

CLINICAL PEARL

In the uncommon cases of high lumbar and midlumbar disc prolapse, the pain radiates toward the groin and front of the thigh rather than to the back of the thigh and leg.

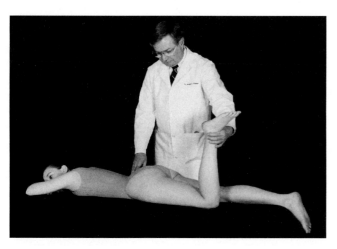

FIG. 8-61   The patient is prone. The legs are fully extended, with the toes hanging over the edge of the table The examiner flexes the knee of the affected leg to 90 degrees.

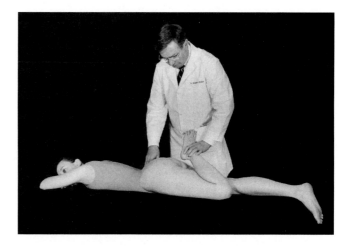

FIG. 8-62   The heel of the affected leg is approximated to the opposite buttock. After flexion of the knee, the thigh can be hyperextended. With irritation of the iliopsoas muscle or its sheath, it will be impossible to extend the thigh to any degree. Pain in the anterior thigh is a positive finding and indicates inflammation of the lumbar nerve roots.

FAJERSZTAJN'S TEST

ALSO KNOWN AS WELL-LEG-RAISING TEST OF FAJERSZTAJN
PROSTRATE LEG-RAISING TEST
SCIATIC PHENOMENON
CROSS-OVER SIGN

Assessment for Lumbar Nerve Root Lesion Caused by Intervertebral Disc Syndrome or Dural Sleeve Adhesion

Comment

Although it is clearly evident in most advanced imaging tests, spinal stenosis is the cause of many cases of low back problems that are refractory to conservative treatment. Lumbar stenosis can occur at the central spinal canal or at the peripheral canal where the nerve root exits. Two major conditions, both of which compromise the vertebral canal and its neural contents, contribute to lumbar stenosis: facet disease and discogenic spondylosis. Degenerative arthritis of the facets has the potential to cause stenosis by encroaching on the lateral recess of the spinal canal.

Patients with discogenic spondylosis develop multidirectional pain in addition to flexion discomfort.

ORTHOPEDIC GAMUT 8-5

LUMBAR CENTRAL CANAL STENOSIS

Structural causes for lumbar central canal stenosis follow:

1. *Osseous:* inferior facet arthrosis
2. *Discogenic:* central disc herniation
3. *Ligamentous:* ligamentum flavum buckling in degenerative spinal disease (Fig. 8-63)

Patients with central lumbar canal stenosis exhibit neurogenic claudication with pain upon walking and feel as if their legs "give way." Temperature changes and weakness of the legs are common. Night pain and sciatic tension signs are equally common.

Patients with lateral lumbar canal stenosis have nerve root entrapment. Pain occurs intermittently over years, with exacerbations. Pain may be referred to the hips, buttocks, or posterior thigh. Pain is rarely referred to the foot or toes. Sensory changes at the calf are common.

Limitation of motion is usually noted during the symptomatic phase of disc disease. The range of motion should be noted, not only in flexion and extension but also in rotation. The examiner must not equate flexion of the hips with flexion of the lumbar spine, and attention should be directed to whether reversal of the normal lumbar lordosis occurs. Even in patients who have only sciatica, marked restriction of motion may be present in the lumbar spine.

When acute sciatica is present, the patient usually lists away from the side of the sciatica, producing the sciatic scoliosis. When the disc herniation is lateral to the nerve root, the patient will incline away from the side of the irritated nerve root in an attempt to draw the nerve root away from the disc fragment. On the contrary, when the herniation is in an axillary position, medial to the nerve root, the patient will list toward the side of the lesion to decompress the nerve root.

When doing a unilateral straight-leg raising test, 80 to 90 degrees of hip flexion is normal. If one leg is lifted and the patient complains of pain on the opposite side, it is an indication of a space-occupying lesion (herniated disc). This finding indicates a rather large intervertebral disc protrusion, usually medial to the nerve root. The test causes stretching of the ipsilateral as well as the contralateral nerve root, pulling laterally on the dural sac.

PROCEDURE

- Straight leg raising and dorsiflexion of the foot are performed on the asymptomatic side of a sciatic patient (Figs. 8-64 and 8-65).
- When this test causes pain on the symptomatic side, Fajersztajn's sign is present.
- The sign indicates sciatic nerve root involvement, such as a disc syndrome or dural root sleeve adhesions.

Confirmation Procedures

Bechterew's sitting test, Bragard's sign, Deyerle's sign, Lasègue differential sign, Lasègue rebound test, Lasègue sitting test, Lasègue test, Lewin standing test, Lindner's sign, Sicard's sign, straight-leg-raising test, and Turyn's sign

DIAGNOSTIC STATEMENT

Fajersztajn's test is positive on the left at 3 degrees of elevation. This result indicates nerve root compression by a space-occupying mass in or near the axilla of the nerve root on the right.

CLINICAL PEARL

There are several causes of pain in the back or lower extremities. Some of these causes are (1) tumors of the spinal cord or cauda equina, (2) tumors of the spinal column, (3) tuberculosis of the spine, (4) osteoarthritis, (5) tumors of the ilium or sacrum, (6) spondylolisthesis, (7) prolapsed intervertebral disc, (8) ankylosing spondylitis, (9) vascular occlusion, (10) intrapelvic mass, and (11) arthritis of the hip. All of these possible causes must be considered in differential diagnosis.

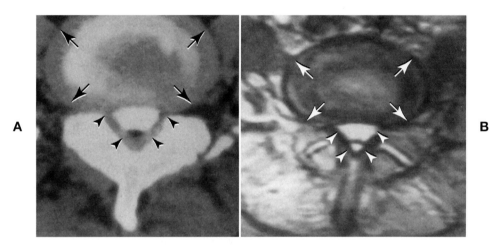

FIG. 8-63 Central canal stenosis attributable to a diffusely bulging disc and hypertrophy of the ligamentum flavum. **A,** Axial computed tomography. **B,** Magnetic resonance imaging. *(From Brier SR:* Primary care orthopedics, *St Louis, 1999, Mosby.)*

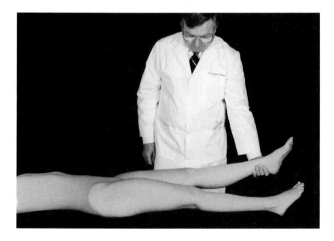

FIG. 8-64 The patient is supine with both legs fully extended. The examiner performs a straight-leg-raising test on the unaffected leg.

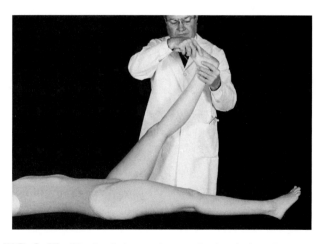

FIG. 8-65 The leg is lowered to a point just below that which produces sciatic symptoms in the affected leg. The examiner sharply dorsiflexes the foot (Bragard's sign). If this maneuver causes pain on the symptomatic side, the test is positive. A positive test indicates sciatic nerve root involvement, such as medial disc protrusion syndrome or dural root sleeve adhesions.

FEMORAL NERVE TRACTION TEST

Assessment for Midlumbar
Nerve Root Involvement (L2, L3, and L4)

Comment

Redundant nerve roots refers to roots of the cauda equina that bend (undulate within the vertebral canal) or buckle during their course through the cauda equina. Degenerative spinal stenosis is thought to be the usual cause of this condition. The vertebral column decreases in superior-to-inferior length with age (an average of 14 mm). Shortening of the vertebral canal forces the roots of the cauda equina to become redundant. The pressure from compressive elements over time results in friction neuritis. Friction neuritis results in the large redundant roots. With walking and extension, increased pressure is placed on the nerve roots (Fig. 8-66), which causes ischemia of the neural elements. Nerve root ischemia results in the signs and symptoms of neurogenic claudication pain. Weakness in the lower extremities during standing and walking is often associated with spinal stenosis and redundant nerve roots. These changes are often permanent.

When a herniated annulus fibrosus compresses a nerve root, the irritation produces pain and motor and sensory loss of the lower extremities. As the nerve root becomes irritated, it becomes inflamed and even more sensitive to pressures. The patient will notice a lancinating pain that begins in the thigh and progresses distally in a pattern typical of a dermatome. The onset of pain may be gradual or extremely sudden and may be associated with a popping or tearing in the spine. This may represent the extrusion of disc material against the nerve root. When this occurs, the back pain often resolves and the patient is left with the radicular symptoms.

Usually, the disc rupture is lateral to the nerve root, and the patient lists or leans away from the side of the sciatica to release the pressure. Occasionally, the disc presents medially or in the axilla of the nerve root, and the patient will list toward the side of the sciatica. The pain is increased by any maneuver that suddenly increases intraspinal pressures, such as a Valsalva maneuver or the triad of Dejerine (coughing, sneezing, or bearing down with defecation). The pain may be so severe as to paralyze the patient in a fixed position.

It is rare that the major presenting symptom is motor weakness, particularly if the fourth or fifth lumbar nerve is affected. Weakness of the quadriceps with later buckling of the knee (fourth lumbar) or a complete foot drop (fifth lumbar), without pain, may present a confusing picture.

A large, midline disc herniation can compress several nerve roots of the cauda equina and can mimic an intraspinal tumor. Usually, lower back and perineal symptoms predominate, with radicular symptoms being masked. Difficulty with urination, such as frequency or overflow incontinence, may develop early. In males, a recent history of sexual impotence may be elicited. The patients experience pain down the posterior thighs to the soles of the feet accompanied by weakness of the legs and feet. L2, L3, and L4 radiculopathies are less common than the L5 and S1 radiculopathies, probably because of their relatively short course within the cauda equina, which makes them less susceptible to compression (Table 8-10).

TABLE 8-10

DIFFERENTIAL ELECTRODIAGNOSIS OF UPPER LUMBAR RADICULOPATHY

	Femoral Neuropathy	Lumbar Plexopathy	Lumbar Radiculopathy
Thigh adductors	Normal	Denervation	Denervation
Tibialis anterior	Normal	Denervation*	Denervation*
Saphenous SNAP†	Low or absent‡	Low or absent‡	Normal
Paraspinal fibrillations	Absent	Absent	Usually present

From Katirji B: *Electromyography in clinical practice: a case study approach,* St Louis, 1998, Mosby.
SNAP, Sensory nerve action potential.
*Abnormal in L4 radiculopathy/plexopathy only.
†May be technically difficult, particularly in the elderly patients or if there is leg edema.
‡Normal in purely demyelinating lesions.

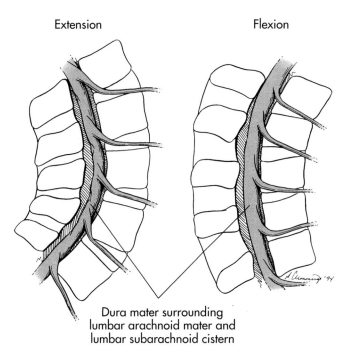

Extension   Flexion

Dura mater surrounding
lumbar arachnoid mater and
lumbar subarachnoid cistern

FIG. 8-66   Changes that occur within the lumbar vertebral canal
during flexion and extension.   *(From Cramer GD, Darby SA:* Basic
and clinical anatomy of the spine, spinal cord, and ANS, *St Louis, 1995,
Mosby.)*

ORTHOPEDIC GAMUT 8-6

UPPER LUMBAR RADICULOPATHY

The electrophysiologic confirmation of an upper lumbar radiculopathy is challenging for the following reasons:

1. The exact compressed root is difficult to identify among upper lumbar roots. This is because of the limited number of muscles innervated by the roots (Fig. 8-67).
2. The myotomal representation of these roots occurs in proximally situated muscles, mostly above the knee (except for the tibialis anterior).
3. There is a lack of available sensory nerve action potential (snap) for confirming that the upper lumbar lesion is preganglionic.

It is sometimes difficult to separate upper lumbar radiculopathies from lumbar plexopathy, especially in chronic situations in which fibrillation potentials are less common in the paraspinal muscles. This is most relevant in diabetic patients in whom diabetic amyotrophy (diabetic proximal neuropathy) also is in question.

PROCEDURE

- The side-lying patient slightly flexes the hip and knee on the unaffected side (Fig. 8-68).
- With neck slightly flexed, the patient's back is straight (not hyperextended).
- The affected limb is extended at the hip 15 degrees.
- The affected knee is flexed, stretching the femoral nerve (Fig. 8-69).
- If the test is positive, pain radiates into the anterior thigh.

Confirmation Procedures
Ely's sign and prone knee-bending test

DIAGNOSTIC STATEMENT

Femoral nerve traction testing on the left is positive and accompanied by radiating pain to the groin. This positive result indicates an L3 nerve root radiculopathy.

Femoral nerve traction testing on the left is positive, with pain extending to the midtibia. This positive result indicates an L4 nerve root radiculopathy.

CLINICAL PEARL

With upper lumbar disc disturbances, there may be weakness of the quadriceps muscle and a diminished or absent patellar reflex. The straight-leg-raising tests and signs may be negative. Pinwheel examination usually reveals hyperesthesia or hypoesthesia of the L4 dermatome.

Anterior primary rami	L2	L3	L4	L5	S1	S2
PROXIMAL NERVES						
Iliacus	■	■				
Adductor longus (obturator)		■	■			
Vastus lateralis/medialis (femoral)		■	■			
Rectus femoris (femoral)		■	■			
Tensor fascia lata (gluteal)				▨	■	
Gluteus medius (gluteal)				▨	■	
Gluteus maximus (gluteal)				▨	■	■
SCIATIC NERVES						
Semi tendinosus/membranosus (tibial)				■	■	
Biceps femoris (sht. hd) (peroneal)					■	▨
Biceps femoris (long hd) (tibial)					■	▨
PERONEAL NERVES						
Tibialis anterior			■	■		
Extensor hallucis			▨	■		
Peroneal longus				■	■	
Extensor digitorum brevis				■	■	
TIBIAL NERVES						
Tibialis posterior				▨	■	
Flexor digitorum longus				■	■	
Gastrocnemius lateral				▨	■	
Gastrocnemius medial					■	▨
Soleus					■	■
Abductor hallucis					■	■
Abductor digiti quinti pedis					■	■

Posterior primary rami	L2	L3	L4	L5	S1	S2
Lumbar paraspinals	■	■	■	■		
High sacral paraspinals				■	■	■

FIG. 8-67   Chart of lower extremity muscles useful in the electromyographic recognition of lumbosacral radiculopathy. *(From Brown WF, Bolton CF:* Clinical electromyography, *ed 2, Philadelphia, 1993, Butterworth-Heinemann.)*

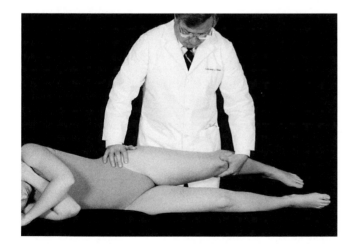

FIG. 8-68   The patient lies on the unaffected leg and slightly flexes the hip and knee. The patient straightens the back and flexes the neck. The affected leg is extended at the hip approximately 15 degrees.

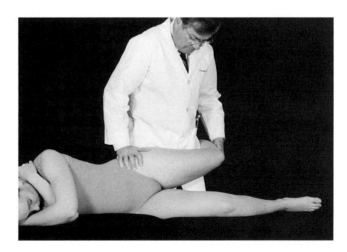

FIG. 8-69   The affected knee is flexed. This stretches the femoral nerve. The test is positive if pain radiates down the anterior thigh. A positive test indicates a radiculopathy that involves L2, L3, and L4.

HEEL/TOE WALK TEST

Assessment for L5 or S1 Nerve Root Motor Deficiency

Comment

Muscle weakness, atrophy, or the inability to perform functional testing maneuvers all suggest the presence of nerve root compression that is more significant than the alteration of sensation (Table 8-11).

When lower extremity weakness is apparent, atrophy may signify a lower motor neuron lesion or muscular disorder. However, disuse of a muscle from any cause—whether pain, immobilization, or paralysis of central origin—will result in some loss of muscle mass. The quadriceps are prone to disuse atrophy, which happens quite rapidly.

The patient who can hop well does not have a serious weakness of the gastrocnemius, which is a strong muscle and is difficult to evaluate through direct testing. The examiner observes the patient walk on the toes, during which the patient's body weight is completely supported on one foot and then the other. If weakness exists, the heel will drop while the patient is walking. The contours of the musculature may demonstrate atrophy or hypertrophy. A patient who has had a stroke and who has a moderate degree of spasticity and increased tone in antigravity muscles may still be able to rise on the toes. When weakness is evident while attempting this maneuver, the disorder is usually a primary lesion of the nerve root, peripheral nerve, or muscle.

Having the patient walk on the heels is an especially valuable screening test because dorsiflexion of the ankles and toes is weakened in many muscular and neural disorders. If necessary, the examiner may help the patient maintain balance in this maneuver. A normal patient can hold the foot and toes anteriorly off the floor, while strongly dorsiflexing the great toe, during walking on the heels. If the patient can do this, foot drop does not exist. However, the patient could still have minor weakness of the muscles of the anterior compartment, and these should be tested directly. Foot drop may be of either central or peripheral origin. Severe foot drop of peripheral origin is clearly revealed by the abnormal nature of the gait and by an observable loss of dorsiflexion of the ankle and toes. If foot drop of a peripheral origin (lower motor neuron) has been present for several weeks, shrinkage and softness of the anterior compartment also will be apparent. When the leg is shaken, such as during the test for alternating motion rate, the foot will be unstable and flop about. The foot is less floppy with central disorders (upper motor neuron lesions) and may be fixed in plantar flexion. When dorsiflexion of the ankles and toes is weak, the toes of the spastic leg are dragged during walking. Before the examiner concludes that there is weakness of dorsiflexion, the foot should be passively dorsiflexed to be certain that previous weakness, now healed, did not permanently shorten the gastrocnemius.

TABLE 8-11

SPECIFIC DUSOLUMBAR RADICULOPATHY PATTERNS

Nerve	HNP	Foramen	Muscle	Reflex	Sensation
T10					Umbilicus
T12					Pubis
L1	T12-L1	L1-L2			Upper anterior thigh
L2	L1-L2	L2-L3			Midanterior thigh
L3	L2-L3	L3-L4	Quadriceps femoris		Lower anterior thigh
L4	L3-L4	L4-L5	Quadriceps femoris Anterior tibial	Patella	Anterior thigh Medial leg Foot (occasionally)
L5	L4-L5	L5-S1	Anterior tibial EHL	Posterior tibial	Lateral leg Dorsum of foot Big toe
S1	L5-S1		Heel raise Peroneal	Achilles' tendon	Posterior leg Sole of foot Lateral foot Little toe

Adapted from Brier SR: *Primary care orthopedics,* St Louis, 1999, Mosby.
HNP, Herniated nucleus pulposus; *EHL,* extensor hallicus longus.

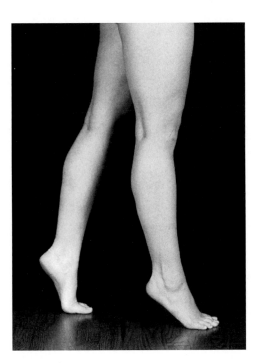

FIG. 8-70   The patient is standing and is instructed to walk on the toes. Weakness is evident if the heel drops while walking.

It is not unusual for patients with severe L5 radiculopathy, in whom significant motor axon loss has occurred, to present with foot drop (Table 8-12).

PROCEDURE

- The examiner observes the patient walking on the toes, which requires each foot, one at a time, to completely support the patient's body weight (Fig. 8-70).
- If weakness exists, the heel will drop while the patient is walking.
- The contours of the musculature may demonstrate atrophy or hypertrophy.
- Having the patient walk on the heels is an especially valuable screening test because many muscular and neural disorders result in weakened dorsiflexion of the ankles and toes (Fig. 8-71).
- The patient may need help maintaining balance during this maneuver.

- The normal patient can hold the foot and toes anteriorly off the floor, while strongly dorsiflexing the great toe during walking on the heels.
- If the patient can do this, foot drop does not exist.

Confirmation Procedures
Antalgia sign, bowstring sign, Cox sign, Kemp's test, Lewin punch test, Lewin snuff test, Milgram's test, and Neri's sign

---

DIAGNOSTIC STATEMENT

The toe walk test is positive on the left and demonstrates weakness in the S1 dermatome.

The heel walk test is positive on the left and demonstrates weakness in the L5 dermatome.

TABLE 8-12

ELECTROPHYSIOLOGIC DIFFERENCES BETWEEN L5 RADICULOPATHY AND PERONEAL NEUROPATHY

	L5 Radiculopathy	Peroneal Neuropathy
Nerve conduction studies		
Peroneal CMAP, recording extensor digitorum brevis	Normal or low amplitude	Conduction block at fibular head, low amplitude, or both
Peroneal CMAP, recording tibialis anterior	Normal or low amplitude	Conduction block at fibular head, low amplitude, or both
Superficial peroneal SNAP	Normal	Low or absent; normal in deep peroneal or purely demyelinating lesions
Needle EMG		
Tibialis anterior	Abnormal	Abnormal
Extensor digitorum brevis	Abnormal	Abnormal
Extensor hallucis	Abnormal	Abnormal
Peroneus longus	Abnormal	Abnormal; normal in selective deep peroneal lesions
Tibialis posterior	Abnormal	Normal
Flexor digitorum longus	Abnormal	Normal
Gluteus medius	May be normal	Normal
Tensor fasciae latae	May be normal	Normal
Lumbar paraspinals	May be normal	Normal

From Katirji B: *Electromyography in clinical practice: a case study approach,* St Louis, 1998, Mosby.
CMAP, Compound muscle action potential; *EMG,* electromyography; *SNAP,* sensory nerve action potential.

CLINICAL PEARL

The inability to walk on the toes indicates an L5-S1 disc problem based on weakness of the calf muscles supplied by the tibial nerve. The inability to walk on the heels indicates an L4-L5 disc problem based on weakness of the anterior leg muscles supplied by the common peroneal nerve.

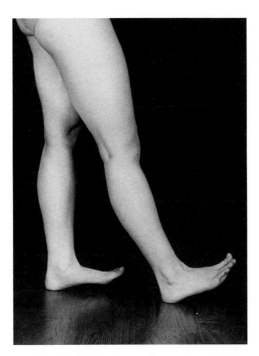

FIG. 8-71   The patient then walks on the heels. If necessary the examiner may help the patient maintain balance during this maneuver. If the patient cannot walk on the heels, foot drop exists.

Assessment for L3 and L4 Nerve Root Inflammation

Comment

Spondylolisthesis in the adult, with the exception of traumatic and pathologic spondylolisthesis, typically presents with a long history of back pain that may be punctuated with waxing and waning symptoms. It is unusual for spondylolisthesis in the adult to present with acute neurologic loss. A more common scenario is the onset of intermittent radicular or neurogenic claudicatory-type symptoms that slowly become a more prominent part of the history. Traumatic spondylolisthesis is caused most typically by a fall from a height. The fractures generally are not simply through the pars interarticularis, as is seen in isthmic spondylolisthesis, but may include the facets, the pedicles, and/or the pars interarticularis. Degenerative spondylolisthesis is based on the advancement of the degenerative cascade with disc degeneration and facet degeneration over time, presenting with incompetence of the facet joint and anterior listhesis of the proximal on the distal vertebra. This most commonly occurs at the L4-L5 level (Fig. 8-72) and to a lesser degree at L3-L4 and L5-S1. Isthmic spondylolisthesis (Fig. 8-73) occurs in two varieties: subtype A, a lytic pars defect, and subtype B, an elongation of the pars interarticularis. The elongation occurs with repetitive stress fractures and healing over time. Pathologic fractures consist of a defect in the posterior arch because of abnormalities of the bone itself, either underlying metabolic bone disease or neoplasia.

Congenital spondylolisthesis consists of structural anomalies of the lumbosacral junction resulting in inadequate mechanical support to prevent forward slippage of L5 on S1 (Fig. 8-74).

During the third through the fifth decades of life, changes that occur in the lumbar spine can be quite pronounced, with the first manifestations of aging reflected in the intervertebral disc. Biochemical changes can be produced by one of three different phenomena: degeneration of the annulus with disc nuclear herniation through posterolateral annular rents, nuclear degeneration with intact annulus, or simultaneous degeneration of both the annulus and the nucleus.

The biomechanical insufficiency of the involved disc compels the posterior elements, or the facets and capsules, to assume a more compressive, tensile, and shear load, resulting in capsular strain, hypermobility, and articular cartilage degeneration. The hypermobility can produce traction spurs. The ligamentum flavum also will be compelled to assume more tensile loads while becoming redundant as the total spine length decreases with disc degeneration. The vertebrae themselves tend toward a lowering and broadening in the superior, inferior, and midbody transverse breadth, a total change that, in static terms, begins to acutely or insidiously affect the neural elements.

If a disc lesion occurs in a spinal canal that is small, compression of the neural elements will result and the patient will experience symptoms. In pure terms, this can be thought of as a relative spinal stenosis. The stenosis occurs secondarily to the herniated nucleus pulposus occupying space in a small spinal canal. On the other hand, a similarly sized disc herniation in a large spinal canal will cause no symptoms because the neural elements have enough room to escape the pressure. Thus symptoms in persons of this age group are not only a result of a disc herniation itself but also the size of the spinal canal with which the individual is born.

Patients in the fifth decade of life and older can manifest the hypermobile end-stage changes of the aging process. Degeneration of both facet joints and the intervertebral disc leads to a narrowing of the spinal canal. The canal is rimmed by large osteophytes, which develop to diminish the load on the now incompetent intervertebral disc. The facets are hypertrophic and deformed by the osteophytic spurs that are encased within the thickened joint capsule. The ligamentum flavum becomes redundant, and in combination with the changes just mentioned, the spinal canal and foramina are affected. Changes in the lumbar spinal canal occur to some degree in all active people as they age. However, not everyone suffers from significant impairment. The symptoms a person will have depend on the original size of the spinal canal. If the individual's spinal canal is small, the changes that are caused by aging and that occur in the disc and facet joints will lead to an absolute spinal stenosis with compression of the neural elements. If the spinal canal is large, the normal changes of aging will lead to a relative spinal stenosis with no neural compression.

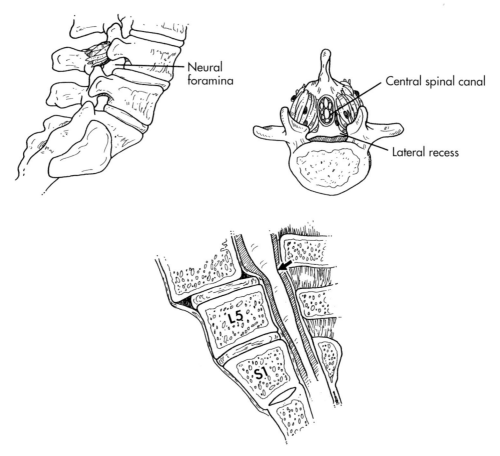

FIG. 8-72 Degenerative spondylolisthesis most commonly occurs at the L4-L5 level. *(From Bucholz RW: Orthopaedic decision making, ed 2, St Louis, 1996, Mosby.)*

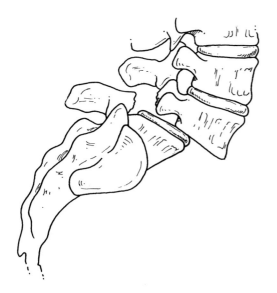

FIG. 8-73 Isthmic spondylolisthesis. *(From Bucholz RW: Orthopaedic decision making, ed 2, St Louis, 1996, Mosby.)*

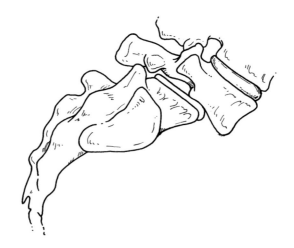

FIG. 8-74 Congenital spondylolisthesis caused by inadequate development of the L5-S1 facet complexes. *(From Bucholz RW: Orthopaedic decision making, ed 2, St Louis, 1996, Mosby.)*

PROCEDURE

- The patient is prone, and the legs are fully extended (Fig. 8-75).
- The examiner anchors the patient's lumbosacral spine with one hand.
- With the other hand, the examiner slowly extends the hip of the affected leg (Fig. 8-76).
- The test is positive if the patient experiences radiating pain in the anterior thigh.
- A positive test indicates inflammation of the L3 and L4 nerve roots.

Confirmation Procedures

Bilateral leg-lowering test, Demianoff's sign, double leg-raise test, Lewin supine test, matchstick test, Mennell's sign, Minor's sign, Nachlas test, Quick test, Schober's test, sign of the buttock, skin pinch test, spinal percussion test, and Vanzetti's sign

---

DIAGNOSTIC STATEMENT

The hyperextension test is positive on the right and elicits anterior thigh pain. This pain suggests inflammation of the L3 and L4 nerve roots.

CLINICAL PEARL

There are five criteria for diagnosis of sciatica caused by a herniated intervertebral disc. (1) Leg pain is the dominant symptom when compared with back pain, and it affects only one leg and follows a typical sciatic or femoral nerve distribution. (2) Paresthesia is localized to a dermatomal distribution. (3) Straight leg raising is reduced to 50% of what is considered normal, and pain is elicited in the symptomatic leg when the unaffected leg is elevated. This pain radiates proximally or distally with digital pressure on the tibial nerve in the popliteal fossa. (4) Two of four neurologic signs (atrophy, motor weakness, diminished sensory appreciation, and diminution of reflex activity) are present. (5) A contrast study or other diagnostic imaging is positive and corresponds to the clinical level.

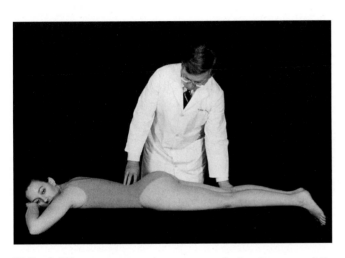

FIG. 8-75 The patient is prone, and the legs are fully extended. The examiner anchors the patient's lumbosacral spine with one hand.

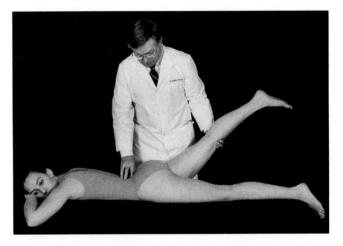

FIG. 8-76 With the other hand, the examiner slowly extends the hip of the affected leg. The test is positive if the patient experiences radiating pain in the anterior thigh. A positive test indicates inflammation of the L3 and L4 nerve roots.

KEMP'S TEST

Assessment for Intervertebral Nerve Root Encroachment, Muscular Strain, Ligamentous Sprain, or Pericapsular Inflammation

Comment

Patients with chronic facet syndrome develop adhesions of the synovial joint, which is innervated by the primary dorsal rami. When facet disease is advanced, bony encroachment on a susceptible spinal canal can occur (Fig. 8-77). Lateral mass stenosis and neuroforaminal impingement can produce symptoms commonly seen in patients with lumbar stenosis.

Disc prolapse occurs in three stages, and it occurs only if the disc has deteriorated as a result of repeated microtrauma and if the annulus fibers have started to degenerate.

ORTHOPEDIC GAMUT 8-7

DISC PROLAPSE

Disc prolapse usually follows lifting or twisting while the trunk is in flexion:

1. During the first stage, trunk flexion flattens the discs anteriorly and opens out the intervertebral space posteriorly.
2. During the second stage, as soon as the weight is lifted, the increased axial compression force crushes the whole disc and violently drives the nuclear substance posteriorly until it reaches the deep surface of the posterior longitudinal ligament.
3. During the third stage, when the trunk is nearly straight, the path taken by the herniating mass is closed by the pressure of the vertebral plateaus, and a hernia remains trapped under the posterior longitudinal ligament.

The hernia causes acute pain, which is felt in the lower back. This occurrence corresponds to the initial phase of the lumbar sciatica complex. This initial acute lower back pain can regress spontaneously or with treatment, but as a result of repeated trauma, the herniation grows in size and protrudes more and more into the vertebral canal. Once this protrusion occurs, the herniation meets with a nerve root, often one of the roots of the sciatic nerve. In fact, the herniation progressively pushes on the nerve root until the latter is jammed against the posterior wall of the intervertebral foramen. The posterior wall is formed by the joint between the articular processes, its anterior capsular ligament, and the lateral border of the ligamentum flavum. The compressed nerve root causes pain in the spinal segment that corresponds to the root and, finally, impairs reflexes and creates motor disturbances, such as those that occur in sciatica with paralysis.

The clinical picture depends on the spinal level of disc prolapse and nerve root compression. If prolapse occurs at L4-L5, the root of L5 is compressed, and pain is felt in the posterolateral aspect of the thigh, the knee, the lateral border of the calf, the lateral border of the instep of the foot, and the dorsal surface of the foot to the great toe. If the prolapse lies at L5-S1, S1 is compressed, and pain is referred to the posterior aspect of the thigh, knee, and calf; the heel; and the lateral border of the foot to the fifth toe. However, this correlation of clinical picture and lesion level is not absolute. A herniation at L4-L5 may lie closer to the midline and compress L5 and S1 simultaneously, or even occasionally, S1 alone. Surgical exploration at L5-S1, performed on the strength of the S1 root pain, may fail to recognize that this lesion lies one level above.

PROCEDURE

- While in a seated position, the patient is supported by the examiner, who reaches around the patient's shoulders and upper chest from behind (Fig. 8-78).
- The patient is directed to lean forward to one side and then around until the patient is eventually bending obliquely backward (Figs. 8-79 and 8-80).
- The maneuver is similar to that used for cervical compression.
- If this compression causes or aggravates a pattern of radicular pain in the thigh and leg, the sign is positive and indicates nerve root compression.
- Local back pain should be noted, but it does not constitute a positive test.
- However, local back pain may indicate a strain or sprain and thus be present when the patient leans obliquely forward or at any point in motion.

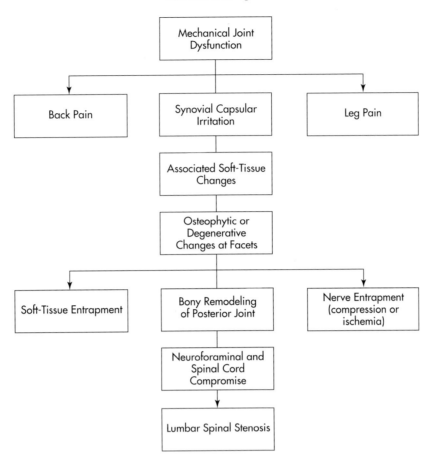

FIG. 8-77   Pathogenesis of the lumbosacral Z joints. *(From Brier SR:* Primary care orthopedics, *St Louis, 1999, Mosby.)*

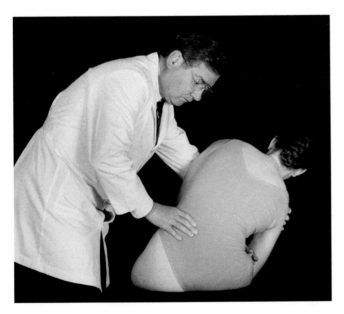

FIG. 8-78   While in a seated position, the patient is supported by the examiner, who reaches around the patient's shoulders and upper chest from behind. The patient is directed to lean obliquely forward and away from the affected side.

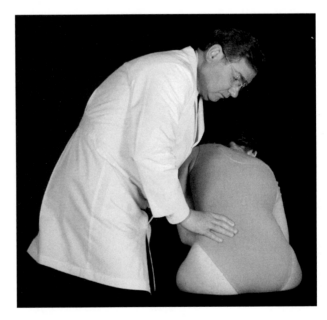

FIG. 8-79   The examiner actively rotates the patient's trunk from the original position and circumducts the trunk toward the affected side.

- Because the elderly are less prone to an actual herniation of a disc because of lessened elasticity involved in the aging process, other reasons for nerve root compression are usually the cause.
- Degenerative joint disease, exostoses, inflammatory or fibrotic residues, narrowing from disc degeneration, and tumors must all be considered.
- This test must elicit a more positive finding when the patient is standing than when sitting (Figs. 8-81 and 8-82).

Confirmation Procedures
Antalgia sign, bowstring sign, Cox sign, heel/toe walk test, Lewin punch test, Lewin snuff test, Milgram's test, and Neri's sign

---

DIAGNOSTIC STATEMENT

Kemp's test (seated) is positive on the left and results in pain that radiates into the left side S1 dermatome. This pain indicates S1 nerve root compression syndrome.

Kemp's test (standing) is positive on the right and elicits pain that radiates into the right side L5 dermatome. This result indicates L5 nerve root compression syndrome.

Kemp's test (standing) is inconclusive on the right and elicits nonradiating pain at the L5-S1 area. This result suggests facet or pericapsular inflammation.

CLINICAL PEARL

Kemp's test can be performed when the patient is either standing or sitting. Sitting increases intradiscal pressure and therefore maximizes stress on the disc. Standing increases weight bearing and maximizes stress to the facets. The test should be performed in both positions.

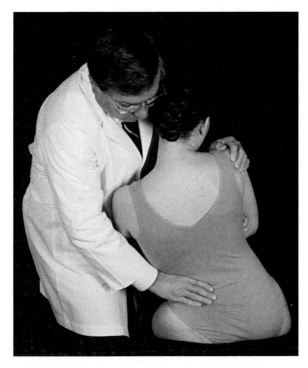

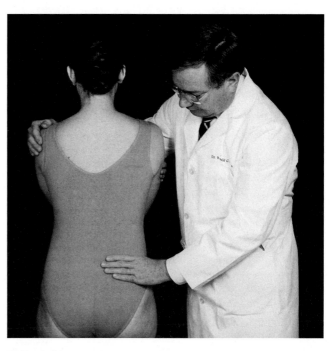

FIG. 8-80 Circumduction of the trunk toward the affected side occurs to the point at which the spine is posterolaterally extended. If this compression causes or aggravates a pattern of radicular pain in the thigh and leg, the test is positive and indicates nerve root compression. Local pain should be noted, but it does not constitute a positive test. Degenerative joint disease, exostoses, inflammatory or fibrotic residues, narrowing from disc degeneration, and tumors must be evaluated.

FIG. 8-81 An alternative is to have the patient assume a standing position. The examiner anchors the pelvis on the affected side with one hand. With the other hand, the examiner grasps the patient's opposite shoulder.

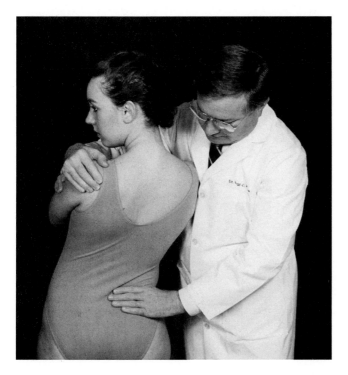

FIG. 8-82 While fixing the pelvis, the examiner firmly moves the patient's opposite shoulder obliquely backward, toward the affected side. This maneuver rotates the trunk, extends it, and exerts downward pressure over the affected lumbosacral area. The test is positive if this compression causes or aggravates a pattern of radicular pain in the thigh and leg. A positive test indicates nerve root compression. In the standing position, the test must elicit a more positive finding than is elicited in the seated position.

KERNIG/BRUDZINSKI SIGN

Assessment for Meningeal Irritation or Inflammation

Comment

With treatment, the fatality rate of adult bacterial meningitis is usually less than 10%, but severe neurologic sequelae are possible. The two leading causes of these sequelae in the adult are pneumococci *(Streptococcus pneumoniae)* and meningococci *(Neisseria meningitidis)*.

Pneumococcal meningitis usually is preceded by pneumonia and often is associated with alcoholism, debilitation, and old age. This type of meningitis usually occurs sporadically, except in developing countries.

Meningococcal meningitis occurs in epidemics (serogroup A or C) in the pediatric age group and may be acquired by susceptible adults.

Meningitis caused by gram-negative enteric bacteria is always a disease of the hospitalized or nursing home patient and often follows bacteremia from other foci, such as cellulitis or urinary tract infection.

The possibility of bacterial meningitis must be considered in any patient with fever and even minimal mental or neurologic symptoms.

Whenever the diagnosis is suspected, a referral for lumbar puncture must be accomplished immediately and bacterial cultures obtained. When the cerebrospinal fluid is abnormal, tuberculous and fungal cultures should be obtained.

Prognosis depends on the interval between the onset of the illness and the institution of therapy.

If severe backache, stiff neck, and the Kernig/Brudzinski sign are absent, but mental symptoms are prominent, and the cerebrospinal fluid shows normal sugar, a low number of cells, or a mononuclear pleocytosis (lymphocytosis), then encephalitis must be suspected. Patients with herpes simplex encephalitis classically present with an acute onset of mental and behavioral symptoms and often with an amnestic syndrome. The patients may have lateralized findings, such as hemiparesis or aphasia.

PROCEDURE

- For the Brudzinski part of the sign, the patient is in the supine position and the examiner passively flexes the patient's head (Fig. 8-83).
- The sign is present if flexion of both knees occurs (Fig. 8-84).
- The sign is often accompanied by flexion of both hips and is present with meningitis.
- For the Kernig part of the sign, the patient is supine.
- The examiner flexes the hip and knee of either leg to 90 degrees, respectively (Fig. 8-85).
- The examiner attempts to completely extend the leg (Fig. 8-86).
- If pain prevents this, the sign is present.
- The sign is often accompanied by involuntary flexion of the opposite knee and hip and is present in meningitis.

Confirmation Procedure

Cerebrospinal fluid examination

DIAGNOSTIC STATEMENT

The Kernig/Brudzinski sign is present. This sign indicates meningeal irritation or inflammation.

CLINICAL PEARL

Following myelography, a percentage of patients experience general malaise, headache, nausea, pain, and stiffness for a week or longer, and the symptoms are strikingly aggravated by the erect position or activity. These conditions may be signs of arachnoiditis. Subarachnoid fibrosis typically affects the lowermost segment of the thecal sac. This whole process represents meningismus or the apparent irritation of the spinal cord, in which the symptoms simulate meningitis. However, no actual infectious agent—such as bacteria, fungi, or viruses—can be found.

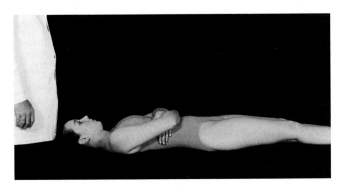

FIG. 8-83   For the Brudzinski sign, the patient is in the supine position.

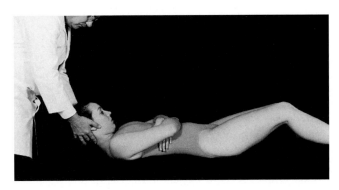

FIG. 8-84   The patient's head is passively flexed by the examiner. The sign is present if flexion of both knees occurs. The sign is often accompanied by flexion of both hips. The sign is present in meningitis.

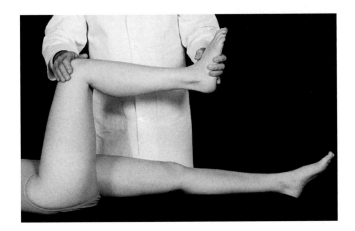

FIG. 8-85   For the Kernig sign, the patient is supine. The examiner flexes the hip and knee of either leg to 90 degrees, respectively.

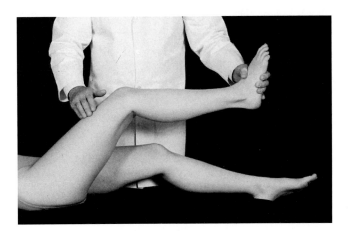

FIG. 8-86   The examiner attempts to completely extend the leg. If pain prevents this extension, the sign is present. The sign is often accompanied by involuntary flexion of the opposite knee and hip. The sign is present in meningitis.

LASÈGUE DIFFERENTIAL SIGN

Assessment for Intervertebral Radiculopathy vs Hip Joint Disease

Comment

The intervertebral disc is the source of most low back pain. Of disc lesions in the lumbar spine, 95% occur at the fourth and fifth spaces. With normal aging and repetitive trauma, progressive degeneration of the nucleus pulposus occurs. Protrusion of nuclear material usually occurs in the area of greatest weakness at the posterolateral aspect of the disc (Fig. 8-87).

Examination often reveals restriction of low back motion. Bending toward the affected side typically exacerbates the pain. Variable degrees of local tenderness and muscle guarding are present. In an attempt to relieve tension on the nerve root, the patient may list or bend away from the painful side and stand with the affected hip and knee slightly flexed. A characteristic clinical picture may be present, depending on the level of nerve root involvement (Table 8-13).

With lower lumbar compression, attempted forward bending is limited by pain and inflexibility of the lumbar spine, and percussion by a fist or reflex hammer over the lower segments may aggravate the complaint in the thigh or leg (doorbell sign). The motor deficits that ensue from paresis of these roots are most apparent below the knee. Seldom is weakness of the calf so severe that the patient cannot walk on the toes, but atrophy of the gastrocnemius may be seen. Heel walking is especially revealing. Severe foot drop is unlikely, but toe drop is common with some atrophy of the anterior compartment. Nevertheless, dorsiflexion of the foot and toes should be tested directly for minor weakness. The straight-leg-raising test often demonstrates marked limitation in range of thigh flexion on the painful side. Squeeze tenderness of the calf is common. The ankle jerk reflex is a stretch reflex of the gastrocnemius-soleus. It is commonly diminished or absent when S1 root impingement occurs but may be normal in L5 root syndromes.

Neoplasms or inflammation of the spine or cauda equina may produce a syndrome similar to that produced by compression of the lower lumbar root, as may a retroperitoneal tumor and invasive neoplasm in the pelvis.

PROCEDURE

- If the examiner flexes the hip of a patient with sciatica while the knee is extended and this movement elicits pain (Fig. 8-88), but flexing the thigh on the pelvis while the knee is flexed produces no sciatic pain, the sign is present (Fig. 8-89).
- This sign rules out hip joint disease.

Confirmation Procedures

Bechterew's sitting test, Bragard's sign, Deyerle's sign, Fajersztajn's test, Lasègue rebound test, Lasègue sitting test, Lasègue test, Lewin standing test, Lindner's sign, Sicard's sign, straight-leg-raising test, and Turyn's sign

TABLE 8-13

LUMBAR DISC SYNDROME PATTERNS

Level	Pain	Sensory	Motor Weakness Atrophy	Reflex
L3-L4 (L4 root)	Low back, posterolateral aspect of thigh, across patella, anteromedial aspect of leg	Anterior aspect of knee, anteromedial aspect of leg	Quadriceps (knee extension)	Knee jerk
L4-L5 (L5 root)	Lateral, posterolateral aspect of thigh, leg	Lateral aspect of leg, dorsum of foot, first web space, great toe	Great toe extension, ankle dorsiflexion, heel walking difficult (foot drop may occur)	Minor (posterior tibial jerk depressed)
L5-S1 (S1 root)	Posterolateral aspect of thigh, leg, heel	Posterior aspect of calf, heel, lateral aspect of foot (3 toes)	Calf, plantar flexion of foot, great toe; toe walking weak	Ankle jerk
Cauda equina syndrome (massive midline protrusion)	Low back, thigh, legs; often bilateral	Thighs, legs, feet, perineum; often bilateral	Variable; may be bowel, bladder incontinence	Ankle jerk (may be bilateral)

Adapted from Mercier LR, Pettid FJ: *Practical orthopedics,* ed 4, St Louis, 1995, Mosby.

DIAGNOSTIC STATEMENT

The Lasègue differential sign is present on the right. This result indicates radiculopathy rather than hip articular disease.

CLINICAL PEARL

Lasègue described how painful it is for patients with sciatica when the sciatic nerve is stretched by extending the knee while the hip is flexed. He also described the pain relief that occurs when the knee was then flexed. This is the classic leg-raising sign. Variations of this sign, with interpretations of its meaning, lend much more knowledge to the examining physician than merely noting at what degree of leg raise the patient experiences either back pain, leg pain, or both.

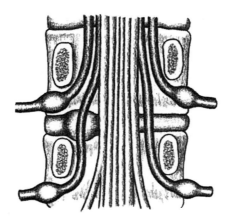

FIG. 8-87 Lumbar disc protrusion. *(From Mercier LR, Pettid FJ: Practical orthopedics, ed 4, St Louis, 1995, Mosby.)*

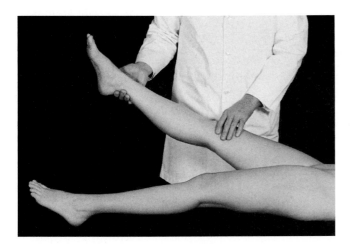

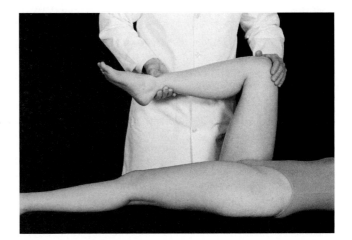

FIG. 8-88 The patient is supine with the legs fully extended. The examiner performs a straight-leg-raising test on the affected leg and notes the angle at which sciatic pain is produced.

FIG. 8-89 The examiner flexes the thigh and the knee, relieving the stretch on the sciatic nerve. The sign is present if the pain is relieved. The presence of the sign indicates neural pain rather than hip articular pain.

LASÈGUE REBOUND TEST

Assessment for Intervertebral Nerve Root Lesion, Piriformis Muscular Spasm, Ischiotrochanteric Groove Adhesion, or Intervertebral Disc Syndrome

Comment

Patients with chronic postural or mechanical problems in the lumbar spine or individuals who are vulnerable to repetitive injury may develop a chronic lumbar strain.

Hip flexion with rotation causes pain in an individual with this problem because it stretches the piriformis muscle, thereby compromising or irritating the sciatic nerve. Activities that externally rotate the thigh can strain the piriformis muscle and can refer pain to the buttocks; toward the hip, posterior thigh, and calf; and even to the sole of the foot, on occasion, as in typical cases of "sciatica" in radiculopathies.

Spasm of the posterior trunk muscles, sometimes accompanied by functional scoliosis and often by pain, usually indicates an underlying strain of the posterior joints, disc, or both. Unilateral spasm suggests a unilateral posterior joint strain. Lesions involving both disc and posterior joints are often accompanied by spasm of the spinal flexors, producing a straight or slightly kyphotic lumbar spine. Psoas spasm produces flexion deformity at the hip, and this may be missed at the initial examination. Spasm of the piriformis muscle, a common cause of buttock pain, can be diagnosed by palpation medial to the lower part of the neck of the femur.

Sciatic nerve entrapment usually occurs at the sciatic notch as the nerve exits from the pelvis. The nerve is compressed against the bony edge as it traverses the belly of the piriformis muscle. The syndrome is characterized by pain that is behind the greater trochanter and is referred down the thigh, the outer side of the leg, and the sole of the foot. Diagnostic findings include a positive Lasègue test, hypoesthesia of the lateral half of the sole of the foot, and pain behind the greater trochanter when the hip and knee joints are flexed to a right angle and the thigh is forced into adduction and internal rotation.

Pain during hip movement is emphasized as the diagnostic feature that differentiates sciatica because of a disc (when only straight leg raising is painful) from peripheral entrapment of the nerve as it traverses the sciatic notch. When the nerve is stretched by straight leg raising, pain is aggravated by internal rotation and relieved by external rotation.

Sensory changes, when present, are below the buttock and in the sole of the foot. Pressure on the nerve roots by a disc may involve the peroneal distribution above the ankle and the buttock itself. The condition is not common and may coexist with a prolapsed disc. The diagnosis of nerve entrapment is often missed initially and recognized only when sciatica persists after excision of the disc.

ORTHOPEDIC GAMUT 8-8

DISC HERNIATION VERSUS OTHER CAUSES OF BACK PAIN

The following elements apply when early disc herniation is difficult to differentiate from other causes of back pain:

1. Plain roentgenograms are indicated within 2 to 4 weeks of onset.
2. Electromyography, CT, MRI, or myelography confirm the diagnosis (Fig. 8-90).
3. Electromyography (EMG), CT, and MRI are not usually indicated for at least 4 to 6 weeks from onset.
4. EMG, CT (if surgical intervention is being contemplated), or MRI is indicated if other, more serious spinal pathology is suspected.
5. Discography is considered to be of only limited value.

PROCEDURE

- To continue a differential after the straight-leg-raising test, the examiner fixes the pelvis on the same side by pressing heavily with a hand on the region of the ipsilateral anterosuperior iliac spine and repeats that straight-leg-raising test (Fig. 8-91).
- Any undue pain experienced is associated with sciatic involvement resulting from a nerve root disorder, piriform spasm, or ischiotrochanteric groove adhesions (Fig. 8-92).
- Differentiation of piriformis spasm from other causes can be accomplished by reproducing the pain during internal rotation of the femur when it is at a lower level than the original point of pain.
- After a positive Lasègue test, the examiner may permit the leg to drop to the examination table without warning the patient (Fig. 8-93).
- If this Lasègue rebound test causes a marked increase in the back pain, sciatic neuralgia, and muscle spasm, then disc involvement is suspected.

Confirmation Procedures
Bechterew's sitting test, Bragard's sign, Deyerle's sign, Fajersztajn's sign, Lasègue differential sign, Lasègue sitting test, Lasègue test, Lewin standing test, Lindner's sign, Sicard's sign, straight-leg-raising test, and Turyn's sign

CLINICAL PEARL

The relationship of the lumbar roots and the lumbar discs is of major clinical importance. A massive posterior extrusion of one of the lumbar discs may severely injure the cauda equina (both intrathecal and extrathecal roots). Although these lesions are rare, they do occur. In these instances, the size and shape of the spinal canal and the size of the extruded mass are major factors in the severity of the clinical syndrome.

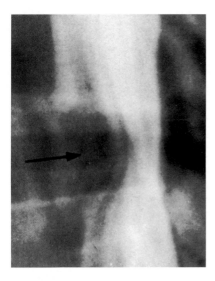

FIG. 8-90   Abnormal myelogram revealing a large extradural defect in the dye column that is consistent with disc herniation. *(From Mercier LR, Pettid FJ:* Practical orthopedics, *ed 4, St Louis, 1995, Mosby.)*

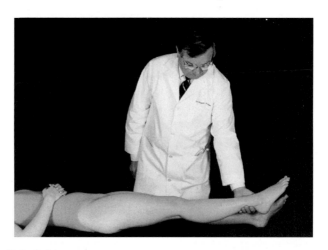

FIG. 8-91   The patient is in a supine position with both legs fully extended. The examiner performs a straight-leg-raising test on the affected leg.

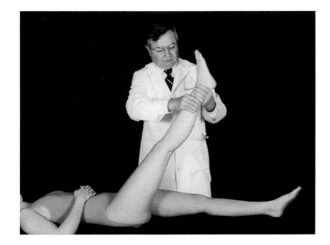

FIG. 8-92   The leg is elevated to the point at which pain is produced.

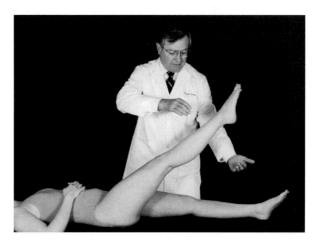

FIG. 8-93   Without warning, the examiner removes support from the elevated leg, allowing it to drop to the examination table If the test causes marked increase in back pain, sciatic neuralgia, and muscle spasm, the test is positive. A positive test indicates disc involvement.

LASÈGUE SITTING TEST

Assessment for Sciatic Nerve Inflammation

Comment

The lumbar spinal canal is bounded anteriorly by lumbar discs, vertebrae bodies, and the posterior longitudinal ligament; laterally by the lamina and facet joints; and posteriorly by the ligamentum flavum (Fig. 8-94).

The epidemiology of lumbar spinal stenosis is unclear. The prevalence of narrowing of the lumbar spinal canal rises with increasing age. Midsagittal narrowing to less than 12 mm has been proposed as being probably pathologic and less than 10 mm unequivocally pathologic. Clinical recognition of the syndrome is very much age related, with few cases diagnosed in patients younger than 50.

The most characteristic symptom is neurogenic claudication. *Neurogenic claudication* is any discomfort that occurs in the buttock, thigh, or leg on standing or walking that is relieved by rest. Neurogenic claudication is not produced by peripheral vascular insufficiency.

Sciatica resulting from lumbar spinal stenosis is distinct from the sciatica that typically follows herniation of the nucleus pulposus. Objective neurologic signs are often absent. Restriction of straight leg raising (Lasègue's test) is present in only 10% of cases of sciatica resulting from

lumbar spinal stenosis. Deep tendon reflexes at the ankle are absent in 40%, deep tendon reflexes at the knee are absent in 10%, and a small percentage have sensory loss or weakness. A condition identical to meralgia paresthetica can be produced by stenosis at the upper lumbar levels.

ORTHOPEDIC GAMUT 8-9

LUMBAR CANAL STENOSIS

The EMG findings in lumbar canal stenosis include the following:

1. An entirely normal EMG
2. Absent H-reflex only, unilaterally or bilaterally
3. Denervation in a single root distribution (single radiculopathy), unilaterally or bilaterally and asymmetrically
4. Occurrence of bilateral and asymmetric lumbosacral radiculopathies, affecting the L5, S1, and S2 roots (the most common EMG finding associated with lumbar canal stenosis) (Table 8-14)

TABLE 8-14

ELECTROPHYSIOLOGIC DIFFERENTIATION OF CHRONIC S1/S2 RADICULOPATHY

	Chronic S1/S2 Radiculopathy	Tarsal Tunnel Syndrome	Peripheral Polyneuropathy
Nerve conduction studies			
Sural sensory study*	Normal	Normal	Usually abnormal
Peroneal motor study	Normal or low amplitude	Normal	Low amplitude and/or slow latency
Tibial motor study	Normal or low amplitude	Low amplitude and/or slow latency	Low amplitude and/or slow latency
Motor conduction velocities	Normal or slowed	Normal	Slowed
Plantar studies*	Normal	Slow latencies or absent	Slow latencies or absent
H-reflex*	Abnormal	Normal	Abnormal
Upper extremity conductions	Normal	Normal	Can be abnormal
Needle EMG			
AH/ADQP	Denervated	Denervated	Denervated
EDB†	Denervated	Normal	Denervated
Medial gastrocnemius	Denervated	Normal	Denervated
Tibialis anterior	Normal	Normal	Denervated
Paraspinal muscles	Normal or fibs	Normal	Normal or fibrillations
Symmetry of findings (when bilateral)	Asymmetric	Asymmetric	Symmetric

From Katirji B: *Electromyography in clinical practice: a case study approach*, St Louis, 1998, Mosby.

AH, Abductor hallucis; *ADQP,* abductor digiti quinti pedis; *EDB,* extensor digitorum brevis; *EMG,* electromyography.

*Commonly absent in asymptomatic elderly subjects.

†May be denervated, selectively, in healthy subjects.

ORTHOPEDIC GAMUT 8-10

LUMBOSACRAL RADICULOPATHY

Following are EMG limitations in lumbosacral radiculopathy:

1. If the dorsal root is the only root compressed and if the ventral root is normal, the EMG examination is normal. This occurs in a significant number of patients whose symptoms are limited to pain and/or paresthesia. Thus a normal EMG does not exclude a root compression.

2. Fibrillation potentials can be absent from the paraspinal muscles, particularly in chronic radiculopathies. This is likely caused by reinnervation. In contrast, fibrillation potentials can be present in the paraspinal muscles after lumbar laminectomy because of denervation during surgical exposure.

3. The lower extremity sensory nerve action potentials (SNAPs) often are unevocable bilaterally in elderly patients. When this occurs, it often is difficult to differentiate a preganglionic lesion (i.e., lumbosacral radiculopathy) from a postganglionic lesion (i.e., lumbosacral plexopathy), unless fibrillation potentials are evident in the paraspinal muscles.

4. No SNAPs have been devised to assess the L2 or L3 fibers up to the dorsal root ganglion, and the saphenous SNAP is not technically reliable (especially in elderly and obese patients) to assess the L4 fibers. Thus it often is difficult to separate an upper lumbar radiculopathy (especially L2 and L3) from lumbar plexopathy, unless there are fibrillations in the paraspinal muscles.

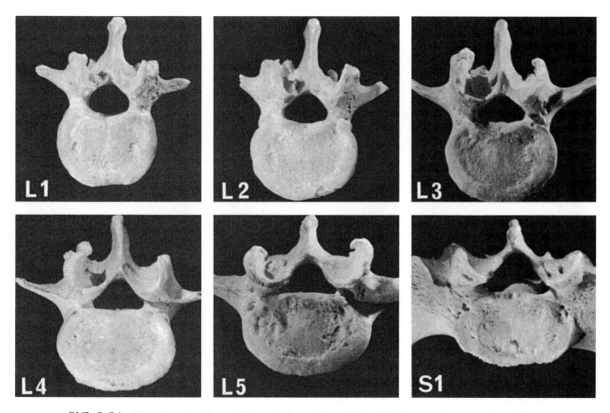

FIG. 8-94   The changing shape of the spinal canal from L1 to S1. The vertebrae are viewed from above. From L1 to S1, the spinal canal changes from an oval on its side to a more trefoil shape as the posterior wall of the vertebrae changes from concave to convex and the pedicles grow shorter and broader, migrate more laterally, and project more posterolaterally.   *(From Kirkaldy WH:* Managing low back pain, *ed 4, Philadelphia, 1999, Churchill Livingstone.)*

Restless leg syndrome produces a predominantly nocturnal discomfort that profoundly disturbs sleep and is relieved only by moving the legs either in bed or forcing the patient to arise and walk around to settle the discomfort. The cause of this condition is uncertain, but it has been attributed to lumbar spinal stenosis syndrome.

Traumatic lumbar intervertebral disc prolapse is found in young adults who are most often male and usually employed in work that involves the lifting of heavy weights. Furniture movers, dockers, miners, truck drivers (who have to load their own trucks), and medical and nursing workers are particularly vulnerable.

The patient develops acute pain in the back immediately after lifting a weight or unexpectedly bearing a heavy load, such as when the worker slips or helpers release their grip prematurely. The sudden force is taken by the flexed and rotated spine. The patient develops immediate, midline lumbar pain that is severe enough to stop motion. The patient is afraid to move and feels as if the back is locked by the pain.

The pain may extend into the leg in the sciatic distribution, and there may be a loss of nerve root function. The pain is severe enough to drive the sufferer to bed after the first attack. Recumbency relieves the symptoms.

PROCEDURE

- The patient is seated upright on the edge of a table with the legs dangling (Fig. 8-95).
- The examiner faces the patient and extends the patient's leg at the knee.
- The lower extremity from the hip to the foot is made parallel with the floor (Fig. 8-96).
- When radiculoneuropathy is not present, the patient should not experience discomfort from this action.

- Initially, the significance of the test is the same as the Lasègue test.
- However, the modification of performing the straight leg raise while the patient is in the seated position provides several advantages.
- In the supine position, straight leg raising may be difficult because the patient may squirm and shift the pelvis, making the leg abduct and rotate.
- The apprehensive patient may attempt to ward off anticipated pain and make the test positive sooner than is warranted.
- When the test is performed in the seated position, the patient faces the examiner, feels more secure and at ease, and is less likely to even know the part is being tested.
- The test has excellent, objective values when the examiner is able to determine immediately the slightest attempt on the part of the patient to withdraw by leaning back from the induced pain.

Confirmation Procedures

Bechterew's sitting test, Bragard's sign, Deyerle's sign, Fajersztajn's test, Lasègue differential sign, Lasègue rebound test, Lasègue test, Lewin standing test, Lindner's sign, Sicard's sign, straight-leg-raising test, and Turyn's sign

---

DIAGNOSTIC STATEMENT

Lasègue sitting test is positive on the left. This result indicates sciatic nerve inflammation.

CLINICAL PEARL

By raising the foot, the examiner has performed a modified straight-leg-raising test. Because the thigh is already flexed to 90 degrees in this position, straightening the knee to the horizontal places stretching forces on the nerve roots. The results of this seated tension should correspond to the results obtained from the tests done in the supine position.

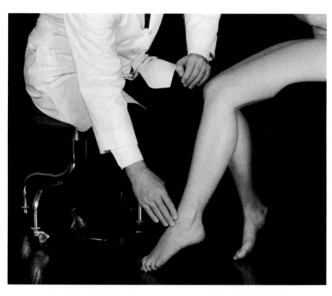

FIG. 8-95   The patient is seated with the legs hanging over the edge of the examination table.

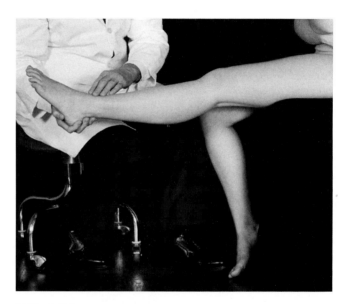

FIG. 8-96   The examiner faces the patient and extends the patient's affected leg at the knee. The lower extremity, from the hip to the foot, is brought up until parallel with the floor. Pain in the sciatic distribution is a positive finding. A positive test indicates radiculoneuropathy.

LASÈGUE TEST

ALSO KNOWN AS LASÈGUE SIGN

Assessment for Sciatica Resulting from Lumbosacral or Sacroiliac Lesions, Lumbar Subluxation Syndrome, Intervertebral Disc Lesion, Spondylolisthesis, Dural Sleeve Adhesions, or Intervertebral Foramen Occlusion (Encroachment)

Comment

A high percentage of adults older than 40 have degenerative disc disease at one or more levels on roentgenographic examination (Fig. 8-97). Significant thinning of the disc accompanied by osteophyte formation is often present. Degenerative changes in the adjacent facet joints and surrounding soft tissues often lead to intermittent low back pain and even nerve root irritation.

The Lasègue test is the pain induced by stretching the sciatic nerve or one of its roots. The sign is elicited by gradual and slow extension of the knee of the elevated lower limb, which is performed while the patient is supine. The pain that is induced is similar to that felt spontaneously by the patient.

The nerve root glides freely through the IVF and during extension of the knee. The nerve roots are pulled out of the foramen for several millimeters at the L5 level.

One point deserves emphasis. During extension of the knee while the leg is elevated, the force of the traction on the nerve roots can reach 3 kg. The resistance to traction of the nerve roots is 3.2 kg.

If a root is trapped or shortened by a prolapsed disc, any rough manipulation of the leg can cause rupture of some axons and may result in paralysis. This is usually short lived, but occasionally, it may take a long time to disappear.

ORTHOPEDIC GAMUT 8-11

LASÈGUE TEST

Following are the interpretations of the Lasègue test:

1. When the patient is supine and the lower limbs are resting on the examination table, the sciatic nerve and its roots are under no tension.
2. When the lower limb is raised while the knees are flexed, the sciatic nerve and its roots are still under no tension.
3. If the knee is extended while the leg is elevated, the sciatic nerve—which must cover a longer distance—is subjected to increasing tension. In the normal patient, the nerve roots slide freely through the IVF, and no pain results. When the lower limb is nearly vertical for people with diminished flexibility, pain is felt on the posterior aspect of the thigh as a result of stretching the hamstrings. However, this pain does not constitute a positive Lasègue sign.
4. When one nerve root is trapped in the foramen or when the root must cover a longer distance because of a prolapsed disc, any stretching of the nerve will become painful with moderate elevation of the lower limb. This result constitutes a positive Lasègue sign, which is evident before 60 degrees of flexion is attained. Pain may be elicited at 10, 15, or 20 degrees of flexion, which allows a rough quantification of the severity of the lesion.

ORTHOPEDIC GAMUT 8-12

PRECAUTIONS FOR LASÈGUE TEST

The following two precautions must be observed in performing Lasègue test:

1. The examiner must always elicit the Lasègue sign cautiously and stop when the patient feels pain.
2. The examiner must never attempt to elicit the Lasègue sign when the patient is under general anesthesia because the protective pain reflex is absent. The reflex can occur when the patient is being placed prone on an operating table and the hips are allowed to flex while the knees are extended. Hip flexion must always be associated with knee flexion, which relaxes the sciatic nerve and the trapped root.

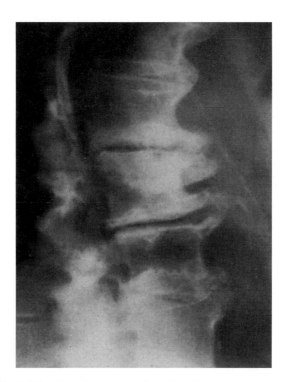

FIG. 8-97 Chronic degenerative disc disease. *(From Mercier LR, Pettid FJ:* Practical orthopedics, *ed 4, St Louis, 1995, Mosby.)*

PROCEDURE

- The patient lies supine with legs extended.
- The examiner places one hand under the ankle of the affected leg and the other hand on the knee and flexes the thigh on the pelvis while the knee is flexed (Fig. 8-98).
- The examiner then slowly extends the knee while the leg is elevated (Fig. 8-99).
- If this maneuver is markedly limited because of pain, the test is positive and suggests sciatica from lumbosacral or sacroiliac lesions, subluxation syndrome, disc lesions, spondylolisthesis, adhesions, or IVF occlusion.

Confirmation Procedures

Bechterew's test, Bragard's sign, Deyerle's sign, Fajersztajn's test, Lasègue differential sign, Lasègue rebound test, Lasègue sitting test, Lewin standing test, Lindner's sign, Sicard's sign, straight-leg-raising test, and Turyn's sign

---

DIAGNOSTIC STATEMENT

Lasègue test is positive on the right. This result indicates sciatica associated with nerve root inflammation or compression.

CLINICAL PEARL

Whenever the presence of the Lasègue sign is questionable, the examiner should combine it with flexion of the cervical spine (Lindner's sign). This combination places the greatest pull and stretch on the nerve roots behind the intervertebral discs and often elicits pain.

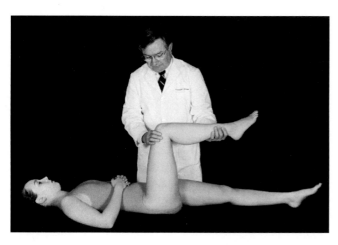

FIG. 8-98   The patient is supine, with both legs fully extended. The examiner places one hand under the ankle of the affected leg and the other hand at the knee. The hip and knee are flexed to 90 degrees, respectively. The nerve roots are under no tension, and pain should not be elicited.

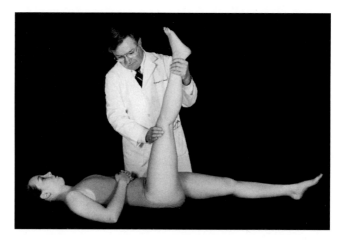

FIG. 8-99   The knee is extended by the examiner. If this maneuver is limited by pain, the Lasègue test is positive. The test suggests sciatica from lumbosacral or sacroiliac lesions, subluxation syndrome, disc lesions, spondylolisthesis, adhesions, or interventricular foramen occlusion.

LEWIN PUNCH TEST

Assessment for Generalized Spinal Lesion or Intervertebral Disc Protrusion

Comment

A defect in the pars interarticularis with no forward displacement is termed *spondylolysis*. Defects can be dysplastic, isthmic, degenerative, traumatic, or pathologic. In Western world cultures, spondylolysis is believed to occur in approximately 6% of the population, with 80% to 90% of these defects occurring at the L5 level. Lumbosacral spine films with additional oblique views help the examiner investigate or confirm defects of the pars interarticularis (Fig. 8-100).

The symptomatic patient has low back pain, which may radiate into the buttocks or leg. Early extension of the lumbar spine causes pain over the affected vertebra. Having the patient stand on the ipsilateral leg and extend the spine (Jackson test) is a unilateral weight-bearing posture in extension that usually evokes pain over the defect or fracture.

When compressed axially, the substance of the nucleus pulposus can stream out in various directions. If the annulus is still strong, the increase in pressure within the disc can cause the vertebral plateaus to give way. This corresponds to intravertebral prolapse.

The annulus fibers begin to degenerate after 25 years of age, allowing the tearing of fibers within each of its layers. Therefore, under axial stress, the nuclear material can stream out through the torn annulus. This streaming of nuclear material can be concentric but is more often radial.

Anterior prolapse is the rarest. Posterior prolapse is the most common, especially posterolateral prolapse. Thus, when the disc is crushed, part of the nuclear substance may stream out anteriorly but more often it streams out posteriorly and can thus reach the posterior edge of the disc to touch the posterior longitudinal ligament. At first, the streamer, which is still attached to the nucleus, gets trapped under the posterior longitudinal ligament. When this happens, it is still possible to bring the streamer back into its fibrous casing by using vertebral traction. Very often, the streamer breaks through the posterior longitudinal ligament and may lie within the vertebral canal, which produces the so-called free type of disc prolapse. In other cases, the nuclear streamer is trapped under the posterior longitudinal ligament and gets nipped off by the annulus fibers, which precludes any restoration to normal because the fibers snap back into position. In some cases, the streamer, after reaching the deep aspect of the posterior longitudinal ligament, slides either superiorly or inferiorly. This is a case of subligamentous prolapse.

It is only when the herniating nucleus presses against the deep surface of the posterior longitudinal ligament that the nerve endings of the ligament are stretched, which causes lower back pain. Finally, compression of the nerve roots by the herniating disc causes nerve root pain, or sciatica.

PROCEDURE

- Punching the buttock produces a referred pain in the back.
- While the patient is standing, the examiner punches the side of the buttock with the lesion (Fig. 8-101).
- If this punch elicits pain, the test is positive.
- Punching the opposite buttock should not elicit pain.
- The test is significant for a spinal lesion, usually involving a protruded disc.

Confirmation Procedures

Antalgia sign, bowstring sign, Cox sign, heel/toe walk test, Kemp's test, Lewin snuff test, Milgram's test, and Neri's sign

---

DIAGNOSTIC STATEMENT

Lewin punch test is positive on the right. This result suggests an intervertebral disc protrusion.

CLINICAL PEARL

In some instances of an acute attack, even light fist percussion over the lumbar spine in the midline will produce such severe accentuation of the local and radiating pain that the patient's knees may buckle. There may be some evidence of a vasovagal response.

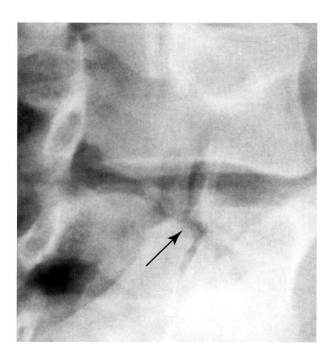

FIG. 8-100 Bony defect in the isthmus or neck of the Scottie dog in oblique view of spondylosis. *(From Brier SR: Primary care orthopedics, St Louis, 1999, Mosby.)*

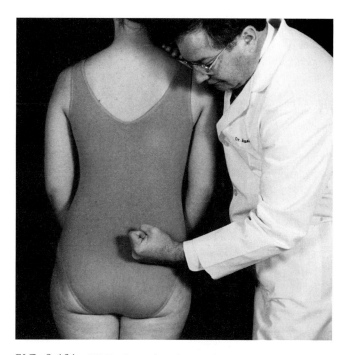

FIG. 8-101 While the patient is standing, the examiner firmly percusses the patient's buttock on the affected side. If the "punch" produces a referred pain in the back, the test is positive. Punching the opposite buttock does not produce pain. The positive test indicates a spinal lesion, usually a protruded disc.

LEWIN SNUFF TEST

Assessment for Intervertebral Disc Rupture or Space-Occupying Mass

Comment

Tumors of the spinal canal are traditionally categorized as to location as follows: intramedullary, intradural, extramedullary, and extradural. With the exception of the rare primary bone tumor, MRI is the method of choice in evaluation of tumors of the spinal column. In intramedullary spinal cord lesions, myelography and CT myelography may demonstrate cord enlargement or contour irregularities. Intradural extramedullary tumors and extradural tumors are more completely demonstrated on MRI than on CT (Fig. 8-102).

The most common extradural or bony neoplastic disease of the spine is metastatic disease, commonly involving bone marrow because of its rich vascularity. The lumbar spine is most commonly affected, followed by the thoracic and cervical spine. The most common primary tumors are breast, prostate, and lung.

The intervertebral discs are not solid lumps of inert gristle, as patients often think, but rather are living structures that flatten during the day and reexpand at night. The discs consist of a firm nucleus pulposus surrounded by the annulus fibrosus, a ring of fibrocartilage, and fibrous tissue that links two vertebrae together. The disc is a symphysis between each pair of vertebrae and, with the two posterior facet joints, allows movement between the vertebrae.

The tension within the disc is maintained by fluid imbibition at the cellular level. If imbibition fails, the pressure within the disc falls, and the disc collapses. Increased movement occurs between the adjacent vertebrae, and the annulus fibrosus is exposed to increased stress. This condition is accompanied by vague lower back pain.

As the degeneration proceeds, the annulus fibrosus softens, and the degenerative disc bulges the annular ligament backward, usually just lateral to the midline. If this bulge occurs in a tight spinal canal opposite a nerve root, the function of the root is affected.

Of all lumbar disc protrusions, 90% involve the lowest two spaces, L4-L5 or L5-S1. Lesions that press on the L5 nerve root cause altered sensibility on the outer side of the calf and weakness of the peronei and ankle extensors, whereas those lesions affecting the S1 nerve root produce altered sensibility on the foot or back of the calf, weak ankle flexors, and a depressed ankle jerk. The resting muscle tone of the glutei, hamstrings, calf muscles, and other posterior muscle groups also may be reduced, and these muscles may atrophy.

Unless there are neurologic symptoms and signs below the knee, the patient probably does not have a true prolapsed intervertebral disc. If the disc presses on a nerve root, the postural reflexes work to diminish the pressure on the root. The spine is held curved to produce a sciatic scoliosis, and straight leg raising, which stretches the nerve, is restricted by pain.

PROCEDURE

- An aromatic substance is introduced, and the patient is instructed to sniff it up the nostril in order to induce sneezing (Fig. 8-103).
- The test is positive when sneezing elicits an exacerbation of well-localized spinal and radicular pain (Fig. 8-104).
- The test is significant for intervertebral disc rupture.

Confirmation Procedures

Antalgia sign, bowstring sign, Cox sign, heel/toe walk test, Kemp's test, Lewin punch test, Milgram's test, and Neri's sign

---

DIAGNOSTIC STATEMENT

Lewin snuff test is positive and reproduces the radiating pain. This result indicates an intervertebral disc rupture.

CLINICAL PEARL

The sneeze produces a sudden Valsalva maneuver. If it is assumed that motion of an irritated nerve root over a disc bulge is one of the causes of pain, any production of a Valsalva effect abruptly increases the patient's pain as the defect appears and disappears and thereby moves the nerve root over the disc.

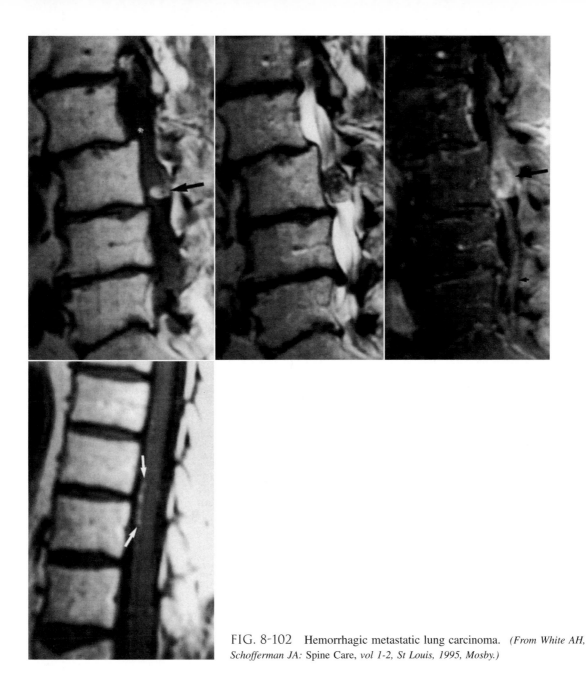

FIG. 8-102   Hemorrhagic metastatic lung carcinoma.   *(From White AH, Schofferman JA: Spine Care, vol 1-2, St Louis, 1995, Mosby.)*

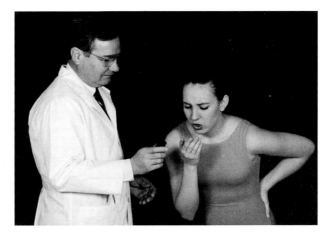

FIG. 8-103   The patient is introduced to a pungent, aromatic substance and instructed to inhale it through a nostril to induce sneezing.

FIG. 8-104   The test is positive when sneezing elicits an exacerbation of well-localized spinal and radicular pain. The test indicates intervertebral disc rupture.

LEWIN STANDING TEST

Assessment for Unilateral or Bilateral Hamstring Spasm

Comment

Rupture of a muscle is felt as a tearing sensation. Swelling and tenderness at the site of the rupture follow within hours, and bruising appears about 24 hours later. The bruising, which is caused by bleeding from the ends of the ruptured muscle, can be dramatic and even alarming.

During examination, a defect can be felt in the muscle belly, and the belly becomes prominent as the muscle contracts. The swelling can occasionally be mistaken for a soft-tissue mass. The rectus femoris and hamstrings are the muscles most often affected.

A hematoma in a muscle is a serious lesion that is sometimes called a charley horse. The lesion usually follows direct trauma or, more rarely, a tear of the central fibers of the muscle.

As the blood in the hematoma becomes organized, it interferes with normal muscle function. In some patients, the hematoma becomes ossified, which restricts muscle movement severely.

If a child has tight hamstrings that prevent flexion of the trunk or hip, spondylolisthesis should be suspected. Radiographs of the lumbosacral spine are essential in any child with tight hamstrings or calf muscles.

The sciatic nerve is considered to supply the posterior aspect of the hip and thigh.

The innervation to the short muscles of the hip and thigh (the obturator, sciatic, and sacral plexuses) also supplies the sensory branches from the hip joint capsule. The cutaneous branches around the hip originate at a higher level than the motor and capsular nerves. The lateral femoral cutaneous nerve that covers the anterolateral thigh is L2.

The anterior of the thigh is covered by the continuation of the femoral nerve by L2 to L4, the upper portion of the thigh is covered by the iliohypogastric, and the buttocks are covered by the posterior primary division of T12 to L3. Superficial cutaneous abnormality is referred from higher spinal levels.

PROCEDURE

- The patient is standing.
- From behind, the examiner stabilizes the pelvis with one hand while sharply pulling the knee on that side into extension (Figs. 8-105 and 8-106).
- The examiner then repeats this move on the opposite side and braces a shoulder against the patient's sacrum and sharply pulls both of the patient's knees into extension.
- The test is positive when pulling one or both knees into extension elicits pain that is followed by one or both knees snapping back into flexion.
- This positive finding represents unilateral or bilateral hamstring spasm.

Confirmation Procedures

Bechterew's sitting test, Bragard's sign, Deyerle's sign, Fajersztajn's test, Lasègue differential sign, Lasègue rebound test, Lasègue sitting test, Lasègue test, Lindner's sign, Sicard's sign, straight-leg-raising test, and Turyn's sign

---

DIAGNOSTIC STATEMENT

Lewin standing test is positive on the right. This result indicates a hamstring spasm.

CLINICAL PEARL

Tight or contracted hamstrings pull eccentrically on the pelvis. The patient with suspected tight hamstring disorder (THD) can be examined in the supine position. Keeping the hips and buttocks in contact with the table, straight leg raising is performed bilaterally. The comparison will indicate any hamstring contracture or tightness.

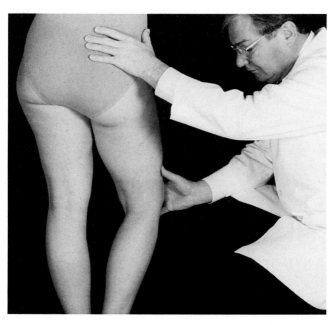

FIG. 8-105   While the patient is standing, the examiner stabilizes the patient's pelvis on the affected side with one hand.

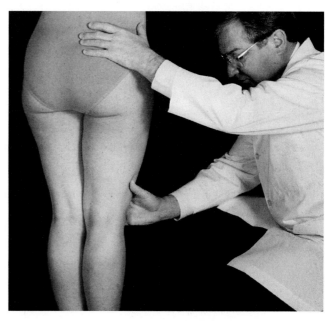

FIG. 8-106   The examiner then sharply pulls the knee of the affected leg into extension. This maneuver is repeated on the unaffected side. Next, the examiner braces a shoulder against the patient's sacrum and pulls both knees sharply into extension. The test is positive if pulling the knee into extension causes pain and is followed by a snapping back, of either knee, into flexion. This positive finding represents unilateral or bilateral hamstring spasm, as seen in sciatic radiculopathy.

LEWIN SUPINE TEST

Assessment for Lumbar Arthritis, Lumbar Fibrosis, Spondylosis, Sacroiliac or Lumbosacral Arthrosis, or Sciatica

Comment

Approximation of the spinous processes (kissing spines) and the development of a bursa between them have been indicated as a cause of low back pain after hyperextension injuries. *Sprung back* is a term describing rupture of the supraspinous ligament following a sudden flexion strain applied to the spine with the pelvis fixed, as in falling on the buttocks with the legs outstretched (Fig. 8-107).

Normally, on flexion of the spine, the discal borders of the vertebral bodies become parallel above the level of L5. This is the maximal movement permitted. In the stage of segmental instability, excessive degrees of extension and flexion are permitted, and a certain amount of backward and forward gliding movement also occurs (Fig. 8-108). This abnormal type of movement can be shown clinically by roentgenograms taken with the patient holding the spine in full extension and in full flexion. There are two radiologic changes that are indicative of instability: the Knutsson phenomenon (vacuum sign) of gas in the disc and the "traction spur" (Fig. 8-109).

ORTHOPEDIC GAMUT 8-13

DISC DEGENERATION

In disc degeneration, the following is observed:

1. Disc degeneration may occur and may remain asymptomatic.
2. Disc degeneration may be associated with changes within the disc itself, which may produce pain.
3. Disc degeneration may give rise to mechanical instability that renders the spine vulnerable to trauma.

Lumbar spondylosis is a condition in which there is progressive degeneration of the intervertebral discs leading to changes of the adjacent vertebrae and ligaments and to osteoarthritis.

Most patients with lumbar spondylosis are older than those with primary disc lesions. A chief symptom is lower back pain, which is often described as both generalized and specific aching, involving certain areas of point tenderness.

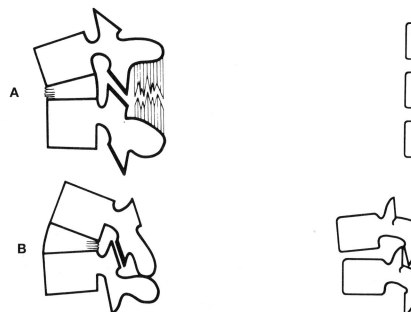

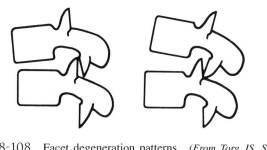

FIG. 8-107 **A,** "Sprung back." **B,** "Kissing spines." *(From Torg JS, Shephard RJ: Current therapy in sports medicine, ed 3, St Louis, 1995, Mosby.)*

FIG. 8-108 Facet degeneration patterns. *(From Torg JS, Shephard RJ: Current therapy in sports medicine, ed 3, St Louis, 1995, Mosby.)*

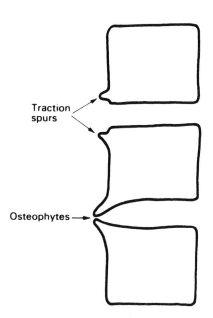

Traction spurs

Osteophytes

FIG. 8-109 The traction spur projects horizontally from the vertebral body about 1 mm away from the discal border. *(From Torg JS, Shephard RJ: Current therapy in sports medicine, ed 3, St Louis, 1995, Mosby.)*

Activity increases the discomfort, and rest eases it. Sciatic pain is rare. When present, sciatic pain is generalized, it involves one or both lower extremities, and it often reflects root compression at several levels.

Examination reveals moderate paraspinal muscle spasm in the lumbar region with some limitation of the lumbar spine mobility in most movements. Extension is usually a bit more restricted than flexion. There is some flattening of the normal lumbar lordosis. A moderate paraspinal muscle spasm usually is present. Straight leg raising is not as painful with spondylosis as with a herniated lumbar disc. Deep tendon reflex changes are elicited but are somewhat vague, which reflects nerve root compression at several levels.

The patient with lumbar spondylosis and a stenotic canal has a long history of intermittent lower back pain that is often related to specific positions and activities. The patient is often unable to sleep in a prone position (which tends to increase the lumbar lordosis). The patient finds it necessary to sleep on a side with the hips and knees flexed to maintain a strong lumbar flexion.

With lumbar spondylosis accompanied by a stenotic lumbar spinal canal, the physical examination is unrevealing despite intermittent symptoms that are often severe. Flexion and straight leg raising are often performed without difficulty. Severe pain during lumbar extension may be the only positive result.

PROCEDURE

- While the patient is supine, the examiner supports the patient's legs on the table (Fig. 8-110).
- The patient is directed to sit up without using the hands (Fig. 8-111).
- The test is positive if the patient is unable to do this.
- A positive test is often associated with lumbar arthritis, lumbar fibrosis, degenerative disc thinning with protrusion, sacroiliac or lumbosacral arthritis, and sciatica.
- The patient is often able to localize the site of the complaint.

Confirmation Procedures
Bilateral leg-lowering test, Demianoff's sign, double leg-raise test, hyperextension test, matchstick test, Mennell's sign, Minor's sign, Nachlas test, Quick test, Schober's test, sign of the buttock, skin pinch test, spinal percussion test, and Vanzetti's sign

---

DIAGNOSTIC STATEMENT

Lewin supine test is positive. This result indicates a pathologic condition of lumbosacral origin, which precludes the patient from completing the test.

CLINICAL PEARL

The security and comfort of the back depend not only on the lumbar muscles and ligaments but also on the strength of the abdominal wall and prevertebral muscles. The abdomen should be palpated to determine whether divarication of the rectus abdominis muscle is present. The clinical test for diagnosis of rectus divarication involves instructing the supine patient to raise the head from the examination table. The examining hand can easily feel the gap between the contracted pillars of the rectus, and the fingers will sink into the soft abdominal wall. The width of the gap may vary from 1 cm to a hand's breadth.

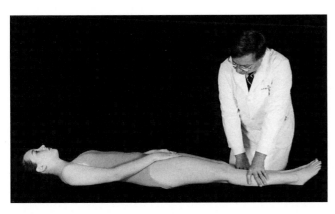

FIG. 8-110 The patient is supine, with both legs fully extended. The examiner firmly applies downward pressure to the patient's legs.

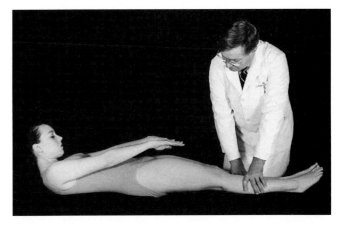

FIG. 8-111 The patient is directed to sit up without using the hands. The test is positive if the patient is unable to do this. A positive test indicates lumbar arthritis, lumbar fibrosis, a degenerative disc with protrusion, sacroiliac or lumbosacral arthritis, or sciatica. The patient is often able to localize the site, or origin, of the pain.

LINDNER'S SIGN

Assessment for Lumbar
Nerve Root Irritation or Inflammation

Comment
Before the development of signs and symptoms compatible with a diagnosis of a herniated lumbar disc, most patients have previously experienced lower back pain and other symptoms, which in retrospect can be related to the ensuing disc syndrome. Often, the preexisting lower back pain is not severe and does not cause impairment. When the back pain becomes associated with pain radiating down the course of the sciatic nerve, the possibility of lumbar disc disease should be seriously considered. Position is usually a factor in intensifying or decreasing the pain.

Most patients report that weight bearing, prolonged standing, walking, and sometimes sitting aggravate the pain. Resting in bed eases the pain. Symptoms may be aggravated by coughing, sneezing, or straining at the stool. Physical activity aggravates the pain, particularly flexion activities or postures.

The various nerve roots, when compressed by the protruding disc, produce characteristic signs and symptoms.

Whenever the straight-leg-raising test produces a questionable result of pain, it should be combined with flexion of the cervical spine (Lindner's sign). This combination places pull and stretch on the nerve roots behind the intervertebral disc and often elicits pain. The simultaneous flexion of the neck and elevation of the contralateral leg can produce pain in the ipsilateral sciatic notch in patients with either free fragments or herniated discs. Raising the contralateral leg alone might not elicit pain in either leg.

ORTHOPEDIC GAMUT 8-14

UNILATERAL DISC HERNIATION BETWEEN L3 AND L4

Unilateral disc herniation between L3 and L4 usually compresses the fourth lumbar root as it crosses the disc before exiting at the L4 intervertebral foramen with the following results:

1. Pain may be localized around the medial side of the leg.
2. Numbness may be present over the anteromedial aspect of the leg.
3. The quadriceps and hip adductor group, both innervated from L2, L3 and L4, may be weak and, in extended ruptures, atrophic.
4. Reflex testing may reveal a diminished or absent patellar tendon reflex (L2, L3, and L4) or tibialis anterior tendon reflex (L4).
5. Sensory testing may show diminished sensibility over the L4 dermatome, the isolated portion of which is the medial leg, and the autonomous zone, which is at the level of the medial malleolus.

ORTHOPEDIC GAMUT 8-15

UNILATERAL DISC HERNIATION BETWEEN L4 AND L5

Unilateral disc herniation between L4 and L5 results in compression of the fifth lumbar root with the following results:

1. Fifth lumbar root radiculopathy should produce pain in the dermatomal pattern.
2. Numbness, when present, follows the L5 dermatome along the anterolateral aspect of the leg and the dorsum of the foot, including the great toe.
3. The autonomous zone for this nerve is the first web of the foot and the dorsum of the third toe. Weakness may involve the extensor hallucis longus (L5), gluteus medius (L5), or extensor digitorum longus and brevis (L5).
4. Reflex change usually is not found.
5. A diminished tibialis posterior reflex is possible but difficult to elicit.

ORTHOPEDIC GAMUT 8-16

UNILATERAL DISC HERNIATION BETWEEN L5 AND S1

In a unilateral disc herniation between L5 and S1, the findings of an S1 radiculopathy are noted as follows:

1. Pain and numbness involve the dermatome of S1.
2. The S1 dermatome includes the lateral malleolus and the lateral and plantar surface of the foot, occasionally including the heel.
3. There is numbness over the lateral aspect of the leg and, more important, over the lateral aspect of the foot, including the lateral three toes.
4. The autonomous zone for this root is the dorsum of the fifth toe.
5. Weakness may be demonstrated in the peroneus longus and brevis (S1), gastrocnemius-soleus (S1), or gluteus maximus (S1).
6. In general, weakness is not a usual finding in S1 radiculopathy.
7. Occasionally, mild weakness may be demonstrated by asymmetrical fatigue with exercise of these motor groups.
8. The ankle jerk usually is reduced or absent.

PROCEDURE

- Passive flexion of the patient's head onto the chest can be accomplished in either a supine, seated, or standing position (Figs. 8-112 and 8-113).
- If pain occurs in the lumbar spine and along the sciatic nerve distribution, the test is positive and, according to Lindner, is an indication of root sciatica (Figs. 8-114 and 8-115).

Confirmation Procedures

Bechterew's sitting test, Bragard's sign, Deyerle's sign, Fajersztajn's test, Lasègue differential sign, Lasègue rebound test, Lasègue sitting test, Lasègue test, Lewin standing test, Sicard's sign, straight-leg-raising test, and Turyn's sign

---

DIAGNOSTIC STATEMENT

Lindner's sign is present and reproduces radiating leg pain on the right or left in the L5 dermatome. This result indicates L5 nerve root irritation or inflammation.

CLINICAL PEARL

Flexion of the head upon the chest increases the traction of the nerve root against the disc bulge. When the disc is a contained disc, in which the annulus is not ruptured, the flexion or maintenance of a flexed position of the trunk obliterates the disc bulge. Motion of an irritated nerve root over a bulging disc is often the source of the patient's back and leg pain. Relief of pain with trunk flexion occurs only because the disc bulge has disappeared.

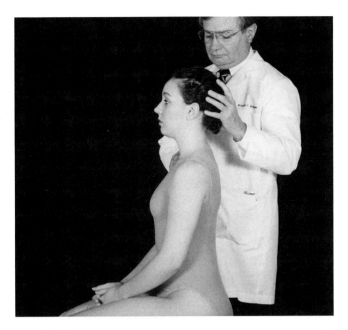

FIG. 8-112   The patient is seated with the arms in a comfortable position.

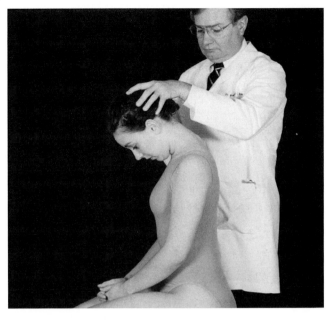

FIG. 8-113   The examiner passively flexes the patient's head onto the chest. If pain occurs in the lumbar spine and the sciatic nerve distribution, the test is positive. A positive test is an indication of root sciatica.

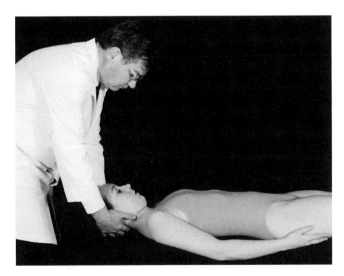

FIG. 8-114   A supine version of this test can also be performed.

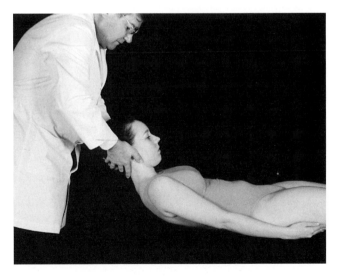

FIG. 8-115   For the supine version, the head is passively flexed toward the chest. If pain occurs in the lumbar spine and the sciatic nerve distribution, the test is positive. A positive test is an indication of root sciatica. This result should be differentiated from Brudzinski sign and the Soto-Hall maneuver. These tests are similar but have slightly different significance.

MATCHSTICK TEST

Assessment for Denervation Hypersensitivity

Comment

Many cases of acute low back pain that are not correctly identified evolve into a chronic spinal problem with significant disability at the muscular level (Table 8-15). Patients with muscular dysfunction of the lumbar spine can have varying types of clinical findings and case histories.

The sensory distribution of each nerve root, or dermatome, varies from person to person, and there is often overlap. A *dermatome* is the area of skin supplied by a single nerve root.

The examiner must also be aware of the sensory, motor, and sympathetic distribution of peripheral nerves to be able to differentiate between lesions of the nerve roots and peripheral nerves.

Pressure on a peripheral nerve resulting in a neurapraxia leads to temporary nonfunctioning of the nerve. With this type of injury, there is primarily motor involvement. Pressure on a nerve root leads to a loss of tone and muscle mass. Spinal nerve roots have a poorly developed epineurium and lack a perineurium. This makes the nerve root more susceptible to compressive forces, tensile deformations, chemical irritants (e.g., alcohol, lead, arsenic), or metabolic abnormalities. For example, diabetes may cause a metabolic peripheral neuropathy of one or more nerves.

In peripheral nerves, the epineurium consists of a loose areolar connective tissue matrix surrounding the nerve fiber that allows changes in growth length of the bundled nerve fibers (funiculi) without allowing the bundles to be strained. The perineurium protects the nerve bundles by acting as a diffusion barrier to irritants and provides tensile strength and elasticity to a nerve.

In the past, there have been many names given to the condition now known universally as reflex sympathetic dystrophy (RSD). Because this condition may follow trauma, it is called *posttraumatic pain syndrome.*

ORTHOPEDIC GAMUT 8-17

MUSCLE SYNDROMES OF THE LUMBOPELVIC SPINE

Common findings in muscle syndromes of the lumbopelvic spine are as follows:

1. Hip inflexibility, especially hamstring and psoas insufficiency
2. Weakness of the hip and spine extensor mechanism
3. Intersegmental lumbosacral fixation
4. Myofascial trigger points in the spinal erector, quadratus lumborum, gluteal musculature, and psoas muscles
5. Referred zones of pain to the hip, buttocks, thigh and lateral lower leg
6. Severe tightness of the outward rotators of the hip
7. Muscle hypertonicity
8. Palpable tenderness with pressure or stretch
9. Taut, tender, or ropelike muscle fibers

ORTHOPEDIC GAMUT 8-18

MIXED MOTOR PERIPHERAL NERVE LESION

The effects of a mixed motor (motor, sensory, and sympathetic) peripheral nerve lesion include the following:

1. Flaccid paralysis (motor)
2. Loss of reflexes (motor)
3. Muscle wasting and atrophy (motor)
4. Loss of sensation (sensory)
5. Trophic changes in the skin (sensory), loss of secretions from sweat glands (sympathetic)
6. Loss of pilomotor response (sympathetic)

TABLE 8-15

SITES OF LUMBOPELVIC SOFT-TISSUE SYNDROMES/MYOFASCIAL TRIGGER POINTS

Diagnosis	Site of Complaint
Quadratus lumborum syndrome	Gluteal region, anterior iliac spine, greater trochanter of femur
Gluteus maximus or medius syndrome	Sacral and gluteal region, lateral hip
Gluteus minimus syndrome	Lateral hip, thigh, and calf
Chronic lumbar strain (spinal erector muscles)	Laterally to ribs, caudally toward lumbosacral junction
Piriformis syndrome	Sacroiliac region; posterior hip, thigh, calf; possibly sole of foot

Adapted from Brier SR: *Primary care orthopedics,* St Louis, 1999, Mosby.

The most important clinical finding in reflex sympathetic dystrophy is pain. However, the distinguishing feature of the pain in RSD is its severity. The degree of pain is completely out of proportion to the inciting trauma. The nature of the pain varies widely, but early in the condition, the pain is usually described as burning or stinging. Later, the pain is often described as a pressure or cutting pain that becomes constant and unrelenting. Motion severely aggravates the pain, and there is almost a complete cessation of voluntary movement of the involved part. Although the pain may start in one area, it rapidly spreads to adjacent sites and eventually involves the entire extremity. In untreated, severe cases, the pain progresses to the point that the patient may request amputation of the affected part or even consider suicide. The pain is made markedly worse by attempting active or passive movement of the joints. Severe and excruciating paresthesia may be produced by lightly stroking the skin, even in uninjured areas. Tenderness is always present and is much more severe than one would normally expect.

Although pain is the most prominent symptom, swelling is the most common physical finding. The swelling usually starts in the area of greatest involvement, but it soon spreads proximally and distally to the immediate adjacent areas of the extremity. The swelling is soft initially but turns to brawny edema if the condition persists. The brawny edema often gets so severe that it acts as a mechanical block to motion. This fixed edema eventually gives way to periarticular thickening and to fibrous tendon adhesions. Elevation of the extremity is most effective in reducing swelling when used early in the disease, but this elevation is beneficial any time.

Metabolic changes form an important part of any neurologic disorder and may occur in the skin, nails, subcutaneous tissues, muscles, bones, and joints. In addition to a neurologic basis, factors such as activity, blood supply, and lymph drainage are involved in the causation of trophic changes. When a peripheral nerve is completely interrupted, the skin loses its delicate indentations and becomes inelastic, smooth, and shiny. When interruption is partial, trophedema occurs. There is gradual fibrosis of the subcutaneous tissue, and the overlying skin becomes fissured and prone to heavy folds. This alteration in the quality of the skin produces a *peau d'orange* affect similar to that described for malignant lumps in the female breast. This is accentuated when the skin is gently squeezed together or when the back is fully extended.

PROCEDURE

- Trophedema is nonpitting to digital pressure, but when a blunt instrument, such as the end of a matchstick or cotton-tip applicator is used, the indentation produced is clear cut and persists for several minutes, which is distinctly longer than such an indentation would persist in normal skin (Fig. 8-116).
- The matchstick test may be positive and yield deep indentations over an extensive area (commonly over the lower back and hamstrings), or in mild cases, the test may yield only slight indentations of skin overlying a tender motor point or the neurovascular hilus.

Confirmation Procedures

Bilateral leg-lowering test, Demianoff's sign, double leg-raise test, hyperextension test, Lewin supine test, Mennell's sign, Minor's sign, Nachlas test, Quick test, Schober's test, sign of the buttock, skin pinch test, spinal percussion test, and Vanzetti's sign

---

DIAGNOSTIC STATEMENT

Matchstick testing reveals localized trophedema. This result suggests denervation supersensitivity, such as that seen in lumbar sprain.

CLINICAL PEARL

RSD can occur in any disease that produces pain. This type of dystrophy is a likely secondary condition after 4 months of unrelenting pain from the primary disorder. The earliest sign, other than the symptoms of burning or stinging pain, is localized trophedema. The matchstick test can be applied to any cutaneous area of pain because the test is sensitive to the earliest changes in fluid management in the skin by the sympathetically operated cutaneous vascularity. The result of this test becomes the earliest warning sign of the advancing RSD. An intervertebral disc syndrome with protracted nerve root compression is a common onset mechanism.

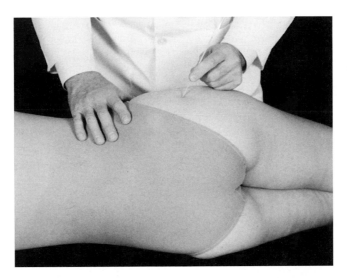

FIG. 8-116   The patient may be in either the prone or side-lying position. The examiner applies the blunt end of a cotton-tipped applicator to the affected area of skin. The indentations produced are clear cut and persist for several minutes, which is distinctly longer than when the test is performed on normal skin. The matchstick test is positive if it yields deep indentations over an extensive area (commonly over the lower back and hamstrings) or, in mild cases, if it yields slight indentations of skin overlying a tender motor point or the neurovascular hilus. A positive test is associated with denervation supersensitivity, as seen with a lumbar sprain.

MENNELL'S SIGN

Assessment for Pathologic Involvement of the Sacroiliac Joint Structures

Comment

Fat nodules, located on the fascia over muscle or bone, may be painful when direct pressure is applied or trunk bending occurs. The aching and radicular sensation that occurs when the nodule is palpated is readily identified with the painful mass. All pain is temporarily relieved with topical anesthesia of the mass.

ORTHOPEDIC GAMUT 8-19

SACROILIAC PAIN

The radicular component of sacroiliac pain is referred pain similar to that associated with the following:

1. The painful tendon attachment
2. Periosteal pain
3. The deep aching associated with compression of a small blood vessel
4. The irritation of a sensory nerve penetrating the fascia

Straight leg raising may be uncomfortable, but it is not radicular.

The findings obtained are different from those associated with nerve root radiculopathy, but they are easy to confuse. All tender areas in the buttock are not fat nodules. Many tender areas may represent pain referral from an irritated nerve root. For example, a nerve root ganglion or cyst may cause pain in the buttock that is similar to that which occurs with a painful fat nodule that is more proximal.

There are 14 local areas in which tenderness during palpation is very constant in certain conditions.

There are five areas on each side of the back to be examined, one in each buttock, and one in the back of each thigh.

S1 radiculopathy is common and is difficult to differentiate from S2 radiculopathy because their myotomal representations overlap almost completely. As with the L5 root, the segmental distribution of the S1 root is diffuse, with both proximal and distal muscle representation.

As with other lumbosacral radiculopathies, bilateral S1/S2 radiculopathies are relatively common, and most are chronic. Because the symptoms usually are bilateral and involve the feet predominantly, these cases imitate a peripheral polyneuropathy or bilateral tarsal syndromes.

Differentiating these three entities requires meticulous EMG examination and is difficult, especially in elderly patients.

ORTHOPEDIC GAMUT 8-20

LUMBOPELVIC TENDERNESS

The following are the local areas of lumbopelvic palpable tenderness:

1. Medial to the posterior superior iliac spine is the most superficial posterior ligament of the sacroiliac joint. Tenderness here suggests a pathologic condition involving the sacroiliac joint.
2. Lateral to the posterior superior iliac spine is the puny part of the gluteal muscle origin that may be torn by minor trauma. Tenderness here suggests a pathologic condition resulting from a muscle tear.
3. Above the posterior superior iliac spine is where the sacrospinalis muscle joins its tendon. Muscle fiber tears frequently occur at this junction during minor lifting trauma.
4. Above and medial to the posterior superior iliac spine is the area over the interlaminar facet joint, where tenderness may be felt if dysfunction is present.
5. Medial and inferior to the posterior superior iliac spine is the area where local tenderness may be felt from a pathologic condition involving a disc.
6. Tenderness lateral to the ischial tuberosity, where the sciatic trunk emerges from beneath the piriformis muscle, suggests either tightness of the muscle or a pathologic condition of a radicular origin.
7. Tenderness elicited by deeply rolling with the fingers over the sciatic trunk in the back of the thigh indicates neuritis.

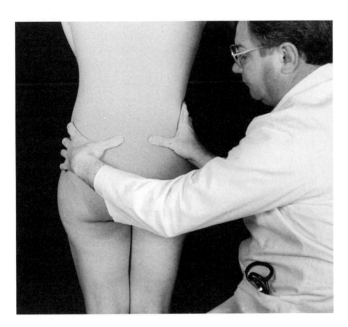

FIG. 8-117 The patient is standing. The examiner places a thumb over the posterior superior iliac spine on the affected side and exerts pressure.

PROCEDURE

- The examiner places a thumb over the posterior superior iliac spine (PSIS), exerts pressure, slides the thumb outward, and then slides it inward (Figs. 8-117 and 8-118).
- The sign is positive if tenderness is increased.
- This result is significant if, when sliding outward, sensitive deposits in structures on the gluteal aspect of the PSIS are noted (Fig. 8-119).
- If, when sliding inward, tenderness is increased, this is a significant result for strain of the superior sacroiliac ligaments.
- Confirmation can be made if tenderness is increased when the examiner posteriorly pulls the anterior superior iliac spine (ASIS) while standing behind the patient or when the examiner pulls the PSIS forward while standing in front of the patient.
- This test is helpful in determining that tenderness is caused by strained superior sacroiliac ligaments.
- A positive result indicates deposits in the structure or adjacent to the structure of the sacroiliac joint.
- These deposits are the result of ligamentous strain or sprain.

Confirmation Procedures

Bilateral leg-lowering test, Demianoff's sign, double leg-raise test, hyperextension test, Lewin supine test, matchstick test, Minor's sign, Nachlas test, Quick test, Schober's test, sign of the buttock, skin pinch test, spinal percussion test, and Vanzetti's sign

DIAGNOSTIC STATEMENT

Mennell's sign is positive on the right. The presence of this sign indicates a pathologic condition involving the sacroiliac joint structures.

CLINICAL PEARL

This method of tissue examination provides pertinent information, providing the results are accurately interpreted. Palpation of the lumbosacral region, with the patient in either the erect or the prone position, may evoke tender areas in the midline, at the level of the disc lesion, and in the paravertebral area on the side of the nuclear extrusion. It is not uncommon to be able to elicit tenderness along the iliac crest or even over the posterior aspect of the sacroiliac joint on the side of an irritated nerve root.

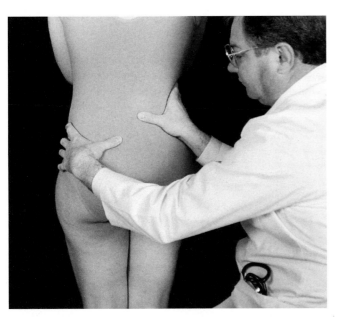

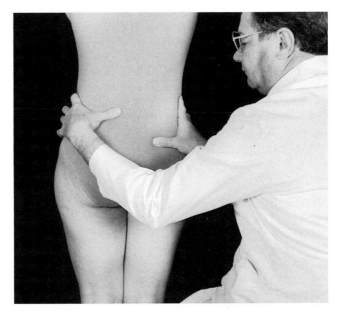

FIG. 8-118   The examiner then slides the thumb upward and inward.

FIG. 8-119   While maintaining the pressure, the examiner moves the thumb downward and outward. The sign is positive if tenderness is increased in either direction. This sign is significant if, when sliding outward, sensitive deposits in structures on the gluteal aspect of the posterior superior iliac spine are noted. An increase in tenderness when sliding inward indicates inflammation or strain in the superior sacroiliac ligaments. A positive sign indicates involvement of the structure or something adjacent to it, involvement of the sacroiliac joint, or a ligamentous sprain.

Assessment for Intervertebral Disc Syndrome or Space-Occupying Mass

Comment

The differential diagnosis of back and leg pain is extremely lengthy and complex. It includes diseases intrinsic to the spine and diseases involving adjacent organs that cause pain referred to the back or leg. Lesions can be categorized as extrinsic or intrinsic to the spine.

Extrinsic lesions include diseases of the urogenital system, gastrointestinal system, vascular system, endocrine system, nervous system not localized to the spine, and the extrinsic musculoskeletal system. These include infections, tumors, metabolic disturbances, congenital abnormalities, and the associated diseases of aging.

Intrinsic lesions involve those diseases that arise primarily in the spine. They include diseases of the spinal musculoskeletal system, the local hematopoietic system, and the local neurologic system. These conditions include trauma, tumors, infections, diseases of aging, and immune diseases affecting the spine or spinal nerves.

The weakest portion of the posterior annulus in the lumbar spine is either side of the midline, where the annulus lacks the reinforcement of the strong central fibers of the posterior longitudinal ligament. Either side of the midline is also the most common site of nuclear protrusions in the lumbar spine. Having penetrated the annulus, the protrusion lodges under the posterior longitudinal ligament. The ligament is stretched commensurate with the size of the fragment and the degree of internal pressure within the disc. In this position, the protrusion is a firm, smooth mound. To accommodate the sequestered fragment, the posterior ligament is lifted off the vertebral bodies. As the nuclear mass increases in size, further stripping of the ligament occurs. The mass may migrate in any direction—cephalad, caudad, medially, or laterally. The mass commonly moves in a lateral direction close to and parallel to a nerve root, and it may even extend into the intervertebral foramen. Under the ligament, the mass lies tightly compressed and folded upon itself. The mass can be completely free, or it may still be attached to material in the nucleus by strands of irregular, stringy, fibrous tissue. This type of protrusion is by far the most common lesion encountered.

Occasionally, a dissecting protrusion may erode through the posterior ligament at a distance from its site of exit from the annulus. More commonly, the fragment is extruded through the annulus and the ligament. These free sequestra, regardless of their mode of origin, may move in any direction in the spinal canal. The usual course for these sequestra is along one of the extrathecal nerve roots, and they may lodge in the IVF.

It becomes apparent that both the dissecting and the extruded nuclear materials can make contact with one of the nerve roots anywhere from the point of exit at the dura

---

ORTHOPEDIC GAMUT 8-21

DISORDERS MIMICKING DISC DISEASE

Common disorders that can mimic disc disease include the following:

1. Ankylosing spondylitis
2. Multiple myeloma
3. Vascular insufficiency
4. Arthritis of the hip
5. Osteoporosis with stress fractures
6. Extradural tumors
7. Peripheral neuropathy
8. Myofascial trigger points and herpes zoster

ORTHOPEDIC GAMUT 8-22

OTHER CAUSES OF SCIATICA

Following are other causes of sciatica not related to disc HNP:

1. Synovial cysts
2. Rupture of the medial head of the gastrocnemius
3. Sacroiliac joint dysfunction
4. Lesions in the sacrum and pelvis
5. Fracture of the ischial tuberosity

to the IVF. In most instances, the nuclear material lodges directly under or slightly to either side of the root, putting it in tension. Because of the lack of elasticity of the roots outside the dura, even a small protrusion is capable of putting tension on the root. In this position, local secondary inflammatory changes bind the root tightly to the underlying nuclear mound, so it is difficult for the root to be displaced to one side or the other of the mass. In cases of long standing, the root may actually become embedded in the heap of local fibrotic tissue that is formed. The root also responds to the abnormal situation by becoming injected, edematous, and cordlike. Within the nerve sheath, granulation tissue appears that, with maturation, is converted to dense fibrous tissue that binds the nerve fasciculi together and in some instances actually destroys the fibers. The neurologic deficits resulting from this process may be permanent.

PROCEDURE

- The patient is lying supine with both lower limbs straight out and is directed to raise the limbs until the heels are 6 inches off the table (Fig. 8-120).
- The patient holds the position for as long as possible.

- The test is positive if the patient experiences lower back pain (Fig. 8-121).
- Because this maneuver increases the subarachnoid pressure, if the patient can hold the position for 30 seconds without pain, a pathologic condition of intrathecal origin can be ruled out.
- If the test is positive, there may be a pathologic condition, such as a herniated disc, in or outside the spinal cord sheath.

Confirmation Procedures
Antalgia sign, bowstring sign, Cox sign, heel/toe walk test, Kemp's test, Lewin punch test, Lewin snuff test, and Neri's sign

---

DIAGNOSTIC STATEMENT

Milgram's test is positive because the patient is unable to lift the legs as a result of lumbosacral pain. This result suggests a herniated intervertebral disc.

CLINICAL PEARL

This test increases thecal pressure. The ability to hold this position for any time rules out a pathologic condition of thecal origin.

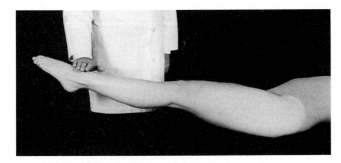

FIG. 8-120   The patient is supine with both legs fully extended. The patient is instructed to raise both legs to a position where the heels are approximately 6 inches from the examination table.

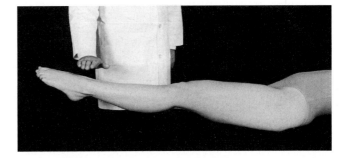

FIG. 8-121   The test is positive if the patient experiences lower back pain that prevents raising of the legs more than 2 to 3 inches, if at all. Because this maneuver increases the subarachnoid pressure, if the patient can hold the position for any length of time without pain, pathologic intrathecal process can be ruled out. A positive test indicates a space-occupying pathologic condition, such as a herniated disc.

MINOR'S SIGN

Assessment for Sacroiliac Lesions, Lumbosacral Strains and Sprains, Lumbopelvic Fractures, Intervertebral Disc Syndrome, Muscular Dystrophy, and Dystonia

Comment

Muscular or ligamentous injury is a common cause of low back pain. It may follow single or multiple traumatic episodes. Incomplete muscular tears or ligament sprains occur and lead to pain and tenderness over the affected area.

Various factors predispose someone to chronic low back pain. Obesity, poor muscular tone, smoking, faulty work habits, the wearing of high-heeled shoes, and the lack of a daily exercise program are among the contributing factors.

Obesity contributes to chronic low back pain. First, it is known that intraabdominal pressure aids the erector spinae muscles in keeping the lumbar spine erect and decreases intradiscal pressure. Obese patients have poor abdominal muscular tone. Obese patients also typically have an increase in their lumbar lordosis, which further adds stress to the lower part of the back.

The most commonly overlooked source of lumbar muscle pain may be the quadratus lumborum. This muscle, which not only contributes to the support of the lumbar spine and abdominal cavity but also is a lateral flexor of the lumbopelvic spine, may be the most active muscle of the lumbar region during activities of daily living. It may possess trigger points that cause localized and referred pain.

The symptom complex of sciatic pain varies widely, and it occurs when a nuclear sequestrum touches one of the nerve roots. In a small percentage of patients, the attack comes on suddenly, and the pain radiates the full length of the limb, along the dermatome of the involved nerve root. In a large percentage of patients, the pain comes on slowly and is often felt as an ache that is in one side of the buttocks and that spreads gradually and distally. In some patients, the pain is localized to the posterior or posterolateral aspects of the thigh, depending on whether S1 or L5 nerve roots are implicated. In some, the pain may extend as far as the calf (the lateral aspect of the lower leg), the sole of the foot, or the dorsum of the outer three toes, depending on the nerve root affected. From time to time, the presenting complaint is pain that is limited to a small but specific area, such as the buttocks, the back of the thigh, the calf, or the sole of the foot. In rare instances, the pattern of pain spread may be reversed. For example, the pain may begin in the calf or sole of the foot and gradually spread cephalad.

In a small percentage of patients, back pain and sciatica appear simultaneously. Two clinical types of this syndrome are discernible. In one type, the symptoms of back pain and sciatica appear suddenly and simultaneously. In the other type, the onset is gradual. The former is associated with some sudden flexion stress that is applied to the lumbar spine and causes rupture of the annulus and retropulsion of the nuclear material. The latter is consistent with gradual extrusion of the nuclear fragments through the annulus fibrosus. The pain in the back and the sciatica may be of almost equal severity, but in most instances, the intensity of one overshadows the other. When pain in both the back and the leg is severe and the onset is sudden, the patient may be incapacitated and may present a dramatic clinical picture. The pain may be so severe that the affected leg is held in the flexed position, and the patient avoids any maneuver that might extend the limb. There is severe spasm of the lumbar paravertebral muscles and often a severe list of the trunk.

PROCEDURE

- Sciatic radiculitis is suggested by how a patient with this condition rises from a seated position (Fig. 8-122).
- The patient supports the body with the uninvolved side by balancing on the healthy leg, placing one hand on the back, and flexing the knee and hip of the affected limb (Fig. 8-123).
- The sign is often present with sacroiliac lesions, lumbosacral strains and sprains, fractures, disc syndromes, dystrophies, and myotonia.

Confirmation Procedures

Bilateral leg-lowering test, Demianoff's sign, double leg-raise test, hyperextension test, Lewin supine test, match stick test, Mennell's sign, Nachlas test, Quick test, Schober's test, sign of the buttock, skin pinch test, spinal percussion test, and Vanzetti's sign

---

DIAGNOSTIC STATEMENT

Minor's sign is present. This sign indicates a pathologic condition of lumbosacral origin.

CLINICAL PEARL

With lumbar disc lesions, all movements of the spine—extension, flexion, lateral flexion, and rotation—are affected. With an acute lesion, extension and flexion are seriously restricted, but lateral flexion and rotation are free. The degree of restriction is governed by the phase and severity of the local pathologic process. During an acute attack, the striking feature of the spine is the complete loss of its inherent flexibility. The patient avoids motion in any direction.

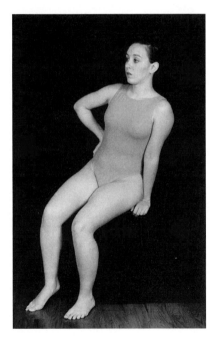

FIG. 8-122   The patient is seated and is asked to stand. The examiner observes how the patient rises from a seated position.

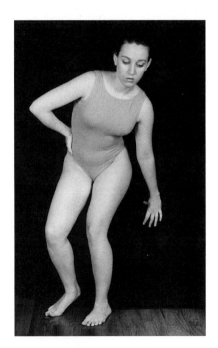

FIG. 8-123   The sign is present if the patient supports weight on the uninvolved side by balancing on the healthy leg, placing one hand on the back, and flexing the knee and hip on the affected side. The sign is often present with sacroiliac lesions, lumbosacral strains and sprains, fractures, disc syndromes, dystrophies, and myotonia.

Assessment for Sacroiliac or Lumbosacral Disorder

Comment

A most comprehensive low back differential diagnosis system based on symptoms is that developed by the Quebec Task Force (Table 8-16).

Acute lumbosacral strain is the most common cause of acute lower back pain. Because of its position in the skeleton, the lumbosacral joint supports the body weight and acts as a fulcrum for this weight in activities that involve bending and lifting. Mechanical damage to this joint is frequent because of the functional demands placed on the lower back area by everyday activities. In this joint, the traumatic force usually involves lifting of a load when the spine is flexed forward. In this position, the lumbosacral joint is functioning as a fulcrum. Acute lumbosacral strain occurs when a load is applied while the spine is twisted or rotated or when a sudden force is applied unexpectedly before the back muscles brace to meet it. The latter instance occurs less often than the former.

The resulting pathologic change is a partial tearing or stretching of the overlying paravertebral muscles, lumbar fascia, and interspinous ligaments. If the injury results in more serious damage to the spine, then by definition it cannot be a lumbosacral strain. Injury to the soft parts initiates paravertebral muscle spasm, which accounts for the clinical picture seen with this condition.

Two facts are basic for understanding an acute lumbosacral strain. First, the stimulus for normal tone of the paravertebral muscles is the upright position. These muscles are in normal postural tone only in the standing or seated positions and are completely flaccid in the prone or supine positions. Spasm of the paravertebral muscles involves markedly exaggerated tone that is initiated by the stimulus of overload and is maintained by the stimulus of the upright position. If the patient were put to bed immediately after sustaining the injury, it is doubtful whether the symptoms and signs associated with an acute lumbosacral strain could develop. It is this basic physiologic fact that accounts for the extreme duration of pain and the impairment that occurs in patients with paraver-

---

TABLE 8-16

DURATION OF SYMPTOMS AND WORKING STATUS CLASSIFICATION OF LOW BACK PAIN DISORDERS

Classification	Symptoms	Duration of Symptoms from Onset	Working Status at Time of Evaluation
1	Pain without radiation	a (<7 days)	W (working)
2	Pain + radiation to extremity, proximally	b (7 days-7 weeks)	I (idle)
3	Pain + radiation to extremity, distally	c (>7 weeks)	
4	Pain + radiation to upper/lower limb neurologic signs		
5	Presumptive compression of a spinal nerve root on a simple roentgenogram (i.e., spinal instability or fracture)		
6	Compression of a spinal nerve root confirmed by Specific imaging techniques (i.e., computerized axial tomography, myelography, or magnetic resonance imaging) Other diagnostic techniques (i.e., electromyography, venography)		
7	Spinal stenosis		
8	Postsurgical status, 1-6 months after intervention		
9	Postsurgical status, >6 months after intervention 9.1 Asymptomatic 9.2 Symptomatic		
10	Chronic pain syndrome		W (working)
11	Other diagnoses		I (idle)

Adapted from Pope MH, Andersson GBJ, Frymoyer JW, Chaffin DB: *Occupational low back pain assessment, treatment and prevention,* St Louis, 1991, Mosby.

tebral muscle spasm who are allowed to remain ambulatory. This explanation also accounts for the rapid subsidence of symptoms that results from absolute bed rest.

Second, in patients with acute lumbosacral strain, there is always a lag period between the time the lower back damage was sustained and the onset of the clinical symptoms. This lag period may vary from hours to days and depends on whether the patient remains upright. It is during this lag period that the paravertebral muscle spasm builds to a point of clinical significance.

The severity of the clinical features of acute lumbosacral strain depends directly on the degree of paravertebral muscle spasm present. The patient gives a history of a twisting or lifting injury to the lower back and states that the onset of symptoms occurred either immediately or, more commonly, after a lag period of several hours or days. The patient walks guardedly and slowly because movement of the spine is painful. The back may be held in flexion or may exhibit a list to one side with a tilted pelvis. The paravertebral muscles feel extremely taut and hard, and the normal lumbar lordotic curve is obliterated. Spinal movements are limited in direct proportion to the amount of muscle spasm present and are associated with a sharp, diffuse, catching type of pain in the lower back, with possible radiation to the buttocks and thighs or upward to the neck.

PROCEDURE

- To eliminate lumbosacral muscular influence in this test, the patient is placed prone and relaxed on a rigid table (Fig. 8-124).
- Pain in the lower back and lower extremity is noted during passive flexion of the knee.
- The test is positive if pain is noted in the sacroiliac area or lumbosacral area or if the pain radiates down the thigh or leg (Fig. 8-125).
- A positive test indicates a sacroiliac or lumbosacral disorder.

Confirmation Procedures

Bilateral leg-lowering test, Demianoff's sign, double leg-raise test, hyperextension test, Lewin supine test, matchstick test, Mennell's sign, Minor's sign, Quick test, Schober's test, sign of the buttock, skin pinch test, spinal percussion test, and Vanzetti's sign

---

DIAGNOSTIC STATEMENT

Nachlas test is positive on the left and elicits pain radiating down the anterior thigh. This result indicates inflammation of the upper lumbar nerve roots.

CLINICAL PEARL

Intermittent prolapse of nuclear material is called a *concealed disc* or *occult disc*. Degenerated nuclear material still within the confines of the annulus, which may be weakened by degenerative process but remains intact, may bulge beyond its normal limits when the spine is subjected to certain stresses. Depending on the stresses, the prolapse appears and then disappears. Extension and hyperextension of the spine favor the prolapse, which can produce a defect in the anterior aspect of a myelographic column of dye. When the spine is relieved of stress, such as when the patient is relaxed and lying in the prone position, the defect disappears.

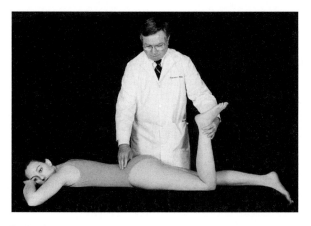

FIG. 8-124   The patient is prone with both legs fully extended. The examiner flexes the knee of the affected leg to 90 degrees.

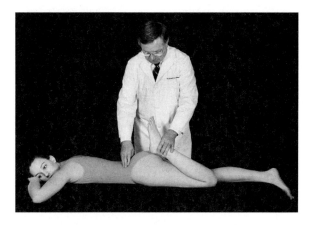

FIG. 8-125   The knee is fully flexed, approximating the heel to the ipsilateral buttock. The test is positive if pain is noted in the sacroiliac area or lumbosacral area or if pain radiates down the thigh or leg. A positive test indicates a sacroiliac or lumbosacral disorder.

Assessment for Lower Intervertebral Disc Syndrome, Lumbosacral and Sacroiliac Strain, and Lumbopelvic Subluxation

Comment

Surgical treatment of a disc rupture is for the symptomatic relief of leg pain. Patients with predominant back pain may not be relieved of their major complaint—back pain. The best results of 99.5% complete or partial pain relief are obtained when the disc is free in the canal or sequestered. Incomplete herniation or extrusion of disc material into the canal results in complete relief for 82% of patients. Excision of the bulging or protruding disc that is not ruptured through the annulus results in complete relief in 63%, and removal of the normal or minimally bulging disc results in complete relief in 38% (Fig. 8-126).

ORTHOPEDIC GAMUT 8-23

LUMBAR NERVE ROOT ANOMALIES

Type I is an intradural anastomosis between rootlets at different levels (Fig. 8-127).

Type II is an anomalous origin of the nerve roots separated into four subtypes (Fig. 8-128):

1. Cranial origin
2. Caudal origin
3. Combination of cranial and caudal origin
4. Conjoined nerve roots

Type III is an extradural anastomosis between roots (Fig. 8-129).

Type IV is the extradural division of the nerve root (Fig. 8-130).

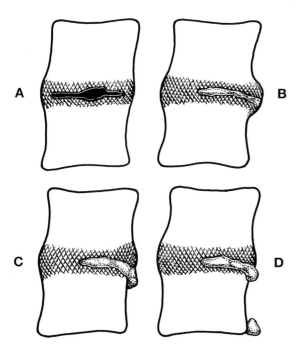

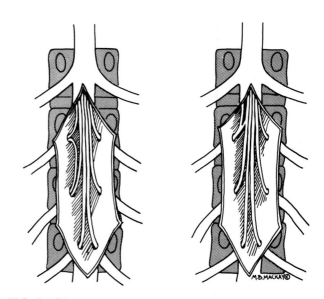

FIG. 8-126   Typical disc herniation. **A,** Normal bulge. **B,** Protrusion. **C,** Extrusion. **D,** Sequestration. *(From Canale ST: Campbell's operative orthopaedics, vol 1-4, ed 9, St Louis, 1998, Mosby.)*

FIG. 8-127   Type I nerve root anomaly: intradural anastomosis. *(From Canale ST: Campbell's operative orthopaedics, vol 1-4, ed 9, St Louis, 1998, Mosby.)*

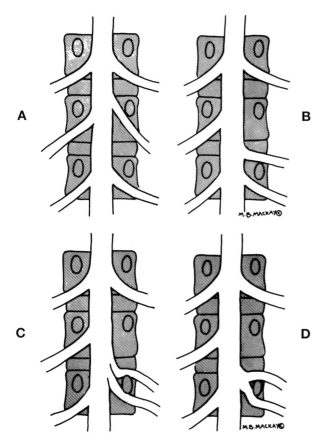

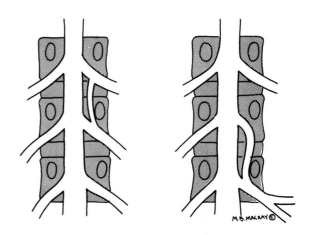

FIG. 8-128   Type II: anomalous origin of nerve roots. **A,** Cranial origin. **B,** Caudal origin. **C,** Closely adjacent nerve roots. **D,** Conjoined nerve roots. *(From Canale ST: Campbell's operative orthopaedics, vol 1-4, ed 9, St Louis, 1998, Mosby.)*

FIG. 8-129   Type III nerve root anomaly: extradural anastomosis. *(From Canale ST: Campbell's operative orthopaedics, vol 1-4, ed 9, St Louis, 1998, Mosby.)*

Traction on anomalous nerve roots has been suggested as a cause of sciatic symptoms without herniation. Sectioning of these roots results in irreversible neurological damage.

Abnormal physical stresses placed on a degenerated disc may exceed the mechanical strength of the degenerated disc and annulus, resulting in rupture of the annulus. Herniation of nuclear material (either wholly or in fragments) into the spinal canal causes either compression of or tension on a lumbar or sacral spinal nerve root as the root prepares to exit from the spinal canal and is the essential pathologic lesion of the condition known as herniated intervertebral disc. The nuclear material may push the posterior longitudinal ligament ahead of it like a sac, or the material may rupture through the posterior longitudinal ligament to extrude directly into the spinal canal.

The general process of intervertebral disc degeneration may extend over a period of years. The clinical picture characteristic of a herniated intervertebral disc does not arise until some of the nuclear material herniates or ruptures the posterior longitudinal spinal ligament. This rupture causes pressure on the adjacent spinal nerve root as it passes by and exits from the spine. The actual contact between disc material and the nerve root may be sudden and commonly follows an acute rise in intrathecal pressure that is triggered by sneezing, lifting, twisting, or straining.

Back pain is associated with disc degeneration, but the predominant symptom is sciatic pain that begins when the nuclear material protrudes posterolaterally into the spinal canal and compresses the nerve root. In most instances, a diagnosis of herniated disc is untenable without sciatic leg pain. Many back conditions may be associated with leg pain, but only nerve root irritation at this level produces pain along the distribution of the sciatic nerve. Pain that follows the distribution of the sciatic nerve is associated with signs of a lumbosacral nerve root compression syndrome.

The patient with a herniated intervertebral disc experiences lower back pain that is accompanied by pain radiating into the posterior buttock and leg or just into the leg. When viewed while standing, the patient may exhibit a list of the pelvis or a sciatic scoliosis.

PROCEDURE

- While in a standing posture, the patient is directed to bow forward (Figs. 8-131 and 8-132).
- The sign is present when the patient flexes the knee on the affected side (Fig. 8-133).
- The trunk flexion action causes pain in the leg.
- This pain is a common sign with lower disc problems as well as lumbosacral and sacroiliac strain subluxations.

Confirmation Procedures

Antalgia sign, bowstring sign, Cox sign, heel/toe walk test, Kemp's test, Lewin punch test, Lewin snuff test, and Milgram's test

---

DIAGNOSTIC STATEMENT

Neri's sign is present on the left. This sign indicates lower lumbar intervertebral disc involvement.

CLINICAL PEARL

Muscle tenderness may be associated with nerve root irritation. With an acute attack, tenderness of the buttock, thigh, and calf on the affected side is often demonstrable. When pain is localized to a specific area along the course of the sciatic nerve, careful regional examination is essential for ruling out local lesions, such as an abscess, neurofibroma, glomus tumor, lipoma, or sterile abscess, that irritate the sciatic nerve.

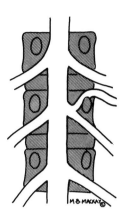

FIG. 8-130 Type IV nerve root anomaly: extradural division. *(From Canale ST:* Campbell's operative orthopaedics, *vol 1-4, ed 9, St Louis, 1998, Mosby.)*

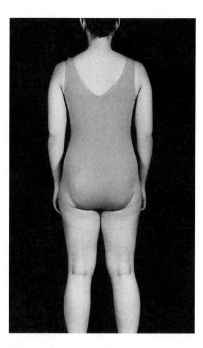

FIG. 8-131   The patient is standing with the arms comfortably at the sides.

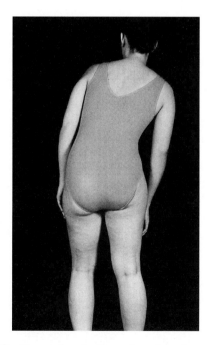

FIG. 8-132   The patient is directed to flex the trunk or bow forward. A lateral antalgic positioning may be noted but does not constitute a positive finding for this test.

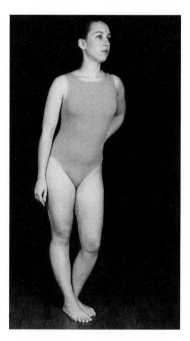

FIG. 8-133   The sign is present if the patient flexes the knee on the affected side and if trunk flexion causes pain in the leg. The sign is present for lower lumbar disc involvement as well as lumbosacral and sacroiliac strains or subluxations.

PRONE KNEE-BENDING TEST

Assessment for L2 or L3 Nerve Root Lesion, Femoral Nerve Inflammation, and Quadriceps Muscular Strain

Comment

ORTHOPEDIC GAMUT 8-24

FRANK DEGENERATION OF THE FACETS

Frank degeneration of the facets may be associated with the following three clinically important conditions:

1. Degeneration of the facets is part of the overall process of spinal degeneration and significantly contributes to pain in patients with multilevel spinal osteoarthritis.
2. Degeneration of the facets, with associated development of osteophytes projecting into the lateral recess and central spinal canal, is a significant part of degenerative spinal stenosis.
3. Degeneration of the facets is sometimes associated with a ventrally projecting synovial cyst, which impinges on the nerve root and thus is part of the differential diagnosis of sciatica.

The femoral nerve arises from the L1, L2, L3, and L4 spinal roots and innervates the iliopsoas, sartorius, and quadriceps femoris muscles. Proximal lesions result in weakness of thigh flexion or, more prominently, loss of extension at the knee. The nerve can be injured by pelvic fractures, by surgery, and by direct, penetrating wounds. The nerve can be paralyzed by pressure during childbirth or by arterial aneurysms, retroperitoneal hemorrhage, pelvic neoplasms, or abscesses.

Probably the most common syndrome involving the femoral nerve is the painful mononeuritis that occurs with diabetes. The quadriceps muscle atrophies quickly, and the knee jerk is lost early. Weakness while stepping up and the inability to rise from a one-legged squat are reliable motor signs of quadriceps paralysis. Quadriceps strength can be tested directly. Sensory distribution includes the anteromedial thigh and the anteromedial leg to the foot. It is appropriate to seek signs of more widespread deficits before concluding that this nerve alone is paralyzed because similar findings may result from a lesion higher in the lumbar plexus.

Femoral nerve injuries fall into two categories, those distal to the inguinal ligament in the femoral triangle and those proximal and, by definition, intrapelvic. Theoretically, injury to the pelvic portion of the femoral nerve should give, in addition to quadriceps paralysis and hypesthesia over the anteromedial thigh, a loss of sartorius muscle function. The branch to the sartorius is somewhat variable in origin and course. One of the clearly intrapelvic femoral nerve lesions appears to spare this muscle, while several thigh-level lesions may have sartorius loss.

Preservation or loss of this muscle's function does not indicate the level of the femoral nerve involvement.

Only sensory function is mediated by the lateral femoral cutaneous nerve. This nerve is not a branch of the femoral nerve, and it follows a different peripheral course. Classic entrapment of the lateral femoral cutaneous nerve occurs where it passes under the inguinal ligament medial to the anterior superior iliac spine. This entrapment results in a syndrome of dysesthesia and pain, called *meralgia paresthetica,* along the lateral thigh. Some loss of sensitivity to pain and touch is often typical in a small area. The skin may become sensitive to touch and pinching. There is no atrophy and no motor or reflex change. Entrapment of the lateral femoral cutaneous nerve is distinguished by its common occurrence, curability, and tendency to be easily mistaken for symptoms of L2 and L3 nerve root compression syndromes. This type of entrapment is initiated by obesity or local trauma caused by a belt or truss. Like other entrapment neuropathies, lateral femoral cutaneous nerve entrapment is apt to occur with metabolic disorders, which may make the peripheral nerves vulnerable to pressure.

PROCEDURE

- The patient is prone as the knees are passively flexed so that the heels touch the buttocks (Fig. 8-134).
- An L2 or L3 nerve root lesion is indicated by unilateral lumbar pain (Fig. 8-135).
- The test stretches the femoral nerve.

Confirmation Procedures
Ely's sign and femoral nerve traction test

DIAGNOSTIC STATEMENT

Prone knee-bending test is positive and elicits pain in the right anterior thigh. This result indicates L2 or L3 nerve root inflammation.

CLINICAL PEARL

Prone knee flexion can provide provocative testing for lumbar disc protrusion. The pathophysiology of this test depends on compression of spinal nerves during hyperextension of the lumbar spine. The compression intensifies intervertebral disc protrusion into the spinal canal. The lumbar intervertebral foramina are narrowed, and the spinal canal cross-sectional area is decreased by lumbar extension. The presence of a protruded disc that has not produced other physical findings may be detected by this test.

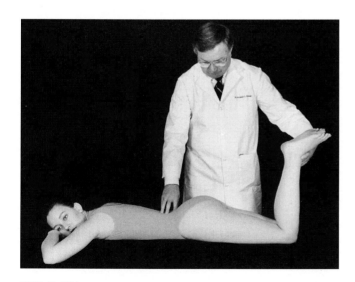

FIG. 8-134   The patient is in the prone position with both knees fully extended. The examiner passively flexes both knees to 90 degrees.

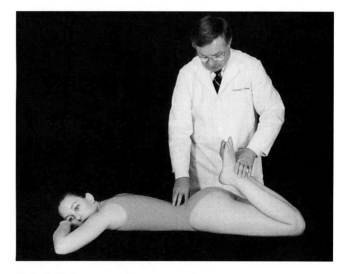

FIG. 8-135   The examiner flexes both knees maximally, approximating the heels to the buttocks. If the examiner is unable to flex the patient's knees past 90 degrees, the test is positive. Unilateral pain in the lumbar area indicates an L2 or L3 nerve root lesion. The test also stretches the femoral nerve. Pain in the anterior thigh indicates tight quadriceps muscles.

QUICK TEST

Assessment for Lower Back or Lower Extremity Screening

Comment

Back pain is the most common and troublesome complaint because its causes are legion and exact diagnosis is often difficult. The impairment, with which back pain is usually associated, is often severe and prolonged.

ORTHOPEDIC GAMUT 8-25

LOW BACK PAIN

It is helpful to consider low back pain under three headings:

1. Back pain may be associated with a spinal pathologic process, such as vertebral infections, tumors, ankylosing spondylitis, polyarthritis, Paget's disease, and primary neurologic disease.
2. Back pain may be associated with nerve root pain. The most common causes are intervertebral disc prolapse and compression of nerve roots within the neural canals.
3. Back pain may be caused by disturbance of the mechanics of the spine (mechanical back pain). This is the largest group of conditions that cause back pain.

The mechanical disturbances are clear (osteoporotic spinal fractures, senile kyphosis, spondylolisthesis, Scheuermann's disease, spinal osteochondrosis, and sometimes osteoarthritis). In other cases, although the symptoms may be identical in character, the cause cannot be determined with any accuracy. These cases of mechanical lower back pain formerly attracted many emotive but valueless names, such as lumbago and lower back strain.

Lumbar spinal stenosis is a syndrome in which narrowing of the lumbar spinal canal occurs; this may lead to vague and unusual symptoms. The disorder occurs secondary to a combination of disc degeneration, facet joint arthritis, and subluxation and occasionally to a congenitally small spinal canal.

Roentgenographic examination of the lumbar spine usually reveals degenerative changes throughout the lower part of the back. Electromyography and myelography may help localize the disorder, and computed axial tomography is often diagnostic (Fig. 8-136). MRI is also helpful.

While taking a history and examining a patient suffering from back pain, the examiner must exhaust the possibility of extraspinal causes; then an attempt should be made to place the patient in one of the three groups described earlier.

PROCEDURE

- The Quick test is accomplished with the patient standing.
- The patient squats down and stands again (Fig. 8-137).
- This action will quickly assess the integrity of the ankles, knees, and hips.
- If the patient can fully squat without any symptoms, these joints are free of pathology related to the pain complaint.

Confirmation Procedures

Bilateral leg-lowering test, Demianoff's sign, double leg-raise test, hyperextension test, Lewin supine test, matchstick test, Mennell's sign, Minor's sign, Nachlas test, Schober's test, sign of the buttock, skin pinch test, spinal percussion test, and Vanzetti's sign

---

DIAGNOSTIC STATEMENT

Quick test demonstrates that the ankles, knees, and hips are free of a pathologic condition associated with the patient's lower back or lower extremity complaints.

CLINICAL PEARL

The Quick test is probably the least demanding screening test for lumbar and lower extremity complaints. In a few, short, and active movements, three major contributors to lower extremity complaints (ankles, knees, and hips) can be ruled in or out of the differential diagnostic process.

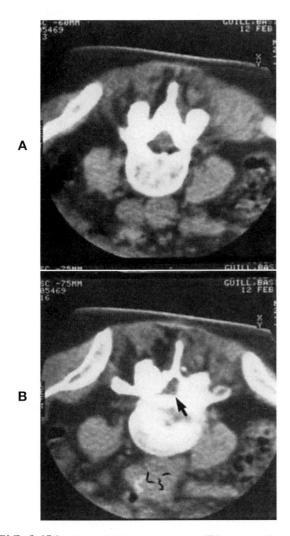

FIG. 8-136   Normal (**A**) and abnormal (**B**) computed tomography scans of the lumbar spine.   *(From Mercier LR, Pettid FJ: Practical orthopedics, ed 4, St Louis, 1995, Mosby.)*

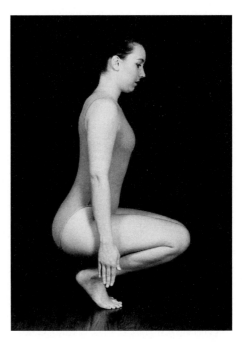

FIG. 8-137   The patient is standing. The patient squats down and stands up again. If the patient can fully squat without any symptoms, the ankles, knees, and hips are free of a pathologic condition. Patients suspected of having arthritis in the lower limb joints should not perform this test. This is also true of pregnant patients and older individuals who exhibit weakness and hypomobility.

SCHOBER'S TEST

Assessment for Lumbar Spine Motion

Comment

Ankylosing spondylitis is often seen in young adults, usually males. This condition is characterized by an inflammatory process that involves primarily the soft-tissue elements of the spine. The synovial membranes, capsules, and ligaments of the joints of the spine become swollen, edematous, and thickened. These changes are followed by calcification and eventually ossification. The result is bony ankylosis of all the affected joints. With ankylosing spondylitis, the pathologic process is confined to the intervertebral joints, the posterior articular joints, the sacroiliac joints, and the surrounding ligaments. The peripheral joints of the extremities are spared.

The proliferative process in the soft tissue in and about the IVF (the capsules of the posterior joints, the ligamentum flavum, and the posterior longitudinal ligament) narrows the outlet and may press and irritate the nerve roots that are traversing the bony canals. In addition, the sheaths of the nerves are involved, so the roots are enmeshed and fixed in a mass of fibrous tissue. It becomes apparent that body movements that stretch the roots, such as flexing the leg when extended at the knee, will accentuate the pain in the back and leg.

Lower back pain and sciatica are common complaints in all stages of this disorder, and the incidence of sciatica is greater than formerly realized. In the early stages, diagnostic imaging is not informative, so making the diagnosis is difficult. At this early stage, the clinical picture may mimic that of a disc lesion in the lumbar spine although the early clinical picture does not unequivocally simulate that of a lumbar disc lesion. Lower back pain is the first manifestation.

The area involved is not only the lumbosacral region but also the regions of the sacroiliac joints. Pain may be referred to the buttocks and the posterior aspects of the thighs. The syndrome is punctuated by remissions. The pain, which is not of a mechanical nature, is influenced by weather changes. The patient experiences considerable stiffness in the dorsal region and in the thoracic cage. Later, sciatica in one or both legs appears, and all movements of the spine are restricted, especially flexion. As time goes on, the lumbar spine is flattened, the patient begins to stoop forward, the cervical curve becomes exaggerated, and flexion contractures of the hips develop. At this point, the clinical picture of ankylosing spondylitis is evident and can be confirmed by diagnostic imaging. Imaging reveals characteristic changes in the posterior articulations and the sacroiliac joints.

Some muscle spasm of the dorsolumbar spine can be demonstrated. Some tenderness can be elicited over the spinous processes and a little to each side of the midline. As the process progresses, the excursions of the thorax become smaller and smaller until the thoracic cage becomes completely rigid and fixed. Throughout the active stages of the disease, the sedimentation rate is always elevated and is a good index to the activity of the process, but serologic tests for rheumatoid factor are usually negative.

Spinal instability (caused by degenerative disc disease) is a clinically symptomatic condition without new injury, in which a physiologic load induces abnormally large deformations at the intervertebral joint. Abnormal motion at vertebral segments with degenerative discs and the transmission of the load to the facet joints are usually present in spinal instability. Instability is demonstrated in the lumbar spine as an anterior slip of 5 mm or more in the thoracic or lumbar spine (Fig. 8-138) or a difference in the angular motion of two adjacent motion segments more than 11 degrees from T1 to L5 and motion greater than 15 degrees at L5-S1 compared with L4-L5.

PROCEDURE

- Schober's test is used to assess lumbar spine flexion.
- A point is marked at the spinous process level of S2. Points 0.5 cm below S2 and 10 cm above the S2 level are marked (Fig. 8-139).
- The distance between the two S2 reference points is measured.
- The patient flexes forward. The distance between the S2 reference points is remeasured.
- The difference between the two measurements indicates the amount of lumbar flexion.
- Normally, the S2 reference points should separate at least 5 to 8 cm (Fig. 8-140).

Confirmation Procedures

Bilateral leg-lowering test, Demianoff's sign, double leg-raise test, hyperextension test, Lewin supine test, matchstick test, Mennell's sign, Minor's sign, Nachlas test, Quick test, sign of the buttock, skin pinch test, spinal percussion test, and Vanzetti's sign

---

DIAGNOSTIC STATEMENT

Schober's test demonstrates that no motion occurs in the lumbosacral spine during flexion.

Schober's test demonstrates that motion greater than the base of 10 cm occurs in the lumbosacral spine during flexion.

CLINICAL PEARL

For a modification of this test, the patient is placed in a maximal flexion position (seated or standing), and starting from the upper sacral spinous prominence, three 10-cm segments are marked up the spine. The distances between the marks are then remeasured while the patient is erect. The lowest segment should shorten by at least 50%, the middle should shorten by 40%, and the upper should shorten by 30%. The shortening effect will be greater in tall subjects.

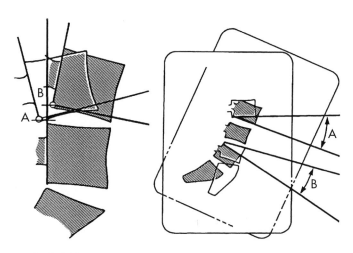

FIG. 8-138   Loss of motion segment integrity. *A,* Translation. *B,* Angular motion. *(From Canale ST:* Campbell's operative orthopaedics, *vol 1-4, ed 9, St Louis, 1998, Mosby.)*

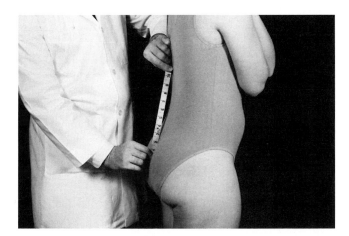

FIG. 8-139   The patient is standing with the arms folded across the chest. Points 0.5 cm below and 10 cm above the S2 level are marked. The span between the two S2 reference points is noted.

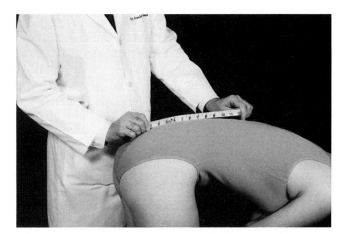

FIG. 8-140   The patient flexes forward. The distances between the two S2 reference points is remeasured. The difference indicates the amount of lumbar flexion. The separation between the S2 reference points should increase at least 5 to 8 cm.

SICARD'S SIGN

Assessment for Sciatic Radiculopathy

Comment

Spondylolisthesis is a disorder, usually in the lumbar spine, in which one vertebra gradually slips on another. Several types have been described (congenital, degenerative, pathologic, traumatic, and spondylolytic). However, most spondylolisthesis is secondary to spondylolysis, which represents a defect in the pars interarticularis or isthmus of the vertebra (Fig. 8-141). Spondylolisthesis is classified according to the amount of forward slippage of the affected vertebra (Fig. 8-142). Low back pain, sometimes radiating into the buttocks, occurs with activity and is relieved by rest. Symptoms of nerve root irritation may also be present, along with radiation of the pain into the extremities. These symptoms often progress in severity, especially in the teenager. Roentgenograms reveal the typical findings of a defect in the pars interarticularis, which may be accompanied by forward slippage (Fig. 8-143).

Characteristic of sciatic pain, increased intraabdominal pressure produced by coughing and sneezing markedly increases the severity of the pain. Patients with a severe attack will walk with the hip and knee slightly flexed and place the foot slowly on the floor. This carefulness is to prevent any undue traction of the nerve root, which normally occurs when the extended leg is flexed at the hip. On the other hand, some of the patients exhibit no external malfunction. They do not experience back pain or muscle spasm. Back motion is free and unrestricted, and in most instances, the patients are able to carry on their daily activities.

A sudden onset of pain usually occurs when a nuclear extrusion touches a nerve root. This phenomenon may occur either during the stage of nuclear sequestration (the intermediate stage) or toward the end of the pathologic process in the nucleus. Fibrosis of the disc is the predominant feature, but fragments of nuclear material that may be extruded may still be present. The distance that the pain spreads along a dermatome is directly proportional to the amount of tension and compression to which the root is subjected.

An interesting phenomenon is observed in patients with severe sciatica. The pain may suddenly disappear, but the motor and sensory deficits remain, which indicates that the physiologic function of the root is completely interrupted. This lack of pain must not be misconstrued as evidence that the patient is getting better.

Any of the patterns of sciatica may be initiated simply by contact with a sensitive nerve root and without actual herniation of nuclear material. Slight bulging, without rupture, of the annulus may be sufficient to precipitate a sciatic syndrome merely because the bulge touches the hypersensitive nerve root.

PROCEDURE

- While the patient is supine, the extended leg is raised to a point just short of that which produces pain (Fig. 8-144).
- When the sign is present, dorsiflexion of the great toe reproduces sciatic pain (Fig. 8-145).
- The test is significant for sciatic radiculopathy.

Confirmation Procedures

Bechterew's sitting test, Bragard's sign, Deyerle's sign, Fajersztajn's test, Lasègue differential sign, Lasègue rebound test, Lasègue sitting test, Lasègue test, Lewin standing test, Lindner's sign, straight-leg-raising test, and Turyn's sign

---

DIAGNOSTIC STATEMENT

Sicard's sign is positive on the left. This sign indicates sciatic radiculopathy.

CLINICAL PEARL

The second, third, and fourth nerve roots do not have an increase in tension during straight leg raising, but they do undergo an increase in tension during the femoral stretch tests.

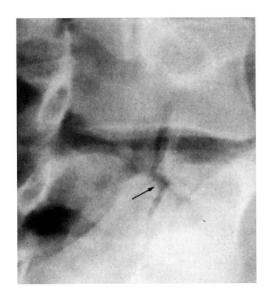

FIG. 8-141 Bony defect in the isthmus or neck of the Scottie dog present in spondylolysis. *(From Mercier LR, Pettid FJ: Practical orthopedics, ed 4, St Louis, 1995, Mosby.)*

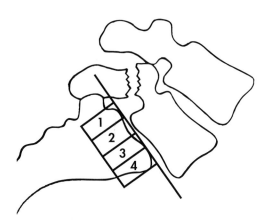

FIG. 8-142 Myerding's classification of spondylolisthesis. *(From Mercier LR, Pettid FJ: Practical orthopedics, ed 4, St Louis, 1995, Mosby.)*

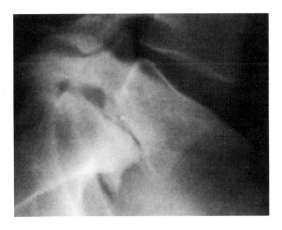

FIG. 8-143 Spondylolisthesis of the lumbosacral junction (note early indication of Knutsson vacuum sign at L5-S1). *(From Mercier LR, Pettid FJ: Practical orthopedics, ed 4, St Louis, 1995, Mosby.)*

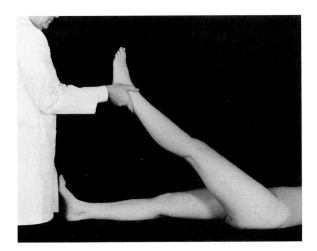

FIG. 8-144 The patient is supine with both legs fully extended. The examiner straight leg raises the affected leg to the point at which symptoms are reproduced.

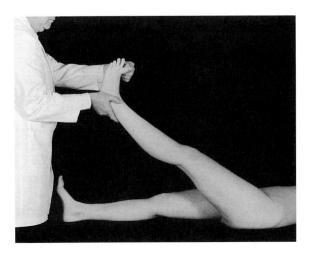

FIG. 8-145 The leg is lowered to a point just below that which produces symptoms, and the examiner sharply dorsiflexes the great toe of the affected foot. The sign is present if toe dorsiflexion reproduces the symptoms. The sign is present with sciatic radiculopathy.

SIGN OF THE BUTTOCK

Assessment for Gluteal Bursitis, Tumor, or Abscess

Comment

Excluding multiple myeloma, primary tumors, benign or malignant, of the spinal column are relatively rare. Of the benign tumors, osteoid osteoma, eosinophilic granuloma, aneurysmal bone cyst, and osteoblastoma occur occasionally. Osteoid osteoma is an interesting benign vascular lesion characterized by night pain that is often relieved by aspirin.

Pain is the most common complaint and usually results from the expanding nature of the lesion and/or a pathologic fracture. There may be a referred or radicular element to the discomfort that gives the problem the appearance of a herniated disc. Night pain, aggravated or not relieved by rest, occurs frequently. With progression of the disease, neurologic dysfunction may progress to complete paralysis.

Plain film radiographs often reveal the lesion, but 30% to 50% of the bone must be destroyed before the lesion is visualized. A bone scan is positive in 90% of patients.

The most common injury to the buttocks is from a direct blow. This does not usually cause injury to the skin because of the ample underlying padding. Contusion of the muscle is a common occurrence, but it usually is of little consequence. In most of the areas of the buttocks, there is a thick muscle mass that is in little danger of being caught between two unyielding objects. As a result, the condition resulting from a blow is diffuse without gross hematoma formation in the muscle. A tender, painful muscle mass results, and although it may be uncomfortable, the condition is not disabling. During athletic competition, the buttocks are usually not protected by any padding other than that inherent in the athlete's anatomy. Superficial contusion is common, and the examiner should be wary of the condition that is unduly severe or that causes something other than local symptoms.

A contusion of the sciatic nerve may result in pain that begins in the buttock and extends down the back of the thigh into the calf and foot in a way that is similar to sciatic pain from other causes. This pain is nonradicular in character and follows the whole distribution of the sciatic nerve rather than any single nerve root. Straight leg raising causes pain in the area of the contusion. During the acute period, hypesthesia (hypoesthesia) of the skin may be evident in the lower portion of the extremity. This contusion of the sciatic nerve will require no particular treatment other than protection against stretch.

Another area of the buttocks in which a complication of contusion may arise is over the ischial tuberosity. Here the bone is subcutaneous, although it is protected by a layer of muscle of greater or lesser thickness. A contusion here may cause a fracture of the tuberosity, in which case there will be severe pain. The pain is increased by straight leg raising or by any local pressure. More commonly, the result of the blow will be periostitis or fibrositis over the roughened surface of the bone. In other cases, there will be involvement of the ischial bursa. It is impossible, in the early stages, to distinguish between these conditions.

PROCEDURE

- A passive unilateral straight-leg-raising test is performed on a supine patient (Fig. 8-146).
- When unilateral restriction is encountered, the knee is flexed to determine if hip flexion increases (Fig. 8-147).
- If the lumbar spine is the source of complaint, hip flexion will increase.
- A positive sign of the buttock occurs when hip flexion does not increase with knee flexion.
- The sign is present in bursitis, tumor, or abscess.

Confirmation Procedures

Bilateral leg-lowering test, Demianoff's sign, double leg-raise test, hyperextension test, Lewin supine test, matchstick test, Mennell's sign, Minor's sign, Nachlas test, Quick test, Schober's test, skin pinch test, spinal percussion test, and Vanzetti's sign

---

DIAGNOSTIC STATEMENT

The sign of the buttock is present on the right. The presence of this sign indicates that a condition affecting the hip or buttock is responsible for the patient's pain complaint.

CLINICAL PEARL

Trochanteric bursitis causes localized pain and tenderness over the trochanter and occasionally causes pain that radiates down the lateral thigh. The pain is particularly strong when lying on the affected side. Pain from ischiogluteal bursitis is felt posteriorly and is particularly exacerbated by sitting.

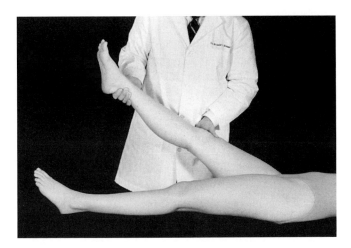

FIG. 8-146 The patient is supine; the examiner performs a straight-leg-raising test on the affected leg.

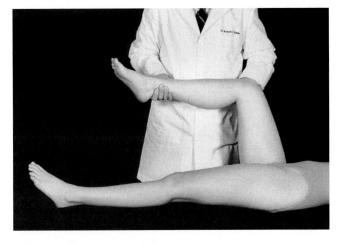

FIG. 8-147 With restriction of the leg movement because of pain or myospasm, the knee is passively flexed. If the disorder is in the lumbar spine, hip flexion increases. If hip flexion does not increase with knee flexion, it is a positive sign of the buttock. A positive sign indicates hip or buttock bursitis, tumor, or abscess.

SKIN PINCH TEST

Assessment for Fibrositic Infiltration

Comment

The most precise definition of true sciatica is pain radiating into the lower limb below the level of the knee in the distribution of a single nerve root, associated with other neurosensory changes such as numbness, tingling, or weakness (Fig. 8-148). Sciatica usually radiates down one leg in the distribution of the L5 or S1 nerve root. In the case of the S1 nerve root, this involves the lateral border of the lower leg and foot, and in the case of the L5 root, the anterolateral aspect of the leg and dorsum of the foot.

Neurologic claudication is another variant of the peripheral manifestations of lumbar disease. In this condition, pain is felt in the distribution of one or more lumbosacral nerve roots, although the pain is often less well localized than the sciatica or femoral neuritis associated with a disc prolapse. It is often accompanied by neurologic symptoms such as numbness or weakness.

A rare but catastrophic type of low back disease is the cauda equina syndrome. This condition may arise from a massive lumbar disc herniation, spinal stenosis, tumors, infections, injuries, or other neurologic disease. It is often preceded or accompanied by symptoms of sciatica or neurologic claudication that may be bilateral.

ORTHOPEDIC GAMUT 8-26

CAUDA EQUINA SYNDROME

Following are the clinical characteristics of cauda equina syndrome:

1. Anesthesia in the distribution of the S2-S4 nerve roots, which supply the perineum in the distribution of a person sitting on a saddle, leading to the term *saddle anesthesia*
2. Disturbance of bladder and bowel control with urinary incontinence or retention and fecal incontinence; any urinary disturbance in a patient with back pain constitutes an emergency and requires urgent investigation

---

Fibromyalgia syndrome or fibromyositis syndrome really does not present a formidable differential diagnosis even though it causes symmetric arthralgia and myalgia, which are usually worse after awakening in the morning. Patients complain of stiffness, but unlike persons with rheumatoid arthritis, they are not stiff. Joint swelling is absent, and tenderness is mild, except over tense muscles. Muscle atrophy is never seen. There are no constitutional symptoms, such as fever and weight loss. The erythrocyte sedimentation rate is normal, and the test for rheumatoid factor is negative. Patients are rarely anemic, and diagnostic imaging of the joints shows normal results. Most patients with the fibromyalgia syndrome are emotionally tense.

Nonarticular (soft tissue) *rheumatism* is a term that encompasses a large group of miscellaneous conditions with a common denominator of musculoskeletal pain and stiffness. This designation is for convenience only and not because of any common etiologic or clinical characteristics. Although some forms of nonarticular rheumatism, such as bursitis and tendinitis, present well-defined features, the causes of others, including fibrositis and myalgia, are not as clear.

Fibrositis is inflammatory hyperplasia of white connective tissue. It is now a term used rarely in the presence of such real tissue inflammation as arthritis, tendinitis, or myositis. Among rheumatologists, fibrositis indicates aching; stiffness; tenderness; and pain around joints, muscle fibers, and subcutaneous tissues without the presence of an inflammatory pathologic process. Fibrositis is a local and diffuse idiopathic condition. The symptom complex of fibrositis, with or without connective tissue inflammation, may be a prominent manifestation of many rheumatic diseases, including systemic lupus erythematosus, rheumatoid arthritis, and subdeltoid bursitis.

PROCEDURE

- The skin pinch test involves smoothly rolling the skin over the spinous process of the vertebrae, by using the forefingers over the advancing thumbs (Fig. 8-149).
- The skin is picked up before rolling it.
- Skin rolling is then performed over each side of the back.
- Fibrositic infiltration and trigger points are demonstrated by tightness and acute tenderness.
- There will be tightness and tenderness, maximally over the level at which a pathologic bone condition exists or

over the vertebra above the level at which a pathologic joint or disc condition exists.

Confirmation Procedures
Bilateral leg-lowering test, Demianoff's sign, double leg-raise test, hyperextension test, Lewin supine test, match stick test, Mennell's sign, Minor's sign, Nachlas test, Quick test, Schober's test, sign of the buttock, spinal percussion test, and Vanzetti's sign

---

DIAGNOSTIC STATEMENT

Skin pinch testing over the lumbosacral area demonstrates trophedematous tissue. A positive test indicates fibrositic infiltration and trigger points in the affected tissue.

CLINICAL PEARL

Trophedematous subcutaneous tissue has a boggy, inelastic texture when rolled between the thumb and finger. This type of tissue is distinguishable from subcutaneous fat. When a patch of skin and subcutaneous tissue a centimeter in diameter is gently squeezed together, instead of immediately forming a fold of flesh, trophedematous tissue does not budge, or it finally yields altogether, with a sudden expanding movement similar to that of inflating a rubber dinghy or air mattress.

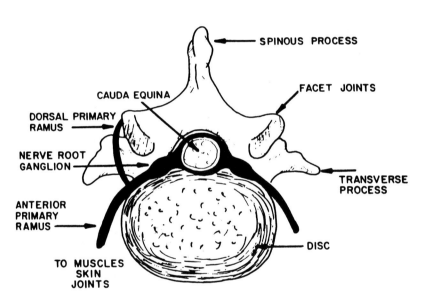

FIG. 8-148   Normal relationships of lumbar nerve roots. *(From Pope MH, et al:* Occupational low back pain assessment, treatment and prevention, *St Louis, 1991, Mosby.)*

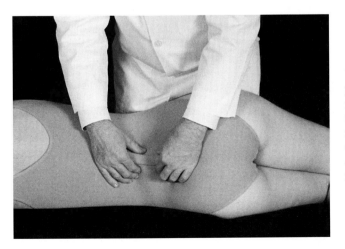

FIG. 8-149   The patient is in either the prone or side-lying position. The examiner picks up an area of skin overlying the affected level of the spine. The examiner performs smooth rolling of the skin over the spinous process of the vertebrae, moving the forefingers over the advancing thumbs. Skin rolling is then performed over each side of the back. The test is positive if tightness and acute tenderness are elicited. A positive test indicates fibrositic infiltration and trigger points.

Assessment for Osseous or Soft-Tissue Injury in the Lumbar Spine

Comment

Vehicular accidents are a common source of trauma to the lumbosacral spine and may cause a wide variety of fractures and dislocations. Compression fractures at the anterior edge of the vertebral bodies may be caused by a hyperflexion motion alone or in combination with a vertical compression. The stability of these fractures depends on the degree of vertebral compression and the presence or absence of posterior ligamentous damage.

The question of cord damage is dominant; spine fractures are classified as stable or unstable. In stable fractures, the cord is rarely damaged, and movement of the spine is safe. In unstable fractures, the cord may have been damaged, but if it has escaped damage, it may still be injured by movement.

Stability depends largely on the integrity of the ligaments and in particular the posterior ligament complex. This complex consists of the supraspinous ligament, the interspinous ligaments, the capsules of the facet joints, and possibly the ligamentum flavum. Fortunately, only 10% of the spinal injuries are unstable, and less than 5% are associated with cord damage.

Injuries usually occur when the spinal column is compressed and collapsed in its vertical axis. This injury typically occurs during a fall from a height or when the patient gets trapped under a cave-in, the direction of the force at any level of the spine is determined by the position of the vertebral column during impact. The flexible lumbar segments also may be injured by violent, free movements of the trunk.

ORTHOPEDIC GAMUT 8-27

SPINAL TRAUMA MECHANISMS

The following are spinal trauma mechanisms:

1. Hyperextension
2. Flexion
3. Flexion combined with rotation
4. Axial displacement (compression)

Hyperextension is rare in the thoracolumbar spine. When hyperextension occurs, the anterior ligaments and the disc may be damaged, or the neural arch may be fractured. Usually, the injury is stable, but fracture of the pedicle is often unstable.

If the posterior ligaments remain intact, forced flexion will crush the vertebral body into a wedge. This is a stable injury and is by far the most common type of vertebral fracture. If the posterior ligaments are torn, the upper vertebral body may tilt forward on the one below. This type of subluxation is often missed because, by the time the diagnostic image is made, the vertebrae have fallen back into place.

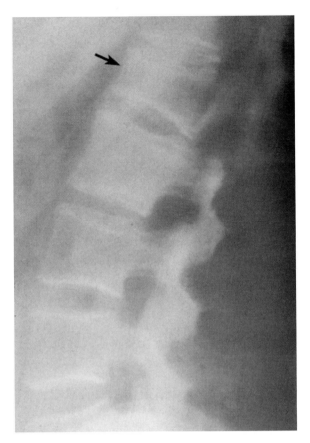

FIG. 8-150 Wedge deformity of the anterior vertebral body height may be indicative of a compression fracture. *(From Deltoff MN, Kogon PL: The portable skeletal x-ray library, St Louis, 1998, Mosby.)*

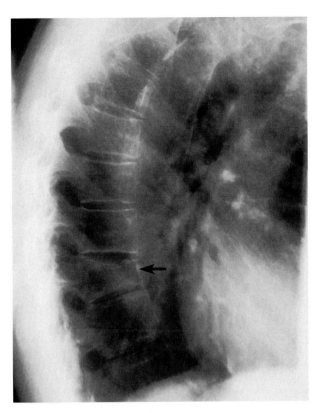

FIG. 8-151 Anterior vertebral body fractures may result in focal or generalized hyperkyphotic angulation of the spine. *(From Deltoff MN, Kogon PL: The portable skeletal x-ray library, St Louis, 1998, Mosby.)*

Most serious injuries of the spine are caused by a combination of flexion and rotation. The ligaments and joint capsules, which are strained to the limit, may tear. The facets may fracture, or the top of one vertebra may be sheared off. The result is a forward shift, or dislocation, of the vertebra above, with or without concomitant bone damage. All fracture-dislocations are unstable.

A vertical force acting on a straight segment of the lumbar spine will compress the vertebral body and may cause a comminuted, or burst, fracture. If the vertebra is split, a large fragment may be driven backwards into the spinal canal. It is this fragment that makes these fractures dangerous. Such fractures are associated with a high incidence of neurologic damage.

Compression defect of the body of a lumbar vertebra may occur with minimal force in osteoporotic or pathologic bone.

ORTHOPEDIC GAMUT 8-28

ANTERIOR VERTEBRAL COMPRESSION FRACTURES

Roentgenographic findings in anterior vertebral compression fractures include the following:

1. Buckling of the anterior vertebral body cortex
2. Wedge deformity of the fractured vertebral body, with loss of the vertebral body height anteriorly compared with its posterior height (Fig. 8-150)
3. Possibility of some focal increase in kyphosis (Fig. 8-151)
4. A zone of condensation, caused by compaction of the trabecular elements of the spongiosa, appearing as a band of increased osseous density through the medullary bone beneath the affected end-plate
5. Vertebral end-plate fractures occur more frequently in the lower thoracic and upper lumbar spines (Fig. 8-152)
6. Vertebral body compression fractures may be suspected when a "frog-face" sign is exhibited on the anteroposterior study (Fig. 8-153)
7. Paraspinal soft-tissue injury is often observed with spinal compression fractures

---

In the Chance fracture, a horizontal line may extend through the spinous process, splitting the neural arch (through the laminae, articular pillars, and pedicles) and extending into the posterior body surface. The fracture line divides the vertebra into upper and lower halves.

ORTHOPEDIC GAMUT 8-29

SPINAL FRACTURES

Other forms of spinal fractures may include the following:

1. Lateral body compression-type fractures
2. Pillar fractures
3. Lamina-pedicle fractures
4. Transverse process fractures (Fig. 8-154)

ORTHOPEDIC GAMUT 8-30

INTRADISCAL PRESSURE

The following are compressive forces that influence intradiscal pressure:

1. *Standing:* Disc pressure is equal to 100% of body weight.
2. *Supine:* Disc pressure is less than 25% of body weight.
3. *Side-lying:* Disc pressure is less than 75% of body weight.
4. *Standing and bending forward:* Disc pressure is approximately 150% of body weight.
5. *Supine with both knees flexed:* Disc pressure is less than 35% of body weight.
6. *Seated in a flexed position:* Disc pressure is approximately 85% of body weight.
7. *Bending forward in a flexed posture and lifting:* Disc pressure is approaching 275% of body weight.

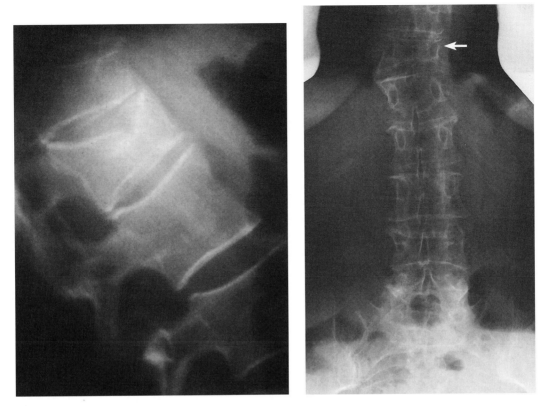

FIG. 8-152   Vertebral body compression fractures occur more often in the upper lumbar or lower thoracic spine.

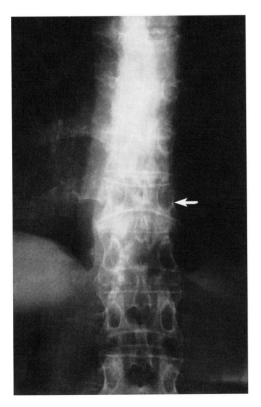

FIG. 8-153   A frog-face sign observed on an anteroposterior radiograph suggests the presence of a vertebral body compression fracture.   *(From Deltoff MN, Kogon PL: The portable skeletal x-ray library, St Louis, 1998, Mosby.)*

PROCEDURE

- While the patient is standing and the trunk is slightly flexed, the examiner uses a neurologic hammer to percuss the spinous processes and the associated musculature of each of the lumbar vertebrae (Fig. 8-155).
- Evidence of localized pain indicates a possible vertebra fracture.
- Evidence of radicular pain indicates a possible disc lesion.
- Because of the nonspecific nature of this test, other conditions will also elicit a positive pain response.
- For example, a ligamentous sprain will cause pain when the spinous processes are percussed.
- Percussing the paraspinal musculature will elicit a positive sign for muscular strain (Figs. 8-156 and 8-157).

Confirmation Procedures

Bilateral leg-lowering test, Demianoff's sign, double leg-raise test, hyperextension test, Lewin supine test, matchstick test, Mennell's sign, Minor's sign, Nachlas test, Quick test, Schober's test, sign of the buttock, skin pinch test, and Vanzetti's sign

DIAGNOSTIC STATEMENT

Spinal percussion elicits pain on the spinous process of L5. This result suggests osseous injury at that level.

Spinal percussion elicits pain at the paraspinals on the left of L5. This result suggests soft-tissue injury at that level.

CLINICAL PEARL

When soft-tissue percussion reproduces the complaint, the examiner may expect the same phenomenon from the use of ultrasound on the tissue. The uses of such therapies may be delayed until the soft tissue is no longer reactive to percussion.

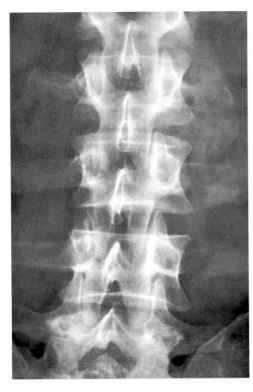

FIG. 8-154   Transverse process fractures at L2, L3, and L4. *(From Deltoff MN, Kogon PL:* The portable skeletal x-ray library, *St Louis, 1998, Mosby.)*

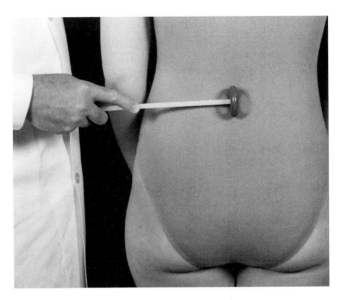

FIG. 8-155   In the standing position, the patient flexes the lumbosacral spine, exposing the spinous processes as much as possible. The examiner percusses the spinous processes of each vertebra. Localized pain is evidence of a fracture or severe sprain. Radiating pain suggests an intervertebral disc syndrome.

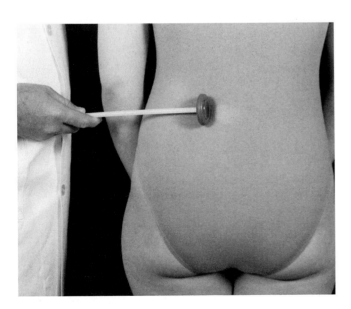

FIG. 8-156   The paravertebral tissues are percussed similarly. Pain elicited in the soft tissues suggests muscular strain and highly sensitive myofascial trigger points.

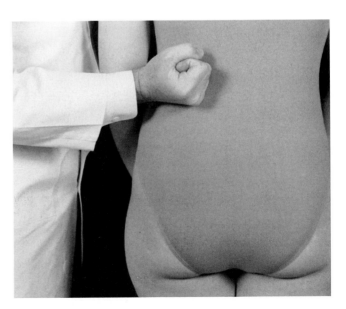

FIG. 8-157   The examiner may perform gross percussion of the lumbar paraspinal tissue. This maneuver is similar to the Lewin punch test. Pain elicited suggests soft-tissue injury.

STRAIGHT-LEG-RAISING TEST

Assessment for Space-Occupying Mass in the Path of a Nerve Root, Sacroiliac Inflammation, and Lumbosacral Involvement

Comment

The straight-leg-raising test assesses irritation of the sciatic nerve (L4, L5, S1). Passively raising the leg with the knee extended stretches the sciatic nerve (Fig. 8-158). When the dura is inflamed and stretched, the patient experiences pain along the dura's anatomic course. Dural movement starts at 30 degrees of elevation. Pain of dural origin should not be felt below that degree of elevation. Pain is maximum between 30 and 70 degrees of elevation. Symptoms at greater degrees of elevation may be of nerve root origin but may also be related to mechanical low back pain secondary to muscle strain or joint disease.

Normal straight leg raising does not preclude the diagnosis of herniated nucleus pulposus. The response to straight leg raising is generally believed to be due in part to the location of the herniation. It has been shown that straight leg raising causes nerve roots to move distally 0.5 to 5 mm, but the nerve roots also move laterally toward the bone and therefore move into a posterolateral herniation and potentially away from a central herniation. Therefore a midline herniation may not cause sciatica during straight leg raising, and the test will be negative.

The L4 nerve root moves less than L5 and S1 during supine straight leg raising.

Obviously, it is important to differentiate sciatica from hamstring tightness during straight leg raising. In a classically positive test, sciatica is produced at 30 degrees or less on one side, while the other side has full range. In hamstring tightness, leg pain occurs at about the same angle on each leg, and pain is confined to the posterior thigh and does not go below the knee.

The straight-leg-raising test will cause traction on the sciatic nerve, lumbosacral nerve roots, and dura mater. Adhesions within these areas may be caused by herniation of the intervertebral disc or to extradural or meningeal irritation. Pain that is felt by the patient comes from the dura mater, nerve root, adventitial sheath of the epidural veins, or the synovial facet joints. The test is positive if pain extends from the back down the leg along the sciatic nerve distribution.

ORTHOPEDIC GAMUT 8-31

UNILATERAL STRAIGHT LEG RAISING

The following are dynamics of unilateral straight leg raising:

1. The slack in sciatic arborization is taken up from 0 to 35 degrees. There is no dural movement.
2. When approaching 35 degrees, tension is applied to the sciatic nerve roots.
3. In the range of 35 to 70 degrees, the sciatic nerve roots tense over the intervertebral disc. The rate of nerve root deformation diminishes as the angle increases.
4. Above 60 to 70 degrees, there is practically no further deformation of the root that occurs during further straight leg raising, and the pain probably originates in the joint.

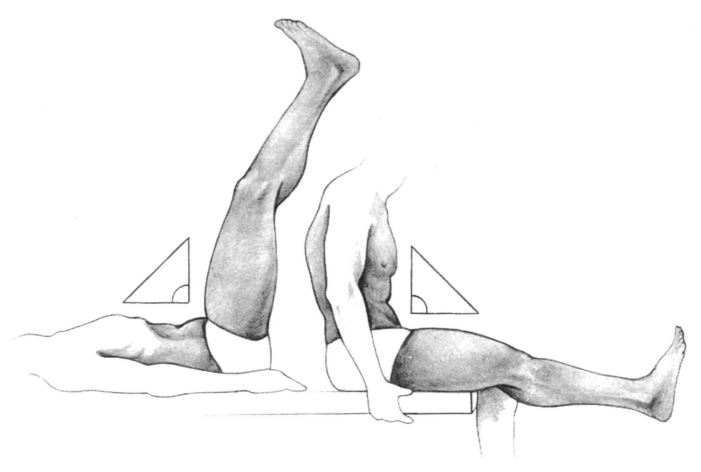

FIG. 8-158   If the examiner suspects the straight-leg-raising test to be unreliable in the supine position, the examiner can surreptitiously raise the leg while the patient is in the sitting position. If the lesion is organic, radiating pain should be experienced in both positions.   *(From Olson WH, et al: Handbook of symptom-related neurology, ed 2, St Louis, 1994, Mosby.)*

PROCEDURE

- The patient lies supine with the legs extended.
- The examiner places one hand under the heel of the affected leg and the other hand on the knee (Fig. 8-159).
- With the limb extended, the examiner flexes the thigh on the pelvis.
- If this maneuver is markedly limited because of pain, the test is positive and may suggest sciatica from lumbosacral or sacroiliac lesions, subluxation syndrome, disc lesions, spondylolisthesis, adhesions, or IVF occlusion.
- The exacerbation of pain by raising the extended leg is further evidence of the effects of traction on a sensitized nerve root (Fig. 8-160).
- Normally, the leg can be raised 15 to 30 degrees before the nerve root is tractioned through the intervertebral foramen.
- Pain, duplicating sciatica, that is elicited by this maneuver indicates a space-occupying lesion—such as lumbar disc protrusion, tumor, adhesions, edema, and tissue inflammation—at the nerve root level.

Confirmation Procedures

Bechterew's sitting test, Bragard's sign, Deyerle's sign, Fajersztajn's test, Lasègue differential sign, Lasègue rebound test, Lasègue sitting test, Lasègue test, Lewin standing test, Lindner's sign, Sicard's sign, and Turyn's sign

---

DIAGNOSTIC STATEMENT

Straight leg raising is positive on the right at 30 degrees. This result indicates stretching of the dura mater because of a space-occupying mass in the path of the nerve root.

Straight leg raising is positive on the right at 45 degrees. This result suggests sciatic irritation because of sacroiliac inflammation.

Straight leg raising on the right produces pain, at 70 degrees, in the lower back. This result indicates lumbosacral involvement.

CLINICAL PEARL

As many authors have pointed out, the nerve roots have a narrow range of movement for stretching. Most authors also conclude that the nerve roots, in normal conditions, are not stretched by the straight-leg-raising test until 35 to 70 degrees of angulation have been reached. However, if the nerve exists with a space-occupying mass (protrusion of disc material) that deflects the nerve's normal pathway, the amount of allowable stretch is already used up by the mass. In this case, the positive sign, pain radiating down the sciatic distribution, occurs at a much lower angulation. This pain has been misconstrued by many to indicate the involvement of the sacroiliac joint instead of the sensitive finding that a nerve root compression syndrome exists. Sciatica that is in the leg and produced from 0 to 30 degrees is caused by nerve root compression. Sciatica that is in the leg and produced from 30 to 60 degrees is probably caused by sacroiliac joint disease. Sciatica that is in the leg and produced above 60 degrees is probably caused by lumbosacral disease.

It is a cardinal point that most, if not all, ranges of movement given for the sciatic nerve roots are based on the absence of a space-occupying mass. The angles change dramatically in the presence of disease. This change is the basis of the Cox sign (which reveals the diseased or compressed nerve root) and Demianoff's sign (which reveals the normal nerve root but diseased sacroiliac or lumbosacral musculature).

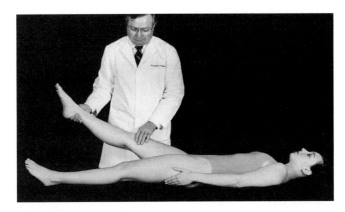

FIG. 8-159   The patient is supine with the legs fully extended. The examiner places one hand under the ankle of the affected leg and the other hand on the knee. The examiner flexes the thigh on the pelvis.

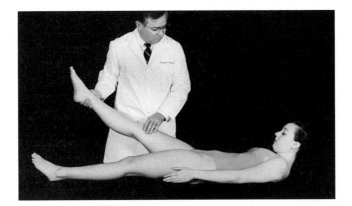

FIG. 8-160   Once the leg reaches the point at which symptoms are reproduced, the patient is instructed to flex the cervical spine and approximate the chin to the chest (Hyndman's sign or Brudzinski sign). If this maneuver is markedly limited because of pain, the test is positive. A positive test suggests sciatica from lumbosacral or sacroiliac lesions, subluxation syndrome, disc lesions, spondylolisthesis, adhesions, or intervertebral foramen occlusion. The angle at which symptoms were reproduced is recorded for future testing.

TURYN'S SIGN

Assessment for Sciatic Radiculopathy

Comment

Various terms are used to describe injuries to the disc. The generally accepted term, *herniated nucleus pulposus,* is rather broad and should be clarified by specific nomenclature to more precisely describe the injury. The three accepted definition categories of herniated nucleus pulposus are protrusion, extruded, and sequestered. In a disc protrusion, the nucleus bulges against an intact annulus (Fig. 8-161). An extruded disc is characterized by the nucleus extending through the annulus, but the nuclear material remains confined by the posterior longitudinal ligament (Fig. 8-162). Finally, in a sequestered disc, the nucleus is free within the canal (Fig. 8-163).

ORTHOPEDIC GAMUT 8-32

LUMBAR DISC DISEASE CLASSIFICATION

Variation of the lumbar disc disease classification model is as follows:

1. Disc protrusion:
   Type I: Peripheral annular bulge
   Type II: Localized annular bulge
2. Disc herniation:
   Type I: Prolapsed intervertebral disc
   Type II: Extruded intervertebral disc
   Type III: Sequestered intervertebral disc

ORTHOPEDIC GAMUT 8-33

CATEGORIES OF LOW BACK PAIN

Following are five categories of low back pain:

1. *Viscerogenic pain:* Pain that originates from the kidneys, sacroiliac, pelvic lesions, and retroperitoneal tumors. This type of pain is neither aggravated by activity nor relieved by rest.
2. *Neurogenic pain:* Pain commonly caused by neurofibromas, cysts, and tumors of the nerve roots in the lumbar spine.
3. *Vascular pain:* Pain characterized by intermittent claudication from aneurysms and peripheral vascular disease.
4. *Spondylogenic pain:* Pain directly related to the pain originating from soft tissues of the spine and sacroiliac joint.
5. *Psychogenic pain:* Pain that is quite uncommon and ascribed to nonorganic causes.

Pain that radiates down the back of the leg is termed sciatica regardless of whether it is associated with lower back pain. The pain can be referred from the back along the thigh to the foot and toe. On the other hand, sciatica also can be caused by referred pain that radiates in the opposite direction, from the foot upward. In some cases of sciatica, the presence of trigger areas in the lower part of the back can be demonstrated. These trigger areas, when compressed, will set off the pain along the sciatic distribution.

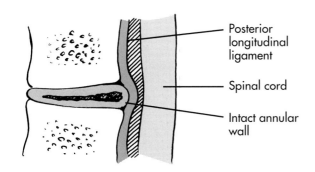

FIG. 8-161 Disc protrusion. *(From Shankman GA:* Fundamental orthopedic management for the examiner, *St Louis, 1997, Mosby.)*

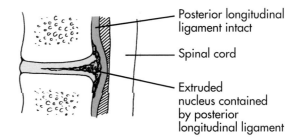

FIG. 8-162 Extruded disc. *(From Shankman GA:* Fundamental orthopedic management for the examiner, *St Louis, 1997, Mosby.)*

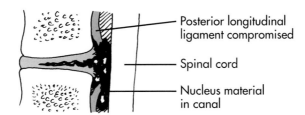

FIG. 8-163 Sequestered disc. *(From Shankman GA:* Fundamental orthopedic management for the examiner, *St Louis, 1997, Mosby.)*

Although herniated intervertebral discs are credited for most cases of sciatica, they do not account for all such symptoms. Diagnosis should be based on careful neurologic evaluation and, when necessary, diagnostic imaging and other tests. The straight-leg-raising test is not pathognomonic. There are instances when, although a disc is central and there are no symptoms of pressure on the nerve root, there is sciatic radiation of the pain and the prolapsed disc is credited as the cause of sciatica.

Sciatica has a variety of causes, some of which produce this type of posterior leg pain without seeming to involve the sciatic nerve or its contributory roots.

PROCEDURE

- When the patient is in the supine position with both lower limbs resting straight out on the table, dorsiflexion of the great toe elicits pain in the gluteal region (Figs. 8-164 and 8-165).
- The sign is significant for sciatic radiculopathy.

Confirmation Procedures

Bechterew's sitting test, Bragard's sign, Deyerle's sign, Fajersztajn's sign, Lasègue differential sign, Lasègue rebound test, Lasègue sitting test, Lasègue test, Lewin standing test, Lindner's sign, Sicard's sign, and straight-leg-raising test

---

ORTHOPEDIC GAMUT 8-34

SCIATICA

The origin of sciatica includes the following:

1. Prolapsed intervertebral disc pressure, infection, and traumatic sciatic neuritis, perineural fibrositis, infections, and tumors of the spinal cord
2. Lumbosacral and sacroiliac sprain and strain, degenerating intervertebral discs, fibrositis, osteomyelitis, hip joint disease, and secondary carcinomatous deposits in bone
3. Nephrolithiasis, prostatic, renal, and anal disease
4. Toxic and metabolic disorders, conversion hysteria, and arterial insufficiency

---

DIAGNOSTIC STATEMENT

Turyn's sign is present on the left. The presence of this sign suggests sciatic radiculopathy.

CLINICAL PEARL

A straight-leg-raising test that is positive under 30 degrees reveals a large disc protrusion. The nerve root is stretched long before it would normally be. The straight-leg-raising test is most useful for identifying L5-S1 disc lesions because the pressures on the nerve root are highest at this level. During straight leg raising, L4-L5 is not as apt to give as much pain as the L5-S1 because the pressure between the disc and the nerve root at L4-L5 is half that at L5-S1. Therefore the L5-S1 disc lesion gives more pain in the lower back and leg than does the L4-L5 disc lesion. No movement on the nerve root occurs until straight leg raising reaches 30 degrees. No movement on L4 occurs during a straight-leg-raising test. From this, the presence of a Turyn's sign indicates a large disc protrusion at the level of the L5-S1 nerve root.

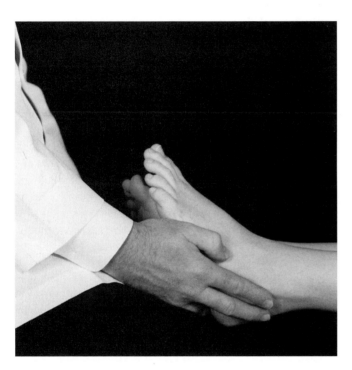

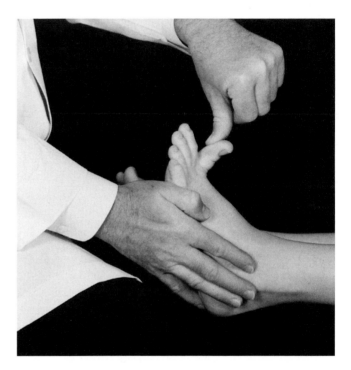

FIG. 8-164   The patient is in the supine position, with both lower limbs fully extended on the examination table.

FIG. 8-165   The examiner sharply dorsiflexes the great toe of the affected leg. Pain elicited in the gluteal region is a positive sign. The sign is present in sciatic radiculopathy.

VANZETTI'S SIGN

Assessment for Sciatic Scoliosis

Comment
An unlevel sacral base is not synonymous with pelvic tilt. Although sacral unleveling may accompany pelvic obliquity to varying degrees, they are different postural and structural imbalances. It is common for patients with sacral unleveling to have a concomitant or resultant lumbar scoliosis, although a certain percentage of individuals with spinal curvatures have compensated through their lumbopelvic articulation (Fig. 8-166).

Scoliosis is a lateral curvature of the spine. For the management of any case, the first and most important decision to make is whether there is any deformity of the vertebrae (structural scoliosis).

ORTHOPEDIC GAMUT 8-35

SCOLIOSIS

In scoliosis, the deformity is usually one of the following:

1. Compensatory, resulting from tilting of the pelvis from real or apparent shortening of one leg
2. Sciatic, resulting from a unilateral protective muscle spasm, especially accompanying a prolapsed intervertebral disc

---

With sciatic scoliosis, the underlying cause is a prolapsed intervertebral disc that impinges on a lumbar or sacral nerve. The deformity also may be observed in some cases of acute lower back pain, the pathogenesis of which is not clear. For this type of scoliosis, the curve is in the lumbar region. The abnormal posture is assumed involuntarily in an attempt to reduce the painful pressure upon the affected nerve or joint. The predominant feature is severe back pain, or sciatica, that is aggravated by movements of the spine. The onset of this pain is usually sudden. The scoliosis is poorly compensated, and the trunk may be tilted markedly to one side. The curvature is not associated with rotation of the vertebrae.

With structural scoliosis, there is alteration in vertebral shape and mobility, and the deformity cannot be corrected by alteration of posture. A careful history and examination are required to find a cause and give a prognosis. Structural scoliosis may be congenital and may be caused by a hemivertebra, fused vertebrae, or absent or fused ribs.

With paralytic scoliosis, the deformity is secondary to loss of the supportive action of the trunk and spinal muscles, which is almost always a sequel to anterior poliomyelitis.

Neuropathic scoliosis is seen as a complication of neurofibromatosis, cerebral palsy, spina bifida, syringomyelia, Friedreich's ataxia, and neuropathic conditions. Primary disorders of the supportive musculature (muscular dystrophy, arthrogryposis) are responsible for myopathic scoliosis.

Metabolic scoliosis is uncommon but occurs in cystine storage disease, Marfan's syndrome, and rickets.

Idiopathic scoliosis is the most common and by far the most important of the structural scolioses. The cause of idiopathic scoliosis remains obscure. Several vertebrae at one or, less commonly, two distinct levels are affected and cause a primary curve. In the area of the primary curve, there is loss of mobility (the fixed curve) and rotational deformity of the vertebrae (the spinous processes rotate into the concavity, and the bodies, which carry the ribs in the thoracic region, rotate into the convexity). Above and below the fixed primary curves, secondary curves that are mobile develop to maintain the normal position of the head and pelvis.

The spinal deformity is accompanied by shortening of the trunk, and there is often impairment of respiratory and cardiac function. In severe cases, this may lead to invalidism and a shortened life expectancy.

PROCEDURE
- With sciatica, the pelvis is always horizontal even though scoliosis exists (Fig. 8-167).
- When scoliosis is present with other spinal lesions, the pelvis will be tilted.

Confirmation Procedures
Bilateral leg-lowering test, Demianoff's sign, double leg-raise test, hyperextension test, Lewin supine test, matchstick test, Mennell's sign, Minor's sign, Nachlas test, Quick test, Schober's test, sign of the buttock, skin pinch test, and spinal percussion test

---

DIAGNOSTIC STATEMENT

Vanzetti's sign is present in the presentation of a left-sided antalgia. The presence of this sign suggests a sciatic scoliosis.

CLINICAL PEARL

Vanzetti's sign allows quick observation of the patient to determine the source of the patient's antalgia before performing the more aggressive assessments of the lumbosacral spine.

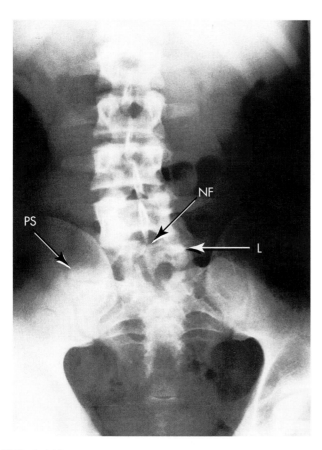

FIG. 8-166 Levorotatory scoliosis with mild pelvic obliquity. *L,* Lumbarization; *NF,* nonfusion defect; *PS,* pseudoarthrosis. *(From Brier SR: Primary care orthopedics, St Louis, 1999, Mosby.)*

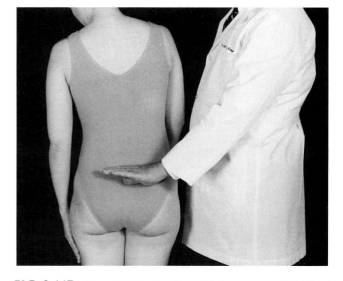

FIG. 8-167 The patient is standing with the arms comfortably at the sides. The examiner assesses the level of the pelvis and sacrum. Despite the antalgia, the pelvis is always horizontal in sciatic conditions. For other spinal lesions, when scoliosis is present, the pelvis is tilted.

CRITICAL THINKING

What is a cauda equina syndrome?

Cauda equina syndrome is a large midline disc herniation that compresses several roots of the cauda equina.

What are the physical findings of disc herniation at the L3-L4 disc?

Herniation at L3-L4 compresses the L4 nerve root. There are sensory deficits in the posterolateral thigh, anterior knee, and medial leg. Motor weakness is in the quadriceps and hip adductors. Patellar reflex is diminished or absent.

What are the physical findings of disc herniation at the L4-L5 disc?

The L5 nerve root is compressed with herniation at L4-L5. Sensory deficit noted in the anterolateral leg, dorsum of the foot, and great toe. Motor weakness is of the extensor hallucis longus, gluteus medius, and extensor digitorum longus and brevis. No reflex changes are present.

What are the physical findings of disc herniation at the L5-S1 disc?

Herniation at L5-S1 compresses the S1 nerve root. Sensory deficits are in the lateral malleolus, lateral foot, heel, and web of the fourth and fifth toes. Motor weakness involves the peroneus longus and brevis, gastrocnemius-soleus complex, and gluteus maximus. The Achilles' reflex is usually diminished.

List "tension" signs associated with lumbar disc herniation.

1. Lasègue test
2. The bowstring sign
3. The Lasègue sitting test
4. Fajarsztajn's test
5. Femoral nerve traction

What is antalgia in the lumbar spine?

Herniation of a disc lateral to the nerve root produces antalgia posture away from the side of the irritated nerve root. Herniation of the disc medial to the nerve root produces a list toward the side of the irritated nerve root.

What imaging techniques are used in evaluating lumbar disc disease?

1. Plain film radiography
2. Magnetic resonance imaging
3. Computed axial tomography
4. Myelography

What is lumbar spinal stenosis?

Lumbar spinal stenosis is an abnormal narrowing of the osseoligamentous vertebral canal or vertebral foramina.

What is the most common cause for neurologic pain in the aging lumbar spine?

Spinal stenosis

What is the hallmark symptom of spinal stenosis?

Pain that increases with walking or standing and that is relieved by sitting and leaning forward or lying down

What is spondylolisthesis?

Spondylolisthesis is the forward slippage of one vertebral body on another.

What is spondylolysis?

Spondylolysis is the clinical entity in which the pars interarticularis is not intact or is separated.

List the five classes of spondylolisthesis.

1. Congenital
2. Isthmic
3. Traumatic
4. Pathologic
5. Degenerative

BIBLIOGRAPHY

Abrams WB, Berkow R: *The Merck manual of geriatrics,* Rahway, NJ, 1990, Merck Sharp & Dohme Research Laboratories.

Adams JC, Hamblen DL: *Outline of orthopaedics,* ed 11, Edinburgh, 1990, Churchill Livingstone.

Agency for Health Care Policy and Research, Public Health Service, US Department of Health and Human Services: Diagnostic imaging for low back pain gets mixed review, *Research Activities* 12:3, 1990.

Agency for Health Care Policy and Research, Public Health Services, US Department of Health and Human Services: Acute low back pain in adults, *Clinical Practice Guideline,* Number 14, Rockville, 1994, AHCPR Publication No. 95-0642, The Agency.

Alaranta H, et al: A prospective study of patients with sciatica: a comparison between conservatively treated patients and patients who have undergone operation, III, results after one year follow-up, *Spine* 15:1245, 1990.

Alario AJ: *Practical guide to the care of the pediatric patient,* St Louis, 1997, Mosby.

Albeck MJU, et al: A controlled comparison of myelography, computed tomography, and magnetic resonance imaging in clinically suspected lumbar disc herniation, *Spine* 20:443, 1995.

Allison D, Strickland N: *Acronyms & synonyms in medical imaging,* Oxford, 1996, ISIS Medical Media.

Allman LF: Back school program, *The Atlanta Sports Medicine Clinic, PC, Introduction to Back Injuries,* 1990.

Altman RD: Musculoskeletal questions and answers, *J Musculoskeletal Med* 7:10, 1990.

American Medical Association: *Guides to the evaluation of permanent impairment,* ed 4, Chicago, 1993, American Medical Association.

American Medical Association: *How to use guides to the evaluation of permanent impairment,* ed 4, Falmouth, Conn, 1993, SEAK.

Ammann W, Matheson GO: Radionuclide bone imaging in the detection of stress fractures, *Clin J Sport Med* 1:115, 1991.

Amundsen T: Lumbar spinal stenosis: clinical and radiologic features, *Spine* 10:1178, 1995.

Anderson KN, Anderson LE: *Mosby's pocket dictionary of medicine, nursing, & allied health,* ed 2, St Louis, 1994, Mosby.

Andersson G: The epidemiology of spinal disorders. In Frymoyer J, editor: *The adult spine,* New York, 1991, Raven.

Apley AG, Solomon L: *Concise system of orthopaedics and fractures,* London, 1988, Butterworth-Heinemann.

Aprill C: Diagnostic disc injection. In Frymoyer JW, editor: *The adult spine: principles and practice,* New York, 1991, Raven.

Avioli LV: Significance of osteoporosis: a growing national health care problem, *Orthop Rev* 21:1126, 1992.

Avramov AI, et al: The effects of controlled mechanical loading on group II, III, and IV afferent units from the lumbar facet joint and surrounding tissue: an in vitro study, *J Bone Joint Surg* 74A:1465, 1992.

Ballinger PW, editor: *Merrill's atlas of roentgenographic positions and standard radiologic procedures,* ed 8, St Louis, 1995, Mosby.

Barkauskas VH, et al: *Health & physical assessment,* ed 2, St Louis, 1998, Mosby.

Batson OV: The function of the vertebral veins and their role in the spread of metastasis, *Ann Surg* 112:138, 1940.

Battie MC, Bigos SJ: Industrial back pain complaints, *Orthop Clin North Am* 22:273, 1991.

Bauer DC, et al: Factors associated with appendicular bone mass in older women, *Ann Intern Med* 118:657, 1993.

Beaman D, et al: Substance P innervation of lumbar facet joints, *Proceedings of the seventh annual meeting of North American Spine Society,* Boston, July 9-11, 1991.

Bednar DA, Orr FW, Simon GT: Observations on the pathomorphology of the thoracolumbar fascia in chronic mechanical back pain: a microscopic study, *Spine* 20:1161, 1995.

Bell GR, Modic MT: Radiology of the lumbar spine. In Rothman RA, Sinecone FA, editors: *The spine,* ed 3, Philadelphia, 1992, WB Saunders.

Bellah RD, et al: Low-back pain in adolescent patients: detection of stress injury to the pars interarticularis with SPECT, *Radiology* 180:509, 1991.

Berquist T: *MRI of the musculoskeletal system,* ed 3, Philadelphia, 1996, JB Lippincott.

Bischoff RJ, et al: A comparison of computed tomography-myelography, magnetic resonance imaging and myelography in the diagnosis of herniated nucleus pulposus and spinal stenosis, *J Spinal Disord* 6:289, 1993.

Boden S, et al: Abnormal magnetic resonance scans of the spine in asymptomatic patients, *J Bone Joint Surg* 72A:403, 1990.

Boden SD, et al: *The aging spine,* Philadelphia, 1991, WB Saunders.

Bogduk N: Pathology of lumbar disc pain, *Manual Med* 5:72, 1990.

Bogduk N: *Pathogenesis of degenerative disc disease,* Toronto, 1991, American Back Society.

Bogduk N, Macintosh JE, Pearcy MJ: A universal model of the lumbar back muscles in the upright position, *Spine* 17:897, 1992.

Bogduk N, Twomey LT: *Clinical anatomy of the lumbar spine,* London, 1991, Churchill Livingstone.

Bond MR: *Pain: its nature, analysis and treatment,* Edinburgh, 1979, Churchill Livingstone.

Borenstein D: Prevalence and treatment outcome of primary and secondary fibromyalgia in patients with spinal pain, *Spine* 20:1055, 1995.

Borenstein DG, Burton JR: Lumbar spine disease in the elderly, *J Am Geriatr Soc* 41:167, 1993.

Borenstein DG, et al: *Low back pain: medical diagnosis and comprehensive management,* ed 2, Philadelphia, 1995, WB Saunders.

Bough B, et al: Degeneration of lumbar facet joints, *J Bone Joint Surg* 72B:275, 1990.

Bowlus B: *Mosby's regional atlas of human anatomy,* St Louis, 1997, Mosby.

Bozzae A, et al: Lumbar disc herniation: MR imaging assessment of natural history in patients treated without surgery, *Radiology* 185:135, 1992.

Bradford FK: Low back sprain and ruptured intervertebral disc, *Med Times* 88:797, 1960.

Breig A, Troup JDG: Biomechanical considerations in straight-leg-raising test: cadaveric and clinical studies of the effects of medial hip rotation, *Spine* 4:242, 1979.

Breen A: The reliability of palpation and other diagnostic methods, *J Manipulative Physiol Ther* 15:54, 1992.

Brier SR: *Primary care orthopedics,* St Louis, 1999, Mosby.

Brody IA, Williams RH: The signs of Kernig and Brudzinski, *Arch Neurol* 21:215, 1969.

Brudzinski J: A new sign of the lower extremities in meningitis of children (neck sign), *Arch Neurol* 21:216, 1969.

Brooks M, Evans R, Fairclough J: *Sports injuries,* ed 2, London, 1992, Gower Medical.

Brotzman SB: *Clinical orthopaedic rehabilitation,* St Louis, 1996, Mosby.

Brown DE, Neumann RD: *Orthopedic secrets,* Philadelphia, 1995, Hanley & Belfus.

Bucholz RW: *Orthopaedic decision making,* ed 2, St Louis, 1996, Mosby.

Buckwalter J: Spine update: aging and degeneration of the human intervertebral disc, *Spine* 20:1307, 1995.

Budgell B, Noda K, Sata A: Innervation of posterior structures in the lumbar spine of the rat, *J Manipulative Physiol Ther* 20:359, 1997.

Buirski G: Magnetic resonance signal pattern of lumbar discs in patients with low back pain: a prospective study with discographic correlation, *Spine* 17:1205, 1992.

Burkus JK: Spine. In Loth T, editor: *Orthopaedic boards review,* St Louis, 1993, Mosby.

Butler D: *Mobilisation of the nervous system,* Melbourne, 1991, Churchill Livingstone.

Cailliet R: *Soft tissue pain and disability,* Philadelphia, 1977, FA Davis.

Cailliet R: *Low back pain syndrome,* ed 3, Philadelphia, 1981, FA Davis.

Campbell JB, Campbell JM: *Mosby's survival guide to medical abbreviations & acronyms prefixes & suffixes symbols Greek alphabet,* St Louis, 1995, Mosby.

Canale ST: *Campbell's operative orthopaedics,* vol 1-4, ed 9, St Louis, 1998, Mosby.

Cats A, Linder SM: Spondyloarthropathies: an overview, *Spine* 4:497, 1990.

Chapman S, Nakielny R: *Aids to radiological differential diagnosis,* ed 3, London, 1995, Bailliere Tindall.

Chappuis JL, Johnson GD, Gines AM: *A source guide for spine care,* Atlanta, 1994, Grater Atlanta Spine Center.

Cipriano JJ: *Photographic manual of regional orthopaedic and neurological test,* ed 3, Baltimore, 1997, Williams & Wilkins.

Cloward RB: Lesions of the intervertebral disc and their treatment by interbody fusion methods: the painful disc, *Clin Orthop* 27:51, 1963.

Cohn RE: *Impairment rating examination and disability evaluation,* ed 3, Wilkesboro, NC, 1994, R Ernest Cohn.

Cole AJ, Herring SA: *The low back pain handbook: a practical guide for the primary care examiner,* Philadelphia, 1997, Hanley & Belfus.

Concannon MJ: *Common hand problems in primary care,* Philadelphia, 1999, Hanley & Belfus.

Connelly C: Easing low back pain, *Postgrad Med* 100, 1996.

Conwell TD: *Documenting patient progress "daily office charting seminar" thorough accurate quick procedures,* ed 11, Lakewood, Colo, 1990, Timothy D. Conwell.

Coppes MH, et al: Innervation of annulus fibrosis in low back pain, *Lancet* 336:189, 1988.

Cox JM: *Low back pain mechanism, diagnosis and treatment,* ed 5, Baltimore, 1990, Williams & Wilkins.

Cramer G, et al: Comparison of computed tomography to magnetic resonance imaging in the evaluation of the lumbar intervertebral foramina, *Clin Anat* 7:173, 1994.

Cramer GD, Darby SA: *Basic and clinical anatomy of the spine, spinal cord, and ANS,* St Louis, 1995, Mosby.

Crisco JJ, Panjabi MM: The intersegmental and multisegmental muscles of the lumbar spine: a biomechanical model comparing lateral stabilizing potential, *Spine* 16:793, 1991.

Cullinan AM: *Optimizing radiographic positioning,* Philadelphia, 1992, Lippincott.

Cyrias JH: Lesions discals lombaires, *Acta Orthop Belg* 27:442, 1961.

Cyriax J: *Textbook for orthopaedic medicine, vol 1: diagnosis of soft tissue lesions,* London, 1975, Bailliere Tindall.

Daffner RH: Thoracic and lumbar vertebral trauma, *Orthop Clin North Am* 21:463, 1990.

Daffner RH: *Clinical radiology: the essentials,* Baltimore, 1993, Williams & Wilkins.

Daffner RH, et al: The radiology assessment of post-traumatic vertebral stability, *Skeletal Radiol* 19:103, 1990.

Dambro MR, Griffith JA: *Griffith's 5 minute clinical consult,* Baltimore, 1997, Williams & Wilkins.

D'Ambrogio KJ, Roth GB: *Positional release therapy assessment & treatment of musculoskeletal dysfunction,* St Louis, 1997, Mosby.

D'Ambrosia RD: *Musculoskeletal disorders: regional examination and differential diagnosis,* Philadelphia, 1977, JB Lippincott.

Dandy DJ: *Essential orthopaedics and trauma,* Edinburgh, 1989, Churchill Livingstone.

Daniels L, Worthingham C: *Muscle testing: techniques of manual examination,* Philadelphia, 1980, WB Saunders.

Day MO: Spondylolytic spondylolisthesis in an elite athlete, *Chiro Sports Med* 5:91, 1991.

Deen HG, et al: Assessment of bladder function after lumbar decompressive surgery for spinal stenosis: a prospective study, *J Neurosurg* 80:971, 1994.

Delamarter RB, et al: Experimental lumbar spinal stenosis, *J Bone Joint Surg* 72A:110, 1990.

Delauche-Cavallier MC, et al: Lumbar disc herniation: computed tomography scan changes after conservative treatment of nerve root compression, *Spine* 17:927, 1992.

Deltoff MN, Kogon PL: *The portable skeletal x-ray library,* St Louis, 1998, Mosby.

Demeter SL, Andersson GBJ, Smith GM: *Disability evaluation,* St Louis, 1996, Mosby.

DePalma AF, Rothman RH: *The intervertebral disc,* Philadelphia, 1970, WB Saunders.

DeRosa C, Porterfield JA: A physical therapy model for the treatment of low back pain, *Phys Ther* 72:261, 1992.

Deshpande JK, Tobias JD: *The pediatric pain handbook,* St Louis, 1996, Mosby.

Dettenmeier PA: *Radiographic assessment for nurses,* St Louis, 1995, Mosby.

Deyerle WM, May VR: Sciatic tension test, *South Med J* 49:999, 1956.

Deyo R: Nonoperative treatment of low back disorders: differentiating useful therapy. In Frymoryer JW, editor: *The adult spine: principles and practice,* New York, 1991, Raven.

Deyo RA, Rainville J, Kent DL: What can the history and physical examination tell us about low back pain? *JAMA* 268:760, 1992.

Doherty M: *Color atlas and text of osteoarthritis,* London, 1994, Wolfe.

Doherty M, Doherty J: *Clinical examination in rheumatology,* London, 1992, Wolfe.

Doherty M, George E: *Self-assessment picture tests in rheumatology,* London, 1995, Mosby-Wolfe.

Dommisse GF, Grobler L: Arteries and veins of the lumbar nerve roots and cauda equina, *Clin Orthop* 115:22, 1976.

Dommisse GF, Louw JA: Anatomy of the lumbar spine. In Floman Y, editor: *Disorders of the lumbar spine,* Rockville and Tel Aviv, 1990, Aspen and Freund Publishing House.

Donelson R, McKenzie R: Mechanical assessment and treatment of spinal pain. In Frymoyer JW, editor: *The adult spine: principles and practice,* New York, 1991, Raven.

Dussault R, Lander P: Imaging of the facet joints, *Radiol Clin North Am* 28:1033, 1990.

Dvorak J, Dvorak V: *Manual medicine: diagnostics,* New York, 1990, Thieme.

Dyck P: The femoral nerve traction test with lumbar disc protrusion, *Surg Neurol* 6:163, 1976.

Dyck P: The stoop-test in lumbar entrapment radiculopathy, *Spine* 4:89, 1979.

Edgar MA, Ghadially JA: Innervation of the lumbar spine, *Clin Orthop* 115:35, 1976.

Edgar MS, Park WM: Induced pain patterns on passive straight-leg-raising in lower lumbar disc protrusion, *J Bone Joint Surg* 56B:658, 1974.

Ellenberg ME, et al: Prospective evaluation of the course of disc herniation in patients with radiculopathy, *Arch Phys Med Rehabil* 74:3, 1993.

Elster AD: *Questions and answers in magnetic resonance imaging,* St Louis, 1994, Mosby.

Epstein BS: *The spine, a radiological text and atlas,* ed 3, Philadelphia, 1969, Lea & Febiger.

Epstein O, et al: *Clinical examination,* ed 2, London, 1997, Mosby.

Ericksen MF: Aging in the lumbar spine, *Am J Phys Anthropol* 48:241, 1974.

Fahrni WH: Observations on straight-leg raising with special reference to nerve root adhesions, *Can J Surg* 9:44, 1966.

Farfan HF: *Mechanical disorders of the low back,* Philadelphia, 1973, Lea & Febiger.

Farrar WE: *Atlas of infections of the nervous system,* London, 1993, Wolfe.

Feldmann E: *Current diagnosis in neurology,* St Louis, 1994, Mosby.

Ferezy JS: *The chiropractic neurological examination,* Gaithersburg, Md, 1992, Aspen.

Fernstrom U, Goldie I: Does granulation tissue in the intervertebral disc provoke back pain? *Acta Orthop Scand* 30:202, 1960.

Fomby EW, Mellion MB: Identifying and treating myofascial pain syndrome, *Phys Sports Med* 25, 1997.

Forbes CD, Jackson WF: *A colour atlas and text of clinical medicine,* Aylesbury, 1993, Wolfe.

Fornage B: *Musculoskeletal ultrasound,* New York, 1995, Churchill Livingstone.

Frymoyer J: *The adult spine,* New York, 1991, Raven.

Frymoyer JW, Cats-Baril WI: An overview of the incidences and costs of low back pain, *Orthop Clin North Am* 22:263, 1991.

Fulton M: *Lower-back pain: a new solution for an old problem,* Rolling Meadows, NJ, 1992, MedX.

Garcia JH: *Neuropathology: the diagnostic approach,* St Louis, 1997, Mosby.

Gartland JJ: *Fundamentals of orthopaedics,* Philadelphia, 1974, WB Saunders.

Gianakopoulos G, et al: Inversion devices: their role in producing lumbar distraction, *Arch Phys Med Rehabil* 66:100, 1985.

Giles LGF, Kaveri MJP: Some osseous and soft tissue causes of lumbar stenosis, *J Rheumatol* 17:1374, 1990.

Gilkey DP: Injury prevention in the workplace: a closer look at OSHA's proposed ergonomic standard, *J Am Chiropractic Assoc* 33:25, 1996.

Gillis L: *Diagnosis in orthopaedics,* London, 1969, Butterworths.

Goddard BS, Reid JD: Movements induced by straight-leg-raising in the lumbo-sacral roots, nerves, and plexus and in the intra pelvic section of the sciatic nerve, *J Neurol Neurosurg Psychiatry* 28:12, 1965.

Goldstein JD, et al: Spine injuries in gymnasts and swimmers, *Am J Sports Med* 19:463, 1991.

Gracovetsky S: The spine as a motor in sports: application to running and lifting, *Spine* 4:267, 1990.

Greenspan A: *Orthopedic radiology,* ed 2, Philadelphia, 1992, JB Lippincott.

Greenspan A, Montesano P: *Imaging of the spine in clinical practice,* London, 1993, Wolfe.

Greenstein GM: *Clinical assessment of neuromusculoskeletal disorders,* St Louis, 1997, Mosby.

Grobler LS, Wiltse LC: Classification, non-operative, and operative treatment of spondylolisthesis. In Frymoyer JW, editor: *The adult spine: principles and practice,* New York, 1991, Raven.

Groen GJ, Baljet B, Drukker J: Nerves and nerve plexuses of the human vertebral collum, *Am J Anat* 188:282, 1990.

Grossman ZD, et al: *Cost-effective diagnostic imaging: the examiner's guide,* ed 3, St Louis, 1995, Mosby.

Gunn CC, Milbrandt WE: Early and subtle signs in low-back sprain, *Spine* 3:267, 1978.

Haher TR, Felmly WT, O'Brien M: Thoracic and lumbar fractures: diagnosis and management. In Bridwell KH, DeWald RL, editors: *The textbook of spinal surgery,* Philadelphia, 1991, JB Lippincott.

Hansson T, et al: The lumbar lordosis in acute and chronic low-back pain, *Spine* 10:154, 1985.

Hammer WI: *Functional soft tissue examination and treatment by manual methods: the extremities,* Gaithersburg, Md, 1991, Aspen.

Hammerberg KW: Kyphosis. In Bridwell DH, DeWald RL, editors: *The textbook of spinal surgery,* Philadelphia, 1991, JB Lippincott.

Hanley EN, Phillips ED: Profiles of patients who get spine infections and the type of infections that have a predilection for the spine. In Wiesel SW, editor: *Seminars in spine surgery,* vol 2, Philadelphia, 1990, WB Saunders.

Hardy RW, editor: *Lumbar disc disease,* ed 2, New York, 1992, Raven.

Hawkins RJ: *An organized approach to musculoskeletal examination and history taking,* St Louis, 1995, Mosby.

Helfet AJ, Gruebel Lee DM: *Disorders of the lumbar spine,* Philadelphia, 1978, JB Lippincott.

Hellstrom M, et al: Radiologic abnormalities of the thoracolumbar spine in patients, *Acta Radiol* 31:127, 1990.

Herkowitz HN, Kurz LT: Degenerative lumbar spondylolisthesis with spinal stenosis: a prospective study comparing decompression with decompression and intertransverse process arthrodesis *J Bone Joint Surg* 73A:802, 1991.

Herlin L: *Sciatic and pelvic pain due to lumbosacral nerve root compression,* Springfield, Ill, 1966, Charles C Thomas.

Herno A, Alraksinen O, Saari T, Miettiner H: The predictive value of preoperative myelography in lumbar spinal stenosis, *Spine* 19:1335-8, 1994.

Herron LD, Pheasant HC: Prone knee-flexion provocative testing for lumbar disc protrusion, *Spine* 5:65, 1980.

Hinkle CZ: *Fundamentals of anatomy & movement: a workbook and guide,* St Louis, 1997, Mosby.

Hochschuler SH, editor: Spinal injuries in sports, *Spine* 4, 1990.

Hoffman RM, Kent DL, Deyo RA: Diagnostic accuracy and clinical utility of thermography for lumbar radiculopathy: a meta-analysis, *Spine* 16:623, 1991.

Hollinshead WH: *Anatomy for surgeons, vol 3, the back and limbs,* ed 3, Philadelphia, 1982, Harper & Row.

Hopwood MB, Abram SE: Factors associated with failure of lumbar epidural steroids, *Reg Anesth Pain Med* 18:238, 1993.

Hornberger JP: *Exercise physiology therapeutic exercise,* Sarasota, Fla, 1991, Joseph P Hornberger.

Hubbard DR, Berkoff GM: Myofascial trigger points show spontaneous needle EMG activity, *Spine* 18:1803, 1993.

Hudgins WR: The crossed-straight-leg-raising test, *N Engl J Med* 297:1127, 1977.

Hutton WC: The forces acting on a lumbar intervertebral joint, *J Manual Med* 5, 66, 1990.

Jablonski S: *Dictionary of medical acronyms & abbreviations,* ed 3, Philadelphia, 1998, Hanley & Belfus.

Jackson HC, Winkelman KK, Bichel WH: Nerve endings in the human lumbar spine column and related structures, *J Bone Joint Surg* 48A:1272, 1966.

Jensen MC, et al: Magnetic resonance imaging of the lumbar spine in people without back pain, *N Engl J Med* 331:69, 1994.

Johnson RJ: Low-back pain in sports: managing spondylolysis in young patients, *Physician Sports Med* 21:53, 1993.

Johnson RM, Murphy MJ, Southwick WO: Surgical approaches to the spine. In Rothman RH, Simeone FA, editors: *The spine,* ed 3, Philadelphia, 1992, WB Saunders.

Johnsson KE, Rosen I, Uden A: The natural course of lumbar spinal stenosis, *Clin Orthop* 279:82, 1992.

Jonsson B, Stromquist B: Symptoms and signs in degeneration of the lumbar spine, a prospective consecutive study of 300 operated patients, *J Bone Joint Surg* 75B:272, 1993.

Jonsson B, Stromquist B: Symptoms and signs in degeneration of the lumbar spine, *J Bone Joint Surg* 75B:381, 1993.

Kanner R: *Pain management secrets,* Philadelphia, 1997, Hanley & Belfus.

Kapandji IA: *The physiology of the joints, vol 3, the trunk and the vertebral column,* Edinburgh, 1974, Churchill Livingstone.

Katirji B: *Electromyography in clinical practice: a case study approach,* St Louis, 1998, Mosby.

Katirji B, Weissman JD: The ankle jerk and the tibial H-reflex: a clinical and electrophysiological correlation, *Electromyogr Clin Neurophysiol* 34:331, 1994.

Katz WA: *Rheumatic diseases diagnosis and management,* Philadelphia, 1977, JB Lippincott.

Katznelson A, Nerubay J, Level A: Gluteal skyline (G.S.L.): a search for an objective sign in the diagnosis of disc lesions of the lower lumbar spine, *Spine* 7:74, 1982.

Keats TE: *An atlas of normal roentgen variants that may simulate disease,* ed 2, Chicago, 1973, Year Book Medical Publishers.

Keats TE, Lusted LB: *Atlas of roentgenographic measurements,* ed 6, St Louis, 1990, Mosby.

Keim HA: *The adolescent spine,* ed 2, New York, 1976, Springer-Verlag.

Kelsey JL: An epidemiological study of acute herniated lumbar intervertebral disc, *Rheumatol Rehab* 14:144, 1975.

Kendall HO, Kendall FP, Wadsworth GE: *Muscles testing and function,* ed 2, Baltimore, 1971, Williams & Wilkins.

Kent DL, et al: Diagnosis of lumbar spinal stenosis in adults: a meta-analysis of the accuracy of CT, MR, and myelography, *AJR Am J Roentgenol* 158:1135, 1992.

Kernig W: Concerning a little noted sign of meningitis, *Arch Neurol* 21:216, 1969.

Kettenbach G: *Writing S.O.A.P. notes,* Philadelphia, 1990, FA Davis.

Khan MA, Linder SM: Ankylosing spondylitis: clinical aspects, *Spine* 4:529, 1990.

Kingston RS: Radiology of the spine. In Watkins RG, editor: *The spine in sports,* St Louis, 1996, Mosby.

Klippel JH, Dieppe PA: *Rheumatology,* vol 1-2, ed 2, London, 1998, Mosby.

Kosteljanetz M, Bang F, Schmidt-Olsen S: The clinical significance of straight-leg raising (Lasègue's sign) in the diagnosis of prolapsed lumbar disc: interobserver variation and correlation with surgical findings, *Spine* 13:393, 1988.

Krodel A, Sturtz H, Siebert CH: Indications for and results of operative treatment of spondylitis and spondylodiscitis, *Arch Orthop Trauma Surg* 110:78, 1991.

LaFreniere JG: *The low-back patient, procedures for treatment by physical therapy,* New York, 1985, Masson.

Lancourt J, Kettelhut M: Predicting return to work for lower back pain patients receiving worker's compensation, *Spine* 17:629, 1992.

Lavy CBD, Barrett DS: *Questions and answers on Apley's concise system of orthopaedics and fractures,* Oxford, 1991, Butterworth-Heinemann.

Lecuire J, et al: 641 operations for sciatic neuralgia due to discal hernia, a computerized statistical study of the results, *Neurochirugie (Stuttg)* 19:501, 1973.

Leffs M: *Back pain in the adolescent athlete,* Toronto, 1991, American Back Society.

Lerner AJ: *The little black book of neurology,* ed 3, St Louis, 1995, Mosby.

Lestini WF, Bell GR: Spinal infections: patient evaluation. In *Seminars in spine surgery,* vol 2, Philadelphia, 1990, WB Saunders.

Lewis CB, Knortz KA: *Orthopedic assessment and treatment of the geriatric patient,* St Louis, 1993, Mosby.

Loth TS: *Orthopedic boards review,* St Louis, 1993, Mosby.

Loth TS: *Orthopedic boards review II a case study approach,* St Louis, 1996, Mosby.

Lovett AW: A contribution to the study of the mechanics of the spine, *Am J Anat* 2:457, 1983.

MacNab I: *Backache,* Baltimore, 1977, Williams & Wilkins.

Magee DJ: *Orthopedic physical assessment,* ed 3, Philadelphia, 1997, WB Saunders.

Magora A: Investigation of the relation between low back pain and occupation: 4, physical requirements: bending, rotation, reaching and sudden maximal effort, *Scand J Rehabil Med* 5:186, 1973.

Maigne JY, Maigne R, Guerin-Surville H: The lumbar mamilla-accessory foramen: a study of 203 lumbosacral spines, *Surg Radiol Ant* 13:29, 1991.

Malone TR, McPoil TG, Nitz AJ: *Orthopedic and sports physical therapy,* ed 3, St Louis, 1997, Mosby.

Manaster BJ: *Handbooks in radiology skeletal radiology,* Chicago, 1989, Year Book Medical Publishers.

Mandelbaum BR, Gross MC: Spondylolysis and spondylolisthesis. In Reider B, editor: *Sports medicine: the school-age athlete,* Philadelphia, 1991, WB Saunders.

Marchand F, Ahmed A: Investigation of the laminate structure of lumbar disc anulus fibrosus, *Spine* 15:402, 1990.

Martin JH: *Neuroanatomy text and atlas,* ed 2, Stamford, Conn, 1996, Appleton & Lange.

Mason M, Currey HLF: *Clinical rheumatology,* Philadelphia, 1970, JB Lippincott.

Mathers LH, et al: *Clinical anatomy principles,* St Louis, 1996, Mosby.

Mayo Clinic and Mayo Foundation: *Clinical examinations in neurology,* ed 5, Philadelphia, 1981, WB Saunders.

Mazion JM: *Illustrated manual of neurological reflexes/signs/tests, part I, orthopedic signs/tests/maneuvers for office procedure, part II,* Orlando, 1980, Daniels Publishing.

McGill S: Quantitative intramuscular myoelectric activity of the quadratus lumborum during a wide variety of tasks, *Clin Biomech* 11:170, 1996.

McGill SM: The influence of lordosis on axial trunk torque and trunk muscle myoelectric activity, *Spine* 17:1187, 1992.

McKenzie RA: *The lumbar spine mechanical diagnosis and therapy,* Wikanae, New Zealand, 1981, Spinal Publications.

McNeil, et al: Trunk strengths in attempted flexion, extension, and lateral bending in healthy subjects and patients with low back disorders, *Spine* 5:529, 1980.

McRae R: *Clinical orthopaedic examination,* ed 3, Edinburgh, 1990, Churchill Livingstone.

McRae R: *Practical fracture treatment,* ed 3, New York, 1994, Churchill-Livingstone.

Medical Economics Books: *Patient care flow chart manual,* ed 3, Oradell, NJ, 1982, Medical Economics Books.

Mellion MB: *Sports medicine secrets,* Philadelphia, 1994, Hanley & Belfus.

Mellion MB: *Office sports medicine,* ed 2, St Louis, 1996, Mosby.

Mengel MB, Schwiebert LP: *Ambulatory medicine: the primary care of families,* ed 2, Stamford, Conn, 1996, Appleton & Lange.

Mennell JM: *Back pain,* Boston, 1960, Little, Brown.

Mennell JM: *The musculoskeletal system differential diagnosis from symptoms and physical signs,* Gaithersburg, Md, 1992, Aspen.

Mercier LR, Pettid FJ: *Practical orthopedics,* ed 4, St Louis, 1995, Mosby.

Merkow RL, Lane JM: Paget's disease of bone, *Orthop Clin North Am* 21:171, 1990.

Micheli LJ, Trapman E: Spinal deformities. In Torg S, Welsh RP, Shephard RJ, editors: *Current therapy in sports medicine,* ed 2, St Louis, 1990, Mosby.

Mooney V: Differential diagnosis of low back disorders. In Frymoyer JW, editor: *The adult spine: principles and practice,* New York, 1991, Raven.

Moore KL: *Clinically oriented anatomy,* ed 3, Baltimore, 1992, Williams & Wilkins.

Morris JM, Lucas DB, Bresler B: Role of the trunk in stability of the spine, *J Bone Joint Surg* 43A:327, 1961.

Mosby-Year Book, Inc: *Expert 10-minute physical examination,* St Louis, 1997, Mosby.

Nachemson A: The lumbar spine-an orthopaedic challenge, *Spine* 1:59, 1976.

Nachemson AL: Newest knowledge on low back pain, *Clin Orthop* 279:8, 1992.

Nakamura SI: Afferent pathways of discogenic low back pain: evaluation of L2 spinal nerve infiltration, *J Bone Joint Surg* 78B:606, 1996.

Nettina SM: *The Lippincott manual of nursing practice,* ed 6, Philadelphia, 1996, Lippincott.

Newton RW: *Color atlas of pediatric neurology,* St Louis, 1995, Mosby-Wolfe.

Nicholas JA, Hershman EB: *The lower extremity & spine in sports medicine,* vol 1-2, ed 2, St Louis, 1995, Mosby.

Nishada T, et al: H reflex in S-1 radiculopathy: latency versus amplitude controversy revisited, *Muscle Nerve* 19:915, 1996.

Nitta H, et al: Study on dermatomes by means of selective lumbar spinal nerve block, *Spine* 18:1782, 1993.

Nordin M, Andersson GBJ, Pope MH: *Musculoskeletal disorders in the workplace: principles and practice,* St Louis, 1997, Mosby.

O'Connor MI, Carrier BI: Metastatic disease of the spine, *Orthopedics* 15:611, 1992.

O'Donoghue DH: *Treatment of injuries to patients,* ed 4, Philadelphia, 1984, WB Saunders.

Olmarker K, Rydevik B: Pathophysiology of sciatica, *Orthop Clin North Am* 22:223, 1991.

Olson WH, et al: *Handbook of symptom-oriented neurology,* ed 2, St Louis, 1994, Mosby.

Omer GE, Spinner M: *Management of peripheral nerve problems,* Philadelphia, 1980, WB Saunders.

O'Young B, Young MA, Stiens SA: *PM&R secrets,* Philadelphia, 1997, Hanley & Belfus.

Padley S, et al: Assessment of a single spine radiograph in low back pain, *Br J Radiol* 63:535, 1990.

Pagana KD, Pagana TJ: *Mosby's manual of diagnostic and laboratory tests,* St Louis, 1998, Mosby.

Patten J: *Neurological differential diagnosis,* ed 2, London, 1996, Springer.

Patton KT: *Student survival guide for anatomy and physiology,* St Louis, 1999, Mosby.

Perkin, GD: *Mosby's color atlas and text of neurology,* London, 1998, Mosby-Wolfe.

Perrone C, et al: Pyogenic and tuberculous spondylodiscitis (vertebral osteomyelitis) in 80 adult patients, *Clin Infect Dis* 19:746, 1994.

Pheasant S: *Ergonomics, work and health,* Gaithersburg, Md, 1991, Aspen.

Phillips LH, Parks TS: Electrophysiologic mapping of the segmental anatomy of the muscles of the lower extremity, *Muscle Nerve* 14:1213, 1991.

Pomeranz SJ, Pretorius HT, Ramsingh PS: Bone scintigraphy and multimodality imaging in bone neoplasia: strategies for imaging in the new health care climate, *Semin Nucl Med* 24:188, 1994.

Pope MH, et al: *Occupational low back pain assessment, treatment and prevention,* St Louis, 1991, Mosby.

Porterfield JA, DeRosa C: *Mechanical low back pain: perspectives in functional anatomy,* Philadelphia, 1991, WB Saunders.

Post M: *Physical examination of the musculoskeletal system,* Chicago, 1987, Mosby.

Postacchini F, Cinotti G: Bone regrowth after surgical decompression for lumbar spinal stenosis, *J Bone Joint Surg* 74B:862, 1992.

Rachlin ES: *Myofascial pain and fibromyalgia trigger point management,* St Louis, 1994, Mosby.

Rantanen J, Hurme M, Falck B: The lumbar multifidus muscle five years after surgery for a lumbar intervertebral disc herniation, *Spine* 18:568, 1993.

Ravel R: *Clinical laboratory medicine clinical application of laboratory data,* ed 6, St Louis, 1995, Mosby.

Resnick D, Niwayama G: *Diagnosis of bone and joint disorders,* Philadelphia, 1995, WB Saunders.

Ro CS: Sacroiliac joint. In Cox JM, editor: *Low back pain: mechanism, diagnosis and treatment,* ed 5, Baltimore, 1990, Williams & Wilkins.

Rodnitzky RL: *Van Allen's pictorial manual of neurologic tests: a guide to the performance and interpretation of the neurologic examination,* ed 3, Chicago, 1969, Mosby.

Rossignol M, Suissa S, Abenhaim L: The evolution of compensated occupational spinal injuries: a three-year follow-up study, *Spine* 17:1043, 1992.

Rothman RH, Simeone FA: *The spine,* ed 3, Philadelphia, 1992, WB Saunders.

Rumack CM, Wilson SR, Charboneau JW: *Diagnostic ultrasound,* vol 1-2, ed 2, St Louis, 1998, Mosby.

Saal JA, Saal JS, Herzog RJ: The natural history of lumbar intervertebral disc extrusions treated nonoperatively, *Spine* 15:683, 1990.

Saidoff DC, McDonough AL: *Critical pathways in therapeutic intervention,* St Louis, 1997, Mosby.

Salovy P, et al: Reporting chronic pain episodes on health surveys, *Vital Health Stat* 6, 1992.

Scham SM, Taylor TKF: Tension signs in lumbar disc prolapse, *Clin Orthop* 75:195, 1971.

Schmorl G: *The human spine in health and disease,* ed 2, New York, 1971, Grune & Stratton.

Schofferman J, Wassermann S: Successful treatment of low back pain and/or neck pain due to a motor vehicle accident, *Spine* 19:1007, 1994.

Schofferman J, et al: Childhood psychological trauma and chronic refractory low back pain, *Clin J Pain* 9:260, 1993.

Schumacher HR, Klippel JH, Koopman WJ: *Primer on the rheumatic diseases,* ed 10, Atlanta, 1993, Arthritis Foundation.

Schwarzer AC, et al: Prevalence and clinical features of lumbar zygapophyseal joint pain: a study in an Australian population with chronic low back pain, *Ann Rheum Dis* 54:100, 1995.

Seidel HM, et al: *Mosby's guide to physical examination,* ed 4, St Louis, 1999, Mosby.

Shankman GA: *Fundamental orthopedic management for the examiner,* St Louis, 1997, Mosby.

Simons DG: Muscle pain syndromes, *J Manual Med* 6:3, 1991.

Sledge CB, Poss R: *The year book of orthopedics 1997,* St Louis, 1997, Mosby.

Smith MD, Bohlman HH: Spondylolisthesis treated by a single-stage operation combining decompression with in situ posterolateral and anterior fusion, *J Bone Joint Surg* 72:415, 1990.

Smith SA, et al: Straight leg raising: anatomical effects on the spinal nerve root without and with fusion, *Spine* 18:992, 1993.

Spangfort E: Lasègue's sign in patients with lumbar disc herniation, *Acta Orthop* 42:459, 1971.

Specht NT, Russo RD: *Practical guide to diagnostic imaging,* St Louis, 1998, Mosby.

Spengler DM, Szpalski M: Newer assessment approaches for the patient with low back pain, *Contemp Orthop* 21, 1990.

Starlanyl D, Copeland ME: *Fibromyalgia & chronic myofascial pain syndrome a survival manual,* Oakland, Calif, 1996, New Harbinger Publications.

Stauffer ES, et al: Fractures and dislocations of the spine, part II, the thoracolumbar spine. In Rockwood CA, Green DP, Bucholz RW, editors: *Fractures in adults,* ed 3, Philadelphia, 1991, JB Lippincott.

Stedman TL: *Stedman's medical dictionary,* ed 25, Baltimore, 1990, Williams & Wilkins.

Stewart DL, Abeln SH: *Documenting functional outcomes in physical therapy,* St Louis, 1993, Mosby.

Stinson JT: Spondylolysis and spondylolisthesis in the athlete, *Clin Sports Med* 12:517, 1993.

Stith WJ: Exercise and the intervertebral disc, *Spine* 4:259, 1990.

Stoller DW: *Magnetic resonance imaging in orthopaedics & sports medicine,* Philadelphia, 1993, JB Lippincott.

Sward L: The thoracolumbar spine in young elite patients, *Sports Med* 13:357, 1992.

Sward L, et al: Anthropometric characteristics, passive hip flexion, and spinal mobility in relation to back pain in patients, *Spine* 15:376, 1990.

Sward L, et al: Disc degeneration and associated abnormalities of the spine in elite patients: a magnetic resonance imaging study, *Spine* 16:437, 1991.

Tan JC, Horn SE: *Practical manual of physical medicine and rehabilitation,* St Louis, 1998, Mosby.

Taylor JR: The development and adult structure of lumbar intervertebral discs, *J Manual Med* 5:43, 1990.

Thelander U, et al: Straight leg raising test versus radiologic size, shape, and position of lumbar disc hernias, *Spine* 17:395, 1992.

Thibodeau GA, Patton KT: *Anatomy & physiology,* ed 4, St Louis, 1999, Mosby.

Thompson GH: Back pain in children, *J Bone Joint Surg* 75A:928, 1993.

Thompson JM: *Clinical outlines for health assessment,* St Louis, 1997, Mosby.

Toghill PJ: *Examining patients: an introduction to clinical medicine,* London, 1990, Edward Arnold.

Tollison CD, Satterthwaite JR, Tollison JW: *Handbook of pain management,* ed 2, Baltimore, 1994, Williams & Wilkins.

Torg JS, Shepard RJ: *Current therapy in sports medicine,* ed 3, St Louis, 1995, Mosby.

Traill Z, Richards MA, Moore NR: Magnetic resonance imaging of metastatic bone disease, *Clin Orthop* 312:76, 1995.

Tumeh SS, Tohmeh AG: Nuclear medicine techniques in septic arthritis and osteomyelitis, *Rheum Dis Clin North Am* 17:559, 1991.

Turek SL: *Orthopaedics principles and their application,* ed 3, Philadelphia, 1977, JB Lippincott.

Twomey L, Taylor JR: Structural and mechanical disc changes with age, *J Manual Med* 5:58, 1990.

Uhthoff J: Prenatal development of the iliolumbar ligament, *J Bone Joint Surg* 75:93, 1993.

Urban LM: The straight-leg-raising test: a review, *J Orthop Sports Phys Ther* 2:117, 1981.

Van Holsbeeck M, Introcaso JH: *Musculoskeletal ultrasound,* St Louis, 1991, Mosby.

Vernon-Roberts B, Perie CJ: Degenerative changes in the intervertebral disc of the lumbar spine and their sequela, *Rheum Rehab* 16:13, 1977.

Vleeming A, et al: The posterior layer of the thoracolumbar fascia. Its function in load transfer from spine to legs, *Spine* 20:753, 1995.

Waddell G, et al: Nonorganic physical signs in low back pain, *Spine* 5:177, 1980.

Waddell G, et al: Objective clinical evaluation of physical impairment in chronic low back pain, *Spine* 17:617, 1992.

Wakefield TS, Frank RG: *The examiner's guide to neuro musculoskeletal practice,* Abbotsford, Wisc, 1995, Allied Health of Wisconsin, S.C.

Walsh MJ: Evaluation of orthopedic testing of the low back for non-specific low back pain, *J Manipulative Physiol Ther* 21:232, 1998.

Walsh TR, et al: Lumbar discography in normal subjects, a controlled, prospective study, *J Bone Joint Surg* 72A:1081, 1990.

Watkins RG: *The spine in sports,* St Louis, 1996, Mosby.

Weineck J: *Functional anatomy in sports,* ed 2, St Louis, 1990, Mosby.

Weinerman SA, Bockman RS: Medical therapy of osteoporosis, *Orthop Clin North Am* 21:109, 1990.

Weinstein SL, Buckwalter JA: *Turek's orthopaedics principles and their application,* ed 5, Philadelphia, 1994, JB Lippincott.

Westmark KD, Weissman BN: Complications of axial arthropathies, *Orthop Clin North Am* 21:427, 1990.

White AA III, Panjabi MM: *Clinical biomechanics of the spine,* Philadelphia, 1978, JB Lippincott.

White AA III, Panjabi MM: The basic kinematics of the human spine, a review of past and current knowledge, *Spine* 3:12, 1978.

White AH, Schofferman JA: *Spine care,* vol 1-2, St Louis, 1995, Mosby.

White G: *Regional dermatology,* London, 1994, Mosby-Wolfe.

White G: *Levene's color atlas of dermatology,* ed 2, London, 1997, Mosby-Wolfe.

Whitmore I, Willan PLT: *Multiple choice questions in human anatomy,* London, 1995, Mosby.

Wicke L: *Atlas of radiologic anatomy,* ed 5, Philadelphia, 1994, Lea & Febiger.

Wiesel SW, Bernini P, Rothman RH: *The aging lumbar spine,* Philadelphia, 1982, WB Saunders.

Wilder DG: The biomechanics of vibration and low back pain, *Am J Ind Med* 23:577, 1993.

Wilkins RH, Brody IA: Lasègue's sign, *Arch Neurol* 21:219, 1969.

Willeford G: *Medical word finder,* West Nyack, NY, 1967, Parker Publishing.

Willis Jr WD, Coggeshall RE: *Sensory mechanisms of the spinal cord,* ed 2, New York, 1991, Plenum.

Windsor RE, Lox DM: *Soft tissue injuries: diagnosis and treatment,* Philadelphia, 1998, Hanley & Belfus.

Woodhall R, Hayes GJ: The well-leg-raising test, *N Engl J Med* 297:1127, 1977.

Xu GL, Haughton VM, Carrera GF: Lumbar facet joint capsule: appearance at MR imaging and CT, *Radiology* 177:415, 1990.

Xu GL, et al: Normal variation of the lumbar facet joint capsules, *Clin Anat* 4:11122, 1991.

Yochum TR: *A closer look at spondylolisthesis,* East Rutherford, 1990, NYCC Second Multidisciplinary Symposium.

Yochum TR, Rowe L: *Essentials of skeletal radiology,* ed 2, Baltimore, 1996, Williams & Wilkins.

Yoshizawa H, Kobayashi S, Hachiya Y: Blood supply of nerve roots and dorsal root ganglia, *Orthop Clin North Am* 22:195, 1991.

Zatouroff M: *Diagnosis in color physical signs in general medicine,* ed 2, London, 1996, Mosby-Wolfe.

Zitelli BJ, Davis HW: *Atlas of pediatric physical diagnosis,* ed 2, London, 1992, Wolfe.

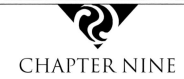

THE PELVIS AND SACROILIAC JOINT

AXIOMS IN PELVIS AND SACROILIAC JOINT ASSESSMENT

- The primary function of the pelvis, including the bones, joints, ligaments, and muscles, is the mechanical transfer of weight.
- A secondary function of the bony pelvis is protection of the viscera.

INTRODUCTION

The pelvis is a uniquely devised mechanism designed to transfer the body weight from the single weight-bearing axis of the trunk to the bipolar weight bearing of the lower extremities. The spine attaches to the pelvis by a single connection to the sacrum. Weight transfers through the bony ring of the pelvis, from the spinal column to the two lower extremities. Enclosed within the pelvis is the bladder, the female genitalia, the rectum, and the great vessels and nerves that extend to the lower extremity.

Narrow, closely fitted, irregularly shaped and cartilage-covered surfaces of the posterior and internal ilium and the lateral border of the sacrum form the sacroiliac articulation. The lumbosacral trunk lies anteriorly in direct relationship to the sacroiliac articulation. An inflammatory neuritis is a common accompaniment of sacroiliac arthritis. The anterior ligaments are thin and easily distended by intraarticular swelling.

The upper two thirds of the joint are covered posteriorly by the posterior end of the ilium. The lower third of the joint is covered by the sacroiliac ligaments but can often be palpated in thin individuals.

The conditions that affect the sacroiliac joints are those that involve any joint. The sacroiliac articulation is a favored site for tuberculous infection and is often the starting point for ankylosing spondylitis. Degenerative arthritic changes often are significant at this joint.

The stability of the sacroiliac joint lies in the nature of its articular surfaces and ligaments (Fig. 9-2). Cardinal in this role are the dense, interosseous ligaments lying dorsal to the joint and the ventral sacroiliac ligament covering its anterior aspect.

In ankylosing spondylitis, the patient complains of spinal pain and stiffness. The sacroiliac joints are affected initially; increasing loss of spinal mobility can lead to loss of the lumbar lordosis (Fig. 9-3).

A common tender fatty nodule in the sacroiliac area is sometimes called the *episacroiliac lipoma* or "back mouse." In this instance, fatty tissue herniates through the normal deep fascia and become edematous and a source of pain. Clinically, the patient complains of pain in the tender nodules that are palpable and often bilateral. The mass is usually palpable as a mobile soft tumor that slips beneath the examining finger.

ESSENTIAL ANATOMY

The two innominate bones (or "hip" bones), the sacrum, and the coccyx (Fig. 9-4) make up the pelvis. The innominate bone consists of the of the ilium, ischium, and pubis (Fig. 9-5).

TABLE 9-1

PELVIS AND SACROILIAC CROSS-REFERENCE TABLE BY ASSESSMENT PROCEDURE

Pelvis

Test/Sign

	Disease Assessed					
	Sacroiliac Pathology	Lumbosacral Syndrome	Sprain	Subluxation	Fracture	Pyogenic Sacroiliitis
Anterior innominate test	●					
Belt test	●	●				
Erichsen's sign	●					
Gaenslen's test	●	●				
Gapping test	●		●			
Goldthwait's sign	●	●				
Hibb's test	●		●	●		
Iliac compression test	●		●	●	●	
Knee-to-shoulder test	●		●	●		●
Laguerre's test	●		●	●		
Lewin-Gaenslen's test	●		●	●		
Piedallu's sign	●		●	●		
Sacral apex test	●		●	●		
Sacroiliac resisted-abduction test			●	●		
Smith-Petersen test	●	●				
Squish test			●			
Yeoman's test	●		●	●		

TABLE 9-2

PELVIS AND SACROILIAC JOINT CROSS-REFERENCE TABLE BY SYNDROME OR TISSUE

Fracture	Iliac compression test
Lumbosacral syndrome	Belt test
	Gaenslen's test
	Smith-Petersen test
Pyogenic sacroilitis	Knee-to-shoulder test
Sacroiliac pathology	Anterior innominate test
	Belt test
	Erichsen's sign
	Gaenslen's test
	Gapping test
	Goldthwait's sign
	Hibb's test
	Iliac compression test
	Knee-to-shoulder test
	Laguerre's test
	Lewin-Gaenslen's test
	Piedallu's sign
	Sacral apex test
	Smith-Petersen test
	Yeoman's test
Sprain	Gapping test
	Hibb's test
	Iliac compression test
	Knee-to-shoulder test
	Laguerre's test
	Lewin-Gaenslen's test
	Piedallu's sign
	Sacral apex test
	Sacroiliac resisted-abduction test
	Squish test
	Yeoman's test
Subluxation	Hibb's test
	Iliac compression test
	Knee-to-shoulder test
	Laguerre's test
	Lewin-Gaenslen's test
	Piedallu's sign
	Sacral apex test
	Sacroiliac resisted-abduction test
	Yeoman's test

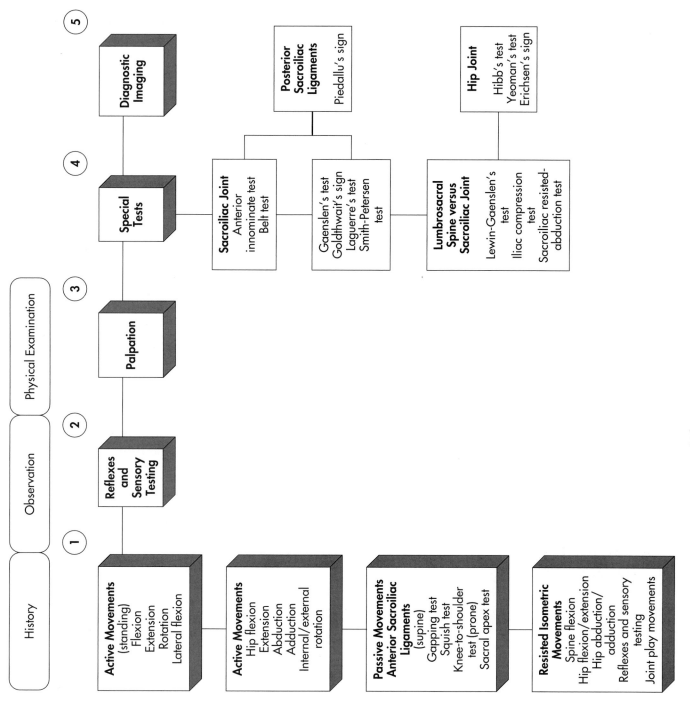

FIG. 9-1 Sacroiliac joint assessment.

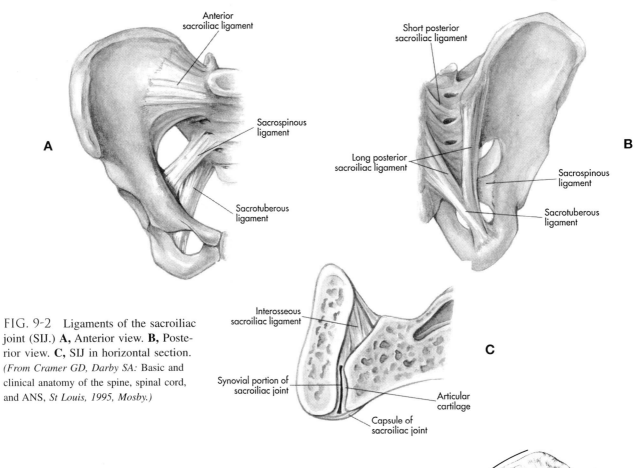

FIG. 9-2   Ligaments of the sacroiliac joint (SIJ.) **A,** Anterior view. **B,** Posterior view. **C,** SIJ in horizontal section. *(From Cramer GD, Darby SA: Basic and clinical anatomy of the spine, spinal cord, and ANS, St Louis, 1995, Mosby.)*

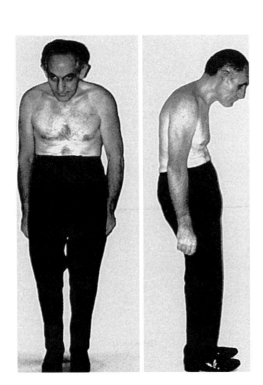

FIG. 9-3   Gross postural changes in man affected by ankylosing spondylitis. *(From Seidel HM, et al: Mosby's guide to physical examination, ed 4, St Louis, 1999, Mosby.)*

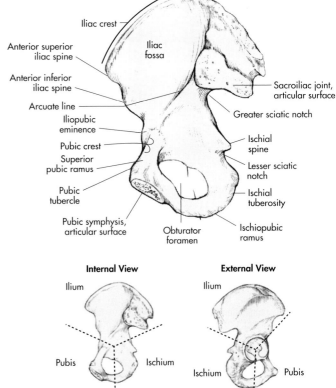

FIG. 9-4   Interior of the pelvis.   *(From Mathers LH, et al: Clinical anatomy principles, St Louis, 1996, Mosby.)*

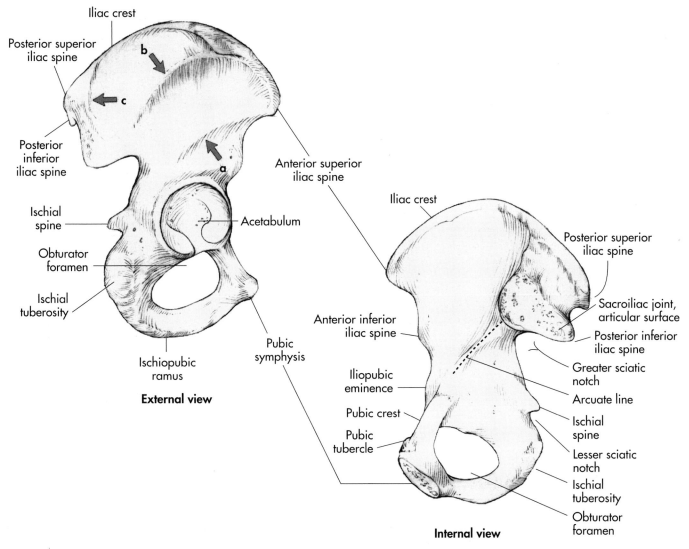

FIG. 9-5 Innominate bone. *(From Mathers LH, et al:* Clinical anatomy principles, *St Louis, 1996, Mosby.)*

ORTHOPEDIC GAMUT 9-1

INNOMINATE BONE

The exterior surface of the innominate bone consists of the following:

1. An upper area, the lateral surface of the ilium
2. A central depressed socket, the acetabulum
3. A lower region, in which curved rami of the pubis and ischium form the obturator foramen

---

ORTHOPEDIC GAMUT 9-2

SUPERIOR HALF OF THE PELVIS

The interior surface of the superior half of the pelvis is as follows:

1. Superiorly, the iliac fossa, a shallow depression in the ilium
2. A posterior roughened articular surface
3. Inferiorly, the medial surface of obturator foramen

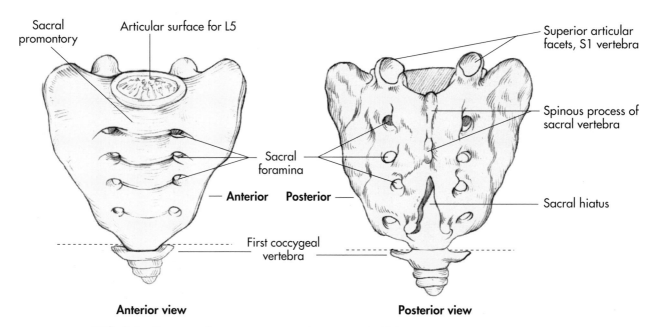

Anterior view   **Posterior view**

FIG. 9-6   Sacrum and coccyx. *(From Mathers LH, et al:* Clinical anatomy principles, *St Louis, 1996, Mosby.)*

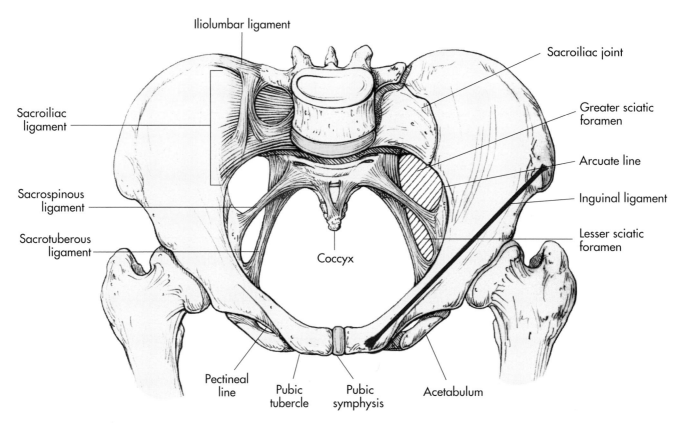

FIG. 9-7   Pelvic ligaments, superoanterior view.   *(From Mathers LH, et al:* Clinical anatomy principles, *St Louis, 1996, Mosby.)*

The sacrum is the fusion of five sacral vertebrae, separate in embryonic life. The fusion of these vertebrae yields a bony shield, shaped like a curved inverted triangle (Fig. 9-6).

The body of vertebra L5 articulates directly with an upward-facing articular surface on the sacrum (forming the lumbosacral joint). The iliolumbar ligaments connect the transverse processes of L5 to the iliac rests on each side (Fig. 9-7).

The lumbosacral plexus (Fig. 9-8) takes shape on the medial surface of the levator ani muscle (Table 9-3).

The sciatic nerve (L4 to S3), the largest peripheral nerve in the body (Fig. 9-9), divides into the common peroneal and tibial nerves. It exits the pelvis through the greater sciatic foramen inferior to piriformis and lies deep to the gluteus maximus.

ESSENTIAL MOTION ASSESSMENT

Although firmly constrained by its ligaments, the sacroiliac joint exhibits movements that are small in magnitude and complex in nature. The amplitude of nutation of the sacrum is normally not more than 2 mm or 2 degrees.

The sacroiliac joint consequently serves as a stress-relieving joint, the tension that otherwise would have been imposed on bone being absorbed by the sacroiliac ligaments, at the expense of slight distracting and sliding movements between the sacrum and ilium.

The pelvis plays an active role in gait, or walking. The femoral heads articulate with the acetabulum on each side, and as one and then the other femur strides forward, the pelvis must "rock" from side to side. Viewed from above,

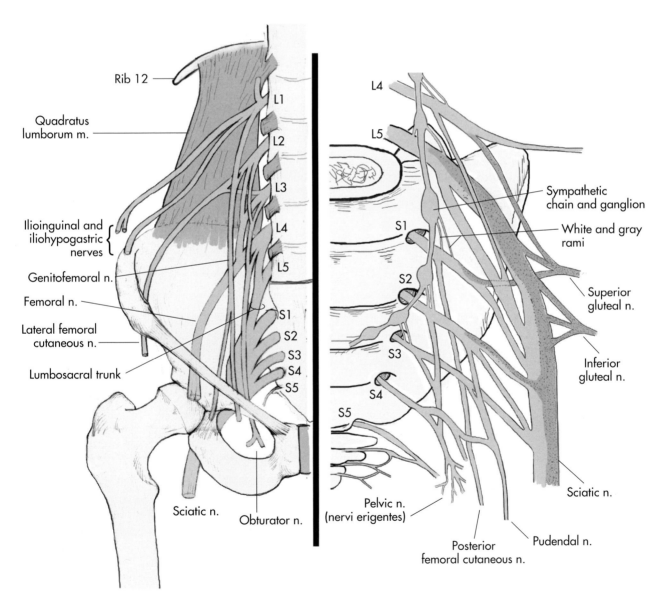

FIG. 9-8 Lumbosacral plexus. *(From Mathers LH, et al:* Clinical anatomy principles, *St Louis, 1996, Mosby.)*

the pelvis appears to rotate its right side anteriorly when the right lower limb strides forward, and the left side of the pelvis moves forward when the left lower limb swings forward.

If the hip joints should become less mobile, as a result of arthritis for example, the head of the femur will not rotate easily within the acetabulum. This condition results in a limitation on the length of the stride and/or in pain accompanying gait.

TABLE 9-3

SACRAL PLEXUS

Anterior Divisions	Posterior Divisions
Nerve to quadratus femoris/ inferior gemellus	Nerve to piriformis
Nerve to obturator internus/ superior gemellus	Superior gluteal nerve
Posterior femoral cutaneous nerve*	Inferior gluteal nerve
Tibial nerve	Posterior femoral cutaneous nerve*
Pudendal nerve	Common peroneal nerve
Pelvic splanchnic nerves	Perforating cutaneous nerve
Nerve to levator ani/coccygeus	—

Adapted from Mathers LH, et al: *Clinical anatomy principles,* St Louis, 1996, Mosby.
*Both divisions contribute to this nerve.

ORTHOPEDIC GAMUT 9-3

LUMBOPELVIC FLEXIBILITY TESTING

Following are lumbopelvic flexibility testing procedures:

1. *Spinal erector muscles:* With the patient in the supine position, the examiner gently bends the patient's knee to the chest.
2. *Hip flexor muscles:* With the patient prone, the examiner places the affected hip into extension, and then abducts the thigh.
3. *Hamstring muscles:* Placing the patient supine and keeping the patient's hips and buttocks down to the table, the examiner performs a straight leg raise with the knee held in extension.
4. *Gluteal muscles:* The patient should be supine and placed in hip flexion with a bent knee. The lower leg can be internally rotated with thigh adduction to facilitate a stretch of the rotator muscles of the hip, such as the gluteus medius and piriformis.
5. *Quadriceps muscles:* With the patient prone and the examiner's inferior hand on the affected knee, the examiner uses his or her shoulder to move the lower leg gently toward the ipsilateral buttock to induce knee flexion.

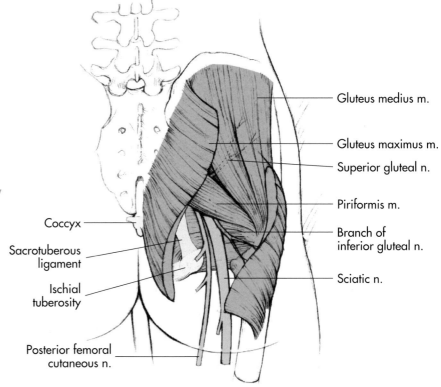

FIG. 9-9   Posterior branches of the sacral plexus.   *(From Mathers LH, et al:* Clinical anatomy principles, *St Louis, 1996, Mosby.)*

Gluteus medius m.

Gluteus maximus m.

Superior gluteal n.

Piriformis m.

Branch of inferior gluteal n.

Sciatic n.

Coccyx

Sacrotuberous ligament

Ischial tuberosity

Posterior femoral cutaneous n.

ESSENTIAL MUSCLE FUNCTION ASSESSMENT

The gluteal and erector muscles aid in stabilizing the spine and provide extension. To evaluate functional strength in spinal extension, the examiner places the patient in a prone position. The patient raises one arm out straight in front and simultaneously lifts the leg on the opposite side out straight. The patient holds this position for 5 to 10 seconds, and the examiner notes any fatigue or inability to gain a healthy contraction, especially on the side of the leg lift. This side activates the hip and spinal extensor mass. The patient repeats the exercise on the opposite side, and the examiner compares the observations.

ESSENTIAL IMAGING

The pelvis can be well visualized by a routine antero-posterior (AP) roentgenogram (Figs. 9-10 and 9-11). In addition, the sacrum and coccyx may be studied by lateral views (Fig. 9-12) and AP views angled 15 degrees cephalad and caudad (Figs. 9-13 and 9-14).

Radiographic evaluation could play an important role in ruling out an inflammatory arthritis. Conditions such as ankylosing spondylitis can have a clinical presentation similar to other spondyloarthropathies, with referral of pain into the hip and gluteal regions. After pregnancy, conditions such as osteitis condensans ilii can also be identified with plain films. In this case, the soft-tissue findings cannot be evaluated with plain films.

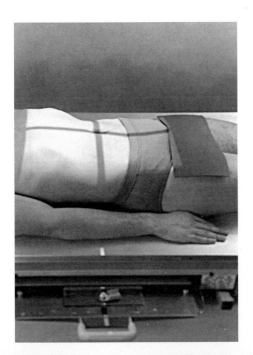

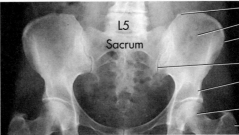

FIG. 9-10   Male anteroposterior abdomen with gonad shield. *(From Ballinger PW:* Merrill's atlas of radiographic positions and radiologic procedures, *vol 1-3, ed 8, St Louis, 1995, Mosby.)*

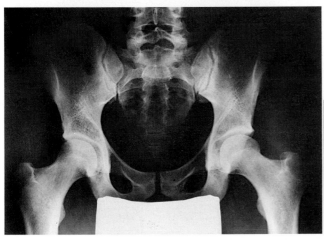

FIG. 9-11   Male anteroposterior pelvis. *(From Ballinger PW:* Merrill's atlas of radiographic positions and radiologic procedures, *vol 1-3, ed 8, St Louis, 1995, Mosby.)*

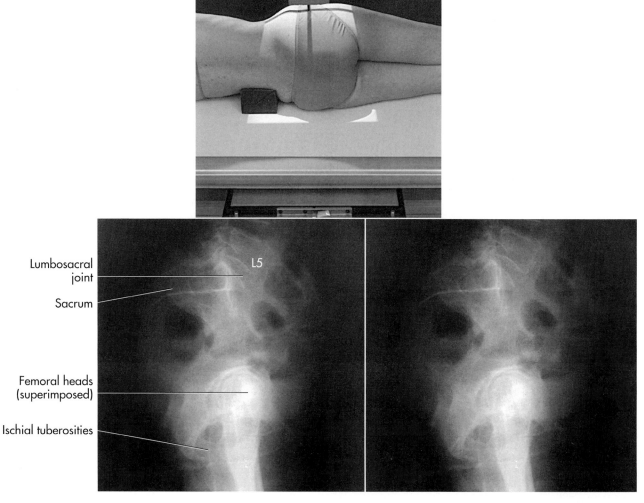

Lumbosacral
joint

Sacrum

Femoral heads
(superimposed)

Ischial tuberosities

L5

FIG. 9-12   Lateral pelvis.   *(From Ballinger PW:* Merrill's atlas of radiographic positions and radiologic procedures, *vol 1-3, ed 8, St Louis, 1995, Mosby.)*

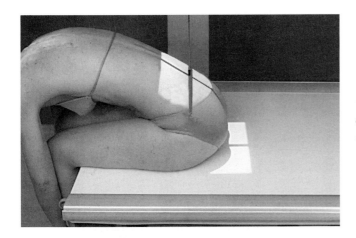

FIG. 9-13   Axial pelvis.   *(From Ballinger PW:* Merrill's atlas of radiographic positions and radiologic procedures, *vol 1-3, ed 8, St Louis, 1995, Mosby.)*

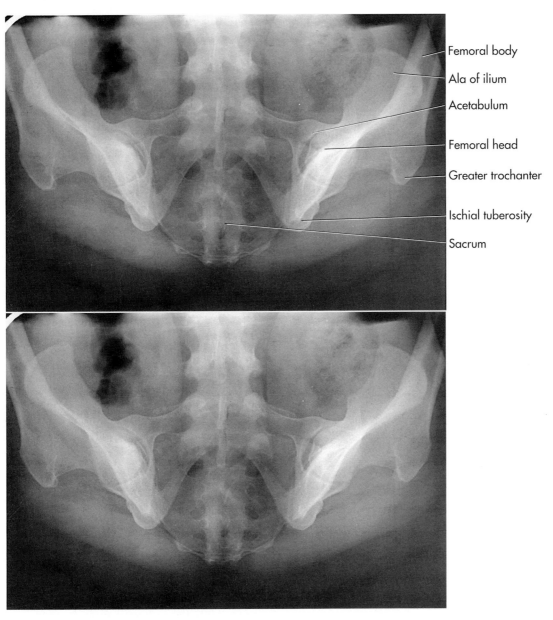

Femoral body

Ala of ilium

Acetabulum

Femoral head

Greater trochanter

Ischial tuberosity

Sacrum

FIG. 9-14   Axial pelvis.   *(From Ballinger PW:* Merrill's atlas of radiographic positions and radiologic procedures, *vol 1-3, ed 8, St Louis, 1995, Mosby.)*

MAZION'S PELVIC MANEUVER

Assessment for Unilateral Forward Displacement of the Ilia on the Sacrum

Comment

Many cases of acute low back pain that are not correctly identified evolve into a chronic spinal problem with significant disability at the muscular level (Table 9-4). Muscular fixation alone can be the cause of spinal joint dysfunction.

ORTHOPEDIC GAMUT 9-4

LUMBOPELVIC MUSCLES

Lumbopelvic muscle contractures result in the following:

1. Contracture of lumbodorsal fascia
2. Anterior pelvic tilt
3. Inappropriate transfer of loads to the lumbar spine
4. Difficulty in attaining the proper biomechanical posture for lifting

---

TABLE 9-4

LUMBOPELVIC SYNDROMES

Diagnosis	Site of Complaint
Quadratus lumborum syndrome	Gluteal region, anterior iliac spine, greater trochanter of femur
Gluteus maximus or medius syndrome	Sacral and gluteal region, lateral hip
Gluteus minimus syndrome	Lateral hip, thigh, and calf
Chronic lumbar strain (spinal erector muscles)	Laterally to ribs, caudally toward lumbosacral junction
Piriformis syndrome	Sacroiliac region; posterior hip, thigh, calf; possibly sole of foot

Adapted from Brier SR: *Primary care orthopedics,* St Louis, 1999, Mosby.

ORTHOPEDIC GAMUT 9-5

LUMBOPELVIC SPINE MUSCULAR SYNDROMES

Following are the clinical findings of lumbopelvic spine muscular syndromes:

1. Hip inflexibility
2. Weakness of the hip and spine extensor mechanism
3. Intersegmental lumbosacral fixation
4. Myofascial trigger points in the spinal erector, quadratus lumborum, gluteal musculature, and psoas muscles
5. Referred zones of pain to the hip, buttocks, thigh and lateral lower leg
6. Severe tightness of the outward rotators of the hip
7. Muscle hypertonicity
8. Palpable tenderness with pressure or stretch
9. Taut, tender, or ropelike muscle fibers

A sprain of the iliosacral ligaments is possible. The injury affects the ligament that extends from the posterior projection of the wing of the ilium to the posterior sacrum. The sprain of this ligament also can have an effect within the pelvis. Many of the conditions identified as sacroiliac sprains were actually other diseases. The sacroiliac ligaments are so strong that ordinary stresses will cause damage to the lumbosacral ligament before they cause damage to the sacroiliac ligaments.

After injury of the sacroiliac joint, pain localizes to the articular structures. There also may be referred pain to the groin, hamstrings, or back of the thigh. Ordinarily, this pain will not be along the sciatic distribution. Many of the tests that will elicit pain in the sacroiliac joint will also be positive in conditions such as ruptured intervertebral disc, sciatic neuritis, and lumbosacral sprain. The fact that the tests cause pain is of little significance. The significance is in the location of the pain. The common tests—such as straight leg raising, which puts torsion force on the sacroiliac joint, or the similar test of forward flexion of the trunk while the knees are straight—will cause pain when

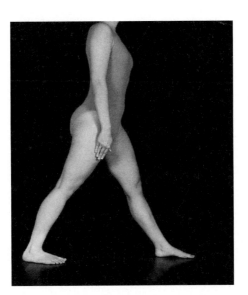

FIG. 9-15   The patient is standing and is instructed to take a big step forward, placing the unaffected leg 2 or 3 feet ahead of the affected leg.

sacroiliac joint involvement exists. Some tests stress the sacroiliac area specifically. Gaenslen's test involves flexing the opposite thigh on the abdomen to immobilize the pelvis in forward flexion. Next, the involved leg is pushed into hyperextension, which causes rotary stress on the sacroiliac joint.

PROCEDURE

- The patient with lower trunk pain is in the standing position and instructed to place the lower extremity that is opposite the painful side approximately 2 or 3 feet in front of the foot of the other extremity (Fig. 9-15).
- This position makes it appear as if the patient is taking a big step forward.
- The patient then bends the upper trunk acutely over the forward extremity, to put all the weight on the front leg (Fig. 9-16).
- The patient flexes to the point at which the heel of the back foot raises from the floor (Fig. 9-17).

- The production or aggravation of lower trunk pain on the side of the posterior leg indicates a positive test.
- A positive test indicates unilateral forward displacement of the ilia (anterior innominate) in relation to the sacrum.

Confirmation Procedures
Knee-to-shoulder test, Lewin-Gaenslen's test, Piedallu's sign, sacral apex test, and sacroiliac resisted-abduction test

---

DIAGNOSTIC STATEMENT

The anterior innominate test is positive on the right. This result indicates unilateral forward displacement of the ilia on the sacrum.

CLINICAL PEARL

The sacroiliac joint, most inaccessible to palpation, is difficult to assess clinically. Only florid inflammation or damage to the fibrous portion is likely to result in local posterior tenderness. This tenderness is probably ligamentous.

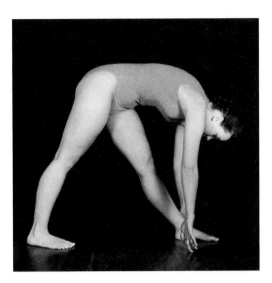

FIG. 9-16   The patient flexes at the waist and tries to touch the floor. This movement places weight onto the forward leg and stretches the affected sacroiliac joint.

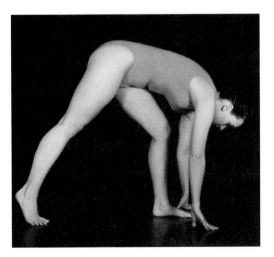

FIG. 9-17   The production of pain in the lower trunk, especially on the affected side, as the heel on the affected side lifts, indicates a positive test. A positive test indicates unilateral forward displacement of the ilium in relation to the sacrum.

BELT TEST

SUPPORTED ADAM'S TEST

Assessment for Sprain of the Sacroiliac Ligaments or Lumbosacral Capsular Sprain

Comment

Sacroiliac sprain denotes painful stretching of the ligaments around the joint. The occurrence of this condition is uncommon because the sacroiliac ligaments are very strong. The movements of bending, lifting, and hyperextension that produce torsion strain of the joint are more likely to cause a sprain of the thinner capsular ligaments surrounding the small lumbosacral joints. However, there can be no question that sacroiliac sprain does occur. It is identifiable by its acute onset during a torsion movement and by tenderness over the joint accentuated by a maneuver that reproduces the sprain.

Certain circumstances favor sprain of the sacroiliac ligaments. The ligaments are softened and elongated by pregnancy, prolonged periods of bending and lifting, or degenerative arthritis. The mechanism of injury usually involves the act of straightening up from a stooped position. It is tempting to suppose that muscular incoordination is at fault. The hip flexors hold the ilium forward while the sacrum is rotated backward, or the hamstrings and the gluteus maximus extend the hip, rotating the ilium backward while the sacrum is held forward by the weight of the trunk. This theory has support because a postural defect of pelvic inclination and excessive lumbar lordosis are associated findings.

Sacroiliac subluxation implies that ligamentous stretching has been sufficient to permit the ilium to slip on the sacrum. An irregular prominence of one of the articular surfaces becomes wedged upon another prominence of the apposed articular surface. The ligaments are taut, reflex muscle spasms are intense, and pain is severe and continuous until reduction is accomplished.

For most of its extent, the sacroiliac joint is inaccessible to invasive diagnostic procedures. The joint cavity lies deep to the rough and corrugated interosseous surfaces of the sacrum and ilium, which are connected by the dense, interosseous sacroiliac ligament (Fig. 9-18).

PROCEDURE

- The patient with lower back symptoms is in the standing position (Fig. 9-19).
- The patient flexes the dorsolumbar spine while the examiner notes the amount of movement necessary to aggravate the pain (Fig. 9-20).
- While positioned behind the patient, the examiner grasps the patient's iliac crests and braces a hip against the patient's sacrum (Fig. 9-21).
- The patient flexes the spine again as the examiner immobilizes the patient's pelvis (Fig. 9-22).
- If the lesion is of a pelvic nature, flexing the spine with the pelvis immobilized will not reproduce the discomfort.
- If the lesion is of a spinal nature, the pain will be aggravated in both instances.

Confirmation Procedures

Gaenslen's test, Goldthwait's sign, and Smith-Petersen test

DIAGNOSTIC STATEMENT

The belt test is positive on the right side of the pelvis and results in significant reduction of sacroiliac pain. This result indicates sprain of the sacroiliac ligaments.

The belt test aggravates both spinal and pelvic complaints. This result suggests lumbosacral capsular sprain.

CLINICAL PEARL

Because of the stabilizing effect of the very strong ligamentous structures, sprain of the sacroiliac ligaments accompanies sacroiliac subluxation and is a subluxation sprain. Posterior subluxation results from a flexion-type injury, which occurs with activities such as lifting or pushing. Anterior subluxation results from extension-type injuries, which occur when falling forward or extending the leg.

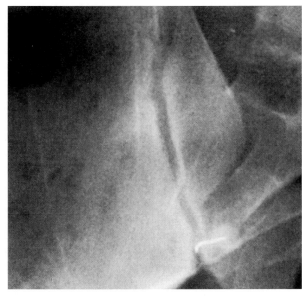

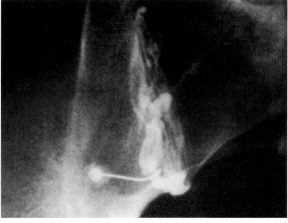

FIG. 9-18   Posterior views of sacroiliac arthrogram. *(From White AH, Schofferman JA: Spine care, vol 1-2, St Louis, 1995, Mosby.)*

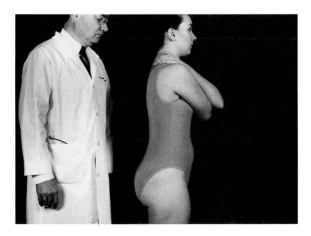

FIG. 9-19   The patient is in the standing position. The examiner, who is positioned behind the patient, notes spinal contours.

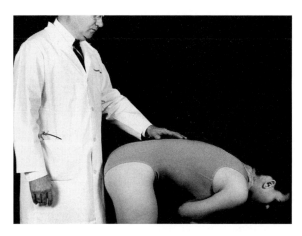

FIG. 9-20   The patient flexes at the waist, as far forward as possible. The examiner notes the amount of flexion necessary to aggravate the lower back or create sacroiliac discomfort.

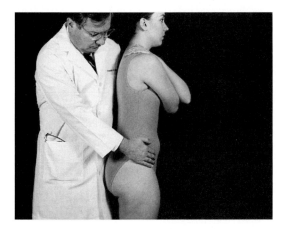

FIG. 9-21   Once the patient stands erect, the examiner grasps the patient's iliac crests and braces a hip against the patient's sacrum.

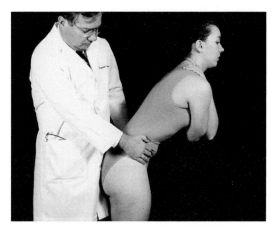

FIG. 9-22   While in this braced position, the patient flexes at the waist. If the source of pain is pelvic, then the move will not reproduce the discomfort because the pelvis is immobilized. Pain of spinal origin will be aggravated in both positions.

ERICHSEN'S SIGN

Assessment for Sacroiliac Disease versus Pathologic Conditions Involving the Hip Joint

Comment

The stability of the sacroiliac joint lies in the nature of its articular surfaces and ligaments (Fig. 9-23). The sacral articular surface is corrugated: a depression occurs opposite the second sacral segment, whereas the first and third segments exhibit prominences.

Movements that do occur in the sacroiliac joint are those of the pelvis as a whole. During extension, each hemipelvis turns downward about this axis, and during flexion, each one turns upward. Extension of the lower limb involves an upward gliding of the ilium on the sacrum coupled with an element of distraction between the two bones superiorly and anteriorly (Fig. 9-24).

The pelvic curve begins at the lumbosacral joint and ends at the termination of the coccyx. The curve is anteriorly concave and is somewhat tilted downward. The thoracic and pelvic curves are primary curves because they are present in the fetus.

The sacrum is a large triangular bone inserted like a wedge between the two iliac bones. The base of the sacrum articulates with L5, producing the rather acute lumbosacral angle, formed by increased anterior width of both the body of L5 and the L5-S1 intervertebral disc.

The coccyx is usually a solid bone formed by the fusion of four rudimentary vertebrae. Occasionally, the first coccygeal vertebra exists as a separate segment, and no vertebral canal exists within the coccyx itself.

Articulation of the pelvis with the vertebral column occurs at the interspace between L5 and the sacrum. This articulation is similar in just about all respects to the articulations that connect the vertebrae with each other. In addition, the iliolumbar ligament connects the pelvis with the vertebral column on either side.

The sacroiliac articulation is an amphiarthrodial, or slightly movable, joint. Cartilaginous plates cover the articular surfaces of the sacrum and ilium. The cartilaginous plates are in close contact with each other and bound together by fibrous strands.

The sacrococcygeal articulation is a joint similar to the articulation between vertebral bodies. The pubic symphysis is an amphiarthrodial joint formed between the two oval symphyseal surfaces of the pubic bones.

ORTHOPEDIC GAMUT 9-6

ACETABULAR FRACTURES

In general, acetabular fractures involve one or more of the following:

1. The posterior rim
2. The posterior column
3. The anterior column
4. The quadrilateral plate

Fractures of the posterior rim are usually caused by posterior dislocation of the femur (Figs. 9-25 and 9-26). Fractures of the posterior column may also be seen with posterior dislocations of the femur (Fig. 9-27). Fractures involving the quadrilateral plate are more commonly associated with lateral compression forces.

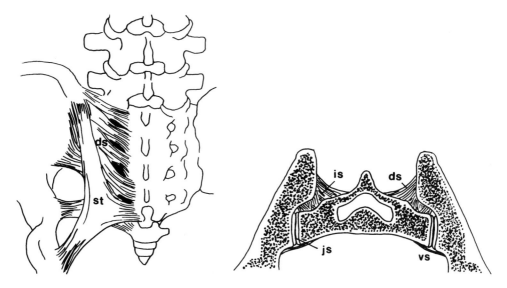

FIG. 9-23 The sacroiliac joints in posterior view and coronal section. *(From White AH, Schofferman JA: Spine care, vol 1-2, St Louis, 1995, Mosby.)*

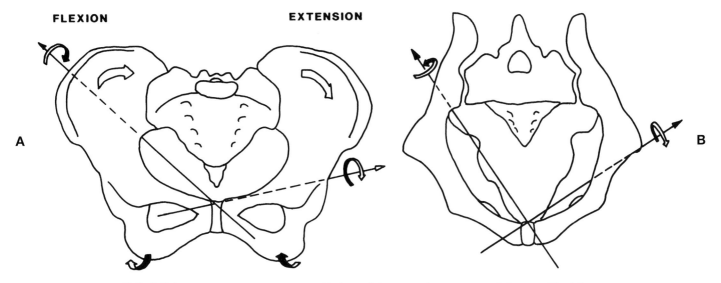

FIG. 9-24 Anterior (**A**) and coronal (**B**) view of the axes of movements of the sacroiliac joints. *(From White AH, Schofferman JA: Spine care, vol 1-2, St Louis, 1995, Mosby.)*

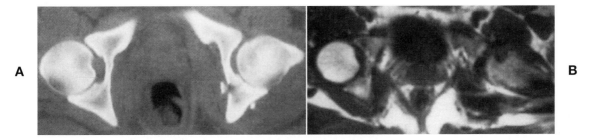

FIG. 9-25 **A,** Left acetabular fracture. **B,** Magnetic resonance imaging scan 3 weeks later reveals grossly abnormal signal within the femoral head. *(From Sutton D, Young JWR: A concise textbook of clinical imaging, ed 2, St Louis, 1995, Mosby.)*

PROCEDURE

- While the patient is prone, the examiner places his or her hands over the dorsum of the ilia and proceeds to give a forceful, sharp, bilateral thrust toward the midline (Fig. 9-28).
- The sign is present when this procedure produces pain over the sacroiliac area.
- Pain is felt in sacroiliac joint disease but not in hip joint disease.

Confirmation Procedures

Hibb's test and Laguerre's test

DIAGNOSTIC STATEMENT

Erichsen's sign is present on the right and suggests sacroiliac disease instead of a pathologic condition involving the hip joint.

CLINICAL PEARL

Patients who possess an anomalous relation of the piriformis muscle to the sciatic nerve are particularly susceptible to developing symptoms of sciatic neuritis when the muscle is hypertonic or spastic. Approximately 10% of the population possess such an anomaly. A reflex spasm of this muscle may occur because of intraarticular sacroiliac subluxation and sacroiliac irritation. Such a spasm is probably the cause of a positive Lasegue test, which is positive in the range of 20 to 45 degrees.

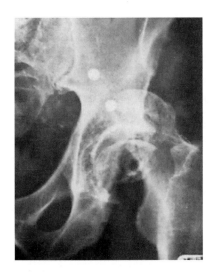

FIG. 9-26   Fracture-dislocation of the left femoral head with a posterior dislocation.   *(From Sutton D, Young JWR:* A concise textbook of clinical imaging, *ed 2, St Louis, 1995, Mosby.)*

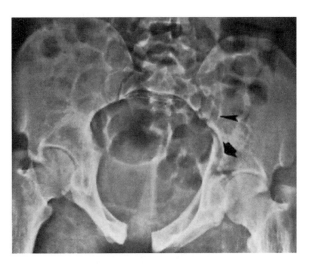

FIG. 9-27   Type II anteroposterior compression fracture.   *(From Sutton D, Young JWR:* A concise textbook of clinical imaging, *ed 2, St Louis, 1995, Mosby.)*

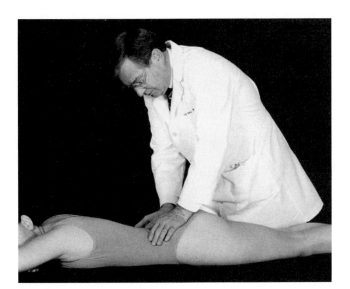

FIG. 9-28   While the patient is lying prone on a firm examining table, the examiner places both hands over the dorsum of the ilia and gives a sharp, forceful thrust toward the midline. The production of pain over the sacroiliac area is a positive sign and indicates sacroiliac joint disease.

GAENSLEN'S TEST

Assessment for Sacroiliac Disease

Comment

Because the pelvic ring is complex and involves a total of eight joints (left and right Z joints, coxals and sacroiliac joints, plus the single lumbosacral joint and the pubic symphysis), any change in the trunk or lower extremity is compensated in some way by the complicated dynamic mechanism of the pelvic ring.

The sacroiliac joint is thought to move only 2 mm and 2 degrees, but this small amount of movement is complex. The sacroiliac joints are the keys of the arch between the two pelvic bones. With the symphysis pubis, the joints help transfer the weight from the spine to the lower limbs. This triad of joints also acts as a buffer to decrease the force of jarring and bumping that occurs within the spine and upper body as the lower limbs make contact with the ground.

Because of this shock-absorbing function, the structure of the sacroiliac and symphysis pubis joints is different from most joints.

The sacroiliac joints are part synovial and part syndesmosis. A syndesmosis is a type of fibrous joint in which the intervening fibrous connective tissue forms an interosseous membrane or ligament. The synovial portion of the joint is C-shaped with the convex iliac surface of the C facing anteriorly and inferiorly. The greater or more acute the angle of the C, the more stable the joint and the less likely it is for a lesion of the joint to occur. The sacral surface is slightly concave.

The size, shape, and roughness of the articular surfaces vary among individuals. In the child, these surfaces are smooth. In the adult, the surfaces become irregular depressions and elevations that fit into one another. By doing so, the articular surfaces restrict movement at the joint and add to the strength of the joint for transferring weight from the lower limb to the spine. Fibrocartilage covers the articular surface of the ilium. Hyaline cartilage covers the articular surface of the sacrum and is three times thicker than the cartilage of the ilium. In older persons, adhesions may obliterate part of the joint surfaces.

The sacroiliac joints, although mobile in young people, become progressively stiffer with age. In some cases, ankylosis results. The movements occurring in the sacroiliac and symphysis pubis are small in relation to the movements in the spinal joints.

The symphysis pubis is a cartilaginous joint. There is a disc of fibrocartilage, called the *interpubic disc,* between the two joint surfaces.

The sacroiliac joints and symphysis pubis have no muscles that directly control their movements. However, the joints are influenced by the action of the muscles that move the lumbar spine and hip because many of these muscles attach to the sacrum and pelvis.

The sacrococcygeal joint is usually a fused line (symphysis) united by a fibrocartilaginous disc. It is between the apex of the sacrum and the base of the coccyx. Occasionally, the joint is freely movable and synovial. The joints fuse and obliterate with advancing age.

PROCEDURE

- The patient is lying supine.
- The examiner acutely flexes the knee and thigh of the unaffected leg to the patient's abdomen.
- This move brings the lumbar spine firmly into contact with the table and fixes both the pelvis and lumbar spine.
- With the examiner standing at a right angle to the

patient, the patient is brought well to the side of the table, and the examiner slowly hyperextends the affected thigh (Fig. 9-29).

- This hyperextension is accomplished by gradually increasing the pressure of one hand on top of the knee, while the examiner's other hand is on the flexed knee.
- The hyperextension of the affected hip exerts a rotating force on the corresponding half of the pelvis.
- The pull is made on the ilium, through the Y ligament, and the muscles attached to the anterior iliac spine.
- The test is positive if pain is felt in the sacroiliac area or referred down the thigh.
- The test is performed bilaterally.

- If the test is negative, a lumbosacral lesion is suspected.
- The test is usually contraindicated in older patients.

Confirmation Procedures
Belt test, Goldthwait's sign, and Smith-Petersen test

DIAGNOSTIC STATEMENT

Gaenslen's test is positive on the left. This result indicates sacroiliac joint disease on the left.

CLINICAL PEARL

Sacroiliac joint involvement produces local pain over the joint, or pain that is referred to (1) the groin on the same side, (2) the posterior thigh on the same side, and (3) down the leg, which is less often. Pain is often increased by lying on the affected side.

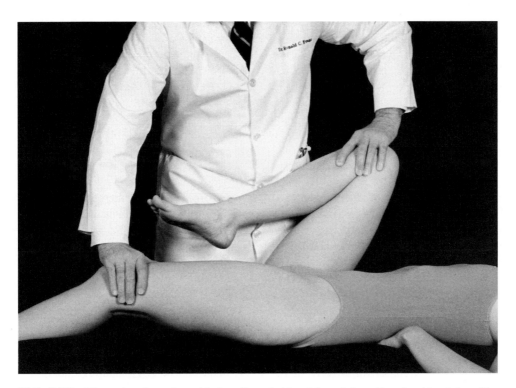

FIG. 9-29   The patient is supine with the affected side of the pelvis well to the side of the table. The unaffected thigh is flexed toward the abdomen. The examiner simultaneously exaggerates the thigh flexion on the unaffected side and the sacroiliac extension on the affected side. The test is positive if pain is felt in the affected sacroiliac joint as it is hyperextended.

GAPPING TEST

Sacroiliac Stretch Test

Assessment for Sprain of the Anterior Sacroiliac Ligaments

Comment

The normal movements that occur at the sacroiliac joints are determined by the direction of the articular surfaces, the muscles acting on the joint, and the symphysis pubis.

The movement is a rotation of the sacrum (or ilia) around the axis of the shortest and strongest part of the posterior interosseous sacroiliac ligament, which is situated in the angle between the posterosuperior and posteroinferior limbs of the auricular surfaces. When anterior rotation of the upper end of the sacrum occurs, the promontory of the sacrum will move in an anteroinferior direction, which narrows the AP diameter of the pelvic inlet. This rotation also increases the coronal width of the pelvic outlet and tightens the sacrotuberous and sacrospinous ligaments. During posterior rotation of the upper end of the sacrum, the reverse movements will occur. These movements produce a widening of the AP diameter of the pelvic inlet, a narrowing of the coronal width of the pelvic outlet, and a relaxation of the sacrotuberous and sacrospinous ligaments. The posterior sacroiliac ligaments will tighten and restrict this posterior rotation of the sacrum on the ilia.

In addition, because the auricular surfaces of the sacrum are inferiorly rather than superiorly closer to the median plane, anterior rotation of the sacrum will result in a slight widening of the symphysis pubis, whereas posterior rotation of the sacrum will result in compression of the symphysis pubis.

When a rotational force is applied to the hip bones in opposite directions—which occurs when extending one thigh while flexing the other, such as in stepping up to a stool—the extended thigh anchors the head of the femur on that side through the iliofemoral and ischiofemoral ligaments and the rectus femoris muscle. The flexed thigh, through the pull of the hamstring muscles, rotates the ilium in a posterior direction. In addition, the sacrum will move with the ilium on the flexed side because the pull of the hamstring muscle is transmitted to it via the sacrotuberous and sacrospinous ligaments. The result is that posterior rotation of the sacrum will occur at the sacroiliac joint on the extended side only.

Although these movements at the sacroiliac joints are small, especially in males, they are definite. The movements are increased when jumping from a height. They are also increased in females, especially toward the end of a pregnancy and up to 3 months after pregnancy because of the action of the hormone relaxin.

The finding that directs immediate attention to the sacroiliac joint as a possible cause of pain in the buttock and thigh is that lumbar movements do not affect the gluteal symptom. With acute arthritis, the lumbar movements sometimes mildly increase the pain because at the extreme of any lumbar motion, an added stress falls on the sacroiliac ligaments. If such an indirect strain on the joint hurts, much more severe pain is produced as soon as the sacroiliac joints are directly tested.

Osteitis pubis is a painful inflammation of the pubic symphysis that is usually self-limited. The cause is unknown, but the condition often develops after urologic procedures or infections, after childbirth, or after repetitive stresses associated with certain athletic activities. Pain and tenderness over the symphysis pubis are usually present. Coughing may aggravate the pain, which radiates along the adductor and rectus abdominis muscles. Stretching these muscles is painful.

Roentgenograms of the pelvis taken early in the disease may be normal. Later, variable amounts of spotty demineralization, widening of the symphysis pubis, and sclerosis are noted (Fig. 9-30).

PROCEDURE

- The patient lies supine, and the examiner places both hands on the anterosuperior spine of each ilium and presses laterally downward.
- Crossing the arms increases the lateral component of the strain on the ligaments (Fig. 9-31).
- The pelvis must not be allowed to rock because the lumbar spine then moves.
- The examiner's hands can cause anterior iliac spine discomfort as a result of compression of the skin against the osseus structures.
- The expected finding is not local pain but rather aggravation of the gluteal symptoms.
- The response to the test is positive only if unilateral gluteal or posterior crural pain is elicited.
- The test is significant for anterior sacroiliac ligament sprain.

Confirmation Procedure

Yeoman's test

DIAGNOSTIC STATEMENT

The gapping test is positive with pain elicited in the right or left gluteal area. This pain suggests sprain of the anterior sacroiliac ligaments on the right.

CLINICAL PEARL

Stretching the anterior ligaments in the manner described is the most delicate test for the sacroiliac joint. Patients recovering from a sacroiliac injury may say that all pain ceased some days before. Patients walk and bend painlessly; yet for 7 to 10 days after subjective recovery, the straining of the joint that occurs in the gapping test still evokes discomfort. It is clear that this test applies more stress to sacroiliac ligaments than ordinary daily activities. If a patient has symptoms referable to the sacroiliac joint, this maneuver will elicit them.

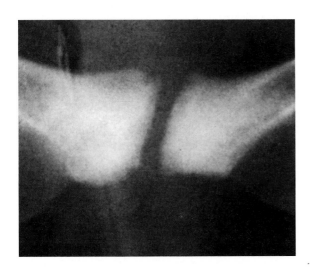

FIG. 9-30   Osteitis pubis. *(From Mercier LR, Pettid FJ: Practical orthopedics, ed 4, St Louis, 1995, Mosby.)*

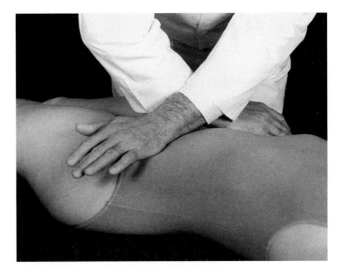

FIG. 9-31   The patient is supine on the examination table. The hips and knees are extended. With crossed arms, the examiner places both hands on the opposite anterosuperior iliac spines of each ilium. A downward and lateral pressure is applied to both ilia. Unilateral gluteal or posterior crural pain is a positive finding and indicates sprain of the anterior sacroiliac ligament.

GOLDTHWAIT'S SIGN

Assessment for Sacroiliac Joint Sprain versus Lumbosacral Spine Pathology

Comment

Because of their position at the juncture of the skeleton of the trunk and the pelvic girdle, sacroiliac articulations are of importance. In recent years, sacroiliac articulations have been the subject of extensive clinical study. It is largely the radiologists who have contributed to the knowledge of these articulations and who have described normal form and pathologic variations.

The radiographic depiction of the sacroiliac synchondrosis is difficult because of its oblique and sinuous form. Severe fractures of the pelvis are sometimes associated with sacroiliac luxations and with marked displacement of the wings of the ilia. The sacroiliac joint may be the site of the infection, especially tuberculosis, with destruction of the articular surfaces and wandering abscess formation. Obliteration or loss of definition of the surface or margins of these joints is an early finding in ankylosing spondylitis.

Sacroiliac joint movement is three dimensional and contains several elements. The primary movements are anteroinferior to posterosuperior nodding called *nutation* of the sacral base in relation to the ilium (Fig. 9-32, *B*). Movement along an axis that passes longitudinally through the iliac ridge of the sacroiliac joint in rotatory (Fig. 9-32, *C*) and gapping of the superior and inferior aspects of the sacroiliac joint is a third type of sacroiliac joint motion (Fig. 9-32, *A*).

The most common morphologic change that is often associated with clinical symptoms is arthrosis deformans, which manifests itself by marginal osteophyte formation, particularly in the inferior portions of the synchondrosis and by subchondral osteosclerosis. These changes are responsible for a considerable degree of pain, especially with certain movements. These changes occur with advancing age in 90% of men and 77% of women. The healing of pelvic fractures that occurs with poor alignment of the sacroiliac articulations has a significant influence on the spine and the changes that are in these joints and are related to back pain.

PROCEDURE

- The patient is supine.
- The patient's affected leg is raised slowly, while one of the examiner's hands is under the lumbar portion of the patient's spine (Fig. 9-33).
- If pain is brought on before the lumbar spine begins to move, a sacroiliac lesion is probably present.
- The lesion may be caused by arthritis or by a sprain of the ligaments that involve the sacroiliac joint (Fig. 9-34).
- If pain does not come on until after the lumbar spine begins to move, the disorder is more likely to have its origin in the lumbosacral area or, less commonly, in the sacroiliac area.
- The test is repeated with the unaffected limb.
- A positive sign of a lumbosacral lesion is elicited if pain occurs at about the same height as it did with the affected limb.
- If the unaffected leg can be raised higher than the affected leg, it signifies sacroiliac involvement of the affected side.

Confirmation Procedures

Belt test, Gaenslen's test, and Smith-Petersen test

DIAGNOSTIC STATEMENT

Goldthwait's sign is present on the left and elicits pain in the sacroiliac joint before lumbosacral movement. This sign indicates sacroiliac joint sprain.

CLINICAL PEARL

This test is similar to the Lasegue test, the straight-leg-raising test, and Smith-Petersen test. All have the use of the affected leg as a lever in common to stretch the suspect tissue, whether neural or ligamentous. The key to differentiation is the determination of the moment of L5-S1 separation, reflecting lumbosacral movement.

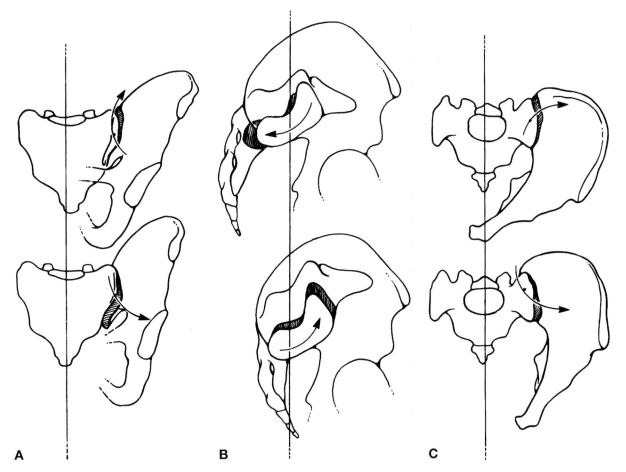

FIG. 9-32   Three types of sacroiliac joint (SIJ) motion. **A,** Superior and inferior aspects of the SIJ are shown gapping. **B,** Anterior and posterior rocking of the sacral base. **C,** Movement of the ilium on the sacrum that takes place in the horizontal plane. The arrows in **A** and **C** show motion of the ilium. The arrows in **B** show sacral motion. These movements are accentuated for demonstrative purposes in this illustration.   *(From Cramer GD, Darby SA: Basic and clinical anatomy of the spine, spinal cord, and ANS, St Louis, 1995, Mosby.)*

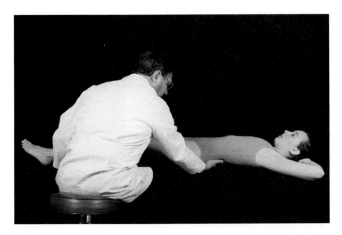

FIG. 9-33   The patient is supine on the examination table. The examiner places one hand under the lumbosacral portion of the patient's spine and palpates the L5 and S1 spinous processes. The examiner maintains contact with these two points.

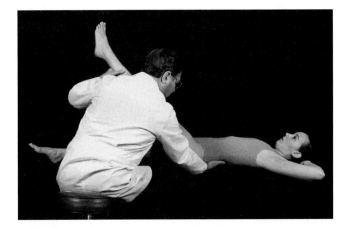

FIG. 9-34   The examiner elevates the affected leg as if performing a straight-leg-raising maneuver. If pain is produced before the L5-S1 spinous processes separate, the lesion involves the sacroiliac joint. If the pain is produced as the L5-S1 spinous processes separate, it is more likely that a spinal lesion exists.

HIBB'S TEST

Assessment for Sacroiliac Disease

Comment

Evaluation of the sacroiliac joint is challenging for many reasons. First, the sacroiliac joint is subject to a wide range of normal anatomic variation. Second, its unusual location and its oblique position make direct palpation almost impossible.

The seronegative spondyloarthropathies, a class of rheumatic disorders, have several factors in common: radiographic presentation, genetic predisposition, and certain clinical features. Included in this group are the so-called reactive arthritides (e.g., ankylosing spondylitis), along with the associated spondylitic disease, psoriatic arthritis, and inflammatory bowel disease. The benchmark of ankylosing spondylitis, a common cause of low back pain and thoracolumbar stiffness, is the presence of sacroiliitis (Fig. 9-35).

Tuberculous infection of the sacroiliac joint often is associated with tuberculosis of the spine at the lumbosacral area and the hip. This association suggests the ease with which tuberculosis spreads from the lumbosacral area to the sacroiliac joint by way of the psoas muscle. Destructive caseous lesions are the rule, and they often destroy the joint and form abscesses. The abscess may present dorsally over the joint or intrapelvically, erupting at the inguinal area. Rupture of the abscess results in a resistant sinus and secondary infection. Severe visceral lesions result in a serious condition. If the patient survives, spontaneous bony ankylosis of the sacroiliac joint occurs after 3 or 4 years. The disease may be bilateral.

The disease affects young adults and is rare in infancy and childhood. The onset of the disease is gradual and may follow trauma or pregnancy.

With this type of ankylosis, pain is felt over the sacroiliac joint. Most of the time, this pain is referred to the groin. Less commonly, the pain is referred to the sciatic distribution. The pain is accentuated by direct pressure, such as during recumbency and particularly when turning over in bed. Sitting on the buttock on the affected side is also painful. Sitting on the opposite buttock relieves the pain. Bending forward with the knee extended is painful, but bending forward while the knees are flexed is painless. Jarring that occurs during walking, coughing, or sneezing accentuates the discomfort.

The patient with this disease lists to the opposite side. With the lower extremities extended, forward bending is limited. When the knees and hips are flexed, the hamstrings are relaxed, tension is removed from the pelvis, and farther forward bending is accomplished. Only the lower end of the joint is posteriorly superficial and displays tenderness and a boggy swelling. The swelling and tenderness may be more easily localized during rectal examination. Compressing the iliac crests together causes direct, painful pressure on the joint. Gaenslen's test for sacroiliac disease depends on twisting the ilium on the sacrum. The strain this move puts on the inflamed ligamentous structures around the sacroiliac joint produces the pain. The low-grade, inflammatory swelling of a cold abscess or sinus may be present.

PROCEDURE

- While the patient is in the prone position, the examiner stabilizes the pelvis on the nearest side by placing one hand firmly on the dorsum of the iliac bone.
- With the other hand around the patient's ankle, the opposite knee is flexed to a right angle (Fig. 9-36).
- The knee is flexed to its maximum without elevating the thigh from the examination table (Fig. 9-37).
- From this position, the examiner slowly pushes the leg laterally, causing strong internal rotation of the femoral head (Fig. 9-38).
- The test is performed bilaterally.
- The production of pelvic pain is a positive finding.
- The test is significant for a sacroiliac lesion.
- In the absence of hip involvement, stress is transmitted through the hip joints into the sacroiliac mechanism, producing pain.

Confirmation Procedures

Erichsen's sign and Laguerre's test

DIAGNOSTIC STATEMENT

Hibb's test is positive on the left. This result suggests sacroiliac disease.

CLINICAL PEARL

Tuberculosis is now rare in developed countries but still a scourge elsewhere. Complications may be serious because of the formation of sinuses. These sinuses may become secondarily infected and may cause paraplegia (Pott's paraplegia) because of (1) pus and intracellular pressure, (2) mechanical injury to the nervous system (cord) caused by bony pressure, or (3) vascular embarrassment of the nervous system where it crosses the bony infection. Hibb's test is not specific for tuberculosis of the sacroiliac joint but is correlated with other systemic findings that may suggest the existence of this type of tuberculosis. At the least, Hibb's test reveals mechanical dysfunction of the sacroiliac joint.

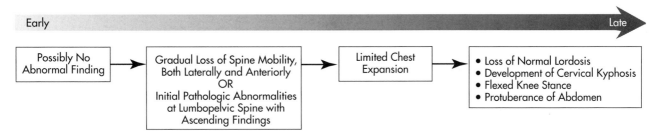

FIG. 9-35   Physical course of ankylosing spondylitis. *(From Brier SR: Primary care orthopedics, St Louis, Mosby, 1999.)*

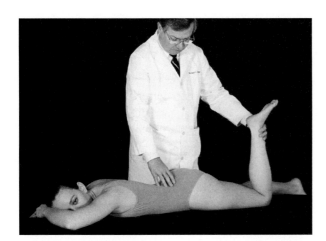

FIG. 9-36   The patient is prone on the examining table. The examiner stabilizes the unaffected side of the pelvis with one hand. With the other hand, the examiner grasps the ankle of the affected leg and flexes the knee to 90 degrees.

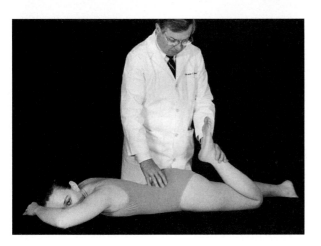

FIG. 9-37   The examiner flexes the patient's knee to its maximum without elevating the thigh from the examination table.

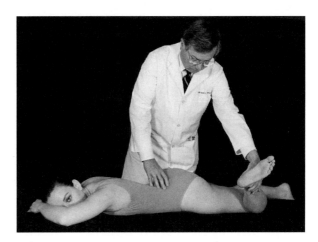

FIG. 9-38   The examiner slowly pushes the leg laterally, causing internal rotation of the femoral head. The production of pelvic pain is a positive finding. Even without a pathologic condition of the hip, the test is significant for a sacroiliac lesion.

ILIAC COMPRESSION TEST

COMPRESSION OF THE ILIAC CRESTS

Assessment for Sacroiliac Lesions, Sprain, Inflammation, Subluxation, and Fracture

Comment

The pelvic ring is essentially a rigid circle with very little motion at the interpubic or sacroiliac areas. Fractures involving the ring are generally classified as stable or unstable. Stable fractures are those in which the ring is completely broken only at one point (e.g., superior and inferior pubic ramus fractures on the same side). With unstable fractures, the ring is broken in two or more areas (e.g., both pubic rami on the same side plus a sacroiliac joint dislocation) (Fig. 9-39). Fractures of the acetabulum occasionally involve the main weight-bearing surface of the hip joint (Fig. 9-40).

Osteoporosis is the usual predisposing cause, but inactivity, long-term steroid use, and other types of metabolic bone disease may also play a role.

Fracture of the wing of the ilium occasionally occurs. When such a fracture occurs, it is usually caused by a direct blow against the wing of the ilium. In most sports in which such an injury is likely, the iliac crest is padded to prevent the occurrence of this injury.

Fracture of the wing of the ilium is a painful injury not only at the time of the blow but also in the period immediately after the injury. This type of fracture is ordinarily recognized as a serious injury. Examination reveals extreme tenderness along the iliac crest and downward onto the wing of the ilium. The area of pain depends on the extent of the fracture. The patient will usually not permit deep enough palpation so that the examiner can actually feel a defect along the rim. Any attempt to use the involved muscles is extremely painful, and involuntary spasms of the abdominal or hip muscles may cause acute distress. It is necessary to have the patient completely relaxed before a definitive examination can be performed. If a lesion of this severity is suspected, an x-ray examination should be made. The fracture can be completely overlooked in the ordinary AP view of the pelvis. The fracture will be well delineated by an AP view of the ilium rather than of the pelvis.

Lateral compression fractures are caused by forces delivered from the side. They are subdivided into several types depending on the severity of the injury and the progressive involvement of the posterior pelvis (Fig. 9-41). Common associations are crush fractures of the sacrum and the medial wall of the acetabulum. The more severe types of AP compression fracture refer to increasing posterior ligamentous injury and subsequent increasing instability (Fig. 9-42). Vertical shear fractures commonly arise from falls from a height. Fractures occur through the pubic rami and posterior pelvis, and they are vertical in orientation (Fig. 9-43). The anterosuperior iliac spine (sartorius), anteroinferior iliac spine (rectus femoris), and ischial tuberosity (hamstrings) are the common sites of avulsion fracture (Fig. 9-44).

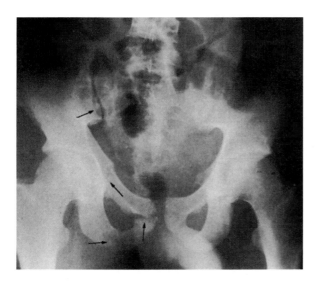

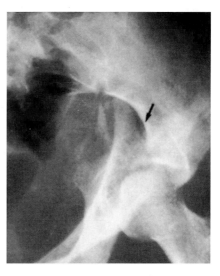

FIG. 9-39   An unstable fracture of the pelvis.   *(From Mercier LR, Pettid FJ:* Practical orthopedics, *ed 4, St Louis, 1995, Mosby.)*

FIG. 9-40   Fracture of the acetabulum.   *(From Mercier LR, Pettid FJ:* Practical orthopedics, *ed 4, St Louis, 1995, Mosby.)*

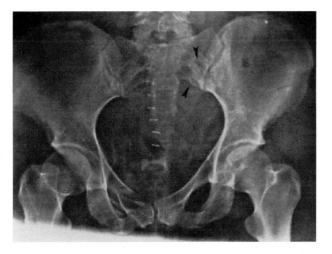

FIG. 9-41   Lateral compression fracture.   *(From Sutton D, Young JWR:* A concise textbook of clinical imaging, *ed 2, St Louis, 1995, Mosby.)*

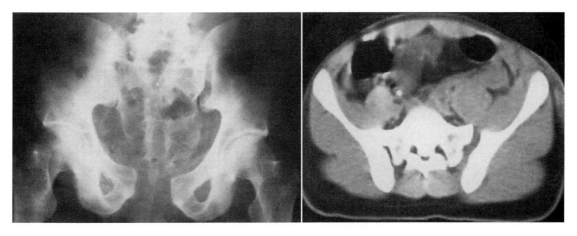

FIG. 9-42   Anteroposterior compression fracture.   *(From Sutton D, Young JWR:* A concise textbook of clinical imaging, *ed 2, St Louis, 1995, Mosby.)*

PROCEDURE

- The patient is in a side-lying position.
- The examiner compresses the superior ilium toward the floor (Fig. 9-45).
- Forward rolling motion of the sacrum occurs.
- Increased pressure in the sacroiliac joint suggests a sacroiliac lesion.
- This may also indicate a sprain of the posterior sacroiliac ligaments.
- A positive finding is significant for sacroiliac lesions.

Confirmation Procedure

Diagnostic imaging

DIAGNOSTIC STATEMENT

The iliac compression test is positive, and pain is elicited at the left ilium, near the crest. This pain suggests fracture of the wing of the ilium.

CLINICAL PEARL

Fractures of the pelvis are serious in themselves and may result in long-term disability. However, even more important is that these fractures are often complicated by damage to the soft tissues, urethra, bladder, bowel, blood vessels, and nerves. These complications can be fatal. Genitourinary complications occur in approximately 20% of pelvic fractures, and the overall mortality is 5%.

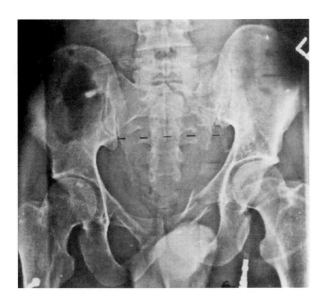

FIG. 9-43   Vertical shear fracture. *(From Sutton D, Young JWR: A concise textbook of clinical imaging, ed 2, St Louis, 1995, Mosby.)*

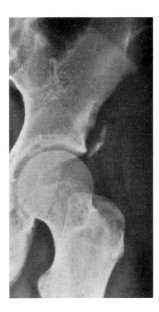

FIG. 9-44   Avulsion of the lateral cortex of the ilium. *(From Sutton D, Young JWR: A concise textbook of clinical imaging, ed 2, St Louis, 1995, Mosby.)*

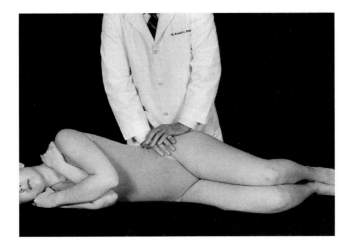

FIG. 9-45   The patient is in the side-lying position on an examination table with a firm surface. The examiner places both hands over the upper part of the superior iliac crest and exerts cautious downward pressure. If the patient experiences an increased feeling of pressure in the sacroiliac joint, the test indicates sacroiliac sprain, inflammation, subluxation, or fracture.

Assessment for Sacroiliac Mechanical Dysfunction and Pyogenic Sacroiliitis (*correlated with systemic findings*)

Comment

Septic arthritis is a disease process caused by the direct invasion of a joint space by infectious agents, usually bacteria. Joints become infected by direct penetration spread from contiguous structures or, more often, by hematogenous invasion through the bloodstream. Septic arthritis occurs more often in large peripheral joints than in the lumbosacral spine. When a joint of the axial skeleton is involved, the sacroiliac joint is the one commonly affected.

Pyogenic sacroiliitis is an uncommon illness. The disease occurs most commonly in young adult men. The range of age is 20 to 66 years, and the male:female ratio is 3:2. Entry of the organisms into the sacroiliac joint is the initial factor that may result in joint infection. Most commonly infectious agents reach the sacroiliac joint by traveling through the bloodstream. They lodge in the vascular synovial membrane that lines the lower portion of the sacroiliac joint. The infectious agents grow in the synovium and invade the joint space. The organisms also might lodge in the ilium, the most commonly infected flat bone in the body, and grow into the sacroiliac joint. The symmetric involvement of the ilium and sacrum in pyogenic sacroiliitis suggests that the joint is the initial area affected. Once an infection is established in the joint, rapid destruction may occur because of both the direct, toxic effects that products or organisms have on joint structures and because of the host's inflammatory response to these products or organisms.

Any factor—such as intravenous drug abuse, skin infections, bone and urinary tract infections, endocarditis, pregnancy, or bowel disease—that promotes blood-borne infection or inhibits the normal defense mechanisms of the synovial joint predisposes the host to infection. Although the role of trauma in the pathogenesis of pyogenic sacroiliitis is unclear, buttock or hip injuries have been reported in patients before development of pyogenic sacroiliitis. Most patients, however, deny a history of trauma, and its importance as a direct cause of the infection is in question. The histocompatibility typing associated with seronegative spondyloarthropathies, HLA-B27, is not associated with pyogenic sacroiliitis.

Another mechanism of joint infection is contamination by local spread from a contiguous suppurative focus. Extension of a pelvic infectious process may cause disruption of the joint capsule or of the periosteum of the ilium or sacrum. Infections spreading beneath the spinal ligaments may gain entry into the sacroiliac joints. Another mechanism of joint infection that is even more uncommon is direct seeding of organisms into the joint during diagnostic or surgical procedures.

PROCEDURE

- The patient is supine. The patient's knee and hip are flexed, and the hip is adducted (Fig. 9-46).
- This rocks the sacroiliac joint (Fig. 9-47).
- The knee is approximated to patient's opposite shoulder (Fig. 9-48).
- A positive test is indicated by pain in the ipsilateral sacroiliac joint.
- A positive test indicates sacroiliac mechanical dysfunction. This may include pyogenic sacroiliitis, when correlated with other system findings.

Confirmation Procedures

Anterior innominate test, Lewin-Gaenslen's test, Piedallu's sign, sacral apex test, and sacroiliac resisted-abduction test

DIAGNOSTIC STATEMENT

The knee-to-shoulder test is positive for the right sacroiliac joint. This result indicates an articular lesion. This afebrile finding implicates mechanical dysfunction.

The knee-to-shoulder test is positive for the right sacroiliac joint. This result, correlated with other systemic findings, implicates pyogenic sacroiliitis.

CLINICAL PEARL

With acute sacroiliac pyogenic infections, the onset is usually rapid and very painful. Swelling is intense, and tenderness is widespread. The patient resists movement and experiences pyrexia and general malaise. Pyogenic infections occurring in patients with rheumatoid arthritis often have a much slower onset. Although the sacroiliac joint is swollen, other inflammatory changes are often suppressed, especially if the patient is receiving steroids. In the early stages, both modes of onset will mimic simple mechanical injury of the sacroiliac joint.

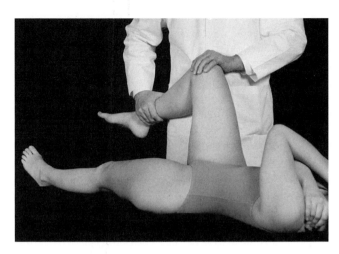

FIG. 9-46   The patient is supine on the examination table. The examiner flexes both the knee and hip of the affected leg to 90 degrees.

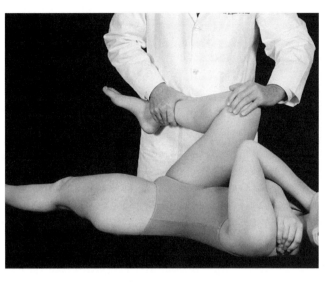

FIG. 9-47   The examiner flexes the patient's hip even farther, toward the patient's abdomen.

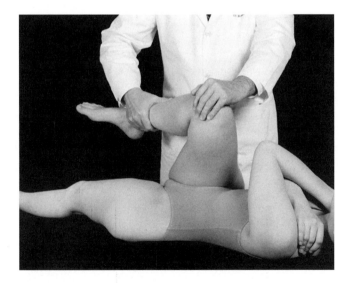

FIG. 9-48   The hip is adducted, approximating the knee of the affected leg to the contralateral shoulder. Pain in the sacroiliac joint indicates a positive test.

LAGUERRE'S TEST

Assessment for Sacroiliac Intraarticular Pathology

Comment

Osteitis condensans ilii is a lesion in which sclerosis of a fairly large area of an ilium adjacent to the sacroiliac joint occurs (Fig. 9-49). It is most common in multiparous women. Its importance lies in distinguishing it from ankylosing spondylitis (Marie-Strumpell disease).

Osteitis condensans ilii is a disease characterized by mild back pain and unilateral or bilateral bony sclerosis of the lower ilium, with sparing of the sacral portion of the sacroiliac joints. The illness is not progressive and is not associated with functional disability. The major difficulty with osteitis condensans ilii is that it is often confused with ankylosing spondylitis.

The prevalence of osteitis condensans ilii has been estimated to be 1.6% in Japanese and 3% in Scandinavians. The typical patient is a female 30 to 40 years old. The female:male ratio is 9:1 or greater.

The pathogenesis of osteitis condensans ilii is unknown. Urinary tract infections, inflammatory diseases of the sacroiliac joint, and abnormal mechanical stresses have been suggested as possible causes in this illness. Urinary tract infection may reach the ilium via nutrient arteries, resulting in reactive sclerosis. The absence of a history of urinary tract infection in many individuals makes this mechanism unlikely. Osteitis condensans ilii may be a subset of ankylosing spondylitis. However, histocompatibility testing for HLA-B27 has not documented increased incidence of this antigen in osteitis patients. In addition, part of the confusion over differentiating osteitis condensans ilii and ankylosing spondylitis is the milder form of the latter illness in females.

A more likely cause of osteitis condensans ilii is mechanical stress across the sacroiliac joint in association with pregnancy and diastasis of the symphysis pubis. A normal physiologic zone of hyperostosis on the anterior iliac margin of the sacroiliac joint may become exaggerated in response to abnormal stresses. Abnormal stresses are placed on the sacroiliac joints during pregnancy. However, these stresses alone would not explain the occasional male with osteitis or female who develops osteitis without having been pregnant. Therefore it must be said that the mechanical stresses that cause osteitis condensans ilii are commonly, but not exclusively, associated with pregnancy. Diastasis of the symphysis pubis may explain this clinical occurrence. Diastasis of the pubis commonly occurs during pregnancy and is secondary to the release of relaxin, a product of the corpus pregnancy, which allows greater laxity of the supporting structures (ligaments) of the pelvis. Patients may actually notice movement or a popping sensation in the sacroiliac joints and pubis. Diastasis is not exclusively related to pregnancy because it may occur secondary to trauma. Individuals, both male and female, with diastasis related to trauma may be at risk of developing osteitis condensans ilii.

PROCEDURE

- The patient is in a supine position (Fig. 9-50).
- The patient's involved hip is flexed, abducted, and laterally rotated (Fig. 9-51).
- An overpressure at the end of the range of motion is applied.
- The opposite anterior-superior iliac spine is stabilized.
- A positive test is sacroiliac joint pain.
- Because this test approximates a Patrick Fabere procedure, the examiner needs to be alert for coxa signs of pathology.

Confirmation Procedures

Erichsen's sign, Hibb's test, and diagnostic imaging

DIAGNOSTIC STATEMENT

Laguerre's test is positive for the right sacroiliac joint and suggests a pathologic condition that is of an intraarticular origin.

CLINICAL PEARL

With osteitis condensans ilii, there is a disturbance of the normal architecture of the ilium, in which increased condensations of bone occur in the auricular portion of the ilium, without a corresponding change in the sacroiliac joint or the sacrum. Osteitis condensans ilii must be differentiated from ankylosing spondylitis, which also causes condensations around the sacroiliac joint. Laguerre's test reveals a mechanical problem of the sacroiliac joint. Involvement of the joint in osteitis condensans ilii can be confirmed only by diagnostic imaging.

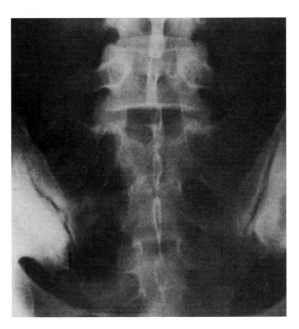

FIG. 9-49   Osteitis condensans ilii.   *(From Mercier LR, Pettid FJ: Practical orthopedics, ed 4, St Louis, 1995, Mosby.)*

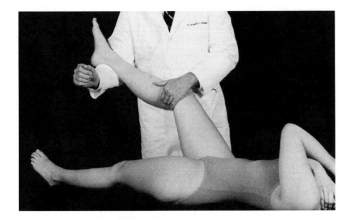

FIG. 9-50   The patient is supine. The examiner flexes and abducts the patient's hip on the affected side. The patient's foot rests on the examiner's forearm.

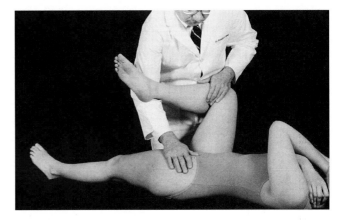

FIG. 9-51   The examiner laterally rotates the hip, applying an overpressure at the end of the range of motion. The contralateral pelvis is stabilized by holding the anterosuperior iliac spine down. Pain in the sacroiliac joint on the affected side constitutes a positive test.

Assessment for Sacroiliac Joint Pathology

Comment

The signs of sacroiliac joint syndrome include tenderness when pressure is applied over the posterior superior iliac spine, in the region of the sacroiliac joint, or in the buttock. Movement of the joint is usually reduced. Normally, the joint moves by rotating in the sagittal plane. Restricted movement can be detected in two ways.

The first way to detect restricted movement is to have the patient stand with one hand resting on the examining table for support. To examine the left sacroiliac joint, the examiner places the thumb of the right hand over the spinous process of L5 and the thumb of the left hand over the left posterior superior iliac spine. The patient then flexes both the left hip and the left knee and lifts the knee toward the chest. As this move is performed, the examiner can detect a small but definite amount of movement. Rotation in the joint causes the iliac spine to move downward in relation to the spinous process of L5. When the sacroiliac joint is fixed in position, this movement of the iliac spine relative to the spinous process is reduced or absent.

Confirmation can be obtained by the second test. To examine the left sacroiliac joint, the examiner places the right thumb over the apex of the patient's sacrum and the left thumb over the ischial tuberosity. In a normal joint, flexing the left knee and hip and bringing the knee toward the chest causes the ischial tuberosity to move laterally, away from the apex of the sacrum. When the joint is fixed in position, the lateral movement does not take place. The sacroiliac joint on the right is examined using the same method.

During forward flexion, the strain falls first on the iliolumbar ligament. Next, the strain is transmitted to the interspinous ligaments from L5 upward and then to the lumbodorsal fascia, particularly to the sacral triangle. During extension, the impingement signs prevail over the tension effects: the articulation comes first and then the interspinous ligaments. The ligamentum flava escapes impingement.

During axial rotation, the iliolumbar ligament becomes strained first and then the intertransverse. During lateral flexion, the sequence is quadratus, ligamentum flava, and the interspinous ligament on the convex side.

For screening ambulation, the patient performs the normal movements of walking. The patient should be observed both coming toward the examiner and walking away.

ORTHOPEDIC GAMUT 9-9

GAIT

Gait observations are as follows:

1. Equality of stride length
2. Excessive pelvic tilt or lean during ambulation
3. Antalgic lean of the lumbopelvic spine
4. Excessive swayback or hyperlordosis
5. Changes in pelvic inclination (tilt)

The sacroiliac joint is subject to several different processes that may damage it. Sprain is common, and sacroiliac joint subluxation can occur. Sprain may occur when heavy loads are placed on the joints, during a fall, or with blows to the sacroiliac joint. The pain that occurs will be felt unilaterally over the sacroiliac joint and can radiate into the ipsilateral hip or buttock. The pain will worsen with movement or axial loading of the joint. During palpation, the joint is extremely tender, particularly near an area just inferomedial to the posterior superior iliac spine. When the patient is being examined for global motions, extending the joint may produce some pain, but flexion is typically not painful. Lateral flexion of the pelvis may be painful but is not universally so, particularly if the motion is very smoothly performed.

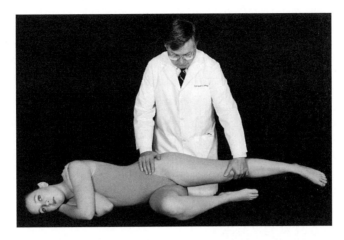

FIG. 9-52   The patient is side-lying on the examination table on the unaffected side. The knee and hip of the unaffected leg are flexed. The examiner abducts the affected leg slightly, supporting its weight with one hand. The examiner's other hand fixes the pelvis to the table with firm downward pressure.

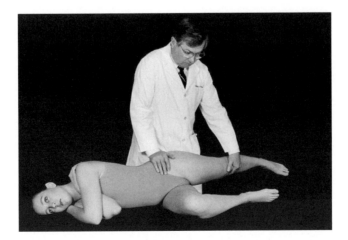

FIG. 9-53   The affected leg is extended by the examiner. Pain elicited during this maneuver constitutes a positive sign and indicates a sacroiliac lesion.

Straight-leg-raising tests produce pain at approximately 70 degrees of flexion. No muscular changes are noted, and reflex testing will be normal.

Pain from sacroiliac joint lesions, other than sprain, will typically be dull in nature and perceived in the region of the buttock. The pain may radiate into the area of the anterior groin, the posterior thigh, the knee, or even the lower abdomen, causing possible misdiagnosis as an intraabdominal lesion. A neurologic symptom is rare, so paresthesia is not often experienced. Patients suffering from mechanical lesions of the sacroiliac joint experience the pain unilaterally. The pain is exacerbated by motions that produce stress on the joint.

ORTHOPEDIC GAMUT 9-10

SACROILIAC JOINT DISORDERS

Disorders of the sacroiliac joint are classified as the following:

1. Inflammatory lesions
2. Infectious lesions
3. Mechanical lesions
4. Degenerative lesions
5. Osteitis condensans ilii

PROCEDURE

- Lewin-Gaenslen's test is a modification of Gaenslen's test.
- The patient lies on the unaffected side and pulls the knee of that side to the chest (Figs. 9-52 to 9-54).
- The patient holds the affected thigh in extension for the examiner.
- The examiner, positioned behind the patient, then provides pressure by hyperextending the affected thigh (Fig. 9-55).
- Pain produced in the sacroiliac joint is a positive finding.
- The test is significant for sacroiliac lesions.

Confirmation Procedures

Anterior innominate test, knee-to-shoulder test, Piedallu's sign, sacral apex test, and sacroiliac resisted-abduction test

---

DIAGNOSTIC STATEMENT

Lewin-Gaenslen's test is positive on the left and indicates an articular pathologic condition of the sacroiliac joint.

CLINICAL PEARL

Because of the strength of the sacroiliac ligaments, sprain of these structures is uncommon. Bending movements—such as lifting and hyperextension, which produce a torsion sprain on the joint—are more likely to cause sprain of the thinner capsular ligaments in the small lumbosacral joints.

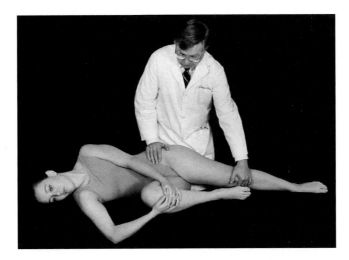

FIG. 9-54   In a slight variation of this test, the patient maximally flexes the thigh of the unaffected leg onto the abdomen and holds it in place.

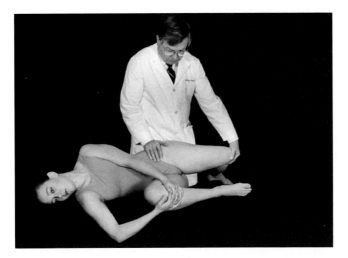

FIG. 9-55   The examiner extends the affected leg, allowing flexion of the knee. With the unaffected thigh in fixed flexion, very little extension motion is required to elicit a pain response in the affected leg.

Assessment for Abnormal Torsion Movement of the Sacroiliac Joint

Comment

Many inflammatory disorders affect the sacroiliac joint. Most of these disorders fall under the general heading of the seronegative arthropathies, such as ankylosing spondylitis, Reiter's syndrome, and psoriatic arthritis. When an inflammatory disorder exists, a combination of radiographic and laboratory tests can be used to confirm the presence of a particular disease. Each disease has it own characteristics, such as a predisposition for ankylosing spondylitis in the sacroiliac joint that migrates superiorly in the spine.

Infections within the sacroiliac joint are most commonly caused by *Staphylococcus* bacteria and also by tuberculous or brucellar infection. X-ray examination can once again be used to show typical changes, and bone scans will be useful in demonstrating the hot-spot appearance of such an infection. Aspiration biopsy is needed to culture the organism.

Mechanical lesions of the sacroiliac joint are common and consist of both hypomobility and hypermobility lesions. Causes of hypomobility lesions include rotational stress on the joint, pregnancy, trauma, and unequal leg length. Hypermobility lesions are due only to an unstable symphysis pubis or to pregnancy, which also affects the symphysis pubis via the release of the hormone relaxin.

Degenerative changes may occur within the sacroiliac joint and also in any other joint in the body. The changes that occur in the joint are similar to those in other joints. There is pitting of the bone accompanied by subchondral sclerosis and osteophytic changes. This condition has a tendency to occur with aging. This is in concert with greater amounts of stress placed upon the joint, such as increasing weight or damage from fracture or biomechanical abnormality.

Osteitis condensans ilii is a condition in which bone condenses along the ilium near the sacroiliac joint. The cause of this condition is not known, but it may be associated with increased stress, ankylosing spondylitis, urinary tract infection, and circulatory problems. Osteitis condensans ilii can lead to lower back pain. During diagnostic imaging, there is a characteristic triangular area of sclerosis located near the medial ilium.

Sacroiliac subluxation may produce irritative microtrauma to the articular structures, induction of spinal curvatures, induction of spinal or pelvic subluxation and fixation, and biomechanical abnormalities in stance and locomotion. Evaluation of the sacroiliac joint for the presence of such subluxation or fixation will need to combine both static and dynamic palpation as well as a plumb-line analysis. There may be tenderness during palpation of the posterior superior iliac spine when there is innominate rotation. A full range-of-motion palpation procedure is needed to evaluate the joint for motion abnormalities or fixation. Both the static and organic procedures need to be performed to evaluate the joint for subluxation or fixation.

In the normal, erect sitting position with weight on the thighs, the coccyx does not have pressure against it. With flattening of the lumbar lordosis and sitting in the slumping position, however, the coccyx can reach the seat, and pain may develop over its tip. In coccydynia, pain on sitting is the most common complaint. This pain is aggravated by slumping, sitting on a hard seat, or activity. Many symptoms begin with an injury and may be aggravated by constipation or rectal disease. The symptoms are more common in females than in males. Fractures, when they occur, usually involve the lower part of the sacrum or first sacrococcygeal segments (Fig. 9-56).

PROCEDURE

- The patient is seated to keep the hamstrings from affecting pelvic-flexion symmetry.
- The posterior superior iliac spines are located and compared for height (Fig. 9-57).
- If one posterior-superior iliac spine (PSIS) is lower than the other, the patient flexes forward.
- If the lower PSIS becomes higher during forward flexion, the test is positive.
- The PSIS migration to a higher prominence is the positive sign (Fig. 9-58).
- An abnormality in the torsion motion of the sacroiliac joint is suggested by the positive finding.

Confirmation Procedures

Anterior innominate test, knee-to-shoulder test, Lewin-Gaenslen's test, sacral apex test, and sacroiliac resisted-abduction test

---

DIAGNOSTIC STATEMENT

Piedallu's sign is present for the right sacroiliac joint and indicates an abnormality in the torsion movement of the joint.

CLINICAL PEARL

In the sacroiliac joint fixation complex, an irregular prominence of one articular surface becomes wedged on another prominence of the opposing articular surface. When reduction is successful, the pain is relieved immediately.

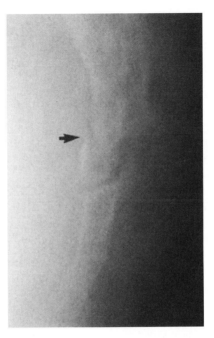

FIG. 9-56   Fracture of the lower portion of the sacrum.   *(From Mercier LR, Pettid FJ:* Practical orthopedics, *ed 4, St Louis, 1995, Mosby.)*

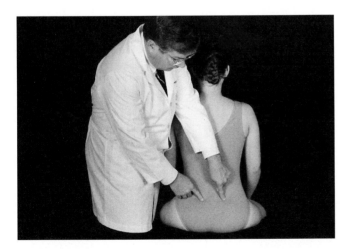

FIG. 9-57   The patient is seated on a hard, flat surface. The examiner notes pelvic symmetry and compares the height of the iliac crests.

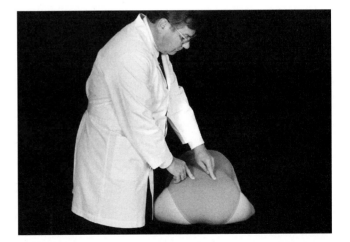

FIG. 9-58   If the posterior superior iliac spine on the affected side is lower than that of the other, unaffected side, the patient flexes forward while remaining seated. If the lower posterior superior iliac spine now becomes higher, the test is positive for an abnormality of torsion motion of the sacroiliac joint.

Assessment for Abnormal Rotational Shifting of the Sacroiliac Joint

Comment

The sacroiliac joint is made up of thin anterior ligaments that blend in with the true anterior joint capsule and a thick posterior ligament complex with interosseous and accessory components (Fig. 9-59).

The forces for sacroiliac joint motion are gravity, ground reaction force, and muscle power. Sacroiliac joint motion is initiated by the muscles of the vertebral column, thighs, and respiratory system. The vertebral column muscles initiate sacroiliac joint motion of the sacrum, relative to the ilium, by changing posture (lying down, sitting, and standing) and by changing the shape of the spinal column (flexion, extension, lateral flexion, and rotation). The movement is caused by change in the center of gravity, with the apex of the lordotic curve moving up or down, which causes the sacrum to nutate and the ilium to flare. As a result, the articular surfaces move anterosuperiorly to posteroinferiorly and superomedially to inferolaterally. The two posterior superior iliac spines will approximate and separate. During lateral flexion, both iliac and sacral auricular surfaces move together but gap at different times in the anterior or posterior part of the joint and the upper or lower margins.

The thigh muscles initiate sacroiliac joint motion of the ilium, relative to the sacrum, again by altering posture and causing motion of the thigh rather than the spine. Here, motions will include thigh flexion, extension, supination, pronation, abduction, and adduction. The two thighs can act together or independently. Abduction and adduction create sacroiliac joint gapping but no shearing of cartilage.

Respiration aids sacroiliac joint motion during inspiration and expiration. During inspiration, the erector spinae muscles contract, and the rectus abdominis relaxes by decreasing abdominal pressure. The pelvic diaphragm also relaxes and decreases abdominal pressure. When the erector group pulls the posterior part of the pelvic ring up and the rectus abdominis is relaxed, the pelvic ring will be tilted anteriorly. This tilt causes the sacral promontory to move backward and superiorly. During expiration, the erector group relaxes, the rectus abdominis contracts, and the pelvic diaphragm contracts. Action of the rectus abdominis pulls the symphysis pubis up and tilts the pelvic ring posteriorly. Abdominal pressure is increased, which causes the sacral promontory to move anteriorly and inferiorly.

PROCEDURE

- The patient is prone.
- The examiner places pressure at the apex of the sacrum.
- Pressure is increased, causing a shear of the sacrum on the ilium (Fig. 9-60).
- If pain is produced over the joint, the test is positive.

Confirmation Procedures

Anterior innominate test, knee-to-shoulder test, Lewin-Gaenslen's test, Piedallu's sign, and sacroiliac resisted-abduction test

DIAGNOSTIC STATEMENT

The sacral apex test is positive and indicates an abnormal rotational shifting of the right or left sacroiliac joint.

CLINICAL PEARL

Sciatic neuritis is a term used to describe pain or other discomfort that is experienced anywhere along the distribution of the sciatic nerve and is due to a primary disease of the nerve or, more commonly, a mechanical disorder affecting the nerve. A sacroiliac subluxation-sprain may be the true cause of sciatic neuritis. The piriformis muscle is most often affected, and it may involve the L5-S1 and S2 distribution.

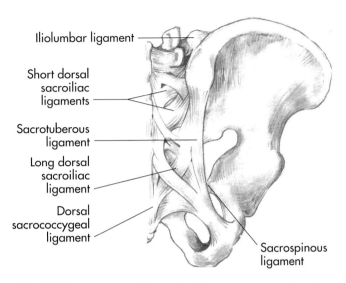

Iliolumbar ligament

Short dorsal sacroiliac ligaments

Sacrotuberous ligament

Long dorsal sacroiliac ligament

Dorsal sacrococcygeal ligament

Sacrospinous ligament

FIG. 9-59 L5 sacrum-iliac articulation, posteroanterior view.
(From Brier SR: Primary care orthopedics, *St Louis, 1999, Mosby.)*

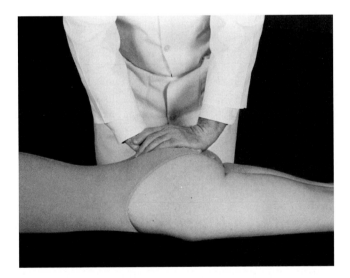

FIG. 9-60 The patient is prone. The examiner places pressure on the apex of the sacrum. Pressure is increased, causing a shear stress of the sacrum on the ilium. Pain produced in a sacroiliac joint is a positive test.

SACROILIAC
RESISTED-ABDUCTION TEST

HIP-ABDUCTION STRESS TEST

Assessment for Generalized Abductor Muscular Weakness or Sprain or Subluxation of the Sacroiliac Joint

Comment

The sacroiliac joint has well-developed cartilage surfaces, a synovial membrane, strong anterior and posterior ligaments, and a large internal sacroiliac ligament. After the fifth decade of life, fibrosis takes place between the cartilage surfaces. By the sixth or seventh decade, the joint has usually undergone fibrous ankylosis. Bony ankylosis is a rare phenomenon late in life. The joint surfaces can rotate 3 to 5 degrees in the younger, symptom-free patient. The joint has two functions: to provide elasticity to the pelvic ring and to serve as a buffer between the lumbosacral and hip joints.

The sacroiliac syndrome causes pain over one sacroiliac joint in the region of the posterior superior iliac spine. This pain may be accompanied by referred pain in the leg.

The mechanism of injury is not well understood. Until late in middle age, a small amount of movement (3 to 5 degrees) is usually present in the sacroiliac joint. After that age, movement is reduced by articular cartilage degeneration, fibrosis, and rarely, ankylosis. It is possible that minor dysfunction in the sacroiliac joint leads to pain, but it is more reasonable to suppose that pain results from sustained contraction of the muscle overlying the joint. This hypertonicity may accompany dysfunction in the sacroiliac joint or in the L4-L5 or L5-S1 posterior lumbar joints.

A typical symptom is pain that varies in its degree of severity and is over the back of the sacroiliac joint. Another typical symptom is referred pain in the groin, over the greater trochanter; down the back of the thigh to the knee; and, occasionally, down the lateral or posterior calf to the ankle, foot, and toes.

One of the more common results of the peripheral entrapment of the sciatic nerve at the pelvis is the piriformis syndrome. A fairly perplexing diagnostic problem, patients with this syndrome have buttock pain in the region of the sciatic notch and down the back of the thigh and leg. The lack of orthopedic and motion findings locally at the spine distinguishes this peripheral entrapment from a lumbar disc lesion. In a small segment of the population, the sciatic nerve splits the piriformis muscle.

Hip flexion with rotation causes pain in an individual with piriformis syndrome because it stretches the piriformis muscle, thereby compromising or irritating the sciatic nerve. Activities that externally rotate the thigh can strain the piriformis muscle, eventually leading to local swelling and irritation of the sciatic nerve sheath and, eventually, sciatic neuritis.

ORTHOPEDIC GAMUT 9-11

PIRIFORMIS MUSCLE

Trigger points in the piriformis muscle refer pain to the following:

1. The buttocks
2. Toward the hip
3. Posterior thigh
4. Calf
5. The sole of the foot

PROCEDURE

- The patient lies on the unaffected side with the affected leg extended and slightly abducted (Fig. 9-61).
- The unaffected limb can be flexed at the hip and knee to provide stability.
- The examiner then exerts downward pressure on the abducted leg against the patient's resistance (Fig. 9-62).
- The test is repeated on the opposite side.
- If the test elicits pelvic pain near the posterior superior iliac spine, it is positive (Fig. 9-63).
- The test is specific for a sacroiliac sprain or subluxation.

Confirmation Procedures

Anterior innominate test, knee-to-shoulder test, Lewin-Gaenslen's test, Piedallu's sign, and sacral apex test

---

DIAGNOSTIC STATEMENT

Sacroiliac resisted-abduction test is positive on the left and indicates generalized abductor muscular weakness. The pain elicited implicates the sacroiliac joint and indicates sprain or subluxation of the joint.

CLINICAL PEARL

Slight, unilateral hip-abductor weakness is found in association with lateral pelvic tilt. The abductors are weak on the slightly elevated side of the pelvis. The beginning weakness in the abductors, as seen in nonparalytic individuals, is usually associated with handedness and is a strain weakness from postural or occupational causes.

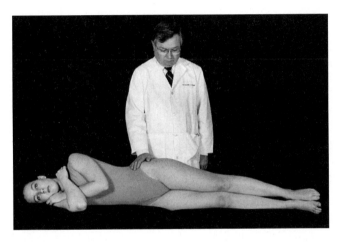

FIG. 9-61   The patient is in a side-lying position on the unaffected side.

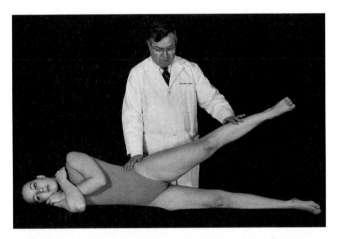

FIG. 9-62   The patient actively abducts the affected leg. At the end of the range of movement, the examiner applies downward pressure on the affected limb. The patient tries to resist this pressure. When it is positive, the test elicits pain at the posterior superior iliac spine. The test is specific for sacroiliac sprain or subluxation.

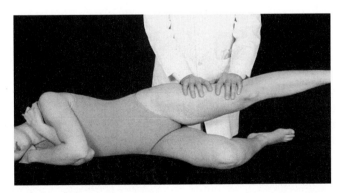

FIG. 9-63   In a slight modification that is only for more stability of the pelvis, the patient may flex the knee of the unaffected leg.

SMITH-PETERSEN TEST

The Smith-Petersen test is often confused with and thought to be synonymous with the Goldthwait's sign or Lasegue test.

Assessment for Sacroiliac Joint Involvement versus Lumbosacral Spine Involvement

Comment

Patients with chronic postural or mechanical problems in the lumbar spine or those individuals who are vulnerable to repetitive injury may develop a chronic lumbar strain. Similar to the acute traumatic sprain, the sacroiliac syndrome commonly causes disability and associated mechanical problems. The patient has sacroiliac tenderness, various fixation patterns, and discomfort or limitation in lumbar flexion and rotation.

ORTHOPEDIC GAMUT 9-12

SACROILIAC JOINT INJURIES

Following are four forms that sacroiliac joint injuries may take:

1. Dislocation, where the articular surfaces are completely displaced from each other
2. Subluxation, where the articular surfaces remain in contact although they are displaced
3. Sprain, in which there is a tear of the capsular ligament without a disturbance in its relationship to the opposing surfaces
4. Fracture-dislocation, where a fracture of part of one of the bones has taken place for the articular surfaces to be completely displaced from each other

---

For complete separation of the articular surfaces in a normal sacroiliac joint to be possible, the capsule of the joint must be completely torn through. Therefore this is an injury that resulted from considerable violence having been applied to the joint. The soft-tissue damage may cause some residual stiffness because of scarring. At certain sites, where the cavity is shallow, residual capsular laxity may leave an unstable joint. There also may be an unhealed rent that leads to recurrent dislocation. Pathologic dislocations may occur where there is some inherent ligamentous laxity or abnormal muscle pull, such as in certain neurologic disorders leading to paralytic dislocations. Pathologic dislocations also may occur where the joint lining has been destroyed by an infective process.

Partial displacement of the articular surfaces of the sacroiliac joint, when the bones remain in contact with each other, is a subluxation. In these cases, residual laxity usually persists.

Tears of the capsular lining of the sacroiliac joint may be of a trivial nature, or they may be severe, involving a complete disruption of one of the posterior ligaments. In the latter case, momentary subluxation will have taken place, and unless the ligamentous rent heals, recurrent sprains from minor violence occurs.

The fracture of the bony margin of the sacroiliac joint, as it is dislocated, is most commonly seen in the more severe rotational injuries.

PROCEDURE

- The Smith-Petersen test is performed with the patient in the supine posture (Fig. 9-64).
- Straight leg raising is performed slowly, while one hand is placed under the lower part of the patient's spine.
- As the hamstrings tighten, leverage is progressively applied to the sacroiliac joint and then to the lumbosacral articulation.
- If pain is brought on before the lumbar spine begins to move, Smith-Petersen considers that a sacroiliac condition is present (Fig. 9-65).
- If, however, pain does not come on until after the lumbar spine begins to move, either sacroiliac or lumbosacral involvement may be present.
- Straight leg raising of both sides should be accomplished.
- If, on the unaffected side, the leg can be raised much higher, sacroiliac involvement is likely.
- If discomfort is elicited when both legs are brought to the same level, lumbosacral involvement is likely.

Confirmation Procedures

Belt test, Gaenslen's test, and Goldthwait's test

DIAGNOSTIC STATEMENT

Smith-Petersen test is positive on the right and strongly indicates sacroiliac joint involvement on that side.

Smith-Petersen test is positive bilaterally and indicates lumbosacral involvement.

CLINICAL PEARL

An acute sacroiliac flexion sprain is caused by lifting heavy objects. Often, however, the patient with chronic sacral pain has also sustained an ancient fall or flexion sprain. In cases of partial tearing of the sacroiliac ligaments, where poor healing has taken place, a painful fibrous area persists, and this results in a chronic, weak area of the joint. This area becomes symptomatic when placed under tension and stress.

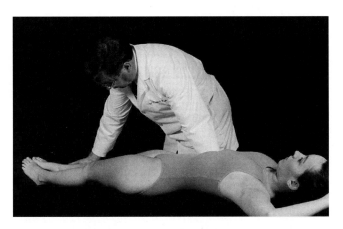

FIG. 9-64 The patient is supine on the examination table. The examiner stands at the side of the table next to the affected leg. The examiner places one hand under the patient's lumbar spine and palpates the L5-S1 spinous processes.

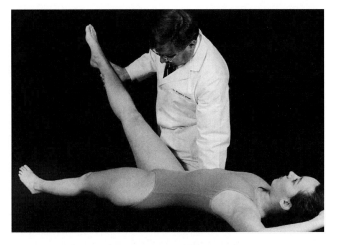

FIG. 9-65 While maintaining contact with the lumbosacral bony landmarks, the examiner performs a straight-leg-raising maneuver on the affected leg. If pain occurs before the L5-S1 spinous processes separate, a sacroiliac lesion is present. If pain occurs as the L5-S1 spinous processes separate, either a sacroiliac or lumbosacral lesion may be present. The test is performed bilaterally.

Assessment for Posterior Sacroiliac Ligament Damage

Comment
Pelvic fractures comprise a spectrum of injuries ranging from stress or insufficiency fractures in osteoporotic bone to life-threatening disruptions of the pelvis ring.

ORTHOPEDIC GAMUT 9-13

BONY PELVIS

Injuries to the bony pelvis are of the following two types:

1. Isolated fractures of the pubic rami or ilium
2. Double fractures of the pelvic ring

ORTHOPEDIC GAMUT 9-14

PELVIC RING

The double fractures of the pelvic ring may occur in the following three forms:

1. With the first type, the anterior portion of the ring may be broken if all four pubic rami are broken, and the loose portion of the ring will get driven posteriorly.
2. With the second type, one side of the pubis may be fractured anteriorly and posteriorly and may roll laterally.
3. With the last type, one side of the pelvic ring may be fractured and not only may it roll laterally but also it may be superiorly displaced.

As with all bony injuries of the trunk, the possibility of visceral damage must be constantly borne in the examiner's mind. With pelvic injuries, this possibility is particularly applicable because the rectum, bladder, and urethra are contained within the pelvic cavity. As the membranous urethra passes through the pelvic diaphragm, this structure is especially vulnerable. A blow hard enough to disrupt the pubic bones is also very capable of rupturing a distended bladder.

Isolated pelvic fractures follow direct blows and therefore occur rather more readily in the more osteoporotic bones of the elderly. Fractures of the ilium alone, although less common than fractures of the pubic rami, usually result from greater trauma and therefore cause more constitutional upset to the patient. Fractures of the pubic rami on one side are of little significance unless they extend into the hip joint.

Detachment of the whole anterior segment of the pubis follows a severe blow on the front of the pelvis. This injury usually results from road accidents or sometimes from falls from a height when the patient lands prone and strikes this region on some hard object.

With lateral disruption of the pelvic ring, the pelvic ring is broken both posterior and anterior to the hip. The natural tendency for the lower limb to roll laterally will open the pelvis anteriorly. The plane of cleavage in the anterior will be either through both pubic rami on the affected side or through the pubic symphysis (diastasis of the symphysis pubis). Posteriorly, the break may be through the ilium, at the sacroiliac joint, or through the ala of the sacrum itself.

The most severe fracture is a combined lateral and superior displacement. With this form of pelvic fracture, the displaced fragment, which is attached to the lower limbs, not only has rolled laterally but also is displaced superiorly.

PROCEDURE

- The patient is supine.
- Pressure is placed on the patient's anterosuperior iliac spines. The examiner pushes down at a 45-degree angle (Fig. 9-66).
- Pain indicates a positive test and suggests injury of the posterior sacroiliac ligaments.

Confirmation Procedures
Gapping test and Yeoman's test

DIAGNOSTIC STATEMENT

The squish test is positive on the right or left. This result indicates damage to the posterior sacroiliac ligaments.

CLINICAL PEARL

In the elderly, fractures of the pubic rami and ischial rami are often caused by a trivial fall. The fractures usually occur in pairs. Fracture of one ramus alone is unusual. A positive squish test in an elderly patient indicates a possible fracture of a ramus and a posterior sacroiliac sprain. The fracture can be confirmed with diagnostic imaging.

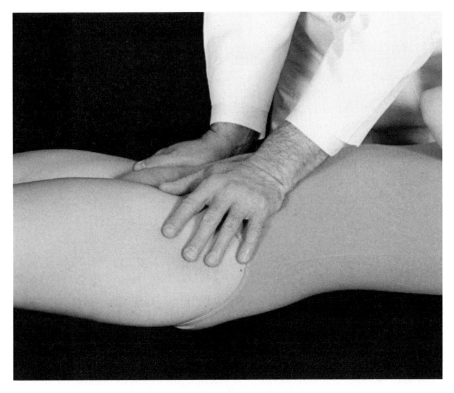

FIG. 9-66 The patient is supine. Pressure is placed on the patient's anterior superior iliac spines. The examiner pushes inferior and caudal at a 45-degree angle. A positive test indicates sprain of the posterior sacroiliac ligaments.

YEOMAN'S TEST

Assessment for Anterior Sacroiliac Ligament Injury

Comment

When certain lumbosacral spinal mesodermal structures—such as ligaments, periosteum, joint capsule, and the annulus—are subjected to abnormal stimuli—such as excessive stretching—a deep, ill-defined, and dull aching is noted. This aching may be referred into areas of the lumbosacral spine, sacroiliac joint, buttocks, and legs. The referral pattern is to the area designated as the sclerotome, which has the same embryonic origin as the mesodermal tissues stimulated. Although this peripheral pathway can explain the referred pain pattern, the significant individual variations that are encountered necessitate the consideration of central neural pathways. Referred pain distribution depends not only on segmental innervation but also on the severity of pain and the extent to which an individual is cognizant of the stimulated components of the axial skeleton.

Pain of this type can often present concurrently with radicular pain that results from nerve root tension. The deeper, penetrating pain is usually attributed to distribution along the myotome and sclerotome. The sharper and more localized superficial pain is conveyed via the dermatomes.

The two types of pain may easily be confused. Moreover, sympathetic dystrophic signs and symptoms caused by nerve root encroachment can further confuse the presentation because the causalgia may exist with or without the more classic complaints associated with radiculopathy.

Thus all lower extremity pain is not a result of nerve root compression.

PROCEDURE

- The patient is lying prone.
- With one hand, the examiner applies firm pressure over the suspect sacroiliac joint, fixing the pelvis to the table (Fig. 9-67).
- With the other hand, the examiner flexes the patient's leg on the affected side and hyperextends the thigh by lifting the knee off the examining table (Fig. 9-68).
- If pain is increased in the sacroiliac area, this increase in pain indicates a sacroiliac lesion.
- This pain is caused by the strain placed on the anterior sacroiliac ligaments.
- In a patient without a sacroiliac lesion, pain will not be felt during this maneuver.

Confirmation Procedures

Gapping test and Squish test

DIAGNOSTIC STATEMENT

Yeoman's test is positive for the left sacroiliac joint. This result indicates injury of the anterior sacroiliac ligaments.

CLINICAL PEARL

Ruptured sacroiliac ligaments do not heal soundly, even if they are accurately repaired, because the scar tissue, which forms at the site of the repair, stretches and is never as tough as the original. Surgical repair is often attempted after severe rupture of these ligaments, but conservative management may be equally effective.

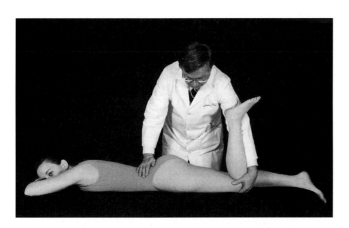

FIG. 9-67   The patient is prone on the examination table. With one hand, the examiner stabilizes the affected sacroiliac joint. The examiner flexes the knee of the affected leg to 90 degrees.

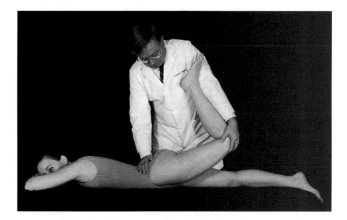

FIG. 9-68   The examiner hyperextends the thigh of the affected leg by lifting it off the examination table. Pressure is maintained over the affected sacroiliac joint. Increased sacroiliac pain constitutes a positive test and indicates a sacroiliac joint lesion.

CRITICAL THINKING

What are the seronegative spondyloarthropathies?
Ankylosing spondylitis, psoriatic arthritis, reactive arthritis (Reiter's syndrome), juvenile ankylosing spondylitis, and arthropathies that complicate inflammatory bowel diseases (regional enteritis and ulcerative colitis)

How is sacroiliitis best demonstrated radiographically?
An anteroposterior radiograph of the pelvis usually suffices to demonstrate the bilateral sacroiliitis of ankylosing spondylitis.

What is osteitis condensans ilii (OCI)?
OCI is characterized by a triangular area of dense sclerotic bone limited to iliac bones of the pelvis adjacent to the lower half of normal sacroiliac joints.

What are Malgaigne fractures?
Malgaigne fractures usually refer to unstable fracture-dislocations of the pelvis, of both the superior and inferior pubic rami.

BIBLIOGRAPHY

Abrams WB, Berkow R: *The Merck manual of geriatrics,* Rahway, NJ, 1990, Merck Sharp & Dohme Research Laboratories.

Adams JC, Hamblen DL: *Outline of orthopaedics,* ed 11, Edinburgh, 1990, Churchill Livingstone.

Alario AJ: *Practical guide to the care of the pediatric patient,* St Louis, 1997, Mosby.

Allison D, Strickland N: *Acronyms & synonyms in medical imaging,* Oxford, 1996, ISIS Medical Media.

Altman RD: Musculoskeletal questions and answers, *J Musculoskeletal Med* 7:10, 1990.

American Medical Association: *Guides to the evaluation of permanent impairment,* ed 4, Chicago, 1993, The Association.

American Medical Association: *How to use guides to the evaluation of permanent impairment,* ed 4, Falmouth, Conn, 1993, SEAK.

Anderson KN, Anderson LE: *Mosby's pocket dictionary of medicine, nursing, & allied health,* ed 2, St Louis, 1994, Mosby.

Andersson GBJ: The epidemiology of spinal disorders. In Frymoyer JW, editor: *The adult spine: principles and practice,* New York, 1990, Raven.

Andersson GBJ: Occupational biomechanics. In Weinstein J, Wiesel SW, editors: *The lumbar spine,* Philadelphia, 1990, WB Saunders.

Apley AG, Solomon L: *Concise system of orthopaedics and fractures,* London, 1988, Butterworth-Heinemann.

Apps BK, Cohen BB, Steel CM: *Biochemistry, a concise test for medical students,* ed 5, Iowa City, 1992, Bailliere Tindall.

Aston JN: *A short textbook of orthopaedics and traumatology,* Philadelphia, 1967, JB Lippincott.

Bakkum B, Cramer G: Muscles that influence the spine. In Cramer G, Darby S: *Basic and clinical anatomy of the spine, spinal cord, and ANS,* St Louis, 1995, Mosby.

Ballinger PW: *Merrill's atlas of radiographic positions and radiologic procedures,* vol 1-3, ed 8, St Louis, 1995, Mosby.

Barkauskas VH, et al: *Health & physical assessment,* ed 2, St Louis, 1998, Mosby.

Battie MC, Bigos SJ: Industrial back pain complaints, *Orthop Clin North Am* 22:273, 1991.

Beal MC: The sacroiliac problem, review of anatomy, mechanics and diagnosis, *J Am Osteopath Assoc* 82:667, 1982.

Berens DL: Roentgen features of ankylosing spondylitis, *Clin Orthop* 74:20, 1971.

Berghs H, et al: Diagnostic value of sacroiliac joint scintigraphy with 99m technetium pyrophosphate in sacroiliitis, *Ann Rheum Dis* 37:190, 1978.

Bhagavan NV: *Medical biochemistry,* Boston, 1992, Jones and Bartlett.

Boden SD, et al: *The aging spine,* Philadelphia, 1991, WB Saunders.

Bogduk N, Amevo B, Pearcy M: A biological basis for instantaneous centers of rotation of the vertebral column, *Proc Inst Mech Eng* 209:177, 1995.

Bogduk N, Macintosh JE, Pearcy MJ: A universal model of the lumbar back muscles in the upright position, *Spine* 17:897, 1992.

Bogduk N, Twomey LT: *Clinical anatomy of the lumbar spine,* ed 2, Melbourne, 1991, Churchill Livingstone.

Borenstein DG, Wiesel SW: *Low back pain: medical diagnosis and comprehensive management,* Philadelphia, 1989, WB Saunders.

Bowen V, Cassidy JD: Macroscopic and microscopic anatomy of the sacroiliac joint from embryonic life until the eighth decade, *Spine* 6:620, 1981.

Brand C, et al: Cryptococcal sacroiliitis: case report, *Ann Rheum Dis* 44:126, 1985.

Breen A: The reliability of palpation and other diagnostic methods, *J Manipulative Physiol Ther* 15:54, 1992.

Brier SR: *Primary care orthopedics,* St Louis, 1999, Mosby.

Brier SR, Nyfield B: A comparison of hip and lumbopelvic inflexibility and low back pain in runners and cyclists, *J Manipulative Physiol Ther* 18:25, 1995.

Brooks M, Evans R, Fairclough J: *Sports injuries,* ed 2, London, 1992, Gower Medical Publishing.

Brotzman SB: *Clinical orthopaedic rehabilitation,* St Louis, 1996, Mosby.

Brown DE, Neumann RD: *Orthopedic secrets,* Philadelphia, 1995, Hanley & Belfus.

Brunner C, Kissling R, Jacob HAC: The efforts of morphology and histopathologic findings on the mobility of the sacroiliac joint, *Spine* 16:1111, 1991.

Bucholz RW: *Orthopaedic decision making,* ed 2, St Louis, 1996, Mosby.

Budgell B, Noda K, Sata A: Innervation of posterior structures in the lumbar spine of the rat, *J Manipulative Physiol Ther* 20:359, 1997.

Burgess A, et al: Pelvic ring disruptions: effective classification system and treatment protocols *J Trauma* 30:848, 1990.

Campbell JB, Campbell JM: *Mosby's survival guide to medical abbreviations & acronyms prefixes & suffixes symbols Greek alphabet,* St Louis, 1995, Mosby.

Canale ST: *Campbell's operative orthopaedics,* vol 1-4, ed 9, St Louis, 1998, Mosby.

Carrera GF, et al: CT of sacroiliitis, *AJR Am J Roentgenol* 136:41, 1981.

Cassidy JD: *The pathoanatomy and clinical significance of the sacroiliac joints,* Toronto, 1991, World Chiropractic Congress.

Cats A, Linder SM: Spondyloarthropathies: an overview, *Spine* 4:497, 1990.

Cipriano JJ: *Photographic manual of regional orthopaedic and neurological test,* ed 3, Baltimore, 1997, Williams & Wilkins.

Cohn RE: *Impairment rating examination and disability evaluation,* ed 3, Wilkesboro, NC, 1994, R Ernest Cohn.

Colachis SC: Movement of sacroiliac joint in adult male, *Arch Phys Med Rehabil* 44:490, 1963.

Cole AJ, Herring SA: *The low back pain handbook: a practical guide for the primary care examiner,* Philadelphia, 1997, Hanley & Belfus.

Cox JM: *Low back pain, mechanism, diagnosis and treatment,* ed 5, Baltimore, 1990, Williams & Wilkins.

Coy JT, et al: Pyogenic arthritis of the sacroiliac joint: long-term follow-up, *J Bone Joint Surg* 58A:845, 1976.

Craik RL, Oatis CA: *Gait analysis theory and application,* St Louis, 1995, Mosby.

Cramer GD, Darby SA: *Basic and clinical anatomy of the spine, spinal cord, and ANS,* St Louis, 1995, Mosby.

Cullinan AM: *Optimizing radiographic positioning,* Philadelphia, 1992, Lippincott.

Curtis P: In search of the "back mouse," *J Fam Pract* 36:657, 1993.

Cyriax J: *Textbook of orthopaedic medicine, vol. 1, diagnosis of soft tissue lesions,* London, 1982, Bailliere Tindall.

Daffner RH, et al: The radiology assessment of post-traumatic vertebral stability, *Skeletal Radiol* 19:103, 1990.

Dambro MR, Griffith JA: *Griffith's 5 minute clinical consult,* Baltimore, 1997, Williams & Wilkins.

D'Ambrogio KJ, Roth GB: *Positional release therapy assessment & treatment of musculoskeletal dysfunction,* St Louis, 1997, Mosby.

D'Ambrosia RD: *Musculoskeletal disorders: regional examination and differential diagnosis,* Philadelphia, 1977, JB Lippincott.

Dandy DJ: *Essential orthopaedics and trauma,* Edinburgh, 1989, Churchill Livingstone.

deBlecourt JJ, et al: Hereditary factors in rheumatoid arthritis and ankylosing spondylitis, *Ann Rheum Dis* 20:215, 1961.

DeBosset P, et al: Comparison of osteitis condensans ilii and ankylosing spondylitis in female patients: clinical, radiological and HLA typing characteristics, *J Chron Dis* 31:171, 1978.

Delbarre F, et al: Pyogenic infection of the sacroiliac joint, *J Bone Joint Surg* 57A:819, 1975.

Deltoff MN, Kogon PL: *The portable skeletal x-ray library,* St Louis, 1998, Mosby.

Demeter SL, Andersson GBJ, Smith GM: *Disability evaluation,* St Louis, 1996, Mosby.

Deshpande JK, Tobias JD: *The pediatric pain handbook,* St Louis, 1996, Mosby.

Dettenmeier PA: *Radiographic assessment for nurses,* St Louis, 1995, Mosby.

Dihlmann W: *Diagnostic radiology of the sacroiliac joints,* New York, 1980, George Thieme Verlag.

Dilsen N, et al: A comparative roentgenologic study of rheumatoid arthritis and rheumatoid (ankylosing) spondylitis, *Arthritis Rheum* 5:341, 1962.

Doherty M: *Color atlas and text of osteoarthritis,* London, 1994, Wolfe.

Doherty M, Doherty J: *Clinical examination in rheumatology,* London, 1992, Wolfe.

Doherty M, George E: *Self-assessment picture tests in rheumatology,* London, 1995, Mosby-Wolfe.

DonTigny RL: Anterior dysfunction of sacroiliac joint as a major factor in the etiology of idiopathic low back pain syndrome, *Phys Ther* 70:250, 1990.

Dulhunty JA: Sacroiliac subluxation, facts, fallacies and illusions, *J Aust Chiro Assoc* 15:91, 1985.

Dunn DJ, Bryan Dm, Nugent JT, Robinson RA: Pyogenic infections of the sacroiliac joint, *Clin Orthop* 118:113, 1976.

Ebraheim N, et al: Percutaneous computed tomography guided stabilization of posterior pelvis fractures, *Clin Orthop* 307:222, 1994.

Elliott FA, Schutta HS: The differential diagnosis of sciatica, *Orthop Clin North Am* 2:477, 1971.

Elster AD: *Questions and answers in magnetic resonance imaging,* St Louis, 1994, Mosby.

Epstein MC: Cause of low back problem, *Dig Chiro Econ* 26:52, 1983.

Epstein O, et al: *Clinical examination,* ed 2, London, 1997, Mosby.

Failinger MS, McGanety PL: Current concepts review, unstable fractures of the pelvic ring, *J Bone Joint Surg* 74A:781, 1992.

Farfan HF: *Mechanical disorders of the low back,* Philadelphia, 1973, Lea & Febiger.

Farrar WE: *Atlas of infections of the nervous system,* London, 1993, Wolfe.

Feldmann E: *Current diagnosis in neurology,* St Louis, 1994, Mosby.

Ferezy JS: *The chiropractic neurological examination,* Gaithersburg, Md, 1992, Aspen.

Finneson BE: *Low back pain,* ed 2, Philadelphia, 1980, JB Lippincott.

Freeman MD, Fox D, Richards T: The superior intracapsular ligament of the sacroiliac joint: confirmation of Ill's ligament, *J Manipulative Physiol Ther* 13:374, 1990.

Garcia JH: *Neuropathology the diagnostic approach,* St Louis, 1997, Mosby.

Gatterman MI: Disorders of the pelvic ring. In Gatterman MI, editor: *Chiropractic management of spine-related disorders,* Baltimore, 1990, Williams & Wilkins.

Gibbons K, Soloniuk D, Razack N: Neurological injury and patterns of sacral fractures, *J Neurosurg* 72:889, 1990.

Gifford DB, et al: Septic arthritis due to pseudomonas in heroin addicts, *J Bone Joint Surg* 57A:631, 1975.

Giles LGF, Kaveri MJP: Some osseous and soft tissue causes of lumbar stenosis, *J Rheumatol* 17:1374, 1990.

Goldberg, J, Kovarsky J: Tuberculous sacroiliitis, *South Med J* 76:1175, 1983.

Goldie BS: *Orthopaedic diagnosis and management a guide to the care of orthopaedic patients,* ed 2, Oxford, 1998, ISIS Medical Media.

Goldstein MJ, et al: Osteomyelitis complicating regional enteritis, *Gut* 10:264, 1969.

Goldstein TS: Treatment of common problems of the hip joint. In Goldstein TS, Lewis CB, series editors: *Geriatric orthopaedics rehabilitative management for common problems,* Gaithersburg, Md, 1991, Aspen.

Gordon G, Kabins SA: Pyogenic sacroiliitis, *Am J Med* 69:50, 1980.

Gorse GJ, et al: Tuberculous spondylitis: a report of six cases and a review of the literature, *Medicine (Baltimore)* 62:178, 1978.

Goulet J, et al: Comminuted fractures of the posterior wall of the acetabulum: a biomechanical evaluation of fixation methods, *J Bone Joint Surg* 76A:1457, 1994.

Gracovetsky S: Biomechanics of the spine. In White AH, Schofferman JA, editors: *Spine care: diagnosis and conservative treatment,* St Louis, 1995, Mosby.

Greenman PE: Innominate shear dysfunction in sacroiliac syndrome, *J Manual Med* 2:114, 1986.

Greenspan A, Montesano P: *Imaging of the spine in clinical practice,* London, 1993, Wolfe.

Greenstein GM: *Clinical assessment of neuromusculoskeletal disorders,* St Louis, 1997, Mosby.

Groen GJ, Baljet B, Drukker J: Nerves and nerve plexuses of the human vertebral column, *Am J Anat* 188:282, 1990.

Gross ML, Nasser S, Finnerman GAM: Hip and pelvis. In DeLee JC, Drez D, editors: *Orthopaedic sports medicine: principles and practice,* vol 2, Philadelphia, 1994, WB Saunders.

Grossman ZD, et al: *Cost-effective diagnostic imaging: the examiner's guide,* ed 3, St Louis, 1995, Mosby.

Hawkins RJ: *An organized approach to musculoskeletal examination and history taking,* St Louis, 1995, Mosby.

Helfet D, Schmeling G: Management of complex acetabular fractures through single nonextensile exposures, *Clin Orthop* 305:58, 1994.

Hendrix RW, Lin PJP, Kane WJ: Simplified aspiration or injection techniques for the sacroiliac joint, *J Bone Joint Surg* 64A:1249, 1982.

Hinkle CZ: *Fundamentals of anatomy & movement: a workbook and guide,* St Louis, 1997, Mosby.

Hornberger JP: *Exercise physiology therapeutic exercise,* Sarasota, Fla, 1991, Joseph P Hornberger.

Iczkovitz JM, Leek JC, Robbins DL: Pyogenic sacroiliitis, *J Rheumatol* 8:157, 1981.

Isler B: Lumbosacral lesions associated with pelvic ring injuries, *J Orthop Trauma* 4:1, 1990.

Jablonski S: *Dictionary of medical acronyms & abbreviations,* ed 3, Philadelphia, 1998, Hanley & Belfus.

Jenkins DH, Young MH: The operative treatment of sacroiliac subluxation and disruption of the symphysis pubis, *Injury* 10:139, 1978.

Kanner R: *Pain management secrets,* Philadelphia, 1997, Hanley & Belfus.

Kapandji LA: *The physiology of the joints, vol 3: The trunk and vertebral column,* New York, 1974, Churchill Livingstone.

Katirji B: *Electromyography in clinical practice: a case study approach,* St Louis, 1998, Mosby.

Katz WA: *Rheumatic diseases diagnosis and management,* Philadelphia, 1977, JB Lippincott.

Keats TE, Lusted LB: *Atlas of roentgenographic measurements,* ed 6, St Louis, 1990, Mosby.

Kelley WN, et al: *Textbook of rheumatology,* vol 1, ed 4, Philadelphia, 1993, Saunders.

Kellgren JH: The anatomical source of back pain, *Rheumatol Rehab* 16:3, 1977.

Kendall HO, Kendall FP, Wadsworth GE: *Muscles testing and function,* ed 2, Baltimore, 1971, Williams & Wilkins.

Khan MA, Linder SM: Ankylosing spondylitis: clinical aspects, *Spine* 4:529, 1990.

King L: Incidence of sacroiliac joint dysfunction and low back pain in fit college students, *J Manipulative Physiol Ther* 14:333, 1991.

Kingston RS: Radiology of the spine. In Watkins RG, editor: *The spine in sports,* St Louis, 1996, Mosby.

Kirkaldy-Willis WH: *Managing low back pain,* New York, 1983, Churchill Livingstone.

Klippel JH, Dieppe PA: *Rheumatology,* vol 1-2, ed 2, London, 1998, Mosby.

Koenigsberg R: *Churchill's illustrated medical dictionary,* New York, 1989, Churchill Livingstone.

Lavy CBD, Barrett DS: *Questions and answers on Apley's concise system of orthopaedics and fractures,* Oxford, 1991, Butterworth-Heinemann.

Lawrence DJ: Sacroiliac joint, part two, clinical considerations. In Cox JM, editor: *Low back pain: mechanism, diagnosis and treatment,* ed 5, Baltimore, 1990, Williams & Wilkins.

Leffs M: *Back pain in the adolescent athlete,* Toronto, 1991, American Back Society.

Lerner AJ: *The little black book of neurology,* ed 3, St Louis, 1995, Mosby.

LeVeau B: Hip. In Richardson JK, Iglarsh JK, editors: *Clinical orthopaedic physical therapy,* Philadelphia, 1994, WB Saunders.

Lewis CB, Bottomley JM: Orthopaedic treatment considerations. In *Geriatric physical therapy: a clinical approach,* New York, 1994, Appleton & Lange.

Lewis CB, Knortz KA: *Orthopedic assessment and treatment of the geriatric patient,* St Louis, 1993, Mosby.

Lewkonia RM, Kinsella TD: Pyogenic sacroiliitis: diagnosis and significance, *J Rheumatol* 8:153, 1981.

Lisbona R, Rosenthall L: Observation on the sequential use of 99mTc-phosphate complex and 67Gd imaging in osteomyelitis and septic arthritis, *Radiology* 123:123, 1977.

Longoria RK, Carpenter JL: Anaerobic phygenic sacroiliitis, *South Med J* 76:649, 1983.

Loth TS: *Orthopedic boards review,* St Louis, 1993, Mosby.

Loth TS: *Orthopedic boards review II: a case study approach,* St Louis, 1996, Mosby.

Macintosh JE, Pearcy MJ, Bogduk N: The axial torque of the lumbar back muscles; torsion strength of the back muscles, *Aust NZ J Surg* 63:205, 1993.

Magee DJ: *Orthopedic physical assessment,* ed 3, Philadelphia, 1997, WB Saunders.

Maigne R: *Orthopaedic medicine: a new approach to vertebral manipulation,* Springfield, Ill, 1972, Charles C Thomas.

Maitland GD: *Vertebral manipulation,* ed 5, London, 1986, Butterworth.

Malone TR, McPoil TG, Nitz AJ: *Orthopedic and sports physical therapy,* ed 3, St Louis, 1997, Mosby.

Marchiori DM: *Clinical imaging with skeletal, chest, and abdomen pattern differentials,* St Louis, 1999, Mosby.

Martin JH: *Neuroanatomy text and atlas,* ed 2, Stamford, Conn, 1996, Appleton & Lange.

Mathers LH, et al: *Clinical anatomy principles,* St Louis, 1996, Mosby.

Mazion JM: *Illustrated manual of neurological reflexes/signs/tests, part I, orthopedic signs/tests/maneuvers for office procedure, part II,* Orlando, 1980, Daniels Publishing.

McRae R: *Clinical orthopaedic examination,* ed 3, Edinburgh, 1990, Churchill Livingstone.

McRae R: *Practical fracture treatment,* ed 3, New York, 1994, Churchill-Livingstone.

Medical Economics Books: *Patient care flow chart manual,* ed 3, Oradell, NJ, 1982, Medical Economics Books.

Mellion MB: *Sports medicine secrets,* Philadelphia, 1994, Hanley & Belfus.

Mellion MB: *Office sports medicine,* ed 2, St Louis, 1996, Mosby.

Mengel MB, Schwiebert LP: *Ambulatory medicine the primary care of families,* ed 2, Stamford, Conn, 1996, Appleton & Lange.

Mennell JM: *The musculoskeletal system: differential diagnosis from symptoms and physical signs,* Gaithersburg, Md, 1992, Aspen.

Mercier LR, Pettid FJ: *Practical orthopedics,* ed 4, St Louis, 1995, Mosby.

Mirvis SE, Young JWR: *Imaging in trauma and critical care,* Baltimore, 1991, Williams & Wilkins.

Modic MT, Masaryk TJ, Ross JS: *Magnetic resonance imaging of the spine,* ed 2, St Louis, 1994, Mosby.

Mooney V, Robertson J: The facet syndrome, *Clin Orthop* 115:149, 1976.

Mosby-Year Book, Inc: *Expert 10-minute physical examination,* St Louis, 1997, Mosby.

Murphy ME: Primary pyogenic infection of sacroiliac joint, *NY State J Med* 77:1309, 1977.

Nachemson AL: Newest knowledge on low back pain, *Clin Orthop* 2279:8, 1992.

Nettina SM: *The Lippincott manual of nursing practice,* ed 6, Philadelphia, 1996, Lippincott.

Newton RW: *Color atlas of pediatric neurology,* St Louis, 1995, Mosby-Wolfe.

Nicholas JA, Hershman EB: *The lower extremity & spine in sports medicine,* vol 1-2, ed 2, St Louis, 1995, Mosby.

Nordin M, Andersson GBJ, Pope MH: *Musculoskeletal disorders in the workplace: principles and practice,* St Louis, 1997, Mosby.

Norman GF: Sacroiliac disease and its relationship to lower abdominal pain, *Am J Surg* 116:54, 1968.

Numaguci Y: Osteitis condensans ilii, including its resolution, *Radiology* 98:1, 1971.

O'Donoghue DH: *Treatment of injuries to athletes,* ed 3, Philadelphia, 1976, WB Saunders.

Olivieri L, et al: Differential diagnosis between osteitis condensans ilii and sacroiliitis, *J Rheumatol* 17:1504, 1990.

Olmarker K, Rydevik B: Pathophysiology of sciatica, *Orthop Clin North Am* 22:223, 1991.

Olson WH, et al: *Handbook of symptom-oriented neurology,* ed 2, St Louis, 1994, Mosby.

Omer GE, Spinner M: *Management of peripheral nerve problems,* Philadelphia, 1980, WB Saunders.

O'Young B, Young MA, Stiens SA: *PM&R secrets,* Philadelphia, 1997, Hanley & Belfus.

Pagana KD, Pagana TJ: *Mosby's manual of diagnostic and laboratory tests,* St Louis, 1998, Mosby.

Panjabi MM: The stabilizing system of the spine, part II, neutral zone and instability hypothesis, *J Spinal Disord* 5:390, 1992.

Panzer DM, Gatterman MI: Sacroiliac subluxation syndrome. In Gatterman MI, editor: *Foundations of chiropractic: subluxation,* St Louis, 1995, Mosby.

Patten J: *Neurological differential diagnosis,* ed 2, London, 1996, Springer.

Pecina MM, Krmpotic-Nemanic J, Markiewitz AD: *Tunnel syndromes,* Boca Raton, Fla, 1991, CRC Press.

Pheasant S: *Ergonomics, work and health,* Gaithersburg, Md, 1991, Aspen.

Polley HF, Hunder GG: *Rheumatologic interviewing and physical examination of the joints,* ed 2, Philadelphia, 1978, WB Saunders.

Poole G, Ward E: Causes of mortality in patients with pelvic fractures, *Orthopedics* 17:691, 1994.

Pope MH, Frymoyer JW, Krag MH: Diagnosing instability, *Clin Orthop* 279:60, 1992.

Pope MH, et al: *Occupational low back pain assessment, treatment and prevention,* St Louis, 1991, Mosby.

Rachlin ES: *Myofascial pain and fibromyalgia trigger point management,* St Louis, 1994, Mosby.

Ravel R: *Clinical laboratory medicine clinical application of laboratory data,* ed 6, St Louis, 1995, Mosby.

Ro CS: Sacroiliac joint. In Cox JM: *Low back pain: mechanism, diagnosis and treatment,* ed 5, Baltimore, 1990, Williams & Wilkins.

Rogers LR: *Radiology of skeletal trauma,* ed 2, London, 1992, Churchill Livingstone.

Rolak LA: *Neurology secrets,* ed 2, Philadelphia, 1998, Hanley & Belfus.

Rothman RH, Simeone FA, editors: *The spine,* vol 1-2, Philadelphia, 1975, WB Saunders.

Rumack CM, Wilson SR, Charboneau JW: *Diagnostic ultrasound,* vol 1-2, ed 2, St Louis, 1998, Mosby.

Ruwe PA, et al: Can MR imaging effectively replace diagnostic arthroscopy? *Radiology* 183:335, 1992.

Saidoff DC, McDonough AL: *Critical pathways in therapeutic intervention,* St Louis, 1997, Mosby.

Saudek CE: The hip. In Gould JA, editor: *Orthopaedic and sports physical therapy,* ed 2, St Louis, 1990, Mosby.

Schafer RC: *Clinical biomechanics,* ed 2, Baltimore, 1987, Williams & Wilkins.

Schlosstein L, et al: High association of an HL-A antigen W 27 with ankylosing spondylitis and rheumatoid arthritis, *Ann Rheum Dis* 20:47, 1961.

Schmorl G, Junghanns H: *The human spine in health and disease,* Am ed 2, New York, 1971, Grune & Stratton (Translated by EF Bessmann).

Schumacher HR, Klippel JH, Koopman WJ: *Primer on the rheumatic diseases,* ed 10, Atlanta, 1993, Arthritis Foundation.

Shankman GA: *Fundamental orthopedic management for the physical therapist assistant,* St Louis, 1997, Mosby.

Simons DG: Muscle pain syndromes, *J Manual Med* 6:3, 1991.

Singal DP, et al: HLA antigens in osteitis condensans ilii and ankylosing spondylitis, *J Rheumatol* 4(suppl 3):105, 1977.

Sledge CB, Poss R: *The year book of orthopedics 1997,* St Louis, 1997, Mosby.

Smith-Petersen MN: Painful affections of lower back. In Christopher F: *Textbook of surgery,* ed 5, Philadelphia, 1949, WB Saunders.

Specht NT, Russo RD: *Practical guide to diagnostic imaging,* St Louis, 1998, Mosby.

Starlanyl D, Copeland ME: *Fibromyalgia & chronic myofascial pain syndrome: a survival manual,* Oakland, 1996, New Harbinger Publications.

Stedman TL: *Stedman's medical dictionary,* ed 25, Baltimore, 1990, Williams & Wilkins.

Stewart DL, Abeln SH: *Documenting functional outcomes in physical therapy,* St Louis, 1993, Mosby.

Stoller DW: *Magnetic resonance imaging in orthopaedics & sports medicine,* Philadelphia, 1993, JB Lippincott.

Strange FGS: The prognosis in sacro-iliac tuberculosis, *Br J Surg* 50:561, 1963.

Sutton D: *A textbook of radiology and imaging,* ed 5, London, 1993, Churchill Livingstone.

Sutton D, Young JWR: *A concise textbook of clinical imaging,* ed 2, St Louis, 1995, Mosby.

Swezey RI: Non-fibrositic lumbar subcutaneous nodules: prevalence and clinical significance, *Br J Rheumatol* 30:376, 1991.

Szlachter BN, et al: Relaxin in normal and pathologenic pregnancies, *Obstet Gynecol* 59:167, 1982.

Tan JC, Horn SE: *Practical manual of physical medicine and rehabilitation,* St Louis, 1998, Mosby.

Taybi H, Lachman RS: *Radiology of syndromes, metabolic disorders, and skeletal dysplasias,* ed 4, St Louis, 1996, Mosby.

Taylor RW, Sonson RD: Separation of the pubic symphysis, an underrecognized peripartum complication, *J Reprod Med* 31:203, 1986.

Thibodeau GA, Patton KT: *Anatomy & physiology,* ed 3, St Louis, 1996, Mosby.

Thibodeau GA, Patton KT: *Pocket reference to accompany anatomy & physiology,* ed 3, St Louis, 1996, Mosby.

Thompson JM: *Clinical outlines for health assessment,* St Louis, 1997, Mosby.

Toghill PJ: *Examining patients: an introduction to clinical medicine,* London, 1990, Edward Arnold.

Tollison CD, Satterthwaite JR, Tollison JW: *Handbook of pain management,* ed 2, Baltimore, 1994, Williams & Wilkins.

Torg JS, Shepard RJ: *Current therapy in sports medicine,* ed 3, St Louis, 1995, Mosby.

Turek SL: *Orthopaedics principles and their application,* ed 3, Philadelphia, 1977, JB Lippincott.

Van Holsbeeck M, Introcaso JH: *Musculoskeletal ultrasound,* St Louis, 1991, Mosby.

Veys EM, et al: HLA and infective sacroiliitis, *Lancet* 2:349, 1974.

Vleeming A, et al: The posterior layer of the thoracolumbar fascia, its function in load transfer from spine to legs, *Spine* 20:753, 1995.

Wakefield TS, Frank RG: *The examiner's guide to neuro musculoskeletal practice,* Abbotsford, Wisc, 1995, Allied Health of Wisconsin, SC.

Wallace R, Cohen AS: Tuberculous arthritis: a report of two cases with review of biopsy and synovial fluid findings, *Am J Med* 61:277, 1976.

Walsh MJ: Evaluation of orthopedic testing of the low back for non-specific low back pain, *J Manipulative Physiol Ther* 21:232, 1998.

Watkins RG: *The spine in sports,* St Louis, 1996, Mosby.

Weiler PJ, King GJ, Geertzbein SD: Analysis of sagittal plane instability of the lumbar spine in vivo, *Spine* 12:1300, 1990.

Weineck J: *Functional anatomy in sports,* ed 2, St Louis, 1990, Mosby.

Weinstein SL, Buckwalter JA: *Turek's orthopaedics principles and their application,* ed 5, Philadelphia, 1994, JB Lippincott.

White AA, Panjabi MM: *Clinical biomechanics of the spine,* ed 2, Philadelphia, 1990, Lippincott.

White AH, Schofferman JA: *Spine care,* vol 1-2, St Louis, 1995, Mosby.

Wicke L: *Atlas of radiographic anatomy,* ed 5, Philadelphia, 1994, Lea & Febiger.

Wiesel SW, editor: *The lumbar spine,* Philadelphia, 1990, WB Saunders.

Wiesel SW, Bernini P, Rothman RH: *The aging lumbar spine,* Philadelphia, 1982, WB Saunders.

Windsor RE, Lox DM: *Soft tissue injuries: diagnosis and treatment,* Philadelphia, 1998, Hanley & Belfus.

Withrington RH, Sturge RA, Mitchell N: Osteitis condensans ilii or sacro-iliitis? *Scand J Rheumatol* 14:163, 1985.

Wray CC, Eason S, Huskinson J: Coccygodynia, aetiology and treatment, *J Bone Joint Surg* 73B:335, 1991.

Young JWR, Mirvis SE, editors: *Imaging in trauma and critical care,* Baltimore, 1991, Williams & Wilkins.

Zatouroff M: *Diagnosis in color physical signs in general medicine,* ed 2, London, 1996, Mosby-Wolfe.

Zitelli BJ, Davis HW: *Atlas of pediatric physical diagnosis,* ed 2, London, 1992, Wolfe.

THE HIP JOINT

AXIOMS IN HIP ASSESSMENT

- The hip joint is a ball-and-socket synovial joint.
- The hip is an exceptionally strong and stable joint, with a wide range of multiaxial movements.

INTRODUCTION

Hip pain is a common symptom with diverse etiologies. Typically, hip disease manifests itself with pain in the groin. The pain may radiate to the anterior, lateral, or medial thigh and occasionally to the knee. Causes of pain in the groin and anterior thigh area include iliopsoas bursitis, adduction tendinitis, hernias, and pain from retroperitoneal structures.

Pain in the trochanteric area aggravated by lateral decubitus position is highly suggestive of trochanteric bursitis. Pain in the ischiogluteal area aggravated by the sitting position should suggest an ischiogluteal bursitis. Groin pain aggravated by walking and relieved by rest is suggestive of a degenerative hip arthropathy. Pain in the same location, when associated with morning stiffness lasting more than 30 minutes and relieved by activity, is typical of an inflammatory arthropathy. Vascular insufficiency tends to present with buttock pain aggravated by walking and relieved within minutes by rest (Table 10-3).

Hip disease may result in adduction or abduction deformities. An adduction deformity is an upward tilt of the pelvis on the side of the adducted thigh (Fig. 10-2). An abduction deformity is an elevation of the uninvolved side.

ORTHOPEDIC GAMUT 10-1

HIP

Loading forces acting on the hip include the following:

1. Standing transfers one third of the body weight to the hip joint mechanism.
2. Standing on one limb transfers 2.4 to 2.6 times the body weight to the hip joint mechanism.
3. Walking transfers 1.3 to 5.8 times the body weight on the hip joint mechanism.

Pain in the posterior aspect of the hip is most often referred from the lumbar spine.

Sacroiliac disorders can also cause buttock pain. Mechanical disorders of the thoracolumbar junction (T12 and L1) may refer pain to the greater trochanter area and thus may mimic trochanteric bursitis (Fig. 10-3). Thrombosis or aneurysm formation of branches of the aorta or iliac vessels may give rise to buttock, thigh, or leg pain that may be confused with hip pain. The presence of pain at the extremes of abduction and internal rotation suggests early hip disease caused by arthritis or osteonecrosis. Limitation of hip movements in all directions in a diabetic patient suggests an adhesive capsulitis of the hip joint. The presence of systemic symptoms, such as fatigue, fever, weight loss, or worsening of pain at night, requires baseline laboratory tests and a radionuclide bone scan in search of a tumor or an indolent infectious process.

ESSENTIAL ANATOMY

The femur is the longest and strongest bone in the body.

TABLE 10-1

HIP JOINT CROSS-REFERENCE TABLE BY ASSESSMENT PROCEDURE

Hip Joint	Disease Assessed																
Test/Sign	Leg Length	Hip Dislocation	Tibial Dysplasia	Fracture	Coxa Pathology	Tibial/Fibular Fracture	Calcaneal Fracture	Pelvic Obliquity	Meningeal Irritation	Osteoarthritis	Iliotibial Band	Gracilis Contracture	Hip Flexion Contracture	Legg-Calve-Perthes Disease	Poliomyelitis	Coxa Vara	Subluxation
Actual leg-length test	●							●									
Allis' sign		●	●														
Anvil test				●	●	●	●										
Apparent leg-length test	●							●									
Chiene's test				●													
Gauvain's sign					●												
Guilland's sign									●								
Hip telescoping test		●															
Jansen's test					●					●							
Ludloff's sign				●													
Ober's test											●						
Patrick's test					●												
Phelp's test					●							●					
Thomas test					●								●				
Trendelenburg's test		●		●						●				●	●	●	●

TABLE 10-2

HIP JOINT CROSS-REFERENCE TABLE FOR SYNDROME OR TISSUE

Calcaneal fracture	Anvil test	Hip flexion contracture	Thomas test
Coxa pathology	Anvil test	Iliotibial band	Ober's test
	Gauvain's sign	Leg length	Actual leg-length test
	Jansen's test		Apparent leg-length test
	Patrick's test	Legg-Calve-Perthes disease	Trendelenburg's test
	Phelp's test	Meningeal irritation	Guilland's sign
	Thomas test	Osteoarthritis	Jansen's sign
Coxa vara	Trendelenburg's test		Trendelenburg's test
Fracture	Anvil test	Pelvic obliquity	Actual leg-length test
	Chiene's test		Apparent leg-length test
	Ludloff's sign	Poliomyelitis	Trendelenburg's test
	Trendelenburg's test	Subluxation	Trendelenburg's test
Gracilis contracture	Phelp's test	Tibial dysplasia	Allis' sign
Hip dislocation	Allis' sign	Tibial/fibular fracture	Anvil test
	Hip telescoping test		
	Trendelenburg's test		

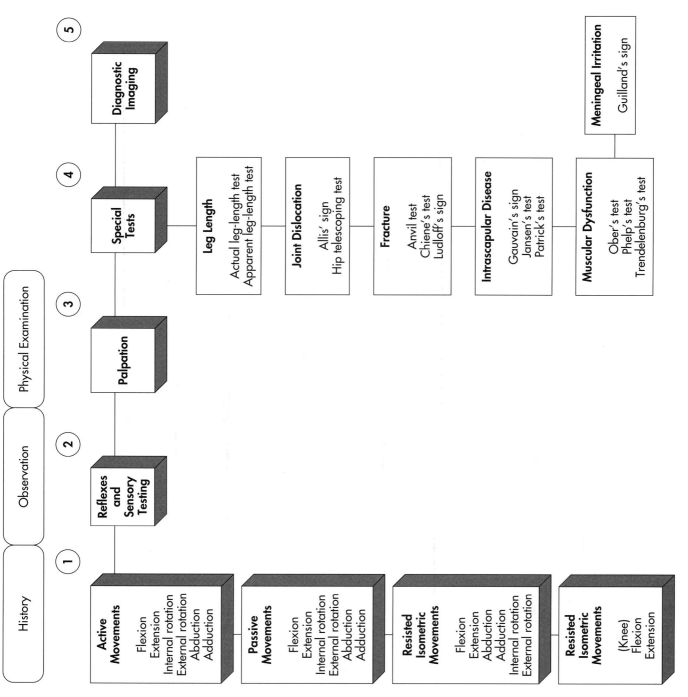

FIG. 10-1 Hip joint assessment.

TABLE 10-3

HIP DIAGNOSTIC CONSIDERATIONS

Articular

Inflammatory joint diseases
  Rheumatoid arthritis
  Spondyloarthropathies
  Polymyalgia rheumatica
Degenerative joint diseases
  Primary osteoarthritis
  Secondary osteoarthritis
Metabolic joint diseases
  Gout
  Pseudogout
  Ochronosis
  Hemochromatosis
  Wilson's disease
  Acromegaly
Infections
Tumors
  Benign
    Pigmented villonodular synovitis
    Osteochondromatosis
  Malignant
    Synovial sarcoma
    Synovial metastasis
Hemarthrosis
Juvenile
  Transient "toxic" synovitis
  Juvenile chronic arthritis

Periarticular

Bursitis
  Trochanteric
  Iliopsoas
  Ischiogluteal
Tendinitis
  Trochanteric
  Adductor
Acute calcific periarthritis
Heterotropic calcifications

Osseous

Bone lesions
  Fractures, neoplasms, infection, osteonecrosis of the
    femoral head, metabolic bone disease (Paget's disease
    of bone, stress fractures, osteomalacia, hyperpara-
    thyroidism, renal osteodystrophy), reflex sympathetic
    dystrophy (transient migratory osteoporosis)
Juvenile
  Congenital dislocation of the hip ⎤
  Acetabular dysplasia   ├ Usually not
  Coxa vara   painful
  Slipped capital femoral epiphysis ⎦
  Legg-Calvé-Perthes disease
  Rickets

Neurologic

Entrapment neuropathies
  Lateral femoral cutaneous nerve (meralgia paresthetica)
Lumbar nerve root compression L2, L3, and L4

Vascular

Atherosclerosis of aorta iliac vessels

Modified from Klippel JH, Dieppe PA: *Rheumatology*, vol 1-2, ed 2, London, 1998, Mosby.

ORTHOPEDIC GAMUT 10-2

PROXIMAL FEMUR

Following are the four major components of the proximal femur:

1. Greater trochanter
2. Lesser trochanter
3. Femoral neck
4. Femoral head

The femoral neck forms an "angle of inclination" with the femoral shaft on the frontal plane. In children, this angle may be up to 150 degrees; in adults, however, it is approximately 125 degrees. Variations in this angle commonly occur. An increase in the angle of inclination is known as *coxa valga*, and a reduction in this angle is coxa vara (Fig. 10-4, *A*). The femoral neck is typically aligned anterior to the femoral shaft on the transverse plane. This "angle of anteversion" is approximately 15 degrees in adults. An increase in this angle is known as *excessive femoral anteversion;* a decrease is often called *femoral retroversion* (Fig. 10-4, *B*).

The ligamentum teres (ligamentum capitis femoris) arises from the transverse acetabular ligament and inserts into the fovea capitus in the head of the femur. Important small blood vessels supplying blood to the epiphyseal region of the head of the femur usually travel with this ligament (Fig. 10-5).

The load-bearing capacity of the femoral neck is enhanced by cancellous bone; the complex trabecular arrangement of that reinforces this structure to withstand compressive, tensile, and bending forces (Fig. 10-6). By

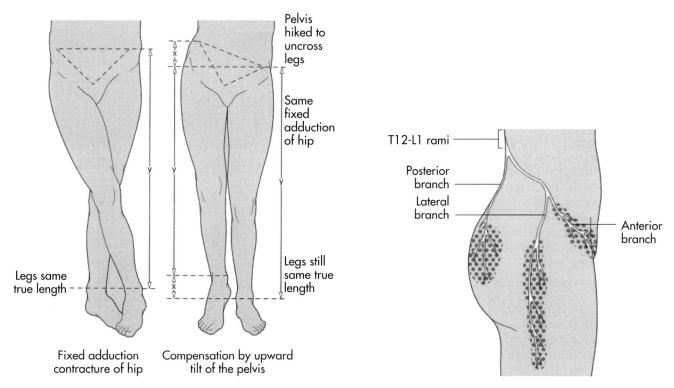

FIG. 10-2 Adduction deformity of the right hip. *(From Klippel JH, Dieppe PA:* Rheumatology, *vol 1-2, ed 2, London, 1998, Mosby.)*

FIG. 10-3 Cutaneous branches originating from the T12-L1 rami. *(From Klippel JH, Dieppe PA:* Rheumatology, *vol 1-2, ed 2, London, 1998, Mosby.)*

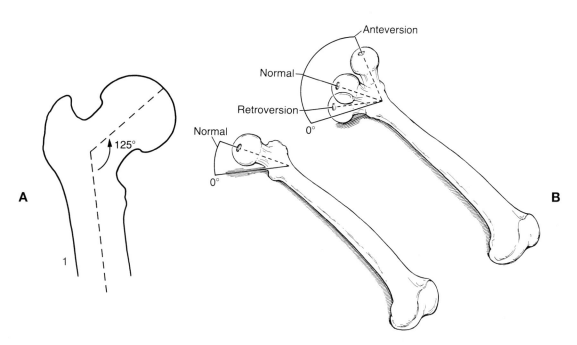

FIG. 10-4 **A,** Angle of inclination. **B,** Representation of retroversion and anteversion of the femoral neck. *(From Malone TR, McPoil TG, Nitz AJ:* Orthopedic and sports physical therapy, *ed 3, St Louis, 1997, Mosby.)*

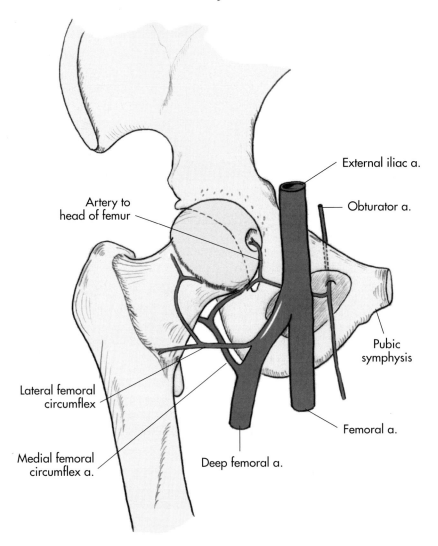

FIG. 10-5   Blood supply to the head of the femur. *(From Mathers LH, et al:* Clinical anatomy principles, *St Louis, 1996, Mosby.)*

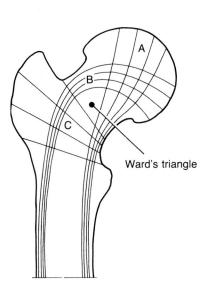

FIG. 10-6   Trabecular structure of the proximal femur, indicating medial system *(A),* arcuate system *(B),* lateral system *(C),* and the weak area of Ward's triangle. *(Modified from Tinver R, editor:* Orthopedics in primary care, *Baltimore, 1979, Williams & Wilkins.)*

virtue of a complex latticework, these bony columns act to reinforce each other to withstand these forces. Ward's triangle often loses its trabecular bone in aged individuals and may be related to hip fractures.

The sciatic nerve (Fig. 10-7) leaves the pelvis via the sciatic notch and then passes, usually, under the piriformis muscle, which is covered by the gluteus maximus. In some individuals, the nerve or its peroneal divisions passes through the piriformis muscle and, more commonly, above it. The superior gluteal nerve, which innervates the gluteus medius and minimus and tensor fascia lata, branches off the sciatic trunk before the piriformis. However, the inferior gluteal nerve, which innervates the gluteus maximus, passes under the muscle (Fig. 10-8). Of the lower extremity mononeuropathies, sciatic mononeuropathy is second in frequency only to peroneal mononeuropathy. The sciatic nerve is predisposed to injury by its proximity to the hip joint and its relatively long course from the sciatic notch to the popliteal fossa.

ESSENTIAL MOTION ASSESSMENT

When measuring the range of hip movement, the examiner must ensure that the pelvis remains stationary. To do this, the examiner keeps a hand on the anterosuperior iliac spine to detect any movement.

To test flexion, the examiner should bend the leg, with the knee flexed, into the abdomen. Standing behind the patient and drawing the leg backward until the point at which the pelvis starts to rotate best assesses extension. Abduction is measured by taking the leg outward, again to the point where, by using the opposite hand, the pelvis is felt to move. Internal and external rotation are tested with the hip and knee flexed to 90 degrees.

Inspection of the hip joint includes an assessment of gait. A smooth and even gait indicates equal leg length and functional hip motion. Antalgic limp is characteristic of

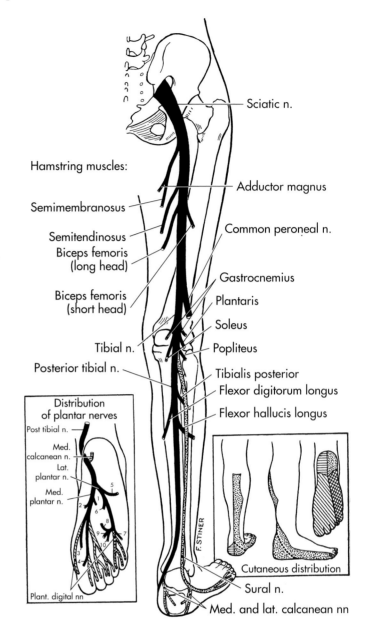

FIG. 10-7 The sciatic nerve and its main branches. *(From Katirji B:* Electromyography in clinical practice: a case study approach, *St Louis, 1998, Mosby.)*

disease that produces pain in a hip joint; the body tilts toward the involved diseased hip in such a way that the weight of the body is directly over the hip. This limp decreases the need for abductor muscle movement and thus may alleviate muscle spasm. If the abductor muscles are weak (i.e., unable to support the pelvis), the unaffected hip may move downward in such a way that the weight is borne on that side. This condition is called *Trendelenburg's limp.*

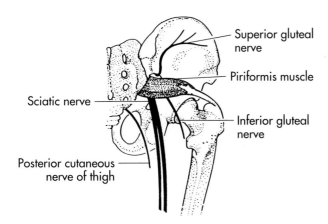

FIG. 10-8   The nerve of the sciatic notch and the piriformis muscle. *(From Stewart JD:* Focal peripheral neuropathies, *ed 2, New York, 1993, Raven Press.)*

ORTHOPEDIC GAMUT 10-4

HIP RANGE OF MOTION

In testing range of motion of the hips, the patient performs the following.

While Supine

1. Raises the leg above the body with the knee extended
2. Brings the knee to the chest while keeping the other leg straight
3. Swings the leg laterally and medially while keeping the knee straight
4. Places the side of the foot on the opposite knee and moves the flexed knee down toward the examination table (external rotation)
5. Flexes the knee and rotates the leg so that the flexed knee moves inward toward the opposite leg (internal rotation)

While Either Prone or Standing

1. Swings the straightened leg behind the body

Among all of the movements of the hip, abduction and internal rotation are usually the first ones to be painful or limited in the presence of hip pathology (Figs. 10-9 to 10-14).

ESSENTIAL MUSCLE FUNCTION ASSESSMENT

Sciatic palsies are associated with pelvic trauma, injuries to the buttock or thigh, and infiltration by tumor. The muscles supplied by the lateral popliteal component of the nerve tend to be more affected than those supplied by the medial popliteal branch (Fig. 10-15).

Muscles acting at the hip joint may have additional actions on the spine or knee. The psoas major passes from the lumbar spine to the lesser trochanter of the femur. In addition to flexing the hip, it flexes the lumbar spine.

The gluteus maximus, the thickest muscle in the body, forms a soft-tissue barrier to protect the posterior hip and large neurovascular structures of the buttock region (Fig. 10-16). Deep to the gluteus maximus, several smaller muscles that act externally to rotate this joint (Fig. 10-17) span the posterior hip. The iliopsoas muscle passes anterior to the hip joint and acts with the rectus femoris, sartorius, tensor fasciae latae, and anterior hip adductors to create a potential for flexion of the hip against strong resistance.

The innervation of the hip joint follows Hilton's law, which states that a joint is innervated by the same nerves that innervate the muscles acting upon it. Thus branches from the femoral, sciatic, obturator, and superior and inferior gluteal nerves innervate the hip joint. The sclerotome reference for the hip joint is generally considered to be L3. The cutaneous innervation of the hip, buttock, and thigh can be referenced to peripheral nerves or dermatomes (Figs. 10-18 to 10-23).

ESSENTIAL IMAGING

The major part of the pelvis is typically visualized with a single anteroposterior (AP) view. Both lower extremities are internally rotated approximately 20 degrees to elongate the femoral necks and take the trochanteric processes out of superimposition with the femoral necks.

ORTHOPEDIC GAMUT 10-5

BASIC HIP STUDY

The basic hip study should include three views:

1. AP pelvic (Figs. 10-24 and 10-25) view
2. AP spot hip (Fig. 10-26) view
3. Lateral (frog leg) spot view of the side of complaint (Figs. 10-27 and 10-28)

The AP pelvic view allows comparative assessment of the various paired structures of the pelvic girdle and hip regions, and the spot AP view brings the central ray to the area of interest, allowing better projection advantage.
Text continued on p. 693

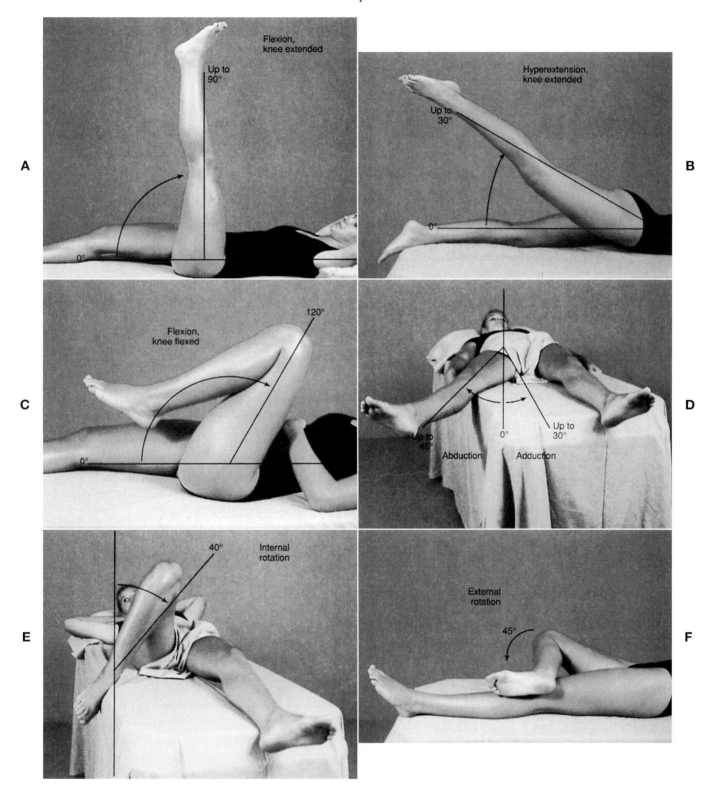

FIG. 10-9 Range of motion of the hip. **A,** Hip flexion with the leg extended. **B,** Hip hyperextension, knee extended. **C,** Hip flexion, knee flexed. **D,** Abduction. **E,** Internal rotation. **F,** External rotation. *(From Barkauskas VH, et al: Health & physical assessment, ed 2, St Louis, 1998, Mosby.)*

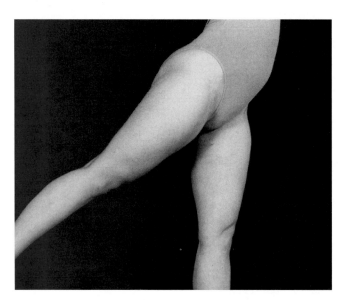

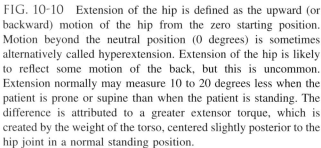

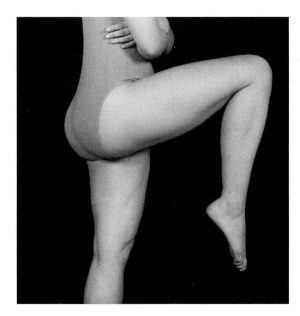

FIG. 10-10   Extension of the hip is defined as the upward (or backward) motion of the hip from the zero starting position. Motion beyond the neutral position (0 degrees) is sometimes alternatively called hyperextension. Extension of the hip is likely to reflect some motion of the back, but this is uncommon. Extension normally may measure 10 to 20 degrees less when the patient is prone or supine than when the patient is standing. The difference is attributed to a greater extensor torque, which is created by the weight of the torso, centered slightly posterior to the hip joint in a normal standing position.

In the usual method of clinical examination for extension of the hip, the patient is prone. The examiner applies downward pressure to the sacrum with a flattened hand. The examiner's other hand, which is placed midway against the anterior aspect of the patient's thigh, is used to lift the thigh on the side that is being examined.

With the available methods of eliminating exaggerated lumbar lordosis and accomplishing fixation of the pelvis, 15 degrees of extension or hyperextension of the hip may be obtained. With less adequate fixation or with abnormal laxity of the ligaments of the hip (a rarity), the thigh may be hyperextended about 30 to 40 degrees. Retained extension range of motion (standing or prone) of 20 degrees or less is an impairment of the hip in the activities of daily living.

FIG. 10-11   The greatest degree of flexion of the hip while in the standing position is possible when the knee is also flexed. The thigh can be flexed to 120 degrees from the neutral or extended position (0 degrees), if the knee has first been flexed to 90 degrees. Sometimes, the hip can be flexed until the anterior surface of the thigh presses against the anterior abdominal wall.

If the knee cannot be flexed, raising the extended leg off the surface of the examination table can test flexion of the hip. If the knee remains extended, tension of the hamstring muscles will limit flexion of the hip. The angle between the thigh and the long axis of the body, when the hip is normal, may not be more than a right angle (90 degrees).

However, some individuals with apparently normal hips are able to flex the hip only to form an angle of about 75 degrees when the leg is extended. In other individuals, the range of motion is much greater than 90 degrees. Retained flexion range of motion of 90 degrees or less is an impairment of hip function in the activities of daily living.

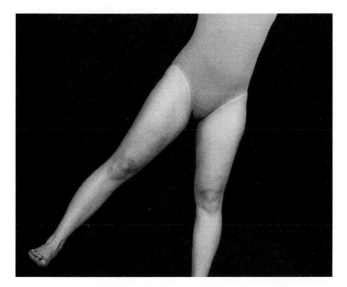

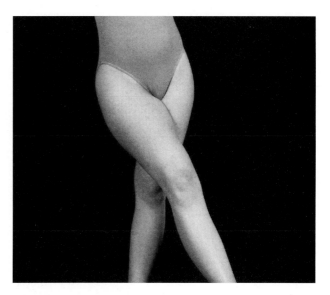

FIG. 10-12   Abduction and adduction are measured while both thighs and legs are in the extended position and are parallel to each other. The patient can be standing or supine. Measurement is made from the angle formed between an imaginary midline that is extended from the long axis of the body and the long axis of the leg. The amount of abduction permitted increases with flexion and decreases with extension of the hip. Normally, when the leg and thigh are extended, the hip abducts to approximately 40 to 45 degrees, from the neutral position, before the pubofemoral and medial portions of the iliofemoral ligaments restrict this abduction. Retained abduction range of motion of 30 degrees or less is an impairment of the hip in the activities of daily living.

FIG. 10-13   Adduction with the leg straight out is limited by the legs and thighs, which come into contact with each other. When it is possible to adduct the hip with enough flexion to permit crossing one leg over the other and then reversing the procedure, the degree of adduction of the hip of the extremity that is on top can be measured. Adduction is usually possible to approximate 20 to 30 degrees from the neutral (starting) position.

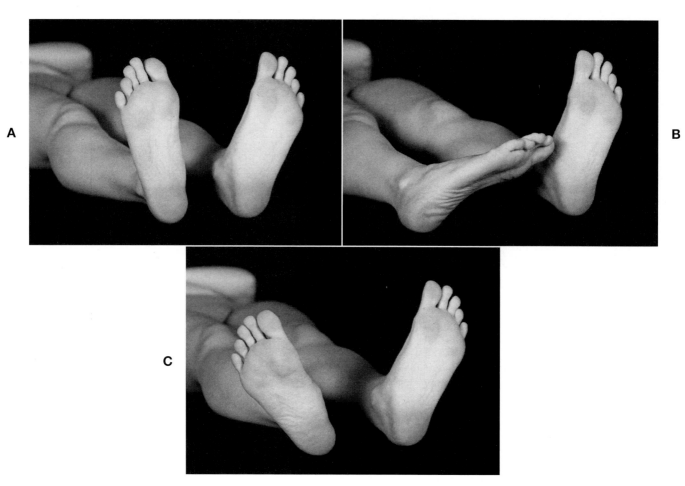

FIG. 10-14   External and internal rotation of the hip can be tested with the patient's hip and knee fully extended while the patient is supine. **A,** Rolling the thigh, leg, and foot inward. **B,** Rolling the thigh, leg, and foot outward. **C,** The hip normally rotates inward approximately 40 degrees and outward approximately 45 degrees. However, the range of motion varies among normal individuals, and both sides should be compared. The lateral band of the iliofemoral ligament limits external rotation. The ischiocapsular ligament limits internal rotation. Rotation of the hip increases with flexion and decreases with extension of the hip. Limitation of internal rotation of the hip is the earliest and most reliable sign of disease of the hip.

Retained internal rotation of 30 degrees or less or retained external rotation range of motion of 40 degrees or less is an impairment of the hip in the activities of daily living.

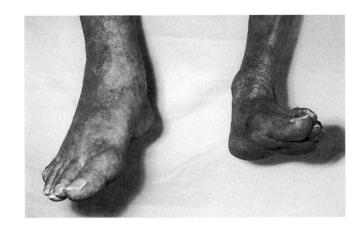

FIG. 10-15   Right sciatic palsy.   *(From Epstein O, et al:* Clinical examination, *ed 2, London, 1997, Mosby.)*

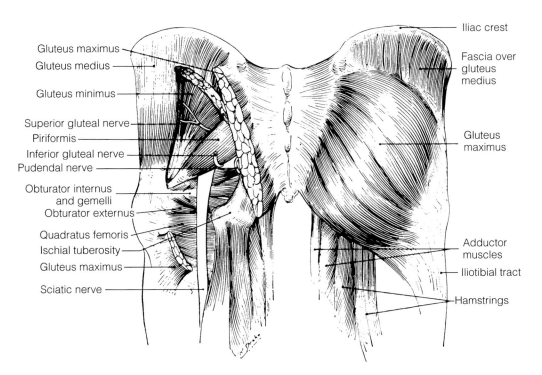

FIG. 10-16   Superficial muscles of the buttock and thigh: lateral.   *(From Malone TR, McPoil TG, Nitz AJ:* Orthopedic and sports physical therapy, *ed 3, St Louis, 1997, Mosby.)*

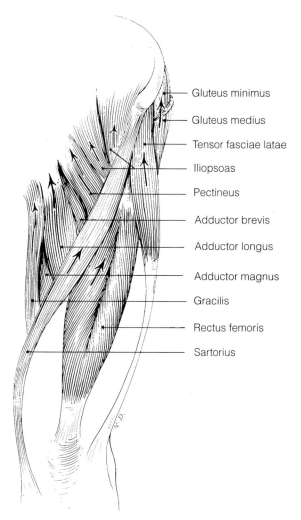

Gluteus minimus

Gluteus medius

Tensor fasciae latae

Iliopsoas

Pectineus

Adductor brevis

Adductor longus

Adductor magnus

Gracilis

Rectus femoris

Sartorius

FIG. 10-17   Muscles of the anterior thigh. *(From Malone TR, McPoil TG, Nitz AJ:* Orthopedic and sports physical therapy, *ed 3, St Louis, 1997, Mosby.)*

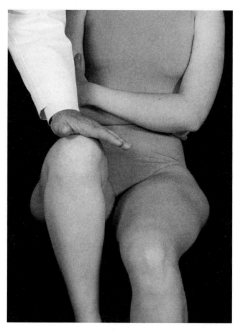

FIG. 10-18   The iliopsoas is the primary flexor of the hip, and it is innervated by the femoral nerve, which contains the L1, L2, and L3 nerve roots. To test the strength of the iliopsoas, the patient is examined while seated on the examination table. The examiner asks the patient to flex the hip against manual resistance, which the examiner provides. Accessory muscles involved are the rectus femoris, sartorius, tensor fasciae latae, pectineus, adductor brevis, adductor longus, and the oblique fibers of the adductor magnus muscle. Flexion of the hip also may be tested while the patient is lying supine with the knee extended. Tension of the hamstring muscles, when they are stretched, may limit flexion and interfere with interpretation of the test.

FIG. 10-19   Prime movers in extension of the hip are the gluteus maximus (inferior gluteal nerve, L5, S1, and S2), semitendinosus (tibial branch of sciatic nerve, L4, L5, S1, and S2), and semi-membranosus (tibial branch of sciatic nerve, L5, S1, and S2) muscles, as well as the long head of the biceps femoris (tibial branch of the sciatic nerve, S1, S2, and S3) muscle. To measure the strength of the gluteus maximus, the patient is placed prone on the examination table and is directed to extend the hip against the examiner's hand, which is placed on the thigh and pelvis.

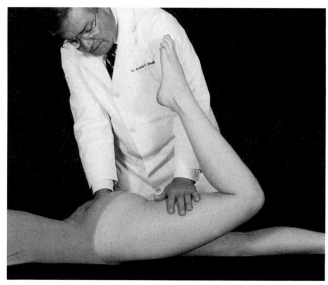

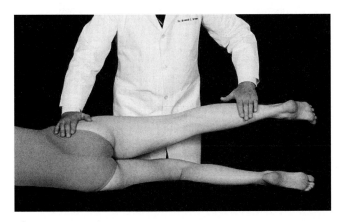

FIG. 10-20   The gluteus medius muscle (superior gluteal nerve, L4, L5, and S1) is the prime mover in abduction of the hip. The gluteus minimus, tensor fasciae latae, and upper fibers of the gluteus maximus muscles are accessory to this motion. The strength of these can be estimated by observing the patient's gait and using Trendelenburg's test. An additional test can be performed by placing the patient in a side-lying position on the examination table and having the patient abduct the hip against resistance provided by the examiner.

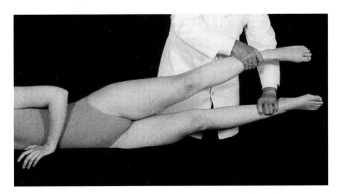

FIG. 10-21   Prime movers in adduction of the hip are the adductor magnus (obturator and sciatic nerves, L3, L4, L5, and S1), adductor brevis (obturator nerve, L3, and L4), adductor longus (obturator nerve, L3, and L4), pectineus (femoral nerve, L2, L3, L4, and occasionally obturator nerve, L3, and L4), and gracilis (obturator nerve, L3, and L4) muscles. Adduction is tested while the patient is lying on one side with the legs extended. The upper leg, which is supported by one of the examiner's hands, is held in approximately 25 degrees of abduction. The patient then adducts the lower leg off the table, toward the elevated leg, without rotating the leg or tipping the pelvis. The examiner's free hand provides graded resistance proximal to the knee joint.

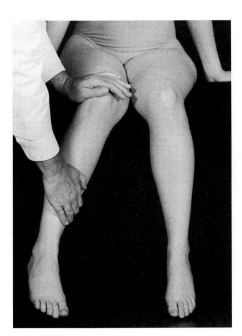

FIG. 10-22   Prime movers in external rotation of the hip are the obturator externus (obturator nerve, L3, and L4), obturator internus (sacral plexus, L4, L5, and S1), piriformis (sacral plexus, S1, and S2), gemellus superior (sacral plexus, L5, S1, and S2), gemellus inferior (sacral plexus, L4, L5, and S1), and the gluteus maximus (inferior gluteal nerve, L5, S1, and S2) muscles. The sartorius muscle is accessory to this motion. Lateral rotation of the hip is tested while the patient sits with the legs hanging over the edge of the table. The examiner places one hand over the lateral aspect of the thigh, just above the knee, and applies counterpressure to the thigh to prevent abduction and flexion of the hip. The patient grasps the edge of the table to help stabilize the pelvis. The patient then rotates the hip and thigh laterally, and the lower leg rotates medially while the examiner's other hand applies graded resistance above the ankle against the motion being tested.

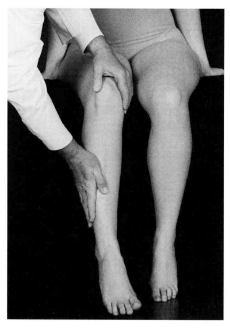

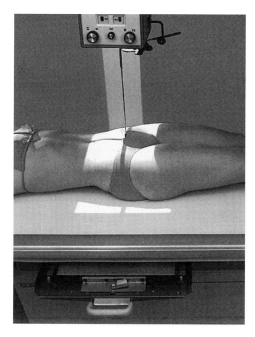

FIG. 10-23   Prime movers in internal rotation of the hip are the gluteus minimus (superior gluteal nerve, L4, L5, and S1) and the tensor fasciae latae (superior gluteal nerve, L4, L5, and S1) muscles. Anterior fibers of the gluteus medius, semimembranosus, and semitendinosus muscles are accessory to this motion. Medial rotation of the hip is tested while the patient sits with the legs over the edge of a table as if testing lateral rotation of the hip. The examiner uses one hand to apply counterpressure above the knee and over the medial aspect of the thigh to prevent adduction of the hip. The patient holds the edge of the table to stabilize the pelvis. The patient then rotates the thigh medially and rotates the lower leg laterally while the examiner's other hand provides graded resistance above the ankle joint.

FIG. 10-24   Female anteroposterior pelvis with gonad (shadow) shield.   *(From Ballinger PW:* Merrill's atlas of radiographic positions and radiologic procedures, *vol 1-3, ed 8, St Louis, 1995, Mosby.)*

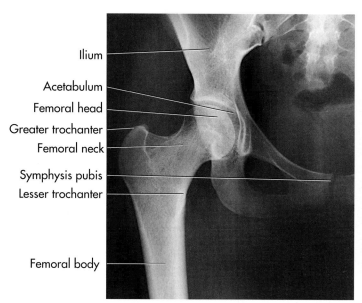

Ilium
Acetabulum
Femoral head
Greater trochanter
Femoral neck
Symphysis pubis
Lesser trochanter

Femoral body

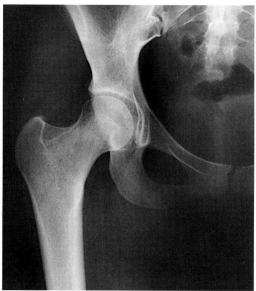

FIG. 10-25   Anteroposterior hip.   *(From Ballinger PW:* Merrill's atlas of radiographic positions and radiologic procedures, *vol 1-3, ed 8, St Louis, 1995, Mosby.)*

The lateral frog-leg spot offers a 90-degree or true lateral analysis of the proximal femur. Occasionally, a bilateral frog projection can be performed as an expedient survey, particularly to rule out slipped capital femoral epiphysis.

ORTHOPEDIC GAMUT 10-6

OSSEOUS DEFORMITIES OF THE PROXIMAL FEMUR

Four common osseous deformities of the proximal femur are the following:

1. Coxa vara
2. Coxa valga
3. Femoral anteversion
4. Femoral retroversion

Whether occurring unilaterally or bilaterally, each of these conditions can result in alterations in load bearing throughout the lower limb and spine and thus are of great importance.

ORTHOPEDIC GAMUT 10-7

COXA VARA

The developmental and acquired conditions that can result in coxa vara include the following:

1. Intertrochanteric fracture
2. Slipped capital femoral epiphysis
3. Legg-Calvé-Perthes disease
4. Congenital hip dislocation
5. Rickets
6. Paget's disease

Excessive femoral anteversion is a condition in which the angle between the femoral neck and the femoral shaft on the transverse plane is greater than approximately 12 degrees in adults. When this deformity is present, the ipsilateral lower limb appears to be excessively internally rotated when the femoral head is in the neutral position within the acetabulum (Fig. 10-30). There is usually a greater range of motion of hip internal rotation than external rotation (Fig. 10-31). Craig's test is typically positive.

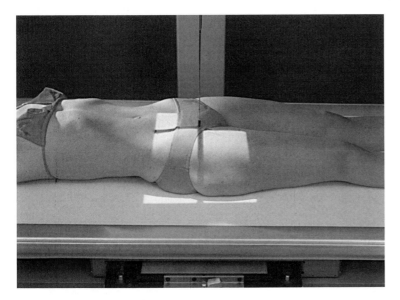

FIG. 10-26   Anteroposterior hip. *(From Ballinger PW: Merrill's atlas of radiographic positions and radiologic procedures, vol 1-3, ed 8, St Louis, 1995, Mosby.)*

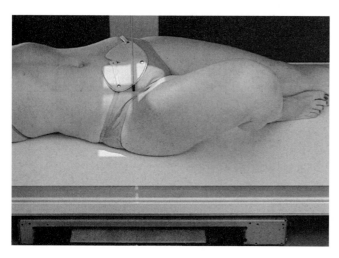

FIG. 10-27 Unilateral anteroposterior oblique femoral neck: modified Cleaves method. *(From Ballinger PW:* Merrill's atlas of radiographic positions and radiologic procedures, *vol 1-3, ed 8, St Louis, 1995, Mosby.)*

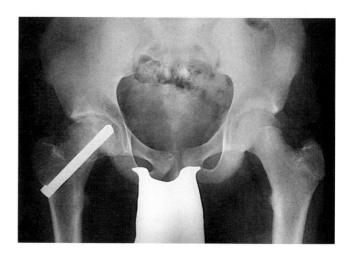

FIG. 10-28 Anteroposterior oblique femoral necks. Note fixation device in right hip and gonad shield. *(From Ballinger PW:* Merrill's atlas of radiographic positions and radiologic procedures, *vol 1-3, ed 8, St Louis, 1995, Mosby.)*

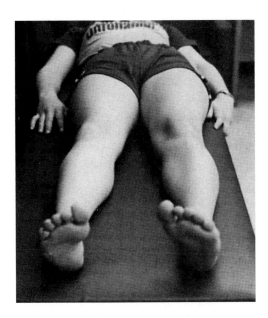

FIG. 10-29   Patient with bilateral femoral anteversion, with the lack of normal toeing out.   *(From Malone TR, McPoil TG, Nitz AJ: Orthopedic and sports physical therapy, ed 3, St Louis, 1997, Mosby.)*

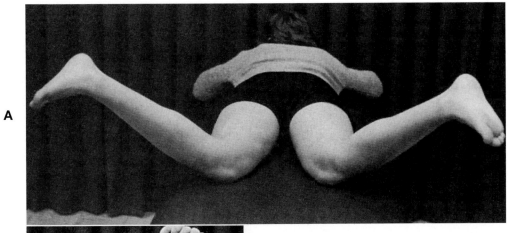

FIG. 10-30   The typical range-of-motion pattern of the hips with bilateral femoral anteversion. **A,** Internal rotation. **B,** External rotation. *(From Malone TR, McPoil TG, Nitz AJ: Orthopedic and sports physical therapy, ed 3, St Louis, 1997, Mosby.)*

ACTUAL LEG-LENGTH TEST

Assessment for True Leg-Length Discrepancy

Comment

Methods of measuring the lower limbs are often confusing. Accuracy in measurement is of more than academic significance. Accurate measurement is of practical importance when corrective operations or adjustments to the shoes are contemplated. Limb length can be measured clinically within an error of 1 cm. If greater accuracy is needed, radiographic measurement (scanography) is recommended (Fig. 10-31).

First, it is necessary to measure the real, or true, length of each limb. Second, it must be determined whether there is any apparent, or false, discrepancy in the length of the limbs as a result of fixed pelvic tilt. It is always necessary to measure the true leg length. It is necessary to measure apparent discrepancy only when there is a correctable pelvic tilt.

The anterosuperior iliac spine is significantly lateral to the axis of hip movement. This positioning does not matter if the angle between the limb and the pelvis is the same on each side. The measurements will be fallacious if the angle between limb and pelvis is not the same for each side. Abduction of a hip brings the medial malleolus nearer to the corresponding anterosuperior iliac spine. Adduction of the hip carries the medial malleolus away from the anterosuperior iliac spine. Thus, if measurements are made while the patient lies with one hip adducted and the other abducted (a common posture in cases of hip disease), inaccurate readings will be obtained. The length will be exaggerated on the adducted side and diminished on the abducted side.

Obtaining an accurate comparison of true length by surface measurement requires that the two limbs be placed in comparable positions relative to the pelvis. If one limb is adducted and cannot be brought out to the neutral position, the other limb must be adducted through a corresponding angle by crossing it over the first limb before the measurements are taken. Similarly, if one hip is in fixed abduction, the other hip must be abducted to the same angle before the measurements of true length are made.

In fixing the tape measure to the anterosuperior iliac spine, a flat metal end is essential. The metal end is placed immediately distal to the anterosuperior iliac spine, and this end is pushed up against the spine. The thumb is then pressed firmly backward against the bone and the tape end. This procedure provides rigid fixation of the tape measure against the bone.

When taking the reading at the medial malleolus, the tip of the index finger should be placed immediately distal to the medial malleolus and should be pushed up against it. The thumbnail is brought down against the tip of the index finger, pinching the tape measure between them. The thumbnail indicates the point of measurement.

If measurements reveal real shortening of a limb, it must be determined whether the shortening is above the trochanteric level (suggesting an affection in or near the hip) or below the trochanteric level (suggesting an affection of the limb bones).

ORTHOPEDIC GAMUT 10-8

LEG SHORTENING

Tests for leg shortening that occurs above the trochanteric level are as follows:

1. Measurement of Bryant's triangle
2. Construction of Nelaton's line
3. Construction of Shoemaker's line

In principle, Bryant's triangle is nothing more than a method of comparing the distance between the greater trochanter and the wing of the ilium on the two sides. While the patient is lying supine, a perpendicular is dropped from the anterosuperior spine of the ilium toward the examination table. A second line is projected upward from the tip of the greater trochanter to meet the first line at a right angle. The second line is the important line of the triangle because it is measured and compared bilaterally. The third side of the triangle is unimportant. This third line joins the anterosuperior iliac spine to the tip of the greater trochanter. Measurement of Bryant's triangle allows for comparison of the distance between the pelvis and the trochanter on each side. Relative shortening on one side indicates that the femur is displaced upward as a result of a lesion in or near the hip. If there is a possibility that both sides are abnormal, measurement of Bryant's triangle is not helpful.

Nelaton's line is measured while the patient is lying on the unaffected side. A tape measure or string is stretched on the affected side from the tuberosity of the ischium to the anterosuperior spine of the ilium. Normally, the greater trochanter lies on or below that tape measure line. If the trochanter lies above the line, the femur has been displaced upward.

Shoemaker's line is a similar test. The test involves projection of two lines, one on each side of the body, from the greater trochanter through and beyond the anterosuperior iliac spine. Normally, the two lines meet in the midline above the umbilicus. If one femur is displaced upward because of shortening above the greater trochanter, the lines will meet away from the midline on the opposite side. If both femora are displaced, the lines will meet at or near the midline but below the umbilicus.

True shortening is sometimes caused by an abnormality such as a congenital defect of development, impaired epiphyseal growth, or previous fracture with overlapping of the fragments that occurs below the trochanteric level. To investigate this possibility, the examiner should obtain measurements of the femur (tip of the greater trochanter to the line of the knee joint) and of the tibia (line of the knee joint to the medial malleolus) on each side.

PROCEDURE

- The patient is lying supine with the feet together, the knees and hips straight, and the anterosuperior iliac spines and the iliac crests exposed.

- The examiner, by way of palpation, marks the apex of the anterior iliac spines and the crests of the ilia.
- The examiner then measures the distance between these features and the medial malleolus (Fig. 10-32).
- The distance is recorded and compared with the opposite side.
- These distances represent the actual leg length.
- Actual leg-length discrepancies are caused by an abnormality above or below the trochanter level.

Confirmation Procedure
Apparent leg-length measurements

DIAGNOSTIC STATEMENT

Leg-length measurements reveal a true leg-length discrepancy on the left. This discrepancy is corroborated by Bryant's triangle as a discrepancy that results from a lesion in or near the hip joint.

CLINICAL PEARL

Causes of true shortening above the trochanter include (1) coxa vara, resulting from neck fractures, slipped epiphysis, Perthes disease, and congenital coxa vara; (2) loss of articular cartilage from infection or arthritis; and (3) dislocation of the hip. It is rare that lengthening of the other limb gives relative, true shortening. This relative, true shortening may be caused by (1) stimulation of bone growth from increased vascularity, which may occur after long bone fracture in children or bone tumor, and (2) coxa valga, which follows polio.

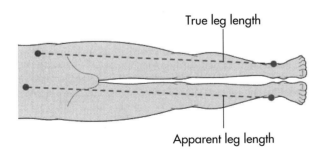

FIG. 10-31 Leg-length measurement. *(From Klippel JH, Dieppe PA: Rheumatology, vol 1-2, ed 2, London, 1998, Mosby.)*

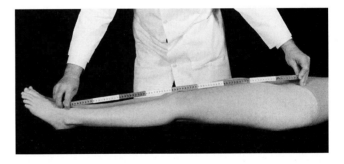

FIG. 10-32 The patient is lying supine with the feet together. The knees and hips are straight. With a tape measure, the examiner measures the length of the affected leg from the apex of the anterosuperior iliac spine to the medial malleolus. The distance is recorded and compared with the opposite leg. Actual leg-length shortening is caused by an abnormality above or below the trochanter level.

ALLIS' SIGN

ALSO KNOWN AS GALEAZZI'S SIGN

Assessment for Femoral Portion Structural Deficiency or Tibial Portion Structural Deficiency

Comment

Legg-Calvé-Perthes disease is an idiopathic form of osteonecrosis (i.e., avascular necrosis) of the femoral head in skeletally immature individuals. Necrotic changes within the epiphysis cause a collapse of the femoral head and alter its articular surface. The incidence of Legg-Calvé-Perthes disease has been reported as 1 in 1200, with 80% of those affected being male and the typical age of onset being 3 to 12 years.

The classic diagnostic findings include an obvious limp and often a complaint of ipsilateral, medial thigh, and knee pain. The affected hip is usually limited in internal rotation and abduction. The radiographic findings vary with the stage of the disorder. The classic crescent is a sign of osteonecrosis (Fig. 10-33).

A slipped capital femoral epiphysis occurs when shear forces lead to a displacement of the epiphysis of the femoral head and cause it to "slip" inferiorly and posteriorly relative to the neck of the femur (Fig. 10-34). This condition is most common in children aged 10 to 16 and seen more often in boys than in girls. Congenital dislocation of the hip can be caused by a variety of conditions that result in dysplasia of the femur or acetabulum.

ORTHOPEDIC GAMUT 10-9

FORMS OF CONGENITAL HIP DISLOCATION

The following are three forms of congenital hip dislocation:

1. Congenital hip dysplasia
2. Acetabular dysplasia
3. Congenital subluxation

ORTHOPEDIC GAMUT 10-10

DIAGNOSIS OF CONGENITAL HIP DYSPLASIA

The following are helpful in diagnosing congenital hip dysplasia:

1. *Neonatal* (birth to 1 month): Barlow's test, Ortolani's test
2. *Infancy* (1 month to 2 years): limited hip abduction with the hips flexed to 45 degrees, shortening on the affected side with hips and knees flexed (Galeazzi's sign), Trendelenburg's sign
3. *Age 2 to 6 years:* obvious limp, Trendelenburg's sign, limb shortening if unilateral
4. *Older than 6 years:* limp, limited hip abduction

Congenital dislocation of the hip is a spontaneous dislocation of the hip that occurs either before, during, or shortly after birth. It is clear that several factors are causative agents. Some of the factors are genetic and some environmental. One such factor, acting alone, may not always be sufficient by itself to bring about dislocation, and it may be that a combination of factors is often at work.

Generalized ligamentous laxity is found in some patients, and it may also be present in a parent or relatives. This laxity leads to a lack of stability at the hip, so dislocation may occur easily in certain positions of the joint.

It is possible that, in females, a ligament-relaxing hormone (relaxin) may be secreted by the fetal uterus in response to estrogen and progesterone that reaches the fetal circulation. This relaxin may cause instability, as does genetically determined joint laxity. It is also possible that laxity of the hip ligaments from this cause might help explain the greater incidence of dislocation in females.

Defective development of the acetabulum and the femoral head can be inherited. The defect appears always to be bilateral and is probably as common in males as in females. Defective development of the acetabulum predisposes a

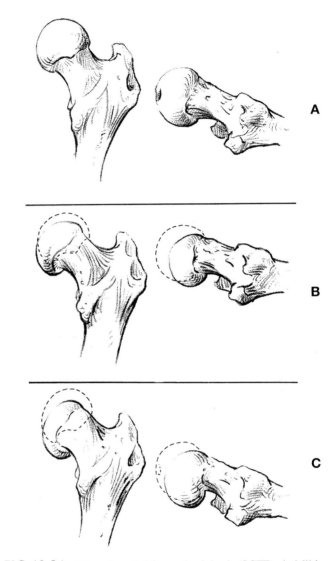

FIG. 10-34 Slipped capital femoral epiphysis (SCFE). **A,** Mild. **B,** Moderate. **C,** Severe. *(From Malone TR, McPoil TG, Nitz AJ: Orthopedic and sports physical therapy, ed 3, St Louis, 1997, Mosby.)*

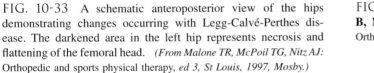

FIG. 10-33 A schematic anteroposterior view of the hips demonstrating changes occurring with Legg-Calvé-Perthes disease. The darkened area in the left hip represents necrosis and flattening of the femoral head. *(From Malone TR, McPoil TG, Nitz AJ: Orthopedic and sports physical therapy, ed 3, St Louis, 1997, Mosby.)*

fetus to hip dislocation, which may indeed occur before birth. If dislocation does not occur, the defect may show itself in adult life in the form of an unduly shallow acetabulum that has a tendency to subluxate. Later, osteoarthritis (acetabular dysplasia) may occur.

The incidence of congenital hip dislocation is slightly higher when an infant is delivered by a breech rather than normal delivery. It is possible that the act of extending the hips during delivery may precipitate dislocation when there is already a predisposition to it from ligamentous laxity or acetabular dysplasia.

There may be two distinct types of congenital dislocation of the hip. The first type of dislocation is caused by ligamentous laxity, whether genetically determined or hormonal. With this type of dislocation, the dislocation occurs almost accidentally when some precipitating movement, such as extension of the hips during delivery, occurs. This dislocation is the type that is often unilateral and readily correctable. The second type of dislocation is caused by genetically determined dysplasia of the acetabulum, which is always bilateral and often much more difficult to treat.

PROCEDURE

- The patient is lying supine with the knees flexed and the soles of the feet flat on the table, the great toes and malleoli being approximated bilaterally.

- The examiner observes the heights of the knees from a viewpoint at the foot of table (Fig. 10-35).
- If one knee is lower than the other, ipsilateral hip dislocation or severe coxa disorder is indicated (Fig. 10-36).
- Tibial length discrepancies are also discerned in this position.
- From viewing the position from the side, the examiner can assess femoral length discrepancies (Figs. 10-37 and 10-38).

Confirmation Procedures
Hip telescoping test and diagnostic imaging

DIAGNOSTIC STATEMENT

Allis' sign is present in the left leg and demonstrates a femoral portion deficiency. The presence of this sign suggests congenital dislocation of the hip joint.

Allis' sign is present in the left leg and demonstrates a tibial portion deficiency. The presence of this sign suggests bone dysplasia of the lower leg.

CLINICAL PEARL

Congenital dislocation of the hip is a condition in which one or both hips are dislocated at birth or are dislocated in the first few weeks of life. There is a familial tendency and a well-established geographic distribution for the disorder. The disorder may occur with other congenital defects.

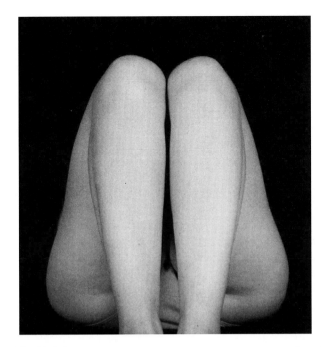

FIG. 10-35   The patient is lying supine. The knees are flexed, and the feet are flat on the examination table. The great toes and malleoli are approximated bilaterally.

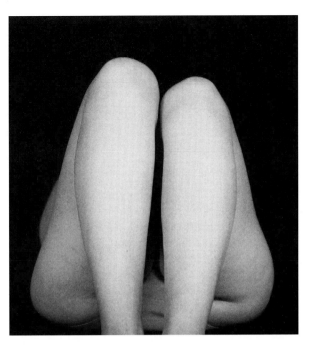

FIG. 10-36   From the foot of the table, the examiner observes the height of the knees. If one is lower than the other, a femoral deficiency that is caused by a pathologic condition of the ipsilateral coxa (dislocation) is indicated. This finding may also indicate a tibial length discrepancy.

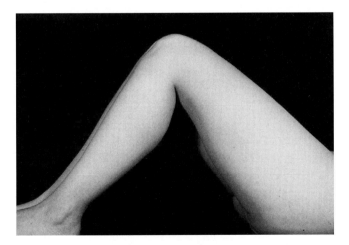

FIG. 10-37   From the side of the table, the examiner observes the position of the patient's knees. Again, the great toes and malleoli are approximated bilaterally.

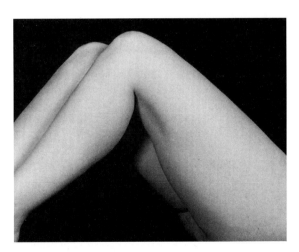

FIG. 10-38   If one knee is ahead of the other, it indicates femoral length discrepancy (dysplasia) or ipsilateral coxa pathology (dislocation).

Assessment for Fracture of the Femoral Neck or Head

Comment

All fracture-dislocations of the hip have a history of severe trauma in common. The type of trauma and the mechanism of injury are extremely important in identifying the fracture-dislocations. Physical examination and simple observation of the attitude of the limp will aid in differentiating the type of fracture-dislocation even before diagnostic imaging. Laboratory data are usually of no help unless there are extremely low hemoglobin and hematocrit counts. When these counts are low, the possibility of pelvic fracture must be a paramount consideration because enormous quantities of blood can be lost in the retroperitoneal area from pelvic fractures.

Fractures of the head of the femur usually occur in association with a dislocation of the head of the femur but have been known to occur without a dislocation. There is nothing unique about the presentation of these fractures that aids in their differentiation. The examiner must rely on diagnostic imaging for help in identifying the type of fracture (Fig. 10-39). The examiner should look for fractures of the superior aspect of the head of the femur with anterior dislocation and fractures of the inferior aspect with posterior dislocations.

Fractures of the neck of the femur may be displaced or undisplaced. The undisplaced fractures are caused by stress, which usually occurs in young athletic individuals; impaction, which usually occurs in instances of minor trauma and associated osteoporosis; or postirradiation of the pelvis, which occurs after treatments for cervical cancer (Fig. 10-40). The patient experiences mild to moderate pain in the groin and no rotational deformity or length discrepancy of the extremity. The patient often is able to walk but has an antalgic gait. Routine AP diagnostic imaging of the hip will often be normal. Oblique x-ray studies and tomograms are indicated.

On the other hand, displaced fractures of the neck of the femur have a usual mode of presentation. These fractures occur in osteoporotic individuals, usually older females, and are associated with a minor fall or severe trauma, although the latter is rare. These patients experience severe pain throughout the hip, and the leg is held in external rotation and mild abduction. Some shortening occurs. Radiographs are diagnostic and make fractures readily apparent with the displacement and disruption of Shenton's line.

In older people, the average age being 70 years, intertrochanteric fractures occur more often than do femoral neck fractures. These neck fractures are more common in females, in a ratio of 8 : 1 over males. Neck fractures usually occur in a major fall or an associated automobile injury,

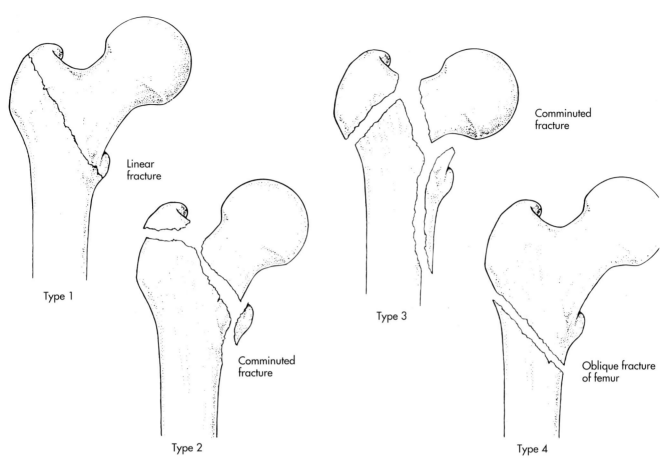

Linear
fracture

Type 1

Comminuted
fracture

Type 2

Comminuted
fracture

Type 3

Oblique fracture
of femur

Type 4

FIG. 10-39   Four common types of trochanteric fractures.   *(From Parker MJ, Pryor GA:* Hip fracture
management, *Boston, 1993, Blackwell.)*

with both direct and indirect forces acting on the hip. The indirect forces are the iliopsoas, with its attachment on the lesser trochanter, and the abductors, with their attachment on the greater trochanter. These indirect forces explain why separate fragments often occur within this type of injury. There will be marked external rotation of the extremity, especially in the comminuted fracture, with the foot often resting on its lateral surface. This rotation occurs because of the attachment of the iliopsoas, which can now rotate the shaft of the femur externally because of the fracture. The leg shortening varies with the degree of comminution.

Patients with subtrochanteric fractures are usually younger than those with femoral neck or intertrochanteric fractures. More force is needed to produce a subtrochanteric fracture than an intertrochanteric fracture. The physical findings are the same, and only diagnostic imaging can make the differentiation.

PROCEDURE

- While the patient is lying supine, the inferior calcaneus is struck with the examiner's fist (Fig. 10-41).

- Localized pain in the thigh indicates a femoral fracture or a severe pathologic condition of the joint.
- Localized pain in the leg indicates a tibial or fibular fracture.
- Pain localized to the calcaneus indicates calcaneal fracture.

Confirmation Procedures
Chiene's test, Ludloff's sign, and diagnostic imaging

DIAGNOSTIC STATEMENT

Anvil test is positive on the left side and elicits a sharp pain in the hip joint. This result suggests fracture of the femoral neck or head.

CLINICAL PEARL

Two questions must be answered in the assessment of a hip fracture. Is there a fracture? Is the fracture displaced? Usually, the break becomes obvious when viewed with diagnostic imaging, but an impacted fracture can be missed. The assessment is important because impacted or undisplaced fractures have a good prognosis. Displaced fractures have a high rate of nonunion and avascular necrosis.

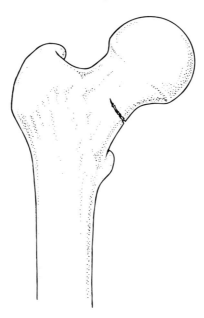

FIG. 10-40   Stress fracture of the femoral neck.   *(From Parker MJ, Pryor GA:* Hip fracture management, *Boston, 1993, Blackwell.)*

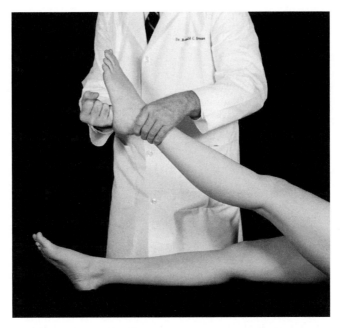

FIG. 10-41   The patient is lying supine. The examiner elevates the affected leg while keeping the knee extended. The inferior calcaneus is struck with the examiner's fist. Localized pain in the thigh indicates a femoral fracture or a severe pathologic condition involving the joint. Localized pain in the leg indicates a tibial or fibular fracture. Pain localized to the calcaneus indicates calcaneal fracture. Markedly reactive patients may be tested with the affected leg resting completely on the examination table.

APPARENT LEG-LENGTH TEST

Assessment for Apparent Leg Length Discrepancy

Comment

Measurements of the patient's leg length can be made while the patient is standing, measuring from the anterior-superior iliac spine to the floor and from the posterior superior iliac spine to the floor bilaterally. If the anterior-superior and posterior-superior iliac spines are lower on one side, an anatomic leg-length difference exists. If the anterior-superior iliac spine is lower and posterior superior iliac spine is higher on the same side, a functional leg-length discrepancy exists.

Apparent, or false, discrepancy in limb length is due entirely to sideways tilting of the pelvis. The usual cause is an adduction deformity in one hip, which gives an appearance of shortening on that side, or an abduction deformity, which gives an appearance of lengthening. An exception is a fixed pelvic obliquity that is caused by severe lumbar scoliosis.

To measure apparent discrepancy, the limbs must be placed parallel to one another and in line with the trunk. Measurement is made from any fixed point in the midline of the trunk (e.g., the xiphisternum) to each medial malleolus. True length must be evaluated when apparent discrepancy is determined.

Measurement is made bilaterally from the umbilicus or xiphisternum to the apex of the medial malleolus. This measurement is an index of the functional length of the lower extremities. An abduction contracture deformity causes apparent lengthening of the limb, and an adduction contracture deformity causes an apparent shortening. Because the pelvis is tilted sideways to make the legs parallel, the heel of the shorter side cannot be placed on the ground when the knees are straight. The difference between the lower limbs is caused only by pelvic obliquity, and measuring for a structural short leg is highly inaccurate when done in this manner.

PROCEDURE

- Measurement is made bilaterally from the umbilicus or xiphisternum to the apex of the medial malleolus (Fig. 10-42).
- This measurement is an index of the functional length of the lower extremities.

Confirmation Procedure
Actual leg-length measurements

DIAGNOSTIC STATEMENT

Measurements of leg length reveal an apparent discrepancy. This discrepancy is corroborated by accurate and equal measurements for true leg length. This result suggests a leg-length discrepancy resulting from pelvic obliquity.

CLINICAL PEARL

Pelvic tilting accompanied by a heel discrepancy indicates apparent shortening of the limb. This apparent shortening may be accompanied by some true shortening. The discrepancy at the heels provides a measure of its degree.

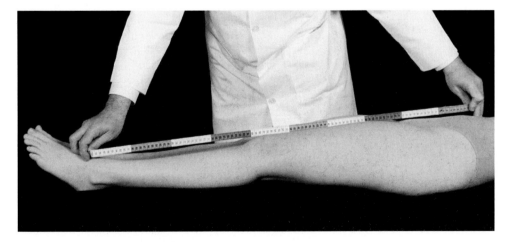

FIG. 10-42   The patient is lying supine with the legs extended on the examination table. With a tape measure, the examiner measures the length of the affected leg from the medial malleolus to the umbilicus. The distance is recorded and compared with the measurement obtained for the opposite leg. The difference in the length of the legs is probably the result of pelvic obliquity.

Assessment for Fracture of the Neck of the Femur

Comment

Although fractures in general occur in all age groups, hip fractures are most common among elderly women.

The vascular supply to the femoral head and neck may be significantly compromised with certain fracture patterns and levels of severity (Fig. 10-43). Generally, hip fractures can be classified by location and described by severity (simple or comminuted).

ORTHOPEDIC GAMUT 10-15

SUBTROCHANTERIC FRACTURE COMPLICATIONS

The following are subtrochanteric fracture complications:

1. Malunion
2. Delayed union
3. Nonunion

ORTHOPEDIC GAMUT 10-14

HIP FRACTURES

Fractures of the hip can be located in the following areas:

1. Extracapsular or trochanteric (Fig. 10-44)
2. Femoral neck or subcapital areas (these are intracapsular) (Fig. 10-45)
3. Proximal femoral shaft or subtrochanteric areas (Fig. 10-46)

ORTHOPEDIC GAMUT 10-16

HIP FRACTURE MALUNION AND NONUNION

Two factors are associated with hip fracture malunion and nonunion:

1. The subtrochanteric area of the proximal femur is cortical bone, with decreased blood supply.
2. The subtrochanteric area is prone to large biomechanical stresses that can lead to loosening of various fixation devices.

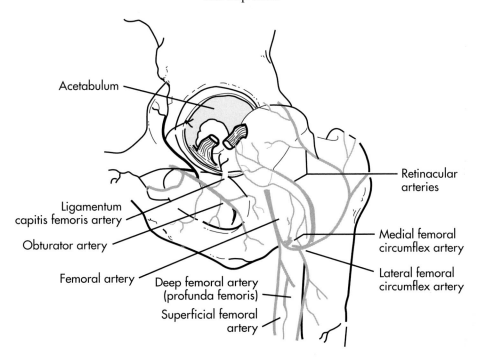

FIG. 10-43 Vascular supply to the femoral head and neck. *(From Shankman GA:* Fundamental orthopedic management for the physical therapist assistant, *St Louis, 1997, Mosby.)*

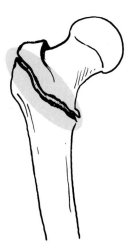

FIG. 10-44 Intertrochanteric hip fracture. *(From Shankman GA:* Fundamental orthopedic management for the physical therapist assistant, *St Louis, 1997, Mosby.)*

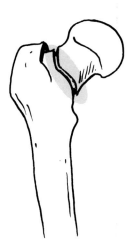

FIG. 10-45 Femoral neck fracture. *(From Shankman GA:* Fundamental orthopedic management for the physical therapist assistant, *St Louis, 1997, Mosby.)*

Fracture about the hip is unusual in the adolescent and young adult because the bone is exceptionally resilient. In young patients, the hip is much more likely to dislocate than it is to break.

If a fracture does occur, it is a major injury and should be treated as a medical emergency. The patient with a broken hip is completely disabled at once. The patient has severe pain in the hip and resists any attempt to manipulate the limb. The extremity is usually held with the thigh internally rotated and adducted while the knee rests above and against its fellow on the opposite side. The trochanter appears prominent. Any attempt to move the thigh from this position of flexion adduction and internal rotation causes pain. Diagnosis is confirmed by diagnostic imaging, and the images should be carefully studied to be sure there is not an accompanying fracture in the femoral shaft or acetabulum. The posterior acetabular margin, vulnerable in the adult, is seldom broken in the adolescent or young adult.

ORTHOPEDIC GAMUT 10-17

FEMORAL NECK FRACTURE NONUNION

Nonunion of femoral neck fractures occurs in approximately 15% of the cases. The reasons for nonunion are the following:

1. Meager blood supply
2. Inaccurate approximation and rigid fixation of the fragments

---

Additional complicating factors that may be present include avascular necrosis of the femoral head, which appears on diagnostic images as density changes and collapse of the head, and osteoarthritis that may restrict the mobility of the head of the acetabulum.

ORTHOPEDIC GAMUT 10-18

MANIFESTATIONS OF NONUNION OF FEMORAL NECK FRACTURES

The outstanding manifestations of nonunion of femoral neck fractures are the following:

1. Pain in the hip when bearing weight
2. Shortening and external rotation of the limb
3. Grating or crepitus in the hip during motion

PROCEDURE

- Determine whether a fracture of the neck of the femur has occurred by using a tape measure.
- The patient is supine with the legs extended on the examination table.
- Using a tape measure, the examiner measures the circumference of the thigh, passing the tape over the level of the greater trochanter (Fig. 10-47).
- The distance is recorded and compared to that of the opposite leg.
- An increased diameter indicates that the trochanter has rolled laterally.
- This increased measurement correlates with fracture of the neck of the femur.

Confirmation Procedures
Anvil test, Ludloff's sign, and diagnostic imaging

DIAGNOSTIC STATEMENT

Chiene's test is positive for the left hip. This result suggests a fracture of the neck of the femur.

CLINICAL PEARL

A fracture of the neck of the femur occurs mainly among elderly females whose bones are osteoporotic. The patient may fall but more often the patient catches a foot on something and ends up twisting the hip. The femoral neck is broken by rotational force. In most cases, the fracture is markedly displaced and completely unstable. In some cases, the fragments are impacted, and the patient may even walk about, albeit with some pain.

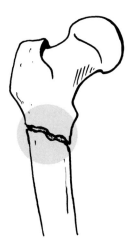

FIG. 10-46 Subtrochanteric hip fracture. *(From Shankman GA:* Fundamental orthopedic management for the physical therapist assistant, *St Louis, 1997, Mosby.)*

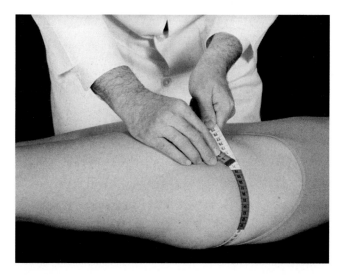

FIG. 10-47 The patient is lying supine with the legs extended on the examination table. Using a tape measure, the examiner measures the circumference of the thigh by passing the tape over the level of the greater trochanter. The distance is recorded and compared with the measurement obtained for the opposite leg. An increased diameter indicates that the trochanter has rolled laterally. This result correlates with fracture of the neck of the femur.

Assessment for Tuberculous Arthritis of the Hip Joint or Adult-Onset Osteonecrosis of the Femoral Head

Comment

Osteonecrosis is a common cause of hip pain in young and middle-aged patients and ultimately results in severe degeneration of the hip joint. The exact pathogenesis of osteonecrosis is unknown, but interference of the blood supply to the femoral head is the common pathway.

ORTHOPEDIC GAMUT 10-19

OSTEONECROSIS

The most common causes of osteonecrosis are the following:

1. Steroid use
2. Alcohol use
3. Trauma
4. Gout
5. Metabolic problems
6. Genetic problems

ORTHOPEDIC GAMUT 10-20

HIP PAIN

Other causes of hip pain that may present with symptoms similar to those of osteonecrosis include the following:

1. Gout
2. Femoral or inguinal hernia
3. Pigmented villonodular synovitis
4. Stress fracture of femoral neck
5. Rheumatoid arthritis

ORTHOPEDIC GAMUT 10-21

CLASSIFICATIONS OF OSTEONECROSIS

Osteonecrosis is classified into several radiographic stages that aid with prognosis and treatment:

Stage 0: No change on plain radiographs, but a positive magnetic resonance imaging (MRI) scan

Stage I: Mottled densities or osteopenia

Stage II: Areas of increased density in the femoral head (Fig. 10-48) crescent sign with subchondral fracture (Fig. 10-49)

Stage III: Depression of femoral head (Fig. 10-50)

Stage IV: Flattening and collapse of femoral head (Fig. 10-51)

Stage V: Degenerative arthrosis

Tuberculosis of the hip joint may appear at any age, but it occurs most commonly in children. An intermittent limp is the first, constant sign. At first, tuberculosis of the hip may come on after exercise, but later it is present after rest, such as in the early morning. Initially, pain may be only a slight discomfort that occurs in the groin or the knee and thigh (referred pain). Startling pain at night occurs at a later stage and is caused by relaxation of the protective muscle contraction. At an even later stage, the patient may experience stiffness of the joint.

In the early stages of the disease, when it is limited to the synovium or bone, the position of the joint is that of slight flexion, abduction, and lateral rotation (greatest fluid capacity). At a later stage, when arthritis supervenes, the leg becomes flexed, adducted, and internally rotated. At an early stage, muscle wasting is not a very pronounced sign, but soon afterward, it becomes obvious. In a longstanding case, atrophy of the quadriceps and glutei becomes very pronounced. At a later stage, swelling that is due to the formation of an abscess may be present. This abscess commonly points anteriorly. Apparent lengthening may be present in the active stage because of fixed abduction. Apparent shortening occurs later and is due to fixed adduction.

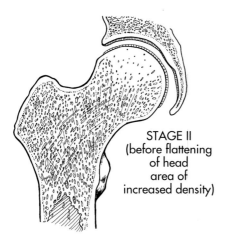

FIG. 10-48   Osteonecrosis stage II; increased density in the area of maximum loading of the femoral head. *(From Bucholz RW: Orthopaedic decision making, ed 2, St Louis, 1996, Mosby.)*

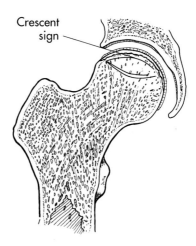

FIG. 10-49   Osteonecrosis stage IIA; the "crescent sign" with subchondral fracture. *(From Bucholz RW: Orthopaedic decision making, ed 2, St Louis, 1996, Mosby.)*

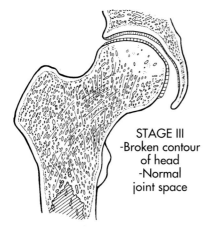

FIG. 10-50   Osteonecrosis stage III; flattening of the femoral head. *(From Bucholz RW: Orthopaedic decision making, ed 2, St Louis, 1996, Mosby.)*

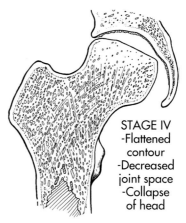

FIG. 10-51   Osteonecrosis stage IV; collapse of the femoral head and loss of normal contour. *(From Bucholz RW: Orthopaedic decision making, ed 2, St Louis, 1996, Mosby.)*

In the early stage, deep tenderness can often be elicited in the groin. At a later stage, if an abscess is present, a soft swelling may be palpable. Atrophy of the muscles occurs later, and the trochanter may be raised on the affected side.

At first, only the extremes of movement are limited and painful. The Thomas test becomes positive at an early stage and reveals concealed flexion contracture. Limitation of extension is also a valuable sign. Later, when arthritis supervenes, movements are restricted by muscular spasm, and attempted movement becomes very painful.

General malaise and pallor accompany tuberculous arthritis, and slight evening pyrexia is not uncommon. In the healing stage, the general condition improves, and the joint is no longer painful.

PROCEDURE

- The patient is lying supine or in a side-lying position with the affected thigh extended (Fig. 10-52).
- The examiner carefully rotates the thigh (Fig. 10-53).

- The sign is positive if contraction of the abdominal muscles is noted on the same side that is being maneuvered (Fig. 10-54).
- The sign is significant for reflex muscle spasm, which is commonly elicited in tuberculosis of the coxa, or adult onset osteonecrosis.

Confirmation Procedures
Jansen's test, Patrick's test, and diagnostic imaging

DIAGNOSTIC STATEMENT

Gauvain's sign is present in the left hip. The presence of this sign suggests tuberculous arthritis of the joint.

CLINICAL PEARL

Tuberculosis of the hip is now rare in the United States. A child infected with this disease walks with a limp and often complains of pain in the groin or knee. Night pain is another feature. In early cases, complete resolution may be hoped for with antituberculous therapy, bed rest, and traction. In the advanced case, joint debridement is carried out with efforts to obtain a bony fusion of the joint.

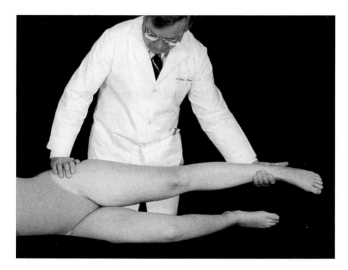

FIG. 10-52   The patient is in a side-lying position on the unaffected hip. The affected leg is extended, and the examiner slightly abducts the affected leg.

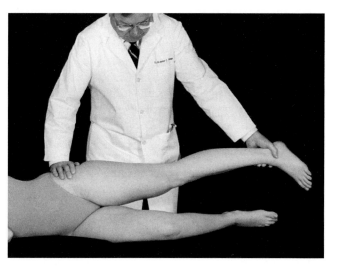

FIG. 10-53   The examiner cautiously externally rotates the leg (internally rotates the femoral head).

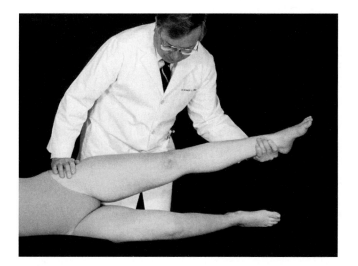

FIG. 10-54   Next, the examiner internally rotates the leg (externally rotating the femoral head). If abdominal muscular contraction occurs on the same side, it is a positive sign. The sign indicates reflex muscle spasm due to tuberculosis of the hip or adult onset osteonecrosis of the femoral head. Tuberculosis of the hip is usually not common after adolescence.

GUILLAND'S SIGN

Assessment for Meningeal Irritation

Comment

Viruses, bacteria, spirochetes, and fungi may infect the meninges and subarachnoid space (Fig. 10-55). The relative incidence of these causes varies enormously in different areas of the world, and viral and bacterial infections sometimes show a seasonal variation.

In senescence, the features that make the diagnosis difficult may include an apyrexial course or neurologic symptoms dominated by confusion and delirium or focal signs caused by cerebral venous thrombosis, mimicking a cerebrovascular accident (Fig. 10-56).

The signs and symptoms of meningitis may develop explosively de novo or may appear in the waning stages of an infection that is localized elsewhere. Headache, backache, nausea, and vomiting are common symptoms, and nuchal rigidity occurs in more than 80% of patients. Kernig/Brudzinski sign is often present (Figs. 10-57 and 10-58). Only in the neonate and very young infant is meningitis often unattended by evidence of increased pressure and meningeal irritation. At this stage, even fever may be absent. Photophobia may be a prominent, early symptom and is related in some way to the meningeal inflammation.

Disturbances in mental status occur in nearly all cases of acute bacterial meningitis. Irritability, confusion, delirium, and stupor are common. Coma occurs in about 10% of the cases and indicates a poor prognosis. Focal or generalized seizures occur in about a fourth of all patients with meningitis. Seizures are encountered much more often in infants, who have a greater susceptibility to them. Signs of cerebral dysfunction, other than altered consciousness and seizures, are uncommon in cases of acute bacterial meningitis. The signs of cerebral dysfunction appear most often when treatment has been delayed. These signs include a disturbed conjugate gaze, dysphagia, paresis of extremities, and visual field defects. Striking and persistent signs are usually due to infarction of tissue as a result of cortical venous thrombosis. The latter complication commonly develops during the second week of the disease, when signs of infection and meningeal irritation are subsiding. Bilateral neurologic signs and convulsions occurring first on one side then on the other always suggest an associated thrombosis of the superior sagittal sinus. Prominent and slowly progressive focal signs appearing early in the meningitis should indicate an associated focus of sepsis such as subdural endocarditis with cerebral embolism.

Between 5% and 20% of the patients with bacterial meningitis will develop cranial nerve palsies during the acute stage of the disease. Impaired ocular movement, deafness, and labyrinthine dysfunction are most frequently seen. Blindness and facial paralysis also occur. Most cranial nerve palsies are probably attributable to the meningeal exudate, but the eighth nerve complex may be damaged by bacteria or their toxins, which act directly on the inner ear. Although the cerebrospinal fluid pressure is usually elevated in patients with bacterial meningitis, papilledema is rare and is more characteristic of a brain abscess, subdural empyema, or venous sinus thrombosis. The uncommon occurrence of papilledema in uncomplicated meningitis is probably explained by the short duration of the increased pressure.

PROCEDURE

- While the patient is in a supine position, there is a brisk flexion of the hip and the knee when the quadriceps muscle on the opposite limb is irritated, such as by a firm pinch (Figs. 10-59 to 10-61).
- The sign is present in cases of meningeal irritation.

Confirmation Procedures

Kernig/Brudzinski sign, clinical laboratory assessment, and neurologic assessment

---

DIAGNOSTIC STATEMENT

Guilland's sign is present on the left. The presence of this sign suggests meningeal irritation.

CLINICAL PEARL

Acute meningitis (associated with cortical encephalitis and often with ventriculitis) is an emergency and should be suspected in any patient with the acute onset of nonlocalizing central nervous system signs. Fever, nuchal rigidity, headache, altered mental status, vomiting, and photophobia are typically present. The absence of fever is not uncommon. Meningeal signs are not usually present in infants younger than 6 months of age. Acute signs may also be less apparent in elderly, alcoholic, immunocompromised, or comatose patients.

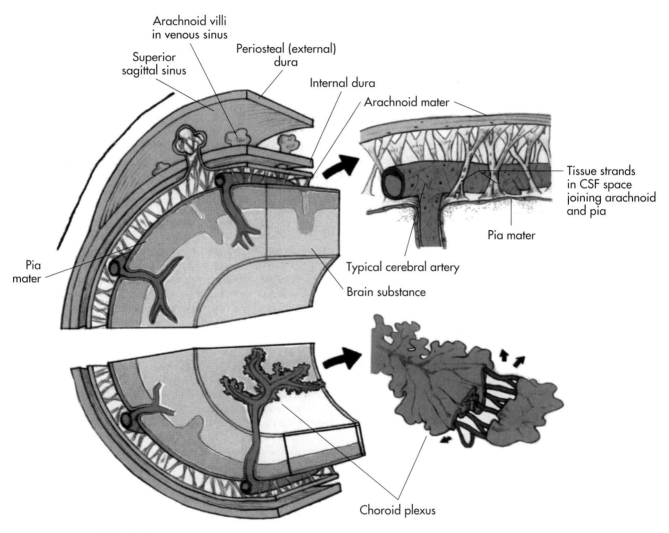

FIG. 10-55   Choroid plexus and arachnoid granulations. *CSF,* Cerebrospinal fluid.   *(From Mathers LH, et al:* Clinical anatomy principles, *St Louis, 1996, Mosby.)*

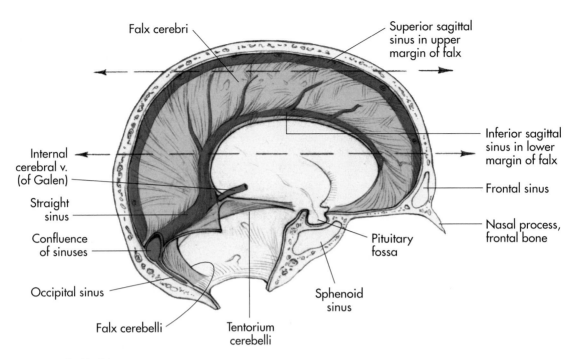

FIG. 10-56 Falx cerebri and sagittal sinuses. *(From Mathers LH, et al:* Clinical anatomy principles, *St Louis, 1996, Mosby.)*

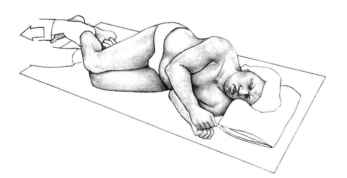

FIG. 10-57 Kernig's sign. *(From Olson WH, et al:* Handbook of symptom-oriented neurology, *ed 2, St Louis, 1994, Mosby.)*

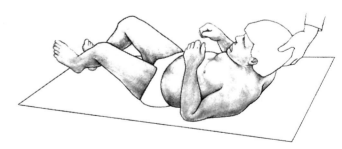

FIG. 10-58 Brudzinski's sign. *(From Olson WH, et al:* Handbook of symptom-oriented neurology, *ed 2, St Louis, 1994, Mosby.)*

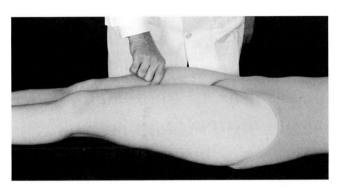

FIG. 10-59   The patient is lying supine with the legs extended on the examination table. The examiner firmly irritates (pinches) one of the quadriceps muscles.

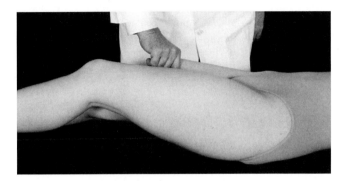

FIG. 10-60   If the sign is present, brisk flexion of the opposite hip and knee occurs. The sign is present only in meningeal irritation.

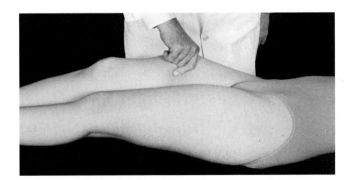

FIG. 10-61   The sign is not exclusive to brisk flexion of the contralateral hip and knee. Ipsilateral flexion, as a function of spasmophilia due to meningeal irritation, can occasionally be observed.

HIP TELESCOPING TEST

Assessment for Congenital Dislocation of the Hip Articulation

Comment

Congenital dislocation of the hip occurs as the result of underlying dysplasia of the joint. There are several theories as to the origin of this type of dislocation, but the precise cause is still unknown. The disorder exhibits familial and racial tendencies and is often seen in Mediterranean and Scandinavian countries.

There are two general degrees of the pathologic condition: complete dislocation and subluxation. Subluxation is the more common type, and if the condition goes untreated, it may develop into complete dislocation.

As a consequence of a defective acetabulum, the roof of the acetabulum slopes vertically instead of lying in its normal horizontal position. The acetabulum is shallow, and the labrum (limbus) may be folded into the cavity. The femoral head is dislocated upward and laterally out of the acetabulum. There is usually marked forward torsion of the axis of the femoral neck (anteversion). Adaptive changes take place in the capsule and muscles, and the acetabulum is filled with fatty tissue.

Dislocation is much more common in females than in males, and it is often bilateral. In the infant, the obvious clinical findings in unilateral cases are the asymmetric skin folds on the medial aspect of the thigh, the exaggerated vertical angle of the inguinal crease, and the shortening of the affected extremity. The lengths of the patient's femurs are compared while the hips and knees are flexed at 90 degrees. Shortening is readily apparent from the lower level of the knee on the involved side. Abduction of the flexed thigh, which is normally possible up to approximately 90 degrees, is sharply limited. While the thigh is flexed to 90 degrees, a telescopic movement may be apparent by a gentle push-pull technique. During palpation, the absence of the femoral head in Scarpa's triangle and its abnormal posterior position are noted. A click may be felt as the femoral head passes in and out of the acetabulum, when the flexed hip is abducted or adducted.

After walking starts, an abnormality of gait is noted. If the condition is unilateral, the child walks with an abduction lurch, and if the condition is bilateral, the child walks with a typical duck-waddling gait.

Congenital subluxation of the hip presents with the clinical findings of asymmetric skin folds and limited abduction of the flexed hip. The diagnosis of congenital subluxation is established by diagnostic imaging. The acetabular roof shows an obliquity and the underdeveloped capital epiphysis, which lies slightly lateral and superior, although in the acetabulum.

Slipped femoral capital epiphysis, which may be chronic, occurs in adolescent children and is probably related to trauma. It represents a variety of Salter-Harris type I fracture of the epiphyseal plate. It is most commonly seen in boys approaching puberty, particularly those who are overweight and sexually immature (Fig. 10-62).

ORTHOPEDIC GAMUT 10-22

SLIPPED FEMORAL CAPITAL EPIPHYSIS

Radiographic signs of slipped femoral capital epiphysis include the following:

1. Blurring of the epiphyseal line
2. Increased width of the epiphyseal plate
3. Prolongation of the superior neck fails to cut epiphysis
4. Loss of height of the epiphysis in comparison with a normal contralateral hip

---

PROCEDURE

- The patient is in a supine position.
- The hip and knee are flexed to 90 degrees, respectively.
- The femur is pushed down toward the examination table (Fig. 10-63).
- The leg is lifted from the examination table.
- There will be considerable movement in hip dislocation.
- This is hip telescoping.

Confirmation Procedures

Allis' sign and diagnostic images

DIAGNOSTIC STATEMENT

The telescoping test is positive in the right hip. This result suggests congenital dislocation of the articulation.

CLINICAL PEARL

When treatment in childhood for congenital dislocation of the hip has been unsuccessful, or even where the condition has not been diagnosed, a patient may seek help during the third and fourth decades of life. Symptoms may arise from the hips or the spine. In the hips, secondary arthritic changes occur in the false joint that may form between the dislocated femoral head and the ilium. In the spine, osteoarthritic changes are the result of longstanding scoliosis. The telescoping test may remain positive for as long as the cause of the dislocation goes untreated.

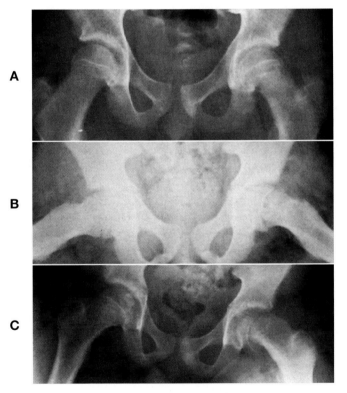

A

B

C

FIG. 10-62   **A,** Slipped capital femoral epiphysis on the left. **B,** In this frog-leg view, the "slippage" is more obvious, with clear superior displacement of the femoral neck. **C,** More obvious slippage on the left.   *(From Sutton D, Young JWR: A concise textbook of clinical imaging, ed 2, St Louis, 1995, Mosby.)*

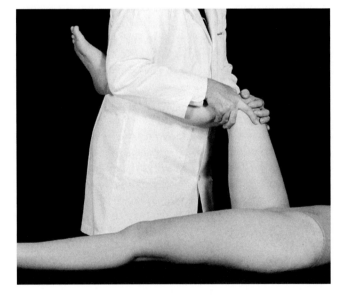

FIG. 10-63   The patient is supine. The examiner flexes the affected hip to 90 degrees and the knee to 90 degrees. The femur is pushed toward the examining table and then pulled up from the table. If the test is positive, a distinct pistoning of the hip is noted. The positive finding indicates dislocation of the hip. Although this test is usually used with neonates, the effect of the test may be observed throughout adult life in individuals with untreated or undiagnosed congenital hip dislocations.

Assessment for Osteoarthritis of the Hip Joint

Comment

Osteoarthritis involves a few joints, so symptoms and signs are localized in nature. Early in the disease, osteoarthritis is associated with few or no symptoms. Pain is usually the earliest symptom, and it comes on with use, particularly after prolonged inactivity of the joint, and is relieved by rest. The pain is usually a low-grade ache that is often difficult for the patient to localize. As the disease progresses in severity, pain occurs even during rest. Cold, damp weather exacerbates the pain. In some patients, pain may be aggravated by heat. The pain that is experienced by patients with osteoarthritis is of multiple origins. The pain may result from periosteal elevation associated with cartilage and bone proliferation, from pressure on exposed bone, from microfractures of bone, or from trauma to the synovium. Synovitis occurs in advanced cases of the disease and may cause pain as a result of inflammation. Spasm of muscles or pressure on nerves in the region of the joint may also be a major source of pain.

Stiffness is another common complaint, and it is usually more severe when a patient awakens in the morning or after inactivity during the day. Pain and stiffness are often worse just before changes in the weather. Although stiffness is an important symptom in other forms of connective tissue disease, the stiffness, or fibrositis, associated with osteoarthritis is short lived and usually lasts less than 15 minutes. Limited joint motion eventually develops, as a result of abnormalities in the joint surface, muscle spasm, contracture of soft tissues, and the interfering effect of spurs and loose bodies.

During physical examination, the joints may show slight tenderness, and pain occurs as the joint is moved. Palpation of the joint will often reveal crepitus—a sensation of grating as the joint is moved. Joint enlargement is seen, primarily as a result of proliferative reactions in cartilage and bone. Later, both deformity and subluxation become more apparent.

Osteoarthritis of the hip usually occurs in older persons, but it may begin at an earlier age. Osteoarthritis is progressive in nature, and bilateral involvement is not uncommon. Pain is often associated with a limp early on in the disease. Hip pain is felt at the side or the front of the joint or along the inner aspect of the thigh. Errors in diagnosis often arise because pain that originates in the hip may be referred to other regions and may present elsewhere. Hip pain may present as pain in the buttocks or sciatic region. Often, pain is referred along the obturator nerve, down the front of the thigh and knee. In some patients, most or all the pain of the hip disease is felt in the knee. The pain in this area may be so

severe that its hip origin is overlooked. Conversely, pain in the region of the hip may originate elsewhere, such as in the lumbosacral spine. Varying degrees of limited hip motion can be noted during examination when osteoarthritis is present. For example, the leg is held in external rotation with the hip flexed and adducted. Functional shortening may occur. Walking is awkward, and the patient finds difficulty sitting, rising from a seated position, and ascending stairs. Sexual intercourse becomes a stressful activity.

A discussion of hip osteoarthritis and subsequent sciatic nerve lesions is not complete without referring to the piriformis syndrome. Leg pain (sciatic) may be caused by compression of the sciatic nerve by the piriformis muscle at the pelvic outlet. In healthy individuals, the sciatic nerve passes underneath the piriformis muscle in 85% to 90% of patients; in 9% to 32% of instances, the peroneal division passes only above or through the muscle; and in 1% to 2% of persons, the entire sciatic nerve pierces the piriformis muscle.

The clinical manifestations of the piriformis syndrome include buttock and leg pain that worsens during sitting (without low back pain) and that is exacerbated by internal rotation or abduction and external rotation of the hip (and the straight-leg-raise test) and exquisite local tenderness in the buttock. These symptoms are caused by sciatic nerve compression by the piriformis muscle.

ORTHOPEDIC GAMUT 10-23

PIRIFORMIS SYNDROME

In piriformis syndrome, the following is true:

1. Symptoms of piriformis syndrome are not substantiated by clinical or electrophysiologic findings.
2. Denervation in the sciatic nerve distribution is usually caused by aberrant fascial bands, rather than piriformis muscle.

The pattern of denervation is useful; the gluteus medius and tensor fascia lata, both innervated by the superior gluteal nerve, which branches from the sciatic trunk before the piriformis muscle, are normal (Fig. 10-64).

PROCEDURE

- In osteoarthritis deformans of the hip, the patient is asked to cross the legs, with a point just above the ankle resting on the opposite knee (Figs. 10-65 and 10-66).

- If significant disease exists, this test and motion are impossible.

Confirmation Procedure

Gauvain's sign, Patrick's test, and diagnostic imaging

DIAGNOSTIC STATEMENT

Jansen's test is positive for the left hip. This result suggests osteoarthritis of the joint.

CLINICAL PEARL

Primary osteoarthritis of the hip occurs in middle-aged and elderly patients and is often associated with obesity and overuse. However, often, no obvious cause can be found. The symptoms of secondary osteoarthritis of the hip are identical to those of primary osteoarthritis. The condition most commonly occurs as a sequel to congenital hip dislocation.

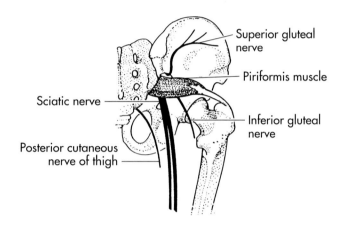

FIG. 10-64   The nerve of the sciatic notch and the piriformis muscle. *(From Stewart JD: Focal peripheral neuropathies, ed 2, New York, 1993, Raven Press.)*

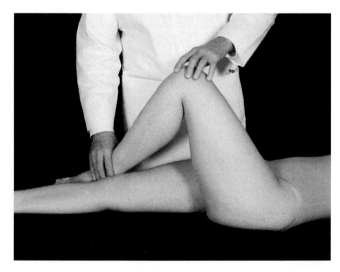

FIG. 10-65   The patient is lying supine. The examiner flexes and externally rotates the affected hip, crossing the patient's ankle over the contralateral knee.

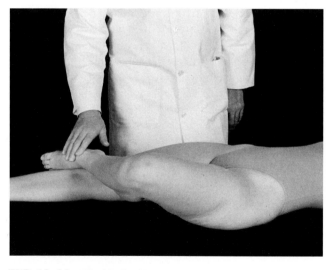

FIG. 10-66   The hip is allowed to abduct and extend passively. The distance between the lateral surface of the thigh and the examination table is noted. The distance is compared with the distance obtained on the opposite side. The test is positive when the motion is impossible to complete. A positive test indicates osteoarthritis of the hip joint.

LUDLOFF'S SIGN

Assessment for Traumatic Separation of the Lesser Trochanter

Comment

Occasionally, the tip of the greater trochanter is cracked as a result of a direct blow. Other than protecting the limb by avoiding weight bearing for a few weeks until the reaction to the trauma has settled down, no specific treatment is required for such a trochanteric crack.

The lesser trochanter may be avulsed by the pull of the psoas muscle. By itself, this avulsion is of no importance, but this avulsion sometimes occurs because the bone at this level is weakened through pathologic change or a secondary neoplastic deposit. The examiner must bear this possibility in mind and should perform a biopsy if necessary.

There are many varieties of malignant tumors. The picture of any of them may vary depending on the age of the patient, the site, and duration of the lesion. A picture common for one tumor at one stage may be similar to that of a different tumor at a different stage. The examiner does not encounter enough examples of a rare tumor to make generalizations.

Two points are imperative for the examiner to remember. There is a constant need to be aware of the possibility that a malignant lesion may be present. There is also a need to simplify the problem. These needs can be accomplished, but even so, the examiner should maintain the attitude that the diagnosis, although highly probable, does not become established until the tissue is actually examined.

Although any metastatic tumor may appear in bone, for many tumors, this is true only when they have existed long enough and are in the terminal stage. Tumors of this type should have been recognized much earlier. Several of the tumors are so rare that the whole group represents less than 2% of the cases involving the structural tissues.

These considerations serve to reduce the list of malignant lesions for practical purposes to approximately 13 varieties, and 2 of these, metastatic carcinomas of the breast and prostate, are differentiated by the sex of the patient.

These few lesions can be separated into conveniently small groups when the usual age of onset of the particular disease is considered.

PROCEDURE

- In traumatic separation of the epiphysis of the lesser trochanter, swelling and ecchymosis are present at the base of Scarpa's triangle, and the patient cannot raise the thigh when in the seated position (Figs. 10-67 and 10-68).

Confirmation Procedures

Anvil test, Chiene's test, and diagnostic imaging

DIAGNOSTIC STATEMENT

Ludloff's sign is present on the left side. The presence of this sign suggests a traumatic separation of the lesser trochanter.

CLINICAL PEARL

As with femoral neck fractures, this fracture is common in elderly, osteoporotic females. However, in sharp contrast to the intracapsular neck fractures, the extracapsular trochanteric fractures unite very easily and seldom cause avascular necrosis.

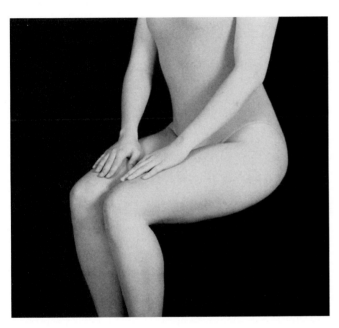

FIG. 10-67 The patient is seated on the edge of the examination table. The feet may touch the floor.

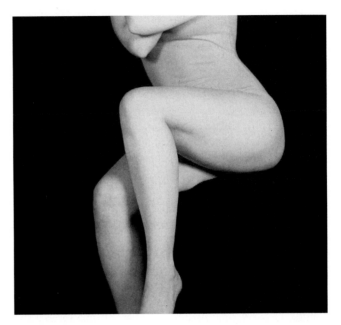

FIG. 10-68 While remaining seated, the patient tries to raise the affected thigh from the table surface. The sign is present when this move cannot be accomplished. When accompanied by swelling and ecchymosis in Scarpa's triangle, this sign indicates fracture of the lesser trochanter.

OBER'S TEST

Assessment for Iliotibial Band Contracture

Comment

Muscle strains commonly occur in the pelvis and thigh. The two primary causes of muscle injury are acute trauma and overuse trauma. A common mechanism is acute trauma. Single traumatic events, which are usually high-velocity eccentric contractions in which the muscle is rapidly forced into an elongated position, cause the so-called pulled muscle.

The greater trochanteric bursa separates the tendon of the gluteus maximus from the superior portion of the greater trochanter; the trochanteric bursa lies between the tendon of the gluteus medius and the anterosuperior portion of the greater trochanter (Fig. 10-69).

During the clinical examination, the patient typically indicates a localized area of tenderness near the superoposterior tip of the greater trochanter. This area is often quite tender, and the patient may be unable to lie on the affected side for prolonged periods. A positive Ober's sign is often present, as is weakness of the hip abductors when tested in an antigravity position.

The iliotibial band is a thickened portion of the tensor fascia latae along its lateral aspect. The tensor fascia latae arises from the coccyx, the sacrum, the iliac crest, Poupart's ligament, and the pubic ramus. Between two layers, the band encloses the gluteus maximus and the tensor fasciae femoris, giving attachment to the latter muscle and most of the former. The fibers of the fasciae converge to form the iliotibial band along the lateral side of the thigh. The iliotibial band is continuous medially with the lateral intermuscular septum, which attaches to the linea aspera. Distally, the band gives origin to the short head of the biceps. At the level of the knee joint, the band spreads out and attaches to the lateral tibial condyle and the head of the fibula. The iliotibial band lies in a plane anterior to the hip joint and posterior to the knee.

Involvement of the attached muscles is responsible for increased tension. The band is placed under the attached muscles during the acute and convalescent stages. The taut band is perceived by deep palpation while adducting and extending the thigh. Resistance to passive flexing of the hip while the knee is fully extended demonstrates spasm in the gluteus maximus. Spasm in the short head of the biceps is demonstrated by flexing the hip, which relaxes the iliopsoas band, and finding resistance to extension of the knee. The patient assumes the most comfortable position in which the thigh is flexed, abducted, and externally rotated at the hip while the knee is flexed. This position relaxes the tension of the band. If tension is not overcome by stretching during the acute stage, band contracture becomes progressive, and permanent deformity ensues.

PROCEDURE

- The patient is in a side-lying position on the unaffected hip and thigh.
- The examiner places one hand on the pelvis to steady it and grasps the patient's ankle lightly with the other hand, holding the knee flexed at a right angle (Fig. 10-70).
- The thigh is abducted and extended in the coronal plane of the body.
- In the presence of iliotibial band contracture, the leg will remain abducted; the degree of abduction depends on the amount of contracture present (Figs. 10-71 and 10-72).
- The sign is present both in the conscious and anesthetized patient.
- Ober calls attention to the frequency of a negative roentgenogram in the presence of clinical signs and symptoms of irritation of the sacroiliac or lumbosacral joints.
- He refers to the importance of the iliotibial band as a factor to consider in the occurrence of lumbosacral spinal disorders with or without associated sciatica.

Confirmation Procedures
Phelp's test, Thomas test, and Trendelenburg's test

DIAGNOSTIC STATEMENT

Ober's test is positive on the left. This result indicates an iliotibial band contracture.

CLINICAL PEARL

Transient synovitis of the hip is the most common cause of an irritable hip and can produce a limp and a positive Ober's test. There is sometimes a history of preceding minor trauma, which in some cases is at least coincidental. Radiographs of the hip sometimes give confirmatory evidence of synovitis, but no other pathologic condition is demonstrable.

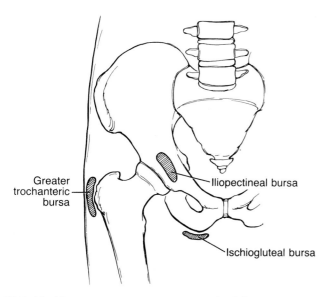

FIG. 10-69 Bursae of the hip and external pelvis. *(From Malone TR, McPoil TG, Nitz AJ:* Orthopedic and sports physical therapy, *ed 3, St Louis, 1997, Mosby.)*

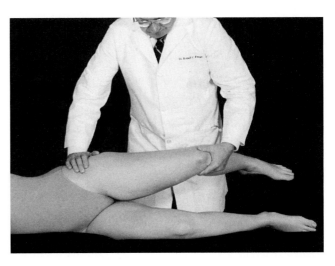

FIG. 10-70 The patient is in a side-lying position on the unaffected hip. The affected leg is extended. The examiner slightly abducts the affected leg.

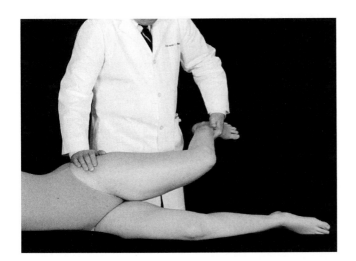

FIG. 10-71 The examiner stabilizes the pelvis with one hand and grasps the ankle of the affected leg with the other hand. The examiner flexes the knee to 90 degrees. The thigh is abducted and extended. The test is positive if the leg remains abducted. A positive test indicates iliotibial band contracture.

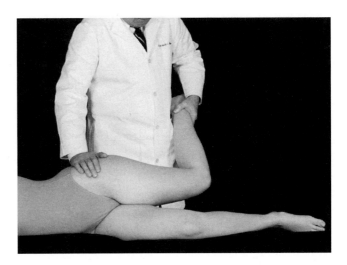

FIG. 10-72 The same procedure used on a normal hip demonstrates the normal adduction movement of the leg.

PATRICK'S TEST

ALSO KNOWN AS FABERE SIGN
(FLEXION, ABDUCTION, EXTERNAL ROTATION, EXTENSION)

Assessment for Intracapsular Coxa Pathologic Conditions

Comment

Death of the subchondral bone of the femoral head as a result of vascular impairment is known as *avascular necrosis* (AVN), *aseptic necrosis,* or *osteonecrosis.* This severely disabling condition can affect individuals of all ages. The clinical picture typically includes persistent inguinal pain and limping. In many cases, the patient is unable to report a recent injury or precipitating event but, when questioned in detail, may report one or more of the risk factors mentioned previously. The diagnosis is confirmed with radiographic evaluation. In many cases, the classic finding of the crescent sign is apparent on AP films (Fig. 10-73).

Articular cartilage is not innervated. As the osteoarthritis progresses, capsular fibrosis and shortening occur; the typical pattern results in limited extension, abduction, and internal rotation of the hip. The capsule can be painfully stretched during the middle and late stance phases of gait, which require the hip to assume these positions. This results in muscle guarding by the hip intrinsic muscles, further restricting motion and causing pain.

ORTHOPEDIC GAMUT 10-25

HIP OSTEOARTHRITIS

Classic radiographic findings of hip osteoarthritis include the following:

1. Loss of joint space
2. Sclerosis of subchondral bone of the femoral head
3. Osteophytes around the joint margins
4. Bone cysts in the subchondral bone (Fig. 10-74)

Rheumatoid arthritis (RA) is a disabling, autoimmune, systemic connective tissue disease that is present to different degrees in more than 3.6 million Americans. This disease is characterized by chronic swelling, pain, and progressive deformity of multiple joints.

Degenerative arthritis that is confined to the hip joint is a common affliction that occurs in the middle and later years of adult life. The cause of degenerative arthritis is not completely understood, but obesity, trauma, congenital hip dysplasia, avascular necrosis of the femoral head, and slipped capital femoral epiphysis are all factors in its onset.

Pathologically, the articular cartilage becomes progressively thinned and worn away. New bone proliferation around the femoral head and acetabulum occurs. The synovium becomes chronically thickened and congested.

The clinical course is gradual, and both hips may be affected. The onset of symptoms may be precipitated by a minor injury. Pain after activity and stiffness after rest are characteristic. The stiffness often subsides with activity, and the pain usually subsides with rest. The pain is often referred to the knee joint region. With the passage of time, the pain increases, sometimes even occurring during rest. Crepitus and grating in the hip may develop, and a painful limp is common.

Numerous special tests can be performed in the supine position to clarify the involved tissues. Gentle, manual spinal distraction may reduce low back pain and assist the examiner in differential diagnosis. The nature of the passive motion of the hip can be further appreciated with inferior glide, lateral glide, and "perimeter" scouring (Fig. 10-75).

Examination reveals tenderness over the anterior and posterior hip joint and restriction of motion, especially internal rotation and abduction. Pain is usually present at the extremes of motion, and a flexion contracture often develops. This contracture can be measured by the Thomas test.

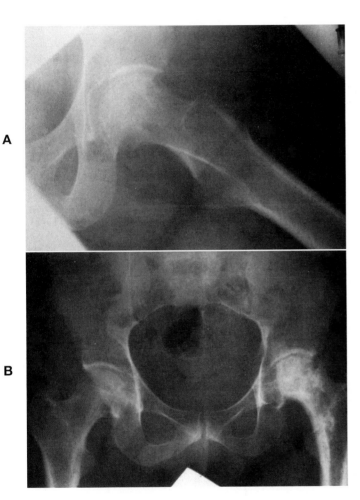

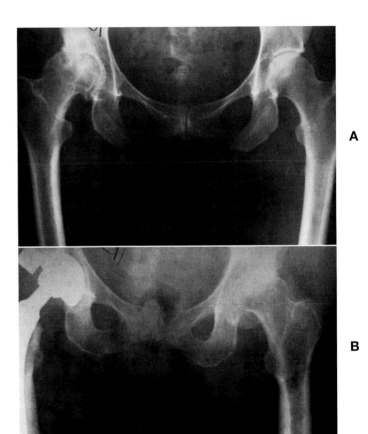

FIG. 10-73 **A,** "Frog-leg" view radiograph of the hip in a patient with early avascular necrosis (AVN) of the femoral head. **B,** An anteroposterior pelvis view of a patient with severe AVN of the left hip. *(From Malone TR, McPoil TG, Nitz AJ: Orthopedic and sports physical therapy, ed 3, St Louis, 1997, Mosby.)*

FIG. 10-74 Arthrosis of the hip. **A,** Early radiographic signs of arthrosis in left hip. Right hip demonstrated advanced signs of arthrosis. **B,** In the anteroposterior pelvis view of a different patient, radiographic signs of severe arthrosis are present in the left hip. *(From Malone TR, McPoil TG, Nitz AJ: Orthopedic and sports physical therapy, ed 3, St Louis, 1997, Mosby.)*

PROCEDURE

- Patrick's test is of particular value in geriatric cases because it indicates hip joint disease.
- The patient lies supine, and the examiner grasps the ankle and the flexed knee (Fig. 10-76).
- The thigh is flexed, abducted, externally rotated, and extended (Figs. 10-77 and 10-78).
- The first letters of these words form the acronym *FABERE.*
- Pain in the hip during the maneuver, particularly on abduction and external rotation, is a positive sign of a coxa pathologic condition.

Confirmation Procedures

Gauvain's sign, Jansen's test, and diagnostic imaging

DIAGNOSTIC STATEMENT

Patrick's test is positive on the right and indicates a coxa pathologic condition.

CLINICAL PEARL

An intracapsular fracture, which can cause a positive Patrick's test, can cut off the blood supply to the femoral head completely, which can lead to aseptic necrosis, nonunion, or both. Because the fracture line is inside the capsule, blood is contained within it. This trapped blood raises the intracapsular pressure, damaging the femoral head still further, and prevents visible bruising because the blood cannot reach the subcutaneous tissues.

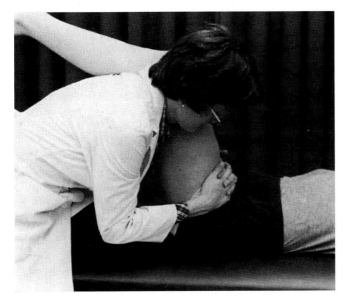

FIG. 10-75 "Perimeter scouring" of the hip. (*From Malone TR, McPoil TG, Nitz AJ:* Orthopedic and sports physical therapy, *ed 3, St Louis, 1997, Mosby.*)

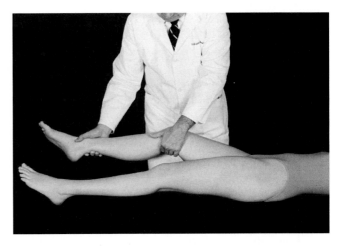

FIG. 10-76 The patient is lying supine on the examination table. The examiner grasps the affected leg.

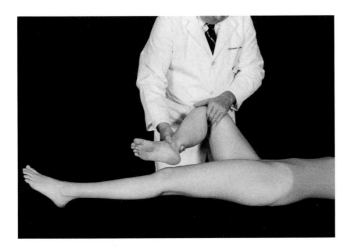

FIG. 10-77 The examiner flexes the hip, abducts the thigh, crosses the ankle over the contralateral knee, and externally rotates the hip.

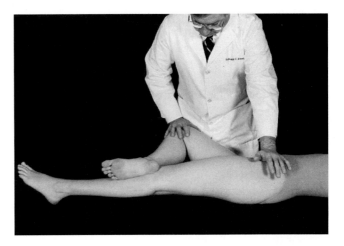

FIG. 10-78 The examiner then extends the hip by applying downward pressure on the knee. The contralateral side of the pelvis is fixed to the table and not allowed to rock upward. Pain during abduction and external rotation is a positive finding and indicates a coxa pathologic condition.

Assessment for Contracture of the Gracilis Muscle, Which Is Associated with a Pathologic Condition of the Hip Joint

Comment

Piriformis syndrome is a condition in which the piriformis muscle contributes to entrapment or irritation of the adjacent nerves. Numerous pain-sensitive structures course in the small interval created by the inferior margin of the piriformis and the superior gemellus muscle (Fig. 10-79). The clinical picture of piriformis syndrome includes a complaint of buttock pain, which often refers posteriorly to the ipsilateral thigh and occasionally to the calf. If a patient has an observable internal rotation of one or both lower limbs, excessive femoral anteversion may be present. There is also usually more range of motion in internal than in external rotation of the hip in these patients.

The presence of excessive femoral anteversion can be corroborated by Craig's test (Fig. 10-80). To perform this procedure, the examiner flexes the prone patient's knee to 90 degrees. The examiner then rotates the hip while palpating the greater trochanter. When the greater trochanter is felt to be in a mid position, such as parallel to the floor, the examiner then views the angle of the tibia relative to the long axis of the body. In a normal adult hip, it should be roughly perpendicular to the floor. Excessive anteversion is present if the tibia is pointing outward, away from the midline of the patient's body.

Most patients seeking help because of a hip-joint problem may do so because of pain, stiffness, a limp, or a deformity.

Pain of a hip-joint origin may be localized to the groin and from there may radiate down the medial or anterior aspect of the thigh. The pain also may arise in the region of the greater trochanter and radiate laterally along the course of the tensor fasciae latae toward the knee. Hip-joint pain may present posteriorly in the region of the ischial tuberosity and must be carefully differentiated from the complaint of sciatica. The pain often is referred to the lower back or knee and can be reproduced or accentuated by movements of the hip joint.

Subjective stiffness of the hip joint may be noted by the patient following periods of immobility, such as after prolonged sitting or upon arising from bed in the morning. In more advanced degenerative states affecting the hip joint, objective stiffness may be noted by the examiner. In degenerative arthritis of the hip joint, for example, the patient will lose hip-joint motion sequentially, with the ability to rotate the hip being lost first, followed by abduction and adduction loss, and finally hip flexion loss. For this reason, many patients with degenerative arthritis of the hip describe difficulty in putting a shoe or stocking on the affected leg because this action usually requires the ability to rotate the hip joint externally.

A limp is a pathologic asymmetric gait, and several mechanisms, singly or in combination, may be operating on the hip joint to produce it. Shortening of the lower extremity and marked stiffness of the hip joint may be sufficient to alter gait pattern. The limp may be protective because of weight-bearing pain. This type of abnormal gait, called an *antalgic gait,* is characterized by a very short stance phase. However, the gait most characteristic of hip-joint disease is called a *gluteal lurch,* and it relates directly to a structural or functional weakness of the gluteus medius on the affected side. Any abnormality of the pelvic-femoral lever arm may weaken the gluteus medius muscle. If this weakening occurs, the muscle can no longer support the pelvis and trunk on the lower extremity, and the patient's trunk lurches to the affected side during weight bearing.

Visible deformity of the lower extremity is often associated with injuries or disease affecting the hip joint. A patient with a fracture of the hip joint usually holds the lower extremity in marked external rotation. A patient who has sustained a traumatic dislocation of the hip joint usually holds the lower extremity in internal rotation. Degenerative arthritis of the hip joint is often associated with flexion-adduction-external rotation contractures. Flexion and adduction contractures about the hip, external rotation position of the lower extremity, shortening of the leg, and a limp are characteristic deformities that may be produced by hip joint disorders.

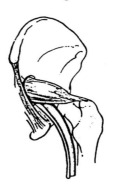

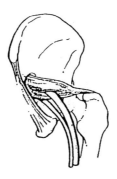

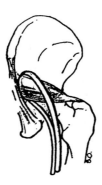

FIG. 10-79 Relationship of the sciatic nerve to the piriformis muscle. *(From Moore K:* Clinically oriented anatomy, *Baltimore, 1980, Williams & Wilkins.)*

PROCEDURE

- The patient is lying prone, the knees are extended, and the thighs are maximally abducted (Fig. 10-81).
- Pain and resistance should be used as criteria for maximum abduction.
- The patient's knees are flexed bilaterally to a right angle (Fig. 10-82).
- The examiner notes if the maneuver allows more hip abduction.
- The test is positive if knee flexion increases or knee extension decreases hip abduction.
- The test indicates contracture of the gracilis muscle.

Confirmation Procedures

Ober's test, Thomas test, and Trendelenburg's test

DIAGNOSTIC STATEMENT

Phelp's test is positive on the right or left. This result suggests contracture of the gracilis muscle, which is associated with a pathologic condition of the hip joint.

CLINICAL PEARL

Two nonspecific gait abnormalities commonly result from hip disease. The antalgic gait usually indicates a painful hip. The patient shortens the stance phase on the affected hip, leaning over the affected side, to prevent painful contraction of the hip abductors. Trendelenburg's gait, or abductor limp, indicates weakness of the abductors on the affected side. During the stance phase, on the affected side, the contralateral pelvis dips down, and the body leans to the unaffected side. If the condition is bilateral, this produces a waddling gait.

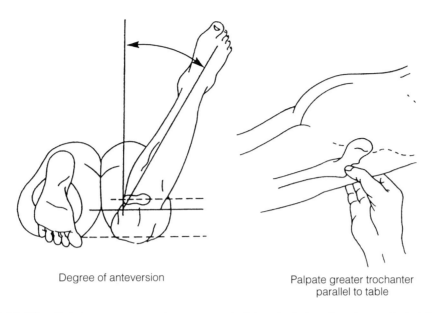

Degree of anteversion

Palpate greater trochanter
parallel to table

FIG. 10-80   Craig's test.   *(From Malone TR, McPoil TG, Nitz AJ:* Orthopedic and sports physical therapy, *ed 3, St Louis, 1997, Mosby.)*

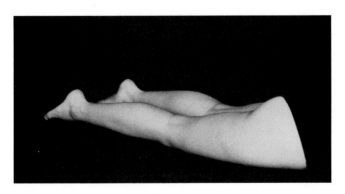

FIG. 10-81   The patient is lying prone with the knees extended. The thighs are maximally abducted as far as the patient can tolerate.

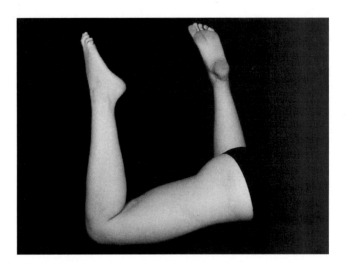

FIG. 10-82   The knees are flexed actively or passively to 90 degrees. If flexion of the knees allows more hip abduction, the test is positive. A positive test indicates gracilis muscle contracture.

THOMAS TEST

Assessment for Flexion Contracture Involving the Iliopsoas

Comment

The Thomas test is designed to evaluate the presence of a flexion contracture of the hip (Fig. 10-83).

Age and sex largely limit osteochondritis deformans juvenilis, or coxa plana. Legg (1910), Perthes (1910), and Calvé (1910) described the disease separately in the United States, Germany, and France. It is seen almost exclusively in children 3 to 12 years old, but the disease has been reported in children as young as 2 and in others as old as 18. More boys than girls are affected, by a ratio of 4:1. The disease is usually unilateral, and a familial history of the disease is present in 20% of the cases.

The most widely accepted cause for the disease is interruption of the blood supply to the head of the femur. This interrupted blood supply is thought to be produced by excessive fluid pressure of a synovial effusion in the hip joint. The head of the femur is at risk between the ages of 3 and 10 because, of the three blood supplies to the femoral head, only the lateral epiphyseal vessels are functional during this period. The blood supply to different segments of the head of the femur varies. For instance, the blood supply to the posterior segment is more generous than the supply to the anterior segment. The posterior portion of the head of the femur is often spared from this disease.

Subchondral fractures occur early in the disease, and these may be the initiating factor in a sequence of events that results in Legg-Calvé-Perthes disease.

Abnormal blood-clotting processes, caused by substances that create a state of hypercoagulability, are thought to result in formation of platelet aggregations and fibrin thrombi that could block the limited vascular supply to the head of the femur.

This process has a relationship with previous transient synovitis or other inflammatory processes because of the presence of thickened blood vessels and capsules.

During physical examination, pain can range from mild to severe and will be felt in the groin, thigh, and often the knee. This pain is associated with a limp or slightly abnormal gait. The gait is an antalgic one, in which the patient tries to protect the hip by rapidly shifting body weight off the foot of the involved side.

With a flexion contracture (positive Thomas test), motion—particularly abduction, internal rotation, extension, and flexion—at the hip is limited. A patient may experience muscle spasm of the adductor and psoas muscle and muscle wasting of the thigh and buttock. The anterior and posterior aspects of the hip joint may also be tender.

The erythrocyte sedimentation rate might be elevated, but the results of other laboratory investigations are normal.

PROCEDURE

- The patient lies supine, and the thigh is flexed with the knee bent upon the abdomen (Fig. 10-84).
- The patient's lumbar spine should normally flatten, or flex.
- If the spine maintains a lordosis, the test is positive and indicates hip flexion contracture, as from a shortened iliopsoas muscle (Fig. 10-85).

Confirmation Procedures

Ober's test, Phelp's test, and Trendelenburg's test

DIAGNOSTIC STATEMENT

Thomas test is positive on the left and indicates a flexion contracture involving the iliopsoas musculature.

CLINICAL PEARL

Restricted hip flexion may be compensated by an increase in lumbar lordosis. This increase masks the fixed flexion deformity. Fixed flexion, external rotation, and abduction accumulate sequentially as the hip disease progresses.

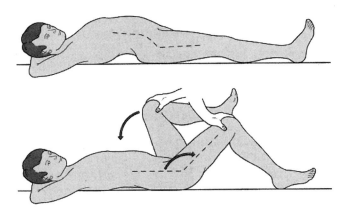

FIG. 10-83 The Thomas test. *(From Klippel JH, Dieppe PA: Rheumatology, vol 1-2, ed 2, London, 1998, Mosby.)*

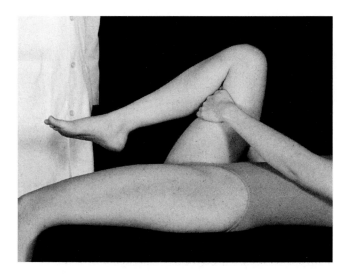

FIG. 10-84 The patient is lying supine on the examination table. The thigh of the unaffected leg is actively flexed toward the abdomen. The patient holds the leg in this position with both hands. The examiner observes the posture of the lower back and the affected leg. The lumbar spine should flatten, and the opposite leg should remain flat on the table.

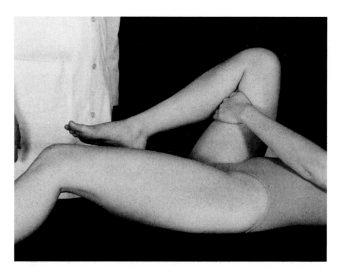

FIG. 10-85 If the lumbar spine maintains a lordosis, if the affected leg flexes, and if the patient is unable to lay the leg flat on the table, the test is positive. A positive test indicates a shortened iliopsoas muscle.

TRENDELENBURG'S TEST

Assessment for Insufficiency of the Hip Abductor System

Comment

The unilateral leg stand or Trendelenburg's test is a useful procedure for detecting hip joint dysfunction. A positive Trendelenburg's sign is identified when the patient is unable to maintain the pelvis horizontal to the floor while standing first on one foot and then on the other foot (Fig. 10-86).

Trendelenburg's test investigates stability of the hip and particularly the ability of the hip abductors (gluteus medius and gluteus minimus) to stabilize the pelvis on the femur.

Normally, when one leg is raised from the ground, the pelvis tilts upward on that side because of the action of the hip abductors of the supporting limb. This automatic mechanism allows the lifted leg to clear the ground while walking. If the abductors are inefficient, they are unable to sustain the pelvis against the body weight. The result is that the pelvis tilts downward instead of rising on the side of the lifted leg.

For instance, in a case of upward dislocation of the hip, there is an unstable fulcrum and also approximation of the origin of the abductor muscles to their insertion.

PROCEDURE

- The patient with a suspected hip involvement stands on one foot, on the side of the involvement, and raises the other foot and leg for thigh flexion and knee flexion.
- If the hip and its muscles are normal, the iliac crest will be low on the standing side and high on the side of the elevated leg (Fig. 10-87).
- If there is hip-joint involvement and muscle weakness, the iliac crest will be high on the standing side and low on the side of the elevated leg (Fig. 10-88).
- The test is commonly positive in a developing Legg-Calve-Perthes disease, poliomyelitis, muscular dystrophy, coxa vara, Otto's pelvis, epiphyseal separation, coxa ankylosis, dislocation, fracture, or subluxation.

Confirmation Procedures

Ober's test, Phelp's test, and Thomas test

DIAGNOSTIC STATEMENT

Trendelenburg's test is positive on the left. This result suggests insufficiency of the hip abductor system.

ORTHOPEDIC GAMUT 10-26

POSITIVE TRENDELENBURG'S TEST

The following are fundamental causes for a positive Trendelenburg's test:

1. Paralysis of the abductor muscles, which can occur with poliomyelitis
2. Marked approximation of the insertion of the muscles to their origin by upward displacement of the greater trochanter causing the muscles to be slack

(This slackening may occur in severe coxa vara or congenital dislocation of the hip.)
3. Absence of a stable fulcrum causes a positive test (This result occurs in the ununited fracture of the femoral neck.)
4. Sometimes, a combination of two of the aforementioned factors

---

CLINICAL PEARL

Trendelenburg's test is positive as a result of (1) gluteal paralysis or weakness (from polio), (2) gluteal inhibition (from pain arising in the hip joint), (3) gluteal insufficiency from coxa vara, or (4) congenital dislocation of the hip. Nevertheless, false-positive results have been recorded in approximately 10% of the patients with hip pain.

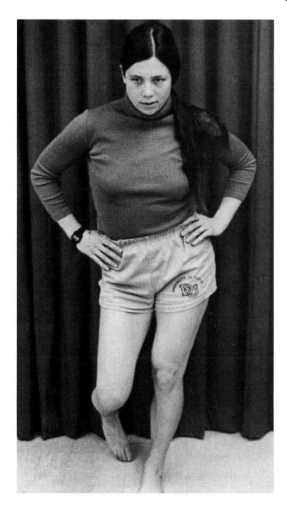

FIG. 10-86   A positive, uncompensated Trendelenburg's test indicates weakness of the left hip abductor mechanism. *(From Malone TR, McPoil TG, Nitz AJ:* Orthopedic and sports physical therapy, *ed 3, St Louis, 1997, Mosby.)*

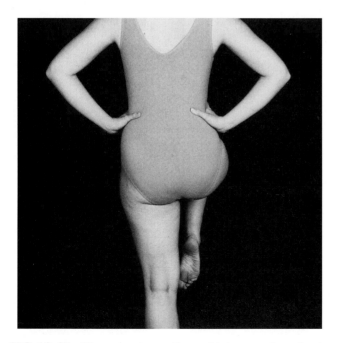

FIG. 10-87   The patient is standing and is instructed to raise the foot of the unaffected leg off the floor. If normal, the iliac crest may be low on the standing side and high on the side of the elevated leg.

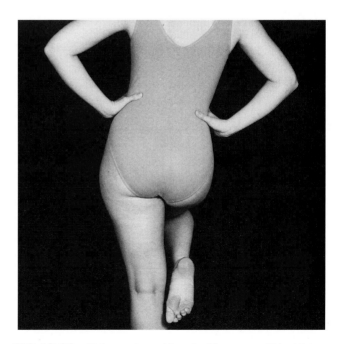

FIG. 10-88   If the test is positive, the iliac crest will be high on the standing side and low on the side of the elevated leg. A positive test indicates a coxa pathologic condition.

CRITICAL THINKING

Where is most of the pain in degenerative arthritis of the hip?
In the groin area, with possible radiation into the anterior portion of the thigh

What is the Thomas test?
The patient holds one leg to the abdomen and lowers the other leg until it is flat on the examination table. Failure of the hip to extend fully indicates a fixed flexion contracture.

What is Trendelenburg's test?
The patient stands on one leg. As the patient stands erect, the gluteus medius muscle on the supported side should contract to keep the pelvis level. If the pelvis remains unsupported and the opposite side drops, the gluteus medius muscle is either weak or nonfunctioning, and the test is positive.

List the three specific tests for hip abnormality in an infant.

1. The Galeazzi sign is a check for apparent thigh length. The Galeazzi sign indicates apparent shortening of one femur in comparison with the normal contralateral femur.
2. Barlow's test assesses the potential for dislocation of the hip.
3. The Ortolani maneuver usually is combined with Barlow's test. If abducting the hip with a little pressure over the trochanter produces a clunk that is felt rather than heard, the Ortolani test is positive.

What is slipped capital femoral epiphysis (SCFE)?
The femoral capital epiphysis of the hip displaces or "slips" on the femoral neck.

What is Legg-Calvé-Perthes (LCP) disease?
LCP disease is necrosis of the bony nucleus of the proximal femoral epiphysis and impairment of the growth of the physis, with subsequent remodeling of regenerated bone in the pediatric patient.

What is a hip dislocation?
Hip dislocation occurs when the femoral head is forcibly dislocated from the acetabulum.

What is the mechanism for an avulsion fracture?
A sudden, violent muscle contraction (eccentric or concentric) or an increased muscular stretch causes an avulsion fracture across an open epiphysis.

What is iliotibial band (ITB) syndrome?
Iliotibial band friction syndrome and iliotibial band tendinitis

When might slipped capital femoral epiphysis be present?
It should be considered when a young athlete (9 to 15 years old) presents with medial thigh pain, hip or knee pain, or a positive Trendelenburg's gait.

What are the causative factors of stress fractures of the femoral neck?
They occur secondary to repetitive microtrauma and often are seen in runners with persistent groin pain.

How can increased femoral anteversion cause problems in the lower extremity?
Excessive anteversion causes a "toe-in" gait. This leads to tight hip internal rotator muscles, internal rotation of the tibia, and flexion at the knee and hip, thus altering normal biomechanics.

How can the presence of femoral anteversion or retroversion be determined?
Craig's test will give an approximation of the degree of anteversion.

BIBLIOGRAPHY

Abrams WB, Berkow R: *The Merck manual of geriatrics,* Rahway, NJ, 1990, Merck Sharp & Dohme Research Laboratories.

Adams JA: Transient synovitis of the hip joint in children, *J Bone Joint Surg* 45B:471, 1963.

Adams JC: *Standard orthopaedic operations,* Edinburgh, 1985, Churchill Livingstone.

Adams JC, Hamblen DL: *Outline of orthopaedics,* ed 11, Edinburgh, 1990, Churchill Livingstone.

Adams RD: *Diseases of muscle,* ed 3, London, 1975, Henry Kimpton.

Alario AJ: *Practical guide to the care of the pediatric patient,* St Louis, 1997, Mosby.

Alexander CJ: The etiology of femoral epiphyseal slipping, *J Bone Joint Surg* 48B:299, 1966.

Allison D, Strickland N: *Acronyms & synonyms in medical imaging,* Oxford, 1996, ISIS Medical Media.

American Academy of Orthopaedic Surgeons: *Atlas of limb prosthetics,* St Louis, 1981, Mosby.

American Academy of Orthopaedic Surgeons: *Instructional course lectures,* vol 37, Chicago, 1988, AAOS.

American Medical Association: *Guides to the evaluation of permanent impairment,* ed 4, Chicago, 1993, American Medical Association.

American Medical Association: *How to use guides to the evaluation of permanent impairment,* ed 4, Falmouth, Conn, 1993, SEAK.

American Orthopaedic Association: *Manual of orthopaedic surgery,* Chicago, 1972, The Association.

Anderson GH, et al: Preoperative skin traction for fractures of the proximal femur, a randomized prospective trial, *J Bone Joint Surg* 75B:794, 1993.

Anderson KN, Anderson LE: *Mosby's pocket dictionary of medicine, nursing, & allied health,* ed 2, St Louis, 1994, Mosby.

Apley AG, Solomon L: *Concise system of orthopaedics and fractures,* London, 1988, Butterworth-Heinemann.

Aston JN: *A Short textbook of orthopaedics and traumatology,* Philadelphia, 1967, JB Lippincott.

Ballinger PW: *Merrill's atlas of radiographic positions and radiologic procedures,* vol 1-3, ed 8, St Louis, 1995, Mosby.

Barkauskas VH, et al: *Health & physical assessment,* ed 2, St Louis, 1998, Mosby.

Barlow TG: Congenital dislocation of the hip, *Hosp Med* 2:571, 1968.

Barnes R: Fracture of the neck of the femur, *J Bone Joint Surg* 49B:607, 1967.

Beattie P, et al: Validity of derived measurements of leg-length differences obtained by the use of a tape measure, *Phys Ther* 70:150, 1990.

Beeson PB, McDermott W: *Textbook of medicine,* ed 13, Philadelphia, 1971, WB Saunders.

Bennett JT, MacEwen GD: Congenital dislocation of the hip: recent advances and current problems, *Clin Orthop* 247:15, 1989.

Benson MKD, Evans DCJ: The pelvis osteotomy of Chiari, *J Bone Joint Surg* 58B:164, 1976.

Berkeley ME, et al: Surgical therapy for congenital dislocation of the hip in patients who are twelve to thirty-six months old, *J Bone Joint Surg* 66A:412, 1984.

Bierbaum BE, et al: Late complications of total hip replacement. In Steinberg ME, editor: *The hip and its disorders,* Philadelphia, 1991, WB Saunders.

Birch R: The place of microsurgery in orthopaedics. In: *Recent advances in orthopaedics,* ed 5, Edinburgh, 1987, Churchill Livingstone.

Blockey NJ: Derotation osteotomy in the management of congenital dislocation of the hip, *J Bone Joint Surg* 66B:485, 1984.

Bombelli R: *Osteoarthritis of the hip: pathogenesis and consequent therapy,* New York, 1976, Springer-Verlag.

Bonalaski JS, Schumacher HR: Arthritis and allied conditions. In Steinberg M, editor: *The hip and its disorders,* Philadelphia, 1991, WB Saunders.

Bowen JR, Foster BK, Hartzell C: Legg-Calve-Perthes disease, *Clin Orthop* 185:97, 1984.

Bradley GW, et al: Resurfacing arthroplasty: femoral head viability, *Clin Orthop* 220:137, 1987.

Brashear HR, Raney RB: *Shands' handbook of orthopaedic surgery,* St Louis, 1978, Mosby.

Bringnall CG, Stainsby GD: The snapping hip: treatment by Z-plasty, *J Bone Joint Surg* 73B:253, 1991.

Brooks M, Evans R, Fairclough J: *Sports injuries,* ed 2, London, 1992, Gower Medical.

Brotzman SB: *Clinical orthopaedic rehabilitation,* St Louis, 1996, Mosby.

Brown DE, Neumann RD: *Orthopedic secrets,* Philadelphia, 1995, Hanley & Belfus.

Bucholz RW: *Orthopaedic decision making,* ed 2, St Louis, 1996, Mosby.

Burnett W: *Clinical science for surgeons,* London, 1981, Butterworth.

Burwell RG, Harrison HM, editors: Perthes disease (symposium), *Clin Orthop* 209:2, 1986.

Butler WT, et al: Diagnostic and prognostic value of clinical and laboratory findings in cryptococcal meningitis, *N Engl J Med* 270:59, 1964.

Caffey J: The early roentgenographic changes in essential coxa plana, their significance in pathogenesis, *Am J Roentgenol* 103:620, 1968.

Callaghan JJ: The clinical results and basic science of total hip arthroplasty with porous coated prosthesis, *J Bone Joint Surg* 75A:299, 1993.

Cameron HU: *The technique of total hip arthroplasty,* St Louis, 1992, Mosby.

Camp WA: Sarcoidosis of the central nervous system: a case with postmortem studies, *Arch Neurol* 7:432, 1962.

Campbell JB, Campbell JM: *Mosby's survival guide to medical abbreviations & acronyms prefixes & suffixes symbols Greek alphabet,* St Louis, 1995, Mosby.

Campbell WC: *Operative orthopaedics,* ed 7, London, 1981, Henry Kimpton.

Campion GV, Dixon A: *Rheumatology,* Oxford, 1989, Blackwell.

Canale ST: *Campbell's operative orthopaedics,* vol 1-4, ed 9, St Louis, 1998, Mosby.

Carney BT, Weinstein SL, Nuhe J: Long term follow up of slipped capital femoral epiphysis, *J Bone Joint Surg* 73A:667, 1991.

Carter CO, Wilkinson JA: Genetic and environmental factors in the etiology of congenital dislocation of the hip, *Clin Orthop* 33:119, 1964.

Catterall A: The natural history of Perthes disease (symposium), *J Bone Joint Surg* 53B:37, 1971.

Catterall A: *Recent advances in orthopaedics,* ed 5, Edinburgh, 1987, Churchill Livingstone.

Catterall M: Perthes disease. In Steinberg ME, editor: *The hip and its disorders,* Philadelphia, 1991, WB Saunders.

Chao EY, et al: Biomechanics of malalignment, *Orthop Clin North Am* 25:379, 1994.

Chapman S, Nakielmy R: *Aids to radiological differential diagnosis,* ed 3, London, 1995, Bailliere Tindall.

Charnley J: Total hip replacement by low-friction arthroplasty, *Clin Orthop* 72:7, 1970.

Chibnall JT, Tait R: The pain disability index: factor structure and normative data, *Arch Phys Med Rehabil* 75:1082, 1994.

Cipriano JJ: *Photographic manual of regional orthopaedic and neurological test,* ed 3, Baltimore, 1997, Williams & Wilkins.

Clarke NMP, Clegg J, Al-Chalabi AN: Ultrasound screening of hips at risk for congenital dislocation, *J Bone Joint Surg* 71B:9, 1989.

Coates CJ, Paterson JM, Woods KR: Femoral osteotomy in Perthes disease: results at maturity, *J Bone Joint Surg* 72B:581, 1990.

Cohn RE: *Impairment rating examination and disability evaluation,* ed 3, Wilkesboro, NC, 1994, R Ernest Cohn.

Collins DN, Nelson CL: Infections of the hip. In Steinberg M, editor: *The hip and its disorders,* Philadelphia, 1991, WB Saunders.

Collo MC, et al: Evaluating arthritic complaints, *Nurse Pract* 16:9, 1991.

Colosimo AJ, Ireland ML: Thigh compartment syndrome in a football athlete: a case report and review of the literature, *Med Sci Sports Exerc* 24:958, 1992.

Cooper DE, Warren RF, Barnes R: Traumatic subluxation of the hip resulting in aseptic necrosis and chondrolysis in a professional football player, *Am J Sports Med* 19:322, 1991.

Copperman DR, Stulberg SD: Ambulatory containment treatment in Perthes disease, *Clin Orthop* 203:289, 1986.

Cormack, DH: *Essential histology,* Philadelphia, 1993, Lippincott.

Craik RL, Oatis CA: *Gait analysis theory and application,* St Louis, 1995, Mosby.

Crenshaw AH editor: *Campbell's operative orthopaedics,* vol 3, ed 8, St Louis, 1992, Mosby.

Cruess RL, Rennie W: *Adult orthopaedics,* New York, 1987, Churchill Livingstone.

Currey HLF: *Essentials of rheumatology,* ed 2, Edinburgh, 1988, Churchill Livingstone.

Cyriax JH: *Textbook of orthopaedic medicine,* ed 8, London, 1983, Bailliere, Tindall.

Daffner RH: *Clinical radiology: the essentials,* Baltimore, 1993, Williams & Wilkins.

Dalinka MK, Neustadter LM: Radiology of the hip. In Steinberg ME, editor: *The hip and its disorders,* Philadelphia, 1991, WB Saunders.

Dambro MR, Griffith JA: *Griffith's 5 minute clinical consult,* Baltimore, 1997, Williams & Wilkins.

D'Ambrogio KJ, Roth GB: *Positional release therapy assessment & treatment of musculoskeletal dysfunction,* St Louis, 1997, Mosby.

D'Ambrosia RD: *Musculoskeletal disorders: regional examination and differential diagnosis,* Philadelphia, 1977, JB Lippincott.

Dandy DJ: *Essential orthopaedics and trauma,* Edinburgh, 1989, Churchill Livingstone.

Deltoff MN, Kogon PL: *The portable skeletal x-ray library,* St Louis, 1998, Mosby.

Demeter SL, Andersson GBJ, Smith GM: *Disability evaluation,* St Louis, 1996, Mosby.

DeRosa GP, Feller N: Treatment of congenital dislocation of the hip, management before walking age, *Clin Orthop* 225:77, 1987.

Deshpande JK, Tobias JD: *The pediatric pain handbook,* St Louis, 1996, Mosby.

Dettenmeier PA: *Radiographic assessment for nurses,* St Louis, 1995, Mosby.

Dickinson WH, Duwelius PJ, Colville MR: Muscle strength following surgery for acetabular fractures, *J Orthop Trauma* 7:39, 1993.

Dixon AS, et al: A double-blind controlled trial of Rumalon in the treatment of painful osteoarthrosis of the hip, *Ann Rheum Dis* 29:193, 1970.

Dobbs HS: Survivorship of total hip replacements, *J Bone Joint Surg* 62B:168, 1980.

Dodge PR, Swartz MN: Bacterial meningitis: special neurologic problems, postmeningitic complications and clinicopathologic correlations, *N Engl J Med* 272:954, 1965.

Doherty M: *Color atlas and text of osteoarthritis,* London, 1994, Wolfe.

Doherty M, Doherty J: *Clinical examination in rheumatology,* London, 1992, Wolfe.

Doherty M, George E: *Self-assessment picture tests in rheumatology,* London, 1995, Mosby-Wolfe.

Duthie RB, Bentley G, editor: *Mercer's orthopaedic surgery,* ed 8, London, 1983, Edward Arnold.

Dutkowski JP: Nontraumatic bone and joint disorders. In Crenshaw AH, editor: *Campbell's operative orthopaedics,* ed 8, vol 3, St Louis, 1992, Mosby.

Eastcott HHG: *Arterial surgery,* ed 2, London, 1973, Pitman.

Echternach J, editor: *Clinics in physical therapy of the hip,* New York, 1990, Churchill Livingstone.

Eftekhar NS, editor: Low friction arthroplasty, *Clin Orthop* 211:2, 1986.

Egund N, Wingstrand H: Legg-Calve-Perthes disease: imaging with MR, *Radiology* 179:89, 1991.

Elster AD: *Questions and answers in magnetic resonance imaging,* St Louis, 1994, Mosby.

Engesaeter LB, et al: Ultrasound and congenital dislocation of the hip, *J Bone Joint Surg* 72B:202, 1990.

Epstein O, et al: *Clinical examination,* ed 2, London, 1997, Mosby.

Esterhai JL, et al: Adult septic arthritis, *Orthop Clin North Am* 22:503, 1991.

Eyre-Brook A: Septic arthritis of the hip and osteomyelitis of upper end of the femur in infants, *J Bone Joint Surg* 42B:11, 1960.

Eyre-Brook AL, Jones DA, Harris FC: Pemberton's acetabuloplasty for congenital dislocation of subluxation of the hip, *J Bone Joint Surg* 60B:18, 1978.

Farrar WE: *Atlas of infections of the nervous system,* London, 1993, Wolfe.

Feldmann E: *Current diagnosis in neurology,* St Louis, 1994, Mosby.

Ferezy JS: *The chiropractic neurological examination,* Gaithersburg, Md, 1992, Aspen.

Ferguson AB Jr: The pathology of degenerative arthritis of the hip and the use of osteotomy in its treatment, *Clin Orthop* 77:118, 1971.

Fisk JW, Balgent ML: Clinical and radiological assessment of leg length, *NZ Med J* 81:477, 1975.

Foldes K, et al: Nocturnal pain correlates with effusions in diseased hips, *J Rheumatol* 19:1756, 1992.

Fornage B: *Musculoskeletal ultrasound,* New York, 1995, Churchill Livingstone.

Fricker PA, Taunton JE, Ammann W: Osteitis pubis in athletes; infection, inflammation, or injury, *Sports Med* 12:266, 1991.

Frost A, Bauer M: Skier's hip: a new clinical entity? proximal femur fractures sustained in cross-country skiing, *J Orthop Trauma* 5:47, 1991.

Frymoyer J, editor: *Orthopedic knowledge update No. 4,* Rosemont, Ill, 1993, American Academy of Orthopedic Surgery.

Fuss FK, Bacher A: New aspects of the morphology and function of the human hip joint ligaments, *Am J Anat* 192:1, 1991.

Gage JR, Winter RB: Avascular necrosis of the capital femoral epiphysis as a complication of closed reduction of congenital dislocation of the hip, *J Bone Joint Surg* 54A:373, 1972.

Galasko CSB, editor: *Neuromuscular problems in orthopaedics,* Oxford, 1987, Blackwell.

Galasko CSB, Nobel J, editors: *Current trends in orthopaedic surgery,* Manchester, UK, 1988, Manchester University Press.

Galpin RD, et al: One-stage treatment of congenital dislocation of the hip in older children, *J Bone Joint Surg* 71A:734, 1989.

Garcia JH: *Neuropathology the diagnostic approach,* St Louis, 1997, Mosby.

Garrick J, Webb DR: Pelvis, hip, thigh injuries. In Garrick J, Webb DR, editors: *Sports injuries: diagnosis and management,* Philadelphia, 1990, WB Saunders.

Gartland JJ: *Fundamentals of orthopaedics,* ed 2, Philadelphia, 1974, WB Saunders.

Gartland JJ: Orthopaedic clinical research, *J Bone Joint Surg* 70A:1357, 1988.

Gerard JA, Kleinfield SL: *Orthopaedic testing,* New York, 1993, Churchill Livingstone.

Gillis L: *Diagnostic in orthopaedics,* London, 1969, Butterworth.

Giuliani G, et al: CT scan and surgical treatment of traumatic iliacus hematoma with femoral neuropathy: case report, *J Trauma* 30:229, 1990.

Glick JM: Hip arthroscopy. In Mcginty JB, et al, editors: *Operative arthroscopy,* New York, 1991, Raven.

Goldie BS: *Orthopaedic diagnosis and management a guide to the care of orthopaedic patients,* ed 2, Oxford, 1998, ISIS Medical Media.

Goldman GA, et al: Idiopathic transient osteoporosis of the hip in pregnancy, *Int J Gynaecol Obstet* 46:317, 1994.

Goldstein TS: Treatment of common problems of the hip joint. In Goldstein TS, Lewis CB, series editors: *Geriatric orthopaedics rehabilitative management of common problems,* Gaithersburg, Md, 1991, Aspen.

Goodman CG, Snyder TE: Systemic origins of musculoskeletal pain: associated signs and symptoms. In *Differential diagnosis in physical therapy,* Philadelphia, 1990, WB Saunders.

Gordon M: *Nursing diagnosis: process and application,* ed 3, St Louis, 1994, Mosby.

Graham S, et al: The Chiari osteotomy, *Clin Orthop* 208:249, 1986.

Grauer JD, et al: Resection arthroplasty of the hip, *J Bone Joint Surg* 71A:669, 1989.

Greenspan A: *Orthopedic radiology,* ed 2, Philadelphia, 1992, JB Lippincott.

Greenstein GM: *Clinical assessment of neuromusculoskeletal disorders,* St Louis, 1997, Mosby.

Greenwald AS: Biomechanics of the hip. In Steinberg ME, editor: *The hip and its disorders,* Philadelphia, 1991, WB Saunders.

Gross ML, Nasser S, Finnerman GAM: Hip and pelvis. In DeLee JC, Drez D, editors: *Orthopaedic sports medicine: principles and practice,* vol 2, Philadelphia, 1994, WB Saunders.

Grossman ZD, et al: *Cost-effective diagnostic imaging the clinician's guide,* ed 3, St Louis, 1995, Mosby.

Gruebel-Lee DM: *Disorders of the hip,* Philadelphia, 1983, JB Lippincott.

Hadlow V: Neonatal screening for congenital dislocation of hip, *J Bone Joint Surg* 70B:740, 1988.

Hall AJ: Perthes disease: progression in aetiological research. In Catterall P, editor: *Recent advances in orthopaedics,* ed 5, Edinburgh, 1987, Churchill Livingstone.

Halland AM, et al: Avascular necrosis of the hip in systemic lupus erythematosus: the role of magnetic resonance imaging, *Br J Rheumatol* 32:972, 1993.

Hammer WI: *Functional soft tissue examination and treatment by manual methods the extremities,* Gaithersburg, Md, 1991, Aspen.

Hansson G: Congenital dislocation of the hip joint: problems in diagnosis and treatment, *Curr Orthop* 2:104, 1988.

Hansson G, et al: Radiographic assessment of coxarthrosis following slipped capital femoral epiphysis, *Acta Radiol* 34:117, 1993.

Hardinge K: The etiology of transient synovitis of the hip in childhood, *J Bone Joint Surg* 52B:100, 1970.

Harris CM, Baum J: Involvement of the hip in juvenile rheumatoid arthritis, *J Bone Joint Surg* 70A:821, 1988.

Harris WH: Etiology of osteoarthritis of the hip, *Clin Orthop* 213:20, 1986.

Hartley A: *Practical joint assessment lower quadrant,* ed 2, St Louis, 1995, Mosby.

Harty M: Hip anatomy. In Steinberg ME, editor: *The hip and its disorders,* Philadelphia, 1991, WB Saunders.

Hawkins RJ: *An organized approach to musculoskeletal examination and history taking,* St Louis, 1995, Mosby.

Heikkila E, Ryoppy S, Louchimo I: The management of primary acetabular dysplasia, *J Bone Joint Surg* 67B:25, 1985.

Heinmann WG, Freiberger RH: Avascular necrosis of the femoral and humeral heads after high-dosage corticosteroid therapy, *N Engl J Med* 263:627, 1960.

Henderson RS: Osteotomy for unreduced congenital dislocation of the hip in adults, *J Bone Joint Surg* 52B:468, 1970.

Hernandez RS, Cornell RG, Hensinger RN: Ultrasound diagnosis of neonatal congenital dislocation of the hip, *J Bone Joint Surg* 76A:539, 1994.

Hernigou P, et al: Deformities of the hip in adults who have sickle-cell disease and had avascular necrosis in childhood, *J Bone Joint Surg* 73:91, 1991.

Hertling D, Kessler R: *Management of common musculoskeletal disorders,* ed 2, Philadelphia, 1990, JB Lippincott.

Hiehle JF, Kneeland JB, Dalinka MK: Magnetic resonance imaging of the hip with emphasis on avascular necrosis, *Rheum Dis Clin North Am* 17:669, 1991.

Hinkle CZ: *Fundamentals of anatomy & movement: a workbook and guide,* St Louis, 1997, Mosby.

Hirsch C, Frankel VH: Analysis of forces producing fractures of the proximal end of the femur, *J Bone Joint Surg* 42B:633, 1960.

Hornberger JP: *Exercise physiology therapeutic exercise,* Sarasota, Fla, 1991, Joseph P Hornberger.

Hughes S, Benson MKD, Colton CL: *The principles and practice of musculoskeletal surgery,* Edinburgh, 1987, Churchill Livingstone.

Hughes SS, et al: Extrapelvic compression of the sciatic nerve, *J Bone Joint Surg* 74A:1533, 1992.

Inerot S, et al: Proteoglycan alterations during developing experimental osteoarthritis in a novel hip joint model, *J Orthop Res* 9:658, 1991.

Jablonski S: *Dictionary of medical acronyms & abbreviations,* ed 3, Philadelphia, 1998, Hanley & Belfus.

Jacobson T, Allen W: Surgical connection of the snapping iliopsoas tendon, *Am J Sports Med* 18:470, 1990.

Jehl J, Crummy P: *Essentials of radiologic surgery,* ed 6, Philadelphia, 1993, JB Lippincott.

Jette AM: Using health-related quality of life measures in physical therapy outcomes research, *Phys Ther* 73:528, 1993.

Johnson KE: *Histology and cell biology,* ed 2, Baltimore, 1991, Williams & Wilkins.

Jones DA: Irritable hip and campylobacter infection, *J Bone Joint Surg* 71B:227, 1989.

Jones JP Jr, Engelman EP: Osseous avascular necrosis associated with systemic abnormalities, *Arthritis Rheum* 5:728, 1966.

Jones M: Clinical reasoning in manual therapy, *Phys Ther* 72:875, 1992.

Junqueira LC, Carneiro J, Kelly RO: *Basic histology,* ed 7, Norwalk, Conn, 1992, Appleton & Lange.

Kampa K: Mortality of hip fracture patients within one year of fracture, an overview, *Geritopics* 14:10, 1991.

Kanner R: *Pain management secrets,* Philadelphia, 1997, Hanley & Belfus.

Katirji B: *Electromyography in clinical practice: a case study approach,* St Louis, 1998, Mosby.

Katirji MB, Wilbourn AJ: High sciatic lesions mimicking peroneal neuropathy at the fibular head, *J Neurosci* 121:172, 1994.

Katz WA: *Rheumatic diseases diagnosis and management,* Philadelphia, 1977, JB Lippincott.

Keats TE: *Atlas of roentgenographic measurement,* ed 6, St Louis, 1990, Mosby.

Keats TE: *Atlas of normal roentgen variants,* ed 6, St Louis, 1996, Mosby.

Kendell RP, McCreary EK, Provance PG: *Muscles: testing and function,* ed 4, Baltimore, 1993, Williams & Wilkins.

Keret D, et al: Coxa plana: the fate of the physis, *J Bone Joint Surg* 66A:870, 1984.

Kessler RM, Hertling D: The hip. In Hertling D, Kessler RM, editors: *Management of common musculoskeletal disorders,* ed 2, Philadelphia, 1990, Lippincott.

Klippel JH, Dieppe PA: *Rheumatology,* vol 1-2, ed 2, London, 1998, Mosby.

Koenigsberg R: *Churchill's illustrated medical dictionary,* New York, 1989, Churchill Livingstone.

Koval KJ, Zuckerman JD: Functional recovery after fracture of the hip, current concepts review, *J Bone Joint Surg* 76A:751, 1994.

Lafforguw P, et al: Early-stage avascular necrosis of the femoral head: MR imaging for prognosis in 31 cases with at least 2 years of follow-up, *Radiology* 187:199, 1993.

Latke PA: Soft tissue afflictions. In Steinberg ME, editor: *The hip and its disorders,* Philadelphia, 1992, WB Saunders.

Lavy CBD, Barrett DS: *Questions and answers on Apley's concise system of orthopaedics and fractures,* Oxford, 1991, Butterworth-Heinemann

Lawrence JS: Generalized osteoarthrosis in a popular sample, *Am J Epidemiol* 90:381, 1969.

Lennox IA, McLauchlan J, Murali R: Failures of screening and management of congenital dislocation of the hip, *J Bone Joint Surg* 75B:72, 1993.

Lerner AJ: *The little black book of neurology,* ed 3, St Louis, 1995, Mosby.

Les RD, Gerhardt JJ:Range-of-motion measurements, *J Bone Joint Surg* 77A:784, 1995.

Letourmeau L, Dessureault M, Carette S: Rheumatoid iliopsoas bursitis presenting as unilateral femoral nerve palsy, *J Rheumatol* 18:462, 1991.

LeVeau B: Hip. In Richardson JK, Iglarsh JK, editors: *Clinical orthopaedic physical therapy,* Philadelphia, 1994, WB Saunders.

Lewis CB, Bottomley JM: Orthopaedic treatment considerations. In Lewis CB, Bottomley JM, editors: *Geriatric physical therapy: a clinical approach,* New York, 1994, Appleton & Lange.

Lewis CB, Knortz KA: *Orthopedic assessment and treatment of the geriatric patient,* St Louis, 1993, Mosby.

Lloyd-Roberts GG: Suppurative arthritis in infancy, *J Bone Joint Surg* 42B:706, 1960.

Lorber J: Long-term follow-up of 100 children who recovered from tuberculous meningitis, *Pediatrics* 28:778, 1961.

Loth TS: *Orthopedic boards review,* St Louis, 1993, Mosby.

Loth TS: *Orthopedic boards review II: a case study approach,* St Louis, 1996, Mosby.

Love BRT, Stevens PM, William PF: A long-term review of shelf arthroplasty, *J Bone Joint Surg* 62B:321, 1980.

Lynch AF: Tuberculosis of the greater trochanter, *J Bone Joint Surg* 64B:185, 1982.

MacAusland WR Jr, Mayo RA: *Orthopedics: a concise guide to clinical practices,* Boston, 1965, Little, Brown.

MacEwen GD: Treatment of congenital dislocation of the hip in older children, *Clin Orthop* 225:86, 1987.

Magee DJ: *Orthopedic physical assessment,* ed 3, Philadelphia, 1997, WB Saunders.

Malone TR, McPoil TG, Nitz AJ: *Orthopedic and sports physical therapy,* ed 3, St Louis, 1997, Mosby.

Marchiori DM: *Clinical imaging with skeletal, chest, and abdomen pattern differentials,* St Louis, 1999, Mosby.

Martin JH: *Neuroanatomy text and atlas,* ed 2, Stamford, Conn, 1996, Appleton & Lange.

Mathers LH, et al: *Clinical anatomy principles,* St Louis, 1996, Mosby.

Maxted MJ, Jackson RK: Innominate osteotomy in Perthe's disease, *J Bone Joint Surg* 67B:399, 1985.

Mazion JM: *Illustrated manual of neurological reflexes/signs/tests, part I, orthopedic signs/tests/maneuvers for office procedure, part II,* Orlando, 1980, Daniels Publishing.

McAndrew MP, Weinstein SL: A long-term follow-up of Legg-Calve-Perthes disease, *J Bone Joint Surg* 66A:860, 1984.

McCarthy GM, McCarthy DJ: Intrasynovial corticosteroid therapy, *Bull Rheum Dis* 43:2, 1994.

McCarty DJ, Koopman WJ, editors: *Arthritis and allied conditions,* ed 12, Philadelphia, 1993, Lea & Febiger.

McDonald D, et al: Total joint reconstruction. In: *Orthopedic boards review,* St Louis, 1993, Mosby.

McGann WA: History and physical examination. In Steinberg ME, editor: *The hip and its disorders,* Philadelphia, 1991, WB Saunders.

McKee GK: Development of total prosthetic replacement of the hip, *Clin Orthop* 72:85, 1970.

McKibbin B: Anatomical factors in the stability of the hip joint in the newborn, *J Bone Joint Surg* 52B:148, 1970.

McKibbin B, editor: *Recent advances in orthopaedics,* ed 4, Edinburgh, 1983, Churchill Livingstone.

McRae R: *Clinical orthopaedic examination,* ed 3, Edinburgh, 1990, Churchill Livingstone.

McRae R: *Practical fracture treatment,* ed 3, New York, 1994, Churchill-Livingstone.

Medical Economics Books: *Patient care flow chart manual,* ed 3, Oradell, NJ, 1982, Medical Economics Books.

Mellion MB: *Sports medicine secrets,* Philadelphia, 1994, Hanley & Belfus.

Mellion MB: *Office sports medicine,* ed 2, St Louis, 1996, Mosby.

Mendez AA, Eyster RL: Displaced nonunion stress fracture of the femoral neck treated with internal fixation and bone graft, *Am J Sports Med* 20:230, 1992.

Menelaus MB: Lessons learned in the management of Legg-Calve-Perthes disease, *Clin Orthop* 209:41, 1986.

Mengel MB, Schwiebert LP: *Ambulatory medicine: the primary care of families,* ed 2, Stamford, Conn, 1996, Appleton & Lange.

Mennell JM: *The musculoskeletal system: differential diagnosis from symptoms and physical signs,* Gaithersburg, Md, 1992, Aspen.

Mercier LR, Pettid FJ: *Practical orthopedics,* ed 4, St Louis, 1995, Mosby.

Meyer HM Jr, et al: Central nervous system syndromes of viral etiology: a study of 713 cases, *Am J Med* 29:334, 1960.

Milgram JW, et al: Resection arthroplasty for septic arthritis of the hip in ambulatory and nonambulatory adult patients, *Clin Orthop* 272:181, 1991.

Miller M: Adult reconstruction and sports medicine. In Miller M, editor: *Review of orthopaedics,* Philadelphia, 1992, WB Saunders.

Modic MT, Masaryk TJ, Ross JS: *Magnetic resonance imaging of the spine,* ed 2, St Louis, 1994, Mosby.

Moll JMH: *Manual of rheumatology,* Edinburgh, 1987, Churchill Livingstone.

Moore FH: Examination of infant's hips: can it do harm? *J Bone Joint Surg* 71B:4, 1989.

Moore FJ, et al: The relationship between head-neck-shaft angle, calcar width, articular cartilage and bone volume in arthrosis of the hip, *Br J Rheumatol* 35:432, 1994.

Moore KL: *Clinically oriented anatomy,* ed 3, Baltimore, 1992, Williams & Wilkins.

Mosby-Year Book, Inc: *Expert 10-minute physical examination,* St Louis, 1997, Mosby.

Mourad LA: *Orthopedic disorders,* St Louis, 1991, Mosby.

Muirhead-Allwood W, Catterall A: The treatment of Perthes disease, *J Bone Joint Surg* 64B:282, 1982.

Nettina SM: *The Lippincott manual of nursing practice,* ed 6, Philadelphia, 1996, Lippincott.

Neumann DA, Hase AD: The electromyographic analysis of the hip abductors during load carriage: implications for hip joint protection, *J Orthop Sports Phys Ther* 19:296, 1994.

Neumann DA, et al: An electromyographic analysis of hip abductor muscle activity when subjects are carrying loads in one or both hands, *Phys Ther* 72:207, 1992.

Newton RW: *Color atlas of pediatric neurology,* St Louis, 1995, Mosby-Wolfe.

Nicholas JA, Hershman EB: *The lower extremity & spine in sports medicine,* vol 1-2, ed 2, St Louis, 1995, Mosby.

Noble HB, Hajek MR, Porter M: Diagnosis and treatment of iliotibial band tightness in runners, *Sports Med* 10:67, 1982.

Nobel J, Galasko CSB: *Recent developments in orthopaedic surgery,* Manchester, UK, 1987, Manchester University Press.

Nordin M, Andersson GBJ, Pope MH: *Musculoskeletal disorders in the workplace: principles and practice,* St Louis, 1997, Mosby.

Noriyasu S, et al: On the morphology and frequency of Weitbrecht's retinacula in the hip joint, *Okajimas Folia Anat Jpn* 70:87, 1993.

Nunn D: The ring uncemented plastic-on-metal total hip replacement, *J Bone Joint Surg* 70B:40, 1988.

Ober FB: The role of the iliotibial and fascia lata as a factor in the causation of low-back disabilities and sciatic, *J Bone Joint Surg* 18:105, 1936.

O'Donoghue DH: *Treatment of injuries to athletes,* ed 3, Philadelphia, 1976, WB Saunders.

Olson WH, et al: *Handbook of symptom-oriented neurology,* ed 2, St Louis, 1994, Mosby.

Omer GE, Spinner M: *Management of peripheral nerve problems,* Philadelphia, 1980, WB Saunders.

Owen R, Goodfellow J, Bullough P, editors: *Scientific foundations of orthopaedics and traumatology,* London, 1980, Heinemann.

O'Young B, Young MA, Stiens SA: *PM&R secrets,* Philadelphia, 1997, Hanley & Belfus.

Pagana KD, Pagana TJ: *Mosby's manual of diagnostic and laboratory tests,* St Louis, 1998, Mosby.

Parker MJ, Pryor GA: *Hip fracture management,* Boston, 1993, Blackwell.

Paterson D, Salvage JP: The nuclide bone scan in the diagnosis of Perthes disease, *Clin Orthop* 209:23, 1986.

Patten J: *Neurological differential diagnosis,* ed 2, London, 1996, Springer.

Patterson RJ, Bickel WH, Dahlin DC: Idiopathic avascular necrosis of the head of the femur: a study of fifty-two cases, *J Bone Joint Surg* 42A:267, 1964.

Persselin JE: Diagnosis of rheumatoid arthritis, medial and laboratory aspects, *Clin Orthop* 265:73, 1991.

Polley HF, Hunder GG: *Rheumatologic interviewing and physical examination of the joints,* Philadelphia, 1978, WB Saunders.

Post M: *Physical examination of the musculoskeletal system,* Chicago, 1987, Mosby.

Poul J, et al: Early diagnosis of congenital dislocation of the hip, *J Bone Joint Surg* 53B:56, 1971.

Pratt NE: *Clinical musculoskeletal anatomy,* Philadelphia, 1991, JB Lippincott.

Radin EL: The physiology and degeneration of joints, *Arthritis Rheum* 2:245, 1972.

Ranawat CS: Surgery for rheumatoid arthritis: the hip, *Curr Orthop* 3:146, 1989.

Ranawat CS, Figgie MP: Early complications of total hip replacement. In Steinberg ME, editor: *The hip and its disorders,* Philadelphia, 1991, WB Saunders.

Rang M, editor: *The growth plate and its disorders,* Edinburgh, 1969, Livingstone.

Rao JP, Bronstein R: Dislocation following arthroplasties of the hip: incidence, prevention and treatment, *Orthop Rev* 20:261, 1991.

Ratliff AHC: Perthes disease: a study of thirty-four hips observed for thirty years, *J Bone Joint Surg* 49B:102, 1967.

Ravel R: *Clinical laboratory medicine: clinical application of laboratory data,* ed 6, St Louis, 1995, Mosby.

Reid DC: *Problems of the hip, pelvis, and sacroiliac joint, sports injury assessment and rehabilitation,* New York, 1992, Churchill Livingstone.

Reid DC: *Sports injury assessment and rehabilitation,* New York, 1992, Churchill Livingstone.

Reikeras O: Is there a relationship between femoral anteversion and leg torsion? *Skeletal Radiol* 10:409, 1991.

Renne JW: The iliotibial band friction syndrome, *J Bone Joint Surg* 57A:1110, 1975.

Renshaw TS: *Pediatric orthopaedics,* Philadelphia, 1987, Saunders.

Resnick D, Niwayama G: *Diagnosis of bone and joint disorders,* Philadelphia, 1995, WB Saunders.

Rhodes I, Matzinger F, Matzinger MA: Transient osteoporosis of the hip, *Can Assoc Radiol J* 44:399, 1993.

Ring PA: Complete replacement arthroplasty of the hip by the ring prosthesis, *J Bone Joint Surg* 50B:720, 1968.

Rizzo PF, et al: Diagnosis of occult fractures about the hip, magnetic resonance imaging compared with bone scanning, *J Bone Joint Surg* 75A:395, 1993.

Roach HI, Shearer JR, Archer C: The choice of an experimental model: a guide for research workers, *J Bone Joint Surg* 71B:549, 1989.

Roach KE, Miles T: Normal hip and knee active range of motion: the relationship to age, *Phys Ther* 71:656, 1991.

Robinson D, On E, Halperin N: Anterior compartment syndrome of the thigh in athletes: indications for conservative treatment, *J Trauma* 32:183, 1992.

Rockwood CA, Green DP, Bucholz RW, editors: *Rockwood and Green's fractures in adults,* vol II, ed 3, Philadelphia, 1991, JB Lippincott.

Rogers AW: *Textbook of anatomy,* New York, 1992, Churchill-Livingstone.

Rolak LA: *Neurology secrets,* ed 2, Philadelphia, 1998, Hanley & Belfus.

Rooser B: Acute compartment syndrome from anterior thigh muscle contusion: report of eight cases, *J Orthop Trauma* 5:55, 1991.

Rumack CM, Wilson SR, Charboneau JW: *Diagnostic ultrasound,* vol 1-2, ed 2, St Louis, 1998, Mosby.

Russotti GM, Conventry MB, Stauffer RN: Cemented total hip arthroplasty with contemporary techniques, *Clin Orthop* 235:141, 1988.

Saidoff DC, McDonough AL: *Critical pathways in therapeutic intervention,* St Louis, 1997, Mosby.

Saji MJ, Upakhyay SS, Leong JCY: Increased femoral neck-shaft angles in adolescent idiopathic scoliosis, *Spine* 20:303, 1995.

Sammarco GJ, Stephens MM: Neuropraxia of the femoral nerve in a modern dancer, *Am J Sports Med* 19:413, 1991.

Saudek CE: The hip. In Gould JA, editor: *Orthopaedic and sports physical therapy,* ed 2, St Louis, 1990, Mosby.

Schapira D: Transient osteoporosis of the hip, *Semin Arthritis Rheum* 22:98, 1992.

Schmalzried TP, Amstutz HC, Dorey FJ: Nerve palsy associated with total hip replacement, risk factors and prognosis, *J Bone Joint Surg* 73A:1074, 1991.

Schulte KR, et al: The outcome of Charnley total hip arthroplasty with cement after a minimum of twenty year follow-up, *J Bone Joint Surg* 75A:961, 1993.

Schumacher HR, Klippel JH, Koopman WJ: *Primer on the rheumatic diseases,* ed 10, Atlanta, 1993, Arthritis Foundation.

Scott JT, editor: *Copeman's textbook of the rheumatic diseases,* ed 6, Edinburgh, 1986, Churchill Livingstone.

Sells LL, German DC: An update on gout, *Bull Rheum Dis* 43:4, 1994.

Shankman GA: *Fundamental orthopedic management for the physical therapist assistant,* St Louis, 1997, Mosby.

Sherlock DA, Gibson PH, Benson MKD: Congenital subluxation of the hip, *J Bone Joint Surg* 67B:390, 1985.

Sledge CB, Poss R: *The yearbook of orthopedics 1997,* St Louis, 1997, Mosby.

Smith ET, Pevey JK, Shindler TO: The erector spinae transplant: a misnomer, *Clin Orthop* 20:144, 1963.

Smith G, et al: Hip pain caused by buttock claudication: relief of symptoms by transluminal angioplasty, *Clin Orthop* 284:176, 1992.

Solomon L: Patterns of osteoarthritis of the hip, *J Bone Joint Surg* 58B:176, 1976.

Somerville EW: A long-term follow-up of congenital dislocation of the hip, *J Bone Joint Surg* 60B:25, 1978.

Specht NT, Russo RD: *Practical guide to diagnostic imaging,* St Louis, 1998, Mosby.

Staheli LT: Medial femoral torsion, *Orthop Clin North Am* 11:39, 1980.

Stedman TL: *Stedman's medical dictionary,* ed 25, Baltimore, 1990, Williams & Wilkins.

Steinberg ME, Steinberg DR: Avascular necrosis of the femoral head. In Steinberg ME, editor: *The hip and its disorders,* Philadelphia, 1991, WB Saunders.

Steinbert ME, Steinberg DR: Evaluation and staging of avascular necrosis, *Semin Arthroplasty* 2:175, 1991.

Stevens A, Lowe J: *Histology,* New York, 1992, Gower Medical.

Stewart DL, Abeln SH: *Documenting functional outcomes in physical therapy,* St Louis, 1993, Mosby.

Stewart JDM, Hallett JP: *Traction and orthopaedic appliances,* Edinburgh, 1983, Churchill Livingstone.

Stock G: *The book of questions,* New York, 1985, Workman Publishing.

Stoller DW: *Magnetic resonance imaging in orthopaedics & sports medicine,* Philadelphia, 1993, JB Lippincott.

Strickland E, et al: In vivo contact pressures during rehabilitation, part 1: acute phase, *Phys Ther* 72:691, 1992.

Susuke S, et al: Diagnosis by ultrasound of congenital dislocation of the hip joint, *Clin Orthop* 217:171, 1987.

Sutton D, Young JWR: *A concise textbook of clinical imaging,* ed 2, St Louis, 1995, Mosby.

Swartout R, Compere EL: Ischiogluteal bursitis: the pain in the arse, *JAMA* 227:551, 1974.

Swartz MN, Dodge PR: Bacterial meningitis: general clinical features, special problems and unusual meningeal reactions mimicking bacterial meningitis, *N Engl J Med* 272:725, 1965.

Swointkowski MF: Intracapsular fractures of the hip, *J Bone Joint Surg* 76A:129, 1994.

Tachdjian MO: *Pediatric orthopedics,* Philadelphia, 1972, WB Saunders.

Tan JC, Horn SE: *Practical manual of physical medicine and rehabilitation,* St Louis, 1998, Mosby.

Taybi H, Lachman RS: *Radiology of syndromes, metabolic disorders, and skeletal dysplasias,* ed 4, St Louis, 1996, Mosby.

Terjesen T: Ultrasonography in the primary evaluation of Perthe's disease, *J Pediatr Orthop* 13:437, 1993.

Terjesen T, Berdland T, Berg V: Ultrasound for hip assessment in the newborn, *J Bone Joint Surg* 71B:767, 1989.

Teshima R, Otsuka T, Yamamoto K: Effects of nonweight bearing on the hip, *Clin Orthop* 279:149, 1992.

Tetsworth K, Paley D: Malalignment and degenerative arthropathy, *Orthop Clin North Am* 25:367, 1994.

Thibodeau GA, Patton KT: *Anatomy & physiology,* ed 3, St Louis, 1996, Mosby.

Thibodeau GA, Patton KT: *Pocket reference to accompany anatomy & physiology,* ed 3, St Louis, 1996, Mosby.

Thompson JM: *Clinical outlines for health assessment,* St Louis, 1997, Mosby.

Toalt V, et al: Evidence for viral aetiology of transient synovitis of the hip, *J Bone Joint Surg* 75B:973, 1993.

Toghill PJ: *Examining patients: an introduction to clinical medicine,* London, 1990, Edward Arnold.

Tollison CD, Satterthwaite JR, Tollison JW: *Handbook of pain management,* ed 2, Baltimore, 1994, Williams & Wilkins.

Toohey AK, et al: Iliopsoas bursitis; clinical features, radiographic findings, and disease associations, *Semin Arthritis Rheum* 10:41, 1990.

Torg JS, Shepard RJ: *Current therapy in sports medicine,* ed 3, St Louis, 1995, Mosby.

Tronzo RG, editor: *Surgery of the hip joint,* Philadelphia, 1973, Lea & Febiger.

Turek SL: *Orthopaedics principles and their application,* ed 3, Philadelphia, 1977, JB Lippincott.

Van Holsbeeck M, Introcaso JH: *Musculoskeletal ultrasound,* St Louis, 1991, Mosby.

Viere RG, et al: Use of the Pavlik harness in congenital dislocation of the hip, an analysis of failures of treatment, *J Bone Joint Surg* 72A:238, 1990.

Vingard E, et al: Sports and osteoarthritis of the hip: an epidemiologic study, *Am J Sports Med* 21:195, 1993.

Vrahas MS, et al: Contribution of passive tissues to the intersegmental moments at the hip, *J Biomech* 23:357, 1990.

Wainwright D: The shelf operation for hip dysplasia in adolescence, *J Bone Joint Surg* 58B:159, 1976.

Wakefield TS, Frank RG: *The clinician's guide to neuromusculoskeletal practice,* Abbotsford, Wisc, 1995, Allied Health of Wisconsin, SC.

Weineck J: *Functional anatomy in sports,* ed 2, St Louis, 1990, Mosby.

Weinstein SL, Buckwalter JA: *Turek's orthopaedics principles and their application,* ed 5, Philadelphia, 1994, JB Lippincott.

Weir J, Abrahams PH: *CD-ROM, Imaging atlas of human anatomy, version 2.0,* London, 1997, Mosby.

Weisl H: Intertrochanteric osteotomy for osteoarthritis, *J Bone Joint Surg* 62B:37, 1980.

Weiss W, Flippen HJ: The changing incidence and prognosis of tuberculous meningitis, *Am J Med Sci* 250:46, 1965.

Wenger DR, Ward WT, Herring JA: Legg-Calve-Perthes disease, *J Bone Joint Surg* 73A:778, 1991.

Whitmore I, Willan PLT: *Multiple choice questions in human anatomy,* London, 1995, Mosby.

Williams PF, editor: *Orthopaedic management in childhood,* Oxford, 1982, Blackwell.

Windsor RE, Lox DM: *Soft tissue injuries: diagnosis and treatment,* Philadelphia, 1998, Hanley & Belfus.

Wingstrand H, Wingstrand A, Krantz P: Intracapsular and atmospheric pressure in the dynamics and stability of the hip, *Acta Orthop Scand* 61:231, 1990.

Winter D: *Biomechanics and motor control of human movement,* ed 2, New York, 1990.

Winternitz WA, et al: Acute compartment syndrome of the thigh in sports related injuries not associated with femoral fractures, *Am J Sports Med* 20:476, 1992.

Woerman AL, Binder-Macleod SA: Leg-length discrepancy assessment: accuracy and precision in five clinical methods of evaluation, *J Orthop Sports Phys Ther* 5:230, 1984.

Wynne-Davis R: Acetabular dysplasia and familial joint laxity: two etiological factors in congenital dislocation of the hip, *J Bone Joint Surg* 52B:704, 1970.

Yang RS, Tsuang YH, Liu TK: Traumatic dislocation of the hip, *Clin Orthop* 265:218, 1991.

Yochum TR, Rowe LJ: Measurements in skeletal radiology. In Yochum TR, Rowe LJ, editors: *Essentials of skeletal radiology,* vol 1, Baltimore, 1987, Williams & Wilkins.

Yuen EC, Olney RK, So YT: Sciatic neuropathy: clinical and prognostic features in 73 patients, *Neurology* 44:1669, 1994.

Yuen EC, So YT, Olney RK: The electrophysiologic features of sciatic neuropathy in 100 patients, *Muscle Nerve* 18:414, 1995.

Zitelli BJ, Davis HW: *Atlas of pediatric physical diagnosis,* ed 2, London, 1992, Wolfe.

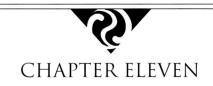

CHAPTER ELEVEN

THE KNEE

AXIOMS IN KNEE ASSESSMENT

- The knee consists of two joints: the patellofemoral and the tibiofemoral.
- Knee pain may arise from the joint itself, from periarticular tissues, or from the hip or femur.

INTRODUCTION

Pain is the most common presenting symptom of knee pathology. The causes of knee pain tend to be age related. A convenient way to classify knee pain complaints is by age group and by whether the pain is intraarticular, periarticular, or referred (Table 11-3).

ORTHOPEDIC GAMUT 11-1

KNEE STABILITY

Knee stability depends on the following four ligaments:

1. Tibial collateral
2. Fibular collateral
3. Anterior cruciates
4. Posterior cruciates

Little stability is furnished by the rounded contour of the femoral condyles and the flat tibial plateaus, which are deepened by the semilunar cartilages. The quadriceps muscle and its tendinous expansions are great contributors to the stability and function of the knee. The earliest clinical indication of internal knee derangement is atrophy of the quadriceps.

The knee is not a hinge joint. The tibia navigates a helical course on the condyles of the femur. Most traumatic arthritis of the knee in middle-aged and elderly people results from minor derangements of the soft tissues, especially the menisci.

The knee lacks the stability of the hip, which has its ball and socket, or the ankle, which has its mortise and tendon. Both the hip and ankle have structures that give some degree of bony stability. In the knee joint, the socket of the top of the tibia is so minimal that the lateral tibial plateau may be flat or even convex. The little bit of buffering provided by the menisci gives minimal increase in stability because the menisci are unstable themselves. For stability, the knee must depend largely on the soft tissues, ligaments, capsule, and muscles. It is extremely important to make an accurate diagnosis about the exact nature of the patient's knee injury. It is vital that a definitive diagnosis be made early so treatment can be started early. Examination must determine what part of the knee is injured and how bad the injury is.

TABLE 11-1

Knee Joint Cross-Reference Table by Assessment Procedure

Disease Assessed

Knee

Test/Sign

Test/Sign	Medial Collateral Ligament	Lateral Collateral Ligament	Medial Meniscus	Lateral Meniscus	Patellar Dislocation	Chondromalacia Patellae	Anterior Cruciate Ligament	Posterior Capsule	Iliotibial Band	Posterior Cruciate Ligament	Arcuate-Popliteus Complex	Posterior Oblique Ligament	Patellar Fracture	Patellar Syndromes (Soft Tissue)	Anterolateral Rotary Syndrome	Effusion	Valgus Deformity	Quadriceps	Osteochondritis
Abduction stress test	•																		
Adduction stress test		•																	
Apley's compression/distraction test			•	•															
Apprehension test for the patella					•														
Bounce home test																			
Childress duck waddle test			•	•															
Clarke's test			•	•		•								•					
Drawer test	•						•	•	•	•	•	•							
Dreyer's sign													•						
Fouchet's sign						•								•					
Lachman test							•				•	•							
Lateral pivot shift maneuver		•					•	•	•			•							
Losee test															•				
McMurray sign			•	•															
Noble compression test									•										
Patella ballottement test																•			
Payr's sign			•																
Q-angle test					•	•								•	•		•		
Slocum's test	•	•					•	•	•	•	•	•							
Steinmann's sign			•	•															
Thigh circumference test																		•	
Wilson's sign																			•

TABLE 11-2

KNEE CROSS-REFERENCE TABLE BY SUSPECTED SYNDROME OR TISSUE

Anterior cruciate ligament	Drawer test	Medial collateral ligament	Abduction stress test
	Lachman test		Drawer test
	Lateral pivot shift maneuver		Slocum's test
	Slocum's test	Medial meniscus	Apley's compression/distraction test
Arcuate-popliteus complex	Drawer test		Bounce home test
	Lachman test		Clarke's test
	Lateral pivot shift maneuver		McMurray sign
	Slocum's test		Payr's sign
Anterolateral rotary syndromes	Losee test		Steinmann's sign
	Q-angle test	Osteochondritis	Wilson's sign
Chondromalacia patella	Clarke's test	Patellar dislocation	Apprehension test for the patella
	Fouchet's sign		Q-angle test
	Q-angle test	Patellar fracture	Dreyer's sign
Effusion	Patella ballottement test	Patellar syndromes	Clarke's test
Iliotibial band	Drawer test		Fouchet's sign
	Lateral pivot shift maneuver		Q-angle test
	Noble compression test	Posterior capsule	Drawer test
	Slocum's test		Lateral pivot shift maneuver
Lateral collateral ligament	Adduction stress test		Slocum's test
	Lateral pivot shift maneuver	Posterior cruciate ligament	Drawer test
	Slocum's test		Slocum's test
Lateral meniscus	Apley's compression/ distraction test	Posterior oblique ligament	Drawer test
	Bounce home test		Fouchet's sign
	Clarke's test		Slocum's test
	McMurray sign	Quadriceps	Thigh circumference test
	Steinmann's sign	Valgus deformity	Q-angle test

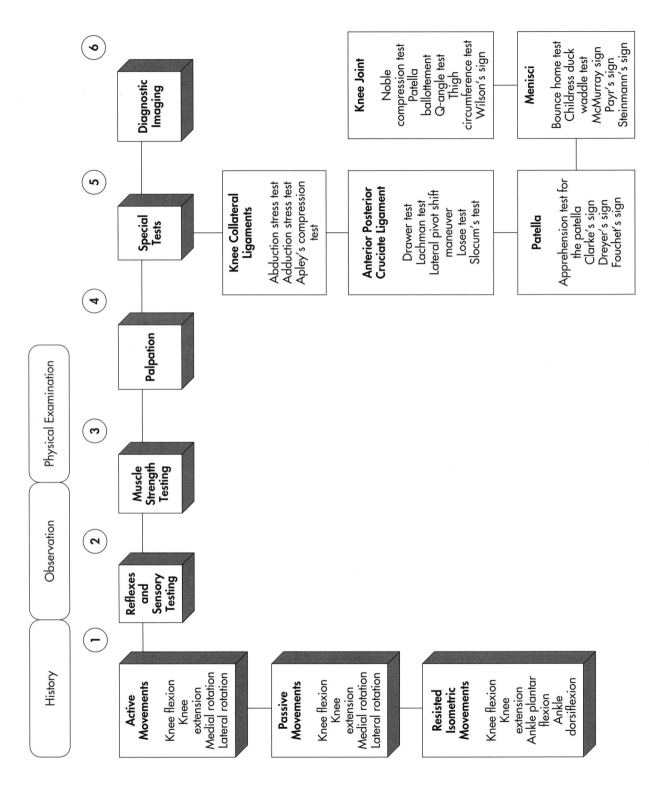

FIG. 11-1 Knee-joint assessment.

TABLE 11-3

INTRAARTICULAR KNEE PAIN DIFFERENTIATED BY AGE

Age	Intraarticular
Juvenile (2-10 years)	Juvenile chronic arthritis
	Osteochondritis dissecans
	Septic arthritis
	Torn discoid lateral meniscus
Adolescence (10-18 years)	Osteochondritis dissecans
	Torn meniscus
	Anterior knee pain syndrome
	Patellar malalignment
Early adult (18-30 years)	Torn meniscus
	Instability
	Anterior knee pain syndrome
	Inflammatory conditions
Adult (30-50 years)	Degenerate meniscal tears
	Early degeneration following injury or meniscectomy
	Inflammatory arthropathies
Mature (>50 years)	Osteoarthritis
	Inflammatory arthropathies

Adapted from Klippel JH, Dieppe PA: *Rheumatology,* vol 1-2, ed 2, London, 1998, Mosby.

ORTHOPEDIC GAMUT 11-2

KNEE

The parts of a knee that may be injured include the following:

1. Ligaments
2. Muscle tendon
3. Capsule
4. Meniscus
5. Cartilage
6. Bone
7. Bursae
8. Any combination of these

ESSENTIAL ANATOMY

The knee joint is the articulation of the femur, patella, and tibia (Fig. 11-2). The fibula is not involved in this articulation. The knee allows for flexion and extension and for rotation when the knee is already flexed (but not if the knee is fully extended).

In both the lateral and medial compartments of the joint is a C-shaped flattened cartilaginous meniscus (Fig. 11-3), loosely attached to the superior surface of the tibial plateau.

The anterior cruciate ligament (ACL) prevents excessive anterior "sliding" of the tibia with respect to the femur; the posterior cruciate ligament (PCL) prevents excessive posterior "sliding" of the tibia on the femur.

The patella enhances quadriceps strength. The articulating surface is divided by a median ridge into lateral and medial facets. Six types of patella are described based upon shape (Wiberg types) (Fig. 11-4). Types I and II are considered most stable, whereas the other types, because of unbalanced forces, are prone to lateral subluxations.

ESSENTIAL MOTION ASSESSMENT

The flexion-extension movement of the knee is not a simple hinge motion (Figs. 11-5 and 11-6). As the knee passes through its degrees of flexion and extensions, the imaginary mediolateral axis through which the movement occurs shifts up and down on the femur (Fig. 11-7).

With the foot planted on the ground and the knee fully extended, the knee is said to be "locked" in such a way that muscles of the thigh and leg can relax for short periods without making the joint too unstable.

ESSENTIAL MUSCLE FUNCTION ASSESSMENT

Test the muscles responsible for knee flexion and extension, the hamstrings and quadriceps, respectively (Figs. 11-8 and 11-9).

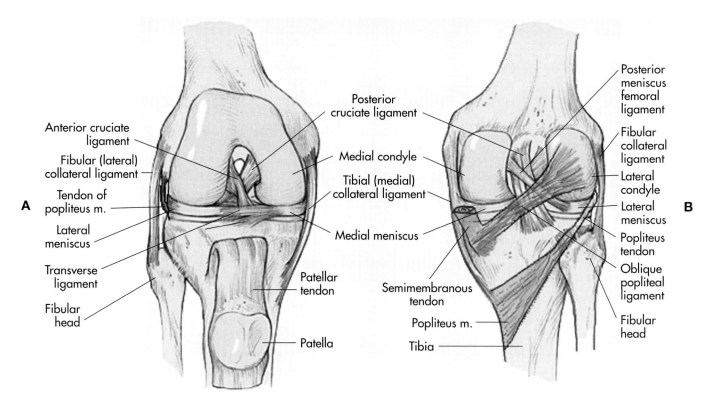

FIG. 11-2   Knee joint opened, anterior (**A**) and posterior (**B**) view.   *(From Mathers LH, et al:* Clinical anatomy principles, *St Louis, 1996, Mosby.)*

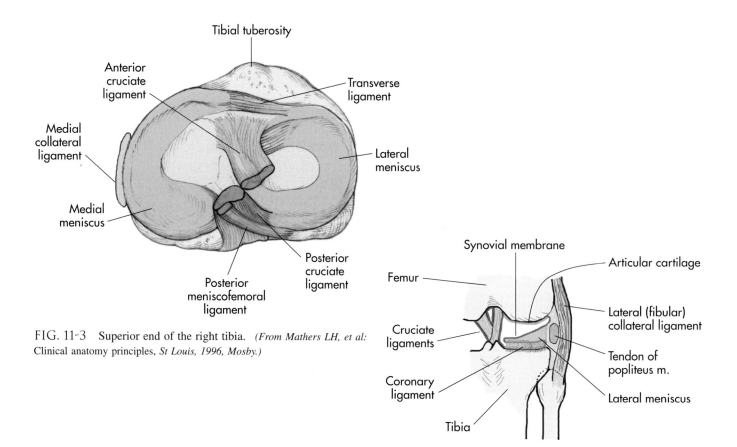

FIG. 11-3   Superior end of the right tibia.   *(From Mathers LH, et al:* Clinical anatomy principles, *St Louis, 1996, Mosby.)*

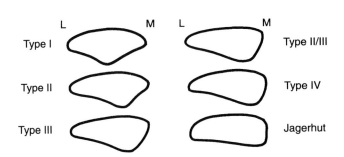

FIG. 11-4 Wiberg's and Baumgartl's patellar types. *(From Scott WN: The knee, vol 1-2, St Louis, 1994, Mosby.)*

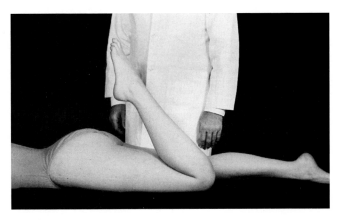

FIG. 11-5 The normal angle of knee flexion ranges from 130 to 150 degrees. A simple and useful but less-precise method for comparing the flexion of both knees can be used. This method involves comparing the distance between the heel and buttock when both knees are maximally flexed. Less than 140 degrees of retained active flexion range of motion is an impairment of the knee joint in the activities of daily living.

Flexion contractures (limitation of extension) of the knee often complicate chronic involvement of the joint. Varying degrees of subluxation or dislocation of the knee are most often the result of posterior displacement of the tibia on the femur or are occasionally from destruction of one condyle and the supporting plate of the tibia. When, as a result of such destruction, the tibia is dislocated laterally or medially, abnormal lateral or medial mobility is present, although the range of flexion and extension of the knee is limited.

A catch or jerky motion sometimes can be felt or seen during passive flexion and extension of the knee when the joint space harbors loose bodies. When the motion is repeated, the catch occurs at the same position in the arc of movement. The knee may lock or become suddenly fixed in partial extension while flexion from the point of limitation may remain unrestricted. A catching or jerky motion also may result from the absence of both menisci, whether from surgical removal or from disintegration that is secondary to articular inflammatory diseases, such as rheumatoid arthritis.

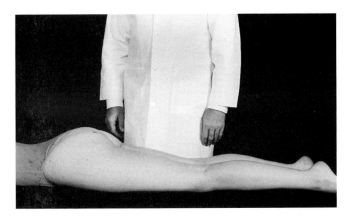

FIG. 11-6 The knee should normally extend to a straight line (0 degrees) and occasionally can be hyperextended up to 15 degrees. The degree of extension is determined by measuring the angle formed between the thigh and the leg. A flexion angle that is 10 degrees or greater in the fully extended knee is an impairment of the knee in the activities of daily living.

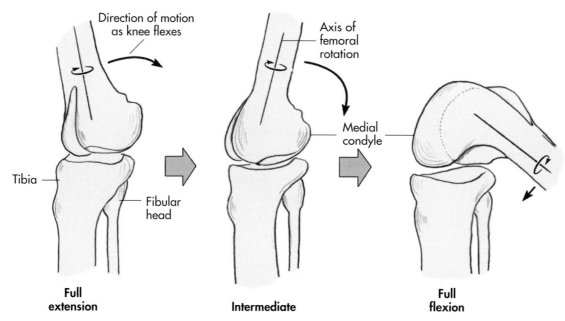

FIG. 11-7   Rotation at the knee.   *(From Mathers LH, et al:* Clinical anatomy principles, *St Louis, 1996, Mosby.)*

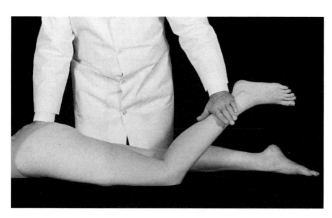

FIG. 11-8   The prime movers involved in flexion of the knee are the biceps femoris (sciatic nerve, tibial branch, S1, S2, and S3 to the long head; peroneal branch, L4, L5, S1, and S2 to the short head), semitendinosus (sciatic nerve, tibial branch, L4, L5, S1, S2, and S3), and the semimembranosus (sciatic nerve, tibial branch, L4, L5, S1, S2, and S3) muscles. Accessory muscles to this motion are the popliteus, sartorius, gracilis, and gastrocnemius. Flexion of the knee is tested while the patient is lying in a prone position with the knees extended. The examiner places one hand over the lateral aspect of the pelvis to immobilize it and applies graded resistance just proximal to the ankle with the other hand. The patient flexes the knee through its range of motion. If knee flexion is tested with the ankle rotated laterally, the biceps femoris is tested more directly because it is placed in better alignment. If knee flexion is tested with the ankle rotated medially, the semimembranosus and semitendinosus muscles are tested more directly during flexion. To prevent substitution by the gastrocnemius muscle, plantar flexion of the foot should not be allowed during knee flexion.

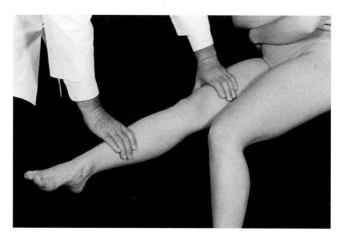

FIG. 11-9   The prime mover involved in extension of the knee is the quadriceps femoris (rectus femoris, vastus intermedius, vastus medialis, and vastus lateralis) muscle (innervated by the femoral nerve, L2, L3, and L4). Extension of the knee is tested while the patient sits with the legs hanging over the edge of a table. The examiner stabilizes the thigh by placing one hand over the pelvis or the proximal part of the thigh. The examiner should not exert pressure over the origin of the rectus femoris or induce pain. While the examiner provides stabilization, the patient then extends the knee through its range of motion. The examiner's free hand applies graded resistance proximal to the leg or ankle. As an alternative, the examiner can observe quadriceps femoris weakness if the patient is not able to rise from a low chair (height less than 65 cm) or from a squatting to a standing position without using the hands or other supports.

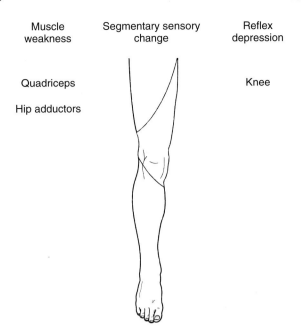

FIG. 11-10 L3 root syndrome. Motor, sensory, and reflex abnormalities. *(From Epstein O, et al: Clinical examination, ed 2, London, 1997, Mosby.)*

ORTHOPEDIC GAMUT 11-3

THIGH MUSCLES

The three thigh muscles that attach to the medial side of the tibia (supplied by three different nerves) are the following:

1. Gracilis (obturator nerve)
2. Sartorius (femoral nerve)
3. Semitendinosus (tibial nerve)

Quadriceps weakness and wasting can accompany joint disease. In a normal joint, unilateral quadriceps weakness suggests either a femoral neuropathy or an L3 root syndrome (Fig. 11-10). Femoral neuropathy leads to weakness and wasting of the quadriceps, loss of the knee jerk, and sensory change over the anterior thigh and the medial aspect of the lower leg (Fig. 11-11).

ORTHOPEDIC GAMUT 11-4

SCIATIC NERVE

The sciatic nerve innervates the following:

1. Hip joint
2. Biceps femoris
3. Semitendinosus
4. Semimembranosus
5. Ischial head of the adductor magnus

ESSENTIAL IMAGING

The typical knee study consists of an anteroposterior (AP) (or posteroanterior [PA]) and a lateral view (Figs. 11-12 to 11-15). Many examiners will include tangential, tunnel, or oblique views for further evaluation. The tangential view provides an axial depiction of the patella and its relationship with the femur. The tunnel allows excellent visualization of the intercondylar region of the femoral-tibial articulation (Figs. 11-16 and 11-17).

Typically, an AP knee radiograph is taken, but if the patella is the primary area of concern, a PA view would be useful (Figs. 11-18 and 11-19).

The lateral film is most sensitive for evaluating effusion of the joint (Fig. 11-20).

Text continued on p. 760

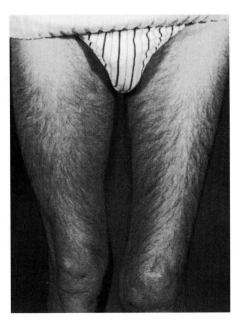

FIG. 11-11 Left femoral neuropathy after profundoplasty. *(From Epstein O, et al: Clinical examination, ed 2, London, 1997, Mosby.)*

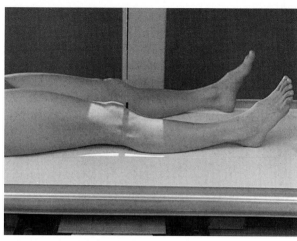

FIG. 11-12   Anteroposterior knee. *(From Ballinger PW: Merrill's atlas of radiographic positions and radiologic procedures, vol 1-3, ed 8, St Louis, 1995, Mosby.)*

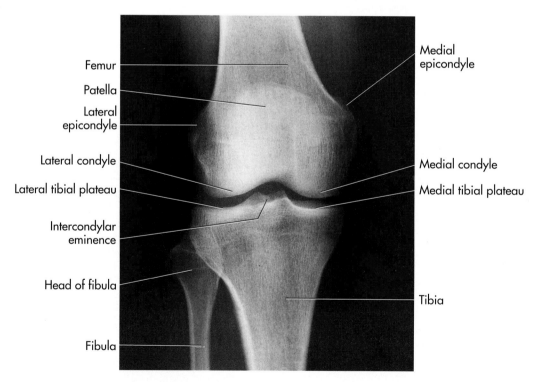

FIG. 11-13   Anteroposterior knee. *(From Ballinger PW: Merrill's atlas of radiographic positions and radiologic procedures, vol 1-3, ed 8, St Louis, 1995, Mosby.)*

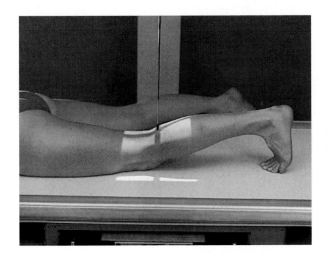

FIG. 11-14 Posteroanterior knee. *(From Ballinger PW: Merrill's atlas of radiographic positions and radiologic procedures, vol 1-3, ed 8, St Louis, 1995, Mosby.)*

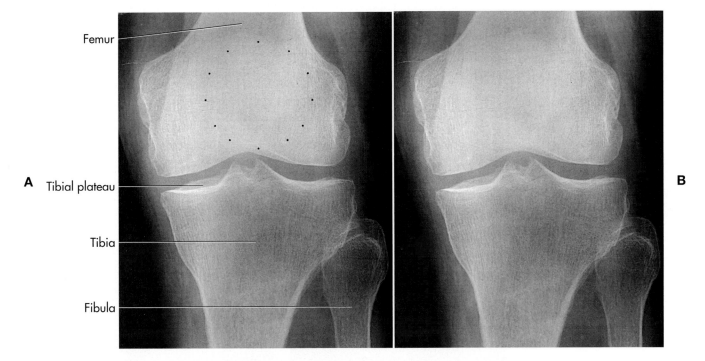

FIG. 11-15 **A,** Posteroanterior knee (patella outlined by dots). **B,** Posteroanterior knee showing epiphyses of teenager. *(From Ballinger PW: Merrill's atlas of radiographic positions and radiologic procedures, vol 1-3, ed 8, St Louis, 1995, Mosby.)*

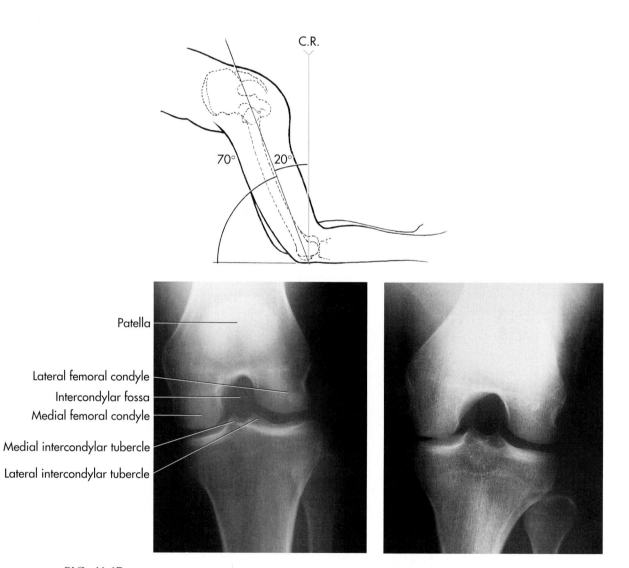

FIG. 11-16   Posteroanterior axial intercondylar fossa: kneeling on radiographic table. *(From Ballinger PW:* Merrill's atlas of radiographic positions and radiologic procedures, *vol 1-3, ed 8, St Louis, 1995, Mosby.)*

C.R.

70°   20°

Patella

Lateral femoral condyle
Intercondylar fossa
Medial femoral condyle

Medial intercondylar tubercle

Lateral intercondylar tubercle

FIG. 11-17   Alignment relationships for any of three intercondylar fossa approaches. *(From Ballinger PW:* Merrill's atlas of radiographic positions and radiologic procedures, *vol 1-3, ed 8, St Louis, 1995, Mosby.)*

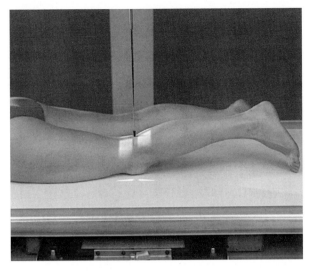

FIG. 11-18   Posteroanterior patella.   *(From Ballinger PW:* Merrill's atlas of radiographic positions and radiologic procedures, *vol 1-3, ed 8, St Louis, 1995, Mosby.)*

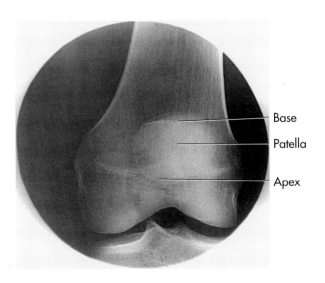

Base

Patella

Apex

FIG. 11-19   Posteroanterior patella.   *(From Ballinger PW:* Merrill's atlas of radiographic positions and radiologic procedures, *vol 1-3, St Louis, 1995, Mosby.)*

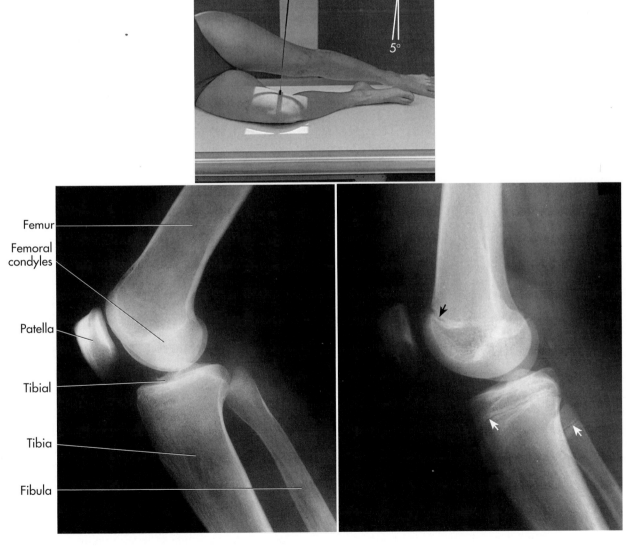

Femur

Femoral condyles

Patella

Tibial

Tibia

Fibula

FIG. 11-20   Lateral knee showing 5 degrees cephalad angulation of central ray.   *(From Ballinger PW:* Merrill's atlas of radiographic positions and radiologic procedures, *vol 1-3, ed 8, St Louis, 1995, Mosby.)*

ABDUCTION STRESS TEST

ALSO KNOWN AS VALGUS STRESS TEST

Assessment for Medial Collateral Ligament Injury

Comment

Injuries to the medial collateral are the most common ligament injuries seen in the knee. There is an intimate anatomic relationship between the medial collateral ligament (MCL) and the medial meniscus of the knee. O'Donoghue is credited with describing the "unhappy triad" as combined injury to the MCL, ACL, and medial meniscus. Because the MCL and medial meniscus are strongly attached to one another, it is clear that the meniscus may become injured along with more severe MCL injuries (Fig. 11-21). However, the more common triad is the MCL, ACL, and lateral meniscus.

ORTHOPEDIC GAMUT 11-5

MEDIAL COLLATERAL LIGAMENT

The severity of MCL injury can be classified as follows:

Grade I: 0 to 5 mm of joint opening with no instability
Grade II: 5 to 10 mm of joint opening with some degree of instability
Grade III: 10 to 15 mm of joint opening with moderate instability
Grade IV: Greater than 15 mm of joint opening with gross ligament instability

---

The medial ligament is the main strut of the capsular tissues of the knee. The deep portion of the ligament is a thickened part of the capsule itself and is adherent to the medial meniscus. The superficial part forms a strong, broad, and triangular strap. Originating from a point just distal to the adductor tubercle, the ligament keeps free of the meniscus and the joint margins and has an extensive insertion into the medial surface of the tibia—at least 1.5 inches below the joint level. The posterior border of the ligament has continuity with the strong posterior capsule of the knee joint. Anteriorly, there are fibrous connections with the quadriceps expansion and the patellar ligament. The whole medial capsule, which is accompanied by its ligament, is adequately designed to take strong control of the tibia in all movements of the knee, both by structure and by the intimate connections that the capsule forms with the anterior and posterior muscles of the thigh.

A ligament is a fibrous structure designed to prevent abnormal motion of a joint. Any ligamentous injury that is caused by an abnormal motion may be defined as a sprain. A sprain can vary from a complete dislocation of the joint, accompanied by total loss of ligament integrity, to a slight tearing of a few isolated fibers with no loss of function. A sprain should include avulsion of the ligament from the bone, with or without a small fragment (sprain-fracture); partial avulsion of the ligament from the bone; or tearing (transversely, obliquely, or longitudinally) of the ligament within its substance. In the last instance, the ligament will be elongated although it will still be intact. The function of the ligament depends not only on its strength but also on its length. A ligament that is elongated does not carry out its function of preventing abnormal motion of the joint. The severity of the injury is of more significance than the exact location or type of tear.

Medial ligament syndrome is an ill-defined syndrome in which the patient complains of pain at the site of insertion of the medial ligament. Examination reveals tenderness over the insertion of the ligament, and valgus stress may exacerbate the pain. It is more common in females than in males and is associated with valgus knees and the pain amplification syndrome. It may be difficult to differentiate from anserine bursitis and pes anserinus tendinitis. The cause is obscure, but in some cases, an inflammatory arthropathy, such as ankylosing spondylitis, is present.

PROCEDURE

- While the patient is lying supine and the knee is in complete extension, the examiner, who is on the ipsilateral side, places one palm against the lateral aspect of the patient's knee, at the joint line.
- While the other hand is gripping the ankle, the examiner laterally draws the leg to open the medial side of the joint (Fig. 11-22).
- If the patient is indifferent to this action, the examiner repeats it while the knee is in approximately 30 degrees of flexion, a position of lesser stability.

- This maneuver makes the medial joint vulnerable to torsion stress.
- The production or increase of pain, especially below, above, or at the joint line, is evidence of MCL injury.

Confirmation Procedures
Adduction stress test and Apley's compression/distraction test

---

CLINICAL PEARL

The knee is an unusual joint because it contains ligaments deep within the joint. There are also medial and lateral collateral menisci that can be damaged. Finally, the normal motions of the knee are very complex, including two planes of rotation. It is very common to see multiple and complex injuries.

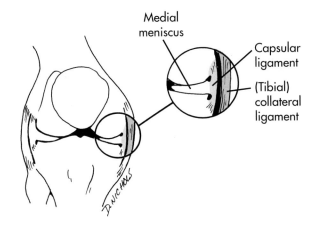

FIG. 11-21 The medial meniscus can also become injured in conjunction with the medial collateral ligament (MCL) because of its intimate anatomic relationship with the MCL. *(From Shankman GA:* Fundamental orthopedic management for the physical therapist assistant, *St Louis, 1997, Mosby.)*

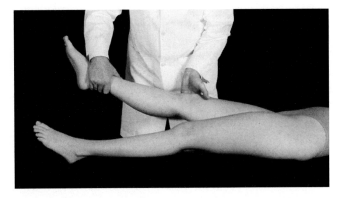

FIG. 11-22 The patient is lying supine, and the knee is in complete extension. The examiner, who is on the ipsilateral side, places one palm against the lateral aspect of the patient's knee at the joint line. With the other hand gripping the ankle, the examiner draws the leg laterally, to open the medial side of the knee joint. The production or increase of pain—especially below, above, or at the joint line—is evidence of medial collateral ligament injury.

ADDUCTION STRESS TEST

ALSO KNOWN AS VARUS STRESS TEST

Assessment for Lateral Collateral Ligament Injury

Comment

The lateral ligament extends in two layers from the lateral condyle of the femur to the head of the fibula, where the ligament inserts on the biceps tendon. The tendon of the popliteus and often a bursa separates the ligament from the knee joint and the lateral meniscus. The only connection the ligament has with the fibrous capsule is at the posterior border of the lateral ligament, which is continuous with the fascia covering the popliteus and therefore is continuous with that muscle's attachments to the posterior horn of the lateral meniscus. The lateral ligament plays its part in stability of the leg on the thigh through the superior tibiofibular joint. The lateral ligament is independent of rotary movements of the tibia. Where the ligament attaches to the lateral meniscus, rotation is prevented, and flexion of the knee is restricted. The lateral capsule is thinner and weaker than the one on the medial side.

Ligament instability may be defined as abnormal rotational or translational motion of the tibial plateaus in relation to the femoral condyles. This rotational or translational motion occurs around one or more axes or in one or more planes of motion and results in a functional deficit. The key to evaluating ligament instability is the term *functional deficit*. Although two patients may have identical degrees of ligamentous instability, the functional deficit in each is not the same because the demands each patient places on the knees are different. A moderate amount of instability in an individual who wants to take part in vigorous physical activity may create a serious handicap, but a more sedentary patient may find that the same degree of instability is not a serious problem.

Stability of the knee is provided by static and dynamic elements that work together as an integrated mechanism. Static support is a function of the ligaments, capsule, menisci, and bony contour of the joint. Dynamic support is the function of the surrounding muscles. Attempting to assign a specific function to each ligament has led to confusion in evaluating ligamentous instability. The examiner must bear in mind that the static stabilizers are an integral part of a mechanism that must provide support to an inherently unstable joint that is subject to a variety of forces. It is rare for an injury to affect only one element in this complex system. An injury usually influences more than one other structure either directly or indirectly. The knee joint is not merely a hinge joint that allows flexion and extension. The joint also has the element of rotation and even some valgus and varus motion.

Even with normal ligaments, knee stability is a rather tenuous situation because the knee does not have the dynamic support of the various thigh and calf muscles, which protect the static elements. The static structures define the limits of motion, and the musculotendinous structures control the motion through voluntary and kinesthetic mechanisms. These structures create appropriate motion and simultaneously serve as energy-absorbing mechanisms for extrinsic and intrinsic forces that might otherwise injure the static structures.

The lateral collateral ligament is rarely injured in isolation but is usually torn in association with damage to the posterolateral ligament complex (lateral capsule, arcuate ligament, and popliteus tendon). The cruciate ligaments may also be damaged. The mechanism of injury is usually a varus force on a flexed knee. The ligament usually ruptures at its fibular insertion, or it may avulse the fibular styloid. A peroneal nerve palsy may be associated with a lateral collateral ligament tear and should be looked for at the time of the injury. Little functional instability arises from an isolated tear of the lateral collateral ligament.

PROCEDURE

- While the patient is lying supine and the knee is in complete extension, the examiner, who is on the ipsilateral side, places one palm against the medial aspect of the patient's knee, at the joint line.
- While the examiner's other hand grips the ankle, the examiner draws the leg medially to open the lateral side of the joint (Fig. 11-23).
- If the patient is indifferent to this procedure, the examiner repeats it with the knee in approximately 30 degrees of flexion.
- An initiation or increase of pain above, below, or at the joint line is evidence of lateral collateral ligament injury.

Confirmation Procedures

Abduction stress test and Apley's compression/distraction test

DIAGNOSTIC STATEMENT

Adduction stress test is positive for the right knee. This result indicates lateral collateral ligament injury.

CLINICAL PEARL

There is little congruency between the articular surfaces of the tibia and the femur. As a result, there is a well-developed system of ligaments for stability and an arrangement of intraarticular menisci that reduce the contact loading between the femur and tibia.

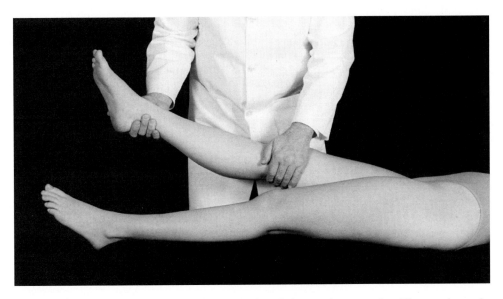

FIG. 11-23 The patient is lying supine, and the knee is in complete extension. The examiner, who is standing on the ipsilateral side, places one palm against the medial aspect of the patient's knee at the joint line. With the other hand gripping the ankle, the examiner draws the leg medially to open the lateral side of the knee joint. The production or increase of pain that is above, below, or at the joint line is evidence of lateral collateral ligament injury.

APLEY'S COMPRESSION TEST

ALSO KNOWN AS APLEY'S DISTRACTION TEST AND APLEY'S GRINDING TEST

Assessment for Collateral Ligament Injury and Meniscus Tears

Comment

When bearing weight, the tibia rotates laterally as the knee joint extends, and it rotates medially as the knee flexes. If this synchrony is forcibly prevented, such as by the weight of the patient's falling body, the rotator mechanism of the knee is injured. Certain cartilage tears are caused by this disruption of the rotator mechanism of the knee. In a geriatric patient, the transverse fracture of the fibrotic medial meniscus, which takes place at the junction of the anterior two-thirds and the posterior one-third, may be due to pressure and grinding between the femur and the tibia. All other tears can be explained by the violent stretching that must occur if medial rotation of the tibia is prevented when the knee is flexed or if lateral rotation is prevented when the knee is extended. Similar forces are brought into play when weight is taken on while squatting or kneeling. For example, a sudden twisting may occur without extension or further flexion, or the tibia may twist laterally while the body lurches backward and increases flexion of the knee.

At first the meniscus straightens. To allow it to do so, a transverse or oblique split forms in the shorter or free edge. This minor split is the most common finding and is usually deeper in the lateral meniscus than in the medial meniscus because of the longer curve of the latter. If no more damage occurs, the knee might be symptomless after recovery from the acute injury, but the split itself would not heal. However, the split occasionally extends obliquely to form a mobile tag, which causes an irritating, recurring, and painful catch in the knee.

The split usually occurs at the apex of the curve or in the anterior portion of the meniscus. This location is to be expected because the straightening under tension would take place first in the more mobile portion. The posterior segments are more firmly fixed to the capsule.

Should the range of unaccommodated movement be greater, it is achieved either by pulling the cartilage away from its attachments to the anterior cruciate and from its capsular moorings at the back or by splitting the cartilage longitudinally to allow the free border to bowstring across the joint.

ORTHOPEDIC GAMUT 11-6

MENISCUS

Indications of pathologic conditions of the meniscus include the following:

1. Pain or tenderness on the lateral surfaces of the knee joint
2. Popping, snapping, or grating sounds with movement
3. Inability to fully extend the knee ("locking")

The medial meniscus is more often injured than the lateral. The two tests commonly used to aid in the diagnosis of a torn meniscus are Apley's test and the McMurray test.

PROCEDURE

- The test involves four steps, and if any or all of them elicit knee pain or clicking, the test is positive.
- The patient is lying prone with the lower limbs straight and the ankles hanging over the end of the examination table.
- The examiner grasps the foot of the involved lower extremity, strongly rotates the leg internally, and flexes the knee past 90 degrees (Fig. 11-24).
- This maneuver is repeated with the leg strongly rotated in external rotation (Fig. 11-25).

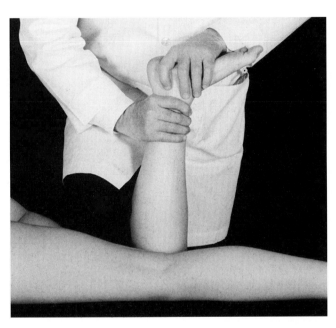

FIG. 11-24   The patient is lying prone with the leg extended and the ankles hanging over the table edge. The examiner grasps the foot and strongly and internally rotates the leg and then flexes the knee to 90 degrees.

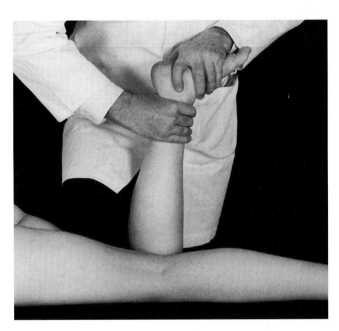

FIG. 11-25   The examiner repeats the maneuver described in Fig. 11-24 while the leg is strongly rotated externally and strong downward pressure is applied to the patient's foot. The production of pain is significant for meniscus tear.

- The examiner anchors the patient's thigh to the examination table by placing a knee in the patient's popliteal space.
- A small pillow or towel should be used for cushioning.
- The examiner strongly distracts the patient's knee joint by lifting the foot (Fig. 11-26).
- This move is followed by rapidly rotating the leg, both internally and externally (Fig. 11-27).
- This procedure is repeated with strong downward pressure on the patient's foot.
- An intermediate maneuver may be performed.
- The examiner flexes the patient's knee to 90 degrees and rapidly rotates the foot and leg, both internally and externally, without anchorage to rule out a rotational strain or collateral ligament tear.
- The test is significant for meniscus tear.

Confirmation Procedures

Abduction stress test, adduction stress test, bounce home test, Childress duck waddle test, McMurray sign, Payr's sign, and Steinmann's sign

DIAGNOSTIC STATEMENT

Apley's compression test is positive on the right and indicates injury to the medial meniscus.

Apley's knee compression testing is positive on the right and indicates injury to the lateral meniscus.

Apley's distraction test is positive on the right and indicates injury to the lateral collateral ligaments.

Apley's distraction test is positive on the right and indicates injury to the MCL.

CLINICAL PEARL

The phrase *internal derangement of the knee* is a common provisional diagnosis for any patient with mechanical symptoms of the knee. The initials of this phrase, *IDK,* also stand for "I don't know," and the temptation to use these initials, instead of making a complete diagnosis, must be avoided.

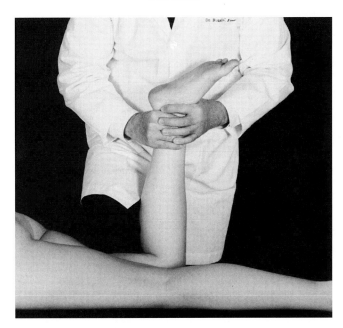

FIG. 11-26 The examiner anchors the patient's thigh to the table by placing a knee in the patient's popliteal space. The maneuver can be cushioned by a small pillow or towel. The examiner strongly distracts the patient's knee joint by lifting the foot.

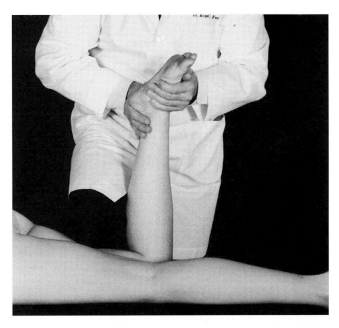

FIG. 11-27 This maneuver is followed by rapid rotation, both internally and externally, of the leg. Pain elicited is significant for collateral ligament tear.

APPREHENSION TEST
FOR THE PATELLA

Assessment for Vulnerability to Recurrent Dislocation of the Patella

Comment

Disorders of the patellofemoral joint are common in children and adolescents.

Recurrent subluxation of the patella is a common disorder that is often undiagnosed because the symptoms are similar to other derangements of the knee. The patella usually subluxates or dislocates laterally. The condition may follow an acute patellar dislocation that fails to heal properly. The disorder is often bilateral and is more common in females.

Roentgenographic studies are usually helpful. A "sunrise" view taken with the knee relaxed in slight flexion will often reveal lateral displacement (Fig. 11-28).

Congenital dislocation occurs in infancy and involves irreducible lateral displacement of the patella. It is associated with genu valgum, a small patella, hypoplasia of the lateral femoral condyle, and tethering of the lateral capsule.

In habitual dislocation, lateral displacement of the patella occurs every time the knee is flexed. It is due to contracture of the vastus lateralis and iliotibial band, with an abnormal insertion of the iliotibial band into the patella.

Recurrent dislocation, or subluxation, of the patella that occurs to the lateral side while the knee is flexed is commonly encountered in adolescents. This type of dislocation is often bilateral, and it occurs in females more often than in males.

The first dislocation is initiated by trauma. A mild hypoplasia of the anterior surface of the lateral femoral condyle and genu valgum are predisposing factors. This type of trauma usually occurs while the patient is engaged in an active sport. The patient falls and strikes the medial aspect of the patella, forcing it laterally over the condyle. Pain is severe, and the patient is unable to straighten the leg. The displacement may be reduced immediately, either by the patient or a companion or spontaneously.

After this type of fall, some patients have no further difficulty. In other cases, dislocation occurs more and more frequently, and the patient complains that the knee is unstable and gives way. Occasionally, a patient is able to describe the maneuver by which the dislocation can be reduced. This maneuver involves straightening the knee and forcing the lateral border of the patella in a medial direction. Following reduction, the knee is usually painful for 2 or 3 days. There may also be mild effusion. With recurrent episodes, degenerative changes develop on the undersurface of the patella and on the femoral condyle.

When the patient is examined after recurrent episodes of dislocation, tenderness occurs along the medial aspect of the patella and suggests a partial tear of the insertion of the vastus medialis. Effusion of the knee and slight quadriceps atrophy also occurs. The range of knee motion is normal.

PROCEDURE

- The apprehension test for the patella is a test for vulnerability to recurrent dislocation of the patella.
- For the test, the patient is either supine or seated with the quadriceps muscles relaxed (Fig. 11-29).
- The knee is flexed to 30 degrees.
- The examiner carefully and slowly pushes the patella laterally (Fig. 11-30).
- If the patella feels as if it is about to dislocate, the patient will contract the quadriceps muscles and bring the patella back into line.
- This action indicates a positive test.
- The patient will also exhibit a look of apprehension.

Confirmation Procedures

Clarke's sign, Dreyer's sign, and Fouchet's sign

DIAGNOSTIC STATEMENT

The apprehension test for the patella is positive on the left. This result indicates a vulnerability to recurrent dislocation of the patella.

CLINICAL PEARL

The examiner should observe for genu recurvatum and the position of the patella in relation to the femoral condyles. A high patella (patella alta) is a predisposing factor to recurrent lateral dislocation of the patella. The recurrent dislocation of the patella is also most common in females with the genu valgum deformity.

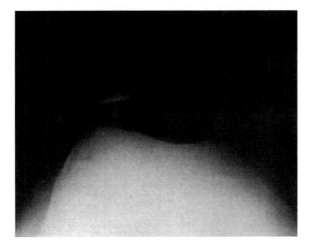

FIG. 11-28 A "sunrise" view of the knee reveals abnormal lateral displacement of the patella. *(From Mercier LR, Pettid FJ: Practical orthopedics, ed 4, St Louis, 1995, Mosby.)*

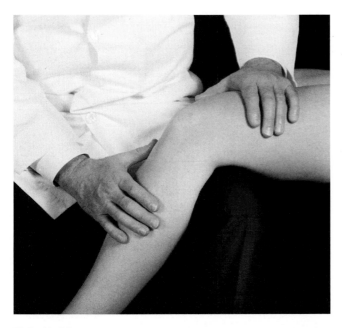

FIG. 11-29 The patient is seated, with the quadriceps muscles relaxed and the knee flexed to approximately 30 degrees over the examiner's leg.

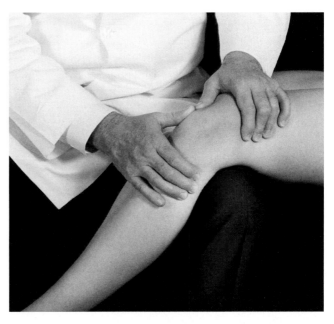

FIG. 11-30 The examiner carefully and slowly pushes the patella laterally. If the patella feels as if it is about to dislocate, the patient will contract the quadriceps muscle to bring the patella back into line. This action indicates a positive test. A positive test indicates a vulnerability or predisposition for recurrent dislocation of the patella.

Assessment for Meniscal Tears

Comment

The congenital discoid meniscus typically involves the lateral meniscus, and it often presents symptoms in childhood. With this defect, the meniscus is not in the usual semilunar form but rather shaped more like a D, with its central edge extending toward the tibial spines. The meniscus may produce a very pronounced clicking from the lateral compartment, a block to the extension of the joint, and other derangement signs.

The most common cause of meniscal tears in young adults is a sporting injury, such as when a twisting strain is applied to the flexed, weight-bearing leg. In this case, the entrapped meniscus often splits longitudinally, and its free edge may displace inward, toward the center of the joint. This is called a *bucket-handle tear* (Fig. 11-31). This type of tear prevents full extension (locking), and if an attempt is made to straighten the knee, a painful, elastic resistance (a springy block to full extension) is felt. The injury of the medial meniscus, which involves prolonged loss of full extension, may lead to stretching and eventual rupture of the ACL. Lateral meniscus tears are often associated with cysts that restrict the mobility of the meniscus. Major meniscus tears are treated by excision of the meniscus, but with bucket-handle tears, the removal of only the central portion may decrease the risk of late, secondary osteoarthritis. In some lesions involving the periphery of the meniscus, repair by direct suture is sometimes attempted.

Loss of elasticity in the menisci through degenerative changes associated with the aging process may cause horizontal cleavage tears within the substance of the meniscus. These tears may not be associated with any remembered incident. Sharply localized tenderness in the joint line is a common feature.

Ganglion-like cysts occur in both menisci. However, these cysts are much more common in the lateral meniscus. There is often a history of a blow on the side of the knee, over the meniscus. The cysts are tender, and because they restrict mobility of the menisci, the cysts render them more susceptible to tears. Medial meniscus cysts must be carefully differentiated from ganglion cysts that arise from the pes anserinus (the insertion of the sartorius, gracilis, and semitendinosus).

PROCEDURE

- The patient is supine.
- The patient's knee is flexed completely (Fig. 11-32).
- The knee is allowed to drop into extension (Fig. 11-33).
- If the extension is not complete, the test is positive.
- The positive finding suggests a torn meniscus.

Confirmation Procedures

Childress duck waddle test, McMurray sign, Payr's sign, and Steinmann's sign

---

DIAGNOSTIC STATEMENT

The bounce home test is positive for the left knee and indicates a torn meniscus.

CLINICAL PEARL

Meniscus lesions are the most common internal derangement. Although the menisci are damaged by trauma, the incident is often so trivial that the patient cannot remember any injury at all. Because of this, patients with meniscal injuries are rarely seen in emergency rooms.

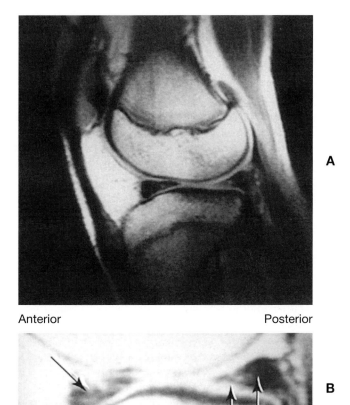

Anterior   Posterior

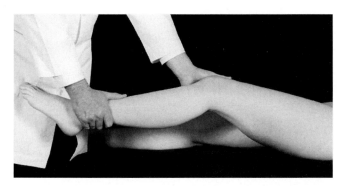

FIG. 11-31 Magnetic resonance image of a 14-year-old male hockey player's knee. **A,** Linear tear of the anterior horn of the lateral meniscus. **B,** Complex tear of the posterior horn. *(From Brier SR: Primary care orthopedics, St Louis, 1999, Mosby.)*

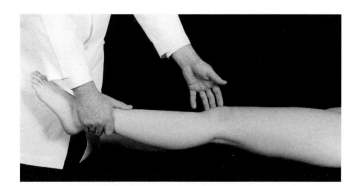

FIG. 11-32 The patient is supine. The examiner grasps the patient's leg at the ankle. The patient's knee is flexed.

FIG. 11-33 The knee is allowed to drop into extension. If the extension is not complete, the finding is positive. This finding indicates a torn meniscus.

CHILDRESS DUCK WADDLE TEST

Assessment for Medial or Lateral Meniscus Tears

Comment

The term *internal derangement* is used to group a variety of knee joint conditions, usually of traumatic origin, in which the internal structure of the joint is affected to such an extent that its function and mechanics are compromised.

A rotary force applied to the knee joint may trap a meniscus between the femur and the tibia and produce the familiar torn-cartilage lesion. A meniscus cannot be torn while the knee is in extension. To produce a tear, the knee joint must be first rotated in the flexed position to trap the meniscus and then extended to produce the tearing force on the tissue. This combination of motions is commonly encountered on the football field or basketball court.

Tears of the medial meniscus are encountered about nine times more frequently than tears of the lateral meniscus. This difference in frequency is believed to be because the medial meniscus is attached to the deep layer of the MCL and because the mechanisms that cause the tearing are more frequently applied to the medial aspect of the joint.

A tear of the medial meniscus is associated with pain that is referred to the medial side of the joint and is accompanied by synovial effusion. The pain caused by the torn meniscus is often aggravated by forced rotation of the foot and leg. Pain or a clicking may be produced by testing for the McMurray sign. Locking of the joint may or may not be present, depending on the location of the tear.

ORTHOPEDIC GAMUT 11-7

MENISCAL TEARS

The following two types of meniscal tears occur most often:

1. The first type is the splitting of the meniscus, along its longitudinal axis, producing the so-called bucket-handle tear.
2. The second type is the tear along its transverse axis.

Tears similar to those seen in the medial meniscus may involve the lateral meniscus, but these tears are less common. On the other hand, cystic degeneration is much more common in the lateral meniscus than in the medial meniscus. In this condition, multiple cysts containing gelatinous material appear within the peripheral border of the meniscus. Repeated trauma causes the appearance of these cysts. Once developed, cartilage cysts may cause pain and often can be seen and palpated along the lateral border of the knee joint.

A discoid meniscus is a congenitally abnormal lateral meniscus, in which the structure assumes a thickened and rounded shape. Because of its thickness, the meniscus does not glide smoothly between the femur and the tibia. Rather, the meniscus must force its way through. As a result, a loud clicking noise is heard when the knee flexes or extends, but locking does not occur.

PROCEDURE

- The patient stands with the feet somewhat apart and the legs in maximal internal rotation (Fig. 11-34).
- A full squat is attempted (Fig. 11-35).
- During this maneuver, the patient's heels may come up from the floor, with weight bearing passing to the balls of the feet.
- The maneuver is repeated, with the lower limbs in maximal external rotation (Figs. 11-36 and 11-37).
- A positive test consists of pain, inability to fully flex the knee, or a clicking sound on either posterior side of the joint.
- The test is significant during internal rotation for a medial meniscus tear or during external rotation for a lateral meniscus tear.

Confirmation Procedures

Bounce home test, McMurray sign, Payr's sign, and Steinmann's sign

---

DIAGNOSTIC STATEMENT

Childress duck waddle test is positive for the right (or left) knee in external rotation. This result indicates a lateral meniscus tear.

Childress duck waddle test is positive for the right knee in internal rotation. This result indicates a medial meniscus tear.

CLINICAL PEARL

The menisci are important parts of the load-bearing mechanism of the knee because they absorb the downward thrust of the convex femoral condyles. The menisci are so effective that if they are removed, the force that is taken by the articular cartilage during peak loading increases about five times. Therefore a meniscectomy exposes the articular cartilage to much greater forces than normal. Evidence of degenerative osteoarthritis is seen in 75% of patients 10 years after a total meniscectomy.

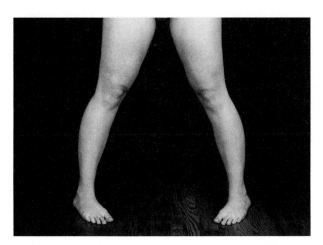

FIG. 11-34   The patient stands with the feet apart and the legs in maximum internal rotation.

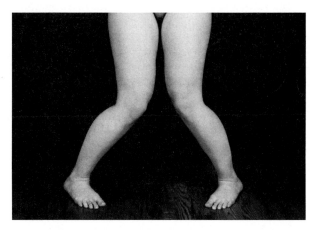

FIG. 11-35   The patient attempts a full squat. During this maneuver, the patient's heels may come up from the floor and weight may be shifted to the balls of the feet.

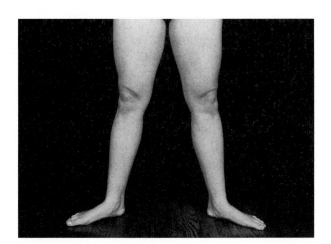

FIG. 11-36   The maneuver is repeated with the lower limbs in maximum external rotation.

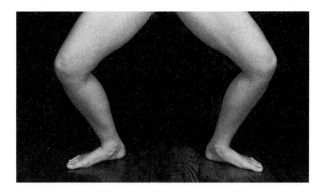

FIG. 11-37   A full squat is attempted again. A positive test consists of pain, inability to fully flex the knee, or a clicking sound on either posterior side of the joint. With internal rotation, the test is significant for a medial meniscus tear. During external rotation, the test is significant for a lateral meniscus tear.

CLARKE'S SIGN

Assessment for Chondromalacia Patellae

Comment

The term *patellar malacia* has been used as a catchall to include the many processes that involve the undersurface of the patella. True malacia is a softening or breaking down of a part of the tissue. When chronic synovitis of the knee causes the patellar cartilage to break down and the bed to eburnate so that denuded bone is exposed, the condition is called *malacia*. This is the same condition that occurs in a young individual who has fragmentation of the patellar cartilage with no signs of arthritis. Patellar malacia falls into three groups.

Group I is trauma related. There may be a chondral fracture or infraction that is caused either by acute trauma or by repeated, lesser traumata to the patella. Infraction of the patellar cartilage causes irritation of the patellar groove on the femur, and gradual changes supervene with fissuring, absorption, and fragmentation of the cartilage.

Group II is associated with a disturbance of the rhythm of the patellar function. These disturbances are commonly called *tracking disorders*. This is the type of malacia that accompanies intrinsic injury to the knee. Any condition that causes a disturbance in the rhythm of the knee action often results in involvement of the undersurface of the patella. The knee is checked abruptly, motion is reversed, and the patella is driven against the femur. There is a relationship between the locking of the knee and the degree of malacia present. These two factors are much more important for indicating the amount of malacia present than is the age of the patient. The exact mechanism of the breakdown of the patella has never been wholly explained. This condition also probably occurs as the result of various other causes, including direct trauma, synovitis of the joint, and general chondrolytic changes. The particular pathologic changes described usually accompany other intrinsic conditions of the knee.

Group III is primary malacia of the patella, usually a bilateral condition, without any demonstrable etiologic factor. These cases are puzzling. The examiner cannot rule out the effect of repeated trauma because the young patients are usually very physically active. These patients should be expected to traumatize the patella repeatedly. However, the simultaneous involvement of both knees, with relative lack of involvement of other chondral surfaces equally susceptible to trauma, prompts the examiner to seek a cause other than a simple contusion.

ORTHOPEDIC GAMUT 11-8

CHONDROMALACIA PATELLA

Factors that may cause chondromalacia patella include the following:

1. Any injury or anatomic abnormality that predisposes to an irregular pattern of movement of the patella
2. Meniscus injuries that alter normal tibiofemoral motion
3. Recurrent subluxation of the patella
4. Quadriceps imbalance
5. Patella alta
6. Angular deformities of the knee
7. Direct trauma to the patella

Careful evaluation of the anatomic development of the knee may give a definite indication of the cause of the idiopathic malacia. Patella alta is prone to alter the mechanism of the gliding surface of the patella on the trochlear groove and to contribute to the malacia. Lateral subluxation of the patella, as the knee comes into complete extension, may cause malacia of the patella without actually giving any evidence of gross displacement.

PROCEDURE

- The patient's knee is extended fully (Fig. 11-38).
- The examiner compresses the quadriceps muscles, at the superior pole of the patella (Fig. 11-39).
- The patient gently contracts the quadriceps muscles as the examiner resists the movement of the patella (Fig. 11-40).
- Retropatellar pain and failure to hold the contraction is considered positive.
- A positive test suggests chondromalacia patella.
- To test different parts of the patella, the knee should be tested in 30, 60, and 90 degrees of flexion and in full extension.

Confirmation Procedures

Apprehension test for the patella, Dreyer's sign, and Fouchet's sign

DIAGNOSTIC STATEMENT

Clarke's sign is present at the left knee. The presence of this sign indicates patellar chondromalacia.

CLINICAL PEARL

In examining the patella, the examiner should note any tenderness over the anterior surface and whether a bipartite ridge is present. Upper and lower pole tenderness occurs in Sinding-Larsen-Johannson disease and jumper's knee (an extensor apparatus traction injury).

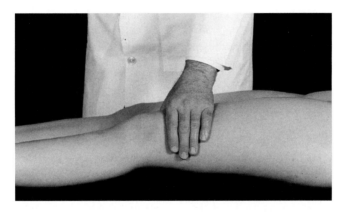

FIG. 11-38 The patient is lying supine with the affected knee extended. The examiner presses down with the web of the hand at a site that is slightly proximal to the upper pole or base of the patella.

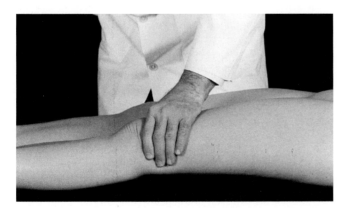

FIG. 11-39 The examiner pushes the patella into an inferior position, which stretches the quadriceps muscle and tendon.

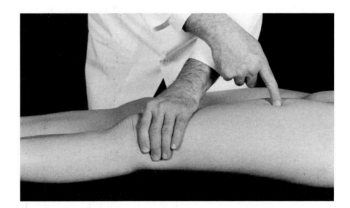

FIG. 11-40 The patient is instructed to contract the quadriceps muscle as the examiner restricts the movement of the patella by continuing to push down. If this maneuver causes retropatellar pain and the patient cannot hold the contraction, the test is positive. A positive test is significant for chondromalacia patellae.

DRAWER TEST

Assessment for Injury to Some Degree of (1) the Anterior Cruciate Ligament, Especially the Anteromedial Bundle; (2) the Posterolateral Capsule; (3) the Posteromedial Capsule; (4) the Medial Collateral Ligament, Especially the Deep Fibers; (5) the Iliotibial Band; (6) the Posterior Oblique Ligament; (7) the Arcuate-Popliteus Complex; and (8) the Posterior Cruciate Ligament (in Testing Posterior Drawer Movements)

Comment

Ligament injuries of the knee refers to various degrees of sprains that may lead to frank ruptures of the ligament, manifested by loss of joint function. Knee ligament sprains and joint instability are complex and sophisticated problems involving various degrees of straight-plane and/or combined rotatory instability.

ORTHOPEDIC GAMUT 11-9

KNEE LIGAMENT SPRAINS

Knee ligament sprains may be defined as follows:

1. Mild—grade I, first-degree ligament sprain: An incomplete stretching of collagen ligament fibers resulting in minimal pain, minimal or no swelling, no loss of joint function, and no clinical or functional instability.
2. Moderate—grade II, second-degree ligament sprain: A partial loss of ligament fiber continuity. A few collagen ligament fibers may be completely torn; however, most of the ligament remains intact. This degree of sprain is characterized by moderate (more intense than first-degree) pain, moderate swelling, some loss of joint function, and some loss of joint stability.
3. Severe—grade III, third-degree sprain (rupture): The entire collagen ligament fiber bundles are completely torn. There is no continuity within the body of the ligament. This is usually characterized by profound pain, intense swelling, loss of joint function, and instability.

Degrees of anterior cruciate instability are graded similarly to degrees of ligament sprains.

Damage to the ACL most commonly occurs as a sequel to tears of the medial meniscus. Many longitudinal meniscus

---

ORTHOPEDIC GAMUT 11-10

HUGHSTON INSTABILITIES

The following are Hughston joint instability indexes:

1. Mild instability: graded 1+; 5 mm or less of joint surface separation
2. Moderate instability: graded 2+; joint surface separation of 4 to 10 mm
3. Severe instability: graded 3+; joint surface separation of 10 mm or more

---

tears produce a block to extension of the joint. Attempts to obtain full extension lead to attrition rupture of the ligament. ACL tears also may accompany severe collateral ligament injuries.

Isolated ruptures of the ACL are uncommon and are not usually treated surgically unless they are accompanied by avulsion of the bone at the anterior tibial attachment. When the tear accompanies a meniscus lesion, the meniscus is preserved, if possible, to reduce the risks of tibial subluxation and secondary osteoarthritic changes. Nevertheless, the damage may be such that excision cannot be avoided. When an acute tear is associated with damage to the collateral ligaments, a combined repair or reconstruction is usually attempted. Problems from tibial subluxation are common, particularly when anterior cruciate tears are accompanied by damage to the medial or lateral structures. When anterior tibial subluxation is the main source of symptoms, surgical reconstruction may be indicated if simple measures, such as quadriceps strengthening, are not successful.

ORTHOPEDIC GAMUT 11-11

POSITIVE ANTERIOR DRAWER TEST

In a positive anterior drawer test, the following structures may have been injured to some degree:

1. ACL, especially the anteromedial bundle
2. Posterolateral capsule
3. Posteromedial capsule
4. MCL, especially the deep fibers
5. Iliotibial band
6. Posterior oblique ligament
7. Arcuate-popliteus complex

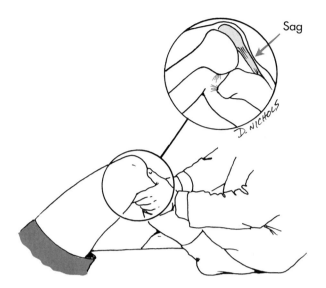

FIG. 11-41   Starting position of the anterior drawer test. If the posterior cruciate ligament is torn, the proximal tibia will be in a posterior tibial sag initial reference position. *(From Shankman GA: Fundamental orthopedic management for the physical therapist assistant, St Louis, 1997, Mosby.)*

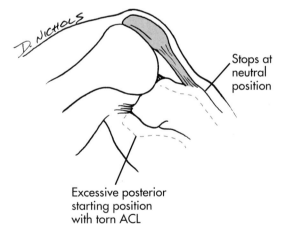

FIG. 11-42   A false-positive anterior drawer test can be seen when the tibia translates forward during the drawer test. *ACL*, Anterior cruciate ligament. *(From Shankman GA: Fundamental orthopedic management for the physical therapist assistant, St Louis, 1997, Mosby.)*

PCL tears are produced when the tibia is forcibly pushed backward while the knee is flexed (e.g., in a car accident in which the upper part of the leg strikes the dashboard). Surgical repair is always advised if the injury is seen at the acute stage. The persisting instability and osteoarthritis are the usual sequelae in the untreated case.

In this group of conditions, which are characterized by rotary instability in the knee, the tibia may subluxate forward or backward on either the medial or lateral side when the knee is stressed. This subluxation may cause pain and a feeling of instability in the joint.

Clinical examination of the PCL can be confusing. In the first test, the anterior and posterior drawer test, the tibia "sags" or subluxates posteriorly relative to the femur if the PCL is torn (Fig. 11-41). The examiner may produce a "false-positive" anterior drawer sign, wherein the posterior tibial sag is actually being reoriented to the neutral position rather than a true anterior translation occurring (Fig. 11-42).

The second test is more sensitive and is the Godfrey posterior tibial sag test. The patient is supine with the hip and knee of the affected limb held at 90 degrees. The examiner holds the heel of the affected limb and allows the tibia to translate, subluxate, or sag posteriorly by gravity (Fig. 11-43).

ORTHOPEDIC GAMUT 11-12

POSTERIOR CRUCIATE LIGAMENT TEARS

The following are the main forms of PCL tears:

1. The medial tibial condyle subluxates anteriorly (anteromedial instability).
2. The lateral tibial condyle subluxates anteriorly (anterolateral rotary instability).
3. The lateral tibial condyle subluxates posteriorly (posterolateral rotary instability).
4. Combinations of these lesions may be found.

ORTHOPEDIC GAMUT 11-13

POSITIVE POSTERIOR DRAWER TEST

In a positive posterior drawer test, the following structures may have been injured to some degree:

1. PCL
2. Arcuate-popliteus complex
3. Posterior oblique ligament
4. ACL

PROCEDURE

*   The patient's knee is flexed to 90 degrees.
*   The patient's foot is held on the table by the examiner.
*   The tibia is pulled forward on the femur, by placing hands around the tibia (Fig. 11-44).
*   Normal movement is approximately 6 mm.
*   When the tibia moves forward more than 6 mm on the femur, the test is positive.
*   To test the PCL, the tibia is pushed back on the femur (Fig. 11-45).
*   The test is positive when excessive movement is noted.

Confirmation Procedures
Lachman test, Lateral pivot shift maneuver, Losee test, and Slocum's test

---

DIAGNOSTIC STATEMENT

The Drawer test is positive for the left knee, and anterior instability is greater than 6 mm. This result indicates insufficiency of the ACL.

The Drawer test is positive for the left knee, and a posterior instability is greater than 6 mm. This result indicates insufficiency of the PCL.

CLINICAL PEARL

A tibia that is already displaced backward, as a result of a posterior cruciate tear, may give a false-positive result when the examiner is testing the anterior cruciate. This false-positive test may also occur with the Lachman test.

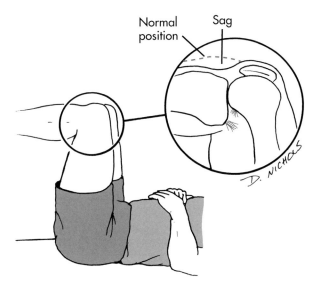

FIG. 11-43   Godfrey tibial sag. This is a clinically sensitive test to view the reference of the proximal tibia in relation to the distal femur with the leg flexed to 90 degrees. *(From Shankman GA: Fundamental orthopedic management for the physical therapist assistant, St Louis, 1997, Mosby.)*

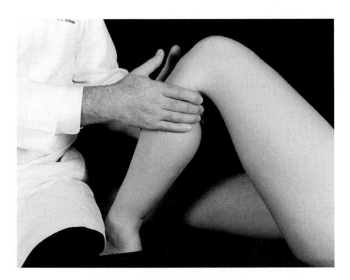

FIG. 11-44   The patient is lying supine; the knee is flexed to 90 degrees. The patient's foot is held on the table by the examiner. The tibia is pulled forward on the femur. Normal movement is approximately 6 mm. If the tibia moves forward more than 6 mm on the femur, the test is positive.

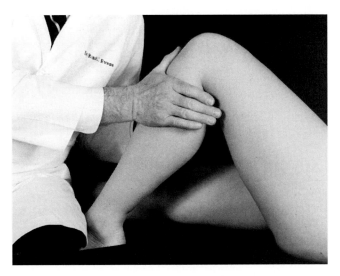

FIG. 11-45   Posterior movement of the tibia on the femur is assessed when the tibia is pushed posterior on the femur. If the test is positive, which is demonstrated by a large amount of posterior movement, (1) the posterior cruciate ligament, (2) the arcuate-popliteus complex, (3) the posterior oblique ligament, or (4) the anterior cruciate ligament may have been damaged.

DREYER'S SIGN

Assessment for Fracture of the Patella

Comment

Fractures of the patella usually result from a direct blow to the knee. They are classified as undisplaced or displaced (Fig. 11-46).

Fracture of the patella is not as common as chondral fractures of the patella. Fractures of either the superior or inferior pole or along the medial or lateral margins are usually either strain fractures or sprain fractures. The examiner should suspect chondral fracture to accompany stellate fracture of the patella without displacement.

Fracture of the patella by direct contusion is not uncommon. The fracture usually involves the lateral portion of the patella because the bone is thinner in this area. A fracture of the patella differs from the avulsion type, in which the fragment is torn away by the tension on the fragment. The avulsion fracture is usually on the medial side and occurs as the patella is forced laterally. A patellar fracture also differs from the explosive type of fracture that is caused by a forceful blow against the patella while the quadriceps are in violent contraction. This situation may occur when the knee hits the dashboard in a car accident. The contusion fracture results from to a sharp blow in a localized area. This same force may cause chondral damage.

The bipartite or tripartite patella should not be confused with acute injury. The partite patella is usually bilateral and symmetric and is asymptomatic. Careful examination will demonstrate that the symptoms are not in the area of the anomaly. It is possible for the quadriceps lateralis to avulse or partially avulse the separate piece, in which the condition will be symptomatic.

Bipartite patella occurs when the ossification centers of the patella fail to fuse. The defect is seen as a lucent line usually at the superolateral corner of the patella, where it may be mistaken for a fracture. Occasionally, the synchondrosis may fracture as a result of repetitive stress and cause pain and tenderness.

PROCEDURE

- While lying supine with the knee extended, the patient is unable to raise the leg (Fig. 11-47).
- When the examiner applies compression to the thigh, by using the hands to give anchorage to the quadriceps, the patient is able to lift the leg (Fig. 11-48).
- When this force is removed, the patient is again unable to raise the leg.
- The test is significant for a fracture of the patella.

Confirmation Procedures

Apprehension test, Clarke's sign, Fouchet's sign, and diagnostic imaging

---

DIAGNOSTIC STATEMENT

Dreyer's sign is positive for the left knee. The presence of this sign indicates a fracture of the patella.

CLINICAL PEARL

The quadriceps muscle gains insertion into the tibia through the medium of the patella, which is enclosed within the quadriceps expansion and the patellar tendon. Complete rupture may occur as a disruption through the patella. This area is the usual site of rupture for a common variety of fractured patella. The injury occurs mainly in adults of middle age.

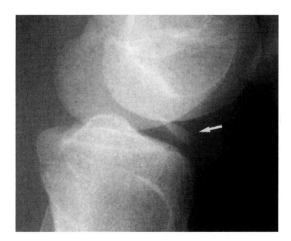

FIG. 11-46   Displaced fracture of the patella.   *(From Mercier LR, Pettid FJ:* Practical orthopedics, *ed 4, St Louis, 1995, Mosby.)*

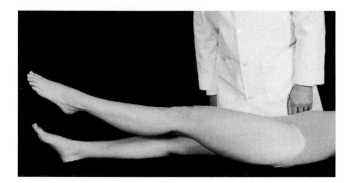

FIG. 11-47   The patient is lying supine with the knee extended. The patient attempts to raise the leg. In the presence of patellar fracture, this raising motion is painful and difficult to accomplish.

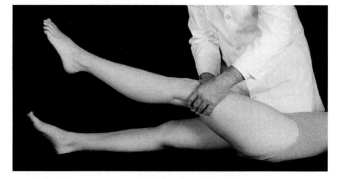

FIG. 11-48   The examiner applies forceful, circumferential grasp to the thigh with the hands, which give anchorage to the quadriceps. The patient attempts to lift the leg. The sign is present when the patient can lift the leg with minimal distress with the force applied, but when this force is removed, the inability to raise the leg recurs. The presence of the sign is significant for a fracture of the patella.

FOUCHET'S SIGN

Assessment for Patellar Tracking Disorder, Peripatellar Syndrome, or Patellofemoral Dysfunction

Comment

Pain arising from the anterior aspect of the knee joint is common in adolescence. Specific conditions, such as patella malalignment, osteochondritis dissecans, Osgood-Schlatter's disease, and trauma, may be responsible.

The patella is a pulley, and its excursion is controlled by the direction of action of the quadriceps group of muscles and the position of the tibial tubercle, which carries the patellar ligament.

The articular surface of the patella is divided into a large lateral and a small medial area. These areas are separated by a vertical, rounded ridge. During full extension, the shape of the patella fits into the trochlear surface of the femur. The ridge then lies in the hollow, or trough, of the trochlear surface. When the knee is flexed, the patella is carried downward and backward on the under aspect of the femur, where the trochlear surface is prolonged onto the inner condyle. During flexion, the patella tilts away from the lateral condyle, so only the inner part of its articular surface rests against the medial condyle.

So long as the tibial tubercle rotates smoothly, the patella travels its short course smoothly and under even tension. However, any derangement of the joint that prevents lateral rotation of the tibia during extension of the knee would affect the normal tension because contraction of the quadriceps would force the inner border of the patella against the medial condyle of the femur. This forced meeting explains the patellar symptoms and signs produced by certain cartilage injuries. Some of these symptoms and signs include retropatellar pain experienced during climbing and descending stairs, tenderness of the medial border of the patella, and the pattern of cartilage erosion that develops only on the medial surfaces of the patella and the femur. This pattern differs from that produced by retropatellar arthritis, which complicates recurring dislocation, when the lateral surface of the patellar cartilage undergoes fibrillation. Later, the medial surface is damaged from repeated drag over the lateral condyle of the femur during reduction. This repeated dragging results in erosion of the articular cartilage. By this time, both sides of the patella are tender.

ORTHOPEDIC GAMUT 11-14

PATELLOFEMORAL DISORDERS

Following are the pathomechanics of patellofemoral disorders:

1. Q angle (Fig. 11-49)
2. Lateral retinacular tightness (Fig. 11-50)
3. Vastus medialis obliquus deficiency (Fig. 11-51)
4. Lateral deviation of the patella at terminal extension (J sign) (Fig. 11-52)
5. Patella alta or infera (Fig. 11-53)
6. Trochlear depth (Fig. 11-54, *A*)
7. Congruence of the patellofemoral joint (Fig. 11-54, *B*)

PROCEDURE

- While the patient is lying supine and the knee is in full extension, the examiner uses the flat of a hand to compress the patella against the femur (Fig. 11-55).
- If this produces point tenderness and pain at the patellar margin, the sign is present.
- If pain is not produced by this maneuver, the examiner then rubs the patella transversely, against the femur.
- Audible or palpable grating and pain confirm the presence of the sign.
- When the patella has peripheral tenderness upon medial or lateral displacement, this is known as *Perkins' sign.*
- Perkins' sign is significant for patellar tracking disorder, peripatellar syndrome, or patellofemoral dysfunction.

Confirmation Procedures

Apprehension test for the patella, Clarke's sign, Dreyer's sign, and diagnostic imaging

DIAGNOSTIC STATEMENT

Fouchet's sign is present in the left knee. The presence of this sign indicates a patellar tracking disorder, peripatellar syndrome, or patellofemoral dysfunction.

CLINICAL PEARL

Placing a palm of the hand over the patella and the thumb and index finger along the joint line as the joint is flexed and extended will distinguish the source of the crepitus from damaged articular surfaces.

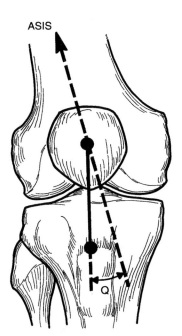

FIG. 11-49 The Q angle. Measure the Q angle *(Q)* with the knee straight, limb in neutral rotation, quadriceps relaxed, and the patella centered to the trochlea. It is the complementary angle of the angle formed from a line drawn from the anterosuperior iliac spine (ASIS) and a second line from the center of the patella to the center of the tibial tubercle. *(From Scott WN: The knee, vol 1-2, St Louis, 1994, Mosby.)*

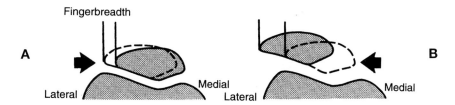

FIG. 11-50 Medial and lateral glide of the patella. **A,** Test for lateral retinacular contracture with knee flexed about 30 degrees and quadriceps relaxed. Push the patella medially; it should move at least one finger-width. **B,** For medial laxity, push the patella laterally. If the patient has experienced prior dislocation, excursion is excessive, and an apprehension response is likely. *(From Scott WN: The knee, vol 1-2, St Louis, 1994, Mosby.)*

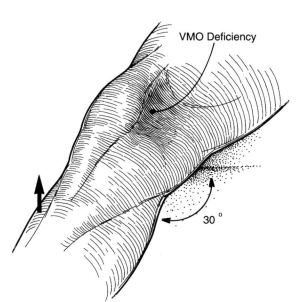

FIG. 11-51 Vastus medialis obliquus *(VMO)* deficiency is best seen as a hollow depression at the superomedial corner of the patella when the patient tries to extend the knee against resistance at about 30 degrees of flexion. *(From Scott WN: The knee, vol 1-2, St Louis, 1994, Mosby.)*

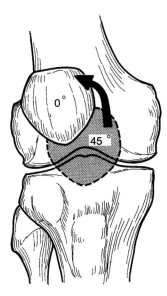

FIG. 11-52   The J sign. Normally, the patella remains centered during active terminal extension. If it deviates laterally in the shape of a J during its excursion from 45 degrees of flexion to 0 degrees of extension, it is abnormal. *(From Scott WN:* The knee, *vol 1-2, St Louis, 1994, Mosby.)*

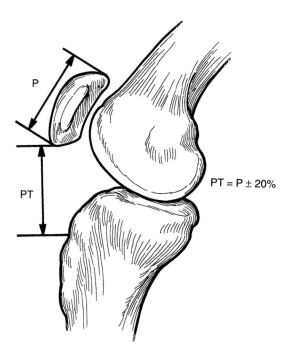

FIG. 11-53   Patella alta or infera. The length of the patellar tendon *(PT)* should equal the length of the patella *(P)* plus or minus 20%. *(From Insall J, Salvati E:* Radiology *101:101, Radiological Society of North America, 1971.)*

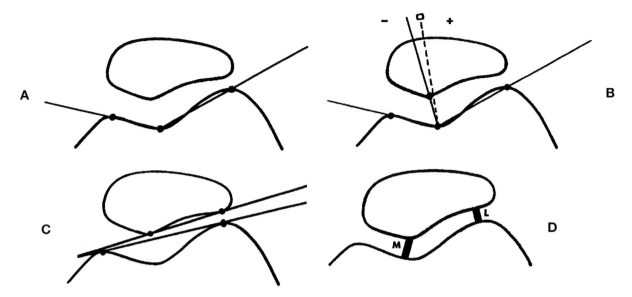

FIG. 11-54 Radiographic measurement of patellofemoral congruence. **A,** The sulcus angle, formed by the condyles and sulcus. Mean, 138 degrees; SD, 6 degrees. This measurement correlates well with instability. **B,** Congruence angle. A zero reference line bisects the sulcus angle; the angular distance of the articular ridge from that line is the congruence angle. Mean, –6 degrees; SD, 6 degrees. It measures subluxation. **C,** The lateral patellofemoral angle is the angle between the intercondylar line and the lateral facet. It should open laterally. It measures tilt with subluxation. **D,** Patellofemoral index. *M,* Closest distance between articular ridge and medial condyle; *L,* closest distance between lateral facet and condyle; *M/L ratio,* ≤1.6. The ratio measures tilt and subluxation. *(From Scott WN: The knee, vol 1-2, St Louis, 1994, Mosby.)*

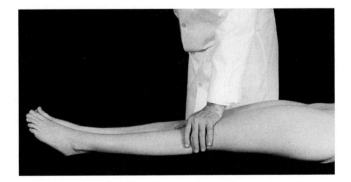

FIG. 11-55 The patient is lying supine, and the affected knee is in full extension. With the flat of a hand, the examiner compresses the patella against the femur. If this produces point tenderness and pain at the patellar margin, the sign is present. If no pain is produced, the patella is then rubbed transversely, against the femur. Audible or palpable grating and pain confirm the presence of the sign. The sign is significant for patellar tracking disorders, peripatellar syndrome, or patellofemoral dysfunction.

LACHMAN TEST

Assessment for Injury to Some Degree of (1) the Anterior Cruciate Ligament, Especially the Posterolateral Bundle, (2) the Posterior Oblique Ligament, and (3) the Arcuate-Popliteus Complex

Comment

Ligamentous injuries to the knee are among the most serious of all knee disorders. Because of the importance of the ligaments in stabilizing the joint, early diagnosis of the injury is mandatory. Any delay in diagnosis and treatment may lead to a chronically unstable knee, which predisposes the individual the knee to early traumatic arthritis.

The mechanism is usually one of forceful stress against the knee while the extremity is bearing weight. A valgus stress against the knee may sprain or tear the MCL; a varus stress will injure the lateral collateral ligament. Tears of the cruciate ligaments, menisci, and capsule also may occur with the collateral ligament injury.

The history of a ligamentous injury is often difficult to reconstruct, but it will provide clues to the type of force applied to the knee. After the injury, the extremity's ability to bear weight is often lost. Swelling from an acute ligament or capsular tear is usually immediate and results from hemorrhage. A pop or tearing sensation may be heard or felt. Incomplete tears or sprains are often more painful than complete ligamentous ruptures.

Patients with chronically unstable knees from old injuries often complain of the knee going out or giving way or crepitus when walking and of not being able to depend on the extremity. These symptoms are always most noticeable during vigorous activities. A chronic effusion is often present.

With an acute injury, the examination is of utmost importance. Any swelling or discoloration is noted. The lesion can often be localized by palpation alone. The palpation should begin away from the suspected area to promote patient cooperation. A point of maximum tenderness is often present along the course of the collateral ligament or capsule.

The knee should always be tested for stability while the patient is in a relaxed, supine position. If the examination cannot be adequately performed because of pain or hamstring spasm, it may have to be repeated while the patient is under local or general anesthesia. The injured knee is always compared with the opposite, uninvolved knee.

The Lachman test is similar to the anterior drawer test, But in this test, the knee is held in 20 degrees of flexion, and the tibia is pulled forward on the femur. An increase in this anterior translation suggests an ACL tear (Fig. 11-56). The Lachman test is thought to be a better indicator of injury to the ACL. If there is a soft or "mushy" feel and the infrapatellar slope disappears when the tibia is moved forward on the femur, the Lachman test is positive. This sign indicates damage to the ACL, especially the posterolateral band.

PROCEDURE

- The patient is supine.
- The patient's knee is held between full extension and 30 degrees of flexion.
- The patient's femur is stabilized with one hand as the tibia is moved forward (Fig. 11-57).
- A mushy, or soft, end-feel when the tibia is moved forward on the femur and the infrapatellar tendon slope disappears is a positive sign.
- A positive sign suggests damage to (1) the ACL, especially the posterolateral bundle; (2) the posterior oblique ligament; and (3) the arcuate-popliteus complex.

Confirmation Procedures

Drawer test, lateral pivot shift maneuver, Losee test, and Slocum's test

---

DIAGNOSTIC STATEMENT

Lachman test is positive for the right knee. This result indicates injury to the ACL.

CLINICAL PEARL

When both medial and lateral or both anterior and posterior, as well as the medial and lateral, compartments are torn, combined complex instability exists. Transitory dislocation, or at least subluxation of the knee, is a preliminary symptom. In many instances, the peroneal nerve has been injured.

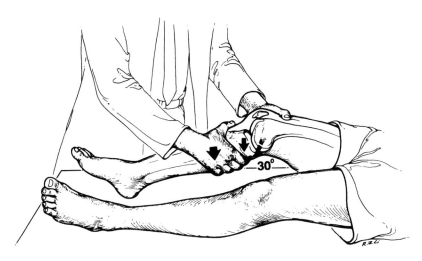

FIG. 11-56   The posterior Lachman test.   *(From Tria AJ, Klein KS:*
Illustrated guide to the knee, *New York, 1991, Churchill Livingstone.)*

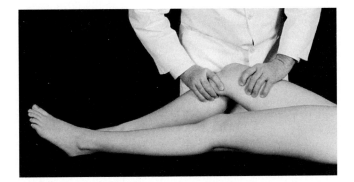

FIG. 11-57   The patient is supine. The patient's knee is held
between full extension and 30 degrees of flexion. The patient's
femur is stabilized with one hand as the tibia is moved forward.
A mushy or soft end-feel when the tibia is moved forward on
the femur and the infrapatellar tendon slope disappears is a
positive sign.

LATERAL PIVOT SHIFT MANEUVER

ALSO KNOWN AS TEST OF MCINTOSH

**Assessment for Injury to Some Degree
of (1) the Anterior Cruciate Ligament,
(2) the Posterolateral Capsule,
(3) the Arcuate-Popliteus Complex,
(4) the Lateral Collateral Ligament,
and (5) the Iliotibial Band**

Comment

Lateral instabilities of the knee may involve both varus and rotational instabilities. The rotation instabilities are anterolateral rotary instability, which involves a lateral tibial plateau that displaces anteriorly, and posterolateral instability, which involves a lateral tibial plateau that displaces posteriorly. The most commonly encountered lateral instability is the anterolateral rotary instability. A lateral rotary instability is called the *lateral pivot shift,* which should not be confused as something other than anterolateral rotary instability. Clinically, this instability is characterized by a sensation that the knee "gives way" as the patient decelerates suddenly and pivots on the involved extremity.

Anterolateral instability is created by incompetency of the ACL, incompetency of the midlateral capsule, some degree of laxity of the arcuate ligament, and occasionally laxity of the iliotibial tract. If the iliotibial tract has been stretched or injured, the McIntosh-type testing for anterolateral rotary instability will not be positive in eliciting the classic jumping sensation. With most anterolateral instabilities, the iliotibial tract is intact, and the instability can be more graphically demonstrated with some form of the McIntosh test. The lateral pivot shift maneuver is the primary test used to assess anterolateral rotary instability of the knee. During this test, the tibia moves away from the femur on the lateral side and moves anteriorly in relation to the femur.

The McIntosh test (lateral pivot shift maneuver) is a duplication of the anterior subluxation-reduction phenomenon that occurs during the normal gait cycle when the ACL is torn. The test illustrates a dynamic subluxation. This shift occurs at between 20 and 40 degrees of flexion. (Zero degrees occurs when the knee is in the extended position.)

It is this phenomenon that gives the patient the clinical description of feeling that the knee gives way.

The pivot shift test of Galway begins with the knee in full extension. The tibia is held in internal rotation with valgus force. The thumb is placed behind the fibular head, and the knee is brought into flexion. As flexion occurs, the tibia is brought forward on the anterolateral side. With further flexion, the tibia reduces with a clunk (Fig. 11-58).

Losee modified the jerk test in an attempt to accentuate the subluxation (Fig. 11-59). The knee begins in flexion but with the tibia externally rotated. The valgus force is applied, and then the knee is extended with gradual internal rotation of the tibia (Fig. 11-60). The clunk of the reduction occurs in the last few degrees from full extension.

PROCEDURE

- The patient is supine.
- The examiner flexes the knee slightly (5 degrees) (Fig. 11-61).
- A valgus stress is applied to the knee while maintaining a medial rotation torque on the tibia and at the ankle (Fig. 11-62).
- The leg is flexed 30 to 40 degrees. The tibia reduces or jogs backward.
- The patient experiences the sensation of the knee "giving way" (Fig. 11-63).
- This is the positive finding.
- To some degree (1) the ACL, (2) the posterolateral capsule, (3) the arcuate-popliteus complex, (4) the lateral collateral ligament, or (5) the iliotibial band has been injured.

Confirmation Procedures

Drawer test, Losee test, and Slocum's test

DIAGNOSTIC STATEMENT

The lateral pivot shift maneuver is positive for the right knee. This result indicates injury to the ACL.

CLINICAL PEARL

Normally, the knee's center of rotation changes constantly through its range of motion as a result of the shape of the femoral condyles, the ligamentous restraint, and the muscle pull. A positive pivot shift test usually suggests damage to the anterior cruciate, the posterior capsule, or the lateral collateral ligament.

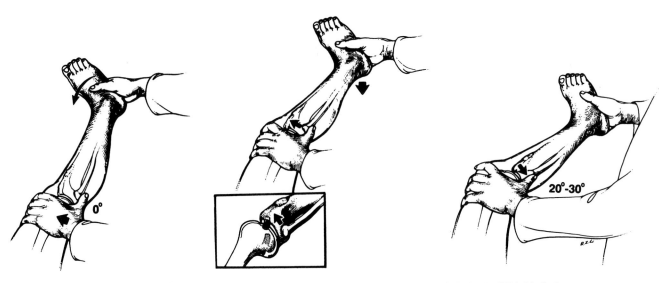

FIG. 11-58 The pivot shift test. *(From Scott WN: The knee, vol 1-2, St Louis, 1994, Mosby.)*

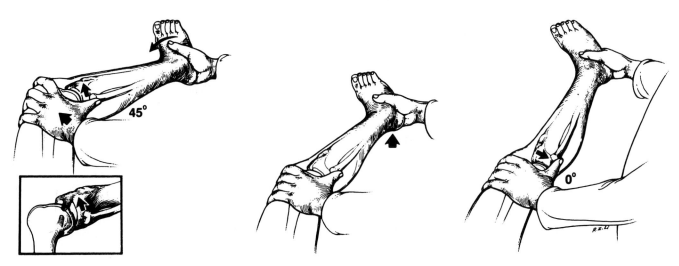

FIG. 11-59 The jerk test begins with the knee in flexion. *(From Scott WN: The knee, vol 1-2, St Louis, 1994, Mosby.)*

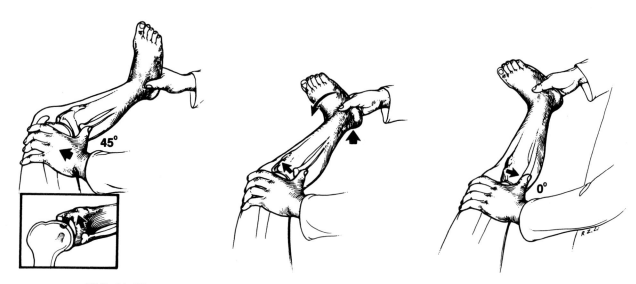

FIG. 11-60   The Losee test begins with the knee in flexion.   *(From Scott WN: The knee, vol 1-2, St Louis, 1994, Mosby.)*

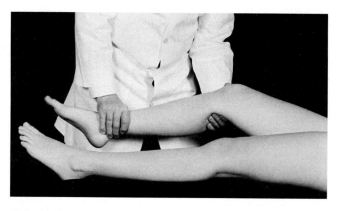

FIG. 11-61   The patient is supine. The examiner flexes the knee slightly (5 degrees).

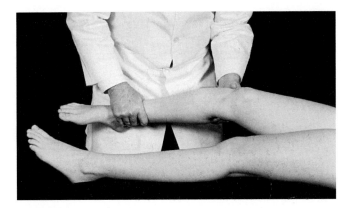

FIG. 11-62   A valgus stress is applied to the knee while maintaining medial rotation torque on the tibia and the ankle.

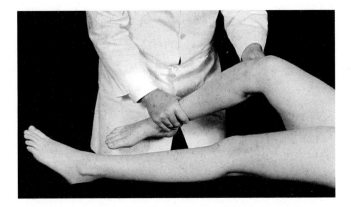

FIG. 11-63   The leg is flexed 30 to 40 degrees. The tibia reduces or jogs backward. The patient experiences the knee "giving way." If the test is positive, the following structures have been injured: (1) the anterior cruciate ligament, (2) the posterolateral capsule, (3) the arcuate-popliteus complex, (4) the lateral collateral ligament, or (5) the iliotibial band.

LOSEE TEST

Assessment for Anterolateral Rotary Instability of the Knee

Comment

There are four primary mechanisms of injury to the ligaments of the knee. Valgus stress with the knee in slight flexion is by far the most common pattern (Fig. 11-64). The ACL is torn in the midsubstance in 75% of cases (Fig. 11-65). The next most common injury is hyperextension. The third most common pattern occurs with the knee flexed and with a posteriorly directed force to the anterior aspect of the knee (Fig. 11-66). The fourth pattern is the varus stress (Fig. 11-67).

The most serious injuries to the knee involve instability. Forceful overrotation of the flexed knee while the leg is fixed may disrupt many parts of the knee.

Simple instability denotes that only one compartment of the knee is involved. The medial complex structures, such as the MCL, can be torn without involving the posterior capsule and can produce a valgus deformity or one-plane laxity. This laxity can result from a blow to the side of the leg or from a fall from a height. Immediate pain, a feeling of weakness, and valgus laxity are the cardinal signs. The MCL usually tears at its upper pole. Motion may not be particularly affected for the first 12 hours, but motion is later impeded by hemarthrosis. Clinically, medial laxity of the joint is what determines the diagnosis.

Lateral instability of the simple type involves primarily varus rather than rotational laxity. However, pure lateral instability is unusual. When present, the lateral ligament and usually the iliotibial band and the popliteal tendon are torn. In both instances, the patient feels a pop, and the knee becomes quite wobbly. Pain during flexion is localized to the upper end of the fibula and over the joint line. The lateral side of the knee is slightly lax in flexion.

Acute anterolateral instability occurs when the leg is hit from the posterior side, while the foot is planted, with the tibia internally rotated and the strain placed on the lateral side. A part of the lateral complex, the anterior cruciate, and the lateral meniscus are torn. Internal-external rotation is increased, but an intact PCL prevents backward tibia displacement. An anterior Drawer test will be positive, and lateral laxity is present.

PROCEDURE

- The patient is in a supine position.
- The patient's leg is externally rotated.
- The patient's knee is flexed to 30 degrees (Fig. 11-68).
- The examiner hooks a thumb behind the fibular head.
- A valgus force is applied to the knee.
- The knee is extended, and forward pressure is applied behind the fibular head with the examiner's thumb (Fig. 11-69).
- The leg moves into medial rotation.
- If there is a "clunk" forward just before full extension of the knee, the test is positive.
- This clunk means that the tibia has subluxed anteriorly and indicates injury to the same structures listed with the lateral pivot shift maneuver.
- The Losee test assesses anterolateral rotary instability.

Confirmation Procedures

Drawer test, lateral pivot shift maneuver, and Slocum's test

DIAGNOSTIC STATEMENT

The Losee test is positive for the left knee. This result indicates anterolateral rotary instability of the knee.

CLINICAL PEARL

If rotary instability is present, then as full extension is reached, a dramatic clunk will occur as the lateral tibial condyle subluxates forward. The patient should relate this to the sensations experienced during activity.

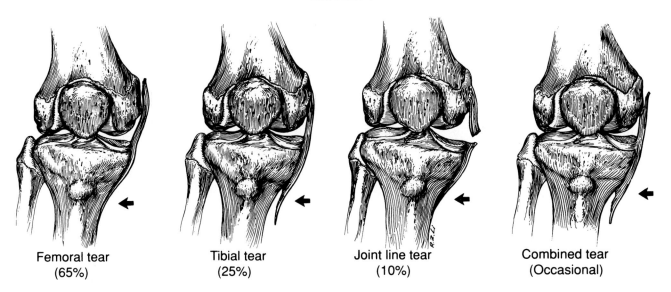

Femoral tear
(65%)

Tibial tear
(25%)

Joint line tear
(10%)

Combined tear
(Occasional)

FIG. 11-64   The distribution of medial collateral ligament disruptions.   *(From Scott WN: The knee, vol 1-2, St Louis, 1994, Mosby.)*

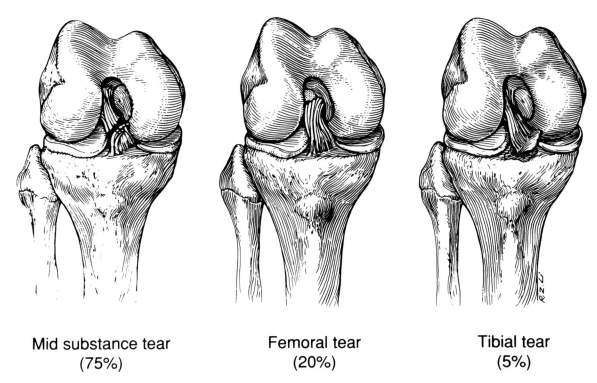

Mid substance tear
(75%)

Femoral tear
(20%)

Tibial tear
(5%)

FIG. 11-65   The distribution of anterior cruciate ligament disruptions.   *(From Scott WN: The knee, vol 1-2, St Louis, 1994, Mosby.)*

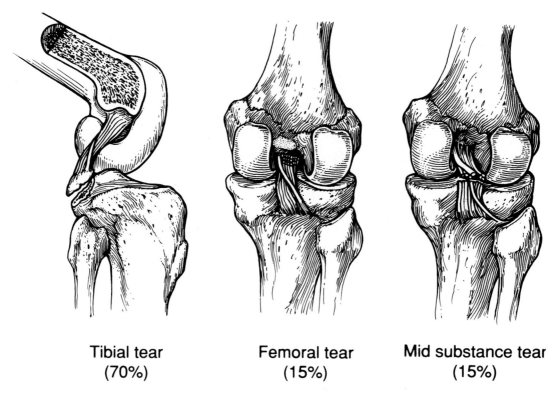

Tibial tear
(70%)

Femoral tear
(15%)

Mid substance tear
(15%)

FIG. 11-66   The distribution of posterior cruciate ligament disruptions.   *(From Scott WN: The knee, vol 1-2, St Louis, 1994, Mosby.)*

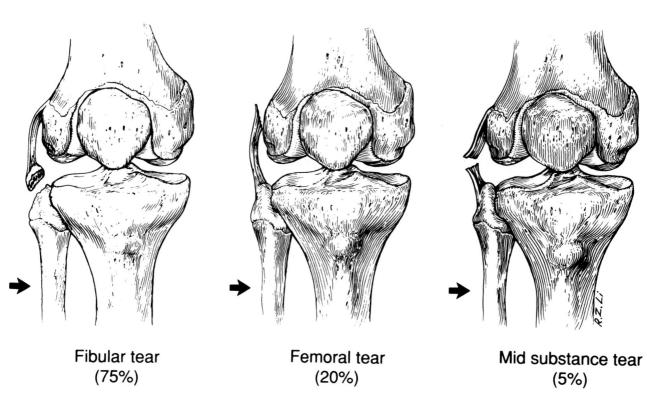

Fibular tear
(75%)

Femoral tear
(20%)

Mid substance tear
(5%)

FIG. 11-67   The distribution of lateral collateral ligament disruptions.   *(From Scott WN: The knee, vol 1-2, St Louis, 1994, Mosby.)*

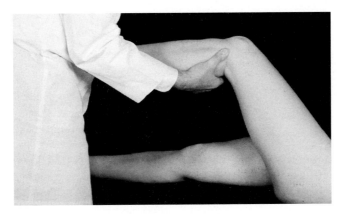

FIG. 11-68 The patient is lying supine, and the knee is extended and relaxed. The examiner holds the patient's leg externally rotated. The knee is then flexed to 30 degrees.

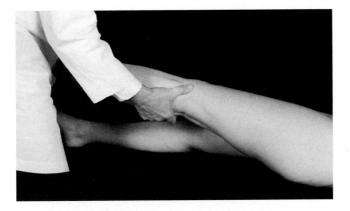

FIG. 11-69 The examiner hooks a thumb behind the fibular head. A valgus force is applied to the knee. The examiner extends the patient's knee and applies forward pressure behind the fibular head with the thumb. The leg is allowed to move into medial rotation. If a "clunk" is heard or felt just before full extension of the knee, the test is positive. This clunk means that the tibia has subluxed anteriorly.

McMURRAY SIGN

Assessment for Medial or Lateral Meniscus Injury

Comment

Injuries of the menisci are common in males younger than 45. A tear is usually caused by a twisting force while the knee is semiflexed or flexed. This tear is usually the result of an athletic injury, but it is also common among males who work in a squatting position, such as coal miners and flooring installers. The medial meniscus is torn much more often than the lateral.

There are three types of tears. All of these tears begin as longitudinal splits. If this split extends throughout the length of the meniscus, it becomes a bucket-handle tear, in which the fragments remain attached at both ends. This tear is the most common type. The bucket handle, the central fragment, is displaced towards the middle of the joint, so the condyle of the femur rolls upon the tibia through the rent in the meniscus. Because of the shape of the femoral condyle, it requires the most space when the knee is straight. The main effect of a displaced bucket-handle fragment is that it limits full extension (locking).

If the initial longitudinal tear emerges at the concave border of the meniscus, a pedunculated tag is formed. With a posterior horn tear, the fragment remains attached at the posterior horn. With an anterior horn tear, the fragment remains attached to the anterior horn. A transverse tear through the meniscus is nearly always an artifact.

The menisci are almost avascular. Consequently, when the menisci are torn, there is not an effusion of blood into the joint. However, there is an effusion of synovial fluid, which is secreted in response to the injury. Major tears of the menisci do not heal spontaneously, probably because the torn surfaces are separated by fluid (Fig. 11-70).

The patient is usually 18 to 45 years old. This history is characteristic, especially with bucket-handle tears. In consequence of a twisting injury, the patient falls and has pain at the anteromedial aspect of the joint. The patient is either unable to continue the activity or does so with difficulty. The patient is unable to straighten the knee fully. The next day, the patient notices swelling of the whole knee. The knee is rested, and during the next 14 days, the swelling decreases. The knee straightens, and the patient resumes activities. Within weeks or months, the knee suddenly gives way again during a twisting movement. Pain and swelling occur as before. Similar incidents occur repeatedly.

Locking means inability to extend the knee fully and is not a true jamming of the joint because there is free range of flexion. Locking is a common feature of a torn medial meniscus, but the limitation of extension is often so slight that the patient does not notice it. Persistent locking can occur only in bucket-handle tears. Tag tears cause momentary catching, but not locking in the true sense.

The meniscal tears described are uncommon in patients older than 50, which is when the menisci begin to show degenerative changes. A degenerative meniscus suffers a different type of lesion. The medial meniscus, in particular, may split horizontally, at a point that is often near the middle of its convexity. Such a split is usually of small dimensions. Because there is no separation of the fragments, natural healing can occur.

Clinically, there is troublesome and persistent pain at the medial aspect of the knee at the joint level. The pain may be noticed after a minor injury, but it often comes on spontaneously, without any preceding incident. In the early stages, there is usually a small effusion of fluid into the joint.

PROCEDURE

- The patient is lying supine, and the thigh and leg are flexed until the heel approaches the buttock (Fig. 11-71).
- One of the examiner's hands is on the knee, and the other is on the heel (Fig. 11-72).
- The examiner internally rotates and slowly extends the leg (Fig. 11-73).
- The examiner then externally rotates and slowly extends the leg.
- McMurray sign is present if, at some point in the arc, a painful click or snap is heard.
- This sign is significant in meniscal injury.
- The point in the arc where the snap is heard locates the site of injury of the meniscus.
- If noted with internal rotation, the lateral meniscus will be involved.
- The higher the leg is raised when the snap is heard, the more posterior the lesion is in the meniscus.
- If noted with external rotation, the medial meniscus will be involved.

Confirmation Procedures

Bounce home test, Childress duck waddle test, Payr's sign, and Steinmann's sign

---

DIAGNOSTIC STATEMENT

McMurray sign is present in the left knee. The presence of this sign indicates injury to the medial meniscus.

McMurray sign is present in the left knee. The presence of this sign indicates injury to the lateral meniscus.

CLINICAL PEARL

The examiner should observe for tenderness in the joint line and test for a springy block to full extension of the knee. These two signs, in association with evidence of quadriceps atrophy, are the most consistent and reliable signs of a torn meniscus.

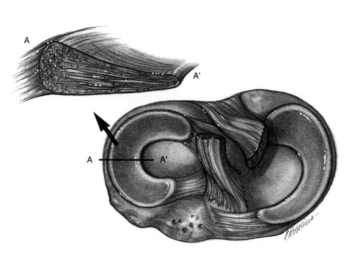

FIG. 11-70   Diagrammatic representation of the cross-sectional anatomy of the meniscus. *(From Scott WN: The knee, vol 1-2, St Louis, 1994, Mosby.)*

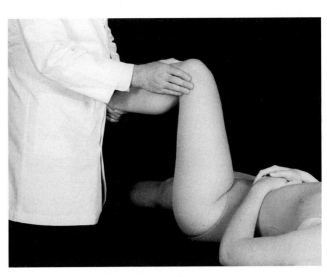

FIG. 11-71   The patient is lying supine. The examiner flexes the thigh and leg to 90 degrees, respectively.

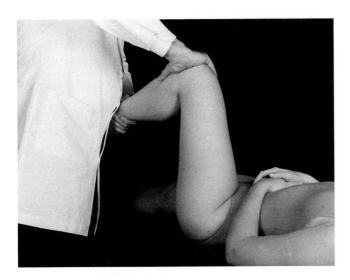

FIG. 11-72   The examiner places one hand on the knee; the other hand grasps the patient's heel.

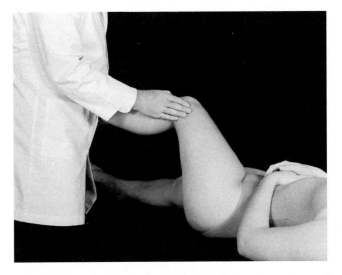

FIG. 11-73   The examiner internally rotates the lower leg and then slowly extends the knee, applying valgus pressure to the joint. The examiner then externally rotates the leg and slowly extends it. The test is positive if, at some point in the arc, a click or snap that causes pain is heard. This test is significant for a meniscal injury. If the click is noted with internal rotation, the lateral meniscus is involved. If the click is noted with external rotation, the medial meniscus is involved. The higher the leg is raised when the snap is heard, the more posterior the lesion is.

Assessment for Iliotibial Band Friction Syndrome

Comment

The biceps femoris and the iliotibial band are both active in stabilizing the fully extended knee. Contraction of these muscles is a preliminary to strong action by the extensors of the knee. In the initial stages of contraction, until the quadriceps group of muscles has shortened sufficiently to exert full power, the position and stability of the knee must be controlled by the action of the biceps femoris and the iliotibial band. The biceps femoris tendon is inserted into the head of the fibula with the fibular collateral ligament, but the iliotibial band finds insertion into the tibia through the lateral capsule and into the fibula through the lateral ligament. The biceps femoris muscle is also a flexor of the knee, and both the biceps femoris and iliotibial band play a part in external rotation of the tibia. With paralytic contracture of the knee, the iliotibial band may indeed be the main contributor to the flexion-external rotation deformity.

However, the most important function of the biceps femoris and iliotibial band is probably to stabilize the fibular component of the leg during weight bearing. Through their attachments, the biceps femoris and iliotibial band exert control on the superior tibiofibular joint. When the knee is fully extended, rotation of the tibia on the femur is impossible. Also the weight-bearing knee cannot indulge in any change of its exact ratio of flexion-extension to rotation. The flexion and extension movements of the ankle and inversion and eversion of the foot do not take place in isolation in the ankle and the subtalar and midtarsal joints. The foot and ankle movements require a component of rotation in the leg. This necessary movement must take place in the inferior and superior tibiofibular joints, a factor more easily appreciated when it is realized that the increasing width of the articular surface of the talus needs posterior changing accommodation in the ankle mortise. Indeed, one might generalize by saying that most actions of the weight-bearing leg are accomplished by adaptive movements of all the joints of the leg, from the hip downward. The coordination of the joints, whether stationary or in motion, is a fundamental part of bodily posture and movement.

Iliotibial band friction syndrome (runner's knee) occurs in runners as a result of overuse. It tends to occur in patients with genu varum and planus feet. The symptoms are of pain over the lateral epicondyle of the femur during running and are thought to be caused by friction between the iliotibial band and the femur and may be caused by an inflamed bursa.

Tenderness is found over the lateral epicondyle. The symptoms usually settle with rest, but in resistant cases, a corticosteroid injection into the tender site may help.

In sports in which repetitive knee flexion past 30 degrees is required, the iliotibial band is especially susceptible to irritation. Therefore this syndrome is typically observed in runners and has been described as the "jogger's knee," but football players and cyclists also present this exertional pain syndrome. Most often, the initiation of the pain syndrome is related to running or cycling as part of training.

ORTHOPEDIC GAMUT 11-15

ILLIOTIBIAL BAND FRICTION SYNDROME

Following are illiotibial band friction syndrome extrinsic and intrinsic factors.

Extrinsic Factors

1. Running or cycling on an oblique surface causing a pelvic tilt
2. Sudden increase in running or cycling distance
3. Improper seating with cleats too far internally rotated or a saddle that is not well positioned

Intrinsic Factors

1. Varus knee deformity that predisposes for this friction syndrome between the lateral femoral epicondyle and the overriding iliotibial band
2. Leg-length discrepancy
3. Forefoot pronation

PROCEDURE

- The patient is in a supine position.
- The patient's hip and knee are flexed 90 degrees (Fig. 11-74).
- The examiner applies thumb pressure to the lateral femoral condyle (Fig. 11-75).
- The patient's knee is extended as the thumb pressure is maintained.
- In the positive test, the patient will complain of severe pain over the lateral femoral condyle, near 30 degrees of flexion (Fig. 11-76).
- This indicates iliotibial band syndrome.

Confirmation Procedures

Patella ballottement test, Q-angle test, thigh circumference test, and Wilson's sign

CLINICAL PEARL

This syndrome produces a line of tenderness that extends from the anterolateral tibia, across the joint line, and up the side of the thigh. Tenderness is usually maximal over the lateral femoral condyle, and a painful arc occurs at about 30 degrees of flexion.

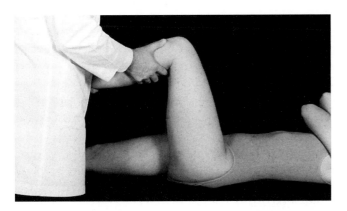

FIG. 11-74   The patient is supine. The patient's knee and hip are flexed to 90 degrees.

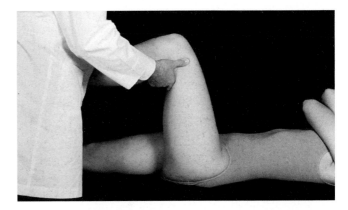

FIG. 11-75   The examiner applies thumb pressure to the lateral femoral condyle.

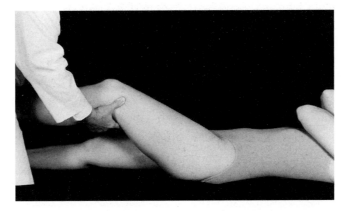

FIG. 11-76   The patient's knee is extended as thumb pressure is maintained. In the positive test, the patient will complain of severe pain over the lateral femoral condyle near 30 degrees of flexion. This indicates iliotibial band syndrome.

PATELLA BALLOTTEMENT TEST

Assessment for Joint Effusion

Comment

The swollen knee is the result of conditions that create an inflammatory response of the synovial membrane. The basic inflammatory process in each condition is similar, and if left to proceed unhindered, the process results in secondary degenerative changes of the joint. The differential diagnosis of these conditions is difficult at the onset, but with sufficient information, the diagnosis usually becomes apparent.

Undoubtedly, trauma is the most common cause of effusion within the knee joint. Effusion is caused by intrinsic factors, such as internal derangements that damage the synovial membrane, creating bleeding within the joint, or from extrinsic factors, such as a direct blow to the knee or a twisting injury. In most instances of trauma, the history is sufficient to make a diagnosis of a traumatic effusion or hemarthrosis. However, such a history may not be apparent in the infant or young child, who is unable to communicate. It also is not apparent in the adult in whom the effusion is secondary to microtrauma. The microtrauma may be secondary to some activity related to the patient's occupation, such as one requiring the repeated use of the knee to perform a certain maneuver or repeated minor blows to the knee, which may not be of any significance to the patient.

Effusion can have its beginnings as a traumatic synovitis, which creates synovial effusion that leads to rest and immobility with resultant quadriceps atrophy. The loss of muscle protection makes the knee more susceptible to the minor trauma of everyday use. Recurring injury creates repeated synovial effusions and sets up a vicious cycle that promotes chronic synovitis. A patient with this condition experiences a painful, swollen knee that is held in a semiflexed position, the position of maximum comfort. The suprapatellar pouch may be distended and quite tense. The patella is ballottable. The knee may be somewhat warm, but it does not give the appearance of a septic joint. Motion is resisted because attempts at flexion or extension create more tension, which causes pain within the joint.

The test for small effusions in the knee joint is called the *bulge sign*. The medial aspect of the knee is "milked" upward two to three times to displace fluid. The lateral margin of the knee is pressed (Fig. 11-77). A positive bulge sign will demonstrate a swelling or bulge of fluid in the area medial to the patella. The bulge sign, useful for assessing small effusions, is often absent in large effusions.

Differentiation of traumatic hemarthrosis from traumatic synovitis can be a diagnostic problem. Swelling from a traumatic hemarthrosis begins within a few minutes after the injury, whereas a traumatic synovial effusion begins several hours after the injury and progresses more slowly. The aspiration of blood from the joint confirms a traumatic hemarthrosis, and fat globules that float in the blood indicate an interarticular fracture as well. A traumatic synovial reaction may have synovial fluid that appears normal but, in some instances, is tinged with blood. The joint is somewhat warmer to the touch than usual but does not have the warmth or redness of the skin that is found with acute septic arthritis.

Rheumatoid arthritis of the knee should be evaluated and treated in the context of a systemic disease involving multiple organs and joints (Fig. 11-78). Rarely are the knee symptoms the initial presentation, and patients most often are taking medication for rheumatoid arthritis.

Other causes of acute inflammation should be excluded. These include crystal arthropathy, hemophilia, and infection. Acute infection is not uncommon in the knee joint in patients taking immunosuppressive medication for rheumatoid arthritis, and knee aspiration with culture of the joint fluid may be indicated.

PROCEDURE

- The patient's knee is extended.
- A slight tap or pressure is applied over the patella (Fig. 11-79).
- This test is positive if a large amount of swelling in the knee is detected.

Confirmation Procedures

Fouchet's test, Q-angle test, thigh circumference test, and Wilson's sign

---

DIAGNOSTIC STATEMENT

Patella ballottement confirms the existence of intraarticular swelling in the left knee.

CLINICAL PEARL

If popliteal swelling is found, it is possible to confirm communication with the joint by massaging its contents back into the main synovial cavity while the knee is in flexion. The examiner maintains pressure on the popliteal fossa, extends the knee, and then removes the pressure. The swelling will not reappear until the patient flexes the knee several times, confirming a valvelike communication between the main cavity and the "cyst."

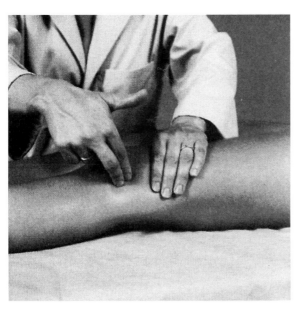

FIG. 11-77 Testing for the bulge sign. After "milking" the medial aspect of the knee, the lateral side of the patella is tapped. The medial side is then observed for the presence of a bulge. *(From Barkauskas VH, et al:* Health & physical assessment, *ed 2, St Louis, 1998, Mosby.)*

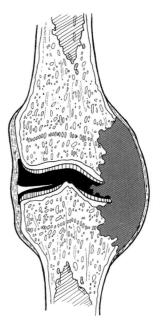

FIG. 11-78 Diagram of the knee showing hypotrophy of the synovium and bony erosion and osteoporosis seen in rheumatoid arthritis. *(From Bucholz RW:* Orthopaedic decision making, *ed 2, St Louis, 1996, Mosby.)*

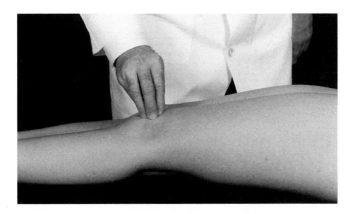

FIG. 11-79 The patient is supine with the knee extended. Pressure is applied over the patella. A floating sensation of the patella is a positive finding and indicates a large amount of swelling in the knee.

PAYR'S SIGN

Assessment for Injury of the Posterior Horn of the Medial Meniscus

Comment

The medial meniscus is shaped like a C. Its anterior attachment is on top of the tibia near the midline and in front of the tibial spines. The posterior attachment is on top of the tibia, behind the tibial spines. In each case, the attachment is near the periphery of the tibia, so the two ends are widely separated from each other. The meniscus is attached by the coronary ligament (which has its origins around the top of the tibia) to the MCL and then to the tibia. This attachment is firm, and although it does allow a little movement, extensive motion is not permitted in the normal medial meniscus.

In sprain of the MCL, the tibia and femur separate on the medial side, and stress is applied in the area of the attachment of the meniscus to the MCL. The cartilage may be forced to accompany either the femur or the tibia, depending on the location of the ligament injury. Because the structure of the meniscus does not allow much flexion stress, it will tear transversely or, more commonly, split around its periphery. If the tear is actually in the attachment to the ligament, it may heal. If the tear is within the substance of the meniscus, it will not. Meniscus injury accompanies repeated sprains of the knee more often than it does the initial, single sprain. With an acute injury, there is no way to determine whether the meniscus is torn unless the knee is locked. If the knee is locked and the ligaments are stable, the episode is the first. If the meniscus has been detached at its periphery, this attachment may heal. This possibility is much more likely if the meniscus has slipped into the knee, locked, and then immediately unlocked.

PROCEDURE

- The patient is in the Turkish Pasha seated position, with the feet and ankles crossed (Fig. 11-80).
- The examiner applies downward pressure on the knee joint (Fig. 11-81).
- Pain is elicited on the medial side of the joint when the sign is present.
- The test is significant when a lesion of the posterior horn of the medial meniscus is present.

Confirmation Procedures

Bounce home test, Childress duck waddle test, McMurray sign, and Steinmann's sign

---

DIAGNOSTIC STATEMENT

Payr's sign is present in the right knee. This sign indicates injury to the posterior horn of the medial meniscus.

CLINICAL PEARL

Meniscal cysts lie in the joint line, feel firm during palpation, and are tender to deep pressure. Cysts of the menisci may be associated with tears. Lateral meniscus cysts are by far the most common. Cystic swellings on the medial side are sometimes caused by ganglions that arise from the pes anserinus (insertion of the sartorius, gracilis, and semitendinosus).

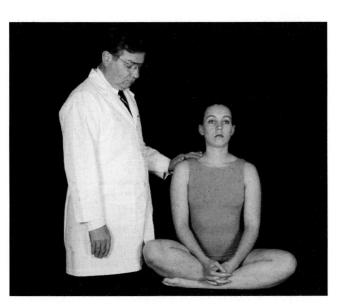

FIG. 11-80   The patient is in the Turkish Pasha seated position, with the feet and ankles crossed.

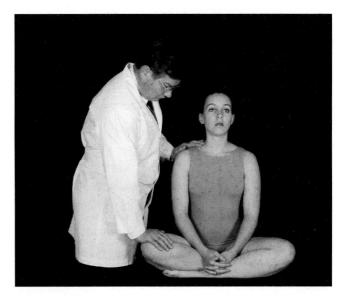

FIG. 11-81   The examiner applies downward pressure on the affected knee joint. Pain is elicited on the medial side of the joint when the sign is present. The sign is present when there is a lesion of the posterior horn of the medial meniscus.

Q-ANGLE TEST

Assessment for Patellofemoral Dysfunction, Patella Alta, Subluxating Patella, Increased Femoral Anteversion, Genu Valgum, or Increased Lateral Tibial Torsion

Comment

The true, congenital dislocation of the patella implies actual and constant dislocation of the patella. This dislocation is usually lateral to the femoral condyle. If fully developed, this condition will interdict athletic participation. Of much greater importance is the dislocation that occasionally occurs under certain circumstances. This type of dislocation results from repeated episodes of acute dislocation in a normal knee. There is no true congenital dislocation, but certain physical characteristics predispose an individual to subluxation or luxation. One predisposing anatomic condition is an abnormally acute angle between the axis of the patellar tendon and the axis of the quadriceps mechanism, the Q angle.

The angle formed by a line drawn from the anterosuperior iliac spine to the center of the patella and a line drawn from the center of the patella to the tibial tubercle is called the Q angle (Fig. 11-82). In a normal knee, the Q angle measures approximately 15 degrees, and an angle exceeding 20 degrees is abnormal.

If the patellar tendon tends to angulate sharply and laterally to reach its tibial attachment, this angulation, combined with a quadriceps mechanism that tends to angulate medially at the knee, results in an increased angle between the patellar tendon and the long axis of the quadriceps tendon. As the quadriceps muscle is contracted, there is a tendency for this angle to straighten by slipping the patella laterally. This action may be inhibited anteriorly by the prominence of the lateral femoral condyle. The general tendency is for the patella to slide laterally with each forceful extension of the knee. The female, with a widened pelvis and internally angulated femora, is much more prone to patellar subluxation or dislocation than the male. A similar situation arises in patients with tibial torsion or genu valgum. A dislocated patella in a patient with genu varum is uncommon, because in such a patient, the axis of the patellar tendon and the quadriceps muscle is parallel. However, in some genu varum patients, this bow is part of the internal torsion of the femur, so the femoral condyles are rotated toward the midline. Such a patient often has an associated external rotation of the tibia to compensate and straighten the long axis of the leg. In this instance, the Q angle may be markedly more acute as the patellar tendon moves from the internally rotated patella down to the externally rotated patellar tubercle.

PROCEDURE

- To determine the Q angle, a line is drawn from the anterosuperior ilial spine to the midpoint of the patella and from the tibial tubercle to the midpoint of the patella (Fig. 11-83).
- The angle formed by the intersection of these two lines is the Q angle (Fig. 11-84).
- Normally, the Q angle is 13 to 18 degrees. The normal angle for males is 13 degrees, and for females it is 18 degrees.
- Less than 13 degrees suggests patellofemoral dysfunction or patella alta.
- Greater than 18 degrees suggests patellofemoral dysfunction, subluxating patella, increased femoral anteversion, genu valgum, or increased lateral tibial torsion.

Confirmation Procedures

Noble compression test, patella ballottement test, thigh circumference test, and Wilson's sign

---

DIAGNOSTIC STATEMENT

The Q angle of the right knee is less than 13 degrees and suggests patellofemoral dysfunction or patella alta.

The Q angle of the right knee is greater than 18 degrees and suggests patellofemoral dysfunction, subluxating patella, or increased tibial torsion.

CLINICAL PEARL

In children, an increased Q angle presents as genu valgum. The examiner must note whether the genu valgum is unilateral or, as is usual, bilateral. The severity of the deformity is recorded by measuring the intermalleolar gap. The examiner grasps the child's ankles and rotates the legs until the patellae are vertical. The legs are brought together to touch lightly at the knees. A measurement is made between the malleoli. Serial measurements, often every 6 months, are used to check progress. Note that with growth, a static measurement is an angular improvement.

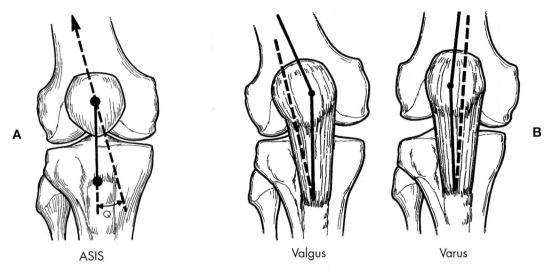

FIG. 11-82 **A,** The Q angle, which may indicate patellar tracking problems, is formed by two lines, one drawn from the anterior superior iliac spine through the center of the patella, and the second line drawn from the tibial tubercle to the center of the patella. **B,** Valgus and varus measurement of the Q angle. *(From Scott WN: The knee, vol 1, St Louis, 1994, Mosby.)*

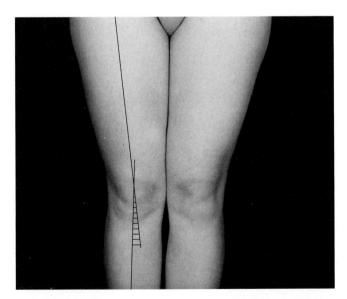

FIG. 11-83 To determine the Q angle, a line is drawn from the anterosuperior iliac spine to the midpoint of the patella and from the tibial tubercle to the midpoint of the patella. The angle formed by the intersection of these two lines is the Q angle. Normally, the Q angle is 13 to 18 degrees (13 degrees for males and 18 degrees for females). Less than 13 degrees suggests patellofemoral dysfunction or patella alta.

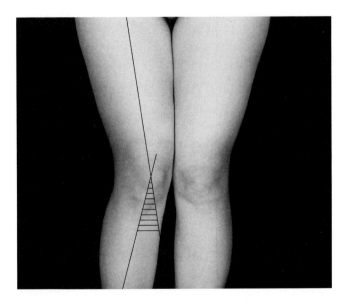

FIG. 11-84 Greater than 18 degrees suggests patellofemoral dysfunction, subluxating patella, increased femoral anteversion, genu valgum, or increased lateral tibial torsion.

SLOCUM'S TEST

Assessment for Anterolateral Rotary Instability, with Injury to Some Degree of (1) the Anterior Cruciate Ligament, (2) the Posterolateral Capsule, (3) the Arcuate-Popliteus Complex, (4) the Lateral Collateral Ligament, (5) the Posterior Cruciate Ligament, and (6) the Iliotibial Band (Tensor Fascia Lata)

Comment

Anterolateral rotatory instability is the most common type of instability to occur with ACL rupture. When the ligament is ruptured, the tibia is able to move forward and internally rotate on the femur. This subluxation of the lateral tibial condyle occurs at between 15 and 20 degrees of knee flexion, causing the pivot shift phenomenon. *Pivot shift* is simply the term used to describe the phenomenon of subluxation or reduction of the tibia on the femur in a knee with anterolateral rotary instability. This subluxation is what the patient describes as the knee "giving way."

The cruciate ligaments are valuable stabilizers of the knee. These ligaments not only assist in knee flexion and extension but also limit rotation, extension, and flexion. The ACL varies in length. The ligament is taut when the knee is in full extension and when the knee is externally rotated at the femorotibial joint. The ligament remains taut until 5 to 20 degrees of flexion, at which point it relaxes. The ligament is most relaxed at 40 to 50 degrees of flexion and becomes taut again when the knee flexes to 70 to 90 degrees.

Internal rotation increases the tension of the ACL even when the knee is flexed to 40 or 50 degrees. External rotation increases the tautness of the ligament as does abduction of the knee. Anterior shear of the tibia upon the femur is permitted to 5 mm of distance, but then is checked. Excessive external rotation can tear the ACL, especially if there is added abduction. Hyperextension and anterior shear may tear this ligament. With the knee flexed to 90 degrees and externally rotated, the first limiting soft tissue that tears is the medial capsular ligament. With further rotation and abduction, the next tissue to tear is the tibial MCL, and then the ACL tears. Isolated tears of the ACL, when they do happen, probably occur from a posterior force, which causes shear stress but also may occur from internal rotation.

The ACL can be torn as an isolated injury that is the result of an acute deceleration from a sharp stop-and-cut movement. As the forward motion of the patient is abruptly halted, the quadriceps muscle decelerates the leg and simultaneously pulls the tibia forward upon the femur. This shearing disrupts the ACL. With the abrupt stop, the patient often makes a rapid rotation, or cut, to form the direction of movement. This rotation places anterior shear and rotatory stress on the knee. The rotational stress depends on the direction of the cut. After a jump, the knee absorbs the impact by being slightly flexed. Thus shear also occurs at this point because of deceleration. The patient who makes the stop and cuts or jumps feels a pop as the knee gives way. Swelling occurs within 3 or 4 hours.

PROCEDURE

- The patient is in a supine position.
- The knee is flexed to 80 or 90 degrees; the hip is flexed to 45 degrees.
- The foot is internally rotated.
- The foot is held as the tibia is pulled anteriorly.
- Movement will occur on the lateral side of the knee if the test is positive.
- This indicates anterolateral rotatory instability.
- Excessive movement suggests injury to (1) the ACL, (2) the posterolateral capsule, (3) the arcuate-popliteus complex, (4) the lateral collateral ligament, (5) the PCL, or (6) the iliotibial band.
- The test also may be performed while the patient is seated with the knees flexed over the edge of the examination table (Fig. 11-85).
- The examiner pulls or pushes the tibia to the knee while medially or laterally rotating the foot (Fig. 11-86).
- Pulling the tibia tests for anterior rotary instability. Pushing the tibia tests for posterior rotary instability.

Confirmation Procedures

Drawer test, lateral pivot shift maneuver, Losee test, and Lachman test

---

DIAGNOSTIC STATEMENT

Slocum's test is positive on the right. This result indicates anterolateral rotary instability of the knee.

Slocum's test is positive on the right. This result indicates anteromedial instability of the right knee.

CLINICAL PEARL

This maneuver tightens the lateral capsule, giving enough stability to eliminate the anterior drawer sign. If the anterior drawer sign is still positive while the patient is in this position (most anterior movement occurring on the lateral side), it is likely that the lateral capsule (or lateral collateral ligament) is also damaged.

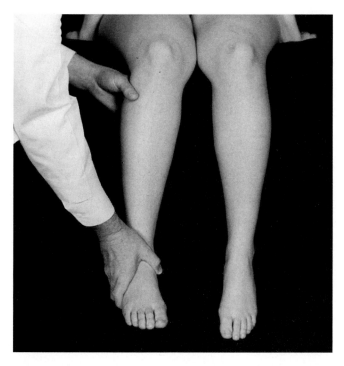

FIG. 11-85 The patient is seated with the knees flexed and hanging over the edge of the examination table.

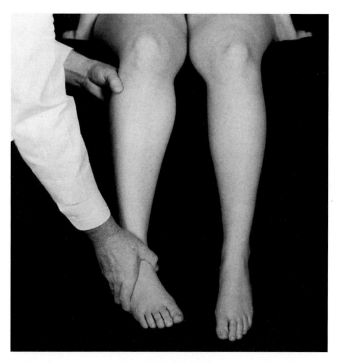

FIG. 11-86 The examiner pulls or pushes the tibia while the foot is medially or laterally rotated. Anterior tibial force tests for anterior rotary instability. Posterior tibial force tests for posterior rotary instability. Excessive movement is a positive test, which indicates cruciate ligament instability.

STEINMANN'S SIGN

ALSO KNOWN AS STEINMANN'S TENDERNESS DISPLACEMENT TEST

Assessment for Lateral or Medial Meniscus Tear

Comment

During normal movements of the knee, the anterior mobile portion of the medial semilunar cartilage slides slightly backward, into the interior of the joint, as flexion occurs. If the joint is simultaneously abducted, the medial side of the joint is opened, and the mobility of the cartilage is increased further. Turning of the trunk toward the opposite side produces a movement of external rotation on the fixed tibia in relation to the femur. The medial meniscus is forced toward the back of the joint, and the MCL becomes taut.

The ligament initially steadies the posterior part of the cartilage. If the MCL can withstand the strain, the anterior mobile part of the meniscus is injured, and either of the following may occur. The anterior part of the ligament may be detached where it joins with the fixed posterior portion. The ligament may sustain any variety of transverse or oblique tears.

A fragment may slip into the interior of the joint. When the knee is extended and an attempt is made to screw the condyle home, the fragment is impacted between the condyles, and the joint locks. When the medial rotator strain is more severe, the collateral ligament is stretched to such an extent that the attachment between it and the meniscus is destroyed. With even more severe strain, the ligament may become avulsed from its tibial attachment and from the cartilage. In either of the two cases, the whole cartilage slips into the interior of the joint. When the knee is extended, the free border is trapped between the condyles, and a longitudinal split occurs in the substance of the meniscus to form the bucket-handle tear.

Detachment or longitudinal tears of the posterior horn are caused by forceful lateral rotation of the femur on the fixed tibia, when the rotation is combined with flexion.

Although the lateral semilunar cartilage is much less frequently injured than the medial cartilage, tears and displacements do occur. The mechanism is the opposite of that which damages the medial cartilage.

ORTHOPEDIC GAMUT 11-16

MENISCUS TEAR

The following are three factors leading to meniscus tear:

1. The knee must be bearing weight.
2. The knee must be flexed.
3. There must be a rotation strain.

PROCEDURE

- Knee pain moves anteriorly when the knee is extended (Fig. 11-87) and moves posteriorly when the knee is flexed (Fig. 11-88).
- The movement of pain is the positive sign.
- This indicates a meniscus tear.
- Medial pain is elicited by lateral rotation.
- Lateral pain is elicited by medial rotation.

Confirmation Procedures

Bounce home test, Childress duck waddle test, McMurray sign, and Payr's sign

---

DIAGNOSTIC STATEMENT

Steinmann's sign is present in the left knee. The presence of this sign indicates a medial meniscus tear.

Steinmann's sign is present in the left knee. The presence of this sign indicates a lateral meniscus tear.

CLINICAL PEARL

Patients use "locking" to describe episodes of severe pain in the knee or even collapsing of the knee. It is curious that the word is not applied in this way to any other joints. "Locking" denotes mechanical jamming of the knee joint and nothing more.

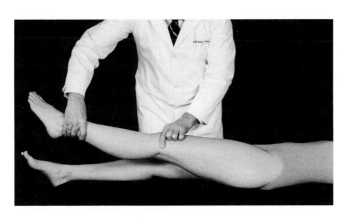

FIG. 11-87   The patient is lying supine with the knee extended. With one hand, the examiner grasps the leg at the ankle and palpates for tenderness at the knee joint with the other hand.

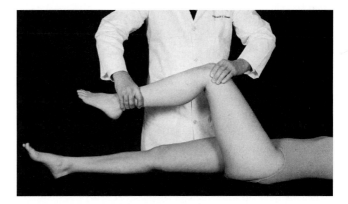

FIG. 11-88   If the pain is found during initial palpation while the knee is extended and if the pain moves posteriorly as the knee is flexed, the sign is present. The sign indicates a meniscal tear.

THIGH CIRCUMFERENCE TEST

Assessment for Muscle Hypertonicity or Hypotonicity of the Thigh

Comment

The quadriceps and, to a lesser extent, the hamstrings rapidly atrophy after injury to the cartilage and the ligaments of the knee. This reaction varies in degree and is caused by disturbance of the neurotrophic relationships between the joint and its controlling musculature. Muscle bulk, tone, and control are diminished rapidly and in some instances severely. This diminishment is not caused by muscle inactivity alone, although this factor does aggravate both atrophy and weakness. Conscientious muscle exercise cannot prevent but does minimize muscle atrophy. Although effusion remains, atrophy is generalized, but the tendency is for the medial vasti to show greater atrophy in sympathy with a medial meniscus injury. Lateral ruptures are associated with atrophy of the lateral vastus.

The vastus medialis obliquus is often the first part of the muscle to waste. The circumference of the thigh 10 cm above the upper pole of the patella should be measured and compared with the other side; this gives an objective measure of thigh wasting. The presence of swellings around the knee should be noted. Swelling within the synovial cavity is seen above the patella and on either side of the patella and patella tendon (Fig. 11-89).

Although muscle weakness is present, effusion persists and is increased with any activity beyond the power and the endurance of the residual muscle bulk. In turn, the effusion affects the trophic reflexes and further atrophy occurs.

Displacement of a meniscus remains and, despite arduous exercise, muscle bulk and tone cannot recover significantly. If the cartilage is reduced or removed so that the knee recovers full movement, then exercise will increase both power and bulk of the muscle.

The bulk of the quadriceps muscle is a sensitive guide to the presence of knee-joint pathology. If necessary, measure the thigh of each leg at a comparable distance from the joint margin. In effusion, swelling will extend from the suprapatellar region down either side of the patella (Fig. 11-90). In osteoarthritis, bony swellings around the joint and secondary quadriceps wasting are common (Fig. 11-91). The popliteal fossa is the site for posterior synovial protrusions (Baker's cysts) (Fig. 11-92).

A varus deformity means that the distal component of a joint is deviated toward the midline. In contrast, a valgus deformity means that the distal member of a joint is deviated away from the midline (Fig. 11-93).

PROCEDURE

- An area of the thigh 10 cm above the patella is identified (Fig. 11-94).
- The circumference of the leg at that point is measured and compared with the opposite leg (Fig. 11-95).

Confirmation Procedures

Noble compression test, patella ballottement test, Q-angle test, and Wilson's sign

---

DIAGNOSTIC STATEMENT

The thigh circumference test indicates increased muscle bulk dimension on the left when compared with the right.

The thigh circumference test indicates decreased muscle bulk dimension on the left when compared with the right.

CLINICAL PEARL

Although all the quadriceps muscle atrophies uniformly, atrophy of the bulky vastus medialis (particularly in a fit young male) may be the most conspicuous. Quadriceps atrophy is a difficult sign to detect, particularly in the middle-aged, elderly, and female patients. Some asymmetry of muscle bulk is common.

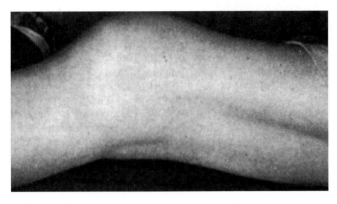

FIG. 11-89 Synovitis of the knee. *(From* Mosby's medical, nursing, and allied health dictionary, *ed 5, St Louis, 1998, Mosby.)*

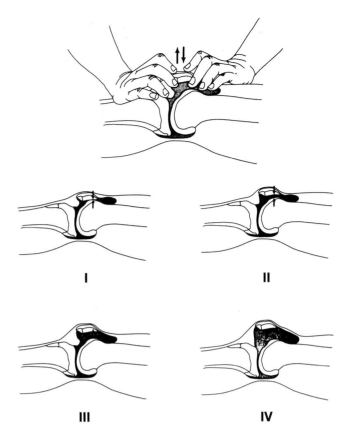

FIG. 11-90 Effusions of the knee can be graded from I to IV. *(From Scott WN:* The knee, *vol 1, St Louis, 1994, Mosby.)*

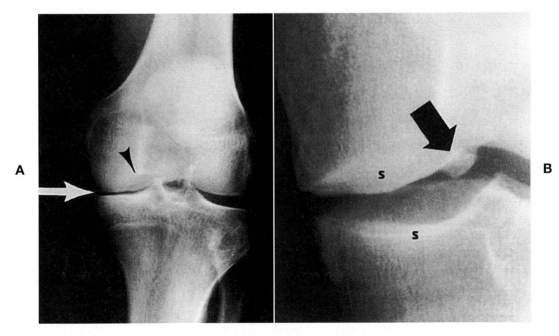

FIG. 11-91 **A** and **B,** Osteoarthritis of the knee is characterized by predominant narrowing of the medial femorotibial compartment *(white arrow)* with genu varus, marginal osteophytosis *(black arrow),* subchondral sclerosis *(s),* and cyst formation *(arrowhead).* *(From Sartoris DJ:* Musculoskeletal imaging: the requisites, *St Louis, 1996, Mosby.)*

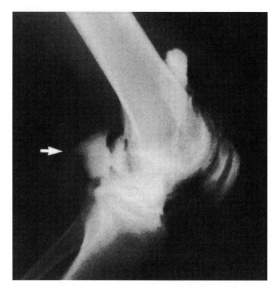

FIG. 11-92   Arthrogram revealing a large popliteal cyst.   *(From Mercier LR:* Practical orthopedics, *ed 5, St Louis, 2000, Harcourt Health Sciences.)*

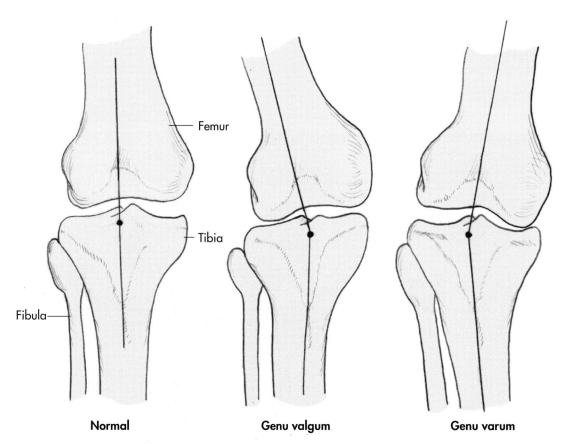

FIG. 11-93   Valgus and varus deformities at the knee joint. A valgus deformity is one in which the distal element of a joint is deviated laterally (away from the midline). A varus deformity is one in which the distal element of a joint is deviated medially (toward the midline).   *(From Mathers LH, et al:* Clinical anatomy principles, *St Louis, 1996, Mosby.)*

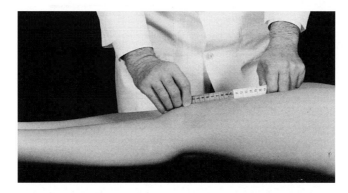

FIG. 11-94   An area of the thigh 10 cm above the patella is identified.

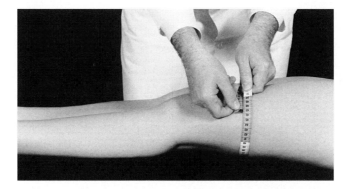

FIG. 11-95   The circumference of the muscle at that point is measured and recorded. This is compared with the uninvolved leg.

WILSON'S SIGN

Assessment for Osteochondritis Dissecans of the Knee

Comment

Loose bodies, or joint mice, are most commonly osteocartilaginous fragments of traumatic origin. They are typically from tangential osteochondral fractures. However, joint mice can also originate from pathologic processes, such as osteochondritis dissecans. Other types of loose bodies may consist of chondral fragments (pieces of articular cartilage), remnants of menisci, foreign bodies, fibrous tissues, and interarticular tumors. Some loose bodies may obtain a synovial attachment, but it is more common for them to remain loose in the joint. A tangential osteochondral fragment, with its normal bone, is more likely to become attached to the synovium than is a fragment from osteochondritis dissecans, with its necrotic bone fragment. Fragments of articular cartilage can enlarge as these are nourished by the synovial fluid. Small, loose bodies are more likely to cause symptoms than larger ones because the former may be more easily impinged between the articular surfaces.

ORTHOPEDIC GAMUT 11-17

LOOSE BODY IN THE KNEE

The most likely origins for a loose body in the knee are the following:

1. Osteochondritis dissecans at the lateral border of the medial femoral condyle (males).
2. Marginal fracture that is from the lateral margin of the lateral femoral condyle and is secondary to direct trauma or patellar dislocation (males).
3. Medial tangential osteochondral fracture of the patella from dislocation (males).
4. This order is reversed in the female patient.

On diagnostic imaging, a fragment of avascular bone is seen that is demarcated from the adjacent femur by a radiolucent line. Occasionally, a loose body may be present (Fig. 11-96).

Osteochondritis dissecans is an ischemic condition that involves the subchondral bone and is probably either the result of or in association with repeated trauma to the area. The involved area of ischemic bone demarcates and may eventually separate with the overlying articular cartilage. This separation leaves behind a defect, a fragment that becomes a loose body within the joint. The knee is the most commonly involved joint, and the incidence is higher in males than in females.

ORTHOPEDIC GAMUT 11-18

OSTEOCHONDRITIS DISSECANS

The most common sites for osteochondritis dissecans in the knee are the following:

1. The lateral border of the medial femoral condyle
2. The inferior, central area of the lateral femoral condyle
3. The inferior, central region of the medial femoral condyle

---

Osteochondritis dissecans occurs at the classic site and is caused by repeated trauma to the area from contact with a prominent medial tibial spine. The central lesions in the femoral condyles are usually associated with a meniscal lesion that traumatizes the area. Often, there is a family history of osteochondritis dissecans, and it is not unusual for both knees to be involved.

Classically, the problem occurs in a teenage male, who complains of pain and a giving way of the knee. There may be effusion and transient episodes of locking as opposed to the more persistent locking that is seen with a torn meniscus. Before the fragment separates, there is nothing diagnostic about the complaints. After the fragment separates, episodes of transient locking are frequent, and the patient may be aware of something loose in the knee.

PROCEDURE

- The patient is in a supine position.
- The knee is flexed to 90 degrees by the examiner.
- The knee is extended with the tibia medially rotated.
- Near 30 degrees of flexion, pain in the knee increases (the patient often stops the rotating movement) (Fig. 11-97).
- If the tibia is rotated laterally, the pain disappears (Fig. 11-98).
- This is a positive test.
- The positive test indicates osteochondritis dissecans of the femur.

814

Confirmation Procedures

Noble compression test, patella ballottement test, Q-angle test, and thigh circumference test

---

DIAGNOSTIC STATEMENT

Wilson's sign is present in the right knee. The presence of this sign indicates osteochondritis dissecans of the knee.

CLINICAL PEARL

Patients with loose bodies give a classic account of a loose fragment in the knee and will usually be able to describe its size and shape. Loose bodies are sometimes called *joint mice,* which is an appropriate description because these loose bodies can be recognized instantly, but they disappear and may be impossible to find again. Loose bodies should not be called *foreign bodies.* Foreign bodies, including bullets and bits of gravel, come from outside the body and are rare in joints.

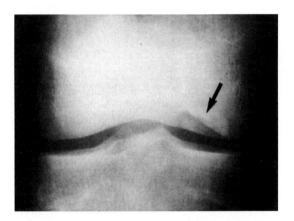

FIG. 11-96   Osteochondritis dissecans of the knee.   *(From Mercier LR, Pettid FJ:* Practical orthopedics, *ed 4, St Louis, 1995, Mosby.)*

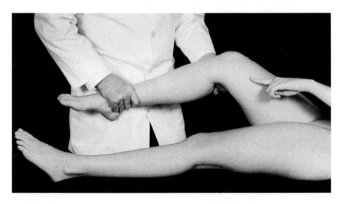

FIG. 11-97   The patient is supine. The knee is flexed to 90 degrees by the examiner. The knee is extended with the tibia medially rotated. Near 30 degrees of flexion, the pain in the knee increases. The patient attempts to stop the movement.

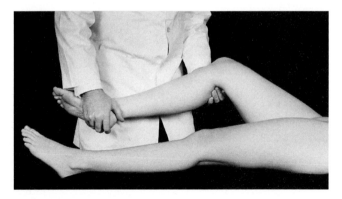

FIG. 11-98   The tibia is rotated laterally, and the pain disappears. This disappearance of pain indicates that the sign is present, which suggests osteochondritis dissecans of the femur.

CRITICAL THINKING

Classify disruptions of knee ligamentous structures.
Grade I: mild sprain—microscopic disruption of the ligamentous structure but no loss of integrity
Grade II: moderate sprain—partial disruption of ligamentous fibers with structures still intact
Grade III: severe sprain—complete disruption of ligamentous integrity

What is the triad of O'Donoghue?
Medial meniscus tear, rupture of the anterior cruciate ligament, rupture of the medial collateral ligament

How is the Q angle measured?
The quadriceps angle is formed by two lines, one projecting from the anterosuperior iliac spine to the midpatella and the second from the midpatella to the tibial tubercle.

How is posterior cruciate ligament injury tested?
A posterior drawer test is performed in a similar fashion to the anterior drawer test, except that a posterior force is applied on the proximal tibia.

What is the usual mechanism of injury for a meniscal tear?
Rotational force as the flexed knee moves toward an extended position

What is the most common meniscal tear?
Longitudinal tear of the posterior horn of the medial meniscus

How is McMurray test performed?
With the knee completely flexed, the leg is externally rotated as far as possible; then the knee is slowly extended. As the femur passes over a tear in the medial meniscus, a painful click or pop is felt or heard if the test is positive. The lateral meniscus is checked by palpating the posterolateral margin of the joint, internally rotating the leg as far as possible, and slowly extending the knee while listening and feeling for a click.

What is the most common congenital meniscal anomaly?
A discoid lateral meniscus

How is the Lachman test performed?
The Lachman test is performed in approximately 15 to 30 degrees of flexion. The femur is stabilized with the examiner's hand. The opposite hand is used to apply an anteriorly directed force to the posterior tibia while stabilizing the femur. The examiner senses any tibial displacement and compares it with the uninvolved knee.

What is the posterior sag test?
The posterior sag test detects the amount of posterior displacement caused by gravity when the knee and hip are flexed to 90 degrees.

What is varus deformity?
The clinical appearance is bow-leggedness, which causes the mechanical axis to go through or inside the medial compartment of the knee.

What is valgus deforming of the knee?
The weight-bearing axis falls outside the lateral compartment of the knee. The patient appears knock-kneed.

What is osteochondritis dissecans?
Osteochondritis dissecans is a disorder of one or more ossification centers with sequential degeneration and/or aseptic necrosis and recalcification.

List the common sites of osteochondritis dissecans in the body.
Medial femoral condyle of the knee
Capitellum of the distal humerus
Talus

Describe the etiology of patellar fracture.
The fracture usually results from a direct blow to the knee sustained in a fall or a motor vehicle or pedestrian accident.

BIBLIOGRAPHY

Abrams WB, Berkow R: *The Merck manual of geriatrics,* Rahway, NJ, 1990, Merck Sharp & Dohme Research Laboratories.

Adams JC, Hamblen DL: *Outline of orthopaedics,* ed 11, Edinburgh, 1990, Churchill Livingstone.

Aegerter E, Kirkpatrick JA: *Orthopaedic diseases,* ed 3, Philadelphia, 1968, WB Saunders.

Alario AJ: *Practical guide to the care of the pediatric patient,* St Louis, 1997, Mosby.

Allison D, Strickland N: *Acronyms & synonyms in medical imaging,* Oxford, 1996, ISIS Medical Media.

American Medical Association: *Guides to the evaluation of permanent impairment,* ed 4, Chicago, 1993, American Medical Association.

American Medical Association: *How to use guides to the evaluation of permanent impairment,* ed 4, Falmouth, Conn, 1993, SEAK.

Anderson KN, Anderson LE: *Mosby's pocket dictionary of medicine, nursing, & allied health,* ed 2, St Louis, 1994, Mosby.

Aniel DM, Fritschy D: Anterior cruciate ligament injuries. In DeLee JC, Drez D, editors: *Orthopaedic sports medicine: principles and practice,* vol 2, Philadelphia, 1994, WB Saunders.

Apley AG, Solomon L: *Concise system of orthopaedics and fractures,* London, 1988, Butterworth-Heinemann.

Arnbjornson A, et al: The natural history of recurrent dislocation of the patella, long-term results of conservative and operative treatment, *J Bone Joint Surg* 74B:140, 1992.

Assimakopoulos A, et al: The innervation of the human meniscus, *Clin Orthop* 275:232, 1992.

Baker CL, Norwood LA, Hughston JC: Acute combined posterior and posterolateral instability of the knee, *Am J Sports Med* 12:204, 1984.

Ballinger PW: *Merrill's atlas of radiographic positions and radiologic procedures,* vol 1-3, ed 8, St Louis, 1995, Mosby.

Barkauskas VH, et al: *Health & physical assessment,* ed 2, St Louis, 1998, Mosby.

Barnett CH, Davies DV, MacConaill MA: *Synovial joints: their structure and mechanics,* New York, 1961, Longmans Green.

Barrack RL, Skinner HB: The sensory function of knee ligaments. In Daniel D, et al, editors: *Knee ligaments: structure, function, injury and repair,* New York, 1990, Raven.

Bennett JG: Rehabilitation of patellofemoral joint dysfunction. In Greenfield BH, editor: *Rehabilitation of the knee: a problem solving approach,* Philadelphia, 1994, FA Davis.

Beynnon BD, et al: Anterior cruciate ligament strain behavior during rehabilitation exercises in vivo, *Am J Sports Med* 23:24, 1995.

Brooks M, Evans R, Fairclough J: *Sports injuries,* ed 2, London, 1992, Gower Medical.

Brotzman SB: *Clinical orthopaedic rehabilitation,* St Louis, 1996, Mosby.

Brown DE, Neumann RD: *Orthopedic secrets,* Philadelphia, 1995, Hanley & Belfus.

Bucholz RW: *Orthopaedic decision making,* ed 2, St Louis, 1996, Mosby.

Butler DL, Noyes FR, Grood ES: Ligamentous restraints to anterior-posterior drawer in the human knee, *J Bone Joint Surg* 622A:259, 1980.

Cailliet R: *Knee pain and disability,* ed 2, Philadelphia, 1983, FA Davis.

Campbell JB, Campbell JM: *Mosby's survival guide to medical abbreviations & acronyms prefixes & suffixes symbols Greek alphabet,* St Louis, 1995, Mosby.

Canale ST: *Campbell's operative orthopaedics,* vol 1-4, ed 9, St Louis, 1998, Mosby.

Childress HM: Popliteal cysts associated with undiagnosed posterior lesions of the medial meniscus, *J Bone Joint Surg* 52A:1487, 1970.

Cipriano JJ: *Photographic manual of regional orthopaedic and neurological test,* ed 3, Baltimore, 1997, Williams & Wilkins.

Clancy WG: Tendon trauma and overuse injuries. In Leadbetter WB, Buckwalter JA, Gordon SL, editors: *Sports-induced inflammation: clinical and basic science concepts,* Park Ridge, Ill, 1990, AAOS.

Clancy WG: Repair and reconstruction of the posterior cruciate ligament. In Chapman MW, editor: *Operative orthopaedics,* vol 2, Philadelphia, 1993, JB Lippincott.

Cohn RE: *Impairment rating examination and disability evaluation,* ed 3, Wilkesboro, NC, 1994, R Ernest Cohn.

Cormack, DH: *Essential histology,* Philadelphia, 1993, Lippincott.

Corso SJ, Thal R, Forman D: Locked patellar dislocation with vertical axis rotation, *Clin Orthop* 279:190, 1992.

Covey DC, Sapega AA: Current concepts review, injuries of the posterior cruciate ligament, *J Bone Joint Surg* 75A:1376, 1993.

Crawford EJ, Emery RJ, Archrogh PM: Stable osteochondritis dissecans-does the lesion unite? *J Bone Joint Surg* 72B:320, 1990.

Crenshaw AH, editor: *Campbell's operative orthopedics,* ed 8, St Louis, 1992, Mosby.

Crosby EB, Insall J: Recurrent dislocation of the patella, *J Bone Joint Surg* 58A:9, 1976.

Dambro MR, Griffith JA: *Griffith's 5 minute clinical consult,* Baltimore, 1997, Williams & Wilkins.

D'Ambrogio KJ, Roth GB: *Positional release therapy: assessment & treatment of musculoskeletal dysfunction,* St Louis, 1997, Mosby.

D'Ambrosia RD: *Musculoskeletal disorders: regional examination and differential diagnosis,* Philadelphia, 1977, JB Lippincott.

Dandy DJ: *Essential orthopaedics and trauma,* Edinburgh, 1989, Churchill Livingstone.

Dandy DJ, Jackson RW: The impact of arthroscopy on the management of disorders of the knee, *J Bone Joint Surg* 57B:346, 1975.

Daniels DM, Stone ML: KT-1000 anterior-posterior displacement measurements. In Daniels DM, Akeson WH, O'Connor JJ, editors: *Knee ligament: structure, function, injury and repair,* New York, 1990, Raven.

DeLee JC, Drez D, editors: *Orthopedic sports medicine: principles and practice,* Philadelphia, 1994, WB Saunders.

Deltoff MN, Kogon PL: *The portable skeletal x-ray library,* St Louis, 1998, Mosby.

Demeter SL, Andersson GBJ, Smith GM: *Disability evaluation,* St Louis, 1996, Mosby.

Deshpande JK, Tobias JD: *The pediatric pain handbook,* St Louis, 1996, Mosby.

Detenbeck LC: Function of the cruciate ligaments in knee stability, *Am J Sports Med* 2:217, 1974.

Dettenmeier PA: *Radiographic assessment for nurses,* St Louis, 1995, Mosby.

Dinham, JM: Popliteal cysts in children, *J Bone Joint Surg* 57B:69, 1975.

Doherty M: *Color atlas and text of osteoarthritis,* London, 1994, Wolfe.

Doherty M, George E: *Self-assessment picture tests in rheumatology,* London, 1995, Mosby-Wolfe.

Doucette SA, Goble EM: The effect of exercise on patellar tracking in lateral patellar compression syndrome, *Am J Sports Med* 20:434, 1992.

Ehrlich M, Hulstyn M, D'Amoto C: Sports injuries in children and the clumsy child, *Pediatr Clin North Am* 39:433, 1992.

Eifert-Mangine M, et al: Patellar tendinitis in the recreational athlete, *Orthopedics* 15:1359, 1992.

Elster AD: *Questions and answers in magnetic resonance imaging,* St Louis, 1994, Mosby.

Engle RP, Meade TD, Canner BC: Rehabilitation of posterior cruciate ligament injuries. In Greenfield BH, editor: *Rehabilitation of the knee: a problem solving approach,* Philadelphia, 1993, FA Davis.

Epstein O, et al: *Clinical examination,* ed 2, London, 1997, Mosby.

Federico DJ, Lynch JK, Jokl P: Osteochondritis dissecans of the knee: a historical review of etiology and treatment, *Arthroscopy* 6:190, 1990.

Fetto JF, Marshall JL: Injury to the anterior cruciate ligament producing the pivot shift sign: an experimental study on cadaver specimens, *J Bone Joint Surg* 61A:710, 1979.

Ficat RP, Hungerford DS: *Disorders of the patello-femoral joint,* Baltimore, 1977, Williams & Wilkins.

Firer P: Aetiology and results of treatment of iliotibial band friction syndrome, *J Bone Joint Surg* 72B:742, 1990.

Franz WB III: Overuse syndromes in runners. In Mellion MB, Walsh WM, Shelton GL, editors: *Sports injuries and athletic problems,* Philadelphia, 1990, Hanley & Belfus.

Fu FH, Baratz M: Meniscal injuries. In DeLee JC, Drez D, editors: *Orthopaedic sports medicine: principals and practice,* vol 2, Philadelphia, 1994, WB Saunders.

Fulkerson JP, Hungerford DS: *Disorders of the patellofemoral joint,* Baltimore, 1990, Williams & Wilkins.

Fulkerson JP, Shea KP: Current concepts review disorders of patellofemoral alignment, *J Bone Joint Surg* 72A:1424, 1990.

Furman W, Marshall JL, Girgis FG: The anterior cruciate ligaments: a functional analysis based on postmortem studies, *J Bone Joint Surg* 58A:179, 1976.

Galland O, et al: An anatomical and radiological study of the femoropatellar articulation, *Surg Radiol Anat* 12:119, 1990.

Galway HR, MacIntosh DL: The lateral pivot shift: symptoms and sign of anterior cruciate ligament insufficiency, *Clin Orthop* 147:45, 1980.

Garret JC: Osteochondritis dissecans, *Clin Orthop Sports Med* 10:569, 1991.

Garth WB: Current concepts regarding the anterior cruciate ligament, *Orthop Rev* 21:565, 1992.

Gartland JJ: *Fundamentals of orthopedics,* ed 2, Philadelphia, 1974, WB Saunders.

Gerard JA, Kleinfield SL: *Orthopaedic testing,* New York, 1993, Churchill Livingstone.

Gillis L: *Diagnosis in orthopaedics,* London, 1969, Butterworths.

Girgis FG, Marshall JL, Al Monajem ARS: The cruciate ligaments of the knee joint: anatomical, functional and experimental analysis, *Clin Orthop* 106:216, 1975.

Goldie BS: *Orthopaedic diagnosis and management: a guide to the care of orthopaedic patients,* ed 2, Oxford, 1998, ISIS Medical Media.

Goldstein RS: Geriatric orthopaedics, rehabilitative management of common problems. In Lewis CB, editor: *Aspen series in physical therapy,* Gaithersburg, Md, 1991, Aspen.

Goodfellow J, Hungerford DS, Woods C: Patello-femoral joint mechanics and pathology: chondromalacia patella, *J Bone Joint Surg* 58B:291, 1976.

Goodfellow J, Hungerford DS, Zindel M: Patello-femoral joint mechanics and pathology: functional anatomy of the patello-femoral joint, *J Bone Joint Surg* 58B:287, 1976.

Greenstein GM: *Clinical assessment of neuromusculoskeletal disorders,* St Louis, 1997, Mosby.

Grelsamer RP, Meadows S: The modified Insall-Salvati ratio for assessment of patellar height, *Clin Orthop* 282;170, 1992.

Grelsamer RP, Proctor CS, Bazos AN: Evaluation of patellar shape in the sagittal plane: a clinical analysis, *Am J Sports Med* 22:61, 1994.

Grelsamer RP, Tedder JL: The lateral trochlear sign: femoral trochlear dysplasia as seen on a lateral view roentgenograph, *Clin Orthop* 281:159, 1992.

Grossman ZD, et al: *Cost-effective diagnostic imaging: the clinician's guide,* ed 3, St Louis, 1995, Mosby.

Guzzanti V, et al: Patellofemoral malalignment in adolescents: computerized tomographic assessment with or without quadriceps contraction, *Am J Sports Med* 22:55, 1994.

Hammer WI: *Functional soft tissue examination and treatment by manual methods: the extremities,* Gaithersburg, Md, 1991, Aspen.

Handelberg FM, Shahabpour M, Casteleyn PP: Chondral lesions of the patella evaluated with computed tomography, magnetic resonance imaging, and arthroscopy, *Arthroscopy* 6:24, 1990.

Harner CD, et al: Loss of motion after anterior cruciate ligament reconstruction, *Am J Sports Med* 20:499, 1992.

Hartley A: *Practical joint assessment: lower quadrant,* ed 2, St Louis, 1995, Mosby.

Hawkins RJ: *An organized approach to musculoskeletal examination and history taking,* St Louis, 1995, Mosby.

Hede A, Hempel-Poulson S, Jensen JS: Symptoms and level of sports activity in patients awaiting arthroscopy for meniscal lesions of the knee, *J Bone Joint Surg* 72A:550, 1990.

Helfet AJ: *Disorder of the knee,* Philadelphia, 1974, JB Lippincott.

Henigan SP, et al: The semimembranosus-tibial collateral ligament bursa, *J Bone Joint Surg* 76A:1322, 1994.

Henry JH: Conservative treatment of patellofemoral subluxation, *Clin Sports Med* 8:261, 1989.

Hinkle CZ: *Fundamentals of anatomy & movement: a workbook and guide,* St Louis, 1997, Mosby.

Hornberger JP: *Exercise physiology therapeutic exercise,* Sarasota, 1991, Joseph P Hornberger.

Hughston J: *Knee ligaments: injury and repair,* St Louis, 1993, Mosby.

Hughston JC, Norwood LA: The posterolateral drawer and external rotational recurvatum test for posterolateral rotary instability of the knee, *Clin Orthop* 147:82, 1980.

Hughston JC, Walsh WM, Puddu G: *Patellar subluxation and dislocation,* Philadelphia, 1984, WB Saunders.

Hughston JC, et al: The classification of knee ligament instabilities: I. the medial compartment and cruciate ligaments, *J Bone Joint Surg* 58A:159, 1976.

Hughston JC, et al: The classification of knee ligament instabilities: II. the lateral compartment, *J Bone Joint Surg* 58A:173, 1976.

Indelicato PA, et al: Clinical comparison of freeze-dried/fresh frozen patella tendon allografts for anterior cruciate ligament reconstruction of the knee, *Am J Sports Med* 18:335, 1990.

Indelicato PA, Hermansdorfer J, Huegel M: The nonoperative management of complete tears of the medial collateral ligament of the knee in intercollegiate football players, *Clin Orthop* 256:174, 1990.

Ingebretsen L, et al: A prospective, randomized study of three surgical techniques for treatment of acute ruptures of the anterior cruciate ligament, *Am J Sports Med* 18:585, 1990.

Insall J, Falvo KA, Wise DW: Chondromalacia patella, *J Bone Joint Surg* 58A:1, 1976.

Jablonski S: *Dictionary of medical acronyms & abbreviations,* ed 3, Philadelphia, 1998, Hanley & Belfus.

Jackson RW, Kunkel SS, Taylor GJ: Lateral retinacular release for patellofemoral pain in the older patient, *Arthroscopy* 7:283, 1991.

Jakob RP, Hassler H, Staeubli HU: Observations on rotary instability of the lateral compartment of the knee, *Acta Orthop Scand Suppl* 191:1, 1981.

James SL: Running injuries to the knee, *J Am Acad Orthop Surg* 3:309, 1995.

Johansson H, Sjolander P, Sojka P: A sensory role for the cruciate ligaments, *Clin Orthop* 268:161, 1991.

Johnson DP, Eastwood DM, Witherow PJ: Symptomatic synovial plicae of the knee, *J Bone Joint Surg* 75A:1485, 1992.

Jonsson T, et al: Clinical diagnosis of ruptures of the anterior cruciate ligament: a comparative study of the Lachman test and the anterior drawer sign, *Am J Sports Med* 10:100, 1982.

Junqueira LC, Carneiro J, Kelly RO: *Basic histology,* ed 7, Norwalk, Conn, 1992, Appleton & Lange.

Kalebo P, et al: Ultrasonography in the detection of partial patellar ligament ruptures (jumper's knee), *Skeletal Radiol* 20:285, 1991.

Kanner R: *Pain management secrets,* Philadelphia, 1997, Hanley & Belfus.

Karlson J, et al: Partial rupture of the patellar ligament, *Am J Sports Med* 19:403, 1992.

Katirji B: *Electromyography in clinical practice: a case study approach,* St Louis, 1998, Mosby.

Katz WA: *Rheumatic diseases diagnosis and management,* Philadelphia, 1977, JB Lippincott.

Keats TE: *Atlas of roentgenographic measurement,* ed 6, St Louis, 1990, Mosby.

Kendall HO, Kendall RP, Wadsworth GE: *Muscles: testing and function,* ed 3, Baltimore, 1992, Williams & Wilkins.

Kennedy JC: *The injured adolescent knee,* Baltimore, 1979, Williams & Wilkins.

King JB, et al: Lesions of the patellar ligament, *J Bone Joint Surg* 72B:46, 1990.

Klippel JH, Dieppe PA: *Rheumatology,* vol 1-2, ed 2, London, 1998, Mosby.

Koenigsberg R: *Churchill's illustrated medical dictionary,* New York, 1989, Churchill Livingstone.

Kolowich PA, et al: Lateral release of the patella: indications and contraindications, *Am J Sports Med* 18:359, 1990.

Koshino T: Changes in patellofemoral compressive force after anterior or anteromedial displacement of tibial tuberosity for chondromalacia patellae, *Clin Orthop* 266:133, 1991.

Koskinen SK, Hurme M, Kujala UM: Restoration of patellofemoral congruity by combined lateral release and tibial tuberosity transposition as assessed by MRI analysis, *Int Orthop* 15:363, 1991.

Krauspe R, Schmidt M, Schaible H: Sensory and innervation of the anterior cruciate ligament, *J Bone Joint Surg* 74A:390, 1992.

Kujula UM, et al: Scoring of patellofemoral disorders, *Arthroscopy* 9:159, 1993.

Kursunoglu-Brahme S, Resnick D: Magnetic resonance imaging of the knee, *Orthop Clin North Am* 21:561, 1990.

Laskin RS: Total condylar knee replacement in patients who have rheumatoid arthritis, *J Bone Joint Surg* 72A:529, 1990.

Laurin CA, et al: The abnormal lateral patellofemoral angle: a diagnostic roentgenographic sign of recurrent patellar subluxation, *J Bone Joint Surg* 60A:55, 1978.

Lavy CBD, Barrett DS: *Questions and answers on Apley's concise system of orthopaedics and fractures,* Oxford, 1991, Butterworth-Heinemann.

Lerner AJ: *The little black book of neurology,* ed 3, St Louis, 1995, Mosby.

Lewallen DG, et al: Effects of retinacular release and tibial tubercle elevation in patellofemoral degenerative joint disease, *J Orthop Res* 8:856, 1990.

Lewis CB, Knortz KA: *Orthopedic assessment and treatment of the geriatric patient,* St Louis, 1993, Mosby.

Linton RC, Indelicato PA: Medial ligament injuries. In DeLee JC, Drez D, editors: *Orthopedic sports medicine: principles and practice,* vol 1, Philadelphia, 1994, WB Saunders.

Lipscomb PR Jr., Lipscomb PR Sr., Bryan RS: Osteochondritis dissecans of the knee with loose fragments, *J Bone Joint Surg* 60A:235, 1978.

Losee RE, Ennis TRJ, Southwick WO: Anterior subluxation of the lateral tibial plateau: a diagnostic test and operative review, *J Bone Joint Surg* 60A:1015, 1978.

Loth TS: *Orthopedic boards review II: a case study approach,* St Louis, 1996, Mosby.

MacAusland WR, Mayo RA: *Orthopedics: a concise guide to clinical practices,* Boston, 1965, Little, Brown.

Magee DJ: *Orthopedic physical assessment,* ed 3, Philadelphia, 1997, WB Saunders.

Main WK, Scott WN: Knee anatomy. In Scott WN, editor: *Ligament and extensor mechanism injuries of the knee, diagnosis and treatment,* St Louis, 1991, Mosby.

Malone TR, McPoil TG, Nitz AJ: *Orthopedic and sports physical therapy,* ed 3, St Louis, 1997, Mosby.

Maquet PGJ: *Biomechanics of the knee: with application of the pathogenesis and the surgical treatment of osteoarthritis,* New York, 1976, Springer-Verlag.

Marchiori DM: *Clinical imaging with skeletal, chest, and abdomen pattern differentials,* St Louis, 1999, Mosby.

Martin AF: The pathomechanics of the knee joint, *J Bone Joint Surg* 42A:13, 1960.

Martin JH: *Neuroanatomy text and atlas,* ed 2, Stamford, Conn, 1996, Appleton & Lange.

Mathers LH, et al: *Clinical anatomy principles,* St Louis, 1996, Mosby.

Mazion JM: *Illustrated manual of neurological reflexes/signs/tests, part I, orthopedic signs/tests/maneuvers for office procedure, part II,* Orlando, 1980, Daniels Publishing.

McMurray TP: The semilunar cartilages, *Br J Surg* 29:407, 1942.

McMurray TP: *The Robert joint birthday volume,* London, 1928, Humphrey Milford.

McRae R: *Clinical orthopaedic examination,* ed 3, Edinburgh, 1990, Churchill Livingston.

McRae R: *Practical fracture treatment,* ed 3, Edinburgh, 1994, Churchill-Livingstone.

Medical Economics Books: *Patient care flow chart manual,* ed 3, Oradell, NJ, 1982, Medical Economics Books.

Mellion MB: *Sports medicine secrets,* Philadelphia, 1994, Hanley & Belfus.

Mellion MB: *Office sports medicine,* ed 2, St Louis, 1996, Mosby.

Mengel MB, Schwiebert LP: *Ambulatory medicine: the primary care of families,* ed 2, Stamford, Conn, 1996, Appleton & Lange.

Mennell JM: *The musculoskeletal system: differential diagnosis from symptoms and physical signs,* Gaithersburg, Md, 1992, Aspen.

Merchant AC: Patellofemoral malalignment and instabilities. In Ewing JW, editor: *Articular cartilage and knee joint function: basic science and arthroscopy,* New York, 1990, Raven.

Merchant AC: Patellofemoral disorders, biomechanics, diagnosis, and non-operative treatment. In McGinty JB, editor: *Operative arthroscopy,* New York, 1991, Raven.

Merchant AC: Radiologic evaluation of the patellofemoral joint. In Aichroth PM, Cannon WD, editors: *Knee surgery,* London, 1992, Martin Dunitz.

Mercier LR, Pettid FJ: *Practical orthopedics,* ed 4, St Louis, 1995, Mosby.

Miller M: *Review of orthopaedics,* Philadelphia, 1992, WB Saunders.

Mirkopulos N, Myer TJ: Isolated avulsion of the popliteus tendon, *Am J Sports Med* 19:417, 1991.

Moore KL: *Clinically oriented anatomy,* ed 3, Baltimore, 1992, Williams & Wilkins.

Mori Y, et al: Lateral retinaculum release in adolescent patellofemoral disorders: its relationship to peripheral nerve injury in the lateral retinaculum, *Bull Hosp J Dis Orthop* 51:218, 1991.

Mosby-Year Book, Inc: *Expert 10-minute physical examination,* St Louis, 1997, Mosby.

Muller W: *The knee: form, function and ligament reconstruction,* New York, 1983, Springer-Verlag.

Munetea T, et al: Computerized tomographic analysis of tibial tubercle position in the painful female patellofemoral joint, *Am J Sports Med* 22:67, 1994.

Munuera L, Reinoso F, Martinez-Moreno E: *The innervation of the anterior cruciate ligament and the patellar ligament of the knee, thesis,* Madrid, 1992, Universidad Autonoma.

Myllymaki T, et al: Ultrasonography of jumper's knee, *Acta Radiol* 31:47, 1990.

Neumann RD: Traumatic knee injuries. In Mellion MB, editor: *Sports medicine secrets,* Philadelphia, 1994, Hanley & Belfus.

Neuschwander D, Drez D, Finney T: Lateral meniscal variant with absence of the posterior coronary ligament, *J Bone Joint Surg* 74A:1186, 1992.

Nicholas JA: The five-one reconstruction for anteromedial instability of the knee, *J Bone Joint Surg* 55A:899, 1973.

Nicholas JA, Hershman EB: *The lower extremity & spine in sports medicine,* vol 1-2, ed 2, St Louis, 1995, Mosby.

Niitsu M: Moving knee joint: technique for kinematic MR imaging, *Radiology* 174:569, 1990.

Noble HB, Hajek MR, Porter M: Diagnosis and treatment of iliotibial band tightness in runners, *Sports Med* 10:67, 1984.

Nordin M, Andersson GBJ, Pope MH: *Musculoskeletal disorders in the workplace: principles and practice,* St Louis, 1997, Mosby.

Noyes FR, et al: Clinical paradoxes of anterior cruciate instability and a new test to detect its instability, *Orthop Trans* 2:36, 1978.

Noyes FR, et al: The anterior cruciate ligament-deficient knee with varus alignment, *Am J Sports Med* 20:707, 1992.

Noyes FR, et al: Posterior subluxations of the medial and lateral tibiofemoral compartments: an in vitro ligament sectioning study in cadaveric knees, *Am J Sports Med* 21:407, 1993.

O'Connor J, et al: Geometry of the knee. In Daniel D, editor: *Knee ligaments: structure, function, injury and repair,* New York, 1990, Raven.

O'Donoghue DH: *Treatment of injuries to athletes,* ed 3, Philadelphia, 1976, WB Saunders.

Ogilvie-Harris DJ, Basinski A: Arthroscopic synovectomy of the knee for rheumatoid arthritis, *Arthroscopy* 7:91, 1991.

Olson WH, et al: *Handbook of symptom-oriented neurology,* ed 2, St Louis, 1994, Mosby.

Omer GE, Spinner M: *Management of peripheral nerve problems,* Philadelphia, 1980, WB Saunders.

Pagana KD, Pagana TJ: *Mosby's manual of diagnostic and laboratory tests,* St Louis, 1998, Mosby.

Pagnani M, Cooper D, Warren R: Extrusion of the medial meniscus: case report, *Arthroscopy* 7:297, 1991.

Palumbo RC, et al: Ligamentous injuries to the knee: a retrospective analysis, *Orthop Trans* 16:321, 1992.

Patten J: *Neurological differential diagnosis,* ed 2, London, 1996, Springer.

Pecina MM, Krmpotic-Nemanic J, Markiewitz AD: *Tunnel syndromes,* Boca Raton, Fla, 1991, CRC.

Pfeiffer WH, Gross JL, Seeger LL: Osteochondritis dissecans of the patella, *Clin Orthop* 271:207, 1991.

Pheasant S: *Ergonomics, work and health,* Gaithersburg, Md, 1991, Aspen.

Polley HF, Hunder GG: *Rheumatologic interviewing and physical examination of the joints,* ed 2, Philadelphia, 1978, WB Saunders.

Pope CF: Radiologic evaluation of tendon injuries, *Clin Sports Med* 11:579, 1992.

Ravel R: *Clinical laboratory medicine: clinical application of laboratory data,* ed 6, St Louis, 1995, Mosby.

Renne JW: The iliotibial band friction syndrome, *J Bone Joint Surg* 57A:1110, 1975.

Ricklin P, Ruttiman A, Del Buono MA: *Meniscus lesions: practical problems of clinical diagnosis, arthrography and therapy,* New York, 1971, Grune & Stratton.

Rockwood CA, Green DP, Bucholz R, editors: *Rockwood and Green's fractures in adults,* vol 2, ed 3, Philadelphia, 1991, JB Lippincott.

Rolak LA: *Neurology secrets,* ed 2, Philadelphia, 1998, Hanley & Belfus.

Royle SC, et al: The significance of chondromalacic changes on the patella, *Arthroscopy* 7:158, 1991.

Rumack CM, Wilson SR, Charboneau JW: *Diagnostic ultrasound,* vol 1-2, ed 2, St Louis, 1998, Mosby.

Saidoff DC, McDonough AL: *Critical pathways in therapeutic intervention,* St Louis, 1997, Mosby.

Schenck RC, Heckman JD: *Injuries of the knee,* Presented at clinical symposia, 1993, Ciba-Geigy.

Schumacher HR, Klippel JH, Koopman WJ: *Primer on the rheumatic diseases,* ed 10, Atlanta, 1993, Arthritis Foundation.

Scott WN: *The knee,* vol 1-2, St Louis, 1994, Mosby.

Scranton PE, et al: Mucoid degeneration of the patellar ligament in athletes, *J Bone Joint Surg* 74A:435, 1992.

Sebast C, Denelli WJ: Osteochondrosis. In DeLee JC, Drez D, editors: *Orthopedic sports medicine: principles and practice,* vol 1, Philadelphia, 1994, WB Saunders.

Sebastianelli WJ, et al: Isolated avulsion of the biceps femoris insertion, *Clin Orthop* 259:200, 1990.

Seto JL, Brewster CE: Rehabilitation of meniscal injuries. In Greenfield BH, editor: *Rehabilitation of the knee: a problem-solving approach,* Philadelphia, 1993, FA Davis.

Shankman GA: *Fundamental orthopedic management for the physical therapist assistant,* St Louis, 1997, Mosby.

Shelbourne KD, et al: Arthrofibrosis in acute anterior cruciate ligament reconstructions, *Am J Sports Med* 19:332, 1991.

Shelbourne KD, Nitz PA: The O'Donoghue triad revisited, *Am J Sports Med* 19:474, 1991.

Shelbourne KD, Porter DA: Anterior cruciate ligament-medial collateral ligament injury: non-operative management of medial collateral ligament tears with anterior cruciate reconstruction, *Am J Sports Med* 20:283, 1992.

Shellock FG, et al: Evaluation of patients with persistent symptoms after lateral retinacular release by kinematic magnetic resonance imaging of the patellofemoral joint, *Arthroscopy* 6:226, 1990.

Shelton GL, Thigpen LK: Rehabilitation of patellofemoral dysfunction: a review of literature, *J Orthop Sports Phys Ther* 14:243, 1991.

Shino K, et al: Reconstruction of the anterior cruciate ligament using allogenic tendon, *Am J Sports Med* 18:457, 1990.

Simmons E, Cameron JC: Patella alta and recurrent dislocation of the patella, *Clin Orthop* 274:265, 1992.

Sisk TD: Knee realignment and replacement in the recreational athlete. In DeLee JC, Drez D, editors: *Orthopaedic sports medicine: principals and practice,* vol 2, Philadelphia, 1994, WB Saunders.

Slocum DB, Larson RL: Rotary instability of the knee, *J Bone Joint Surg* 50A:211, 1968.

Slocum DB, et al: A clinical test for anterolateral rotary instability of the knee, *Clin Orthop* 118:63, 1976.

Smillie IS: *Injuries of the knee joint,* Edinburgh, 1970, E & S Livingstone.

Smillie IS: *Diseases of the knee joint,* New York, 1974, Longmans.

Solomonow M, D'Ambrosia R: Neural reflex arcs and muscle control of knee stability and motion. In Scott NW, editor: *Ligament and extensor mechanism injuries of the knee, diagnosis and treatment,* St Louis, 1991, Mosby.

Specht NT, Russo RD: *Practical guide to diagnostic imaging,* St Louis, 1998, Mosby.

Spring H, et al: *Stretching and strengthening exercises,* New York, 1991, Thieme.

Stanitski CL: Anterior knee pain syndromes in the adolescent, *J Bone Joint Surg* 75A:1407, 1993.

Staubli HU, Birrer S: The popliteus tendon and its fascicles at the popliteal hiatus: gross anatomy and functional arthroscopic evaluation with and without anterior cruciate ligament deficiency, *Arthroscopy* 6:209, 1990.

Stedman TL: *Stedman's medical dictionary,* ed 25, Baltimore, 1990, Williams & Wilkins.

Steinkamp LA, et al: Biomechanical consideration in patellofemoral joint rehabilitation, *Am J Sports Med* 21:438, 1993.

Stewart DL, Abeln SH: *Documenting functional outcomes in physical therapy,* St Louis, 1993, Mosby.

Stoller DW: *Magnetic resonance imaging in orthopaedics & sports medicine,* Philadelphia, 1993, JB Lippincott.

Strum GM, et al: Acute anterior cruciate reconstructions, *Clin Orthop* 253;184, 1990.

Sutton D, Young JWR: *A concise textbook of clinical imaging,* ed 2, St Louis, 1995, Mosby.

Tamea CD, Henning CD: Pathomechanics of the pivot shift maneuver, *Am J Sports Med* 9:31, 1981.

Tan JC, Horn SE: *Practical manual of physical medicine and rehabilitation,* St Louis, 1998, Mosby.

Taybi H, Lachman RS: *Radiology of syndromes, metabolic disorders, and skeletal dysplasias,* ed 4, St Louis, 1996, Mosby.

Taylor JC: Fractures of the lower extremity. In Crenshaw AH, editor: *Campbell's operative orthopedics,* ed 8, St Louis, 1992, Mosby.

Tenuta JJ, Arciero RA: Arthroscopic evaluation of meniscal repairs: factors that affect healing, *Am J Sports Med* 22:797, 1994.

Thibodeau GA, Patton KT: *Anatomy & physiology,* ed 3, St Louis, 1996, Mosby.

Thibodeau GA, Patton KT: *Pocket reference to accompany anatomy & physiology,* ed 3, St Louis, 1996, Mosby.

Timm K: Knee. In Richardson JK, Iglarsh ZA, editors: *Clinical orthopaedic physical therapy,* Philadelphia, 1994, WB Saunders.

Toghill PJ: *Examining patients: an introduction to clinical medicine,* London, 1990, Edward Arnold.

Tollison CD, Satterthwaite JR, Tollison JW: *Handbook of pain management,* ed 2, Baltimore, 1994, Williams & Wilkins.

Torg JS, Shepard RJ: *Current therapy in sports medicine,* ed 3, St Louis, 1995, Mosby.

Turek SL: *Orthopaedics principles and their application,* ed 3, Philadelphia, 1977, JB Lippincott.

Vail TP, Malone TR, Basset FH: Long-term functional results in patients with anterolateral rotatory instability treated by iliotibial band transfer, *Am J Sports Med* 20:274, 1992.

Van Holsbeeck M, Introcaso JH: *Musculoskeletal ultrasound,* St Louis, 1991, Mosby.

Van Kampen A, Huiskes R: The three-dimensional tracking pattern of the human patella, *J Orthop Res* 8:372, 1990.

Voight ML, Wieder DL: Comparative reflex response times of vastus medialis obliquus and vastus lateralis in normal subjects and subjects with extensor mechanism dysfunction: an electromyographic study, *Am J Sports Med* 19:131, 1991.

Waldron VD: A test for chondromalacia patella, *Orthop Rev* 12:103, 1983.

Walsh WM: Patellofemoral joint. In DeLee JC, Drez D, editors: *Orthopaedic sports medicine: principles and practice,* vol 2, Philadelphia, 1994, WB Saunders.

Walsh WM, Helzer-Julin MJ: Patellar tracking problems in athletes, *Prim Care* 19:303, 1992.

Watanabe Y, et al: Functional anatomy of the posterolateral structures of the knee, *Arthroscopy* 9:57, 1993.

Waters P, Kasser J: Infection of the infrapatellar bursa, *J Bone Joint Surg* 72A:1095, 1990.

Weineck J: *Functional anatomy in sports,* ed 2, St Louis, 1990, Mosby.

Weinstein SL, Buckwalter JA: *Turek's orthopaedics principles and their application,* ed 5, Philadelphia, 1994, JB Lippincott.

Whitmore I, Willan PLT: *Multiple choice questions in human anatomy,* London, 1995, Mosby.

Wilk KE: Rehabilitation of medial capsular injuries. In Greenfield BH, editor: *Rehabilitation of the knee: a problem solving approach,* Philadelphia, 1993, FA Davis.

Wilson RM, Fowler P: Arthroscopic anatomy. In Scott WN, editor: *Arthroscopy of the knee: diagnosis and treatment,* Philadelphia, 1990, WB Saunders.

Windsor RE, Lox DM: *Soft tissue injuries: diagnosis and treatment,* Philadelphia, 1998, Hanley & Belfus.

Wiss DA: Supracondylar and intercondylar fractures of the femur. In Rockwood CA, Green DP, Bucholz RW, editors: *Rockwood and Green's fractures in adults,* ed 3, Philadelphia, 1991, JB Lippincott.

Woodland LH, Francis RS: Parameters and comparisons of the quadriceps angle of college-aged men and women in the supine and standing positions, *Am J Sports Med* 20:209, 1992.

Zatouroff M: *Diagnosis in color physical signs in general medicine,* ed 2, London, 1996, Mosby-Wolfe.

Zitelli BJ, Davis HW: *Atlas of pediatric physical diagnosis,* ed 2, London, 1992, Wolfe.

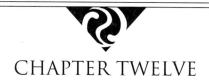

LOWER LEG, ANKLE, AND FOOT

AXIOMS IN LOWER LEG, ANKLE, AND FOOT ASSESSMENT

- Pain in the ankle and foot may arise from the bones and joints, periarticular soft tissues, nerve roots and peripheral nerves, or vascular structures.
- Pain in the foot may also be referred from the lumbar spine or knee joint.
- The greatest majority of painful foot conditions result from inappropriate footwear, weak intrinsic muscles, foot deformities, or static disorders.

INTRODUCTION

The leg, ankle, and foot are subject to static deformities more than any other skeletal unit. The weight-transmitting and propulsive functions of these structures are restricted daily by nonyielding foot coverings. Anatomic variations in the shape and stability of joint surfaces may predispose, resist, or modify the deforming force of common footwear.

Modern civilization disregards the physiology of the ankle and foot. Fashion and eye appeal rather than function determine shoe design, especially in the fore part of the shoe, where most disabilities and deformities of the foot occur.

The restrictive force of poorly fitting shoes produces little deformity on the tarsus because the tarsus is made up of short, heavy bones. Normal movement in the tarsal joints is limited because the articular surfaces of the tarsal joints are flat (Fig. 12-2). However, the phalanges and metatarsals are long thin bones with a normally wide range of joint motion. Restrictive force on these bones produces most of the static deformities of the forefoot. These static deformities include first metatarsophalangeal joint deformities, hammertoe, tailor's bunion, overlapping toes, and many other conditions that are deviations from the normal (Table 12-3).

The human foot is uniquely specialized. The metatarsals and toes enable the body to stand erect. The versatility of the forefoot permits the human to retain an upright stance and allows for grace during walking, dancing, and athletics.

A well-developed and strong foot withstands surprising abuse. Morbid changes take place only when maltreatment becomes excessive. An underdeveloped and frail foot, ankle, and lower-leg mechanism may fail under ordinary stress and strain.

The ankle and foot are inspected in both the resting and standing positions for evidence of swelling (Fig. 12-3), deformity (Fig. 12-4), or skin abnormalities such as edema, erythema, tophi, subcutaneous nodules (Fig. 12-5), or ulcers. Abnormalities of gait are observed while the patient is walking. The gait or walking cycle can be divided into two phases: the stance or weight-bearing phase and the swing or non–weight-bearing phase.

ORTHOPEDIC GAMUT 12-1

ACHILLES' TENDON

Swelling in the region of the Achilles' tendon may be caused by the following:

1. Tendon rupture
2. Calcaneal bursitis
3. Rheumatoid nodules
4. Urate tophi

Text continued on p. 827

TABLE 12-1

LOWER LEG, ANKLE, AND FOOT CROSS-REFERENCE TABLE BY ASSESSMENT PROCEDURE

Lower Leg, Ankle, and Foot Test/Sign	Talofibular Ligament	Vascular	Atrophy	Peroneal Nerve Paralysis	Foot Pronation	Calcaneus Fracture	Thrombophlebitis	Fibular Fracture	Neuroma	Metatarsalgia	Achilles' Tendon	Tarsal Tunnel Syndrome
Anterior drawer sign of the ankle	●											
Buerger's test		●										
Calf circumference test			●									
Claudication test		●										
Duchenne's sign				●								
Foot tourniquet test		●										
Helbings' sign					●							
Hoffa's test						●						
Homans' sign		●					●					
Keen's sign								●				
Morton's test									●	●		
Moszkowicz test		●										
Moses' test		●					●					
Perthes' test		●										
Strunsky's sign										●		
Thompson's test						●					●	
Tinel's foot sign												●

TABLE 12-2

LOWER LEG, ANKLE, AND FOOT CROSS-REFERENCE TABLE BY SYNDROME OR TISSUE

Achilles' tendon	Thompson's test	Tarsal tunnel syndrome	Tinel's foot sign
Atrophy	Calf circumference test	Thrombophlebitis	Homans' sign
Calcaneus fracture	Hoffa's test		Moses' test
	Thompson's test		
Fibular fracture	Keen's sign	Vascular	Buerger's test
Foot pronation	Helbings' sign		Claudication test
Metatarsalgia	Morton's test		Foot tourniquet test
	Strunsky's sign		Homans' sign
Neuroma	Morton's test		Moszkowicz test
Peroneal nerve paralysis	Duchenne's sign		Moses' test
Talofibular ligament	Anterior drawer sign of the ankle		Perthes' test

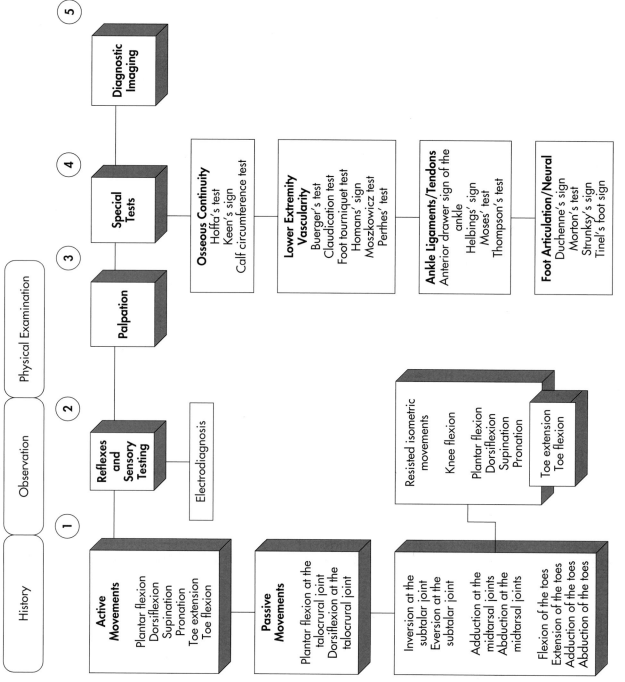

FIG. 12-1 Lower leg, ankle, and foot assessment.

TABLE 12-3

ANKLE AND FOOT DIFFERENTIATION BY ONSET

Articular
Trauma, sprain
Arthritis
Metatarsalgia
Congenital disorders (e.g., clubfoot)

Periarticular
Cutaneous and subcutaneous
Plantar fascia
Tendons and tendon sheaths
Bursitis
Acute calcific periarthritis

Osseous
Fracture
Epiphysitis (osteochondritis)
Bone neoplasms, infection
Painful accessory ossicles

Neurologic
Entrapment of lumbosacral nerve roots form herniated lumbar disc
Entrapment of the lateral popliteal nerve behind the neck of the fibula
Tarsal tunnel syndrome (posterior tibial nerve)
Interdigital (Morton's) neuroma
Peripheral neuropathy and insensitive foot

Vascular
Ischemic foot pain
Vasospastic disorders with Raynaud's phenomenon
Cholesterol embolization with "purple toes"

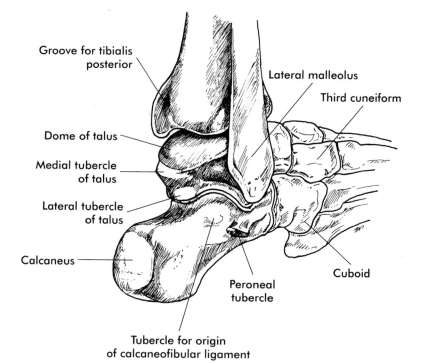

FIG. 12-2   Posterior process of the talus as made up of the posterolateral and posteromedial tubercles separated by the groove for the flexor hallucis longus tendon. *(From Baxter DE: The foot and ankle in sport, St Louis, 1995, Mosby.)*

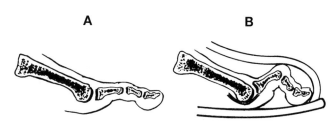

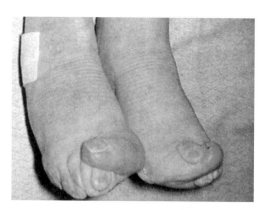

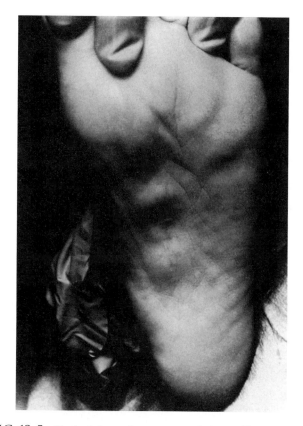

FIG. 12-3   Hallux valgus. *(From Mosby's medical, nursing, and allied health dictionary, ed 5, St Louis, 1998, Mosby.)*

FIG. 12-4   **A,** Phalanx extended to normal length. **B,** Buckling of the phalanx is caused by restriction of the toe box. The interphalangeal joints and MTP joints become subluxed. Over time, dislocation may occur. *(From Coughlin MJ, Mann RA: Surgery of the foot and ankle, vol 1-2, ed 7, St Louis, 1999, Mosby.)*

FIG. 12-5   Typical size and appearance of plantar fibromas along medial border of plantar fascia. *(From Coughlin MJ, Mann RA: Surgery of the foot and ankle, vol 1-2, ed 7, St Louis, 1999, Mosby.)*

In the standing position, the calcaneus normally maintains the line of the Achilles' tendon. Deformities of the subtalar joint, resulting in eversion (calcaneovalgus) or inversion (calcaneovarus) of the heel are best observed from behind (Fig. 12-6). *Equinus* and *calcaneus* refer to angulation of the ankle in plantar and dorsiflexion, respectively. Inspection while the patient is standing may reveal lowering of the longitudinal arch (pes planus) or increased height of the arch (pes cavus).

Essential Anatomy

The leg is divided by fascial septa into posterior, lateral, and anterior compartments (Fig. 12-7). Because they have a common nerve supply, the anterior and lateral compartments often are considered to be one. The posterior compartment is further divided into a superficial and deep area. Although each compartment of the leg has a specialized vascular and nerve supply, the nerves and vessels are sometimes not physically within the compartment they supply (e.g., the lateral compartment is supplied by the peroneal artery, which lies in the posterior compartment).

The anterior leg muscles (Fig. 12-8) attach to the area between the tibia and fibula.

ORTHOPEDIC GAMUT 12-2

ANTERIOR COMPARTMENT

Following are the three muscles of the anterior compartment:

1. Tibialis anterior
2. Extensor hallucis longus
3. Extensor digitorum longus

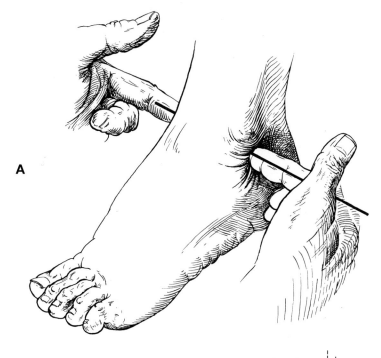

A

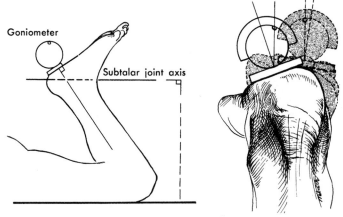

B

Goniometer

Subtalar joint axis

FIG. 12-6   **A,** Estimating location of ankle axis. **B,** Spherical goniometer attached to calcaneus to measure degree of subtalar motion. *(From Coughlin MJ, Mann RA: Surgery of the foot and ankle, vol 1, ed 7, St Louis, 1999, Mosby.)*

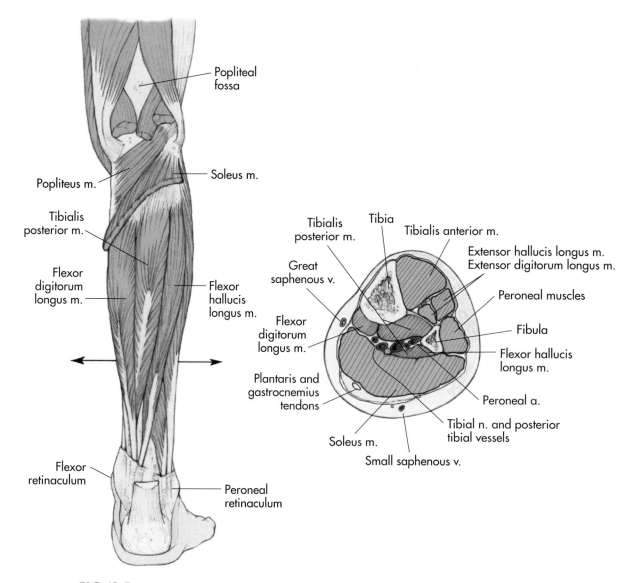

FIG. 12-7   Right leg muscles, posterior view, deep layers.   *(From Mathers LH, et al:* Clinical anatomy principles, *St Louis, 1996, Mosby.)*

The muscles in the anterior and lateral compartments can be injured with a traumatic blow to the lateral leg. This damages the common peroneal nerve. The most noticeable deficits to result from such an injury are weakness in extension (dorsiflexion) of the ankle and a dragging of the toes ("foot drop") in walking. One of the more difficult complications to traumatic injury of the leg is compartment syndrome. The fascial enclosures of the three compartments are so strong that hemorrhage, major tissue injury, and edema within one or another of these compartments cause pressure to increase. This compartmental hyperextension decreases the blood flow. Structures distal to the injury become ischemic and are usually permanently injured.

The ankle is the joint between the malleoli of the tibia and fibula, which combine to form a mortise. The talus is a tarsal bone that fits into this mortise (Fig. 12-9).

The flexor retinaculum connects the medial malleolus to the calcaneus and plantar aponeurosis posteroinferiorly.

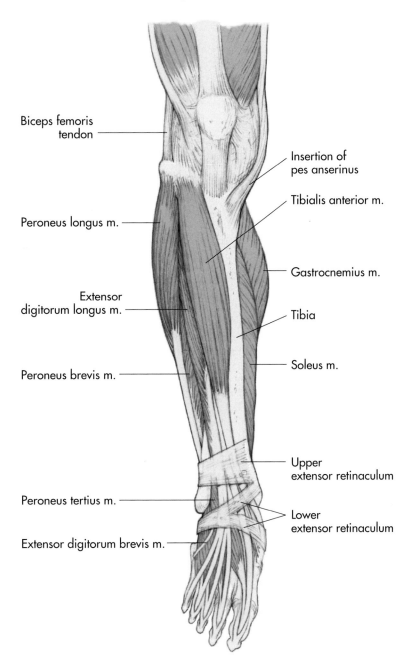

FIG. 12-8 Right leg muscles, anterior view. *(From Mathers LH, et al:* Clinical anatomy principles, *St Louis, 1996, Mosby.)*

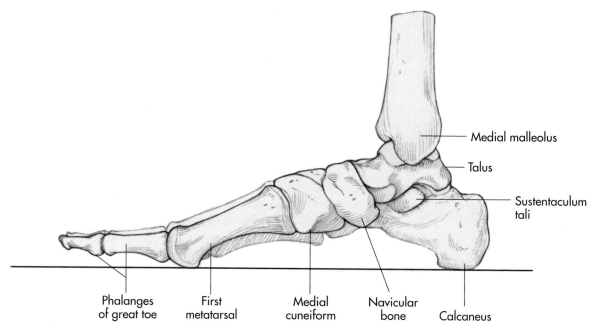

FIG. 12-9　Medial view of ankle and bones of the foot. *(From Mathers LH, et al:* Clinical anatomy principles, *St Louis, 1996, Mosby.)*

This passage is also called the *tarsal tunnel,* and compression and pressure can produce a tarsal tunnel syndrome comparable to the carpal tunnel syndrome of the wrist.

ORTHOPEDIC GAMUT 12-3

ANKLE JOINT

The following important structures cross the ankle joint (Fig. 12-10):

Anteriorly

1. Tendons of the tibialis anterior
2. Extensor hallucis longus
3. Anterior tibial vessels
4. Deep peroneal nerve
5. Extensor digitorum longus
6. Peroneus tertius

Posteromedially

1. Tibial vessels
2. Tibial nerve
3. Flexor hallucis longus

Posterolaterally

1. Tendons of the peroneus longus and brevis

ESSENTIAL MOTION ASSESSMENT

For the sake of simplicity, motions are tested along three different axes. Dorsiflexion and plantar flexion are movements at the ankle joint that occur around a transverse axis that passes through the body of the talus. Inversion and eversion are movements of rotation of the foot along its long axis. Abduction and adduction of the forefoot, occurring along a vertical axis, are movements of the midtarsal joints. Pronation and supination refer to a weight-bearing foot. The complex movements of eversion and inversion indicate changes in the form of the whole foot when it is not bearing weight.

ORTHOPEDIC GAMUT 12-4

ANKLE AND FOOT

The following test range of motion of the ankle and foot (Fig. 12-11):

1. Point the foot up toward the ceiling.
2. Point the foot down toward the floor.
3. With the foot bent at the ankle, point the medial side of the foot toward the floor (eversion) and repeat with the lateral side (inversion).
4. Rotate the ankle, turning the foot away from and then toward the other foot.

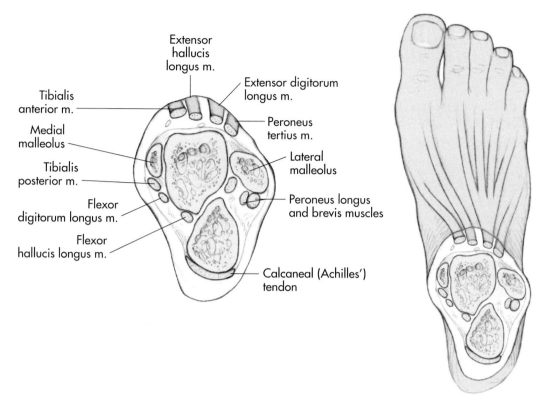

FIG. 12-10 Tendons at the ankle. *(From Mathers LH, et al:* Clinical anatomy principles, *St Louis, 1996, Mosby.)*

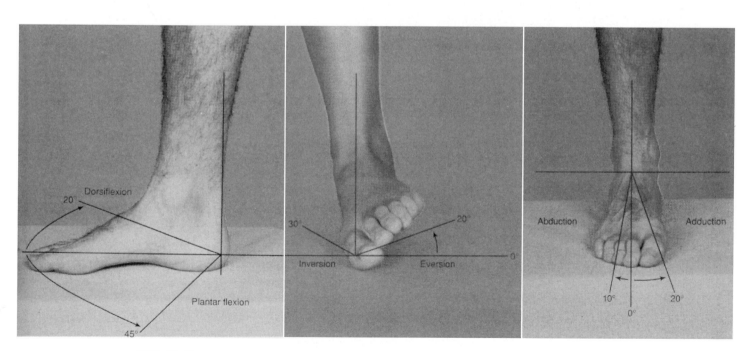

FIG. 12-11 Range of motion of the ankle and foot. *(From Barkauskas VH, et al:* Health & physical assessment, *ed 2, St Louis, 1998, Mosby.)*

Forefoot adduction and abduction occur mainly at the midtarsal joints and are tested passively. The examiner moves the forefoot laterally and medially in relation to the calcaneus and then compares the range of motion with that of the opposite foot.

The other joints that allow significant motion in the forefoot are the metatarsophalangeal and interphalangeal joints. Of particular importance are the joints of the great toe. Normal dorsiflexion of the great toe is approximately 50 degrees. Plantar flexion of the metatarsophalangeal and interphalangeal joints of the great toe is approximately 30 degrees. Retained dorsiflexion of the great toe that is 40 degrees or less is an impairment of the foot in the activities of daily living. Retained plantar flexion of the great toe that is 20 degrees or less is an impairment of the foot in the activities of daily living.

Movements of the lesser toes can be measured in a similar manner. Clinically, it is adequate to note whether there are fixed contractures or if the joints are supple. Restriction of joint motion can be the result of soft-tissue contractures, bony abutment, or intraarticular adhesions. Motion may be restricted because of pain that results from inflammation or injuries (Figs. 12-12 and 12-13).

ESSENTIAL MUSCLE FUNCTION ASSESSMENT

The main muscles of the calf are the soleus and gastrocnemius. The soleus acts purely as a flexor of the ankle, and the gastrocnemius flexes both the ankle and the knee. The flexor digitorum longus and flexor hallucis longus flex the toes and big toe, respectively (Fig. 12-14). The anterior compartment muscles include the tibialis anterior, extensor digitorum longus, and extensor hallucis longus (Fig. 12-15). The tibialis anterior inverts the foot and dorsiflexes the ankle.

The examiner should test the individual muscles concerned with movement at the ankle and foot, starting with the plantar and dorsiflexors of the ankle, then of the toes (Fig. 12-16). The extensor of the big toe, extensor hallucis longus, should be specially tested. Finally, the examiner should test the evertors and invertors of the foot. Variations of the arch need to be assessed (Fig. 12-17).

The motions in the ankle joint are plantar flexion and dorsiflexion. The muscles in the posterior compartment, which are innervated by the tibial nerve, are primarily responsible for plantar flexion motion. The major muscles

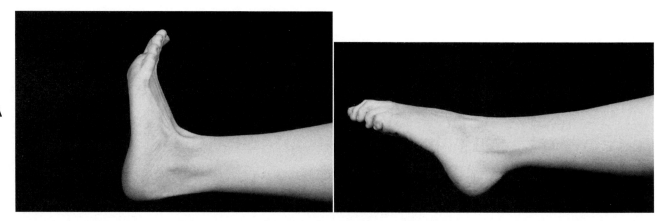

FIG. 12-12   When testing the dorsiflexion and plantar flexion of the ankle joint, neutral position for the ankle is when the lateral border of the foot is at 90 degrees in relation to the leg and the knee is in full extension. A normal ankle allows 20 degrees of dorsiflexion (**A**) and 40 degrees of plantar flexion from this position (**B**). Retained dorsiflexion of 10 degrees or less and retained plantar flexion range of motion of 30 degrees or less are impairments of the ankle for the activities of daily living. The measurements of dorsiflexion and plantar flexion can be repeated while the knee is held in 45 degrees of flexion. If the arc of motion is different from the previous finding, it indicates the presence of Achilles' tendon tightness. For all practical purposes, movements of the ankle joint are considered limited to dorsiflexion and plantar flexion. In some individuals with hypermobility of the ankle joint, medial tilt of the talus can occur within the ankle mortise. This tilt is the result of a congenital laxity of the lateral collateral ligaments and predisposes the patient to recurrent ankle sprains.

A   **B**

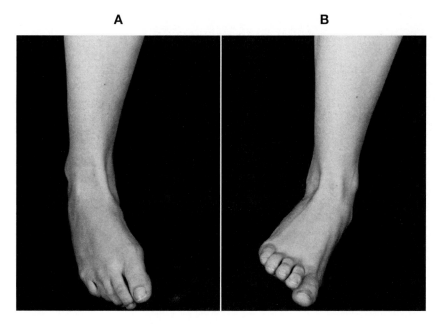

FIG. 12-13   Inversion and eversion of the foot occur mainly at the subtalar joint and are tested while the patient is lying supine. The ankle is first dorsiflexed to a neutral position. The patient rocks the foot into inversion (**A**) and eversion (**B**). A normal joint allows 20 degrees of eversion and about 30 degrees of inversion. Retained inversion range of motion that is 20 degrees or less and retained eversion range of motion that is 10 degrees or less are impairments of the foot-ankle mechanism in the activities of daily living.

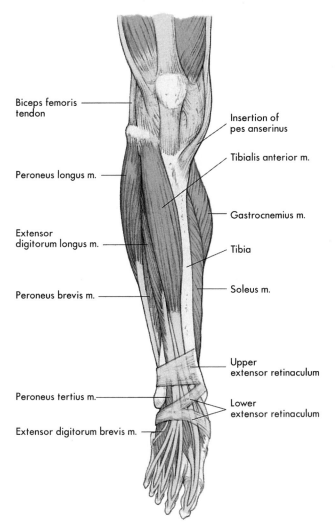

FIG. 12-14   Right leg muscles, lateral view. *(From Mathers LH: Principles of clinical anatomy, St Louis, 1996, Mosby.)*

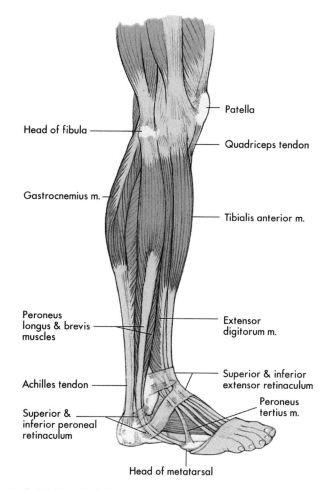

FIG. 12-15   Right leg muscles, anterior view. *(From Mathers LH: Principles of clinical anatomy, St Louis, 1996, Mosby.)*

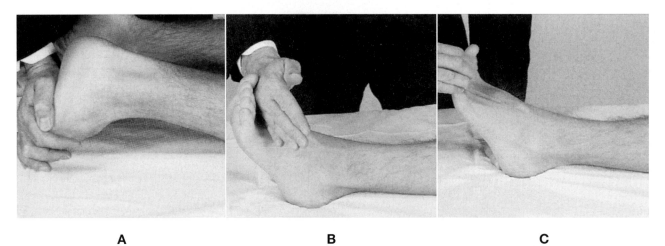

A   **B**   **C**

FIG. 12-16   Testing **(A)** and plantar flexion and dorsiflexion of the ankle **(B)** and dorsiflexion of the toes **(C)**.   *(From Epstein O, et al: Clinical examination, ed 2, London, 1997, Mosby.)*

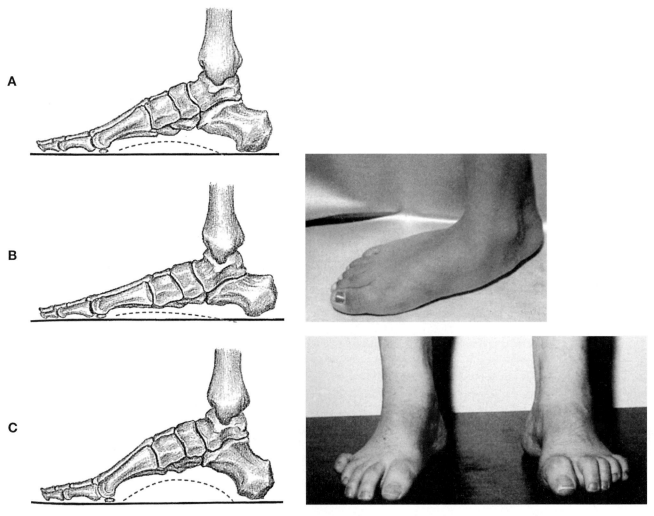

FIG. 12-17   Variations in the longitudinal arch of the foot. **A,** Expected arch. **B,** Pes planus (flatfoot). **C,** Pes cavus (high instep).   *(From Seidel HM: Mosby's guide to physical examination, ed 4, St Louis, 1999, Mosby.)*

for plantar flexion are the gastrocnemius and soleus, and they are supplemented by the tibialis posterior, peroneus longus, flexor digitorum longus, and hallucis longus. The power of the gastrocnemius-soleus group is weakened when the knee is in flexion because the gastrocnemius is a two-joint muscle. However, while the knee is in flexion, the passive range of ankle dorsiflexion increases slightly. The muscles of the anterior compartment, innervated by the deep peroneal nerve, are primarily responsible for dorsiflexion motion. Dorsiflexion is performed by the tibialis anterior and the extensor digitorum longus. When these two muscles act together, their individual actions of inversion and eversion are neutralized. The extensor hallucis longus and peroneus tertius also aid in dorsiflexion (Figs. 12-18 to 12-21).

Essential Imaging

The standard views of the ankle are the anteroposterior (AP) (Figs. 12-22 and 12-23), medial oblique (Mortise view), and lateral views (Figs. 12-24 and 12-25). The AP ankle view includes the collimate field from the distal tibia and fibula through the talocalcaneal junction. The primary purpose of the AP ankle view is to illustrate the coronal relationship of the talocrural articulation and its surrounding bony elements of the tibia, fibula, and talus. The AP and oblique projections of the ankle are sensitive for ruling out sites of injury along the lower tibia and fibula. The lateral ankle view includes the lower tibia and fibula. In cases of suspected ligamentous instability, eversion and inversion stress views can be performed. Inversion will test the lateral collateral ligament, whereas eversion will check the medial collateral (deltoid) ligament (Fig. 12-26).

ORTHOPEDIC GAMUT 12-5

VIEWS OF THE FOOT

The following are three basic views of the foot:

1. AP or dorsoplantar view (Figs. 12-27 and 12-28)
2. Oblique view (Figs. 12-29 and 12-30)
3. Lateral view

Text continued on p. 842

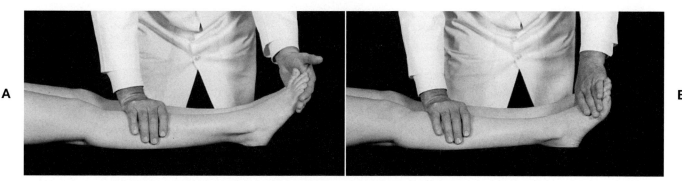

FIG. 12-18   The soleus and gastrocnemius should be evaluated separately. The soleus is evaluated by applying a dorsiflexion force to the foot while the patient plantar flexes the foot **(A).** The maneuver is performed with the knee in extension to evaluate the muscle power of the gastrocnemius. The tibialis anterior is tested by exerting a counter force to the dorsiflexion and inversion movement of the foot and ankle **(B).**

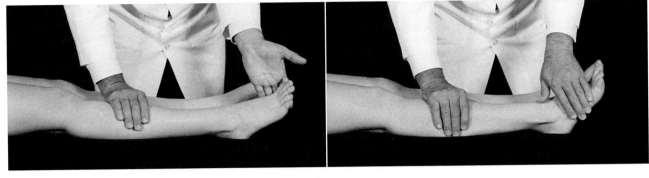

FIG. 12-19   The prime motions at the intertarsal joints are inversion and eversion, and these motions occur primarily at the subtalar joint. Inversion is achieved principally by the tibialis posterior and the tibialis anterior, but it is supplemented by the long toe flexors and gastrocnemius soleus muscle. Eversion is achieved primarily by the peroneus brevis and peroneus longus, which are innervated by the superficial peroneal nerve, and is supplemented by the extensor digitorum longus and peroneus tertius. The tibialis posterior is evaluated by exerting a counter force to the foot while the patient inverts and plantar flexes the foot (**A**). The peroneus longus is tested by exerting a counter force to a foot that is held in plantar flexion while the patient actively everts it (**B**). The peroneus brevis is evaluated the same way, but the foot is held in the neutral position.

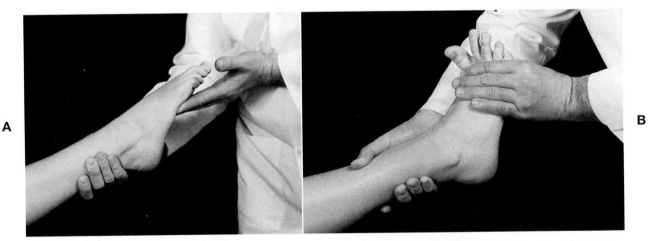

FIG. 12-20   The main motions at the metatarsophalangeal and interphalangeal joints are extension and flexion. Flexion of the metatarsophalangeal joint is achieved primarily by the lumbricales, interossei, and flexor hallucis brevis, which are augmented by the flexor hallucis longus and the flexor digitorum longus and brevis (**A**). Extension of these joints is achieved primarily by the extensor digitorum longus and the extensor hallucis longus, which are supplemented by the extensor digitorum brevis and the extensor hallucis brevis (**B**). The interphalangeal joints are hinge joints that allow flexion and extension but more flexion than extension. Flexion is achieved by the flexor digitorum longus at the distal interphalangeal joint and is supplemented by the flexor digitorum brevis at the proximal interphalangeal joints.

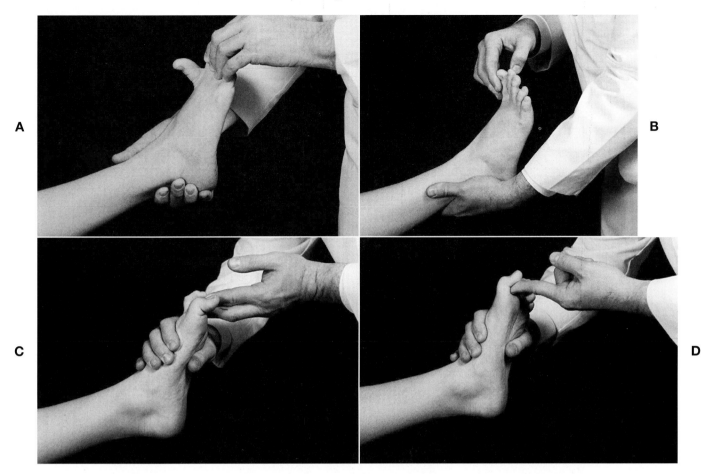

FIG. 12-21   The muscle power of the long toe extensors is tested by exerting a counterforce to the toes while the patient extends the metatarsophalangeal joints (**A** and **B**). The long toe flexors are tested by exerting a counter force to the tip of the toes while the patient flexes the interphalangeal joints (**C** and **D**).

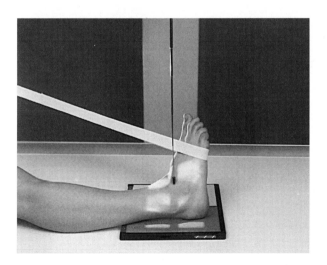

FIG. 12-22   Anteroposterior ankle in neutral position. *(From Ballinger PW:* Merrill's atlas of radiographic positions and radiologic procedures, *vol 1-3, ed 8, St Louis, 1995, Mosby.)*

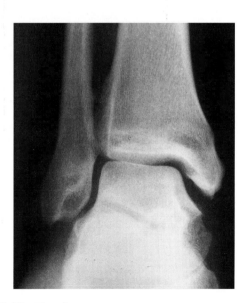

FIG. 12-23   Eversion stress. *(From Ballinger PW:* Merrill's atlas of radiographic positions and radiologic procedures, *vol 1-3, ed 8, St Louis, 1995, Mosby.)*

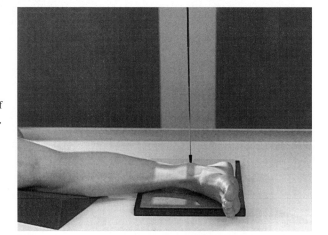

FIG. 12-24   Lateral ankle.   *(From Ballinger PW: Merrill's atlas of radiographic positions and radiologic procedures, vol 1-3, ed 8, St Louis, 1995, Mosby.)*

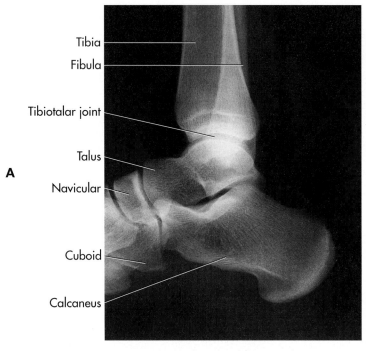

Tibia

Fibula

Tibiotalar joint

Talus

Navicular

Cuboid

Calcaneus

A

B

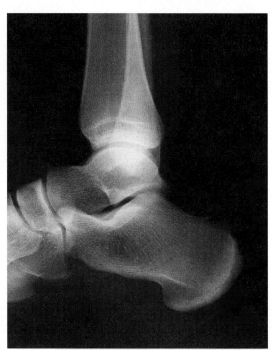

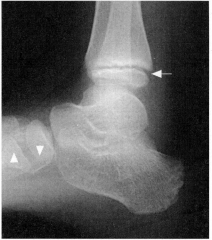

C

FIG. 12-25   **A** and **B,** Lateral ankle. **C,** Lateral ankle of 8-year-old child. *(From Ballinger PW: Merrill's atlas of radiographic positions and radiologic procedures, vol 1-3, ed 8, St Louis, 1995, Mosby.)*

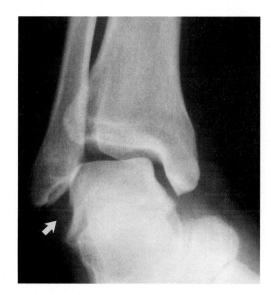

FIG. 12-26   Inversion stress. *(From Ballinger PW:* Merrill's atlas of radiographic positions and radiologic procedures, *vol 1-3, ed 8, St Louis, 1995, Mosby.)*

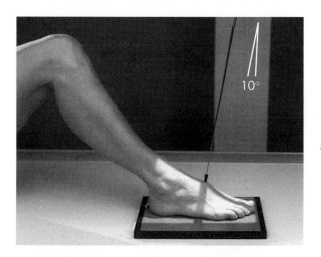

FIG. 12-27   Anteroposterior axial foot with posterior angulation of 10 degrees. *(From Ballinger PW:* Merrill's atlas of radiographic positions and radiologic procedures, *vol 1-3, ed 8, St Louis, 1995, Mosby.)*

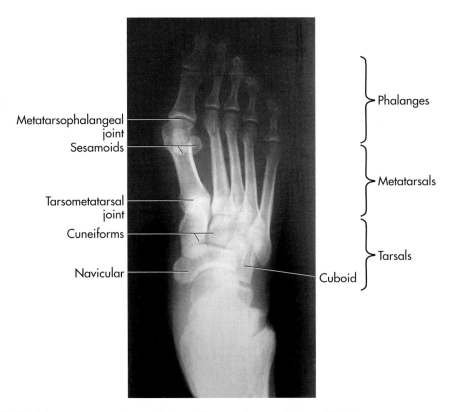

FIG. 12-28   Anteroposterior axial foot with posterior angulation of 10 degrees.   *(From Ballinger PW: Merrill's atlas of radiographic positions and radiologic procedures, vol 1-3, ed 8, St Louis, 1995, Mosby.)*

FIG. 12-29   Anteroposterior oblique foot, medial rotation.   *(From Ballinger PW: Merrill's atlas of radiographic positions and radiologic procedures, vol 1-3, ed 8, St Louis, 1995, Mosby.)*

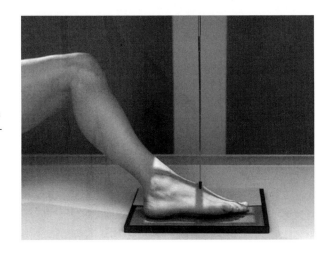

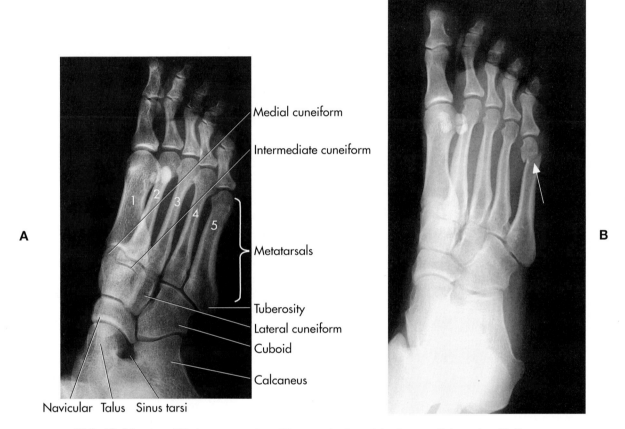

A

Medial cuneiform

Intermediate cuneiform

Metatarsals

Tuberosity

Lateral cuneiform

Cuboid

Calcaneus

Navicular   Talus   Sinus tarsi

B

FIG. 12-30   **A** and **B,** Anteroposterior oblique projection of the foot, medial rotation. **B,** Fracture of the distal aspect of the fifth metatarsal *(arrow).   (From Ballinger PW:* Merrill's atlas of radiographic positions and radiologic procedures, *vol 1-3, ed 8, St Louis, 1995, Mosby.)*

ANTERIOR DRAWER
SIGN OF THE ANKLE

Assessment for Anterior Talofibular Ligament Sprain

Comment

Ankle sprain results from the stretching or tearing of ankle ligaments following inversion or eversion foot injuries. It is the most common injury in athletics but can occur in any age group with trauma not related to sports. Radiographs should be obtained when the ankle injury meets the Ottawa rules for ankle sprain (Fig. 12-31).

ORTHOPEDIC GAMUT 12-6

ANKLE SPRAINS

Following are ankle sprain classifications:

Grade I: Localized tenderness, minimal swelling or ecchymoses, and normal range of motion without instability

Grade II: Moderate to severe pain, swelling or ecchymoses and restricted range of motion, potential mild instability, and painful weight bearing

Grade III: Severe pain, edema, hemorrhage, loss of motion, and inability to ambulate; ankle instability common, with complete functional loss

---

The most common fractures during ankle sprain are avulsions of the malleoli or tarsal bones. Other sites include the anterior process of the calcaneus, the base of the fifth metatarsal (insertion of the peroneus brevis tendon), the talar neck, the cuboid, and the bony epiphyses in children. The strength of the deltoid ligament makes it an uncommon site for injury, but when injury occurs, malleolar fractures of concomitant sprains of the syndesmosis are more likely.

With injuries to the ankle, there is such a close association between sprain dislocation and fracture that it is unwise to place them in separate categories. This is particularly true because the same forces may cause a combination of injuries. Resultant pathologic conditions may be determined more by the strength and duration of the forces that cause the injury than by the exact type of stress. The injury is usually caused by stresses that may result in either a sprain, a dislocation, a fracture, or all three.

Because the ankle is functionally a hinge joint that normally permits only dorsal and plantar flexion, injuries to the ankle are primarily due to lateral stresses that force the ankle through an arc of motion that it does not normally possess. Less commonly, injuries are caused by hyperflexion or hyperextension. The injuries that result from lateral stresses may readily be divided into two categories: inversion injuries and eversion injuries.

Inversion injuries to the ankle are usually not caused by pure inversion. The force consists of inversion, internal rotation, and plantar flexion of the foot in relation to the leg so that the foot is inverted and the ankle and foot are thrown laterally. In this injury mechanism, the push is against the medial malleolus, and the pull is away from the lateral malleolus. As the foot inverts in relation to the leg, strain is put upon the lateral collateral ligament, the ligament primarily constructed to resist this motion. As a result of this overinversion, the ligament will tear slightly, partially, or completely according to the severity of the force. If the inverting force continues as the lateral ligament gives way, the ankle opens on the lateral side, and the talus is forcibly thrust against the medial malleolus. The medial malleolus acts as a fulcrum, and its tip impinges against the central portion of the medial face of the talus. The talus rotates over the malleolus rather than pushes off it. In such a case, the injury will probably be confined to the lateral side, and there will be complete laceration of the lateral collateral ligaments. It is unusual for this type of force to break off the lateral malleolus. In the geriatric patient in whom the bone is osteoporotic, the lateral malleolus may break before the ligament tears.

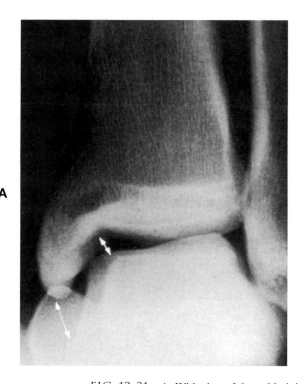

An ankle diagnostic image is required if there is any pain along the lateral malleolus or medial malleolus and any of these findings:

1. Bone tenderness at posterior edge or tip of lateral malleolus

or

2. Bone tenderness at posterior edge or tip of medial malleolus

or

3. Inability to bear weight both immediately and later

A foot diagnostic image is required if there is any pain in the midfoot tarsal area and any of these findings:

1. Bone tenderness at the base of the fifth metatarsal

or

2. Bone tenderness at the navicular

or

3. Inability to bear weight immediately or later

FIG. 12-31 **A,** Widening of the ankle joint space medially *(double-headed arrows)* with eversion stress indicates a deltoid ligament tear. **B,** Ottawa Ankle Rules for foot and ankle imaging in acute ankle injuries. *(A From Sartoris DJ:* Musculoskeletal imaging: the requisites, *St Louis, 1996, Mosby.)*

PROCEDURE

- The patient may be seated or supine.
- The examiner places one hand around the anterior aspect of the lower tibia, just above the ankle, while gripping the calcaneus in the palm of the other hand.
- While the tibia is pushed posteriorly, the calcaneus and talus are drawn anteriorly (Figs. 12-32 and 12-33).
- Normally, there is no movement from this action.
- The sign is present when the talus slides anteriorly under the ankle mortise.
- The test indicates anterior talofibular ligament instability, which is usually secondary to rupture.

Confirmation Procedures

Keen's sign, calf circumference test, and diagnostic imaging

DIAGNOSTIC STATEMENT

Anterior drawer sign of the ankle is positive for the right ankle. The presence of this sign implicates the anterior talofibular ligament and may represent a sprain.

CLINICAL PEARL

The drawer sign is a sensitive indicator of the amount of ligamentous damage in the ankle. Often, ankles with drawer sign present will require casting or rigid immobilization, at the least, in acute-stage management. Instability may sometimes follow tears of the anterior talofibular portion of the lateral ligament. This instability may be confirmed by radiographs after local anesthesia. Support the heel on a sandbag and press firmly downward on the tibia for 30 seconds before exposure. A gap that is between the talus and the tibia and is greater than 6 mm is a pathologic condition.

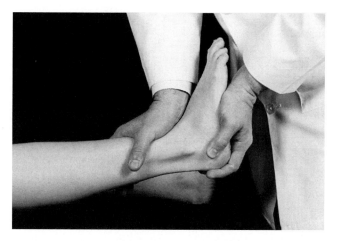

FIG. 12-32 The patient may be seated or supine. The examiner places one hand around the lower tibia, slightly above the ankle mortise. The calcaneus and talus are gripped in the palm of the other hand. The tibia is pushed posteriorly while the calcaneus and talus are drawn anteriorly. The sign is present if any movement of the talus is detected in the ankle mortise. The presence of this sign represents a talofibular ligament instability.

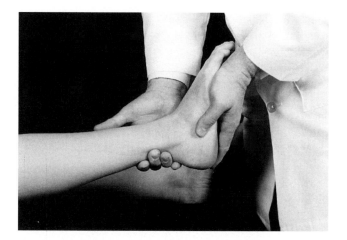

FIG. 12-33 In a reversal of this maneuver, the tibia is drawn anteriorly as the calcaneus and talus are pushed posteriorly. In this maneuver, a positive sign is indicated by a greater degree of mortise definition in the anterior. This may indicate insufficiency of the posterior talofibular portion of the lateral ligament.

BUERGER'S TEST

Assessment for Vascular Compromise of the Lower Extremity

Comment

Peripheral vascular disease in the lower extremity can be considered under two headings: disease of the peripheral arterial system and disease of the peripheral venous system. Peripheral arterial disease is mainly caused by impairment of the blood supply. This may result from atheromatous narrowing of the artery, from thrombosis, or much more rarely, from cardiac embolism.

Chronic arterial insufficiency is much more common in the lower limb and usually presents as intermittent claudication. The patient is aware of pain either in the leg, the thigh, or the buttock that comes on with walking and goes away when stopping to rest. The leg exhibits weak or absent foot, knee, and femoral pulses. The skin tends to become discolored and shiny, and hair is lost from the foot. Gangrene may affect the toes and foot (Fig. 12-34).

Knowledge of the smaller, peripheral, vascular bed structures is important to the understanding of diseases that cause peripheral vascular compromise. After leaving the mainstream artery, the efferent circulatory system branches into smaller and smaller, muscularly walled precapillaries and arterioles. Arterioles can lead directly to venules through arteriovenous anastomoses (thin-walled arterioles that contain contractile smooth muscle for control of shunting). However, more often, arterioles channel into precapillaries, and then capillaries connect to the venules and larger venous system. Fine-tuning of the systemic blood pressure can be controlled by the small, muscularly walled vessels and by shunting blood through collateral channels around the capillary bed. The pressures in capillaries of skeletal muscle range between 20 and 30 mm Hg. Therefore external pressures that exceed this value may occlude these capillaries, which deliver oxygen and remove carbon dioxide during the normal blood flow. It is at this micro-vascular level that increased interstitial fluid pressure first affects compartmental contents and leads to a progressive pathologic condition.

Similar to the varying types of muscles, different patterns of blood supply within the muscles exist. Muscles in general have isolated vascular support systems with limited internal and external anastomoses, and therefore anatomic relationships may be inconsistent. In some muscles, abundant communications between arteriolar systems exist (longitudinal anastomotic chains, such as the soleus and peroneus longus). In other muscles, several mainstream arteries send arterial branches into the muscle, so damage to a single vessel, such as the anterior tibialis and the flexor hallucis longus, may not be critical. However, some muscles, such as the extensor hallucis longus, have a single blood supply with few anastomoses. These latter systems are extremely susceptible to any circulatory compromise by virtue of their single vascular stem.

Tendons have a substantial and constant blood supply that may form an anastomosis with the muscular system. The vascularity of muscles may be isolated from the surrounding tissue and therefore susceptible to arterial injury.

In general, every major artery in a limb has one or two veins traveling with it. Any stasis or engorgement in this system may retard blood flow. This retardation causes increased pressure in the small arteriolar capillary system and leads to an alteration of the Starling equilibrium. The Starling equilibrium or mechanism is the alternation of the energy of cardiac muscle contraction that accompanies changes in the fiber length at the start of contraction. This is an essential component in the dysfunction of cardiac decompensation syndromes. This could then cause fluid extrusion from the capillary walls and add to or create increased pressure in a closed compartment.

Because the venous walls are thinner and less muscular than comparable arterial channels, the venous walls are more compressible and therefore more susceptible to changes surrounding muscle and interstitial fluid pressure. The extremities have two venous flow networks: the superficial and the deep. Deep veins are apparently more efficient in maintaining blood flow.

Through the forces of external muscular pumping and the system of intimal valves and communicating branches, the blood is shunted to and transported through the deep vessels.

PROCEDURE

- While the patient is lying supine, the examiner elevates the leg and extends the knee to a point of comfortable tolerance, approximately 45 degrees, for no less than 3 minutes (Figs. 12-35 and 12-36).
- The examiner lowers the limb, and the patient sits up with both legs dangling side by side over the examining table (Fig. 12-37).
- The test measures arterial blood supply to the lower limbs.
- The blood supply is deficient if the dorsum of the foot blanches and the prominent veins collapse when the leg is initially raised.
- The test is also positive if, when the leg is lowered, it takes 1 to 2 minutes for a ruddy (reddish) cyanosis to spread over the affected part and for the veins to fill and become prominent.

Confirmation Procedures

Claudication test, foot tourniquet test, Homans' sign, Moszkowicz test, Moses' test, Perthes' test, and vascular assessment

CLINICAL PEARL

It is not uncommon in lower extremity vascular disorders for sciatic-like pain to be produced. This test allows a quick determination of neurogenic versus vascular pain. The test demonstrates loss of vascular integrity, but as circulation diminishes, the primary complaint is produced.

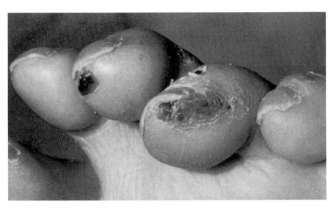

FIG. 12-34 Gangrene of toes in peripheral vascular disease. *(From Epstein O, et al:* Clinical examination, *ed 2, London, 1997, Mosby.)*

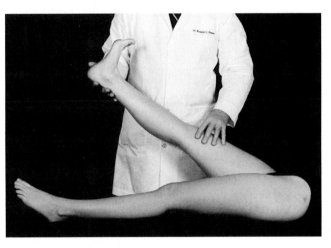

FIG. 12-35 The patient is lying supine. The examiner elevates the patient's leg to 45 degrees while the knee is fully extended. The patient actively dorsiflexes the foot.

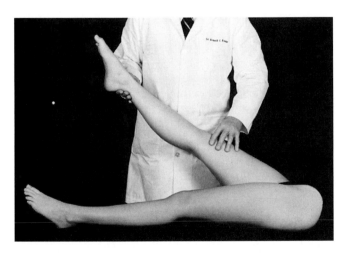

FIG. 12-36 After dorsiflexing the foot, as in Fig. 12-35, the patient plantar flexes the foot for at least 3 minutes. This maneuver diminishes the amount of blood in the distal vessels.

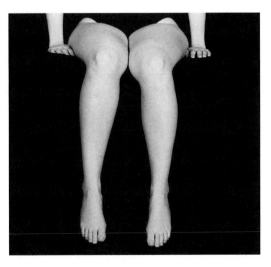

FIG. 12-37 After performing the maneuvers in Figs. 12-35 and 12-36, the patient sits at the edge of the examining table and dangles the legs. The test is positive for circulatory deficiency if the foot is blanched and the veins are collapsed. Also, the test is considered positive if it takes more than 2 minutes for the circulation to return to the dangling leg.

Assessment for Muscular Atrophy
or Hypertrophy of the Lower Extremity

Comment

ORTHOPEDIC GAMUT 12-7

LEG COMPARTMENTS

**The leg is divided into the following five
compartments by the intermuscular septa:**

1. Anterior
2. Lateral
3. Posterior tibial
4. Deep posterior
5. Superficial posterior

In the anterior compartment of the leg, the anterior tibial, the extensor hallucis, and the extensor digitorum longus muscles arise from the sides of the tibia, fibula, and interosseous membrane. These muscles completely fill the anterior compartment. This compartment is tightly roofed by the anterior fascia of the leg. With the anterior tibial syndrome, there is a rapid swelling of the muscle within its compartment. This swelling may come on following active exercise alone. In theory, this is because muscles that have not been previously conditioned are overused, so they respond with swelling and edema. The swelling also may come on following a direct injury in which there is excessive swelling and hemorrhage into the space. The condition also can be caused by localized infection within the space. In fact, anything that causes intractable swelling may cause this syndrome (Fig. 12-38).

At the onset of anterior tibial syndrome, there is severe pain over the involved area and a loss of function. Contraction of the muscles contained in the space rapidly becomes impossible, and foot drop can ensue. Even passive stretching of the muscles quickly becomes painful. However, this condition is not ordinarily preceded by the symptoms of tenosynovitis. The skin over the area becomes red, glossy, warm, and markedly tender. There is a feeling of woody tension over the point of real hardness of the fascia over the space. There may occasionally be involvement of the peroneal nerve with sensory loss (Fig. 12-39). The loss of muscle function is usually not caused by nerve involvement but by pathologic changes within the muscle itself. The muscles develop ischemic necrosis, which is often called *Volkmann's ischemia of the leg.*

ORTHOPEDIC GAMUT 12-8

VOLKMANN'S ISCHEMIA

**Volkmann's ischemia is characterized by the
following:**

1. Swelling
2. Edema
3. Extravasation of red blood cells
4. Destruction of blood cells
5. Replacement of muscle tissue by a fibrous scar

The result is a firm, inelastic, and noncontractile muscle group. This condition can be extremely disabling and defies reconstructive treatment (Fig. 12-40).

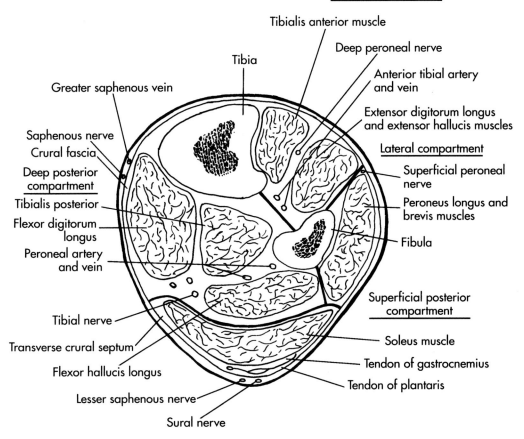

FIG. 12-38   Compartments of the leg.   *(From Nicholas JA, Hershman EB: The lower extremity & spine in sports medicine, vol 1-2, ed 2, St Louis, 1995, Mosby.)*

PROCEDURE

- While the patient is lying supine, the circumference of the bellies of the gastrocnemius and soleus muscles are measured (Figs. 12-41 and 12-42).
- The measurement is compared with the calf circumference of the opposite leg.
- Because the dominance of a leg is not established except in highly specialized sports or occupations, the measurements should be equal.
- A diminished calf circumference may represent simple loss of muscle tone, but it also may represent atrophy of muscle fibers.
- An increased calf circumference, corroborated with other pathologic findings, may indicate a fulminating compartment syndrome.

Confirmation Procedures

Keen's sign, anterior drawer sign of the ankle, vascular assessment, and diagnostic imaging

---

DIAGNOSTIC STATEMENT

Calf circumference measurements reveal a diminished size when compared with the uninvolved leg. This size difference suggests loss of muscular tone or atrophy.

Calf circumference measurements reveal an increased size relative to the uninvolved leg. This difference suggests an increase in muscular bulk, muscular compartment pressures, or hypertrophy.

CLINICAL PEARL

In knee injuries, the first sign of internal joint derangement is loss of tone in the quadriceps. Internal derangement of the ankle joint produces the same phenomenon in its controlling musculature. The gastrocnemius-soleus mechanism weakens and loses tone to a degree sufficient enough to be quantified with a tape measure. This measuring can help differentiate the degree of ankle involvement.

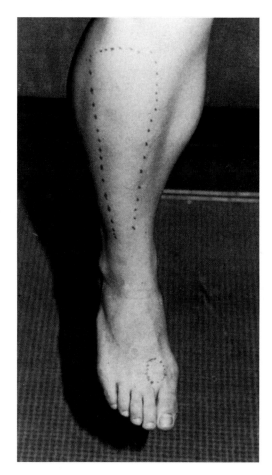

FIG. 12-39 Anterior compartment syndrome with swelling and tenderness in anterior compartment and decreased sensation in first web space of the foot, as outlined. *(From Nicholas JA, Hershman EB:* The lower extremity & spine in sports medicine, *vol 1-2, ed 2, St Louis, 1995, Mosby.)*

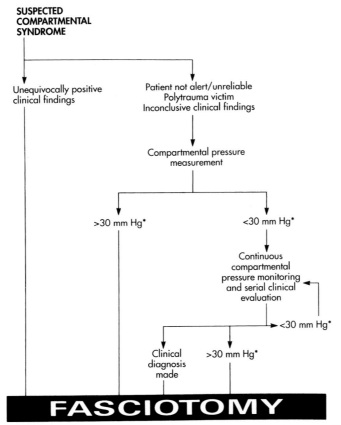

SUSPECTED
COMPARTMENTAL
SYNDROME

Unequivocally positive
clinical findings

Patient not alert/unreliable
Polytrauma victim
Inconclusive clinical findings

Compartmental pressure
measurement

>30 mm Hg*   <30 mm Hg*

Continuous
compartmental
pressure monitoring
and serial clinical
evaluation

<30 mm Hg*

Clinical
diagnosis
made   >30 mm Hg*

FASCIOTOMY

*In patients with hypotension, compartmental syndromes may occur at pressures <30 mm Hg.
Currently, we use 25 mm Hg as the critical pressure in these patients.

FIG. 12-40   Algorithm used in diagnosing and treating acute compartment syndromes of the lower leg.   *(From Bourne RB, Rorabeek CH:* Clin Orthop *240:97, 1989.)*

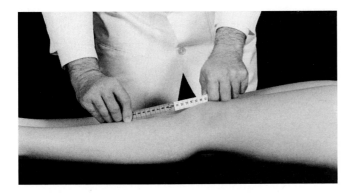

FIG. 12-41   The patient is lying supine with the knees extended. The examiner establishes a point in the leg 6 inches below the midline of the patella.

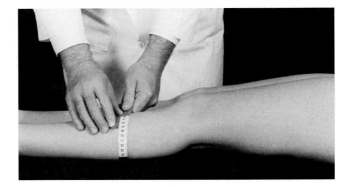

FIG. 12-42   The circumference of the leg is measured at the point selected in Fig. 12-41. The examiner should be cautious when drawing the tape measure tight. The tape should be snug, but no skin depressions should be observed. The measurement is recorded and compared with the circumference of the same point in opposite leg.

CLAUDICATION TEST

Assessment for Chronic Arterial Occlusive Disease

Comment

Many patients with vascular diseases present with signs and symptoms evident at a site distal to the anatomic location of the pathology. Because most of the vessels in the lower limb either terminate or originate in the foot, they are most often affected by circulatory problems.

Arterial diseases usually result in reduction of blood flow to the foot. Most commonly, this is an occlusive process involving the vessel itself or from mechanical obstruction of the vessel lumen by foreign material. The most common cause of occlusion is atherosclerosis and associated embolic atheromatous plaques.

ORTHOPEDIC GAMUT 12-9

POPLITEAL ARTERY

Following are two conditions affecting the popliteal artery:

1. Popliteal artery entrapment syndrome
2. Adventitial cystic disease of the popliteal artery

Popliteal artery entrapment syndrome has a male predilection of 15:1 and typically presents by the second or third decade of life. Symptoms are described as cramping in the calf and foot, often associated with paresthesias and numbness. Adventitial cystic disease of the popliteal artery generally affects males in their fourth or fifth decade. The patient experiences sudden claudication and absent pedal pulses in an otherwise healthy-appearing limb.

Frostbite occurs from freezing of the tissues and resultant vascular injury (Fig. 12-43). Long-term sensitivity to cold with vasospasm and Raynaud's phenomenon is a common sequela of frostbite.

Erythromelalgia is a rare disorder, usually involving the feet, in which paroxysmal vasodilatation, erythema, and burning pain are brought on by exposure to heat. The cause may be primary or may be secondary to concomitant diseases such as diabetes, hypertension, venous insufficiency, or myeloproliferative disorders. Erythromelalgia should be suspected when the patient's subjective complaints of erythema and burning pain are associated with an objective elevation in skin temperature. It often begins as a mild discomfort mimicking neuropathy, but it may slowly progress to the point at which patients are severely disabled.

The most common causes of small vessel diseases are arteriosclerosis and the collagen-vascular diseases. Micro-embolization will produce histologic changes in muscles that are comparable to those seen in myopathic diseases. An acute obstruction of small vessels is an example of such a change. The clinical conditions are chronic and usually progressive. The collagen-vascular diseases may have periods of acute exacerbation. During these periods, the diseases are rapidly progressive. In this case, the electromyographic (EMG) findings would be myopathic in nature and would resemble polymyositis. The nerve conduction studies would show normal or slightly slowed velocities, and the M wave would probably be reduced slightly. With slowly progressive arteriosclerosis, EMG studies are rarely performed. The changes would be very slow and would represent loss of individual muscle fibers from the motor units as well as loss of small nerve fibers. The EMG findings would demonstrate myopathic and neuropathic, large-amplitude and small-amplitude motor units of brief duration. Fibrillation potentials would be a rare finding.

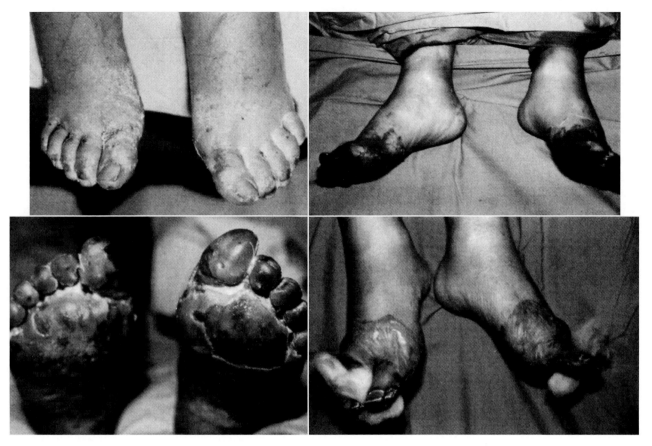

FIG. 12-43   Patients with frostbite.   *(From Baxter DE:* The foot and ankle in sport, *St Louis, 1995,* Mosby.)

PROCEDURE

- The patient walks at a rate of 120 steps per minute for 60 seconds (Fig. 12-44).
- This goal can be accomplished by having the patient walk on a treadmill.
- The time that elapses between the start of the test and the occurrence of leg cramping is the claudication time (Fig. 12-45).
- The site of the cramping and often the color change (pallor) in the tissues identifies the level of the lesion.
- The test indicates peripheral vascular disease of chronic arterial occlusion.

Confirmation Procedures

Buerger's test, foot tourniquet test, Homans' sign, Moszkowicz test, Moses' sign, Perthes' test, and vascular assessment

---

DIAGNOSTIC STATEMENT

The claudication test is positive on the right. This result suggests chronic arterial occlusive disease.

CLINICAL PEARL

The claudication test may be an assumed finding in patients who complain of leg cramps during distance walking. The pain of neurogenic origin is differentiated from pain of arterial origin when the patient relates sitting with almost immediate cramp relief.

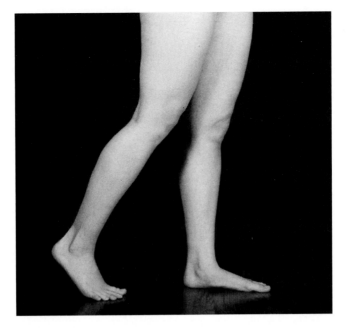

FIG. 12-44   The patient begins marching in place. The pace should be about 120 steps per minute and should be continued for 60 seconds. This maneuver also may be accomplished by using a treadmill.

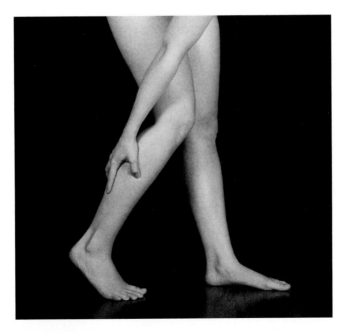

FIG. 12-45   The time elapsing between the start of the test and the onset of the leg cramping is the claudication time. The normal leg should not cramp. When positive, the test indicates chronic arterial occlusion.

DUCHENNE'S SIGN

Assessment for Lesions of the Superficial Peroneal Nerve

Comment

Compression or distortion of the superficial peroneal nerve may occur where the nerve exits the muscular layer of the leg and pierces the crural fascia at the level between the middle and distal third of the leg. Chronic ankle sprains, a major underlying factor, subject the nerve to recurrent stretching (Fig. 12-46).

At the entrance into the peroneal tunnel, near the head of the fibula, the common peroneal nerve divides into two terminal branches: the deep and the superficial peroneal nerve. This terminal branch point and the course of the superficial peroneal nerve may vary. The superficial branch continues distally between the fibula and the peroneus longus muscle, which lies on the intermuscular septum of the anterior compartment. The nerve also lies proximally between the peroneus longus and the extensor digitorum longus muscles and distally between the peroneus longus and brevis muscles. At the level between the middle and distal third of the leg, the nerve pierces the crural fascia and continues subcutaneously as the cutaneous dorsalis medialis and the cutaneous dorsalis intermedius nerves. Before piercing the fascia, the superficial peroneal nerve supplies the peroneus longus and brevis muscles. The cutaneous branches of the superficial nerves supply the skin of the anterolateral side of the leg; the dorsum of the foot; the dorsum of the first, second, and third toes; and the medial side of the fourth toe. The sural nerve, via the cutaneous dorsalis lateralis nerve, supplies the lateral sides of the fourth and fifth toes.

Trauma represents the most commonly proposed cause of this rarely diagnosed syndrome of the superficial peroneal nerve. Surgical trauma, lipomas, muscular hernias, tight boots, repetitive compression of the foot in sports, and dynamic compression of the narrow fascial tunnel have been offered as possible causes. Trauma in this area may lead to local inflammation, reactive swelling, and eventual compression of the fascial tunnel.

Dynamic compression, based on the functional anatomy of the leg, places the nerve at risk. The superficial peroneal nerve is fixed. Therefore forced inversion and extension of the foot further stretches the nerve over the fascial border. Although typically 1 cm long, surgical evidence shows that the tunnel may actually extend up 3 to 11 cm in length. Repetitive activities may cause scarring of the nerve or fascial borders, which narrows the tunnel even further.

Described as mononeuralgia, pain caused by compression or damage to the superficial peroneal nerve appears on the dorsum of the foot and is occasionally accompanied by dysesthesia or complete anesthesia in the nerve's dermatome.

ORTHOPEDIC GAMUT 12-10

ANTEROLATERAL COMPARTMENT SYNDROME

Following are three additional tests for evaluating patients for anterolateral compartment syndrome:

1. Resisted dorsiflexion and eversion with pressure applied over the tunnel
2. Passive plantar flexion and inversion
3. Stretching of the nerve, as in the second test, with percussion over the tunnel

---

A positive result for these provocative tests is the production of pain or paresthesia over the nerve's dermatome. EMG studies of the peroneal and anterior tibial muscles and conduction velocities help in identifying the syndrome.

PROCEDURE

- The examiner pushes up the head of the first metatarsal with the thumb, and the patient plantar flexes the foot (Fig. 12-47).
- The sign is present when the medial border of the foot dorsiflexes, with the lateral border plantar flexing (Fig. 12-48).
- The head of the first metatarsal offers no resistance to the pushing thumb.
- The plantar crease runs laterally from the medial side of the big toe to the heel, and the arch disappears.
- This result is caused by paralysis of the peroneus longus, which results from a lesion of the superficial peroneal nerve or a lesion at or above the L4, L5, and S1 roots.

Confirmation Procedures

Tinel's foot sign and electrodiagnosis

DIAGNOSTIC STATEMENT

Duchenne's sign is positive in the left foot. The presence of this sign suggests a lesion of the superficial peroneal nerve.

CLINICAL PEARL

Before diagnosing pes planus that is caused by structural problems, the examiner should attempt to elicit Duchenne's sign. The presence of this sign indicates a pes planus phenomenon that is caused by neural lesions at a much higher level than the arch itself.

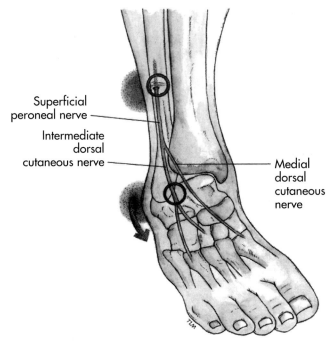

FIG. 12-46 Anterolateral compartment syndrome. *(From Baxter DE: The foot and ankle in sport, St Louis, 1995, Mosby.)*

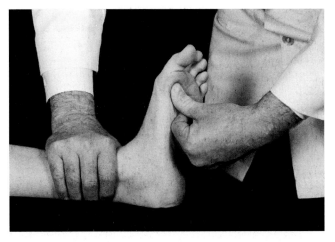

FIG. 12-47 The patient is lying supine, and the leg is extended. The examiner grasps the lower tibia with one hand, slightly above the ankle mortise. With the thumb of the other hand, the examiner applies pressure to the head of the first metatarsal.

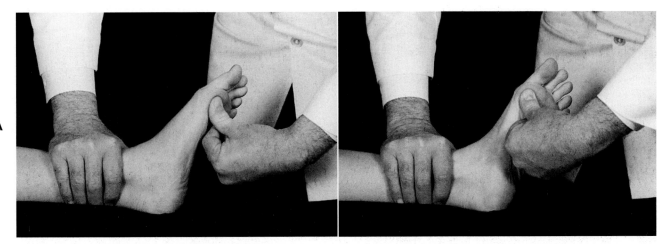

FIG. 12-48 The patient plantar flexes the foot as the examiner maintains pressure on the first metatarsal **(A).** The sign is present when the medial border of the foot dorsiflexes, the lateral border of the foot plantar flexes, and the arch of the foot disappears **(B).** The presence of this sign indicates paralysis of the peroneus longus muscle that is due to a lesion of the superficial peroneal nerve.

Assessment for Arterial Insufficiency of the Lower Extremity

Comment

Chronic compartment syndrome is caused by high pressure within the noncompliant fascial boundaries of the leg with resultant ischemia of muscles and nerves (Fig. 12-49). The elevated pressures are believed to arise from increased muscle volume and from increased intracellular and extracellular fluid accumulation with or without muscular microtears and hemorrhage. These increased pressures may cause venous and lymphatic compromise and further compound the situation (Fig. 12-50).

The diagnosis of chronic compartment syndrome can be made on clinical examination during or after exercise, but confirmation with compartmental pressures is warranted when considering surgical treatment (Fig. 12-51).

ORTHOPEDIC GAMUT 12-11

COMPARTMENT SYNDROME

The diagnosis of compartment syndrome is based on the following:

1. Preexercise compartment pressures of 15 mm Hg or greater
2. One-minute postexercise compartment pressures of 30 mm Hg or greater
3. Compartment pressure measured 5 to 10 minutes after cessation of exercise of 15 mm Hg or greater

---

Pressures can be reproducibly obtained using the Stryker manometer or other handheld devices (Fig. 12-52).

Significant diminution of blood flow to individual toes or to an entire foot results in pale nail beds, slow capillary recovery after skin compression, diminished bleeding after skin puncture, lowering of the skin temperature, and pain of varying intensity. Symptoms and signs of pain, pulselessness, pallor, paresthesia, and paralysis indicate arterial insufficiency or inadequate capillary perfusion. The coexistence of pallor with cyanosis and rubor (mottling) is consistent with vasoconstriction and later vasodilation.

The spectrum of causes for diminished blood flow is made apparent by observing the alterations that occur in the healthy extremity, which is affected temporarily by decreased blood flow as a result of environmental alterations, such as cooling of the feet, contact of a toe with ice, or sympathetic nervous stimulation from anxiety or fear. In each instance, the occurrence of pallor and a significant drop in skin temperature will cause pain that is moderately severe and is described as a deep, aching sensation. As the ischemic state persists, pain becomes more intense.

The phrase *Raynaud's disease* is used to describe the occurrence of vasospasm within an underlying primary disease. If vasospasm is associated with a known connective-tissue disease, Raynaud's phenomenon is implied. Recognition of Raynaud's syndrome and the patient's response to this condition is important in explaining pain and cold tolerance associated with a known pathologic condition. When the symptoms of pain occur in a toe, the foot, or the entire lower extremity, the existence of adequate blood flow in the large and small vessels must be determined.

In patients known to have a nerve compression lesion, such as superficial peroneal nerve compression at the fascial tunnel, diminished blood flow will cause abnormal sensory changes to occur earlier than they would in the normal patient. Motor weakness occurs more quickly when partial or complete ischemia occurs.

Various conditions—such as atherosclerotic stenosis, thromboembolism, or compression of major arteries in the lower abdomen—cause pain, claudication, paresthesia, and intermittent episodes of pallor. The lesions may be partial or complete, and the clinical symptoms may vary according to the degree of ischemia.

Acute occlusion of an artery is associated with unrelenting pain and pallor, followed by rubor and cyanosis. Cold tolerance is diminished, and intrinsic muscle weakness occurs.

Obliteration of the artery results from trauma and the occurrence of an anterior compartment compression of the lower leg muscles, vessels, and nerves. This compression causes pallor of the foot, diminished pulse volume, and severe pain. The effect of diminished arterial inflow and lessened venous outflow during pain has been well calibrated by analyzing the effects of traumatic lesions at various levels of the extremity. Decompression of a tight compartment that is anterior to the leg will diminish pain almost immediately. Elimination of nerve compression syndromes at the ankle will provide a measurable relief of pain.

Causalgia is considered a mixed nerve lesion with accompanying or secondary vascular insufficiency. The residual pain may require direct treatment of the peripheral nerve.

Sympathetic dystrophy is one condition that may occur, although a specific nerve injury cannot be demonstrated. However, there is a vasospastic element that occurs secondary to a major or minor insult of the extremity or an adjacent organ.

PROCEDURE

- Application of a pneumatic tourniquet, with pressure elevated to 20 mm Hg above the patient's resting diastolic blood pressure, to a normal extremity will obliterate arterial inflow and venous outflow, slow motor nerve conduction, decrease sensory conduction, and cause pain in the foot and at the site of tourniquet compression (Fig. 12-53).
- Anoxia and nerve compression occur simultaneously, and muscle weakness is evident within 3 to 5 minutes.

- Digital paresthesia occurs, and sensation diminishes gradually to anesthesia in about 30 minutes.
- These painful sensations are a combination of muscle and nerve ischemia and nerve compression.

Confirmation Procedures
Buerger's test, claudication test, Homans' sign, Moszkowicz test, Moses' test, Perthes' test, and vascular assessment

Text continued on p. 864

DIAGNOSTIC STATEMENT

The tourniquet test is positive for the left leg and ankle. This result indicates arterial insufficiency.

CLINICAL PEARL

Tenderness at the front of the leg is characteristic in (1) Osgood-Schlatter disease, (2) Brodie's abscess (or osteitis), (3) anterior tibial compartment syndrome, (4) stress fracture, and (5) shin splints. Tenderness at the back of the leg is characteristically situated (1) in the plantaris tendon in partial and complete ruptures, (2) over varicosities in superficial thrombophlebitis, and (3) over the tendocalcaneus in partial tears and complete ruptures.

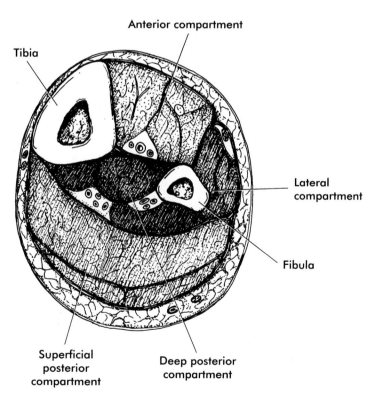

FIG. 12-49   Compartments of the leg in cross section.   *(From Baxter DE: The foot and ankle in sport, St Louis, 1995, Mosby.)*

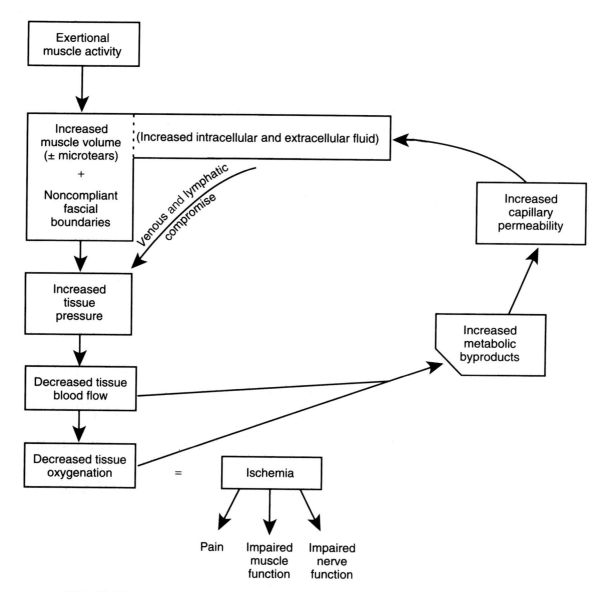

FIG. 12-50   Development of a compartment syndrome. *(From Baxter DE:* The foot and ankle in sport, *St Louis, 1995, Mosby.)*

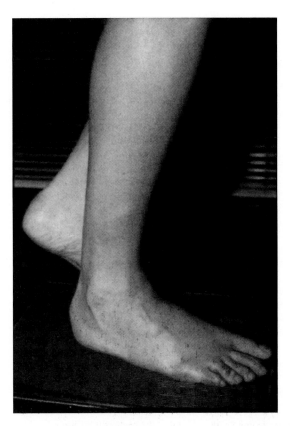

FIG. 12-51 Anterolateral fascial defect and peroneal muscle herniation in a runner. *(From Baxter DE:* The foot and ankle in sport, *St Louis, 1995, Mosby.)*

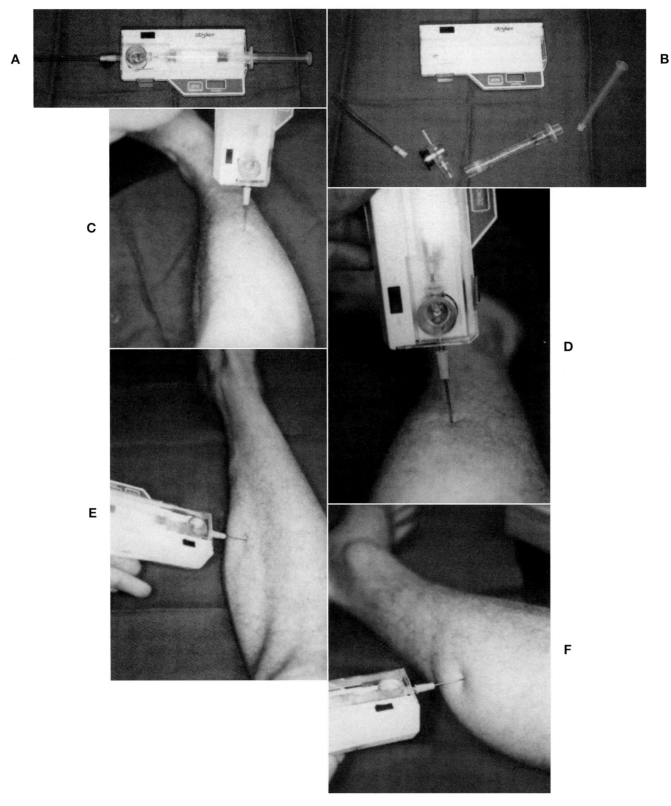

FIG. 12-52   Stryker handheld device for compartment pressure measurement **(A)**, disassembled components **(B)**, measuring anterior **(C)**, lateral **(D)**, deep posterior **(E)**, and superficial posterior compartments **(F)**. *(From Baxter DE: The foot and ankle in sport, St Louis, 1995, Mosby.)*

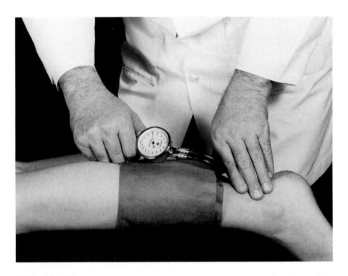

FIG. 12-53 The patient is lying prone on the examination table, and the leg is extended. The foot dangles over the end of the examining table. The calf musculature should be as relaxed as possible. A blood pressure cuff is applied to the leg, near the ankle, above the area of complaint. The cuff is inflated to 20 mm Hg above the patient's resting diastolic blood pressure. Pressure may need to be increased to reach blanching of the distal extremity. Foot pain, paresthesia, and muscle weakness appearing in less than 5 minutes indicate arterial insufficiency.

HELBINGS' SIGN

Assessment for Pes Planus

Comment

Flattening of the longitudinal arch, or flat foot, is often asymptomatic but may result in muscle fatigue with aching and intolerance due to long hours of standing or walking. Physical findings include loss of the medial longitudinal arch on weight bearing with medial and plantar displacement of the navicular and the talar head. In severe cases, the calcaneus is everted (valgus), and the forefoot is abducted with "too many toes" when viewed from behind (Fig. 12-54).

Pes planus is attributed to deficiencies in the structure of the talus and calcaneus. Conversely, strong and well-shaped feet are attributed to tarsal bones so shaped and so integrated into one another that they cannot shift when weight is imposed on them. In symptomatic pes planus that does not involve osseous anomalies, the condition is often related to weak posterior tibial muscle function. This weakness permits an abnormal excursion of the talonavicular joint.

Rupture of the tendon of the posterior tibialis muscle is an etiologic factor in pes planus. These ruptures have occurred in middle-aged individuals who have had one or more injections of a corticosteroid into the sheath of the tendon. Such an injection is used to relieve local discomfort or to alleviate an obvious synovitis. Rupture of the tendon occurs with prompt development of a markedly pronated foot. When the patient, attempting to rise on the toes, has difficulty doing so on the involved side, it is because the heel fails to invert and the longitudinal arch fails to rise during this maneuver. Rupture of the posterior tibial tendon should be suspected in any patient in which unilateral pes planus suddenly appears.

The symptomatic weak foot may be flat or may have a high longitudinal arch, especially when at rest. The flat foot usually has a degree of abduction of the forefoot and eversion of the ankle. The Achilles' tendon may be shortened and pulled at an angle instead of following a plumb line. The long, narrow, flaccid foot with a normal arch is likely to become symptomatic.

PROCEDURE

- Medial curving of Achilles' tendon, when viewed posteriorly, indicates foot pronation (Figs. 12-55 and 12-56).

Confirmation Procedures

Hoffa's test and Thompson's test

DIAGNOSTIC STATEMENT

Helbings' sign is present for the left foot. The presence of this sign suggests pes planus.

CLINICAL PEARL

The arches of the foot do not become fully formed until a child has been walking for some years. The young child's foot is normally flat. If the arches fail to establish, an awkward gait and rapid, uneven wear and distortion of the shoes may occur, but it is rare for pain or other symptoms to develop. Persistent flatfoot may be associated with knock-knees, torsional deformities of the tibia, and valgus deformities of the heel.

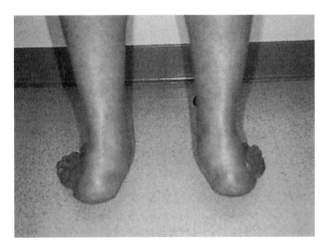

FIG. 12-54   Pronation of heel. Notice that weight bearing is not through the midline of the foot.
(From Seidel HM: Mosby's guide to physical examination, *ed 4, St Louis, 1999, Mosby.)*

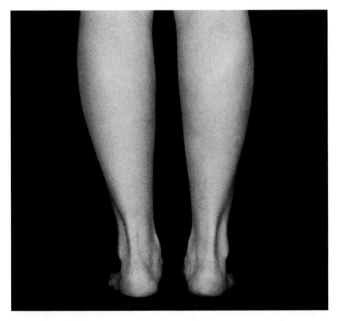

FIG. 12-55   The patient is standing, with the feet resting on a smooth, flat surface. From the posterior, the examiner observes the positions of the Achilles' tendons. Normally, there should be no curving of the tendons as the patient bears weight.

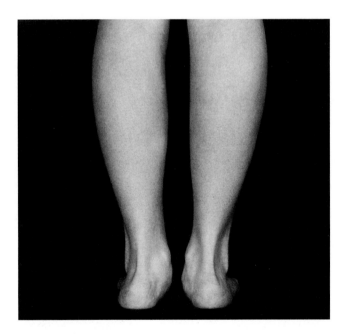

FIG. 12-56   The sign is present when a medial curving of the Achilles' tendon is observed (as on the left). The sign indicates a pes planus condition.

HOFFA'S TEST

ALSO KNOWN AS HOFFA'S SIGN

Assessment for Fracture of the Calcaneus

Comment

The posterior portion of the foot is rarely fractured—if sprain-fractures are excluded. The ordinary fracture of the calcaneus is by direct compression as in a fall from a height or from driving the foot into a hard surface. Fortunately, neither of these causes is common. Certain fractures do occur in special situations. Abnormal, forceful motion may cause avulsion or snubbing fractures of the talus. Also, the sustentaculum tali may be broken by forceful eversion of the foot. It is extremely important to restore the contour of the calcaneus and particularly the integrity of the talocalcaneal joint. Adduction or abduction of the foot may cause a snubbing or avulsion fracture of the superior portion of the calcaneus at the calcaneocuboid joint.

A fracture of the calcaneus usually results from a fall on the heel. It often is associated with a compression fracture of the lumbar spine. The os calcis is usually crushed, and the fragments are displaced in varying amounts (Fig. 12-57). The heel is often so painful that the spine injury may not be noticed initially.

Fractures of the os calcis are painful injuries characterized by severe swelling. The swelling may be so intense that blistering and even skin necrosis may occur.

Fracture of the calcaneus is the most common tarsal bone injury. A fracture involving the body of the calcaneus is the most common calcaneal fracture, and it often extends into the subtalar joint, with the posterior portion of the body displaced upward. This type of fracture is caused by a direct vertical force onto the calcaneus that usually occurs after a fall from a height. The spine should always be examined carefully because a compression fracture of the spine in the dorsolumbar area is often associated with calcaneal fractures.

The other types of calcaneal fractures, such as an avulsion fracture of Achilles' tendon insertion and fracture of the sustentaculum tali or anterior process, are seen less frequently.

AP and lateral diagnostic imaging of the foot are necessary to evaluate the involvement of the subtalar joint. Fracture of the sustentaculum tali is demonstrable only in the axial views.

PROCEDURE

- While the patient is lying prone, the ankles hang well over the edge of the examining table in a symmetric position.
- Hoffa's test is positive if the examiner, using movement and palpation, finds the Achilles' tendon on the injured side less taut than that on the contralateral side.
- There may also be increased dorsiflexion of the foot in the relaxed position on the affected side (Fig. 12-58).
- A loose fragment may be observed and felt behind either malleolus.
- The test is significant for fracture of the calcaneus.

Confirmation Procedures

Helbings' sign, Thompson's test, and diagnostic imaging

DIAGNOSTIC STATEMENT

Hoffa's test is positive for the left foot. This result indicates fracture of the calcaneus.

CLINICAL PEARL

In geriatric patients, the Achilles' tendon insufficiency that is caused by attrition also produces a positive Hoffa's test. In this instance, the calcaneus remains intact.

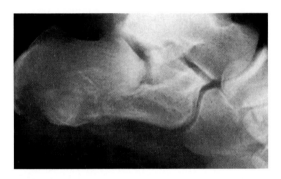

FIG. 12-57 Fracture of the calcaneus with moderate displacement. *(From Mercier LR, Pettid FJ:* Practical orthopedics, *ed 4, St Louis, 1995, Mosby.)*

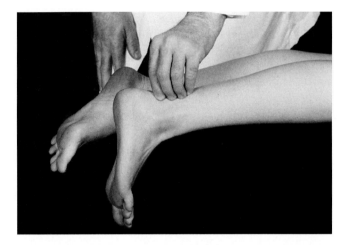

FIG. 12-58 The patient is prone on the examination table. The knees are extended, and the ankles hang well over the end of the table. The sign is present when the affected foot rests in a more dorsiflexed position (as noted on the right) than the opposite foot. The test is positive when the examiner determines by palpation the loss of Achilles' tendon integrity. The sign implicates calcaneal fracture.

HOMANS' SIGN

Assessment for Thrombophlebitis of the Lower Extremity

Comment

Superficial thrombophlebitis is inflammation and thrombosis of a superficial vein. This condition commonly results either from local trauma or from an intravenous infusion, but it may occur spontaneously. Thrombosis of the deep veins in the calf or pelvis usually occurs as a result of a combination of damage to the endothelial lining of the veins, with stasis of the blood within them as a consequence of physical inactivity.

Intermittent claudication is the term applied to a condition that denotes an insufficient blood supply to the muscles of the lower extremities when they are called into activity during locomotion. Intermittent claudication occurs in atheroma, with or without thrombosis, and in embolism, Buerger's disease, and rarely, syphilitic endarteritis. The condition is aggravated by anemia.

The patient complains of pain that occurs in one or both legs and in the calf muscles and comes on after walking a certain distance. The pain disappears during rest. The pain becomes so intolerable that the patient is obliged to stand or sit still until it passes. As time goes on, the distance that the patient can walk in comfort becomes progressively shorter. Examination of the affected limb reveals nothing obvious. The legs are well nourished and normal in sensation and reflexes. The arteries at the ankle will be pulseless, and the popliteal pulsation behind the knee joint may not be felt. The femoral artery can usually be felt to pulsate in a normal manner.

After the patient walks, the foot may appear unduly pale. With rest, normal color returns and spreads gradually over the surface of the foot. The ankle jerk may be diminished or absent as a result of ischemia of the posterior tibial nerve. In later cases, paresthesia and objective sensory loss occur in the toes and foot. Intermittent claudication is not uncommon, and its diagnosis is not difficult.

The importance of recognizing the condition is paramount because of the tendency for the condition to develop into gangrene.

PROCEDURE

- While the patient is lying in the supine position, the examiner dorsiflexes the patient's foot and squeezes the calf (Figs. 12-59 and 12-60).
- Deep-seated pain in the posterior leg or calf indicates thrombophlebitis.

Confirmation Procedures

Buerger's test, claudication test, foot tourniquet test, Moszkowicz test, Moses' sign, Perthes' test, and vascular assessment

---

DIAGNOSTIC STATEMENT

Homans' sign is present in the left leg. The presence of this sign suggests thrombophlebitis.

CLINICAL PEARL

The use of Homans' sign does not aid differentiation between a muscular lesion and thrombophlebitis. The differentiation occurs when the test is concluded. When the pain remits quickly, thrombophlebitis is suspected. When the pain persists or lags as an ache, calf strain is suspected.

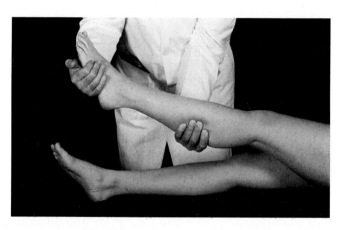

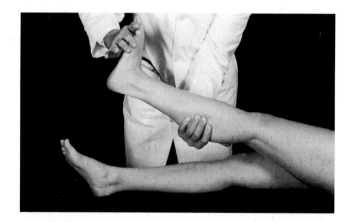

FIG. 12-59   The patient is lying supine with the knees extended and the legs resting on the examination table. The examiner elevates the affected leg to 45 degrees, and the calf is squeezed firmly.

FIG. 12-60   As the calf pressure is maintained, the examiner dorsiflexes the foot. Deep calf or leg pain during this maneuver indicates thrombophlebitis.

Assessment for Distal Fibular Fracture

Comment

Fracture of the tibia is uncommon, but fracture of the fibula is common. In any fracture of the fibula, associated injury of the ankle must be investigated. Whenever there is a complete fracture of the fibula above the level of the tibiofibular syndesmosis, complete rupture of the inferior tibiofibular ligaments must be investigated. The possibility of rupture is the most serious and most important consideration in the fracture of the fibula. The actual fracture of the fibula is usually inconsequential, except that it does require a certain period of healing. If the fracture is accompanied by a rupture of the tibiofibular ligaments and results in instability or separation of the ankle mortise, a serious and permanent disability results.

Fractures of the fibula result from direct blows that usually occur in the lower one third of the fibula. These blows may be caused by contact with a shoe or other hard object. With fracture of the fibula, there is immediate pain but not severe disability. Upon examination, local tenderness will be present at the site of the injury. There may or may not be local crepitus. There is usually prompt swelling with localized hematoma formation. The individual can usually walk quite well. In fact, the patient may be able to complete a walking task because with a fracture of the fibula by direct blow, the integrity of the ankle is not involved, and disability is caused by contraction of the muscle attachments on the fibular shaft. Diagnosis is confirmed by diagnostic imaging, which should always be used in a case of localized tenderness over any bone.

Of all bones, the fibula is particularly prone to stress fracture and is second only to the metatarsals in this respect. This condition arises early in athletic or new job training requiring prolonged standing and first appears as an ache, with some soreness and distress during function. The ache is usually localized near the neck of the fibula. The patient has no history of injury.

ORTHOPEDIC GAMUT 12-12

DISTAL TIBIAL AND FIBULAR FRACTURES

Types of distal tibial or fibular fractures include the following:

1. *Bimalleolar fracture:* fractures of the medial and lateral malleoli (Fig. 12-61)
2. *Boot-top (skier's) fracture:* spiral fracture of the distal diametaphyseal portions of the tibia and fibula
3. *Maisonneuve fracture:* fracture of the proximal fibula, as a result of severe inversion and external rotation of the ankle (often unobserved because of the severity of the ankle injury)
4. *Pott's fracture:* fracture of the metadiaphyseal region of the distal fibula, with associated rupture of the distal tibiofibular ligament (Fig. 12-62); Pott's fracture that involves both the lateral and medial malleolus is highly likely to result in dislocation of the talus from the ankle mortise; isolated lateral (the more common) or medial malleolar fracture is less likely to destabilize the joint (Fig. 12-63)
5. *Toddler's fracture:* spiral fracture of the distal diametaphyseal region of the tibia in a toddler
6. *Trimalleolar (Cotton's) fracture:* fracture of the medial and lateral malleoli, in addition to the posterior tibial lip, often with tibiotalar dislocation

Isolated, undisplaced fractures of either malleolus are usually stable (Fig. 12-64).

Fractures with significant displacement must be reduced, especially if any widening of the ankle joint is present (Fig. 12-65). Fractures with dislocation of the talus should be reduced as rapidly as possible (Fig. 12-66).

PROCEDURE

- If a fracture of the distal fibula exists (as in Pott's fracture), there is an increased diameter around the malleoli area of the affected ankle (Fig. 12-67).

Confirmation Procedures

Calf circumference test, anterior drawer sign of the ankle, and diagnostic imaging

---

DIAGNOSTIC STATEMENT

Keen's sign is present in the left ankle. This sign indicates a distal fibular fracture.

CLINICAL PEARL

Keen's sign is an early indicator of ankle fracture. When it is present, the sign mandates diagnostic imaging of the joint.

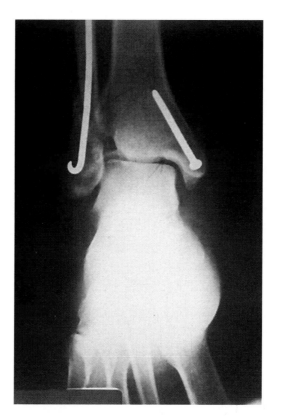

FIG. 12-61 Bimalleolar fracture. *(From Deltoff MN, Kogon PL: The portable skeletal x-ray library, St Louis, 1998, Mosby.)*

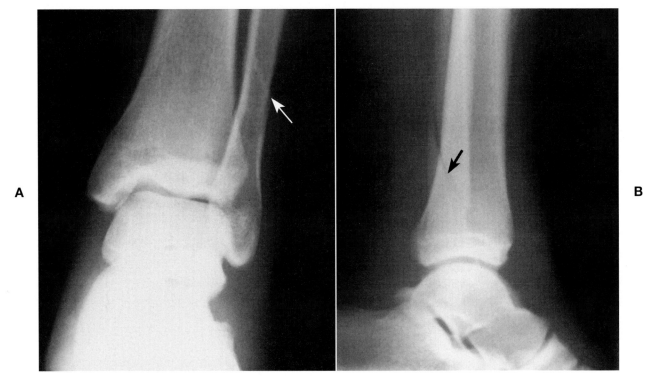

FIG. 12-62 **A** and **B,** Pott's fracture *(arrows).* *(From Deltoff MN, Kogon PL:* The portable skeletal x-ray library, *St Louis, 1998, Mosby.)*

FIG. 12-63   Pott's fracture. *(From Mathers LH, et al:* Clinical anatomy principles, *St Louis, 1996, Mosby.)*

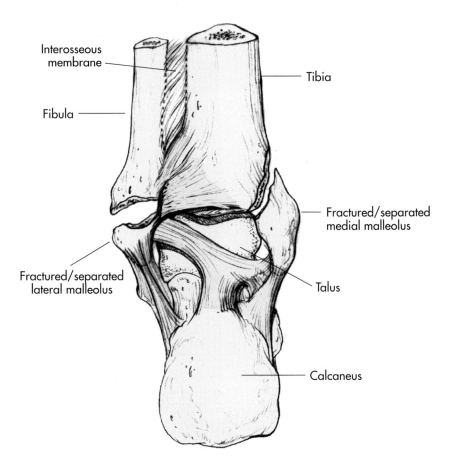

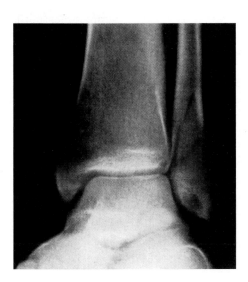

FIG. 12-64 Undisplaced fracture of the lateral malleolus. *(From Mercier LR, Pettid FJ: Practical orthopedics, ed 4, St Louis, 1995, Mosby.)*

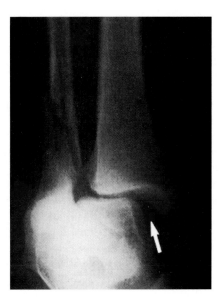

FIG. 12-65 Displaced fracture of the lateral malleolus with widening of the ankle mortise due to lateral shift of the talus. *(From Mercier LR, Pettid FJ: Practical orthopedics, ed 4, St Louis, 1995, Mosby.)*

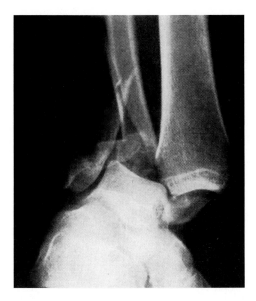

FIG. 12-66 Fracture-dislocation of the ankle. *(From Mercier LR, Pettid FJ: Practical orthopedics, ed 4, St Louis, 1995, Mosby.)*

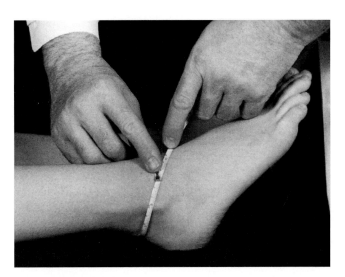

FIG. 12-67 The patient is lying supine on the examination table. The foot and ankle are in a resting position. A tape measure is placed around the ankle, passing over both malleoli. The diameter of the ankle is recorded and compared to the opposite ankle. An increased diameter, correlated with other pathologic findings, indicates a fracture of the distal fibula.

MORTON'S TEST

Assessment for Metatarsalgia or Morton's Neuroma

Comment

As the foot plantar flexes and the toes dorsiflex during push off, the interdigital nerves between the second and third, and third and fourth metatarsal (Fig. 12-68) may be compressed by the intermetatarsal ligament. This causes neuritic radiation of pain into the affected web space and toes. The pain often radiates proximally as well.

Morton's neuroma is a common disorder in the adult. A fibroneuromatous reaction between the third and fourth metatarsal heads, over the deep transverse metatarsal ligaments, affects the lateral terminal branch of the median plantar nerve. The impinging effect on the nerve is accentuated during weight bearing, particularly during the push-off phase of walking or when the metatarsal heads are compressed. Localized tenderness between the third and fourth metatarsal heads on the plantar surface also occurs. Hypesthesia over the lateral and medial side of the third and fourth toes, respectively, may be present. Morton's neuroma can occur in the web spaces that involve the corresponding terminal branch of either the medial or lateral plantar nerve, but this is not a common occurrence.

Metatarsalgia, pain in the metatarsals, is very common in adults. This pain is caused by various foot deformities or arthritis of the metatarsophalangeal joints. This latter type of pain is most commonly due to rheumatoid arthritis. The term *metatarsalgia* is used to refer to a pain syndrome and is not disease nomenclature per se. The disease may occur as an isolated condition or in association with hallux valgus or rigidus. The patient complains of pain in the metatarsal heads or toes when standing during the push-off phase of gait. On examination, there is localized tenderness directly under the plantar surface of the metatarsal head. The most common sites for the pain are the second and third metatarsal heads.

Excessive pressure over the metatarsal heads is a primary cause of the pain. This pain is aggravated by ill-fitting shoes that squeeze the toes into a narrow toe-box and is differentiated from Morton's neuroma by having its most severe tenderness directly under the metatarsal heads with no associated hypesthesia of the involved toes.

PROCEDURE

- Transverse pressure across the heads of the metatarsals causes sharp pain in the forefoot (Fig. 12-69).
- This pressure indicates metatarsalgia or neuroma.

Confirmation Procedures

Strunsky's sign and diagnostic imaging

DIAGNOSTIC STATEMENT

Morton's test is positive for the left foot and indicates a neuroma at the third and fourth interspace.

Morton's test is positive for the left foot and indicates a metatarsalgia at the first through third metatarsal heads.

CLINICAL PEARL

Anterior metatarsalgia is particularly common in the middle-aged female and is also often associated with some splaying of the forefoot. Symptoms may be triggered by periods of excessive standing or by an increase in weight, and there is often concurrent flattening of the medial longitudinal arch. Weakness of the intrinsic muscles is usually present, so there is a tendency for clawing of the toes.

875

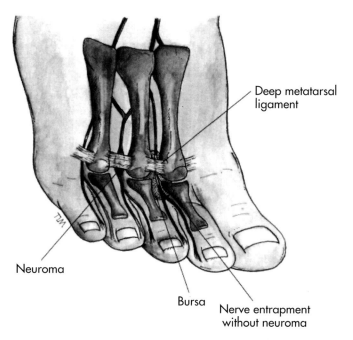

FIG. 12-68   Interdigital neuroma.   *(From Baxter DE:* The foot and ankle in sport, *St Louis, 1995, Mosby.)*

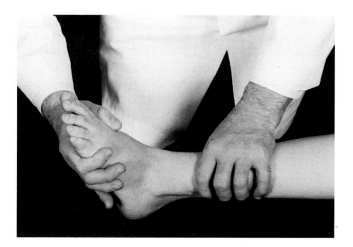

FIG. 12-69   The patient is lying supine on the examination table. The examiner grasps the affected forefoot with one hand and applies transverse pressure to the metatarsal heads. Sharp pain in the foot indicates a positive test and suggests metatarsalgia or neuroma.

MOSZKOWICZ TEST

Assessment for Inadequacy of the Collateral Circulation as in an Arteriovenous Fistula in the Lower Extremity

Comment
Most of the pathologic sequelae from venous diseases develop in the lower extremities.

ORTHOPEDIC GAMUT 12-13

THROMBOPHLEBITIS

Thrombophlebitis, or intravascular coagulation, is usually related to the three factors identified in Virchow's triad:

1. Venous stasis
2. Injury to the vein wall
3. Hypercoagulable state

Deep venous thrombosis carries the threat of potentially fatal consequences and thus requires the immediate institution of bed rest and anticoagulation therapy. Such treatment reduces the likelihood of thrombus propagation and lessens the risk of emboli. Varicose veins are prominent, tortuous, abnormally distended veins that occur in approximately 20% of adults. They are five times more common in women than in men and are often associated with a family history of varicosities. Congenitally absent or defective valves are the usual underlying cause of varicose veins. Obstruction of outflow from venous thrombosis or pregnancy may also precipitate varicosities.

Patients with venous insufficiency complain of heaviness and tightness in the lower limbs with exercise. Exercise may greatly increase the degree of venous congestion and produce a deep-seated discomfort known as *venous claudication*. As the condition progresses, the deep and perforated system valves may fail, resulting in chronic stasis edema, dermatitis, and stasis ulcers.

Another source of edema in the lower extremities is dysfunction of the lymphatic system. The well-known but poorly understood problem of primary lymphedema is related to aberrant development or function of the lymphatic system. This condition is most common in women and is often unilateral. Manifestations may be evident at birth but usually appear not later than age 40. When suspected, the diagnosis may be confirmed with a radioisotope lymphogram and contrast lymphangiography. Chronic lymphedema predisposes patients to skin infections, which may in turn exacerbate fibrosis and obstruction of lymph flow.

Arteriovenous fistulas are abnormal communications, single or multiple, between arteries and veins, by which arterial blood enters the veins directly without traversing a capillary network.

Acquired arteriovenous fistulas, usually single and saccular, may develop after a bullet or stab wound involving an artery and a contiguous vein. Fistulas of the iliac vessels may occur after surgery for intervertebral disc disease. Congenital fistulas, which are present from birth, are usually multiple, and they result from defects in the differentiation of the common embryologic tissue into artery and vein. There is no special sex incidence, and any part of the body may be involved.

Arterial blood, following the path of least resistance, flows directly into the vein and bypasses the corresponding capillary bed. The arterial blood pressure is transmitted to the venous side of the fistula. The distal vein pressure is increased, but the proximal vein pressure may actually be negative. The elevated venous pressure leads to the development of varicose veins and venous stasis changes in the leg. Increased blood flow makes the tissues near the fistula abnormally warm, and diminished flow distal to the fistula may produce peripheral coldness and trophic changes. Large fistulas impose a burden on the heart. The cardiac output must be increased above normal by an amount proportional to the size of the fistula to maintain the general circulation. Total blood volume may be increased. The low peripheral resistance of the involved area decreases diastolic and increases systolic and pulse pressure systemically. Large fistulas may lead to cardiac decompensation.

In the region of the fistula, the intima and the media of the involved veins become thickened, and newly developed elastic fibers appear. The arteries show a thinning of their walls, with a loss of elastic tissue and muscular fibers in the media.

Patients complain of ache, pain, edema, varicosities, or hypertrophied legs. Occasionally, cardiac symptoms—such as palpitations, substernal pain, and dyspnea on exertion—are present.

Examination reveals tortuous, dilated superficial veins in the leg. The venous pulsation can be felt unless the fistula is small and deeply placed. With congenital fistulas, the skin temperature is usually elevated locally but decreased distal to the fistulas, although in acquired lesions, the temperature of the toes may be greater than in the opposite normal foot. Bruits or thrills are common over acquired fistulas. The bruit lasts throughout systole and diastole and has a coarse machinery-like quality. The tissues near the fistula may be tender, edematous, and either red or slightly cyanotic. The circumference of the leg is increased by edema or true hypertrophy, but bony structures are hypertrophied only if the fistula was present before epiphyseal closure. Temporary compression of the artery that supplies the large fistula diminishes the heart rate (Branham's sign) and may be a helpful diagnostic sign.

PROCEDURE

- The patient's lower extremity is elevated, and an elastic bandage is wrapped firmly around the limb (Fig. 12-70).
- The elevated position is maintained for 5 minutes. Then the extremity is placed in a horizontal position, and the examiner quickly removes the applied bandage (Fig. 12-71).

- If the circulation is normal, a hyperemic blush occurs and rapidly flows into the area as the bandage is removed.
- The test is positive when the blush is absent or lags slowly behind the unbandaged area.
- The test demonstrates inadequacy of the collateral circulation as in an arteriovenous fistula.

Confirmation Procedures
Buerger's test, claudication test, foot tourniquet test, Homans' sign, Moses' test, Perthes' test, and vascular assessment

---

DIAGNOSTIC STATEMENT

The Moszkowicz test is positive for the left leg. This result suggests an arteriovenous fistula at the level of the iliac artery.

CLINICAL PEARL

Thrombosis in the superficial veins of the calf and with local inflammatory changes is a common cause of recurrent calf pain, and the presence of tenderness and other inflammatory signs along the course of the calf vein makes diagnosis easy. Thrombosis in the deep veins is often silent, and its importance in the postoperative situation is well known.

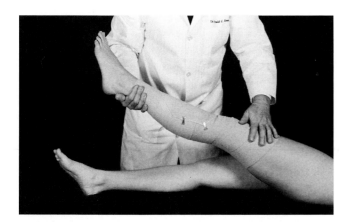

FIG. 12-70   The patient is lying supine on the examination table. The patient's legs are extended at the knees. The affected leg is elevated or flexed at the hip. While maintaining the leg in an elevated position, the examiner wraps the leg firmly with a 6-inch-wide elastic bandage and maintains the elevation of the leg for 5 minutes.

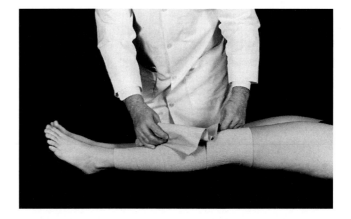

FIG. 12-71   At the end of 5 minutes, the leg is returned to the horizontal position, and the bandage is quickly removed. The test is positive if the area of the leg previously wrapped has no hyperemic blush. The lack of hyperemic blush indicates arteriovenous fistula formation.

MOSES' TEST

Assessment for Arteriosclerosis Obliterans of the Lower Extremity

Comment

Arteriosclerosis obliterans is caused by arteriosclerotic narrowing or obstruction of large and small arteries that supply the extremities. Symptoms and signs are produced by ischemia.

Arteriosclerosis obliterans is the leading cause of obstructive arterial disease of the lower extremities after the age of 30. The superficial femoral artery is affected by stenosis or obstruction in approximately 90% of patients. The aortoiliac and popliteal arteries are the next most common sites. The greatest incidence of superficial femoral and more distal arterial disease occurs in the seventh decade, but aortoiliac disease has its peak a decade earlier. The disease is more common in males than in females, especially before menopause. Patients with diabetes mellitus develop arteriosclerosis obliterans more frequently and at an earlier age than nondiabetic patients.

The most common symptom of arteriosclerosis obliterans is intermittent claudication (intermittent limping). The patient experiences cramping pain, tightness, numbness, or severe fatigue in the muscle group being exercised. The amount of exercise producing the pain is constant in each patient. The pain is relieved promptly by rest. In a few patients, pain may disappear after further walking because of an unconscious slowing of the gait. Intermittent claudication is typically seen in the calf muscles because femoral artery disease is so common. However, the calf is the most common site of claudication because these muscles do the most work during walking. Lower back, buttock, thigh, and foot claudication also may occur. The site of the symptom localizes the obstruction proximally.

Rest pain is the other important symptom of obstructive arterial disease. Rest pain is a grave sign that indicates that the blood supply is not sufficient even for the small nutritional requirements of the skin. Rest pain may be localized to one or more toes, but often has a stocking distribution. The latter distribution means that ischemic neuritis is not usually the cause of rest pain. Rest pain is worse at night and is relieved somewhat by dependency and by cooling.

Other symptoms of arteriosclerosis obliterans include coldness, numbness, paresthesia, and color changes in the involved extremity.

Exercise-induced vascular claudication is unusual in young athletes. A rare cause of arterial occlusion has been reported in the adductor canal. An abnormal musculoskeletal band arising from the adductor magnus and lying adjacent and superior to the adductor tendon may lead to compression of the femoral artery at the adductor hiatus. The band may extend from the adductor magnus to the vastus medialis above and across the outlet of Hunter's canal.

Symptoms in this syndrome are identical to other vascular occlusion problems. Exercise-induced claudication is present. On examination, the pulses distal to the occlusion are diminished or absent. The workup of these patients consists of noninvasive vascular testing, such as Doppler studies and arteriography.

PROCEDURE

- Moses' test is performed by grasping the patient's calf, which creates pain if phlebitis or vascular occlusion is present (Fig. 12-72).

Confirmation Procedures

Buerger's test, claudication test, foot tourniquet test, Homans' sign, Moszkowicz test, Perthes' test, and vascular assessment

---

DIAGNOSTIC STATEMENT

Moses' test is positive for the left leg. This result indicates arteriosclerosis obliterans.

CLINICAL PEARL

Pain in the calf is common for patients suffering from prolapsed intervertebral discs. Claudication pain is a feature of vascular insufficiency and spinal stenosis. Lesions of the foot and ankle that lead to protective muscle spasm during standing and walking often cause marked calf and leg pain.

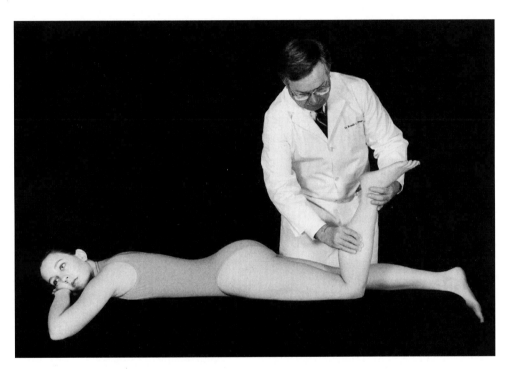

FIG. 12-72   The patient is lying prone on the examining table. The examiner flexes the patient's knee to 90 degrees. The examiner grasps and squeezes the calf of the affected leg. The sign is present if pain is elicited. The pain suggests phlebitis.

PERTHES' TEST

Assessment for Superficial Varicosities (Incompetency of the Valves of the Saphenous Vein) of the Lower Extremity

Comment

Chronic venous insufficiency results in a rise in tissue pressure in the skin and subcutaneous tissues. This increased pressure can interfere with adequate nutrient blood flow and may lead to skin necrosis and ulceration, most commonly at the ankle just above the malleoli. The skin is often dusky and indurated. Scarring as part of the healing process tends to impair the microcirculation further, and the condition may become self-perpetuating (Fig. 12-73).

Varicose veins are distended, tortuous veins with incompetent valves. The postphlebitic syndrome denotes the chronically swollen lower extremity with trophic changes secondary to chronic venous stasis. Despite the name, a history of thrombophlebitis is often not obtainable.

Varicose veins are caused either by congenitally defective valves or by a condition that deforms valves or obstructs venous outflow over a long period. Varicosities that result from congenital defects are most common and may develop early in life. Because increased forearm vein distensibility has been demonstrated in patients with leg varicosities, a generalized abnormality of the veins has been suggested as the predisposing factor. Thrombophlebitis leads to deformation or destruction of venous valves and venous obstruction, and it is the second most common etiologic factor of venous problems. Pregnancy, ascites, abdominal tumor, excessive weight and height, or prolonged weight bearing may lead to increased venous pressure in the legs, distension of the veins, and finally, incompetency of the valves.

Varicose veins are rather common. The condition appears in approximately 40% of all females, but the incidence is less in males. The saphenous veins in the lower extremity are the veins most commonly affected.

The dilated, tortuous, sacculated varices are easily visible. Some patients with extensive superficial varicosities have no other symptoms or signs, but some patients experience aching or easy fatigability of the calf muscles and edema after weight bearing. The edema usually disappears with bed rest overnight. When the communicating or deep veins are incompetent, symptoms and signs are more common. Chronic venous insufficiency is manifested by edema, which may later become fibrosed to produce brawny induration. Extravasation of blood locally may cause a brownish pigmentation. An itchy eczematoid rash may appear in the area. Finally, the skin may ulcerate, which produces an indolent, painless lesion that is usually above the medial malleolus, near a palpable, incompetent communicating vein. This picture of chronic swelling and stasis dermatitis is called the postphlebitic syndrome. Arterial pulses are normal. When the deep venous system is blocked, pain similar to intermittent claudication may rarely occur.

PROCEDURE

- While the patient is supine or standing, an elastic tourniquet is applied around the upper thigh to compress only the long saphenous vein (Fig. 12-74).
- The patient then exercises the limb briskly, by walking, kicking, or twisting, for up to 60 seconds.
- The examiner then notes the prominence of the varicosities.
- Normally, the muscular action of the exercise should empty the blood from the superficial system (long saphenous) through the communicating veins into the deep system.
- If superficial varicosities disappear, the valves of the communicating and deep veins are competent.
- If superficial varicosities remain the same, both the superficial and communicating valves are incompetent.
- If the varicosities become distended and more prominent and pain develops, the deep veins are obstructed, and the valves of the communicating veins are incompetent (Fig. 12-75).

Confirmation Procedures

Buerger's test, claudication test, foot tourniquet test, Homans' sign, Moszkowicz test, Moses' test, and vascular assessment

---

DIAGNOSTIC STATEMENT

Perthes' test is positive for the left leg. This result indicates varicosities that are caused by incompetency of the valves of the saphenous vein.

CLINICAL PEARL

Vascular damage may lead to gangrene of the foot and ankle. The circulation must always be observed if it is likely that the vessels have been traumatized seriously by stretching or contusion, and the findings must be recorded. Neurologic damage often accompanies vascular injury.

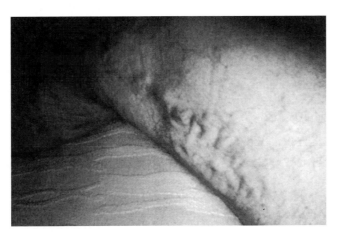

FIG. 12-73   Varicose veins. *(From Barkauskas VH, et al:* Health and physical assessment, *ed 2, St Louis, 1998, Mosby.)*

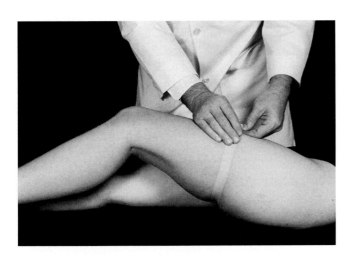

FIG. 12-74   The patient is lying supine on the examination table. A tourniquet is applied at the upper thigh of the affected leg. The tourniquet is only tight enough to compress the long saphenous vein.

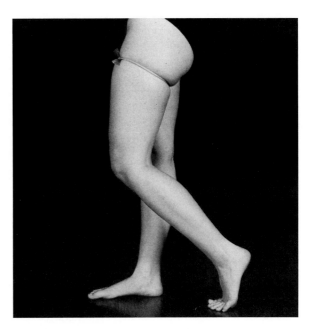

FIG. 12-75   The patient stands and briskly exercises the leg for up to 60 seconds. Prominent varicosities that do not disappear with exercise suggest that the valves of the communicating and deep veins are incompetent.

Assessment for Metatarsalgia

Comment

Metatarsalgia in a patient can be a debilitating disorder leading to loss of athletic competitiveness or even loss of the ability to participate in a recreational fashion.

ORTHOPEDIC GAMUT 12-14

FOREFOOT DISORDERS

Forefoot disorders encompass the following:

*Lesser Toe Abnormalities
Such as the Following:*

1. Claw toes
2. Hammer toes
3. Mallet toes
4. Hard and soft corns

*More Proximally Problems
Can Include the Following:*

1. Intractable plantar keratosis (IPK)
2. Bunionette (Fig. 12-76)
3. Neuromas
4. Metatarsophalangeal joint capsulitis and instability

The complaint of pain in the forefoot must be differentiated to make a correct diagnosis (Fig. 12-77). Most important is the exact location of pain.

The metatarsals are arranged in an arch both in an AP and in a transverse direction. The transverse arch, in which the central three bones lie at a higher level than the peripheral bones, is pronounced proximally at the tarsometatarsal junctions and becomes shallower toward its distal extremity. The term *metatarsal arch* refers to the shallow concavity over the plantar aspect of the metatarsal heads. The central three heads are elevated by the transverse metatarsal ligaments and the transverse head of the adductor hallucis muscle. The mechanism is ineffective during weight bearing, but it transfers pressure toward the medial and lateral tarsal heads when the arch is obliterated. During the push-off movement of a step, the intrinsic muscles flex the toes and help elevate the central metatarsal heads off the ground, thus relieving them of pressure. Paralysis of these muscles results in clawed toes, dropped metatarsal heads, and the inevitable plantar calluses.

Stretching of the transverse metatarsal ligaments is a major cause of pain in the forefoot. This pain is caused by congenital laxity, which typically results in flatfoot, in which the heel is everted, the longitudinal arch depressed, the metatarsals and the toes widely spread (splayfoot), and the forefoot supinated in relation to the hindfoot. An acquired stretching occurs as a result of obesity, prolonged standing, degenerative changes of aging, and acute illness. The three central metatarsal heads drop and are prominent in the sole when palpated through the thinned subcutaneous fat.

Weakness of the intrinsics deprives the toes of strong flexor power, and the metatarsal heads drop. With poliomyelitis, paralysis of the foot dorsiflexors results in equinus that throws the weight forward on the foot. In addition, the common cavus deformity, which follows this disease, causes a downward tilting of the metatarsals, and added pressure is brought to bear distally.

Any form of arthritis can affect the metatarsophalangeal joints. In young and middle-aged patients, rheumatoid arthritis is suspected. Severe degenerative arthritis favors the first metatarsophalangeal articulation. Degenerative changes in a single joint, other than the first, suggest an antecedent osteochondrosis.

An acute exacerbation of gout characteristically develops around the first metatarsophalangeal joint. Pain is severe and continuous and is aggravated by weight bearing and movement of the large toe.

Prolonged walking will cause a sprain of the transverse metatarsal ligament. Pain occurs throughout the distal metatarsal area during weight bearing and is intensified by spreading the toes passively.

Any deformity of the foot that changes the axis of the metatarsal to a more vertical direction throws forward the pressure of weight bearing.

PROCEDURE

- Sudden passive flexing of the toes is painless in a normal foot, but if inflammation exists, pain is experienced in the anterior arch of the foot (Fig. 12-78).

Confirmation Procedures

Morton's test and diagnostic imaging

DIAGNOSTIC STATEMENT

Strunsky's sign is present in the left foot. The presence of this sign indicates metatarsalgia.

CLINICAL PEARL

Pain in the forefoot (called *metatarsalgia*) has many origins. A prominent metatarsal head is a common cause of pain and can follow any operation on the forefoot, including Keller's operation, or dislocation of the second toe.

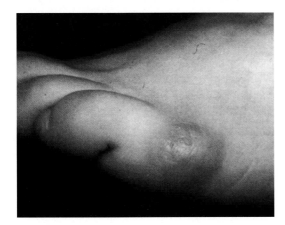

FIG. 12-76   Bunionette with enlarged bursa. *(From Baxter DE: The foot and ankle in sport, St Louis, 1995, Mosby.)*

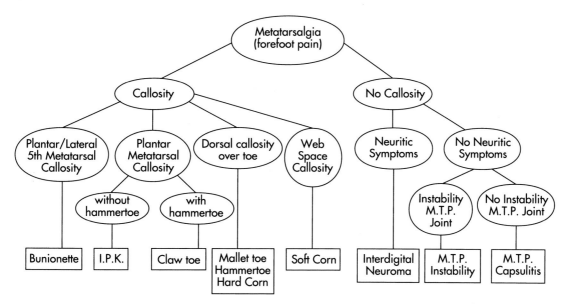

FIG. 12-77   Metatarsalgia algorithm. *I.P.K.,* intractable plantar kelatosis; *M.T.P.,* metatarsophangeal. *(From Baxter DE: The foot and ankle in sport, St Louis, 1995, Mosby.)*

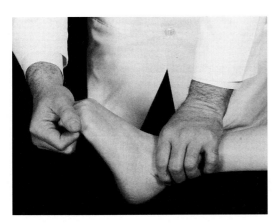

FIG. 12-78   The patient is lying supine, and the affected leg is extended on the examination table. The examiner grasps the toes of the affected foot. The examiner causes a sudden, passive flexion of the toes. The sign is present if the maneuver causes pain. The presence of this sign indicates inflammation of the anterior arch of the foot (metatarsalgia).

THOMPSON'S TEST

Assessment for Achilles' Tendon Rupture

Comment

The history obtained in patients with a ruptured Achilles' tendon is remarkably consistent. Typically, the individual is a middle-aged, weekend, male athlete. A pop is often heard at the time of the rupture. The patient often thinks the heel was hit by an opponent's racquet. Upon turning, the patient realizes that no one is there. Most individuals are disabled enough to seek medical attention immediately, but some are not. Only when the latter group fails to recover from this presumed "sprain" do they then seek help.

ORTHOPEDIC GAMUT 12-15

ACHILLES' TENDON EXAMINATION

Physical examination of a ruptured Achilles' tendon involves the following:

1. The Thompson-Doherty squeeze test
2. Palpation of the medial head of the gastrocnemius
3. Palpation of a gap in the tendon
4. O'Brien's needle test
5. Assessment of heel resistance strength

The Thompson-Doherty squeeze test involves placing the patient prone with the knee at 90 degrees of flexion. A squeeze of the calf musculature normally results in passive plantar flexion. A positive Thompson-Doherty test is the absence of passive plantar flexion.

Calf pain with the Thompson-Doherty test indicates a probable medial gastrocnemius tear. A palpable gap is usually present in an Achilles' rupture, particularly in an acute situation. This is best felt with the patient prone, the foot over the edge of the examination table, and the patient actively dorsiflexing the ankle.

O'Brien's needle test involves placing a needle (acupuncture) 10 cm proximal to the superior border of the calcaneus into the tendon substance. If the needle is seen to swivel on passive motion of the foot, the Achilles' tendon is intact. An absence of motion indicates a positive O'Brien test.

The final assessment is that of heel resistance strength. The examiner grasps the foot in a neutral position and

instructs the patient to plantar flex. With an intact Achilles' tendon, the grasp is easily broken. If the Achilles' tendon is torn, the posterior tibial, peroneal, and flexor tendons will fail to break the grasp. In an acute case, usually palpation of a gap and a positive Thompson-Doherty test will suffice. However, with a delayed presentation, the other three techniques may be indicated.

ORTHOPEDIC GAMUT 12-16

ACHILLES' TENDON RUPTURE

The following three factors predispose the Achilles' tendon to rupture:

1. *Mechanical:* The patient rapidly pushes off with the knee extended.
2. *Vascular:* The tendon that ruptures usually will do so in the zone of relatively diminished blood supply.
3. *Quality of the tissue substance:* Many studies have revealed that the ruptured Achilles' tendon will have preexisting degenerative pathologic changes.

The calf muscle may be partially or completely ruptured at any place, from its origin on the posterior part of the femoral condyles and back of the tibia to its attachment to the calcaneus. The tear may be in the muscle belly, but it occurs more often in the musculotendinous junction between the gastrocnemius and the conjoined tendon with the soleus. The muscle unit may rupture through the tendon or at the attachment to the heel, sometimes avulsing a fragment of bone. As with a muscle rupture anywhere, determination of the location and extent of injury is extremely important. The location is usually determined when the injury is examined early because the tenderness will be quite localized. After several hours, swelling, edema, and inflammation become diffuse, and the exact location may be in doubt. Both active and passive stretching will cause pain. If there is complete severance of the whole muscle-tendon unit from the head of the gastrocnemius or the entire gastrocnemius from the conjoined tendon or rupture of the tendon, then loss of function will be noted and the muscle will bunch up during contraction rather than flatten down, as it normally does. If the rupture is in the distal tendon or musculotendinous junction, a palpable defect often can be felt. The condition is disabling even with a minor degree of tearing, and it interdicts running or any activity that causes the patient to be on the toes. This loss of function may be caused by actual loss of continuity of the tendon, but it more commonly results from muscle spasm and pain.

PROCEDURE

- The patient is in a prone position with the feet hanging over the edge of the examination table.
- The examiner flexes the knee of the affected leg to 90 degrees and squeezes the calf muscles just below the widest level of the posterior portion of the leg (Fig. 12-79).
- Normally, this maneuver causes a reflex plantar flexion motion of the foot (Fig. 12-80).

- The test is positive when the foot does not respond.
- The test indicates a complete rupture of the Achilles' tendon.

Confirmation Procedures
Helbings' sign, Hoffa's test, and diagnostic imaging

DIAGNOSTIC STATEMENT

Thompson's test is positive for the left ankle. This result indicates loss of integrity of the Achilles' tendon.

CLINICAL PEARL

The Achilles' tendon can be torn by the same movements, such as a forward lunge on the sports field or a squash court, that tear the medial head of the gastrocnemius. The patient will feel as though someone has kicked the Achilles' tendon. There are legendary stories, in which the victim of such a tear turns around and punches the person behind, in retribution.

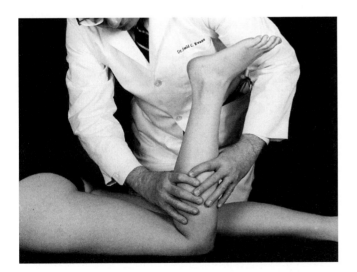

FIG. 12-79 The patient is lying prone on the examination table. The knee of the affected leg is flexed to 90 degrees by the examiner. The examiner grasps the patient's calf with both hands. The patient's musculature is relaxed.

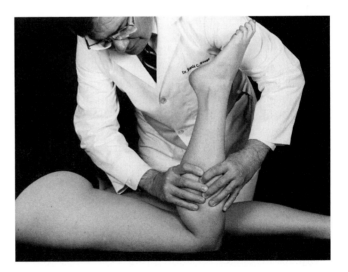

FIG. 12-80 The examiner squeezes the calf musculature at a point just distal to the widest level of the posterior portion of the leg. The test is positive if the foot does not plantar flex with this maneuver. A positive test indicates a rupture of the Achilles' tendon.

TINEL'S FOOT SIGN

Assessment for Tarsal Tunnel Syndrome

Comment

The tarsal tunnel is a fibroosseous tunnel formed by the flexor retinaculum or lacinate ligament, the medial wall of the calcaneus, the posterior portion of the talus, the distal tibia, and the medial malleolus.

ORTHOPEDIC GAMUT 12-17

TARSAL TUNNEL STRUCTURES

The structures within the tarsal tunnel include the following:

1. Posterior tibial nerve and its branches
2. Tendons of the posterior tibialis
3. Flexor digitorum longus
4. Flexor hallucis
5. Posterior tibial artery and vein

The posterior tibial nerve may be compressed at several locations (Fig. 12-81). A high tarsal tunnel syndrome exists when compression of the posterior tibial nerve occurs at the lower edge of the gastrocnemius muscle in the middle aspect of the posteromedial tibia. The traditional tarsal tunnel occurs behind the medial malleolus under the retinacular ligament. The compression may occur from a posterior bony preeminence of the talus (Fig. 12-82).

Accompanied by their corresponding arteries and veins, the tibial nerve's two terminal branches, the medial and the lateral plantar nerves, pass around the medial malleolus through a fibroosseous tunnel, which is the tarsal tunnel.

Although the causes of tarsal tunnel syndrome may be diverse, nerve compression or irritation is a common feature of them all. Mechanical pressure from changes in the tissue relationships within the tunnel remains the common denominator of the proposed causes. Therefore trauma and congenital or acquired anomalies predispose these individuals to a higher risk of nerve compression because their tarsal tunnels are abnormally configured. Rather than change the bony components, autoimmune and inflammatory diseases affect the tunnel's soft tissues and decrease the tunnel's volume. Because the tunnel's neural components remain most sensitive to increased pressure, changes in sensory and motor function are among the first symptoms of tunnel damage. The upper section of the tunnel, containing the medial plantar neurovascular structures, remains more sensitive to volume changes than the lower section, which contains the lateral plantar neurovascular structures.

The tibial nerve, like the median nerve, has a rich vascularity, but it is sensitive to ischemia. Compression of the vasa vasorum, which surrounds the nerve, will lead to ischemia and neurologic symptoms. Increased vascular compromise during standing and walking accounts for the crises that appreciate in patients with tarsal tunnel syndrome. In several idiopathic cases that have been relieved by surgery, the nerves were normal in appearance. These cases have been proposed to be vascular in nature.

PROCEDURE

- Tapping the area over the posterior tibial nerve (medial plantar nerve) with a reflex hammer produces tingling distal to the percussion (Fig. 12-83).
- The paresthesia that radiates into the foot indicates tarsal tunnel syndrome.

Confirmation Procedures

Duchenne's sign and electrodiagnosis

DIAGNOSTIC STATEMENT

Tinel's foot sign is positive on the right. The presence of this sign indicates tarsal tunnel syndrome that involves the medial plantar nerve.

CLINICAL PEARL

The medial plantar nerve enters the foot after passing beneath the medial ligament of the ankle, which it shares with the posterior tibial and flexor tendons. The structure of this feature is comparable to the carpal tunnel of the wrist. The medial plantar nerve is vulnerable to compression by swelling of the tendons or by space-occupying lesions, such as ganglia. Tarsal tunnel syndrome is not common, but it should be considered for patients who have neurologic symptoms in the hindfoot.

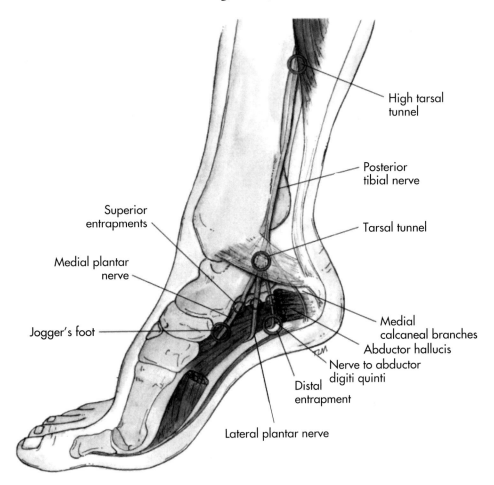

FIG. 12-81 Areas of compression of the posterior tibial nerve and its branches. *(From Baxter DE: The foot and ankle in sport, St Louis, 1995, Mosby.)*

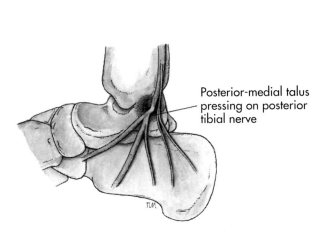

FIG. 12-82 Compression by the talus on the posterior tibial nerve. *(From Baxter DE: The foot and ankle in sport, St Louis, 1995, Mosby.)*

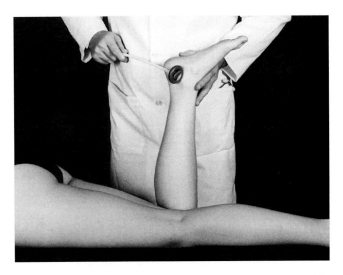

FIG. 12-83 The patient is lying prone on the examination table. The leg may be extended at the knee or flexed. The examiner percusses the posterior tibial nerve (medial plantar nerve) with a reflex hammer. Paresthesia that is elicited distal to the percussion indicates tarsal tunnel syndrome.

CRITICAL THINKING

What is medial tibial stress syndrome?
Medial tibial stress syndrome is an inflammatory condition involving the periosteal attachment of the deep posterior compartment.

What is acute compartment syndrome?
An acute increase in tissue pressure within the enclosed anatomic space (the muscle compartment that is surrounded by semirigid fascia) results in increased local venous pressure, leading to a decrease in the arteriovenous gradient and thus a decrease in arterial inflow.

What are the primary causes of acute compartment syndrome?
Eighty-five percent of cases of acute compartment syndrome are caused by overuse of the musculature (strain).

Who is most at risk for sustaining an Achilles' tendon tear?
Tears are most commonly seen in males between the ages of 30 and 50.

Describe the physical findings in an acute complete Achilles' tendon rupture.
There will be palpable defect in the tendon as the proximal tendon retracts following rupture. The gap is usually 2 to 3 cm long. Within 24 to 48 hours, marked swelling and ecchymosis usually occur. The patient is able to weakly plantar flex the foot. Thompson's test is positive.

What is Thompson's test?
With the patient supine and the affected foot hanging over the end of the table, the examiner squeezes the calf and observes for ankle motion. A positive Thompson's test occurs when there is no plantar flexion of the ankle when the calf is squeezed.

What is the most common musculoskeletal injury?
Sprain of the lateral ankle ligaments

What mechanism of injury most commonly produces an ankle sprain?
Inversion of the supinated, plantar flexed foot produces 85% of ankle sprains.

How is the anterior drawer test performed?
The examiner stabilizes the distal tibia with one hand and then grasps the posterior heel with the opposite hand. The examiner applies anterior force in an attempt to displace the talus anteriorly.

What indicates a positive anterior drawer test?
A "clunk" and increased laxity of the ankle are noted when the examiner attempts to displace the talus anteriorly.

How are ankle sprains graded?
Grade I: no laxity, minimal pain with range of motion, and mild swelling. Grade II: mild to moderate laxity, soft-tissue swelling, and slight laxity on anterior drawer and talar tilt tests. Grade III: moderate to severe swelling and pain. The patient is usually unable to bear weight.

What is metatarsalgia?
It is pain in the region of the metatarsophalangeal joints.

What is Morton's neuroma?
Morton's neuroma is a perineural thickening of the common digital nerves of the second or third interspace of the foot.

What is the tarsal tunnel?
The tarsal is a fibroosseous tunnel formed by the flexor retinaculum or laciniate ligament, the medial wall of the calcaneus and talus, and the medial malleolus.

What are the most common symptoms of tarsal tunnel syndrome?
Patients with tarsal tunnel syndrome complain of plantar numbness, diffuse plantar burning sensations, and tingling pain that increases with activity and decreases with rest.

BIBLIOGRAPHY

Abrams WB, Berkow R: *The Merck manual of geriatrics,* Rahway, NJ, 1990, Merck Sharp & Dohme Research Laboratories.

Adams JC, Hamblen DL: *Outline of orthopaedics,* ed 11, Edinburgh, 1990, Churchill Livingstone.

Agur A, editor: *Grant's atlas of anatomy,* Baltimore, Williams & Wilkins, 1991.

Alario AJ: *Practical guide to the care of the pediatric patient,* St Louis, 1997, Mosby.

Allison D, Strickland N: *Acronyms & synonyms in medical imaging,* Oxford, 1996, ISIS Medical Media.

American Academy of Orthopaedic Surgeons: *Joint motion: method of measuring and recording,* Edinburgh, 1965, British Orthopaedic Association.

American Medical Association: *Guides to the evaluation of permanent impairment,* ed 4, Chicago, 1993, The Association.

American Medical Association: *How to use guides to the evaluation of permanent impairment,* ed 4, Falmouth, Conn, 1993, SEAK.

Anderson KN, Anderson LE: *Mosby's pocket dictionary of medicine, nursing, & allied health,* ed 2, St Louis, 1994, Mosby.

Andrish JT: The leg. In DeLee JD, Drez D editors: *Orthopaedic sports medicine, principles and practice,* vol 2, Philadelphia, 1994, WB Saunders.

Apley AG, Solomon L: *Concise system of orthopaedics and fractures,* London, 1988, Butterworth-Heinemann.

Ballinger PW: *Merrill's atlas of radiographic positions and radiologic procedures,* vol 1-3, ed 8, St Louis, 1995, Mosby.

Barkauskas VH, et al: *Health & physical assessment,* ed 2, St Louis, 1998, Mosby.

Barton NJ: Arthroplasty of the forefoot in rheumatoid arthritis, *J Bone Joint Surg* 55B:126, 1973.

Bassett FH III, et al: Talar impingement by the anteroinferior tibiofibular ligament: a cause of chronic pain in the ankle after inversion sprain, *J Bone Joint Surg* 72A:55, 1990.

Baxter DE: *The foot and ankle in sport,* St Louis, 1995, Mosby.

Baxter DE, Pfeiffer GB: Treatment of chronic heel pain by surgical release of the first branch of the lateral plantar nerve, *Clin Orthop* 279:229, 1992.

Beeson PB, McDermott W: *Textbook of medicine,* ed 13, Philadelphia, 1971, WB Saunders.

Berkowitz JF, Kier R, Rudicel S: Plantar fasciitis: MR imaging, *Radiology* 179:665, 1991.

Binak K, et al: Arteriovenous fistula: hemodynamic effect of occlusion and exercise, *Am Heart J* 60:495, 1960.

Boisen WR, Staples OS, Russell SW: Residual disability following acute ankle sprains, *J Bone Joint Surg* 37A:1237, 1955.

Bordelon RL: Heel pain. In DeLee JD, Drez D, editors: *Orthopaedic sports medicine: principles and practice,* vol 2, Philadelphia, 1994, WB Saunders.

Boytim MJ, Fischer DA, Neuman L: Syndesmotic ankle sprains, *Am J Sports Med* 19:294, 1991.

Bradley JP, Tibone JE: Percutaneous and open surgical repairs of Achilles tendon ruptures, *Am J Sports Med* 18:188, 1990.

Brahms MA: Common foot problems, *J Bone Joint Surg* 49A:1653, 1967.

Brooks M, Evans R, Fairclough J: *Sports injuries,* ed 2, London, 1992, Gower Medical.

Brotzman SB: *Clinical orthopaedic rehabilitation,* St Louis, 1996, Mosby.

Brown DE: Ankle and leg injuries. In Mellion MB, Walsh M, Shelton GL, editors: *The team physician's handbook,* Philadelphia, 1990, Hanley & Belfus.

Brown DE, Neumann RD: *Orthopedic secrets,* Philadelphia, 1995, Hanley & Belfus.

Bucholz RW: *Orthopaedic decision making,* ed 2, St Louis, 1996, Mosby.

Cahill DR: The anatomy and function of the contents of the human tarsal sinus and canal, *Anat Rec* 153:1, 1965.

Calliet R: *Foot and ankle pain,* Philadelphia, 1979, FA Davis.

Campbell JB, Campbell JM: *Mosby's survival guide to medical abbreviations & acronyms prefixes & suffixes symbols Greek alphabet,* St Louis, 1995, Mosby.

Canale ST: *Campbell's operative orthopaedics,* vol 1-4, ed 9, St Louis, 1998, Mosby.

Chapman S, Nakielny R: *Aids to radiological differential diagnosis,* ed 3, London, 1995, Bailliere Tindall.

Cipriano JJ: *Photographic manual of regional orthopaedic and neurological test,* ed 3, Baltimore, 1997, Williams & Wilkins.

Clain MR, Baxter DE: Achilles tendonitis, *Foot Ankle* 13:482, 1992.

Clanton TO, Schon LC: Athlete injuries to the soft tissues of the foot and ankle. In Mann RA, Coughlin MJ, editors: *Surgery of the foot and ankle,* ed 6, St Louis, 1993, Mosby.

Coffman JD, Mannick JA: An objective test to demonstrate the circulatory abnormality in intermittent claudication, *Circulation* 33:177, 1966.

Cohen HL, Brumlik J: *A manual of electroneuromyography,* New York, 1968, Harper and Row.

Cohen MS, et al: Acute compartment syndrome: effect of dermotomy on fascial decompression in the leg, *J Bone Joint Surg* 73A:287, 1991.

Cohn RE: *Impairment rating examination and disability evaluation,* ed 3, Wilkesboro, NC, 1991, R Ernest Cohn.

Colter JM: Lateral ligamentous injuries of the ankle. In Hamilton WC, editor: *Traumatic disorder of the ankle,* New York, 1984, Springer-Verlag.

Cooke TDV, Lehmann PO: Intermittent claudication of neurogenic origin, *Can J Surg* 11:151, 1968.

Coughlin MJ: Conditions of the forefoot. In DeLee JD, Drez D, editors: *Orthopaedic sports medicine: principles and practice,* vol 2, Philadelphia, 1994, WB Saunders.

Craik RL, Oatis CA: *Gait analysis theory and application,* St Louis, 1995, Mosby.

Crenshaw AH, editor: *Campbell's operative orthopedics,* St Louis, 1992, Mosby.

Dambro MR, Griffith JA: *Griffith's 5 minute clinical consult,* Baltimore, 1997, Williams & Wilkins.

D'Ambrogio KJ, Roth GB: *Positional release therapy assessment & treatment of musculoskeletal dysfunction,* St Louis, 1997, Mosby.

D'Ambrosia RD: *Musculoskeletal disorders: regional examination and differential diagnosis,* Philadelphia, 1977, JB Lippincott.

Dandy DJ: *Essential orthopaedics and trauma,* Edinburgh, 1989, Churchill Livingstone.

Dejong RN: *The neurological examination incorporating the fundamentals of neuroanatomy and neurophysiology,* ed 3, New York, 1967, Harper & Row.

Deltoff MN, Kogon PL: *The portable skeletal x-ray library,* St Louis, 1998, Mosby.

DeMaio M, et al: Plantar fasciitis, *Orthopedics* 16:1153, 1993.

Demeter SL, Andersson GBJ, Smith GM: *Disability evaluation,* St Louis, 1996, Mosby.

Deshpande JK, Tobias JD: *The pediatric pain handbook,* St Louis, 1996, Mosby.

Dettenmeier PA: *Radiographic assessment for nurses,* St Louis, 1995, Mosby.

Di Marzo L, et al: Diagnosis of popliteal artery entrapment syndrome: the role of duplex scanning, *J Vasc Surg* 13:434, 1991.

Doherty M: *Color atlas and text of osteoarthritis,* London, 1994, Wolfe.

Doherty M, Doherty J: *Clinical examination in rheumatology,* London, 1992, Wolfe.

Doherty M, George E: *Self-assessment picture tests in rheumatology,* London, 1995, Mosby-Wolfe.

DuVries HL: *Surgery of the foot,* ed 2, St Louis, 1965, Mosby.

DuVries HL: Five myths about your feet, *Today's Health* 45:49, 1967.

Eastwood DM, Gregg PJ, Atkins RM: Intra-articular fractures of the calcaneum, *J Bone Joint Surg* 75B:183, 1993.

Eisele SA, Sammarco GL: Fatigue fractures of the foot and ankle in the athlete, *J Bone Joint Surg* 75:290, 1993.

Elster AD: *Questions and answers in magnetic resonance imaging,* St Louis, 1994, Mosby.

Elstorm, Pankovich A: Muscle and tendon surgery of the leg. In Evarts CM, editor: *Surgery of the musculoskeletal system,* ed 2, New York, 1990, Churchill Livingstone.

Epstein O, et al: *Clinical examination,* ed 2, London, 1997, Mosby.

Farrar WE: *Atlas of infections of the nervous system,* London, 1993, Wolfe.

Fegan WG, Fitzgerald DE, Beesley WH: A modern approach to the injection treatment of varicose veins and its applications in pregnant patients, *Am Heart J* 68:757, 1964.

Feldmann E: *Current diagnosis in neurology,* St Louis, 1994, Mosby.

Ferezy JS: *The chiropractic neurological examination,* Gaithersburg, Md, 1992, Aspen.

Ferkel RD, et al: Arthroscopic treatment of anterolateral impingement of the ankle, *Am J Sports Med* 19:440, 1991.

Fernandez-Palazzi F, Rivas S, Mujica P: Achilles tendinitis in ballet dancers, *Clin Orthop* 257:257, 1990.

Fornage B: *Musculoskeletal ultrasound,* New York, 1995, Churchill Livingstone.

Frey C, Shereff M, Greenridge N: Vascularity of the posterior tibial tendon, *J Bone Joint Surg* 72A:884, 1990.

Friedman SA, Holling HE, Roberts B: Etiologic factors in aortoiliac and femoro-popliteal vascular disease, *N Engl J Med* 271:1382, 1964.

Gamstorp I: Normal conduction velocity of ulnar, median, and peroneal nerves in infancy, childhood and adolescence, *Acta Paediatra Suppl* 146:68, 1963.

Garcia JH: *Neuropathology: the diagnostic approach,* St Louis, 1997, Mosby.

Gardner E, Gray DJ: The innervation of the joints of the foot, *Anat Rec* 161:141, 1968.

Gardner E, Gray DJ, O'Rahilly R: *Anatomy: a regional study of human structure,* ed 4, Philadelphia, 1975, WB Saunders.

Gerard JA, Kleinfield SL: *Orthopaedic testing,* New York, 1993, Churchill Livingstone.

Gibbon WW, Cassar-Pullicino VN: Heel pain, *Ann Rheum Dis* 53:344, 1994.

Gilliatt RW: Normal conduction in human and experimental neuropathies, *Proc R Soc Lond B Biol Sci* 59:989, 1966.

Goldie BS: *Orthopaedic diagnosis and management: a guide to the care of orthopaedic patients,* ed 2, Oxford, 1998, ISIS Medical Media.

Gray H: *Anatomy of the human body,* ed 28, Philadelphia, 1966, Lea & Febiger.

Greenspan A: *Orthopedic radiology,* ed 2, Philadelphia, 1992, JB Lippincott.

Greenstein GM: *Clinical assessment of neuromusculoskeletal disorders,* St Louis, 1997, Mosby.

Grossman ZD, et al: *Cost-effective diagnostic imaging: the clinician's guide,* ed 3, St Louis, 1995, Mosby.

Hamilton WC: Anatomy. In Hamilton WC, editor: *Traumatic disorder of the ankle,* New York, 1984, Springer-Verlag.

Hammer WI: *Functional soft tissue examination and treatment by manual methods: the extremities,* Gaithersburg, Md, 1991, Aspen.

Hart FD: *French's index of differential diagnosis,* ed 10, Baltimore, 1973, Williams & Wilkins.

Hartley A: *Practical joint assessment: lower quadrant,* ed 2, St Louis, 1995, Mosby.

Hawkins RJ: *An organized approach to musculoskeletal examination and history taking,* St Louis, 1995, Mosby.

Hinkle CZ: *Fundamentals of anatomy & movement: a workbook and guide,* St Louis, 1997, Mosby.

Hopkinson WJ, et al: Syndesmotic sprains of the ankle, *Foot Ankle* 10:325, 1990.

Inman VT: *The joints of the ankle,* Baltimore, 1976, Williams & Wilkins.

Jablonski S: *Dictionary of medical acronyms & abbreviations,* ed 3, Philadelphia, 1998, Hanley & Belfus.

Jackson BA, Schwane JA, Starcher BC: Effect of ultrasound therapy on the repair of Achilles tendon injuries in rats, *Med Sci Sports Exerc* 23:171, 1991.

Jahss MH: *Disorders of the foot,* Philadelphia, 1982, WB Saunders.

Jahss MH: Foot and ankle pain resulting from rheumatic conditions, *Curr Opin Rheumatol* 4:233, 1992.

Jehl J, Crummy P: *Essentials of radiologic surgery,* ed 6, 1993, JB Lippincott.

Junqueira LC, Carneiro J, Kelly RO: *Basic histology,* ed 7, Norwalk, Conn, 1992, Appleton & Lange.

Kadel NJ, Teitz CC, Kronmal RA: Stress fractures in ballet dancers, *Am J Sports Med* 20:445, 1992.

Kainberger FM, et al: Injury of the Achilles tendon: diagnosis with sonography, *Am J Roentgenol* 155:1031, 1990.

Kanner R: *Pain management secrets,* Philadelphia, 1997, Hanley & Belfus.

Kannus P, Jozsa L: Histopathologic changes preceding spontaneous rupture of a tendon, *J Bone Joint Surg* 73A:1507, 1992.

Kannus P, Renstrom P: Current concepts review: treatment for acute tears of the lateral ligaments of the ankle, *J Bone Joint Surg* 73A:305, 1991.

Karasick D: Preoperative assessment of symptomatic bunionette deformity: radiologic findings, *Am J Roentgenol* 164:147, 1995.

Karasick D, Schweitzer ME: Tear of the posterior tibial tendon causing asymmetric flatfoot: radiographic findings, *Am J Roentgenol* 161:1237, 1993.

Karr SD: Subcalcaneal heel pain, *Orthop Clinic North Am* 25:161, 1994.

Katirji B: *Electromyography in clinical practice: a case study approach,* St Louis, 1998, Mosby.

Katz WA: *Rheumatic diseases diagnosis and management,* Philadelphia, 1977, JB Lippincott.

Keats TE: *Atlas of roentgenographic measurement,* ed 6, St Louis, 1990, Mosby.

Keene JA: Tendon injuries of the foot and ankle. In DeLee JD, Drez D, editors: *Orthopaedic sports medicine, principals and practice,* vol 2, Philadelphia, 1994, WB Saunders.

Kelikian H, Kelikian AS: *Disorders of the ankle,* Philadelphia, 1985, WB Saunders.

Kendall HP, Kendall RP, Wadsworth GE: *Muscles: testing and function,* ed 3, Baltimore, 1992, Williams & Wilkins.

Kleiger B: Mechanisms of ankle injury, *Orthop Clin North Am* 5:127, 1974.

Klenerman L: *The foot and its disorders,* ed 2, Boston, 1982, Blackwell Scientific.

Klippel JH, Dieppe PA: *Rheumatology,* vol 1-2, ed 2, London, 1998, Mosby.

Koenigsberg R: *Churchill's illustrated medical dictionary,* New York, 1989, Churchill Livingstone.

Konradsen L, Halmer P, Sondergard L: Early mobilizing treatment for grade III ankle ligament injuries, *Foot Ankle* 12:69, 1991.

Kontos HA: Vascular diseases of the limbs. In Wyngaarden JB, Smith LH, Bennett JC, editors: *Cecil textbook of medicine,* ed 19, Philadelphia, 1992, WB Saunders.

Kouchoukos NT, et al: Operative therapy for femoral-popliteal arterial occlusive disease, *Circulation* 35(suppl 1):174, 1967.

Larkin J, Brage M: Ankle, hindfoot, and midfoot injuries. In Reider B, editor: *Sports medicine: the school aged athlete,* Philadelphia, 1991, WB Saunders.

Larsen E, Angermann P: Association of ankle instability and foot deformity, *Acta Orthop Scand* 61:136, 1990.

Lavy CBD, Barrett DS: *Questions and answers on Apley's concise system of orthopaedics and fractures,* Oxford, 1991, Butterworth-Heinemann.

Lee TH, Wapner KL, Hecht PJ: Plantar fibromatosis, current concepts review, *J Bone Joint Surg* 75A:1080, 1993.

Leppilahti J, et al: Overuse injuries of the Achilles tendon, *Ann Chir Gynaecol* 80;202, 1991.

Lerner AJ: *The little black book of neurology,* ed 3, St Louis, 1995, Mosby.

Lewis CB, Knortz KA: *Orthopedic assessment and treatment of the geriatric patient,* St Louis, 1993, Mosby.

Lloyd-Roberts GC, Clark RC: Ball and socket ankle joint in metatarsus adductus varus (S-shaped or serpentine foot), *J Bone Joint Surg* 55B:193, 1973.

Loth TS: *Orthopedic boards review II: a case study approach,* St Louis, 1996, Mosby.

Magee DJ: *Orthopedic physical assessment,* ed 3, Philadelphia, 1997, WB Saunders.

Malone TR, McPoil TG, Nitz AJ: *Orthopedic and sports physical therapy,* ed 3, St Louis, 1997, Mosby.

Mann RA: *Surgery of the foot,* St Louis, 1986, Mosby.

Mann RA, et al: Chronic rupture of the Achilles tendon; a new technique of repair, *J Bone Joint Surg* 73A:214, 1991.

Marchiori DM: *Clinical imaging with skeletal, chest, and abdomen pattern differentials,* St Louis, 1999, Mosby.

Martens MA, Moeyersoons JP: Acute and recurrent effort-related compartment syndrome in sports, *Sports Med* 9:62, 1990.

Martin JH: *Neuroanatomy text and atlas,* ed 2, Stamford, Conn, 1996, Appleton & Lange.

Mathers LH, et al: *Clinical anatomy principles,* St Louis, 1996, Mosby.

Mazion JM: *Illustrated manual of neurological reflexes/signs/tests, part I, orthopedic signs/tests/maneuvers for office procedure, part II,* Orlando, 1980, Daniels Publishing.

McBryde A: Disorders of ankle and foot. In Grana WA, Kalenak A, editors: *Clinical sports medicine,* Philadelphia, 1991, WB Saunders.

McBryde A: Stress fractures of the foot and ankle In DeLee JD, Drez D, editors: *Orthopaedic sport medicine, principles and practice,* vol 2, Philadelphia, 1994, WB Saunders.

McRae R: *Clinical orthopaedic examination,* ed 3, Edinburgh, 1990, Churchill Livingstone.

McRae R: *Practical fracture treatment,* New York, 1994, Churchill Livingstone.

Medical Economics Books: *Patient care flow chart manual,* ed 3, Oradell, NJ, 1982, Medical Economics Books.

Mellion MB: *Sports medicine secrets,* Philadelphia, 1994, Hanley & Belfus.

Mellion MB: *Office sports medicine,* ed 2, St Louis, 1996, Mosby.

Mennell JM: *Foot pain,* Boston, 1969, Little, Brown.

Mennell JM: *The musculoskeletal system: differential diagnosis from symptoms and physical signs,* Gaithersburg, Md, 1992, Aspen.

Mercier LR, Pettid FJ: *Practical orthopedics,* ed 4, St Louis, 1995, Mosby.

Michelson JD, et al: Examination of the pathologic anatomy of ankle fractures, *J Trauma* 32:65, 1992.

Milgram JE: Office measures for relief of painful foot, *J Bone Joint Surg* 46A:1095, 1964.

Miller M: *Review of orthopaedics,* Philadelphia, 1992, WB Saunders.

Moore KL: *Clinically oriented anatomy,* ed 3, Baltimore, 1992, Williams & Wilkins.

Morton DJ: *Biomechanics of the human foot,* American Academy of Orthopaedic Surgeons Instructional Course Lectures, vol 2, Ann Arbor, Mich, 1944, J W Edwards.

Mosby-Year Book, Inc: *Expert 10-minute physical examination,* St Louis, 1997, Mosby.

Mubarak SJ, Hargens AR: *Compartment syndromes and Volkmann's contracture,* vol 3, Philadelphia, 1981, WB Saunders.

Mubarak SJ, et al: The medial tibial stress syndrome: a cause of shin splints, *Am J Sports Med* 10:201, 1992.

Mullark RE: *The anatomy of varicose veins,* Springfield, Ill, 1965, Charles C Thomas.

Myerson MS: Injuries to the forefoot and toes. In Jahss MH, editor: *Disorders of the foot and ankle: medical and surgical management,* vol 2, ed 2, Philadelphia, 1991, WB Saunders.

Myerson MS, Quill GE: Late complications of fractures of the calcaneus, *J Bone Joint Surg* 75A:331, 1993.

Nettina SM: *The Lippincott manual of nursing practice,* ed 6, Philadelphia, 1996, Lippincott.

Newton RW: *Color atlas of pediatric neurology,* St Louis, 1995, Mosby-Wolfe.

Nicholas JA, Hershman EB: *The lower extremity & spine in sports medicine,* vol 1-2, ed 2, St Louis, 1995, Mosby.

Nordin M, Andersson GBJ, Pope MH: *Musculoskeletal disorders in the workplace: principles and practice,* St Louis, 1997, Mosby.

O'Donoghue DH: *Treatment of injuries to athletes,* ed 3, Philadelphia, 1976, WB Saunders.

Olson WH, et al: *Handbook of symptom-oriented neurology,* ed 2, St Louis, 1994, Mosby.

Omer GE, Spinner M: *Management of peripheral nerve problems,* Philadelphia, 1980, WB Saunders.

Orava S, et al: Diagnosis and treatment of stress fractures located at the mid-tibial shaft in athletes, *Int J Sports Med* 12:419, 1991.

O'Reilly MAR, Massouh H: Pictorial review: the sonographic diagnosis of pathology in the Achilles tendon, *Clin Radiol* 48:202, 1993.

O'Young B, Young MA, Stiens SA: *PM&R secrets,* Philadelphia, 1997, Hanley & Belfus.

Pagana KD, Pagana TJ: *Mosby's manual of diagnostic and laboratory tests,* St Louis, 1998, Mosby.

Paley D, Hall H: Intra-articular fractures of the calcaneus, *J Bone Joint Surg* 75A:342, 1993.

Parmar HV, Triffitt PD, Gregg PJ: Intra-articular fractures of the calcaneum treated operatively or conservatively, *J Bone Joint Surg* 75B: 932, 1993.

Patten J: *Neurological differential diagnosis,* ed 2, London, 1996, Springer.

Pecina NM, Krmpotic-Nemanic J, Markiewitz AD: *Tunnel syndromes,* Boca Raton, Fla, 1991, CRC Press.

Pedowitz RA, et al: Modified criteria for the objective diagnosis of chronic compartment syndrome of the leg, *Am J Sports Med* 18:35, 1990.

Peters JW, Trevino SG, Renstrom PA: Chronic lateral ankle instability, *Foot Ankle* 12:182, 1991.

Pfeiffer WH, Cracchiolo A: Clinical results after tarsal tunnel decompression, *J Bone Joint Surg* 76A:1222, 1994.

Pheasant S: *Ergonomics, work and health,* Gaithersburg, Md, 1991, Aspen.

Post M: *Physical examination of the musculoskeletal system,* Chicago, 1987, Mosby.

Prichasuk S: The heel pad in plantar heel pain, *J Bone Joint Surg* 76B:140, 1994.

Prichasuk S, Subhadrabandhu T: The relationship of pes planus and calcaneal spur to plantar heel pain, *Clin Orthop* 306:192, 1994.

Puranen J: The medial tibial syndrome, *Ann Chir Gynaecol* 80:215, 1991.

Quirk R: Common foot and ankle injuries in dance, *Orthop Clin North Am* 25:123, 1994.

Raatikainen T, Mikko P, Puranen J: Arthrography, clinical examination, and stress radiograph in the diagnosis of acute injury to the lateral ligaments of the ankle, *Am J Sports Med* 20:2, 1992.

Rao UB, Joseph B: The influence of footwear on the prevalence of flatfoot, *J Bone Joint Surg* 74B:525, 1992.

Rasmussen O, Tovberg-Jansen I: Anterolateral rotational instability in the ankle joint, *Acta Orthop Scand* 52:99, 1981.

Ravel R: *Clinical laboratory medicine clinical application of laboratory data,* ed 6, St Louis, 1995, Mosby.

Renstrom AFH: Persistently painful sprained ankle, *J Am Acad Orthop Surg* 2:270, 1994.

Renstrom AFH, Kannus P: Injuries of the foot and ankle. In DeLee JD, Drez D, editors: *Orthopaedic sports medicine, principles and practice,* vol 2, Philadelphia, 1994, WB Saunders.

Resnick D, Niwayama G: *Diagnosis of bone and joint disorders,* Philadelphia, 1995, WB Saunders.

Riddle DL: Foot and ankle. In Richardson JK, Iglarsh ZA, editors: *Clinical orthopaedic physical therapy,* Philadelphia, 1994, WB Saunders.

Riehl R: Rehabilitation of lower leg injuries. In Prentice WE, editor: *Rehabilitation techniques in sports medicine,* ed 2, St Louis, 1994, Mosby.

Roberts DK, Pomeranz SJ: Current status of magnetic resonance in radiologic diagnosis of foot and ankle injuries, *Orthop Clin North Am* 25:61, 1994.

Roberts JM, et al: Comparison of unrepaired, primarily repaired, and polygalactin mesh-reinforced Achilles tendon lacerations in rabbits, *Clin Orthop* 181:244, 1993.

Rolak LA: *Neurology secrets,* ed 2, Philadelphia, 1998, Hanley & Belfus.

Rooser B, Bengtson S, Hagglund G: Acute compartment syndrome from anterior thigh muscle contusion: a report of eight cases, *J Orthop Trauma* 5:57, 1991.

Rumack CM, Wilson SR, Charboneau JW: *Diagnostic ultrasound,* vol 1-2, ed 2, St Louis, 1998, Mosby.

Rust M: Achilles tendon injuries in athletes, *Ann Chir Gynaecol* 80:188, 1991.

Saidoff DC, McDonough AL: *Critical pathways in therapeutic intervention,* St Louis, 1997, Mosby.

Salter RB, Harris WR: Injuries involving the epiphyseal plate, *J Bone Joint Surg* 45A:587, 1963.

Schadt DC, et al: Chronic atherosclerotic occlusion of the femoral artery, *JAMA* 175:937, 1961.

Schepsis AA, Leach RE, Gorzyca J: Plantar fasciitis: etiology, treatment, surgical results and review of the literature, *Clin Orthop* 266:185, 1991.

Schneck CD: Mesgarzadeh M, Bonakdarpour A: MR imaging of the most commonly injured ankle ligaments, *Radiology* 184:507, 1992.

Schon LC: Nerve entrapment, neuropathy and nerve dysfunction in athletes, *Orthop Clin North Am* 25:47, 1994.

Schon LC, Glennon TP, Baxter DE: Heel pain syndrome, electrodiagnostic support for nerve entrapment, *Root Ankle* 14:129, 1993.

Schumacher HR, Klippel JH, Koopman WJ: *Primer on the rheumatic diseases,* ed 10, Atlanta, 1993, Arthritis Foundation.

Scioli MW: Achilles tendinitis, *Orthop Clin North Am* 25:177, 1994.

Shankman GA: *Fundamental orthopedic management for the physical therapist assistant,* St Louis, 1997, Mosby.

Smorto MP, Basmajian JV: *Clinical electroneurography: an introduction to nerve conduction tests,* Baltimore, 1972, William & Wilkins.

Specht NT, Russo RD: *Practical guide to diagnostic imaging,* St Louis, 1998, Mosby.

Spittell JA Jr, et al: Arteriovenous fistula complicating lumbar disc surgery, *N Engl J Med* 268:1162, 1963.

Stanley K: Ankle sprains are always more than "just a sprain," *Postgrad Med* 89:251, 1991.

Stedman TL: *Stedman's medical dictionary,* ed 25, Baltimore, 1990, Williams & Wilkins.

Stephens MM: Haglund's deformity and retrocalcaneal bursitis, *Orthop Clinic North Am* 25:41, 1994.

Stevens A, Lowe J: *Histology,* New York, 1992, Gower Medical.

Stewart DL, Abeln SH: *Documenting functional outcomes in physical therapy,* St Louis, 1993, Mosby.

Stiell IG, et al: Implementation of the Ottawa ankle rules, *JAMA* 271:827, 1994.

Stock G: *The book of questions,* New York, 1985, Workman Publishing.

Stoller DW: *Magnetic resonance imaging in orthopaedics & sports medicine,* Philadelphia, 1993, JB Lippincott.

Sutton D, Young JWR: *A concise textbook of clinical imaging,* ed 2, St Louis, 1995, Mosby.

Tachdjian MO: *The child's foot,* Philadelphia, 1985, WB Saunders.

Tan JC, Horn SE: *Practical manual of physical medicine and rehabilitation,* St Louis, 1998, Mosby.

Taybi H, Lachman RS: *Radiology of syndromes, metabolic disorders, and skeletal dysplasias,* ed 4, St Louis, 1996, Mosby.

Thibodeau GA, Patton KT: *Anatomy & physiology,* ed 3, St Louis, 1996, Mosby.

Thibodeau GA, Patton KT: *Pocket reference to accompany anatomy & physiology,* ed 3, St Louis, 1996, Mosby.

Thompson JM: *Clinical outlines for health assessment,* St Louis, 1997, Mosby.

Thompson T, Doherty J: Spontaneous rupture of the tendon of Achilles: a new clinical diagnostic test, *Anat Rec* 158:126, 1967.

Thompson TC: A test for rupture of the tendon of Achilles, *Acta Orthop Scand* 32:461, 1992.

Thompson TC, Doherty JH: Spontaneous rupture of the tendon of Achilles: a nonclinical diagnostic test, *J Trauma* 2:126, 1962.

Toghill PJ: *Examining patients: an introduction to clinical medicine,* London, 1990, Edward Arnold.

Tollison CD, Satterthwaite JR, Tollison JW: *Handbook of pain management,* ed 2, Baltimore, 1994, Williams & Wilkins.

Torg JS, Shepard RJ: *Current therapy in sports medicine,* ed 3, St Louis, 1995, Mosby.

Tranier S, et al: Value of somatosensory evoked potentials in saphenous entrapment neuropathy, *J Neurol Neurosurg Psychiatry* 55:461, 1992.

Turek SL: *Orthopaedics principles and their application,* ed 3, Philadelphia, 1977, JB Lippincott.

Turnipseed WD, Pozniak M: Popliteal entrapment as a result of neurovascular compression by the soleus and plantaris muscles, *J Vasc Surg* 15:284, 1992.

Van Holsbeeck M, Introcaso JH: *Musculoskeletal ultrasound,* St Louis, 1991, Mosby.

Verhaven EFC, et al: The accuracy of three-dimensional magnetic resonance imaging in the diagnosis of ruptures of the lateral ligaments of the ankle, *Am J Sports Med* 19:583, 1991.

Wagner FW Jr: The dysvascular foot: a system for diagnosis and treatment, *Foot Ankle* 2:64, 1981.

Wakefield TS, Frank RG: *The clinician's guide to neuro musculoskeletal practice,* Abbotsford, Wisc, 1995, Allied Health of Wisconsin, SC.

Weineck J: *Functional anatomy in sports,* ed 2, St Louis, 1990, Mosby.

Weinstein SL, Buckwalter JA: *Turek's orthopaedics principles and their application,* ed 5, Philadelphia, 1994, JB Lippincott.

Whitmore I, Willan PLT: *Multiple choice questions in human anatomy,* London, 1995, Mosby.

Wilkerson LA: Ankle injuries in athletes, *Primary Care* 19:337, 1992.

Wilkins RW, Coffman JD: Tests of peripheral vascular efficiency, *Practitioner* 188:346, 1962.

Windsor RE, Lox DM: *Soft tissue injuries: diagnosis and treatment,* Philadelphia, 1998, Hanley & Belfus.

Winter D: *Biomechanics and motor control of human movement,* ed 2, New York, 1990, Wiley-Interscience Publication.

Wood JE: *The veins,* Boston, 1965, Little, Brown.

Yao L, et al: Plantar plate of the foot: findings on conventional arthrography and MR imaging, *Am J Roentgenol* 163:641, 1994.

Yochum T, Rowe L: *Essentials of skeletal radiology,* ed 2, Baltimore, 1996, Williams & Wilkins.

Zatouroff M: *Diagnosis in color physical signs in general medicine,* ed 2, London, 1996, Mosby-Wolfe.

Zitelli BJ, Davis HW: *Atlas of pediatric physical diagnosis,* ed 2, London, 1992, Wolfe.

Zsoter T, Cronin RFP: Venous distensibility in patients with varicose veins, *Can Med Assoc J* 94:1293, 1966.

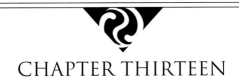

MALINGERING

Pain Qualification and Quantification
Axial trunk-loading test
Burn's bench test
Flexed-hip test
Flip sign
Libman's sign
Magnuson's test
Mannkopf's sign
Marked part pain-suggestibility test
Plantar flexion test
Related joint motion test
Seeligmuller's sign
Trunk rotational test

Sensory Deficit Qualification and Quantification
Anosmia testing
Coordination-disturbance testing
Cuignet's test
Facial anesthesia testing
Gault test
Janet's test
Limb-dropping test (upper extremities)
Lombard's test
Marcus Gunn's sign
Midline tuning-fork test
Optokinetic nystagmus test
Position-sense testing
Regional anesthesia testing
Romberg's sign
Snellen's test
Stoicism indexing

Paralysis Qualification and Quantification
Bilateral limb-dropping test (lower extremities)
Hemiplegic posturing
Hoover's sign
Simulated foot-drop testing
Simulated forearm-and-wrist-weakness testing
Simulated grip-strength-loss testing
Tripod test (bilateral leg-fluttering test)

INTRODUCTION

In a framework for disability, the interaction between the disability and the factors affecting a return to work needs to be understood by examining physicians (Fig. 13-2). In this model of interaction, *pathology* is the disturbance of normal bodily processes at the cellular level. *Impairment* is a specific loss of function. *Functional limitation* is the lack of ability to perform an action or activity. *Disability* is the inability to perform socially defined activities. *Quality of life* refers to the patient's concept of total well-being. *Risk* or *cofactors* include biologic, environmental, lifestyle, and behavioral characteristics that are associated with musculoskeletal conditions (Fig. 13-3). Whether people with specific physical limitations are disabled depends on their expectations, resources, and the demands of their physical environment.

Feigned illness, or malingering, is a sensitive medicolegal issue. Illness or injury that cannot be supported by medical fact confounds the physician's diagnostic procedures and health care delivery and also serves as an element of fraud in the third-party payer system. Patients participating in this behavior are a bane.

Not all patients who feign an illness are completely aware of their actions. Some patients embellish symptoms and physical signs as learned responses or traits, whereas others describe physical problems with hysterical emotional overlays. The latter group is influenced mostly by fear of the unknown. Depression bears a significant relationship to pain (Box 13-1 and Fig. 13-4).

ORTHOPEDIC GAMUT 13-1

DEPRESSION

Predictors of work incapacity and work loss because of depression include the following:

1. Incoherent presentation of pain localization and stable symptoms
2. Inability to influence pain and function by movement or change of position
3. Relapse of a preexisting condition and lack of response in previous episodes
4. Work dissatisfaction
5. Problems of communicating realistic treatment goals
6. Poor self-perceived prognoses with unrealistically high perception of impairment

Text continued on p. 902

TABLE 13-1

MALINGERING CROSS-REFERENCE TABLE BY ASSESSMENT PROCEDURE

Malingering, Hysteria, and Embellishment

Test/Sign	Lower Back	Sciatica	General Pain	Facial Pain	Olfactory Nerve	Trigeminal Nerve	Cerebellar Lesions	Blindness	Facial Anesthesia	Deafness	Anesthesia	Consciousness	Stoicism	Paresis
Pain														
Axial trunk-loading test	●													
Burn's bench test	●													
Flexed-hip test	●													
Flip sign		●												
Libman's sign			●											
Magnuson's test	●													
Mannkopf's sign			●											
Marked part pain-suggestibility test			●											
Plantar flexion test	●	●												
Related joint motion test			●											
Seeligmuller's sign				●										
Trunk rotational test	●													
Sensory														
Anosmia testing					●	●								
Coordination-disturbance testing							●							
Cuignet's test								●						
Facial anesthesia testing									●					
Gault test										●				
Janet's test											●			
Limb-dropping test (upper extremities)												●		
Lombard's test										●				
Marcus Gunn's sign								●						
Midline tuning-fork test											●			
Optokinetic nystagmus test								●						
Position-sense testing							●							
Regional anesthesia testing									●		●			
Romberg's sign							●							
Snellen's test								●						
Stoicism indexing												●	●	
Motor														
Bilateral limb-dropping test (lower extremities)														●
Hemiplegic posturing							●							●
Hoover's sign														●
Simulated foot-drop testing							●							●
Simulated forearm-and-wrist-weakness testing														●
Simulated grip-strength-loss test														●
Tripod test (bilateral leg-fluttering test)	●													

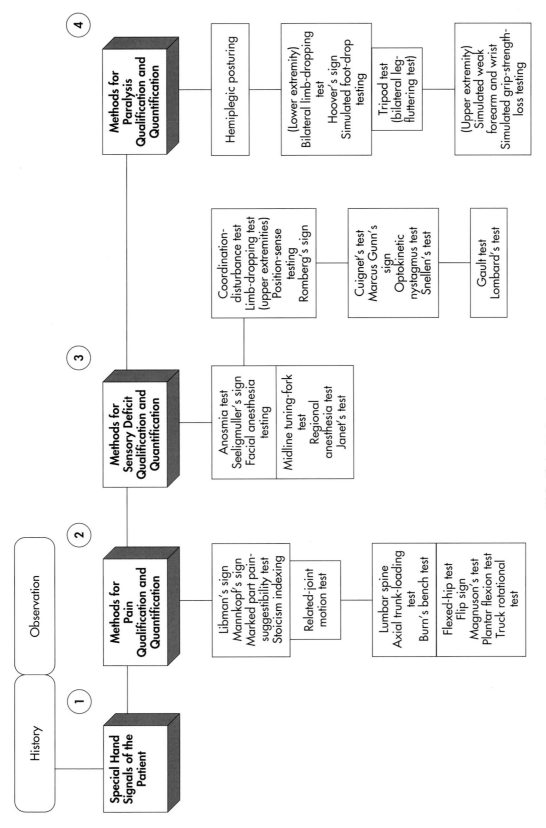

FIG. 13-1 Malingering assessment.

TABLE 13-2

MALINGERING, HYSTERIA, AND EMBELLISHMENT CROSS-REFERENCE TABLE BY SUSPECTED SYNDROME OR TISSUE

Anesthesia	Janet's test	General pain—	Marked part pain-suggestibility test
	Midline tuning-fork test	cont'd	Related joint motion test
	Regional anesthesia testing	Lower back	Axial trunk-loading test
Blindness	Cuignet's test		Burn's bench test
	Marcus Gunn's sign		Flexed-hip test
	Midline tuning-fork test		Magnuson's test
	Snellen's test		Plantar flexion test
Cerebellar lesions	Coordination-disturbance testing		Trunk rotational test
	Position-sense testing		Tripod test (bilateral leg-fluttering test)
	Romberg's sign	Olfactory nerve	Anosmia testing
	Hemiplegic posturing	Paresis	Bilateral limb-dropping test (lower extremities)
	Simulated foot-drop testing		Hemiplegic posturing
Consciousness	Limb-dropping test (upper extremities)		Hoover's sign
	Stoicism indexing		Simulated foot-drop testing
Deafness	Gault test		Simulated forearm-and-wrist-weakness testing
	Limb-dropping test (lower extremities)		Simulated grip-strength-loss testing
Facial anesthesia	Facial anesthesia testing	Sciatica	Flip sign
	Lombard's test		Plantar flexion test
Facial pain	Seeligmuller's sign	Stoicism	Stoicism indexing
General pain	Libman's sign	Trigeminal nerve	Anosmia testing
	Mannkopf's sign		

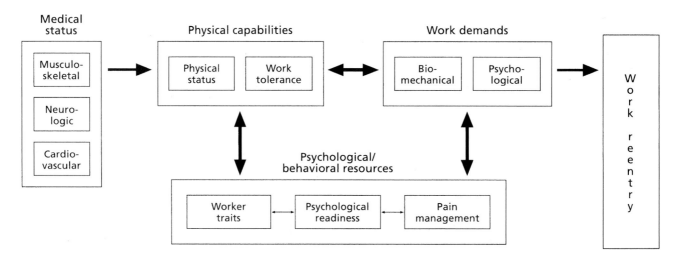

FIG. 13-2 Multiple factors potentially affecting return to work following occupational musculoskeletal injury/illness. Conceptual Model of Work Disability. *(From Demeter SL, Andersson GBJ, Smith GM: Disability evaluation, St Louis, 1996, Mosby.)*

FIG. 13-3 Disability lies at the interface between functional limitations and role demands. *(From Demeter SL, Andersson GBJ, Smith GM: Disability evaluation, St Louis, 1996, Mosby.)*

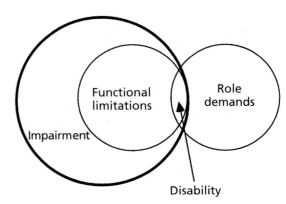

**Psychiatric History
and Mental Status Examination**

(To be completed by attending psychiatrist or psychiatric resident under direct supervision of the attending psychiatrist)

Psychiatric History

Chief Complaint(s)

_____
_____
_____

Present Illness(es) (Presenting symptoms, precipitating events, details of outpatient therapy, medications and pt.'s response)

_____
_____
_____
_____
_____
_____
_____
_____
_____
_____
_____

Past Psychiatric History (Include previous mental illnesses, suicide attempts, hospitalizations, treatments, medications)

_____
_____
_____
_____
_____

Habits (Include use of tobacco, caffeine, laxatives, alcohol and non-prescription drugs)

_____
_____
_____

Personal History (Education, occupational functioning, military, legal, marital, history of childhood abuse, etc.)

_____
_____
_____

Family History (Include all information relevant to this admission)

_____
_____
_____

FIG. 13-4 Psychiatric history and mental status examination. *(Akron Medical Center, 1995.)*

Continued

Mental Status Examination

General Observations
General Appearance   ○ Neat/well-groomed   ○ Casually groomed and dressed   ○ Dishevelled/unkempt
General Demeanor   ○ Spontaneous   ○ Overtly negativistic and hostile   ○ Mistrustful and suspicious
                          ○ Preoccupied   ○ Regressed   ○ Demanding and manipulative
(Behavior/Activity   ○ Hyperactive   ○ Hypoactive   ○ Stuporous   ○ Agitated   ○ Silly
Check all that apply)   ○ Grimaces   ○ Mannerisms   ○ Tics   ○ Compulsions   ○ Hypervigilant
                          ○ Bored   ○ Stooped   ○ Tearful   ○ Elated
                          ○ Facial expression and body posture appropriate to interview   ○ Other (specify)

     Eye Contact: ○ Avoids direct gaze   ○ Most of the time   ○ Often   ○ Occasionally
                          ○ Stares into space   ○ Most of the time   ○ Often   ○ Occasionally
                          ○ Glances furtively   ○ Most of the time   ○ Often   ○ Occasionally

Motor Behavior
   Psychomotor Retardation   ○ None   ○ Mild   ○ Moderate   ○ Marked
   Psychomotor Excitement   ○ None   ○ Mild   ○ Moderate   ○ Marked
   Specific Observations   ○ Posturing   ○ Waxy Flexibility   ○ Catatonic Rigidity   ○ Catatonic Stupor
                                ○ Pacing   ○ Fidgeting   ○ Tremors   Gait: ○ Rigid   ○ Unsteady

Comments on Behavior:
_____

_____

Mood and Affect
Depression   ○ None   ○ Mild   ○ Moderate   ○ Severe
Anxiety   ○ None   ○ Mild   ○ Moderate   ○ Severe
Anger   ○ None   ○ Mild   ○ Moderate   ○ Severe
Anhedonia   ○ None   ○ Mild   ○ Moderate   ○ Severe
Loneliness   ○ None   ○ Mild   ○ Moderate   ○ Severe
Euphoria   ○ None   ○ Mild   ○ Moderate   ○ Severe
Diurnal mood variation ○ None   ○ Worse in a.m.   ○ Worse in p.m.
Affect
   Range   ○ Full   ○ Restricted
   Inappropriate   ○ None   ○ Mild   ○ Moderate   ○ Severe
   Flat   ○ None   ○ Mild   ○ Moderate   ○ Severe
   Labile   ○ None   ○ Mild   ○ Moderate   ○ Severe
Comments on Mood and Affect:
_____

_____

Thought Processes
Ability of speech   ○ Clear, comprehensible   ○ Blocking   ○ Slow   ○ Slurred
                          ○ Rapid   ○ Pressured   ○ Flight of Ideas   ○ Talkative
Incoherence   ○ None   ○ Mild   ○ Moderate   ○ Severe
Irrelevance   ○ None   ○ Mild   ○ Moderate   ○ Severe
Evasiveness   ○ None   ○ Mild   ○ Moderate   ○ Severe
Circumstantiality   ○ None   ○ Mild   ○ Moderate   ○ Severe
Loose associations   ○ None   ○ Mild   ○ Moderate   ○ Severe
Concrete thinking   ○ None   ○ Mild   ○ Moderate   ○ Severe
Other finding: ○ None   ○ Clang Associations   ○ Neologisms   ○ Flight of Ideas
                          ○ Echolalia   ○ Perseverations   ○ Word play   ○ Excessive profanity
                          ○ Unintelligible muttering
Comments on Thought Processes:
_____

_____

_____

FIG. 13-4, cont'd   Psychiatric history and mental status examination.   *Continued*

Mental Status Examination—cont'd

Thought Content

Delusions   ○ Absent   ○ Present

              ○ Grandiose   ○ Persecutory   ○ Somatic   ○ Bizarre   ○ Religious   ○ Nihilistic

Other Findings   ○ Phobic Ideas   ○ Ambivalence   ○ Obsessive Ideas   ○ Autistic Thinking

              ○ Guilt   ○ Self Reproach   ○ Ideas of Reference   ○ Suicidal ideation

              ○ Suspicious   ○ Self-derogatory   ○ Resentful of Others   ○ Preoccupation with death

              ○ Preoccupied w/ self-harm

Comments on Thought Content:

_____

_____

Somatic Functioning and Concern

Appetite Disturbance:	○ None	○ Poor	○ Excessive
Energy Disturbance:	○ None	○ Easily Fatigued	○ Excessively Energetic
Libido Disturbance	○ None	○ Decreased	○ Markedly increased
Insomnia	○ None	○ Diff. falling asleep	○ Early a.m. awakening ○ Awakening at night
Incontinence	○ None	○ Occasional	○ Often ○ Very often
Seizures (past week)	○ None	○ One	○ Several ○ Daily ○ Several/day
Sensory impairment (organic)	○ None	○ Visual	○ Hearing
Preoccup. with physical health	○ None	○ Mild	○ Moderate ○ Marked

Somatic concerns (e.g., constipation, diarrhea, GI disturbance, short of breath, headaches, backaches, sweating, itching, etc):

_____

Perception

Hallucinations	○ Unknown	○ None	○ Suspected	○ Definite
Auditory	○ Slight	○ Mild	○ Moderate	○ Marked
Visual	○ Slight	○ Mild	○ Moderate	○ Marked
Olfactory	○ Slight	○ Mild	○ Moderate	○ Marked
Gustatory	○ Slight	○ Mild	○ Moderate	○ Marked
Tactile	○ Slight	○ Mild	○ Moderate	○ Marked
Visceral	○ Slight	○ Mild	○ Moderate	○ Marked

Belief that hallucinations are real   ○ Knows unreal   ○ Unsure   ○ Convinced they are real

Hallucinatory content (threatening, accusatory, self-derogatory, grandiose, flattering, reassuring, sexual, religious):

_____

Illusions	○ None	○ Mild	○ Moderate ○ Marked
Depersonalization	○ None	○ Mild	○ Moderate ○ Marked
Derealization	○ None	○ Mild	○ Moderate ○ Marked

Misperceptions of Role and Meaning:

_____

Sensorium

Orientation Disturbances	○ Tested	○ Too disturbed to test	
Time	○ None	○ Mild	○ Moderate ○ Marked
Place	○ None	○ Mild	○ Moderate ○ Marked
Person	○ None	○ Mild	○ Moderate ○ Marked
Clouded Consciousness	○ None	○ Mild	○ Moderate ○ Marked
	○ Fluctuating	○ Continuous	
Dissociation	○ None	○ Mild	○ Moderate ○ Marked

Comments on Sensorium:

_____

_____

FIG. 13-4, cont'd   Psychiatric history and mental status examination.   *Continued*

Mental Status Examination—cont'd

Cognitive Functions

Memory Disturbances	○ Tested	○ Too disturbed to test		○ Confabulations	
Immediate	○ Unknown	○ None	○ Mild	○ Moderate	○ Marked
Recent	○ Unknown	○ None	○ Mild	○ Moderate	○ Marked
Remote	○ Unknown	○ None	○ Mild	○ Moderate	○ Marked

Attention Disturbances	○ None	○ Mild	○ Moderate	○ Marked	
Distractibility	○ None	○ Mild	○ Moderate	○ Marked	
Intelligence (estimated)	○ Unknown	○ Retarded	○ Borderline	○ Average	○ Bright

Comments on Cognitive Functions:

_____

_____

Judgment

Family Relations	○ Poor	○ Fair	○ Healthy	
Other social relations	○ Poor	○ Fair	○ Healthy	
Employment	○ Poor	○ Fair	○ Healthy	
Future Plans	○ No Plans	○ Poor	○ Fair	○ Realistic

Comments on Judgment:

_____

_____

Insight and Attitude Toward Illness

Recognition of one's illness   ○ Unknown   ○ Too sick to be tested   ○ Physically ill only
   ○ None   ○ Little   ○ Fair   ○ Full recognition

Awareness of one's contribution to problem
   ○ Unknown   ○ Too sick to be tested   ○ Not applicable
   ○ None   ○ Little   ○ Fair   ○ Full awareness
   ○ Blames others   ○ Blames circumstances

Motivation for getting well   ○ Unknown   ○ Too sick to be tested
   ○ None   ○ Little   ○ Fair   ○ Highly motivated
   ○ Accepts offered treatment   ○ Refuses offered treatment

Comments on Insight:

_____

_____

Potential for Self-Injury, Suicide and Violence

Self-Injury	○ Unknown	○ Absent	○ Minimal	○ Potentially present	○ Marked (specify precautions)
Suicide Risk	○ Unknown	○ Absent	○ Minimal	○ Potentially present	○ Marked (specify precautions)
Assaultiveness	○ Unknown	○ Absent	○ Minimal	○ Potentially present	○ Active (specify interventions)

Comments on self-injury, suicide/violence potential (e.g., plan, history, behavior):

_____

_____

_____

Reliability and Completeness of Information:
   ○ Very good   ○ Good   ○ Only Fair   ○ Poor   ○ Very Poor

FIG. 13-4, cont'd   Psychiatric history and mental status examination.   *Continued*

Mental Status Examination—cont'd

Barriers to Communication/reliability due to (Complete only if reliability rated poor/very poor):

○ Dialect/Foreign language   ○ Quality of speech   ○ Deafness   ○ Physical illness
○ Refuses to give information   ○ Massive Denial   ○ Conscious falsification
○ Pt. psychopathology   Other (explain) _____

_____

_____

Attitude Toward Examiner:

○ Positive   ○ Neutral   ○ Ambivalent   ○ Negative   ○ Unknown

Overall Severity of Illness:

○ Mild   ○ Moderate   ○ Marked   ○ Severe   ○ Extremely Severe

Discussion and Formulation (include description of patient's strengths/assets)

_____

_____

_____

_____

_____

_____

Diagnoses (DSM-IV)

Axis I _____

Axis II _____

Axis III _____

Axis IV (assessment of psychosocial/environmental problems) _____

Axis V (Global Assessment of Functioning score) Current _____ Past year _____

Recommendations:

_____

_____

_____

_____

_____

_____

_____

Examiner's Name, Title   Date

Examining Psychiatrist Signature   Date

FIG. 13-4, cont'd   Psychiatric history and mental status examination.

Symptoms of Depression

1. Depressed mood or irritable mood
2. Markedly diminished interest or pleasure in activities
3. Significant weight loss or weight gain when not dieting
4. Insomnia or hypersomnia nearly every day
5. Psychomotor agitation or retardation—observable by others
6. Fatigue or loss of energy
7. Feelings of worthlessness or excessive or inappropriate guilt, which may be delusional
8. Diminished ability to think or concentrate, or indecisiveness
9. Recurrent thoughts of death, recurrent suicidal ideation without a plan, or a suicide attempt, or a specific plan for committing suicide
10. Lack of reactivity to usually pleasurable stimuli
11. Depression worse in the morning
12. Early morning awakening

From White AH, Schofferman JA: *Spine care,* vol 1-2, St Louis, 1995, Mosby.

Two major categories of hysterical disorders are identified: patients with a fictitious illness, such as in malingering, and patients with Munchausen syndrome. Both types are patients with signs and symptoms that have no organic basis but who are not deliberately attempting to mislead the examiner.

Trivial physical trauma or disease is often at the root of a portrayed illness or injury. Often, by the time symptom embellishment is clinically recognized, the complaints are of such a magnitude that they are completely incongruous with the original illness or injury. A patient who originally experienced a minor, clinically documented upper respiratory infection now describes symptoms and subjective complaints that resemble those for histoplasmosis or black lung disease. Yet another patient may complain of total leg disability following a minor thigh contusion. Both patients have in common the total lack of clinical findings to support the complaints, and some type of secondary gain serves as a driving force behind the medical charade.

Individuals may feign physical symptoms to continue in a less strenuous job at work, or they may receive a parking space closer to their place of employment. These individuals may also fake symptoms to gain control over family members or fellow workers. The injured party may also allow others to do work the patient would ordinarily do.

The diagnosis of hysteria should be established only on the basis of positive evidence. Even if the patient has an obvious hysterical disorder, a serious organic illness may still be present.

Conversion symptoms have a physiologic or pathologic substrate. A conversion disorder denotes a process in which a patient's emotions become transformed into physical (motor or sensory) manifestations. These patients are asking for help but in an inappropriate way. Conversion symptoms often occur in mentally defective individuals or in adolescents as a way of coping (albeit inadequately) with the environment. Common presentations include blindness, deafness, paresis, sensory disturbances, ataxia, seizures, and unconsciousness.

TABLE 13-3

DISTINCTIONS AMONG WORK CAPACITY, WORK TOLERANCE, DEPENDABLE ABILITY, AND TASK DEMAND

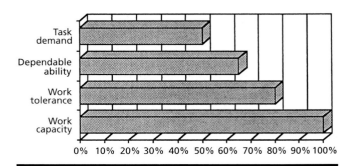

From Demeter SL, Andersson GBJ, Smith GM: *Disability evaluation,* St Louis, 1996, Mosby.

Malingering is the conscious misrepresentation of thoughts, feelings, and facts, and it is a condition in which symptoms and signs associated with pain or dysfunction are either partially or entirely feigned for secondary gain. Most commonly, malingering occurs in the setting of the workplace, where workers' compensation is an issue.

It is difficult to label patients as hysterics, frauds, or malingerers. This is rarely accomplished without reaping the wrath of the patient or substantial legal repercussions.

The actual percentage of patients who are malingerers is undetermined. However, it has been estimated that 2% of all patients seeking health care are malingering. Obviously, the ascertainment of the inaccuracy of a patient's report of pain and disability is a difficult process, but the possibility of malingering should be raised in the mind of the treating physician when major discrepancies or inconsistencies appear in the patient's medical situation. In this effort, outcome measures for the assessment of work capacity, work tolerance, dependable ability, and task demand are useful tools (Table 13-3).

GLOBAL HEALTH STATUS

Global health status is categorized into the following five dimensions—the "5 D's":

1. Death
2. Disability—upper or lower limb functional problems
3. Discomfort—physical or psychologic
4. Drug reactions—or other medical or surgical iatrogenic problems
5. Dollars—both direct and indirect costs

Outcomes Assessments

The Health Assessment Questionnaire (HAQ) is a self-administered instrument that assesses discomfort and disability. It is used to measure outcome in many different neuromusculoskeletal diseases (Fig. 13-5). Disease-specific instruments have been produced to help follow outcome in several other neuromusculoskeletal diseases. This includes a Fibromyalgia Impact Questionnaire (Fig. 13-6). The activity of inflammatory neuromusculoskeletal diseases can be assessed through serologic measures. Separate measures of both tender and swollen joints can be charted on a homunculus (Fig. 13-7). A generic measure of anxiety and depression, such as the Hospital Anxiety and Depression (HAD) scale (Fig. 13-8), allows psychologic variables to be assessed independently from orthopedic disease-related outcomes. The EuroQuol Thermometer is one of the instruments that uses a simple visual technique to allow people to assess their own health status (Fig. 13-9); the Disease Repercussion Profile is another such resource (Box 13-2).

Armed with Borg pain scales, Oswestry disability indices, symptom magnification indexing, Dallas Pain Questionnaire (Fig. 13-10), Waddell indexing (Table 13-4), and neuroorthopedic malingering tests, the physician is able to substantiate or refute the existence of malingering in any given case. These tests and indices are usually used in combination with the more traditional neuroorthopedic physical examinations. A singular positive finding or test does not indicate that the patient is magnifying or faking symptoms. Rather, the malingering diagnosis is based on the preponderance of positive malingering test findings and the absence of findings from traditional neuroorthopedic tests. Any positive findings must be further correlated with the medical history of the patient. It is the constellation of positive malingering tests, normal findings in traditional tests, and medical history discrepancies that form the malingering diagnosis. Malingering and psychogenic rheu-matism patients primarily complain of pain, sensory losses, or paralysis in any combination.

GENERAL PROCEDURES

General Patient Observation

There is consensus among physicians that malingering is readily detected with appropriate medical and psychologic tests. Most patients who have remained conscious during an injury can give an adequate description of what happened. A malingerer is vague and on guard while describing the incidents of an injury or accident. However, some patients who also remain conscious at the time of injury are not as observant as others are, and these patients will be somewhat vague.

A malingerer often appears quarrelsome, nervous, and ill at ease. General observation of the patient before and after the physical examination may reveal that the patient is fully capable of movements or activities that were claimed to be impossible in the physical examination. Note how the patient enters and behaves in the reception room. It is helpful if a nonprofessional staff person takes the patient's history and engages the claimant in conversation.

When hearing loss is the complaint, the examiner should speak to the patient calmly and in a very low tone of voice to test the patient's response. With visual-disturbance complaints, the examiner should give the patient a magazine with fine print to read while waiting, and later ask something about the subject matter.

The patient should be asked to describe the accident in detail. The examiner should encourage the patient to go through as many of the painful motions as possible. Often, the extreme interest of the examiner in the patient's story will cause the patient to move the arms, legs, or back in a normal manner.

The examiner should try to observe the patient tying the shoes, walking down a hallway, bending at the waist, drinking at a fountain, pulling or pushing a door, or many other unguarded activities of daily living.

Detailed History

Occasionally, the physician is called upon to distinguish fraud or exaggeration from organic injury. As should be apparent by now, this is not an easy task. An examination, when deception or exaggeration is suspected, should be completed with a strictly impartial attitude on the part of the examiner. The patient must be accorded all the tact and courtesy that is ordinarily extended to any other patient. If the doctor-patient rapport is compromised, confidence is destroyed, and questions and tests, which are constructed to evoke sincerity on the part of the patient, become unreliable.

In many instances, the patient grudgingly gives the history. The malingering patient may remark, "I've told this to the last doctor, and I don't see any reason to repeat it."

Please check (x) the response which best describes your usual abilities

Over the past week:

Hygiene Are you able to:	Without any difficulty	With some difficulty	With much difficulty	Unable to do	
Wash and dry your body?	☐	☐	☐	☐	
Take a tub bath?	☐	☐	☐	☐	
Get on and off the toilet?	☐	☐	☐	☐	☐ **Hygiene**

Reach Are you able to:					
Reach and get down a 5 pound object (such as bag of sugar) from just above your head?	☐	☐	☐	☐	
Bend down to pick up clothing from the floor?	☐	☐	☐	☐	☐ **Reach**

Grip Are you able to:					
Open car doors?	☐	☐	☐	☐	
Open jars which have been previously opened?	☐	☐	☐	☐	
Turn faucets on and off?	☐	☐	☐	☐	☐ **Grip ARA**

Activities Are you able to:					
Run errands and shop?	☐	☐	☐	☐	
Get in and out of a car?	☐	☐	☐	☐	
Do chores such as vacuuming or yardwork?	☐	☐	☐	☐	☐ **Activity**

Please check (x) any **aids or devices** that you usually use for any of these activities:

☐ Raised toilet seat   ☐ Bathtub bar

☐ Bathtub seat   ☐ Long-handled appliances for reach

☐ Jar opener   ☐ Long-handled appliances in bathroom

☐ (for jars previously opened)   ☐ Other (specify...........................)

Please check (x) any categories for which you usually need **help from another person:**

☐ Hygiene   ☐ Gripping and opening things

☐ Reach   ☐ Errands and chores

We are also interested in learning whether or not you are affected by pain because of your illness. How much pain have you had because of your illness **In the past week:**

Place a vertical (I) mark on the line to indicate the severity of the pain

No pain |————————————————| **Severe pain**
0   100

Name [＿＿＿＿＿＿]   Date [＿＿＿＿]

In this section we are interested in learning how your illness affects your ability to function in daily life. Please feel free to add any comments on the back of this page.

Please check the response which best describes your usual abilities

over the past week:

Dressing & grooming Are you able to:	Without any difficulty	With some difficulty	With much difficulty	Unable to do
Dress yourself, including tying shoelaces and doing buttons?	☐	☐	☐	☐
Shampoo your hair:	☐	☐	☐	☐

Arising Are you able to:				
Stand up from a straight chair?	☐	☐	☐	☐
Get in and out of bed?	☐	☐	☐	☐

Eating Are you able to:				
Cut your meat?	☐	☐	☐	☐
Lift a full cup or glass to your mouth?	☐	☐	☐	☐
Open a new milk carton?	☐	☐	☐	☐

Walking Are you able to:				
Walk outdoors on flat ground?	☐	☐	☐	☐
Climb up five steps?	☐	☐	☐	☐

Please check any **aids or devices** that you usually use for any of these activities:

☐ Cane   ☐ Devices used for dressing (button hook, zipper pull, long-handled shoe horn, etc.)

☐ Walker   ☐ Built up or special utensils

☐ Crutches   ☐ Special or built up chair

☐ Wheelchair   ☐ Other (specify . . . .)

FIG. 13-5   The Health Assessment Questionnaire (HAQ): disability and discomfort scales. *(From Fries JF, et al: Measurement of patient outcomes in arthritis, Arthritis Rheum 23:137, 1980.)*

Fibromyalgia Impact Questionnaire

1. Were you able to:

	Always	Most times	Occasionally	Never
a. Do shopping	0	1	2	3
b. Do laundry with a washer and dryer	0	1	2	3
c. Prepare meals	0	1	2	3
d. Wash dishes/cooking utensils by hand	0	1	2	3
e. Vacuum a rug	0	1	2	3
f. Make beds	0	1	2	3
g. Walk several blocks	0	1	2	3
h. Visit friends/relatives	0	1	2	3
i. Do yard work	0	1	2	3
j. Drive a car	0	1	2	3

2. Of the 7 days in the past week, how many days did you feel good?

1	2	3	4	5	6	7

3. How many days in the past week did you miss work because of your fibromyalgia? (If you don't have a job outside the home leave this item blank.)

1	2	3	4	5

4. When you did go to work, how much did pain or other symptoms of your fibromyalgia interfere with your ability to do your job?

No problem |—————————————| Great difficulty

5. How bad has your pain been?

No pain |—————————————| Very severe pain

6. How tired have you been?

No tiredness |—————————————| Very tired

7. How have you felt when you got up in the morning?

Awoke well rested |—————————————| Awoke very tired

8. How bad has your stiffness been?

No stiffness |—————————————| Very stiff

9. How tense, nervous or anxious have you felt?

Not tense |—————————————| Very tense

10. How depressed or blue have you felt?

Not depressed |—————————————| Very depressed

FIG. 13-6   Fibromyalgia Impact Questionnaire (FIQ). *(From Burkhardt CS, Clark SR, Bennett RM: The Fibromyalgia Impact Questionnaire: development and validation, J Rheumatol 18:728, 1991.)*

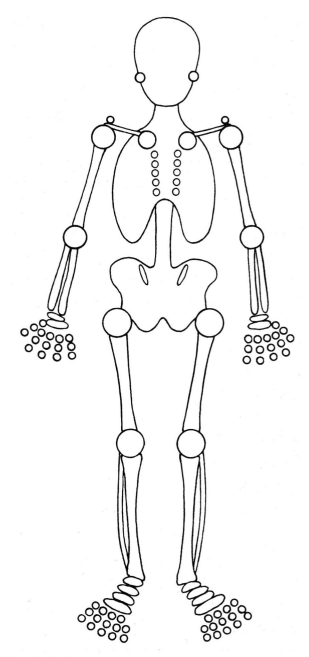

FIG. 13-7   Skeleton diagram for recording joint examination findings. *(From Polley HF, Hunder GG: Rheumatologic interviewing and physical examination of the joints, ed 2, Philadelphia, 1978, WB Saunders.)*

1. Are you basically satisfied with your life?   Yes   No
2. Have you dropped many of your activities and interests?   Yes   No
3. Do you feel that your life is empty?   Yes   No
4. Do you often get bored?   Yes   No
5. Are you hopeful about the future?   Yes   No
6. Are you bothered by thoughts you can't get out of your head?   Yes   No
7. Are you in good spirits most of the time?   Yes   No
8. Are you afraid that something bad is going to happen to you?   Yes   No
9. Do you feel happy most of the time?   Yes   No
10. Do you often feel helpless?   Yes   No
11. Do you often get restless and fidgety?   Yes   No
12. Do you prefer staying at home rather than going out and doing new things?   Yes   No
13. Do you frequently worry about the future?   Yes   No
14. Do you feel that you have more problems with memory than most?   Yes   No
15. Do you think it is wonderful to be alive now?   Yes   No
16. Do you often feel downhearted and blue?   Yes   No
17. Do you feel pretty worthless the way you are now?   Yes   No
18. Do you worry a lot about the past?   Yes   No
19. Do you find life very exciting?   Yes   No
20. Is it hard for you to get started on new projects?   Yes   No
21. Do you feel full of energy?   Yes   No
22. Do you feel that your situation is hopeless?   Yes   No
23. Do you think that most individuals are better off than you are?   Yes   No
24. Do you frequently get upset over little things?   Yes   No
25. Do you frequently feel like crying?   Yes   No
26. Do you have trouble concentrating?   Yes   No
27. Do you enjoy getting up in the morning?   Yes   No
28. Do you prefer to avoid social gatherings?   Yes   No
29. Is it easy for you to make decisions?   Yes   No
30. Is your mind as clear as it used to be?   Yes   No

FIG. 13-8   GDS Form. *(Modified from Yesavage JA, et al: Development and validation of a geriatric depression screening scale: a preliminary report, J Psych Res 17:37, 1983.)*

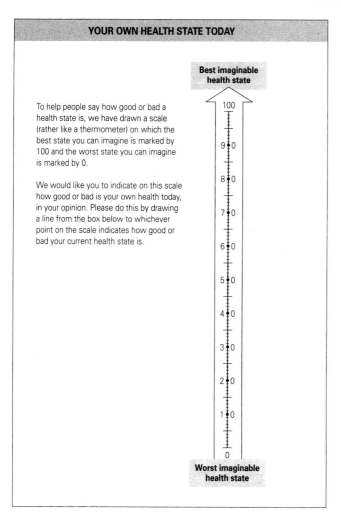

YOUR OWN HEALTH STATE TODAY

To help people say how good or bad a health state is, we have drawn a scale (rather like a thermometer) on which the best state you can imagine is marked by 100 and the worst state you can imagine is marked by 0.

We would like you to indicate on this scale how good or bad is your own health today, in your opinion. Please do this by drawing a line from the box below to whichever point on the scale indicates how good or bad your current health state is.

Best imaginable
health state

100

90

80

70

60

50

40

30

20

10

0

Worst imaginable
health state

FIG. 13-9 The EuroQuol Thermometer for assessing health status. *(From Euroquol Group: Euroquol: a new facility for the measurement of health-related quality of life,* Health Policy *16:199, 1990.)*

The patient also may deny permission to review previous x-ray findings or case histories, stating that the attorney can only grant such permission. The genuine patient usually will not hesitate to furnish all patient information or permissions in this regard.

Malingerers will give an involved and long history, most of which is often discovered to be false. When the patient's history, actions, and examination findings suggest that symptoms are exaggerated, it is the duty of the physician to make the examination so complete that there will be no question as to the actual extent of any organic disease or injury.

The physician's next duty is to decide whether the patient is a malingerer attempting to defraud and deceive or whether hysteria or neurasthenia exists, in which the patient benignly imagines the disability. Many patients become convinced that a certain type of disability is caused by a specific injury. If the physician can establish sufficient confidence with the patient to explain and treat the condition

BOX 13-2

Disease Impact Index

Patients report severity of problems on a 0-10 scale in six dimensions:
- Functional activities
- Social activities
- Relationships
- Emotions
- Socioeconomic factors
- Body image

From Carr AJ, Thompson PW: Towards a measure of patient-perceived handicap in rheumatoid arthritis, *Br J Rheumatol* 33:378, 1994.

effectively, often the exaggerated symptoms will disappear. However, with malingering, any attempt on the part of the physician to confront the patient results in further exaggeration.

To achieve a secondary gain, the malingerer must use subterfuge. Exaggeration usually is obvious no matter how cleverly it is performed. The malingerer exhibits slyness of expression and watches the examiner carefully during the various procedures. The patient may try to impress the examiner with the importance of the case and often reiterates a great degree of personal honesty. The patient appears to be constantly suspicious that detection is likely and attempts to avoid disclosure.

A detailed history is the first essential, and many times, the answers to questions must be requested repeatedly (Fig. 13-11). The patient may give strange stories about the exact nature of an accident or the treatment that was previously administered for the condition (Figs. 13-12 to 13-14).

Psychogenic Rheumatism Profile

Patients with psychiatric disorders may develop pain as part of the symptoms associated with mental illness. Patients with pain also may develop psychiatric disorders as part of the symptoms associated with the physical illness. Pain associated with neurosis is more common than pain associated with schizophrenia or endogenous depression.

ORTHOPEDIC GAMUT 13-3

PSYCHOLOGIC ILLNESS

Reasons for psychologic illness that cause the appearance or exacerbation of pain include the following:

1. Anxiety
2. Psychiatric hallucination
3. Increased tension in the muscles, with associated inadequate circulation and the accumulation of metabolic byproducts (lactic acid)
4. Hysteria with conversion reactions

Text continued on p. 928

DALLAS PAIN QUESTIONNAIRE

Name: _____   Date of Birth: _____

Today's Date: _____   Occupation: _____

PLEASE READ: *Mark an "X" along the line from 0 to 100 for each question that tells your doctor how your pain has affected your life. Be sure to mark your own answers. Do not ask someone else to answer the questions for you.*

For example: I feel bad.

Never				Some				Mostly all the time
0%	0	X 1	2	3	4	5		100%

SECTION I: DAILY ACTIVITIES

1. PAIN AND INTENSITY - to what degree do you rely on pain medications or pain relieving substances for you to be comfortable?

A

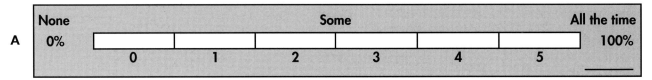

None				Some				All the time
0%	0	1	2	3	4	5		100%

2. PERSONAL CARE - how much does pain interfere with your personal care (getting out of bed, teeth brushing, dressing, etc.)?

None (no pain)				Some			Cannot get out of bed
0%	0	1	2	3	4		100%

3. LIFTING - how much limitation do you notice lifting?

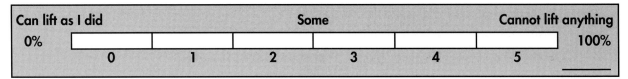

Can lift as I did				Some				Cannot lift anything
0%	0	1	2	3	4	5		100%

4. WALKING - compared to how far you could walk before your injury or back trouble, how much does pain restrict your walking now?

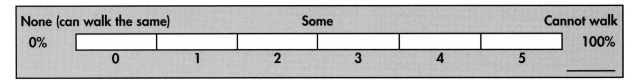

None (can walk the same)				Some				Cannot walk
0%	0	1	2	3	4	5		100%

FIG. 13-10   **A,** Dallas Pain Questionnaire. *(From White AH, Schofferman JA: Spine care, vol 1-2, St Louis, 1995, Mosby.)*   *Continued*

5. SITTING - back pain limits my sitting in a chair to:

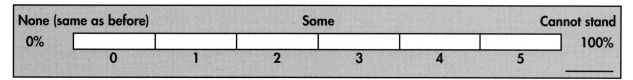

| No pain (same as before) | | | Some | | | Cannot sit at all |
0% 0 1 2 3 4 5 100%

6. STANDING - how much does your pain interfere with your tolerance to stand for long periods of time?

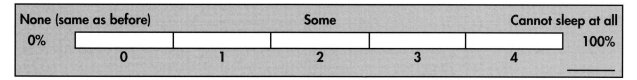

None (same as before) Some Cannot stand
0% 0 1 2 3 4 5 100%

7. SLEEPING - how much does your pain interfere with your sleeping?

None (same as before) Some Cannot sleep at all
0% 0 1 2 3 4 100%

$$D = \underline{\quad} \times 3 = \underline{\quad}\%$$

SECTION II: WORK AND LEISURE

A

8. SOCIAL LIFE - how much does pain interfere with your social life (dancing, games, going out, eating with friends, etc.)?

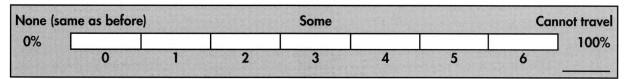

None (same as before) Some No activities (total loss)
0% 0 1 2 3 4 5 6 7 100%

9. TRAVELING - how much does pain interfere with traveling in a car?

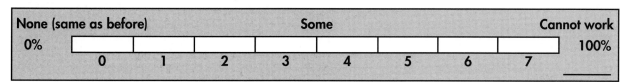

None (same as before) Some Cannot travel
0% 0 1 2 3 4 5 6 100%

10. VOCATIONAL - how much does pain interfere with your job?

None (same as before) Some Cannot work
0% 0 1 2 3 4 5 6 7 100%

$$W = \underline{\quad} \times 5 = \underline{\quad}\%$$

FIG. 13-10, cont'd **A,** Dallas Pain Questionnaire.   *Continued*

SECTION III: ANXIETY/DEPRESSION

11. ANXIETY/MOOD - how much control do you feel that you have over the demands made on you?

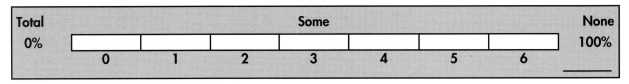

12. EMOTIONAL CONTROL - how much control do you feel you have over your emotions?

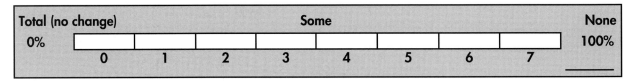

13. DEPRESSION - how depressed have you been since the onset of pain?

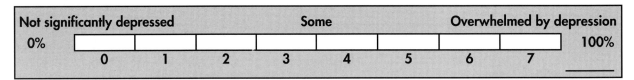

A = ___ × 5 = ___%

SECTION IV: SOCIAL INTERESTS

A 14. INTERPERSONAL RELATIONSHIPS - how much do you think your pain changed your relationship with others?

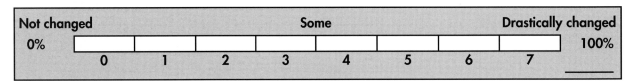

15. SOCIAL SUPPORT - how much support do you need from others to help you during this onset of pain (taking over chores, fixing meals, etc.)?

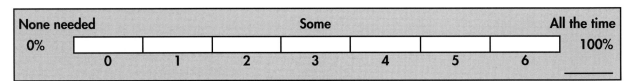

16. PUNISHING RESPONSE - how much do you think others express irritation, frustration, or anger toward you because of your pain?

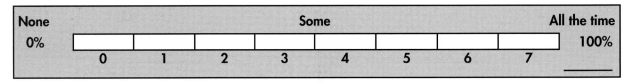

S = ___ × 5 = ___%

FIG. 13-10, cont'd **A,** Dallas Pain Questionnaire. *(From White AH, Schofferman JA: Spine care, vol 1-2, St Louis, 1995, Mosby.)*

Continued

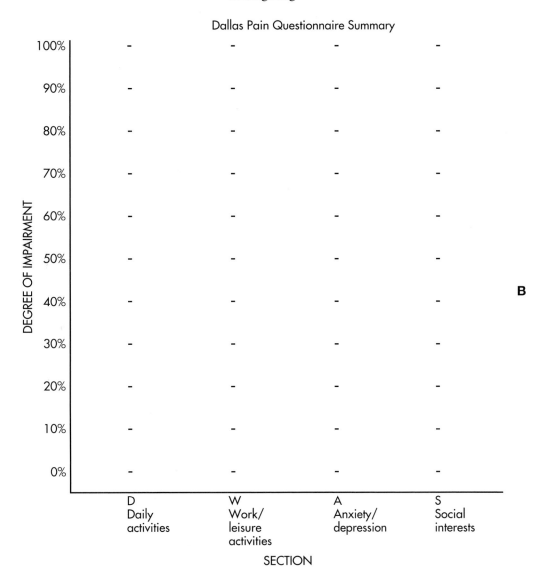

FIG. 13-10, cont'd   **B,** Dallas Pain Questionnaire Summary.

Patient History

Please take time to fill out the appropriate spaces

Name _____ Date _____

Age _____ Medication allergies _____ Current Rx'd medicine _____

Present job _____

Type of work done _____

When did your back or neck pain originally start? _____

When did your arm or leg pain originally start? _____

When did your current episode begin? _____

Did your pain start gradually? _____ Suddenly?_____ Injury _____

What type of injury? _____

What time of day is your pain worse?   Morning _____ Later in the day _____

Middle of the night _____

Do you have numbness or tingling in an arm or leg? Please describe.

_____

Are there any recent changes in bowel or bladder habits? Please describe.

_____

Do you feel stiffness in the morning?_____

My pain is: check the appropriate column:	Better	Worse	No different
With cough or sneeze	_____	_____	_____
With straining	_____	_____	_____
Sitting in straight chair	_____	_____	_____
Sitting in soft, easy chair	_____	_____	_____
Bending forward to brush teeth	_____	_____	_____
Walking up stairs	_____	_____	_____
Walking down stairs	_____	_____	_____
Lying flat on stomach	_____	_____	_____
On side with knees bent	_____	_____	_____
When bending	_____	_____	_____
When lifting	_____	_____	_____
When working overhead	_____	_____	_____
Lying on back	_____	_____	_____
Standing	_____	_____	_____

	Yes	No
My back sometimes gets stuck when I bend forward.	_____	_____
After walking, bending forward relieves my pain.	_____	_____
My back feels like giving way when I bend forward.	_____	_____
Do you have headaches?	_____	_____

FIG. 13-11   Patient history and examination forms.   *(From Watkins RG:* The spine in sports, *St Louis, 1996, Mosby.)*   *Continued*

Patient History—cont'd

	Yes	No
Have you had a change in hearing, vision?	_____	_____
Have you had dizzy spells?	_____	_____
My pain stops me when I walk a certain distance.	_____	_____
Have you been in a hospital for back, leg, or neck pain?	_____	_____

Number of times hospitalized _____ Please give dates. _____

How long can you sit? _____

How long can you walk? _____

If you have to stop walking, how long does the pain last? _____

Have you had myelograms? _____

Number of times _____

Have you had neck or back surgery? _____

Number of times _____ Please give dates and types. _____

Have you been in the hospital with other medical problems? _____

Number of times _____ Please describe. _____

What treatments have made your pain better? _____

What treatments have made your pain worse? _____

Who referred you to this office? _____

Do you have an attorney helping you? _____

Do other members of your family have significant back trouble? _____

Who? _____

Did you have to change jobs? _____ To what? _____

Are you under any pressure at home? _____ At work? _____

Mild _____ Moderate _____ Severe _____

What can you not do because of your pain that you want to do? _____

_____

What was the date of your last physical exam and the name of the doctor? _____

Who did it? _____

Pelvic done? _____ Rectal done? _____

FIG. 13-11, cont'd   Patient history and examination forms.   *Continued*

Patient Pain/Sensation Chart

Date ____________________

Please give this paper to the doctor at the time of examination

Mark the areas on your body where you feel the described sensations. Use the appropriate symbol. Mark areas of radiation. Include all affected areas. Just to complete the picture, please draw in your face.

NUMBNESS	— — —	PINS AND NEEDLES	oooo oooo oooo	BURNING	XXXX XXXX XXXX	STABBING	//// //// ////

Have you had prior back or neck surgery? ( )Yes ( )No

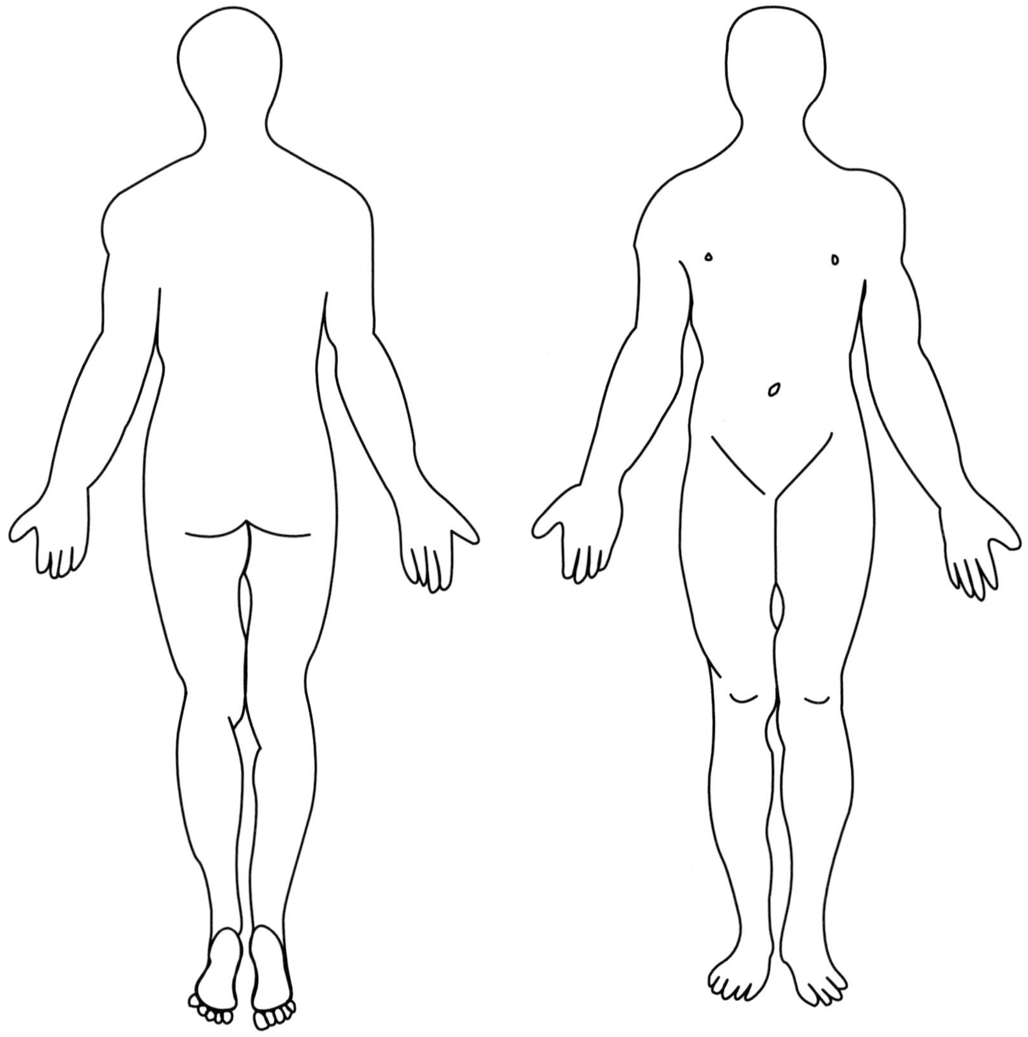

FIG. 13-11, cont'd Patient history and examination forms. *(From Watkins RG:* The spine in sports, *St Louis, 1996, Mosby.)*

Continued

Oswestry Function Test

Please choose one answer only per section

Pain Intensity

1. I can tolerate my pain without having to use pain killers.
2. My pain is bad, but I manage without taking pain killers.
3. Pain killers give me complete relief from my pain.
4. Pain killers give me moderate relief from my pain.
5. Pain killers give me very little relief from my pain.
6. Pain killers have no effect on my pain, and I do not use them.

Personal Care

1. I can look after myself normally without causing extra pain.
2. I can look after myself normally, but it causes extra pain.
3. It is painful to look after myself, and I am slow and careful.
4. I need some help, but I manage most of my personal care.
5. I need help every day in most aspects of self-care.
6. I do not get dressed, wash with difficulty, and stay in bed.

Lifting

1. I can lift heavy objects without causing extra pain.
2. I can left heavy objects, but it gives me extra pain.
3. Pain prevents me from lifting heavy objects off the floor, but I can manage light to medium objects if they are conveniently positioned.
4. I can lift only very light objects.
5. I cannot lift anything at all.

Walking

1. Pain does not prevent me from walking any distance.
2. Pain prevents me from walking more than 1 mile.
3. Pain prevents me from walking more than $1/2$ mile.
4. Pain prevents me from walking more than $1/4$ mile.
5. I can only walk using a cane or crutches.
6. I am in bed most of the time and have to crawl to the toilet.

Sitting

1. I can sit in any chair as long as I like.
2. I can sit only in my favorite chair as long as I like.
3. Pain prevents me from sitting more than 1 hour.
4. Pain prevents me from sitting more than $1/2$ hour.
5. Pain prevents me from sitting more than 10 minutes.
6. Pain prevents me from sitting at all.

Standing

1. I can stand as long as I want without extra pain.
2. I can stand as long as I want, but it gives me extra pain.
3. Pain prevents me from standing more than 1 hour.
4. Pain prevents me from standing more than $1/2$ hour.
5. Pain prevents me from standing more than 10 minutes.
6. Pain prevents me from standing at all.

Sleeping

1. Pain does not prevent me from sleeping well.
2. I can sleep well only by taking medication for sleep.
3. Even when I take medication, I have less than 6 hours' sleep.
4. Even when I take medication, I have less than 4 hours' sleep.
5. Even when I take medication, I have less than 2 hours' sleep.
6. Pain prevents me from sleeping at all.

Sex Life

1. My sex life is normal and gives me no extra pain.
2. My sex life is normal but causes some extra pain.
3. My sex life is nearly normal but is very painful.
4. My sex life is severely restricted by pain.
5. My sex life is nearly absent because of pain.
6. Pain prevents any sex life at all.

Social Life

1. My social life is normal and gives me no extra pain.
2. My social life is normal but increases the degree of pain.
3. Pain has no significant effect on my social life apart from limiting my more energetic interests, like dancing, etc.
4. Pain has restricted my social life, and I do not go out as often.
5. Pain has restricted my social life to my home.
6. I have no social life because of pain.

Traveling

1. I can travel anywhere without extra pain.
2. I can travel anywhere, but it gives me extra pain.
3. Pain is bad, but I manage journeys over 2 hours.
4. Pain restricts me to journeys of less than 1 hour.
5. Pain restricts me to short necessary journeys of less than $1/2$ hour.
6. Pain prevents me from traveling except to the doctor or hospital.

FIG. 13-11, cont'd   Patient history and examination forms.   *Continued*

History and Present Status of the Back/Neck Problem

Patient's name _____ Date _____

CHIEF COMPLAINT (Major items only) _____

_____

_____

ONSET: Time—sudden or gradual—Date and time of day _____

*Cause—injury, sickness, etc. _____

_____

†Immediate symptoms _____

_____

_____

_____

COURSE: Detailed chronologic study of symptoms and medical care and reaction to each procedure

_____

_____

_____

_____

_____

_____

_____

_____

_____

_____

PAST RELEVANT HISTORY: Previous and recent attacks, etc. _____

_____

_____	Pain	1	2	3	4
_____	Function	1	2	3	4
_____	Occupation	1	2	3	4

PROGRESS: Better, worse, stationary _____

Relation to Activity

Lying down—position of greatest comfort: _____

Does rest or activity relieve? _____

Awakened often and why? _____

Sitting—one side, or shifts _____ How most comfortable? _____

Getting up from sitting—need assist? _____ Hard or soft _____ Driving _____

Standing—one side or shifts _____ Time, and what happens? _____

Walking—distance _____ What happens? _____

Stairs, inclines, irregular ground _____

Bending—degree _____ Pain and assist returning to erect position _____

Lifting: Wt. _____ lbs. _____ Fatigue _____

Working _____ Type _____ Date discontinued _____ Returned _____

Effect of manipulation _____ Support: type and effect _____

Effect of exercise _____

*Describe carefully just how forces of the accident affected the patient, how he or she was thrown, fell, landed: twists to back or limbs. Just mechanical factors. (Don't include extraneous material, such as who was to blame.)
†How patient felt immediately: unconscious—how long, ache, severe pain, gradual increase, inability to walk or use certain joints, numbness, and/or paralysis.

FIG. 13-11, cont'd   Patient history and examination forms. *(From Watkins RG:* The spine in sports, *St Louis, 1996, Mosby.)*

Continued

History and Present Status of the Back/Neck Problem—cont'd

Neurologic Effects

Ratio of neck/arm pain: _____ / _____

Radiation of pain: Where? _____ When? _____

Effects of coughing, sneezing, and straining during bowel movements: On back, where? _____

On referred pain, how far? _____

Areas of skin tingling, numbness, coldness _____ Muscle weakness? _____

Chronic Inflammatory Factors

Stiffness after rest: Getting out of bed _____ After sitting _____

Effect of change of weather _____ Cold, damp weather _____ Hot _____

Effect of heat to part _____ Type of heat _____

(Women) Relation to menstrual periods _____

Remarks: _____

Physical Examination

Review of Systems
HEENT

Chest
Cardiovascular
Abdomen
Rectal
Fundi
Prostate

Pulses	Right	Left
Femoral		
Popliteal		
Pedal		
Bruits		

Back and Lower Extremity Examination

Range of motion	Right	Left
Flexion		
Extension		
Left lateral flexion		
Right lateral flexion		

Muscle strength	Right	Left
Hip abduction		
Hip adduction		
Hip flexion		
Hip extension		
Knee flexion		
Knee extension		
Ankle dorsiflexion		
Ankle plantar flexion		
Ankle inversion		
Ankle eversion		

FIG. 13-11, cont'd   Patient history and examination forms.   *Continued*

Physical Examination—cont'd

Muscle strength—cont'd	Right	Left
Toes dorsiflexion		
Toes plantar flexion		
Big toe dorsiflexion		

Reflex grades	Right	Left
Patella		
Achilles		
Posterior tibia		

Pain radiation	Right	Left
Thighs		
Calves		
Feet		
Foot top		
Foot bottom		
Heel		
Big toe		
Little toe		

Sensory function	Right	Left
Light touch		
Pinprick		
Vibratory		

Tests	Right	Left
Leg lengths		
Thighs		
Calves		
Muscle spasm		
Convexity scoliosis		
Kyphosis		
Lordosis		

Tests	Right	Left
Babinski		
Clonus		
Laségue		
Flip		
Bowstring		
Cram		
Foot dorsiflexion		
Neck flexion		
Faber		
Hip range of motion		
Femoral stretch		

Point tenderness

Thoracic spine
L1
L2
L3
L4
L5
S1
S2 to S5
Coccyx
Anterior spine

FIG. 13-11, cont'd   Patient history and examination forms. *(From Watkins RG:* The spine in sports, *St Louis, 1996, Mosby.)*   *Continued*

Physical Examination—cont'd

Point tenderness—cont'd	Right	Left

Sacroiliac joint
Sciatic notch
Greater trochanter
Ischial tuberosity
Paraspinous

Straight leg raising	Right	Left

Supine—leg pain
Sitting—leg pain
Contralateral—leg pain
Sitting—low back pain
Contralateral—low back pain

Neck and Upper Extremity Examination

Muscle strength	Right	Left

Trapezius
Cuff
Deltoid
Rhomboid
Serrant
Pectoralis
Biceps
Triceps
Forearm supination
Forearm pronation
Wrist extension
Wrist flexion
Thumb
Grip
Intrinsics

Sensory function

Light touch
Pinprick
Vibratory

PERRLA

Gag
Tongue
Smile
Hearing
Sight
Thyroid
Neck mass
Bruits:
   Carotids
   Subclavicular
   Axillary
Torticollis

Range of motion	Right	Left

Flexion
Extension
Left flexion
Right flexion
Left rotation
Right rotation

FIG. 13-11, cont'd   Patient history and examination forms.

TABLE 13-4

NONORGANIC PHYSICAL SIGNS INDICATING ILLNESS BEHAVIOR

	Physical Disease/Normal Illness Behavior	Abnormal Illness Behavior
Symptoms		
Pain	Anatomic distribution	Whole leg pain
		Tailbone pain
Numbness	Dermatomal	Whole leg numbness
Weakness	Myotomal	Whole leg giving way
Time pattern	Varies with time and activity	Never free of pain
Response to treatment	Variable benefit	Intolerance of treatments
		Emergency admissions to hospital
Signs		
Tenderness	Anatomic distribution	Superficial
		Widespread nonanatomic
Axial loading	No lumbar pain	Lumbar pain
Simulated rotation	No lumbar pain	Lumbar pain
Straight leg raising	Limited on distraction	Improves with distraction
Sensory	Dermatomal	Regional
Motor	Myotomal	Regional, jerky, giving way

From Waddell G, et al: Symptoms & signs: physical disease or illness behavior? *Br Med J* 289:739, 1984, British Medical Association.

North American Spine Society Back Pain Questionnaire-Baseline Medical History, Expectations and Outcomes*

1. HOW LONG AGO did your *current* episode begine?
   - 1 Less than 2 weeks ago
   - 2 2 weeks to less than 8 weeks ago
   - 3 8 weeks to less than 3 months ago
   - 4 3 months to less than 6 months ago
   - 5 6 to 12 months ago
   - 6 More than 12 months ago

2. HOW did your *current* episode begin?
   - 0 Suddenly
   - 1 Gradually

3. Have you had back symptoms before your current episode?
   - 0 No (IF NO, GO TO QUESTION 6)
   - 1 Yes, one episode
   - 2 Yes, two or more episodes

   Answer #4–5 about your PAST back symptoms.

   ---
   4. Did you receive Worker's Compensation for your PAST back symptoms?
      - 1 No   0 Yes
   5. How much work did you miss because of your worst prior episode?
      - 0 None
      - 1 1 day to 2 weeks
      - 2 More than 2 weeks to 4 weeks
      - 3 More than 4 weeks to 12 weeks
      - 4 More than 12 weeks to 24 weeks
      - 5 More than 24 weeks
   ---

6. Have you had previous back surgery?
   - 0 No (If NO, go to question 9)
   - 1 Yes: How many surgeries? #_____

FIG. 13-12 North American Spine Society Back Pain Questionnaire–Baseline Medical History, Expectations and Outcomes. *(North American Spine Society, 1993.)*   *Continued*

7. After your most recent surgery, did you return to work?
   0 No
   1 Yes, with limitations
   2 Yes, with no limitations
   3 Never stopped working
   4 Did not work: _____ Homemaker
                    _____ Student
                    _____ Retired
                    _____ Other

8. After your most recent surgery, did you return to full function?
   0 No   1 Yes

There will be several questions about leg and back pain in this questionnaire. When we say LEG, we mean your thigh, calf, ankle, and foot. When we say BACK, we mean your low back and buttocks.

9. Which hurts you more, your legs or back?
   1 Legs hurt much more
   2 Legs hurt somewhat more
   3 Legs and back hurt about the same
   4 Back hurts somewhat more
   5 Back hurts much more

Please answer every question in the box below.

In the PAST WEEK, how often have you suffered:	None of the time	A little of the time	Some of the time	A good bit of the time	Most of the time	All the time
10. low back and/or buttock pain	1	2	3	4	5	6
11. leg pain	1	2	3	4	5	6
12. numbness or tingling in leg and/or foot	1	2	3	4	5	6
13. weakness in leg and/or foot (such as difficulty lifting foot)	1	2	3	4	5	6

Please answer every question in the box below.

In the PAST WEEK, how bothersome have these symptoms been?	Not at all bothersome	Slightly bothersome	Somewhat bothersome	Moderately bothersome	Very bothersome	Extremely bothersome
14. low back and/or buttock pain	1	2	3	4	5	6
15. leg pain	1	2	3	4	5	6
16. numbness/tingling in leg and/or foot	1	2	3	4	5	6
17. weakness in leg and/or foot (such as difficulty lifting foot)	1	2	3	4	5	6

FIG. 13-12, cont'd   North American Spine Society Back Pain Questionnaire–Baseline Medical History, Expectations and Outcomes.

Continued

In the LAST WEEK, please tell us HOW PAIN HAS AFFECTED YOUR ABILITY TO PERFORM the following daily activities. Mark the ONE statement that best describes your average ability.

18. Getting Dressed (in the LAST WEEK)
    1   I can dress myself without pain.
    2   I can dress myself without increasing pain.
    3   I can dress myself but pain increases.
    4   I can dress myself but with significant pain.
    5   I can dress myself but with very severe pain.
    6   I cannot dress myself.

19. Lifting (in the LAST WEEK)
    1   I can lift heavy objects without pain.
    2   I can lift heavy objects but it is painful.
    3   Pain prevents me from lifting heavy objects off the floor but I can manage if they are on a table.
    4   Pain prevents me from lifting heavy objects but I can manage light to medium objects if they are on a table.
    5   I can lift only light objects.
    6   I cannot lift anything.

20. Walking (in the LAST WEEK)
    1   Pain does not prevent me from walking.
    2   Pain prevents me from walking more than 1 hour.
    3   Pain prevents me from walking more than 30 minutes.
    4   Pain prevents me from walking more than 10 minutes.
    5   I can only walk a few steps at a time.
    6   I am unable to walk.

21. Sitting (in the LAST WEEK)
    1   I can sit in any chair as long as I like.
    2   I can only sit in a special chair for as long as I like.
    3   Pain prevents me from sitting more than 1 hour.
    4   Pain prevents me from sitting more than 30 minutes.
    5   Pain prevents me from sitting more than a few minutes.
    6   Pain prevents me from sitting at all.

22. Standing (in the LAST WEEK)
    1   I can stand as long as I want.
    2   I can stand as long as I want but it gives me pain.
    3   Pain prevents me from standing for more than 1 hour.
    4   Pain prevents me from standing for more than 30 minutes.
    5   Pain prevents me from standing for more than 10 minutes.
    6   Pain prevents me from standing at all.

23. Sleeping (in the LAST WEEK)
    1   I sleep well.
    2   Pain occasionally interrupts my sleep.
    3   Pain interrupts my sleep half of the time.
    4   Pain often interrupts my sleep.
    5   Pain always interrupts my sleep.
    6   I never sleep well.

24. Social and Recreational Life (in the LAST WEEK)
    1   My social and recreational life is unchanged.
    2   My social and recreational life is unchanged but it increases pain.
    3   My social and recreational life is unchanged but it severely increases pain.
    4   Pain has restricted my social and recreational life.

FIG. 13-12, cont'd   North American Spine Society Back Pain Questionnaire–Baseline Medical History, Expectations and Outcomes. *(From White AH, Schofferman JA:* Spine care, *vol 1-2, St Louis, 1995, Mosby.)*

Continued

North American Spine Society Back Pain Questionnaire-Baseline Medical History, Expectations and Outcomes—cont'd

     5 Pain has severely restricted my social and recreational life.

     6 I have essentially no social and recreational life because of pain.

26. Traveling (in the LAST WEEK)

     1 I can travel anywhere.

     2. I can travel anywhere but it gives me pain.

     3 Pain is bad but I can manage to travel over 2 hours.

     4 Pain restricts me to trips of less than 1 hour.

     5 Pain restricts me to trips of less than 30 minutes.

     6 Pain prevents me from traveling.

26. Sex Life (in the LAST WEEK)

     1 My sex life is unchanged.

     2 My sex life is unchanged but causes some extra pain.

     3 My sex life is nearly unchanged but is very painful.

     4 My sex life is severely restricted by pain.

     5 My sex life is nearly absent because of pain.

     6 Pain prevents any sex life at all.

Please answer every question in the box below.

HOW OFTEN do you need to use the following assistive devices?	Never	Sometimes	About half the time	Often	All the time
27. One or two canes	1	2	3	4	5
28. One or two crutches	1	2	3	4	5
29. Walker	1	2	3	4	5
30. Wheelchair	1	2	3	4	5

31. Which health care providers have you used for your current back condition? (CIRCLE ALL THAT APPLY)

    A Acupuncturist   I Osteopath

    B Chiropractor   J Orthopaedic Surgeon

    C Emergency room   K Pain Clinic

    D General practitioner   L Physical Therapist

    E Immediate care clinic   M Rheumatologist

    F Internist   N Work Hardening Clinic

    G Massage Therapist   O Other: _____

    H Neurosurgeon   P None of the above

32. During the LAST WEEK, how often have you taken narcotic medication such as codeine, Demerol, Percodan, or Vicodin for your back and/or leg pain?

     1 3 or more times a day   4 Once a week

     2 Once or twice a day   5 Not at all

     3 Once every couple of days

33. During the LAST WEEK, how often have you taken non-narcotic medication such as aspirin, Motrin, or Tylenol for your back and/or leg pain?

     1 3 or more times a day   4 Once a week

     2 Once or twice a day   5 Not at all

     3 Once every couple of days

FIG. 13-12, cont'd North American Spine Society Back Pain Questionnaire–Baseline Medical History, Expectations and Outcomes.   *Continued*

34. Have you used alcoholic beverages (beer, wine, liquor) to relieve your current back or leg pain?
    0 No
    1 Yes, once in a while
    2 Yes, often

35. If you had to spend the rest of your life with your *back condition as it is right now*, how would you feel about it?
    1 Extremely dissatisfied
    2 Very dissatisfied
    3 Somewhat dissatisfied
    4 Neutral
    5 Somewhat satisfied
    6 Very satisfied
    7 Extremely satisfied

What expectations do you have for your treatment at this office?

As a result of my treatment, I expect	not likely	slightly likely	somewhat likely	very likely	extremely likely
36. Complete pain relief	1	2	3	4	5
37. Moderate pain relief	1	2	3	4	5
38. To be able to do more everyday household or yard activities	1	2	3	4	5
39. To be able to sleep more comfortably	1	2	3	4	5
40. To be able to go back to my usual job	1	2	3	4	5
41. To be able to do more sports, go biking, or go for long walks	1	2	3	4	5

42. What other results do you expect from your treatment? Please describe:

_____

_____

_____

How important are the following treatment outcomes for you?

How important is...	not important	slightly important	somewhat important	very important	extremely important
43. Pain relief	1	2	3	4	5
44. To be able to do more everyday household or yard activities	1	2	3	4	5
45. To be able to sleep more comfortably	1	2	3	4	5
46. To be able to go back to my usual job	1	2	3	4	5
47. To be able to do more sports, go biking, or go for long walks	1	2	3	4	5
48. Other (see your answer to #42 above): _____	1	2	3	4	5

FIG. 13-12, cont'd   North American Spine Society Back Pain Questionnaire–Baseline Medical History, Expectations and Outcomes.   *Continued*

North American Spine Society Back Pain Questionnaire-Baseline Medical History, Expectations and Outcomes—cont'd

Following are some questions about your general health.

49. In general would you say your health is:
    1 Excellent
    2 Very Good
    3 Good
    4 Fair
    5 Poor
    6 Terrible

50. Have you ever had any of the following conditions?
    (CIRCLE ALL THAT APPLY)

    A Diabetes   F Depression
    B Heart Disease   G High Blood Pressure (hypertension)
    C Stroke   H Colitis
    D Arthritis other than in your back   I Psoriasis
    E Asthma or other lung disease   J None of the above

51. Do you currently smoke cigarettes?
    0 I have never smoked
    1 Yes
    2 No, I quit in the last 6 months
    3 No, I quit more than 6 months ago

52. Has the treatment for your back condition met your expectations so far?
    1 Yes, totally
    2 Yes, almost totally
    3 Yes, quite a bit
    4 More or less
    5 No, not quite
    6 No, far from it
    7 No, not at all

53. Would you have the same treatment again if you had the same condition?
    1 Definitely not
    2 Probably not
    3 Not sure
    4 Probably yes
    5 Definitely yes

54. If you had back pain, how has your back pain been affected by the treatment?
    (CHECK ONLY ONE STATEMENT)
    1 I did not have back pain to start with.
    2 The pain is totally gone.
    3 The pain is much better than before treatment.
    4 The pain is somewhat better than before treatment.
    5 The pain is about the same as before treatment.
    6 The pain is somewhat worse than before treatment.
    7 The pain is much worse than before treatment.

55. If you had leg pain, how has your leg pain been affected by the treatment?
    (CHECK ONLY ONE STATEMENT)
    1 I did not have leg pain to start with.
    2 The pain is totally gone.
    3 The pain is much better than before treatment.
    4 The pain is somewhat better than before treatment.

FIG. 13-12, cont'd   North American Spine Society Back Pain Questionnaire–Baseline Medical History, Expectations and Outcomes.   *Continued*

5 The pain is about the same as before treatment.

6 The pain is somewhat worse than before treatment.

7 The pain is much worse than before treatment.

The following questions are about how you feel and how things have been with you during the last week. For each question, please indicate the one answer that comes closest to the way you have been feeling. Please, CIRCLE ONE ANSWER ON EACH LINE.

How much of the time during the LAST WEEK	All of the time	Most of the time	A good bit of the time	Some of the time	Little of the time	None of the time
56. Have you been a very nervous person?	1	2	3	4	5	6
57. Have you felt so down in the dumps nothing could cheer you up?	1	2	3	4	5	6
58. Have you felt calm and peaceful?	1	2	3	4	5	6
59. Have you felt downhearted and blue?	1	2	3	4	5	6
60. Have you been a happy person?	1	2	3	4	5	6

North American Spine Society Back Pain Questionnaire-Baseline Medical Employment History, and Work Status.*

1. How many jobs have you had in the last 3 years?

    0 None

    1 1 or 2

    2 3 or more

2. Which statements describe your current employment situation? *CIRCLE ALL THAT APPLY*

    A Currently working

    B On paid leave

    C On unpaid leave

    D Unemployed

    E Homemaker

    F Student

    G Retired (not due to health)

    H Disabled and/or retired because of my back problems

    I Disabled due to a health problem not related to my back

    J Other, please specify: _____

3. Are you self-employed?

    0 No   1 Yes

4. If NOT WORKING now, how long has it been since you stopped?

    1 Less than 1 week ago

    2 1 week to less than 3 months ago

    3 3 months to less than 6 months ago

    4 6 months to less than 12 months ago

    5 1 to 2 years ago

    6 More than 2 years ago

    8 Currently working

    9 Never employed

FIG. 13-12, cont'd   North American Spine Society Back Pain Questionnaire–Baseline Medical History, Expectations and Outcomes. *Continued*

North American Spine Society Back Pain Questionnaire-Baseline Medical Employment History, and Work Status—cont'd

5. What is your primary occupation? If you are not working now, what was your primary occupation? (Please be as specific as possible)

   Occupation: _____

6. Is your current job the same one you had when your current back symptoms started?

   1 Yes, exact same job

   2 Yes, but job was modified or hours reduced because of my back

   3 No, I have changed jobs because of my back symptoms

   4 No, I have changed jobs but for reasons unrelated to my back

   5 Not working now

7. How long have you worked at your current job?

   0 less than 6 months

   1 6 to 12 months

   2 more than 12 months

   3 not working now

Please answer each of the following questions about your current job (or the one you plan to go back to if on leave).
CIRCLE ONE ANSWER ON EACH LINE.

	All of the time	Most of the time	A good bit of the time	Some of the time	Little of the time	None of the time
8. How much sitting does your work involve?	1	2	3	4	5	6
9. How much standing or walking does your work involve?	1	2	3	4	5	6
10. How often do you lift 25 lbs. on the job?	1	2	3	4	5	6
11. How often do you lift 50 lbs. on the job?	1	2	3	4	5	6

Please answer each of the following questions about your current job (or the one you plan to go back to if on leave):

	Extremely	Very much	Quite a bit	Somewhat	A little	Not at all
12. Is your current work physically demanding?	1	2	3	4	5	6
13. Is your work stressful to you?	1	2	3	4	5	6
14. How much do you like your job?	1	2	3	4	5	6
15. How much do you like your co-workers?	1	2	3	4	5	6
16. How much do you like your supervisor?	1	2	3	4	5	6

FIG. 13-12, cont'd   North American Spine Society Back Pain Questionnaire–Baseline Medical History, Expectations and Outcomes.

Continued

North American Spine Society Back Pain Questionnaire-Baseline Medical Employment History, and Work Status—cont'd

17. Other than your salary, what other sources of income does your household receive?
CIRCLE ALL THAT APPLY:

A Another person's salary

B State Support

C Social Security

D Disability

E Other (Investments, Retirement Plan, etc.)

F No other source of income

18. Are you experiencing financial difficulties because of your back condition?

0 None at all

1 Only a little

2 Some

3 A lot

Please answer the questions in the box, or check below if none applies.

Are you on or planning to apply for any of the following programs?	Already on it	Applied for it	Planning to apply for it
19. Social Security	1	2	3
20. Disability	1	2	3
21. Workers Compensation	1	2	3
22. Other (please specify): _____	1	2	3

☐ Check here if none of the above applies.

23. Do you think the fault for your current back condition is: (CIRCLE ALL THAT APPLY)

A Yours?

B Your employer's?

C A co-worker's?

D Another person's?

E Nobody's?

24. Have you hired a lawyer because of your back condition?

0 No, I have not hired a lawyer.

1 Yes, I have and the case is in litigation.

2 Yes, I have and the case has been settled.

Thank you for your help. Please take a moment to go over the questionnaire to make sure you have not missed any pages or questions. Then return it to the person who gave it to you or in the envelope provided.

FIG. 13-12, cont'd   North American Spine Society Back Pain Questionnaire–Baseline Medical History, Expectations and Outcomes.

Psychogenic rheumatism is a term used to describe patients who have musculoskeletal psychiatric disorders. An example of psychogenic rheumatism that is associated with back pain is camptocormia, which is a special form of conversion hysteria that occurs mainly in military service personnel and industrial workers. The disease is characterized by the patient's assumption of a posture in which the back is flexed acutely, the arms hang loosely, and the patient's eyes are directed downward. The posture disappears when the patient assumes a recumbent position. The

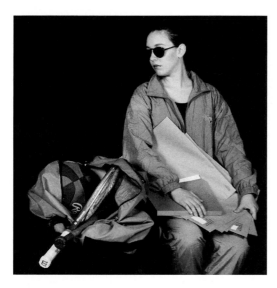

FIG. 13-13   When observing a malingering patient, the examiner will note the following: (1) The patient will fail to make consistent eye contact and may obscure eye contact with sunglasses; (2) the patient may be dressed in clothing that indicates athletic involvement, which is inappropriate for an injury of a supposedly disabled patient; (3) the patient usually carries a voluminous medical file and an aggregation of radiographs from doctor to doctor; (4) the patient may be impatient; (5) the patient may be unwilling to participate in a full examination, not wanting to risk exposure of the feigned illness. Other subtle signs to watch for are appointments—such as a tennis match immediately after the examination of the disabled lower back—that are inappropriate for the disability.

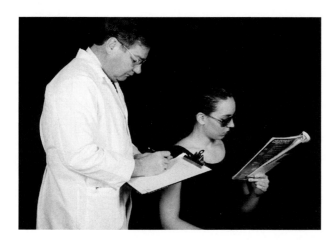

FIG. 13-14   A detailed history from a malingering patient is difficult to acquire and assess. The patient may relate queer and exaggerated stories of the injurious event, or the patient may act disinterested and distant in the history interview. The patient avoids eye contact.

short-form McGill Pain Questionnaire, a pain scale, and pain drawings represent a few of the many methods to document psychogenic rheumatism (Figs. 13-15 to 13-17).

Many of the afflicted individuals are males whose parents have had back disorders. Therapy for the condition involves separation of the individual from the source of stress.

ORTHOPEDIC GAMUT 13-4

PSYCHOGENIC RHEUMATISM

Symptoms and signs of psychogenic rheumatism include the following*:

1. Dramatic urgency for an appointment that is not justified by the severity of the disease
2. A list (in writing) of complaints so long and detailed that no fact is left out
3. Multiple test results, including electrocardiogram (ECG), electromyelogram (EMG), electroencephalogram (EEG), barium enema, upper gastrointestinal (GI) series, computed tomography (CT) scans, myelograms, and magnetic resonance imaging (MRI), with no positive findings
4. Patient demands to review the laboratory data first to determine the cause of the symptoms; patient highlights any minor abnormalities
5. Preoccupation with future disability from minor physical changes
6. Those who accompany the patient may be entirely separated from the patient's condition or intensely supportive; the companion may be highlighting every abnormality, often using the pronoun *we* during the description of tests or treatments
7. Inability of the patient to relax during the examination (Boxes 13-3 and 13-4)
8. Marked theatrical responses to questions concerning pain
9. The patient often holds onto the physician during the examination, as a gesture of seeking support

*From Rotes-Querol J: The syndrome of psychogenic rheumatism, *Clin Rheum Dis* 5:797, 1979.

The malingerer exaggerates or fakes a condition or injury. It is important to believe the history the patient relates even though malingering is suspected.

In many instances, a malingerer can be extremely convincing during the examination. The malingering patient usually complains of sensory loss, paralysis, pain, or a combination of these symptoms. A hysterical patient will claim similar problems. Unlike the hysterical patient, the malingerer consciously attempts to deceive the doctor.

Two separate sets of criteria have been developed to document the likelihood of malingering: the Emory Pain Control Center inconsistency profile and Ellard's profile of inconsistency.

ORTHOPEDIC GAMUT 13-5

EMORY AND ELLARD INCONSISTENCY PROFILES

Combined Emory and Ellard inconsistency profiles are as follows*:

1. Discrepancies become apparent between a patient's complaints of terrible pain and an attitude of calmness and well-being.

2. A complete workup for organic disease by two or more physicians is negative.

3. The patient makes dramatized complaints that are vague or have global implications. "It just hurts," or "I hurt bad." This may be further attested by malingering hand signals.

4. The patient exaggerates a trivial pathologic condition (e.g., a mild strain, muscular cramp, contusion) and embellishes it with medical terms learned from previous contact with physicians. "My back spasms paralyze my legs."

5. The patient overemphasizes gait or posture abnormalities that develop suddenly, persist, and cannot be substantiated objectively. For example, the patient complains of a limp that is not confirmed by a specific pattern of wear on old shoes. Or the patient reports daily use of a cane or back brace, but these items show little wear.

6. The patient resists evaluation or rehabilitation when the stated goal of therapy is a return to gainful employment.

7. The patient exhibits a lack of motivation to learn new coping skills, despite verbal reports of compliance with treatment. (For instance, the patient will show no increase in back motion despite claims of completing range-of-motion exercise daily.)

8. The patient misses appointments for objective studies that measure function, motion, or vocational capabilities.

9. The patient has an unconventional response to treatment, such as reports of increased symptoms following therapy that follows no anatomic or physiologic pattern. For example, the patient may respond to tranquilizers as if they are stimulants and vice versa.

10. The patient shows resistance to treatment procedures, especially in the presence of intense complaints of pain.

11. Psychologic or emotional disturbances are absent (Box 13-5).

12. Psychologic tests are inconsistent and without clinical presentations. For example, the Minnesota Multiphasic Personality Index (MMPI) profile indicates a psychotic disorder, but no clinical signs of psychosis are present (Box 13-6).

13. Discrepancies arise between reports by the patient and spouse or other close relatives.

14. Personal and occupational history appears unstable.

15. The patient's personal history reflects a character disorder that might include drug or alcohol abuse, criminal or compulsive behavior, erratic personal relationships, and violence.

*From Evans RC: Malingering/symptoms exaggeration. In Sweere JJ, editor: *Chiropractic family practice,* Gaithersburg, Md, 1992, Aspen.

BOX 13-3

Clinical Symptoms of Anxiety

Motor tension
1. Trembling, twitching, or feeling shaky
2. Muscle tension, aches, or soreness
3. Restlessness
4. Easy fatigability

Autonomic hyperactivity
5. Shortness of breath or smothering sensation
6. Palpitations or accelerated heart rate
7. Sweating, or cold clammy hands
8. Dry mouth
9. Dizziness or light-headedness
10. Nausea, diarrhea, or other abdominal distress
11. Flushes (hot flashes) or chills
12. Frequent urination
13. Trouble swallowing or "lump in throat"

Vigilance and scanning
14. Feeling keyed up or on edge
15. Exaggerated startle response
16. Difficulty concentrating or "mind going blank" because of anxiety
17. Trouble falling or staying asleep
18. Irritability

From White AH, Schofferman JA: *Spine care,* vol 1-2, St Louis, 1995, Mosby.

SHORT-FORM McGILL PAIN QUESTIONNAIRE

Please tick which of these words describes your pain. Put the tick in the box which gives the intensity of that particular quality of your pain.

	None	Mild	Moderate	Severe
Throbbing	0) ____	1) ____	2) ____	3) ____
Shooting	0) ____	1) ____	2) ____	3) ____
Stabbing	0) ____	1) ____	2) ____	3) ____
Sharp	0) ____	1) ____	2) ____	3) ____
Cramping	0) ____	1) ____	2) ____	3) ____
Gnawing	0) ____	1) ____	2) ____	3) ____
Hot-burning	0) ____	1) ____	2) ____	3) ____
Aching	0) ____	1) ____	2) ____	3) ____
Heavy	0) ____	1) ____	2) ____	3) ____
Tender	0) ____	1) ____	2) ____	3) ____
Splitting	0) ____	1) ____	2) ____	3) ____
Tiring-exhausting	0) ____	1) ____	2) ____	3) ____
Sickening	0) ____	1) ____	2) ____	3) ____
Fearful	0) ____	1) ____	2) ____	3) ____
Punishing-cruel	0) ____	1) ____	2) ____	3) ____

Please put a mark on the scale to show how bad your *usual pain* has been *these days.*

No
pain _____ Worst
possible
pain

How bad is your pain now?

0	No pain	____
1	Mild	____
2	Discomforting	____
3	Distressing	____
4	Horrible	____
5	Excruciating	____

FIG. 13-15   The short-form McGill Pain Questionnaire. *(From Melzack R: Pain 30:191, 1987, Elsevier Science.)*

BOX 13-4

DSM-III-R Criterion for Anxiety

300.02 Generalized Anxiety Disorder—Unrealistic or excessive anxiety and worry more days than not.

Other anxiety disorders
Panic disorder
300.21 with Agoraphobia or
300.01 without Agoraphobia

300.22 Agoraphobia without history of panic disorder
300.23 Social phobia

300.29 Obsessive compulsive disorder
300.89 Posttraumatic stress disorder
300.00 Anxiety disorder Not Otherwise Specified (NOS)

From White AH, Schofferman JA: *Spine care,* vol 1-2, St Louis, 1995, Mosby.

BOX 13-5

Mood Disorders—DSM-III-R Classifications

Bipolar Disorders
296.6x Mixed—both manic and depressed features
296.4x Manic
296.5x Depressed
301.13 Cyclothymia
296.70 Bipolar disorder Not Otherwise Specified (NOS)

Depressive Disorders
Major Depression
296.6x Single episode
296.3x Recurrent

300.40 Dysthymia
311.00 Depressive disorder Not Otherwise Specified (NOS)

Fifth digit x allows coding of current state of disorder: 1 = mild; 2 = moderate; 3 = severe, without psychotic features; 4 = with psychotic features; 5 = in partial remission; 6 = in full remission; 0 = unspecified

From White AH, Schofferman JA: *Spine care,* vol 1-2, St Louis, 1995, Mosby.

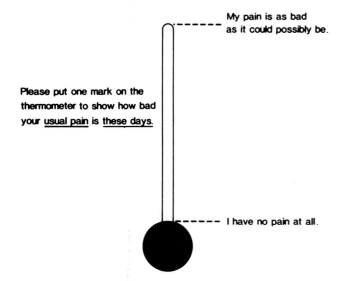

FIG. 13-16   The pain scale. The scale should be exactly 100 mm long, and the level marked by the patient is scored as a percentage. *(From Pope MH, et al:* Occupational low back pain assessment, treatment and prevention, *St Louis, 1991, Mosby.)*

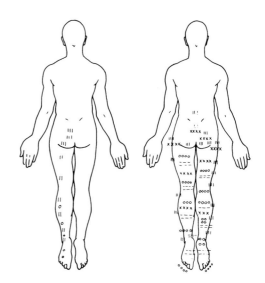

FIG. 13-17   The pain drawing provides information about the physical and emotional aspects of the patient's pain. *(From Pope MH, et al:* Occupational low back pain assessment, treatment and prevention, *St Louis, 1991, Mosby.)*

Description of MMPI-2

L, F, and K are validity scales.

L is called the Lie scale and measures willingness to admit minor social faults. It gives information about social conformity, self-image and self-insight, and denial.

F refers to infrequency and consists of items that are socially unacceptable or have disturbing content. Persons scoring on the low end of this scale are usually conventional and unassuming. Those with elevations are admitting to severe emotional distress and/or psychopathology. Very high scores suggest an invalid profile.

K refers to correction, and the items measure personal resources required to cope with life. Low scores suggest exaggeration of problems or severe emotional distress. Higher scores can result when patients are very confident and in charge or when they are being defensive in their efforts to present themselves as adequate and in control; when in fact their lives are in disarray.

Scales 1 through 10 are the basic clinical scales of the MMPI-2. The information is presented using T scores. A T score of 50 is average; T scores over 65 are in the abnormal range.

Scale 1 is also referred to as the "Hypochondriasis (HS)" scale. This scale consists of items that concern bodily functioning. Many of the items are vague in their content. Persons scoring low on this scale do not have or are denying that they have any physical complaints. Those whose scores are elevated have many physical complaints and concerns. If scores are above 65 physical complaints are often the major focus of the person's life.

Scale 2 is referred to as the "Depression (D)" scale. It consists of items that measure subjective depression, psychomotor slowing and immobilization, physical complaints, mental dullness, and brooding. High scores indicate the presence of depression and low scores indicate those whose affective functioning is within normal limits.

Scale 3 is referred to as "Hysteria (Hy)." It consists of items that indicate whether the individual tends to avoid emotional and social unpleasantness. Those that do may then experience their emotions and stress as somatic complaints. High scorers will often deny psychologic problems and look for concrete solutions to their problems.

Scale 4 is referred to as "Psychopathic Deviate (Pd)." While eight items refer to authority conflicts, the rest of the items deal with family conflicts, denial of social and dependency needs, social alienation, and self-integration. High scorers are often angry, impulsive, in conflict with authority figures in their lives, and are feeling isolated and despondent. High scorers who are not psychopathic are often undergoing stressful transitions in their lives.

Scale 5 is referred to as "Masculinity-Femininity (Mf)." Scores on this reflect traditional versus non-traditional masculine or feminine interests and beliefs, conflicts about sexuality, and interests in aesthetics. Low scores for women suggest feelings of helplessness and dependency, while low scores for men suggest an action-oriented "macho" approach to life. High-scoring males often hold interests in activities usually thought of as feminine and may be experiencing insecurity, helplessness, and conflicts of sexuality. High-scoring females report interest in traditional male patterns, and are often seen as unfriendly, dominating, and aggressive.

Scale 6 is referred to as "Paranoia (Pa)." In addition to paranoia and externalization of blame, this scale contains items related to hypersensitivity, subjectivity, naivete, righteousness, and denial of hostility and distrust. Very high scorers are outright paranoid and may have a thought disorder, while low scorers may be insensitive to others and unaware of other's motives. They may also be denying the presence of paranoid thoughts.

Scale 7 is referred to as "Psychasthenia (Pt)." Items center around the presence of worries, brooding, and rumination. High scorers are seen as anxious and insecure, and may be indecisive. If scores are very high the individual may be compulsive and agitated with feelings of guilt and fear disrupting everyday functioning.

Scale 8 is referred to as "Schizophrenia (Sc)." High scorers are having difficulty with their thinking and feelings. They often feel out of control and unable to take positive action in their own behalf. Extremely high scores are suggestive of severe situational stress. More moderate elevations are seen in those with thought disorders with difficulties in logic concentration, and judgment common.

Scale 9 is referred to as "Hypomania (Ma)." This scale provides information about motivation, physical and emotional activity levels, confidence in social situations, and feelings of self-importance. High scorers are restless, agitated, emotionally labile, and may have racing thoughts. They may also have difficulty delaying gratification and can be impulsive. Manic features appear as scores elevate.

Scale 10 is referred to as "Social Introversion (Si)." This scale provides information about social interests, interpersonal skills, self-consciousness, and feelings of alienation from self or others. High scorers are often depressed. They withdraw from social interactions and feel shy and insecure. Low scorers are usually socially extroverted and outgoing.

From White AH, Schofferman JA: *Spine care,* vol 1-2, St Louis, 1995, Mosby.

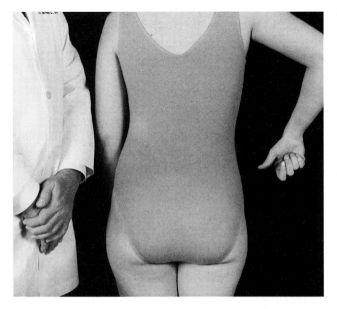

FIG. 13-18   At first, the malingering patient takes care not to touch the area of claimed pain. The complaint is a sham, so the patient allows the examiner to touch the part first. Then the patient simply agrees with the suggested origin of pain.

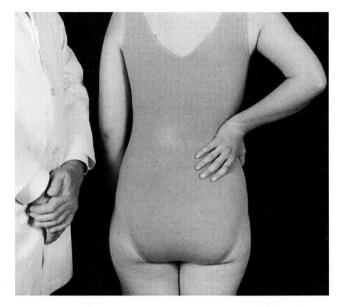

FIG. 13-19   The hysteric patient, or the patient with psychogenic rheumatism, paints the area of complaint with the whole hand. The discomfort is real, but the borders of the complaint exceed the known anatomic distributions. Careful investigation will define the focal triggers.

Special Hand Signals by the Patient

How a patient uses the hands to describe the area of pain is useful in determining the validity of the complaints. At first, malingering patients take care not to touch the area they claim experiences pain. Because the complaint is a sham, touching of the part abets the lie. The examiner often inadvertently aids this process by physically touching the area of complaint before the patient has. The patient now only has to agree with the frustrated examiner concerning the exact location of the pain (Fig. 13-18).

The psychogenic rheumatic patient uses the whole hand to paint the area of involvement with pain. Because this type of patient perceives the lesion abnormally, the distribution is painted to cover a whole body part. This pain crosses more than one dermatome boundary, and this patient's discomfort is real. The discomfort may have origin in an organic lesion, but because of learned responses or fear, the patient rubs the whole part with the hand to indicate its extent. Careful questioning and guidance will help this patient better define the most focal trigger areas (Fig. 13-19).

Patients with organic, pain-producing lesions are concerned that the source of the pain might be missed. When directed to point to the pain, this type of patient will touch the part with one or two fingers, which is representative of a more focal appreciation of the discomfort. In severe expression of the symptoms, this patient also may place the

examiner's hand on the exact location of the pain. These patients do not want to risk having the source missed and not treated (Fig. 13-20).

PAIN QUALIFICATION AND QUANTIFICATION

Overview

Pain disrupts the life of the individual in terms of relationships with others, self-esteem, ability to complete tasks of daily living and to work, and ability to function as a member of the community. Disability is strongly correlated with attitude to illness: these considerations underlie the importance of assessing patients' beliefs regarding the nature and prognosis of their pain (Table 13-5).

Pain is an image that becomes perfected in the sensorium of the cerebral cortex. This pain image is created by stimuli that have passed through a chain of lower centers, in which they are modified and refined. Even at the cortical level, the pain image is subject to changes by associated constitutional and emotional factors. Stimuli coming from the same source and passing through the same modifications by the lower centers will produce in one patient a pain image of bright and burning colors and, in another, a faded out, unimpressive design. The patient's constitution is mirrored in this difference (Fig. 13-21).

TABLE 13-5

ACTIVITIES OF DAILY LIVING AND VISUAL ANALOG QUESTIONNAIRE

A. How often is it *painful* for you to:

	Never	Sometimes	Most of the Time	Always
Dress yourself?	_____	_____	_____	_____
Get in and out of bed?	_____	_____	_____	_____
Lift a cup or glass to your lips?	_____	_____	_____	_____
Walk outdoors on flat ground?	_____	_____	_____	_____
Wash and dry your entire body?	_____	_____	_____	_____
Bend down to pick up clothing from the floor?	_____	_____	_____	_____
Turn faucets on or off?	_____	_____	_____	_____
Get in and out of a car?	_____	_____	_____	_____

B. How much pain have you had in the *past week* (mark the scale):

No pain _____ Pain as bad as it could be

0   100

From Callahan LF, et al: Quantitative pain assessment for routine care of rheumatoid arthritis patients, using a pain scale on activities of daily living and a visual analog pain scale, *Arthritis Rheum* 30:630, 1987.

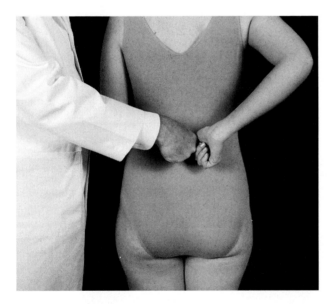

FIG. 13-20   Patients experiencing organic pain for the first time are concerned that the lesion will be missed. This patient will touch the part, precisely locating it with one or two fingers. The patient also may hold the examiner's finger on the spot of worst complaint.

In general, the closer to the axis of the body, the more scant is the distribution of sensory end organs in the tissues and the less precise the allocation of the pain source. There are some exceptions. Some deep-lying structures are intensely sensitive because of their rich endowment with pain-conducting terminal fibers, in contrast to other structures occupying the same anatomic plane. Sensory nerves are obvious exceptions to the rule because they are the conductors of pain.

ORTHOPEDIC GAMUT 13-6

RELAY STATIONS

Following are the three main relay stations for sensory stimuli wandering from the periphery to the sensory cortex:

1. The peripheral sensory nervous system, with its cell station in the spinal ganglia
2. The pathways and centers in the spinal cord and medulla
3. The sensory centers of the diencephalon, especially the thalamus

---

The differential diagnosis and evaluation of pain depend on a description of the intensity of the unpleasant sensation, a comparison by the patient to other known sensations, and an attempted designation of the severity of the pain based on a number system.

The spectrum of pain awareness and severity varies from a minimal pain response that is tolerated and easily overlooked to an unbearable sensation that interferes with the individual's productive activities.

There are physiologic variations of the pain threshold from one person to another. There is an inherent, definable difference in the pain level that varies from congenital insensitivity to pain to a state of hypersensitivity to almost any external stimulus.

Congenital insensitivity to pain is recognized as a true syndrome in which the person does not respond to epicritic stimuli, or even fractures of the extremities, by anything other than a descriptive comment concerning the injury. These patients do not complain of pain.

A high threshold of pain is recognized in many individuals who tolerate painful stimuli—such as heat, cold, sharp prick, or heavy pressure—and who recognize the abnormal sensation and the kind of sensation but are able to accept the stimulus with minimal response.

ORTHOPEDIC GAMUT 13-7

BORG-TYPE PAIN SCALE

The Borg-type pain scale consists of the following*:

*On a Scale of 1 to 10, Place an **X** at Your Current Pain Level.*

Normal	Low	Moderate	Intense	Emergency
( ) 0	( ) 1	( ) 4	( ) 7	( ) 10
( ) 2	( ) 5	( ) 8		
( ) 3	( ) 6	( ) 9		

Scoring: (0-3) Patients at this level may be able to return to work depending on many factors. (4-5) The transitional zone may indicate a significant degree of impairment for a non–symptom-magnifying patient or a low level of impairment for a patient who has a low pain threshold. (6-10) This level indicates a severe pathologic condition or symptom magnification behavior. Above (10) indicates symptom magnification.

---

*From Borg G: Psychophysical bases of perceived exertion, *Med Sci Sports Exerc* 14: 377, 1982.

A temporary, limited awareness of pain occurs immediately after certain severe injuries, such as a tear of major ligaments around the knee during a football game or a severe inversion injury to the ankle resulting in massive ligamentous tear. The individual experiences sudden, exquisite pain at the time of the injury and may become hypotensive, nauseated, and faint. During the recovery phase, the injured part may be manipulated with little or no discomfort in certain instances. However, within several minutes after injury, the pain pattern associated with periosteal injury, distended synovium and capsule, and pressure from hematoma becomes severe.

An average reaction to pain stimuli is the one that most individuals have to a sudden sharp point, to excessive heat, or to a severe rotary injury to a joint. The individual with an

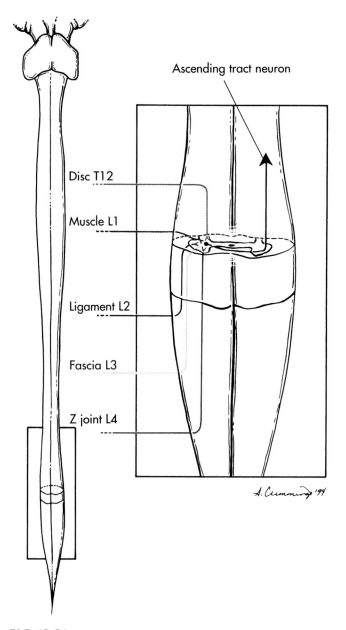

FIG. 13-21 Nociception from a variety of sources may influence the same pool of tract neurons. *(From Cramer CD, Darby SA: Basic and clinical anatomy of the spine, spinal cord, and ANS, St Louis, 1995, Mosby.)*

average pain tolerance will describe pain in the shoulder as dull and aching but compatible with moderate limitation of the activities of daily living. If the pain is more severe, the condition will be described as sharp, lancinating, and intermittently severe. The circadian cycle affects the intensity of the pain. Complaints of pain are usually greater at night and may increase as barometric pressure increases. External modalities—such as excessive heat or cold or an unusual degree of compression or forcible rotation—cause pain to increase.

The individual's personality affects the average reaction to pain. Those with hysterical personalities or with a tendency for hypochondriasis or those who are anxious and depressed respond with more frequent and intense complaints concerning pain, and they overreact to the severity of the stimulus. Sleep deprivation and an unnaturally high anxiety level affect pain. Individuals with a labile personality who have acute pain may overreact to painful stimulus. The same individuals may become dependent and passive and accept chronic pain, although they often complain about the effect of the pain on their personality. For example, they state that the pain lessens their sex drive and performance and alters their disposition. The emotional aspects of pain cannot be separated from the physical aspects. A severe toothache that interferes with sleeping, eating, and working is represented by a much higher degree of pain and responds less readily to medications and external applications than does the acute form of pain that is present for only a short period and does not affect rest and nutrition.

A patient who actually is in pain demonstrates a definite pallor or change in the facial features. Pain often will produce positive evidence, through involuntary muscle spasm and contractures, leading to postural attitudes for relief. The patient who is in genuine pain will perspire freely and flinch consistently. Also, the pulse will increase suddenly, the blood pressure may rise, and the pupils will dilate. In a malingerer, the pulse does not change, the pupils do not dilate abnormally, and the complaints of pain will usually be greater than the clinical findings can support.

Anesthesia denotes a state in which a patient gives no demonstrable recognition of eternal stimuli except for stimuli that involve movement of the part with extreme pressure that causes tendon or bone stimulation.

Hypesthesia (hypoesthesia) is the diminution of the ability to recognize cutaneous stimulation caused by pressure made with a sharp point or a dull object. This description usually designates alteration of a dermatome.

Dysesthesia is an uncomfortable, unpleasant sensation that results from stimulation of a cutaneous region, caused or affected by peripheral nerve trauma or regeneration. Stimulation of one side of a digit may actually be felt in an adjacent digit.

Paresthesia is painful tingling, aching, and/or burning along the course of a peripheral nerve that results from percussion of the involved nerve or stimulation of the skin in the autonomous zone of the involved nerve.

Hyperesthesia is the unpleasant feeling of excessive sensation that results from cutaneous stimulation. When a finger or toe is affected, hair follicles in the geographic dermatome are excessively sensitive to touch, as are the skin and cuticle of that digit.

Cold intolerance is the dull, deep, aching sensation in a segment of the extremity that occurs as the environmental temperature is lowered. The more rapidly the temperature drops, the greater the pain. The pain distribution is not well localized and is not relieved immediately by warming the part. The pain associated with cold intolerance may be minimal if the temperature is dropped slowly but may be severe if warm-up is accomplished too rapidly.

Burning, searing, cutting, and *hot* are terms commonly used by individuals with peripheral dysfunction lesions that result from complete or partial nerve trauma.

ORTHOPEDIC GAMUT 13-8

PAIN PROBLEMS

Pain problems can be categorized as follows:

1. Pure nerve pain
2. Pain associated with nerve and vascular insufficiency
3. Pain related to numerous local alterations, such as inadequate skin coverage, fibrosis, bone pressure, tendon irritation, and collagen fibrosis

---

Determining the most relevant factors, whether biologic or psychologic, should be incorporated into a prospective assessment of each patient. The goal is the identification of individuals who will and will not benefit from medical and surgical management of pain.

ORTHOPEDIC GAMUT 13-9

OSWESTRY-TYPE PAIN-DISABILITY QUESTIONNAIRE

Oswestry-Type Pain-Disability Questionnaire consists of the following*:

This Questionnaire Has Been Designed to Give the Examiner Information About Pain and How It Affects Your Ability to Manage in Everyday Life. Please Circle, in Each Section, Only One Statement That Most Closely Applies to You.

Section 1: Pain intensity

1. I can tolerate the pain I have without having to use painkillers.
2. The pain is bad, but I manage without taking painkillers.
3. Painkillers give complete relief from pain.
4. Painkillers give moderate relief from pain.
5. Painkillers give very little relief from pain.
6. Painkillers have no affect on the pain, and I do not use them.

Section 2: Personal care (e.g., washing, dressing)

1. I can look after myself normally, without causing extra pain.
2. I can look after myself normally, but it causes extra pain.
3. It is painful to look after myself, and I am slow and careful.
4. I need some help, but I manage most of my personal care.
5. I need help every day in most aspects of self-care.
6. I do not get dressed. I wash with difficulty and stay in bed.

Section 3: Lifting

1. I can lift heavy weights without increased pain.
2. I can lift heavy weights, but it gives added pain.
3. Pain prevents me from lifting heavy weights off the floor, but I can manage if they are conveniently positioned, such as on a table.
4. Pain prevents me from lifting heavy weights, but I can manage light to medium weights if they are conveniently positioned.
5. I can lift only very light weights.
6. I cannot lift or carry anything at all.

Section 4: Walking

1. Pain does not prevent me from walking any distance.
2. Pain prevents me from walking more than 1 mile.
3. Pain prevents me from walking more than ½ mile.
4. Pain prevents me from walking more than ¼ mile.
5. I can walk only using a cane or crutches.
6. I am in bed most of the time and have to crawl to the toilet.

Section 5: Sitting

1. I can sit in any chair as long as I like.
2. I can only sit in my favorite chair as long as I like.
3. Pain prevents me from sitting more than 1 hour.
4. Pain prevents me from sitting for more than ½ hour.
5. Pain prevents me from sitting more than 10 minutes.
6. Pain prevents me from sitting at all.

Section 6: Standing

1. I can stand as long as I want without added pain.
2. I can stand as long as I want, but it gives me added pain.
3. Pain prevents me from standing for more than 1 hour.
4. Pain prevents me from standing for more than 30 minutes.
5. Pain prevents me from standing for more than 10 minutes.
6. Pain prevents me from standing at all.

Section 7: Sleeping

1. Pain does not prevent me from sleeping well.
2. I can sleep well only by using sleeping tablets.
3. Even when I take sleeping tablets, I have less than 6 hours of sleep.
4. Even when I take sleeping tablets, I have less than 4 hours of sleep.
5. Even when I take sleeping tablets, I have less than 2 hours of sleep.
6. Pain prevents me from sleeping at all.

ORTHOPEDIC GAMUT 13-9

OSWESTRY-TYPE PAIN-DISABILITY QUESTIONNAIRE—cont'd

Section 8: Sexual activity

1. My sexual activity is normal and causes no extra pain.
2. My sexual activity is normal but causes some extra pain.
3. My sexual activity is nearly normal but is very painful.
4. My sexual activity is severely restricted by pain.
5. My sexual activity is nearly absent because of pain.
6. Pain prevents any sexual activity at all.

Section 9: Social life

1. My social life is normal and gives me no extra pain.
2. My social life is normal but increases the degree of pain.
3. Pain has no significant effect on my social life other than limiting my more energetic interests, such as dancing.
4. Pain restricts my social life, and I do not go out often.
5. Pain has restricted my social life to my home.
6. I have no social life because of pain.

Section 10: Traveling

1. I can travel anywhere without added pain.
2. I can travel anywhere, but it gives me added pain.
3. Pain is bad, but I manage journeys of more than 2 hours.
4. Pain restricts me to a journey of less than 1 hour.
5. Pain restricts me to short, necessary journeys that take no longer than 30 minutes.
6. Pain prevents me from traveling, except to the doctor or hospital.

Scoring

Each item is given a point value ranging from 0 to 5, from top to bottom, for a potential total score of 0 to 50. The score is doubled for a total percentage score. If an item is not answered or the patient makes up an answer, it is dropped from the total potential score, and the total percentage is calculated using the remaining answers. The percentages are interpreted as follows: 0% to 20% indicates minimal disability in the activities of daily living (ADLs), 20% to 40% represents moderate ADL disability, 40% to 60% is severe ADL disability, 60% to 80% is crippled ADL disability, and 80% to 100% represents symptom magnification or bed bound.

*From Fairbank JTC: The Oswestry low back disability questionnaire, *Physiotherapy* 66:271, 1980, Chartered Society of Physiotherapy.

ORTHOPEDIC GAMUT 13-10

PURE MALINGERING

Pure malingering is suggested by the following characteristics:

1. The simulation of a nonexistent illness or injury
2. The voluntary provocation, aggravation, and protraction of disease by artificial means
3. False allegations about the existence of some malady, such as epilepsy

CLINICAL PEARL (ASSESSMENT OF PAIN)

Feigning or pretense of nonexistent symptoms by word, gesture, action, or behavior is simulation (positive malingering) or dissimulation (negative malingering). The deliberate and designed feigning of disease or disability or the intentional concealment of disease, if it exists, is pure malingering. The magnification or intensification of symptoms that already exist is partial malingering or exaggeration. Ascribing morbid phenomena or symptoms to a definite cause, although the cause may be recognized or ascertained to have no relationship to the symptoms, is false imputation.

AXIAL TRUNK-LOADING TEST

Assessment for Lumbar Spine Malingering

Comment

In the valid patient, any antalgic position can be taken as a sign that pain can be alleviated or abolished. The Quebec Task Force Classification System for categorizing spinal disorders lends in the differentiation of spinal pain validity (Table 13-6). An antalgic position, which is assumed automatically, cannot easily be simulated, and it is a protective measure. With uncomplicated lumbosacral strain, the typical antalgic position when standing is slight forward flexion. When maintaining this position, it is not only the abdominal muscles, as forward flexors of the trunk, that are under tension but also the long back muscles, even though they are extensors. The antalgic position does not merely block extension, but it also prevents an excess of forward flexion.

PROCEDURE

- The examiner presses the patient's cranium in a downward direction (Fig. 13-22).

- The existing antalgic positioning must not be disturbed during the axial loading.
- The axial loading may elicit pain in the neck, but it should not elicit pain in the lower back.
- Malingering should be suspected if the patient indicates that pain is felt in the lower back.

Confirmation Procedures

Burn's bench test, flexed-hip test, flip sign, Magnuson's test, plantar flexion test, and trunk rotational test

---

DIAGNOSTIC STATEMENT

The axial trunk-loading test is positive and elicits a complaint of pain in the lumbar spine. This result suggests a lack of organic basis for the lower back complaint.

TABLE 13-6

THE QUEBEC CLASSIFICATION SYSTEM

Classification	Symptoms	Duration of Symptoms from Onset	Working Status at Time of Evaluation
1	Pain without radiation	a (<7 days)	W (working)
2	Pain + radiation to extremity, proximally	b (7 days-7 weeks)	I (idle)
3	Pain + radiation to extremity, distally	c (>7 weeks)	
4	Pain + radiation to upper/lower limb neurologic signs		
5	Presumptive compression of a spinal nerve root on a simple roentgenogram (i.e., spinal instability or fracture)		
6	Compression of a spinal nerve root confirmed by (1) specific imaging techniques (i.e., computed axial tomography, myelography, or magnetic resonance imaging) or (2) other diagnostic techniques (e.g., electromyography, venography)		
7	Spinal stenosis		
8	Postsurgical status, 1-6 months after intervention		
9	Postsurgical status, >6 months after intervention 9.1 Asymptomatic 9.2 Symptomatic		
10	Chronic pain syndrome		W (working)
11	Other diagnoses		I (idle)

From Spitzer WO, et al: Scientific approach to the assessment & management of activity related spinal disorders: a monograph for clinicians. Report of the Quebec Task Force on Spinal Disorders, *Spine* 12(suppl 7):S1, 1987.

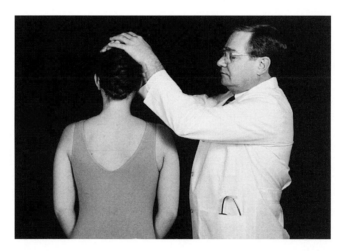

FIG. 13-22 The patient is in the standing position. The examiner presses downward on the patient's head with both hands carefully and not disturbing the existing antalgic posture. The axial loading may elicit pain in the neck, but should not elicit pain in the lower back. Lower back pain is a positive finding and indicates a lack of organic basis for the lower back complaint.

BURN'S BENCH TEST

Assessment for Lumbar Spine Malingering

Comment

A herniated disc can be defined as the herniation of the nucleus pulposus through the fibers of the annulus fibrosus.

The patient's major complaint is a sharp lancinating pain. Often, the patient has a history of intermittent episodes of localized back pain. The pain also radiates down the leg in the anatomic distribution of the affected nerve root, and it is usually described as deep and sharp, progressing from above downward. The onset of pain may be insidious or sudden and may be associated with a tearing or snapping sensation in the spine. Occasionally, when sciatica develops, the back pain resolves. Once the annulus is ruptured, it may no longer be under tension. Disc herniation occurs with sudden physical effort when the trunk is flexed or rotated. The sciatica may vary in intensity, and it may be so severe that a patient is unable to ambulate and feels as if the back is locked.

PROCEDURE

- The patient is instructed to kneel on a stool (Fig. 13-23) and bend the trunk forward (Fig. 13-24) far enough to allow touching of the floor with fingertips or hands (Fig. 13-25).

- Patients who may be expected to perform this test successfully include those afflicted with sciatica, sacralization, spondylolisthesis, compression fractures of vertebra, and so on.
- A malingerer will fail to perform the maneuver and usually states, "I can't do it," or words to that effect, even before attempting the move.

Confirmation Procedures

Axial trunk-loading test, flexed-hip test, flip sign, Magnuson's test, plantar flexion test, and trunk rotational test

---

DIAGNOSTIC STATEMENT

Burn's bench test cannot be accomplished. This result suggests a lack of organic basis for the patient's lower back complaint.

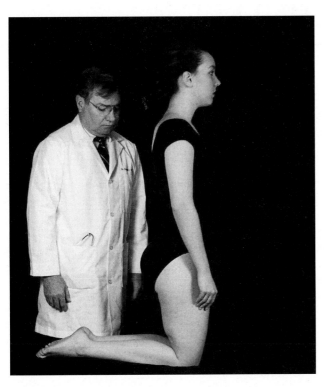

FIG. 13-23   The patient is instructed to kneel on a table or stool, approximately 18 in from the floor.

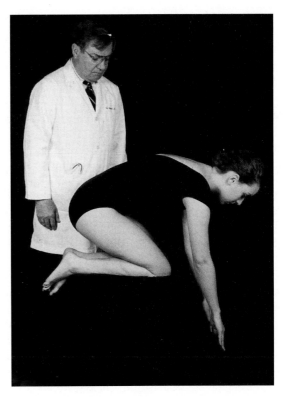

FIG. 13-24   The patient is then instructed to flex the trunk forward.

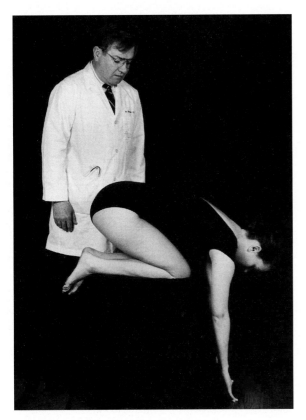

FIG. 13-25   This flexion should be far enough to allow the patient to touch the floor. This maneuver does not affect the lumbar tissues to any significant degree. A malingering patient will fail to perform the maneuver, stating, "I can't do it," or words to that effect.

FLEXED-HIP TEST

Assessment for Lumbar Spine Malingering

Comment

Acute pain in the back that radiates down to the knee but will not radiate beyond this point without neurologic abnormality is usually caused by an acute muscle or ligament injury in the lumbar spine. The symptoms can be precipitated by a sudden violent movement or by a comparatively trivial movement following a period of hard work.

Tall, slim patients with willowy backs and weak muscles are especially prone to acute back strains, as are those in sedentary occupations. Those who sit for a long time and then have to lift heavy weights without an adequate warm-up are very vulnerable. Such occupations include a delivery person, who may drive in a vehicle over bumpy surfaces for more than an hour with the spine flexed and then leap out of the seat to lift a heavy weight from the vehicle.

The sacroiliac joints are also subject to acute strains. Although the joints have a large surface area, they have poor mechanical cohesion, and violent twisting strains can cause severe pain around the joints.

PROCEDURE

- The examiner places one hand under the patient's lumbar spine and the other hand under the patient's knee.
- The examiner lifts the knee while flexing the hip (Fig. 13-26).
- If the patient indicates that lower back and/or leg pain is felt in the lower back before the lumbar spine moves, malingering should be suspected.

Confirmation Procedures

Axial trunk-loading test, Burn's bench test, flip sign, Magnuson's test, plantar flexion test, and trunk rotational test

DIAGNOSTIC STATEMENT

The flexed-hip test elicits pain before movement at the lumbosacral spine occurs. This test demonstrates a lack of organic basis for the patient's complaint.

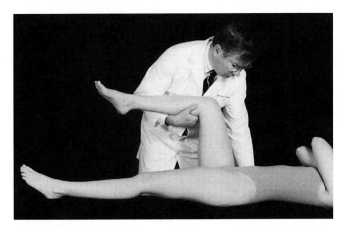

FIG. 13-26   The patient is supine on the examination table. The examiner places one hand under the patient's lumbar spine, palpating the bony landmarks of the L5 and S1 spinous processes. The examiner maintains contact with these landmarks. While the knee is passively held in 90 degrees of flexion, the examiner flexes the hip to 90 degrees. If lower back and/or leg pain is experienced before the L5 and S1 spinosus separate, malingering is suspected.

FLIP SIGN

Assessment for Feigned Low Back Pain

Comment

With the patient who has a valid lower back injury, a full neurologic examination is warranted if there are continued root symptoms. Enhanced imaging (CT, MRI) is indicated if there is continued disabling pain, despite a period of absolute rest, and if the distribution of the pain does not give a clear indication of which root is involved. Enhanced studies are required if there is paralysis of any muscle that does not recover within a few days. Further investigation is required if there is any disturbance of micturition. If the pain is clearly in the distribution of a lumbar root but is not accompanied by any stiffness of the back, enhanced studies are warranted. This situation may be observed in spinal neurofibromata.

PROCEDURE

- While the patient is lying in a supine position on the examining table, the examiner raises the patient's affected leg, keeping the patient's knee straight (Fig. 13-27).

- If this movement is limited by pain or muscle resistance, the examiner then directs the patient to sit up, making sure the legs are kept flat on the table.
- If the patient can sit in this manner without pain, the test is positive.
- Sitting with the legs straight out reproduces the same maneuver as a straight-leg-raising test (Fig. 13-28).

Confirmation Procedures

Axial trunk-loading test, Burn's bench test, flexed-hip test, Magnuson's test, plantar flexion test, and trunk rotational test

DIAGNOSTIC STATEMENT

Flip sign is present and indicates a lack of organic basis for the patient's complaint.

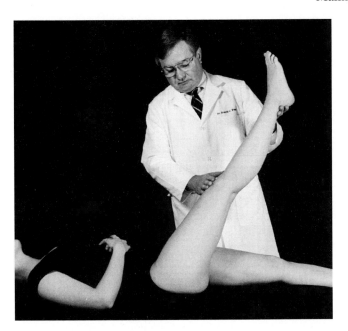

FIG. 13-27   The patient is lying supine on the examination table. The examiner performs a straight-leg-raising test on the affected side, noting the limitation of movement because of pain or muscle spasm.

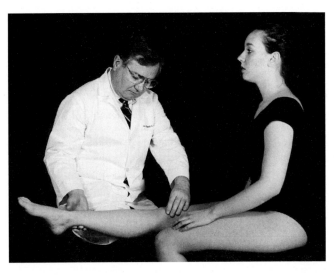

FIG. 13-28   The patient is then directed to sit at the side of the examination table, with the legs dangling over the edge. On pretext of examining an uninvolved joint of the leg, the examiner fully extends the knee of the affected leg, effecting a straight-leg-raising sciatic stretch maneuver. If the maneuver does not elicit pain, the test is positive, and malingering should be suspected. In a modification of this test, the patient is directed to sit up from the position shown in Fig. 13-27, with the legs extended and flat on the examination table. If the patient can sit up in this manner, the test is positive.

LIBMAN'S SIGN

Assessment for Hypersensitivity of Mastoid Process

Comment

Spontaneous pain, hyperpathia, and hyperalgesia usually characterize central pain. The term *spontaneous pain* is used to denote the absence of extrinsic stimuli, which ordinarily produce pain. Spontaneous pain is often differentiated from evoked pain in which the stimuli are obvious. Hyperpathia designates a painful overreaction to different stimuli and is associated with diminished sensibility to the form of stimulation that excites such a reaction. Hyperalgesia is an overreaction without diminished sensibility or sensory loss. In the last two, regardless of the threshold value, the sensation evoked is abnormal. These painful sensations always develop in an explosive manner; are of an excessive, compelling, diffuse, and complex nature; and continue unduly after stimulation has ceased.

PROCEDURE

- The examiner applies finger pressure to the mastoid process (Fig. 13-29).
- The pressure is gradually increased until the patient states that it is becoming noticeably uncomfortable.
- This point is an indication of that patient's pain threshold, which varies from patient to patient.
- The threshold gives the examiner an idea if this patient has a low, high, or moderate pain threshold.
- The threshold is not to be used specifically as a criterion for malingering.
- Identifying a patient's pain threshold will quantify discomfort in this patient and applies to this patient only.
- This testing procedure will be useful during interpretation of palpation findings or subjective statements concerning pain or discomfort.

Confirmation Procedures

Mannkopf's sign, marked part pain-suggestibility test, and related joint motion test

---

DIAGNOSTIC STATEMENT

Libman's sign demonstrates an unusually low threshold for pain in the patient.

Libman's sign demonstrates a normal threshold for pain in this patient.

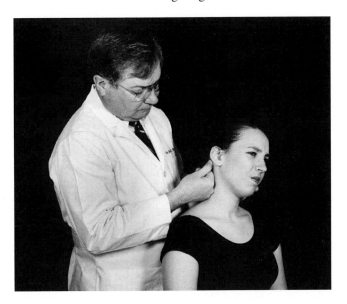

FIG. 13-29   The patient is seated, and the examiner is positioned behind the patient. The examiner applies thumb pressure to the mastoid process and gradually increases the pressure until the patient states that it is becoming noticeably uncomfortable. The test may be repeated for comparison on the opposite mastoid process. This test provides an indication of the patient's pain threshold and is a useful index for interpretation of palpation findings in later examination procedures.

MAGNUSON'S TEST

Assessment for Feigned Low Back Pain

Comment

Cutaneous tenderness is present when pain and discomfort are elicited by a normally innocuous amount of pressure. This tenderness may be related to, but is slightly different from, hyperalgesia. Pain may or may not be concomitantly present. The tenderness may be caused by a direct, underlying pathologic condition, such as occurs with inflammatory lesions or after trauma to the skin, subcutaneous, and muscular tissue. The tenderness may occur as a result of peripheral nerve lesions, or it may occur as a result of a visceral or deep, somatic pathologic condition at some distance from the tenderness. The tenderness may be present over the area where pain is felt, or it may be absent entirely from that area and found at some distant point. The latter condition exists in visceral disease, for example in cholecystitis, in which the pain is felt in the back at the angle of the scapula, while the tenderness is felt in the skin of the upper right quadrant. Cutaneous tenderness may be elicited by pinching the skin or pressing on it, and it should always be compared with a symmetrically identical area on the opposite side.

PROCEDURE

- The patient with lower back pain is directed to point to the site of the pain.
- The examiner marks that site (Fig. 13-30).
- The examiner then distracts the patient by performing an examination away from the marked site of pain and later resumes the examination of the lower back.
- The test is positive with any change in the location of the pain of greater than 1 to 2 cm (Fig. 13-31).
- The test is significant as evidence of simulated pain, hysteria, or malingering.

Confirmation Procedures

Axial trunk-loading test, Burn's bench test, flexed-hip test, flip sign, plantar flexion test, and trunk rotational test

DIAGNOSTIC STATEMENT

Magnuson's test is positive with significant changes between the location of the sites of pain during testing. This result indicates a lack of organic basis for the patient's lower back complaint.

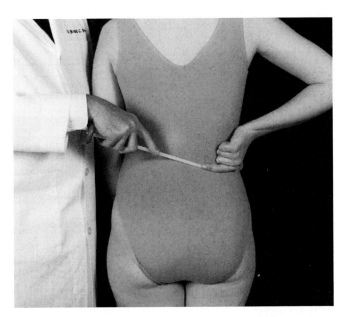

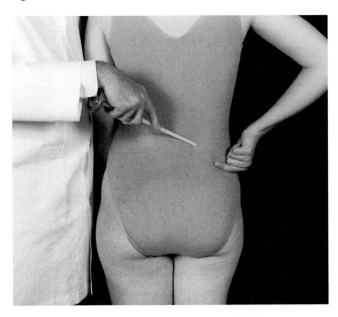

FIG. 13-30   The patient may be standing or seated for this test. The patient is directed to point to the site of lower back pain. The examiner marks the site.

FIG. 13-31   Following distraction by other examination procedures, the patient is instructed to once again point to the location of the lower back pain. The test is positive when the patient identifies any site other than the original. The test is significant for simulated lower back pain, hysteria, or malingering.

MANNKOPF'S SIGN

Assessment for Simulated Pain

Comment

The autonomic nervous system is a division of the peripheral nervous system that distributes to smooth muscle and glands throughout the body. By definition, the autonomic nervous system is entirely a motor (efferent) system and is automatic in the sense that most of its functions are carried out below the conscious level.

The sympathetic division of the autonomic nervous system is thrown into activity in preparing the organism for fight or flight, and it causes a mass response because of the existence of sympathetic ganglion chains or plexuses where the preganglionic synapse occurs. In action, the sympathetic nervous system produces vasoconstriction of the skin and viscera, shifting more blood to the brain, skeletal muscles, and heart.

PROCEDURE

- The examiner establishes the patient's resting pulse rate, and the patient is made as comfortable as possible (Fig. 13-32).

- Then, without changing the patient's position, the examiner applies mechanical pressure or electrical stimulation over the painful area, while monitoring the pulse rate (Fig. 13-33).
- An increase in pulse rate of 10 or more beats per minute constitutes a positive sign.
- The sign is absent in simulated pain.

Confirmation Procedures

Libman's sign, marked part pain-suggestibility test, and related joint motion test

---

DIAGNOSTIC STATEMENT

Mannkopf's sign is present on the right, with an increase in the patient's baseline pulse rate by a factor of 10 beats per minute. This increase indicates that an organic basis exists for the patient's musculoskeletal complaint.

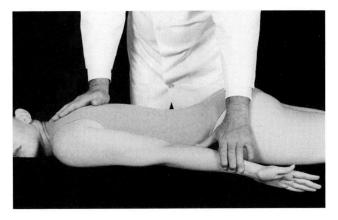

FIG. 13-32 The test may be applied for any area of musculo-skeletal pain. The examiner palpates the patient's resting radial pulse and establishes a baseline index.

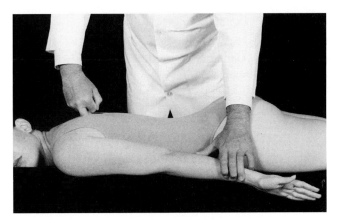

FIG. 13-33 The examiner applies firm pressure, or any form of noxious stimulation, over the area of the pain. The examiner again palpates the patient's radial pulse. An increase of 10 or more beats per minute in the pulse rate is a positive sign. The sign is absent in simulated pain.

MARKED PART
PAIN-SUGGESTIBILITY TEST

Assessment for Pain Exaggeration

Comment

Hypochondriacal neurosis denotes a preoccupation with bodily processes, in which the individual becomes unduly concerned about possible dysfunctions that are largely imagined or exaggerated. Health issues occupy the patient's thoughts, and there is concern that one or more illnesses exist. Contrary facts are not reassuring. The symptoms chosen for expression are often those experienced by close associates. In psychodynamic terms, the hypochondriacal person is immature and never achieved an external object relationship, focusing instead on the body for the major and often sole means of communicating with others. Underlying these complaints is the need for continual reassurance that an illness does not exist and that someone cares and is willing to listen.

PROCEDURE

- The examiner applies pressure to the described painful point and marks it (Figs. 13-34 and 13-35).

- The patient is distracted by examination of some other part of the body and pressing on new, tender areas.
- The examiner returns to the area of original complaint and asks the patient to close the eyes and then locate the tender points (Figs. 13-36 to 13-38).
- If the patient cannot place the points of pain/tenderness closer than 2 in from the marked area, exaggeration is suspected (Fig. 13-39).

Confirmation Procedures

Libman's sign, Mannkopf's sign, and related joint motion test

---

DIAGNOSTIC STATEMENT

The marked part pain-suggestibility test is positive and indicates a lack of organic basis for the patient's pain.

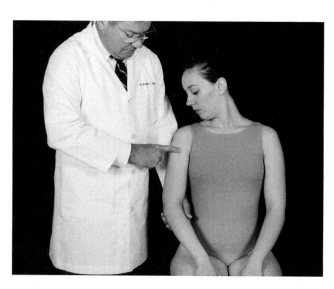

FIG. 13-34 The patient is seated. The examiner instructs the patient to identify the area of pain. The examiner applies pressure to the site, confirming the pain reaction. The site is marked or noted by some nonstimulating method. The patient is distracted with other examination procedures.

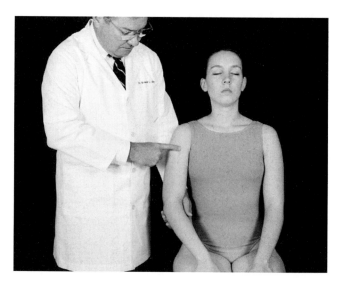

FIG. 13-35 The patient is instructed to close the eyes.

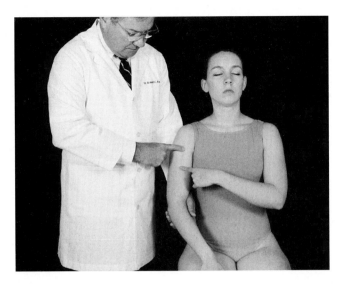

FIG. 13-36 With the eyes closed, the patient is asked to once again identify the site of pain. If the patient cannot place the point of pain within 2 in of the original site, exaggeration is suspected. It is important that the examiner not remind the patient of the original location, especially by touch.

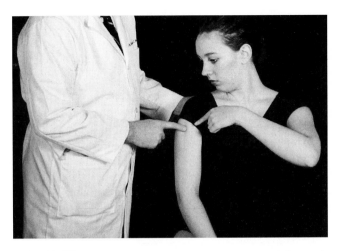

FIG. 13-37 In an alternative method of determining pain suggestibility, the examiner first suggests a certain point as the source of pain and marks it.

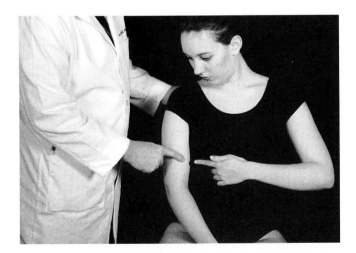

FIG. 13-38 By distracting the patient with different testing procedures, the examiner suggests a nearby but new point of discomfort and notes whether the pain shifts with the suggestion.

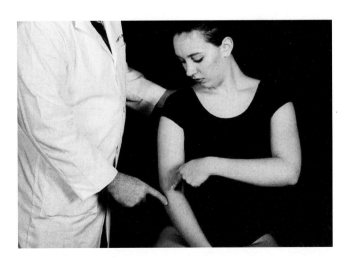

FIG. 13-39 If the site of pain does shift, this suggestibility indicates exaggeration of pain. It is important that the examiner *not* remind the patient of the original location, especially by touch.

PLANTAR FLEXION TEST

Assessment for Feigned Low Back Pain

Comment
There are several maneuvers that tighten the sciatic nerve and, in doing so, further compress an inflamed nerve root against a herniated disc. With the straight-leg raising maneuver, the L5 and S1 nerve roots move 2 to 6 mm at the level of the foramen. The L4 nerve root moves a shorter distance, and the more proximal nerve roots show little motion. Thus the straight-leg-raising test is important and has value in detecting lesions of the fifth lumbar and first sacral nerve root.

PROCEDURE
- The patient is instructed to raise the legs, one at a time, until pain is felt in the lower back or the leg (Fig. 13-40).
- The angle at which the pain occurs is noted, and the patient lowers the leg.
- The examiner places one hand under the patient's knee and one hand under the patient's foot and raises the lower extremity, keeping the patient's knee slightly flexed (Fig. 13-41).
- The leg is raised to half of the height at which the pain was originally elicited.
- The foot is plantar flexed at this point (Fig. 13-42).
- If the patient indicates that this move causes lower back pain, malingering should be suspected.

Confirmation Procedures
Axial trunk-loading test, Burn's bench test, flexed-hip test, flip sign, Magnuson's test, and trunk rotational test

DIAGNOSTIC STATEMENT
The plantar flexion test is positive on the right and indicates a lack of organic basis for the patient's sciatic pain.

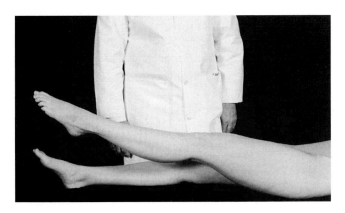

FIG. 13-40   The patient is lying supine on the examination table. The patient is instructed to raise the extended, affected leg until pain is felt in the lower back or in the leg. The examiner notes the angle at which pain occurs. The patient lowers the leg to the table.

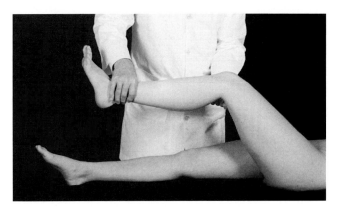

FIG. 13-41   The examiner places one hand under the patient's knee and one hand under the ankle and elevates the leg, keeping the knee slightly flexed. The leg is elevated to a point below the production of the original pain.

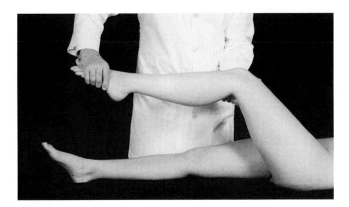

FIG. 13-42   The examiner plantar flexes the foot. If the patient indicates that the final maneuver caused lower back pain, malingering is suspected.

RELATED JOINT MOTION TEST

Assessment for Feigned Pain

Comment
Most orthopedic conditions are associated with some restriction of movement in the related joint. Complete loss of movement follows surgical ablation of a joint (arthrodesis) or may occur during some pathologic process, such as infection, where fibrous or bony tissue binds the articular surfaces together. The joint then cannot be moved, either actively or passively. In many conditions, there is a loss of that part of the range of motion that allows the joint to be brought into its neutral position. The common loss of movement usually prevents the joint from being fully extended. This is known as a *fixed flexion deformity.*

PROCEDURE
- The painful part is either actively or passively moved.
- This move is performed with isometric resistance of a muscle group that is nearby but is in no way associated with the pain (Fig. 13-43).
- If the patient complains of pain, the examiner moves the muscle group or related joint later, judging the inaccuracy of the statements and the correlated reactions (Fig. 13-44).
- This assessment is accomplished by using a flexor group where an extensor group may produce pain in the joint.
- Where the same muscle serves more than one movement, all movements should be tested.

Confirmation Procedures
Libman's sign, Mannkopf's sign, and marked part pain-suggestibility test

---

DIAGNOSTIC STATEMENT

The related joint motion test is positive on the right. This result indicates embellished pain.

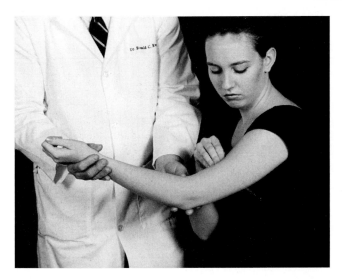

FIG. 13-43   The patient identifies the area of musculoskeletal complaint, especially the point at which motion of the affected joint is uncomfortable. The examiner confirms this reported site of pain with the patient. For example, the patient identifies that flexion of the elbow hurts the biceps musculature.

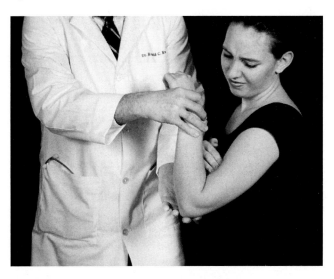

FIG. 13-44   The examiner places the painful joint or part into isometric testing of a muscle group that is nearby, but unrelated to the primary injury group. For example, the examiner isometrically tests the triceps muscle group. If the patient complains of the original pain, the examiner moves the primary muscle group later in the examination, noting the accuracy of statements and reactions to the original findings. Discrepancies suggest exaggeration of symptoms or malingering.

SEELIGMULLER'S SIGN

Assessment for Hysterical Face Pain

Comment
Trigeminal neuralgia is characterized by a sudden attack of excruciating pain of short duration along the distribution of the fifth cranial nerve. The attack is normally precipitated by mild stimulation of a trigger zone in the area of the pain and is characterized by recurrent paroxysms of sharp, stabbing pains in the distribution of one or more branches of the nerve. The onset is usually in middle or late life, and the incidence is higher in females than in males. The pain may be described as a burning or searing pain that occurs in lightninglike jabs, lasting only 1 to 2 minutes or as long as 15 minutes. The frequency of attacks varies from many times a day to several times a month or a year. The patient often tries to immobilize the face during conversation or attempts to swallow food without chewing in order to avoid irritating the trigger zone.

PROCEDURE
- Mydriasis (dilated pupil) is present on the side of the face that is afflicted with neuralgia.
- The sign is present as long as pain is present.
- The sign is absent in cases of hysteria and malingering (Fig. 13-45).

Confirmation Procedures
Anosmia testing and facial anesthesia testing

DIAGNOSTIC STATEMENT
Seeligmuller's sign is absent on the right and indicates hysterical face pain.

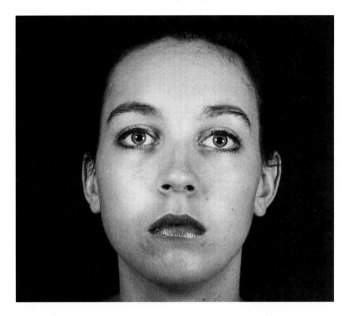

FIG. 13-45   In the patient complaining of facial neuralgia, the examiner observes the pupils for mydriasis. A dilated pupil is a usual finding with facial neuralgia and is absent, as in this photo, in cases of hysteria or malingering.

TRUNK ROTATIONAL TEST

Assessment for Nonorganic Low Back Pain

Comment
During flexion of the trunk, the strain falls first on the iliolumbar ligament. Next, strain is transmitted to the interspinous ligaments, from the fifth lumbar vertebra upward, and then to the dorsolumbar fascia, particularly to the sacral triangle. During extension, the impingement signs prevail over the tension effects. The articulation comes first, and the interspinous ligaments follow. The ligamentum flavum escapes impingement. During axial rotation, the iliolumbar ligament becomes strained first and then the intertransverse.

Confirmation Procedures
Axial trunk-loading test, Burn's bench test, flexed-hip test, flip sign, Magnuson's test, and plantar flexion test

---

DIAGNOSTIC STATEMENT

The trunk rotational test is positive and elicits pain in the lumbar spine on the right. This result indicates a lack of organic basis for the patient's lumbar spine complaint.

ORTHOPEDIC GAMUT 13-11

LATERAL FLEXION

Following is the sequence of strain during lateral flexion on the convex side:

1. Quadratus
2. Ligamentum flavum
3. Interspinous ligament

The legs transmit their effect through the pelvis. Single leg raising causes no pelvic movement, although it does cause contraction of the contralateral gluteus maximus. Double leg raising tilts the pelvis into extension. The ischial tuberosities serve as fulcrums.

PROCEDURE
- The patient rotates the trunk.
- The examiner ensures that the pelvis rotates as well (Fig. 13-46).
- If the patient indicates that this causes lower back pain, malingering should be suspected.
- The lumbar spine is not moving.
- Instead the whole spine is rotated from the hips and thighs.

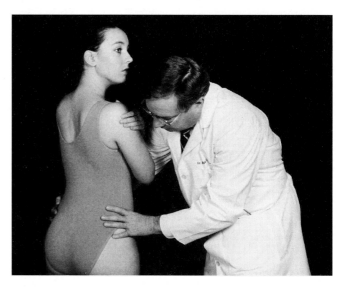

FIG. 13-46   The patient is in the standing position with the arms folded across the chest. The examiner instructs the patient to rotate the trunk, while making sure that the pelvis is rotated simultaneously. If the patient indicates that this move causes pain in the lower back, the test is positive and indicates malingering.

SENSORY DEFICIT QUALIFICATION AND QUANTIFICATION

Overview

The nervous system does not perceive external events directly. Instead, the brain receives an abstract picture that is a composite of nerve impulses that originate at the periphery. The transformation of external stimuli into conductible impulses is called transduction. Sensibility is the reception or encoding of external stimuli and the transmission of impulses along nerve fibers.

ORTHOPEDIC GAMUT 13-12

NEURAL SENSIBILITY

Neural sensibility encompasses the following:

1. Sight
2. Smell
3. Sound
4. Taste
5. Temperature change
6. Pain
7. Touch-pressure
8. Movement or change in position

Sensibility is the modality of prime importance. Touch-pressure is the ability to recognize touch, whether moving across the surface or continually applied to a single spot.

In contrast to sensibility, which is primarily a peripheral phenomenon, sensation is the central reception and conscious recognition of external stimuli. Sensation involves several facets of central nervous system function. Some of these facets are voluntary, and some are involuntary. Among these facets are the orderly reception and integration of impulses from several sources, association with other information (either current or from memory storage), assimilation and interpretation of such data, and finally, elevation to the conscious level. All of these facets may result, at the patient's discretion, in an appropriate response.

The transmission of impulses from skin surface to cerebral cortex requires a chain of three afferent neurons. The cell body of the first-order afferent neuron lies in the dorsal ganglion, and the other two are in the spinal cord and brain. From a practical standpoint, the examiner has access only to the axon of the first-order afferent neuron, its receptors, and the skin that contains them.

ORTHOPEDIC GAMUT 13-13

SENSATION

Sensation is divided into the following three groups:

1. Superficial
2. Deep
3. Combined

Superficial sensation is concerned with touch, pain, temperature, and two-point discrimination; deep sensation is concerned with muscle and joint position sense (proprioception) and deep muscle pain and vibration sense (pallesthesia). The combination of superficial and deep sensory mechanisms is involved in stereognosis, the recognition and naming of familiar objects placed in the hand, and topognosis, the ability to localize cutaneous stimuli. Stereognosis depends on the integrity of the cerebral cortex.

ORTHOPEDIC GAMUT 13-14

CUTANEOUS SENSIBILITY

Cutaneous sensibility is divided into the following two groups:

1. Epicritic
2. Protopathic

Each is served by a different neuron. Epicritic senses are concerned with perception of light touch, two-point discrimination, and small differences in temperature; the protopathic senses are concerned with pain and more marked changes of temperature.

CLINICAL PEARL (SENSORY DEFICIT ASSESSMENT)

In the evaluation of what appears to be psychogenic changes in sensation, it is always essential to recall that there is some variation in the nerve supply in normal individuals. Furthermore, hysterical or malingered changes may be superimposed on organic anesthesia in peripheral nerve lesions and other neurologic disorders. An ipsilateral decrease or loss of the senses of vision, hearing, smell, and taste may occasionally accompany hysterical (or malingered) hemianesthesia, which almost invariably occurs on the left side.

ANOSMIA TESTING

Assessment for Feigned Anosmia

Comment

The central connections of the olfactory nerve are complex. Association fibers to the tegmentum and pons pass directly as third-order neurons from the anterior perforated substance, and indirectly from the hippocampus, via the fornix and olfactory projection tracts, through the mamillary bodies and anterior nuclei of the thalamus. Reflex connections, thus established within the nuclei of the other cranial and spinal nerves, may be functionally significant during swallowing and digestion.

The olfactory nerve may serve as a portal of entry for cryptogenic infections of the brain and meninges (poliomyelitis, epidemic meningitis, and encephalitis).

ORTHOPEDIC GAMUT 13-15

SMELL

Disorders of the sense of smell may by caused by the following:

1. Inflammatory and other lesions of the nasal cavity
2. Fracture of the anterior fossa of the skull
3. Tumors of the frontal lobe and pituitary region
4. Meningitis
5. Hydrocephalus
6. Posttraumatic cerebral syndrome
7. Arteriosclerosis
8. Cerebrovascular accidents
9. Certain drug intoxications
10. Psychoses
11. Neuroses
12. Congenital defects

Anosmia may be of significance. Bilateral anosmia commonly occurs with colds, rhinitis, and so on. Unilateral anosmia may be of diagnostic significance in locating brain lesions, such as tumors, at the base of the frontal lobe.

ORTHOPEDIC GAMUT 13-16

OLFACTORY NERVE

Special syndromes involving the olfactory nerve include the following:

1. Foster-Kennedy syndrome (unilateral optic atrophy, with or without anosmia and contralateral papilledema)
2. Aura of epilepsy

PROCEDURE

- With complaints involving the loss of the sense of smell, the patient is directed to index various odors by smelling aromatics such as peppermint, clove, vanilla, coffee grounds (uncooked), and then finally, spirit of ammonia (Fig. 13-47).
- An individual with psychogenic loss of smell often claims the inability to smell any of these substances.
- Ammonia is extremely pungent and actually irritates the trigeminal nerve endings in the nose, rather than being smelled by the olfactory nerve proper.
- Hence, a damaged olfactory nerve does not impair a patient's ability to notice (smell) the pungent ammonia fumes.

Confirmation Procedures

Seeligmuller's sign and facial anesthesia testing

DIAGNOSTIC STATEMENT

Anosmia testing demonstrates normal function of the olfactory nerve. This result suggests feigned anosmia.

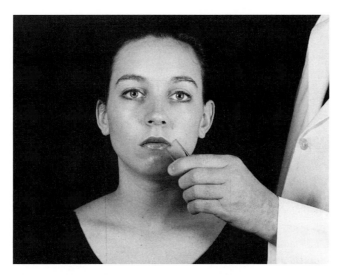

FIG. 13-47 In complaints of loss of smell, the patient is instructed to index various odors by smelling aromatics, such as peppermint, clove, vanilla, coffee grounds, and finally, spirit of ammonia. An individual with feigned anosmia will claim the inability to smell any of the substances. Using spirit of ammonia directly irritates the trigeminal nerve endings in the nose. A damaged olfactory nerve does not impair the patient's ability to notice (smell) pungent ammonia. Anosmia to ammonia suggests a psychogenic or manufactured complaint.

COORDINATION-DISTURBANCE TESTING

Assessment for Nonorganic Loss of Coordination

Comment

Tremors are involuntary movements in one or more parts of the body, produced by rhythmical alternate contractions of opposing muscle groups. Tremors are symptoms of constitutional diseases or disorders rather than clinical entities.

In differentiating tremors, the examiner should note their rate, rhythm, and distribution and the effect of movement or rest. A rapid tremor oscillates 8 to 10 times per second, a slow tremor 3 to 5 times per second. Tremors may be fine or coarse. Intention tremor appears during, or is accentuated by, volitional movements of the affected part. Resting tremors are present when the involved part is at rest, but they diminish or disappear during active movements.

Transient tremors, without particular significance, may occur in healthy individuals during hunger, chilling, or excitement or after physical exertion.

PROCEDURE

- The patient with coordination disturbances is instructed to touch the tip of the nose while the eyes are open.

- The patient is then instructed to close the eyes and again touch the tip of the nose (Fig. 13-48).
- With organic cerebellar lesions, an intention crescendo tremor manifests as the finger approaches the nose.
- The malingerer will move the finger in a guided but devious course toward the nose, without exhibiting the intention tremor (Fig. 13-49).

Confirmation Procedures

Limb-dropping test (upper extremities), position-sense testing, and Romberg test

---

DIAGNOSTIC STATEMENT

Coordination-disturbance testing does not demonstrate involuntary intention crescendo tremors. This result indicates a lack of organic basis for the patient's complaint of a loss of coordination.

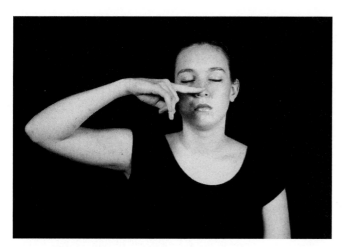

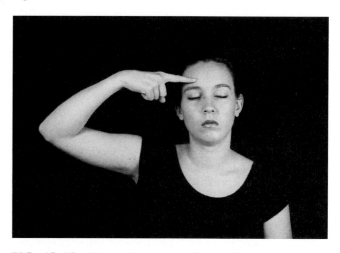

FIG. 13-48 The seated patient is instructed to touch the tip of the nose while the eyes are open. The patient is then instructed to close the eyes and again touch the tip of the nose. With organic cerebellar lesions, an intention crescendo tremor manifests as the finger approaches the nose.

FIG. 13-49 The malingering patient will move the finger toward the nose in a guided, but devious course, without the intention tremor.

CUIGNET'S TEST

Assessment for Simulated Blindness

Comment

Optic atrophy is commonly divided into primary and secondary (or postneuritic) categories. Primary optic atrophy results from a degeneration of the nerve fibers following retrobulbar neuritis that results from syphilis, central retinal artery occlusion, glaucoma, trauma, or any condition or drug that causes injury to the optic nerve along its intracanalicular or intracranial course. With secondary optic atrophy, degeneration of the nerve fibers is accompanied by glial formation on the nerve head and is caused by optic neuritis or severe and prolonged papilledema.

Visual loss is directly proportional to the degree of nerve atrophy. This appreciation of light is demonstrated by the Marcus Gunn phenomenon. With the Marcus Gunn phenomenon, the examiner is able to recognize the quantitative difference in the pupillary light reflex between the two eyes by means of alternately illuminating the pupils of the two eyes and observing the difference in pupillary constriction. In optic atrophy, total blindness and a dilated, fixed pupil may result. In primary optic atrophy, the disc is white or grayish with sharp edges and a saucer-shaped excavation. The lamina cribrosa is clearly visible. The retina is usually normal.

In secondary optic atrophy, the disc is dirty white with irregular and indistinct margins and is covered by glial tissue that conceals the lamina cribrosa. Evidence of previous inflammation, such as sheathed vessels, may be seen in the retina.

PROCEDURE

- Without a positive Marcus Gunn's phenomenon but with continued complaint of unilateral blindness, the examiner places a refractive lens over the "good eye," ostensibly to test it (Fig. 13-50).
- The lens actually deprives the eye of any effective vision.
- The malingering patient is directed to read a Snellen chart (Fig. 13-51).
- This is accomplished perfectly with the blind eye.

Confirmation Procedures

Marcus Gunn's sign, optokinetic nystagmus test, and Snellen's test

---

DIAGNOSTIC STATEMENT

Cuignet's test is positive for simulated blindness in the right eye.

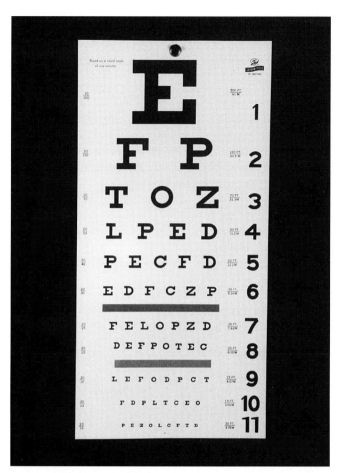

FIG. 13-50 The seated patient is placed at an appropriate distance from a Snellen eye chart. The patient is instructed to read the chart with one eye at a time. With simulated unilateral blindness, the patient will claim that the blind eye cannot read the chart.

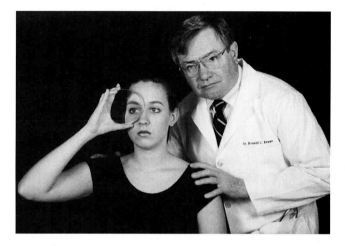

FIG. 13-51 The examiner places a refractive, but myopic lens over the good eye, ostensibly to aid its vision and test it. The patient is again instructed to read the Snellen chart. The lens deprives the eye of any effective vision. If the chart is read, it was done so with the blind eye. If the chart can be read, the test is positive and indicates simulated unilateral blindness.

FACIAL ANESTHESIA TESTING

Assessment for Hysterical or Simulated Face Anesthesia

Comment

Neuritis is a disease of a nerve. As an affectation of a single nerve, it is called *mononeuritis.* As an affectation of two or more nerves in separate areas, the disease is called *mononeuritis multiplex,* and if it affects many nerves simultaneously, it is called *polyneuritis.* The term implies a syndrome of sensory, motor, reflex, and vasomotor symptoms, singly or in combination, produced by lesions of the nerve roots or peripheral nerves.

Sensory symptoms may be prominent. Descriptive terms—such as *tingling, pins-and-needles sensation, burning, boring,* and *stabbing*—are used by the patient. Pain, often worse at night, may be aggravated by touching the affected area or by temperature changes. Numbness and objective loss of sensation occur, in severe cases, in stocking-and-glove distributions. The nerve trunks may be tender. When sensory loss is profound, painless ulcers may appear on the digits or joints may be painlessly enlarged (Charcot joints).

PROCEDURE

- In a patient with symptoms of facial anesthesia, the examiner applies a vibrating tuning fork to the numb side of the patient's forehead, near the midline (Fig. 13-52).
- The malingerer or hysteric will state that there is no sensation.
- When the examiner moves the application of the tuning fork just across the midline, the patient now reports sensing the vibrations immediately.
- The lack of vibration sense on the "numb" side is an impossibility because the bone tissue conducts the vibration that is applied to the area of claimed anesthesia to the normal side.
- This test is valid even for a pathologic bone condition or an organic bone disease.

Confirmation Procedures

Seeligmuller's sign and anosmia testing

DIAGNOSTIC STATEMENT

Facial anesthesia testing is positive on the right for hysterical or simulated facial anesthesia.

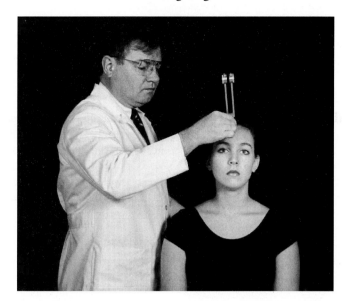

FIG. 13-52 The patient is seated. The examiner applies a vibrating tuning fork to the numb side of the forehead, near the midline of the forehead. The patient is asked to identify sensations of vibration across the forehead. If the patient denies feeling the vibration on the numb side of the forehead, the test is repeated just across the midline, on the normal side of the forehead. If the patient feels the vibration only on the normal side, hysteria or malingering is suspected.

GAULT TEST

Assessment for Simulated Deafness

Comment
Perceptive deafness is impaired hearing caused by disorders of the inner ear, the eighth (auditory) nerve, cerebral pathways, or the auditory center.

ORTHOPEDIC GAMUT 13-17

IMPAIRED HEARING

Causes of impaired hearing include the following:

1. Involvement of the auditory structures in infectious diseases such as meningitis, syphilis, typhoid, mumps, measles, and hemolytic streptococcal infection
2. Tumors of the cerebellopontine angle, temporal lobe, eighth nerve, or cochlea
3. Trauma, such as from skull fracture
4. Injury by such toxic substances as quinine, arsenic, alcohol, salicylates, mercury, or aminoglycoside antibiotics (kanamycin)
5. Psychogenic disturbances
6. Physiologic dysfunction that may occur in senility and from excessive noise

---

Excessive noise is a common cause of hearing loss. The loss is more pronounced in the high frequencies and traditionally has been caused by industrial noise and exposure to heavy gunfire. Recently, the condition has appeared in adolescents, caused by excessive electronic amplification of music.

Deafness is a form of sensory deprivation easily feigned and as easily tested. Although the complaint is the inability to hear any sound, the patient with such a conversion reaction may startle to a loud noise and can be awakened from a sound sleep by the same. A startled response to sound is an important finding when an examiner is testing a noncooperative, hysterical, or malingering patient.

PROCEDURE

- The examiner can gain a crude estimate of the patient's hearing ability by using the auditory-palpebral reflex.
- When a patient hears a loud sound, an involuntary blink is the response.
- With the patient's normal ear covered, an assistant standing behind the patient (out of the patient's line of sight) can clap the hands or pop a bag (Fig. 13-53).
- The examiner observes the patient for blinking or a startled response (Fig. 13-54).
- If the patient has a response, the examiner can be certain that the patient heard something.
- If the patient does not respond, the significance of the test is doubtful.

Confirmation Procedure
Lombard's test

DIAGNOSTIC STATEMENT

The Gault test is positive and elicits an auditory-palpebral reflex. This result indicates simulated deafness.

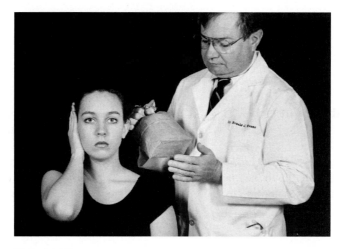

FIG. 13-53 The patient is seated and is instructed to cover the normal ear. The examiner or an assistant is positioned behind the patient, out of the patient's peripheral vision.

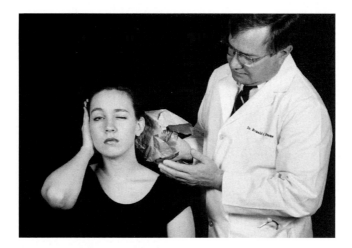

FIG. 13-54 The examiner or an assistant claps hands loudly or pops a bag. The examiner observes the patient for involuntary blinking or a startle response (auditory-palpebral reflex). If the response is present, the test is positive and indicates that the deaf ear heard something. This result suggests malingering.

JANET'S TEST

Assessment for Simulated Anesthesia

Comment
Hysterical paralysis of one limb usually provides little difficulty during diagnosis. The affected limb may be either rigid or flaccid, and there is no true muscular atrophy and no alteration in the muscular response to electrical stimulation. The reflexes provide the most information. With hysterical paralysis, the reflexes may be exaggerated, but they are never lost.

More often than not, a limb that is the seat of hysterical paralysis also presents complete insensibility to all forms of stimulation, and the upper limit of such anesthesia may end abruptly at a level for which there is no anatomic basis.

PROCEDURE

- If anesthesia is the complaint, the patient is instructed to close the eyes (Fig. 13-55).

- The patient is then directed to answer "yes" if a pinprick is felt on the skin or "no" if not (Fig. 13-56).
- Obviously, the only appropriate answer is silence when the supposedly anesthetic area is touched.

Confirmation Procedures
Facial anesthesia testing, midline tuning-fork test, and regional anesthesia testing

---

DIAGNOSTIC STATEMENT

Janet's test indicates simulated anesthesia on the right.

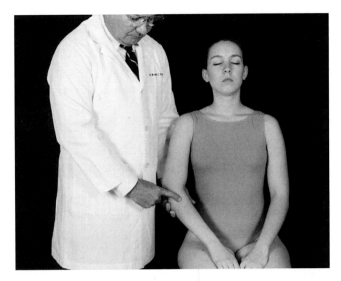

FIG. 13-55   In this test for anesthesia, the patient may be seated or recumbent. The patient is instructed to close the eyes.

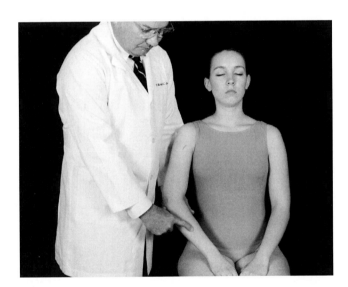

FIG. 13-56   As the examiner touches the involved part, either with a finger or sharp object, the patient is directed to indicate feeling the touch by saying "yes" and not feeling the touch by saying "no." The only appropriate answer, when the anesthetic area is touched, is silence. The test is positive when the patient identifies with the answer "no." The test indicates hysteria or malingering.

LIMB-DROPPING TEST (UPPER EXTREMITIES)

Assessment for Feigned Unconsciousness

Comment

Level of consciousness is a phrase that refers to certain processes that provide awareness of one's self and the environment. Terms used to describe pathologic alterations in the level of consciousness are determined, largely, by the degree of patient arousal. These alterations range from confusion to somnolence, stupor, and coma.

The examiner should be familiar with conditions that, in some respects, resemble stupor or coma. Akinetic mutism is a state of wakeful unresponsiveness in which the patient has no meaningful mental content or purposeful movement but seems to be awake. This condition may follow bilateral cerebral damage (the apallic state), lesions of the upper midbrain or diencephalon, and rarely, hydrocephalus. The locked-in syndrome is a condition in which the patient is conscious and aware but paralyzed and anarthric. Eye movements are preserved and may be of use for communication. The condition is caused by a lesion of the ventral portion of the pons. Disease processes involving two general areas of the central nervous system can alter consciousness. These are lesions, either in both cerebral hemispheres or in the deep midline structures, in the upper brainstem near the central core of the gray matter.

Reduced awareness or faked stoicism is attempted to portray a reduced level of consciousness. In a conversion reaction or malingering, the pupillary and corneal reflexes and plantar responses will be normal, although reduced awareness or increased pain tolerance is exhibited.

PROCEDURE

- Often, when the examiner holds up the hand of a patient who is feigning reduced consciousness and lets the hand drop over the patient's face, the arms will consciously swerve to keep the hand from striking the face.
- A patient with an organically reduced level of consciousness will not make this movement of avoidance and will usually have pupillary abnormalities and other positive neurologic signs (Figs. 13-57 to 13-60).

Confirmation Procedures

Coordination-disturbance testing, position-sense testing, and Romberg test

---

ORTHOPEDIC GAMUT 13-18

LEVEL OF CONSCIOUSNESS

Diseases producing disturbances of the level of consciousness fall into the following four main categories:

1. Supratentorial mass lesions that secondarily compress deep midline structures
2. Infratentorial lesions that directly damage the central brainstem core
3. Metabolic disorders that widely depress or interrupt cortical function
4. Psychiatric disorders resembling coma

DIAGNOSTIC STATEMENT

The limb-dropping test (upper extremities) is positive. This result indicates a reduced level of consciousness that is feigned.

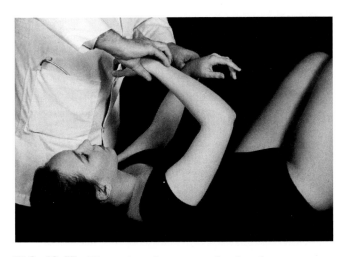

FIG. 13-57 The patient, in a state of reduced awareness or consciousness, is recumbent on the examination table. The examiner elevates the patient's arms by the wrists.

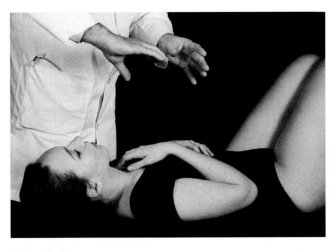

FIG. 13-58 The arms are allowed to drop over the patient's chest.

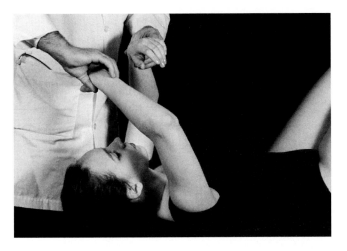

FIG. 13-59 The test is repeated, this time with the examiner holding the arms over the patient's head and face.

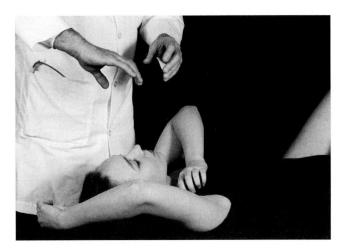

FIG. 13-60 The arms are allowed to drop. The test is positive when the arms are swerved to avoid striking the face. A positive test indicates a lack of organic basis for the reduced level of awareness or consciousness.

LOMBARD'S TEST

Assessment for Simulated Deafness

Comment
Anomalies of the external auditory canal, eardrum, middle ear, or eustachian tube that interfere with the conduction of sound waves to the inner ear may be responsible for conductive deafness. In this category are mechanical obstructions of the external auditory canal from a foreign object, cerumen, furuncle, osteoma, or stenosis. Perforation, scarring, or inflammation of the tympanic membrane also restrict sound-wave movement in the ear. Ankylosis of the ossicles, middle ear inflammation (acute or chronic), tumor, or osteosclerotic involvement of the oval window margin restricts the vibration of the footplate of the stapes. Obstruction of the eustachian tube by inflammation, stenosis, tumor, or lymphoid hypertrophy at the ostium also diminishes conductive hearing.

PROCEDURE
- Lombard's auditory test is a test of hearing that relies on the effect of induced noise on a subject's hearing responses.
- The test is used in the investigation of nonorganic hearing loss.

- The patient with hearing loss is seated for this examination.
- The examiner engages the patient in conversation or has the patient read aloud from a page.
- As the reading progresses or the conversation continues, background noise is induced and amplified (Fig. 13-61).
- If the patient's voice grows louder with the background noise, the testing is positive and indicates nonorganic hearing loss.

Confirmation Procedure
Gault test

DIAGNOSTIC STATEMENT

Lombard's test is positive. This result indicates simulated deafness.

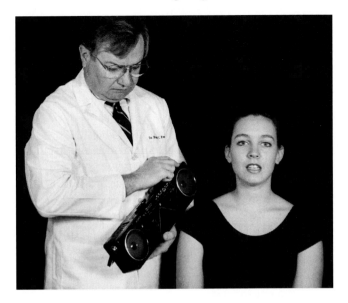

FIG. 13-61 The patient with hearing loss is seated for this examination. The examiner engages the patient in conversation or has the patient read aloud from a page. As the reading progresses or the conversation continues, background noise is induced and amplified. If the patient's voice grows louder with the background noise, the testing is positive and indicates nonorganic hearing loss.

MARCUS GUNN'S SIGN

Assessment for Normal Optic Neural Function

Comment

Optic neuritis is inflammation of that portion of the optic nerve that is ophthalmoscopically visible. This inflammation occurs with meningitis, encephalitis, syphilis, and acute febrile diseases; with foci of infection and multiple sclerosis; and with poisoning by methyl alcohol, carbon tetrachloride, lead, and thallium. Optic neuritis is almost always unilateral. Disturbances of vision are the only symptoms, which vary from minimal contraction of the visual field to enlargement of the blind spot to complete blindness and pain during motion of the globe. The maximum reduction of vision is often reached within 1 or 2 days. The disease can last for months. Ophthalmoscopic examination discloses hyperemia and minimal edema of the disc in the early stages, with more noticeable changes in advanced cases.

The Marcus Gunn's sign represents an afferent pupillary defect caused by a lesion of the optic nerve. Resting pupil sizes are normal. Both direct and consensual pupillary responses are decreased (reduced constriction) with bright illumination of the involved side. Both responses are normal with illumination of the normal side. When moving the light back to the involved eye, both pupils dilate, and both constrict with stimulation on the normal side.

PROCEDURE

- If there is an organic basis for unilateral blindness, the lesion must be situated anteriorly to the optic chiasm, and the pupillary reaction is usually abnormal.

- Marcus Gunn's sign is especially useful for evaluating the existence of unilateral blindness.
- To elicit the Marcus Gunn's sign, the patient's eyes are fixed at a distant point and a strong light shone on the intact eye (Fig. 13-62).
- A crisp, bilateral contraction of the pupils is noted.
- Upon moving the light to the affected eye, both pupils dilate for a brief period (Fig. 13-63).
- When the light is returned to the intact eye, both pupils contract promptly and remain contracted (Fig. 13-64).
- This response indicates damage to the optic nerve on the affected side.

Confirmation Procedures

Cuignet's test, optokinetic nystagmus testing, and Snellen's test

---

DIAGNOSTIC STATEMENT

Marcus Gunn's sign cannot be demonstrated. The absence of this sign indicates normal optic nerve functioning bilaterally.

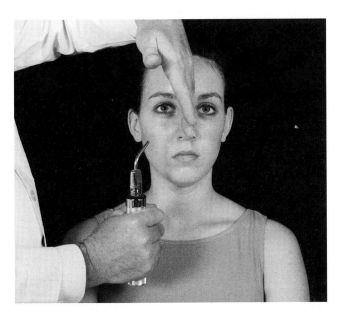

FIG. 13-62 To elicit the Marcus Gunn's sign, the seated patient's eyes are fixed at a distant point. The examination room is dimmed, and a strong light is shone on the normal eye. The examiner notes a crisp bilateral contraction of the pupils.

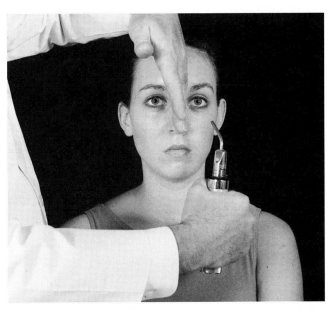

FIG. 13-63 Upon moving the light to the affected eye, both pupils dilate for a brief period.

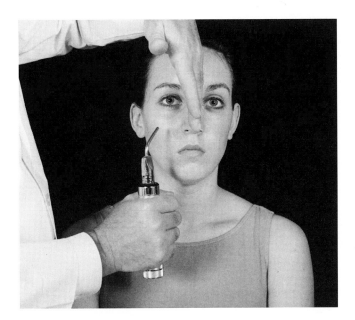

FIG. 13-64 On return of the light to the intact eye, both pupils contract promptly and remain contracted. This response indicates damage to the optic nerve on the affected side. The absence of Marcus Gunn's sign in unilateral blindness indicates a nonorganic basis for the complaint.

MIDLINE TUNING-FORK TEST

Assessment for Simulated Anesthesia

Comment

Fibers conveying touch, superficial pain, and temperature pass via cutaneous nerves to mixed nerves, where they are joined by fibers carrying impulses from joints, ligaments, and muscles. Lesions of cutaneous nerves will not cause proprioceptive sensory loss, but interruption of mixed nerves and pure motor nerves will. All sensory fibers have their cell station in the ganglia of the cranial nerves or the posterior spinal roots. The spinal roots enter the posterolateral aspect of the cord in the root entry zone. Fibers conveying touch and postural sensibility pass upward in the posterior columns to the nuclei gracilis and cuneatus in the medulla. Those from the lower half of the body lie medially, and those from the upper half of the body occupy the lateral portion of the posterior column. These fibers cross the midline of the central nervous system as sensory decussation, form the medial lemniscus, and then pass upward through the brainstem to the thalamus.

Many feigned complaints fall in the category of sensory loss. Complaints of this kind usually manifest as numbness or anesthesia of a body part. The major distinguishing factor between feigned numbness and organic anesthesia is the disregard of the former for anatomic continuity. Indeed feigned numbness includes all levels of sense (e.g., light touch, heat, cold, position, deep pressure) However, such instances of sensory loss are physically impossible without spinal cord transection. Conversion reactions that involve only the sensory systems are difficult to prove. Organic sensory losses follow known anatomic distributions, but conversion reaction sensory disturbances follow the patient's perception of human anatomy.

PROCEDURE

- Patients with organic sensory disturbances are able to perceive a vibrating tuning fork placed on either side of the head or on either side of the sternum because the conduction vibrates through the bone (Fig. 13-65).
- In a conversion reaction, the sternum or head is split.
- For example, vibration is perceived on one side of the midline of the forehead or sternum but not on the other.

Confirmation Procedures

Janet's test and regional anesthesia testing

DIAGNOSTIC STATEMENT

The midline tuning-fork test is positive. This test indicates simulated anesthesia on the right.

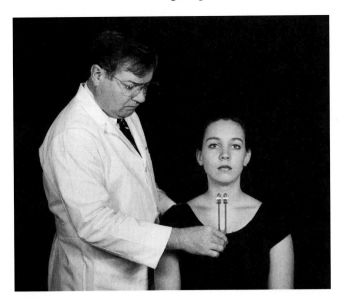

FIG. 13-65 The patient may be seated or recumbent. The examiner places a vibrating tuning fork on the affected side of the sternum, near the midline. The patient is instructed to identify areas of perceived vibration. If the patient does not feel the vibration, the tuning fork is moved across the midline to the normal side. The test is positive if the patient identifies that vibration is felt only on the normal half of the body and not on the affected side. The positive test indicates hysteria, conversion reaction, or malingering.

OPTOKINETIC NYSTAGMUS TEST

Assessment for Feigned Blindness

Comment

Nystagmus is a rhythmic horizontal or vertical oscillation of the eyeballs. This oscillation is more pronounced when the patient is looking in certain directions. Nystagmus is often a sign of cerebellar, vestibular, or labyrinthine disease, and it is a common sign in certain systemic diseases, such as multiple sclerosis. Prolonged use of the eyes with insufficient illumination and in strained positions, such as that maintained by miners, and fatigue of the eye muscles, especially when caused by errors of refraction, also may be causative. Vestibular stimulation causes nystagmus.

PROCEDURE

- With faked blindness, the patient will often avoid personal injury when walking and will blink to unexpected physical threats.
- Pupillary reactions are normal, and optokinetic nystagmus is normal.
- To demonstrate optokinetic nystagmus, the examiner instructs the patient to keep the eyes open.
- The examiner holds a ruler or a tape measure 10 inches in front of the patient's face, ostensibly to measure pupillary distances (Fig. 13-66).

- As the pupils constrict, which demonstrates attempted focusing, the ruler is moved from left to right across the patient's field of vision (Fig. 13-67).
- A patient who can see the ruler will fix the vision on the vertical markings and develop an involuntary eye movement called *optokinetic nystagmus*.
- This is a similar phenomenon to a person riding in a vehicle and looking out the window watching telephone poles go by.
- This test is used when routine eye examination reveals a normal fundus and intact pupillary reactions to light.
- With organic blindness, pupillary reflexes are abnormal and optokinetic nystagmus is absent.
- Hysterical field defects, when plotted out on a tangent screen, will not change with the varying distance between the patient and the screen.

Confirmation Procedures

Cuignet's test, Marcus Gunn's sign, and Snellen's test

DIAGNOSTIC STATEMENT

Optokinetic nystagmus is present and does not support the patient's complaint of blindness.

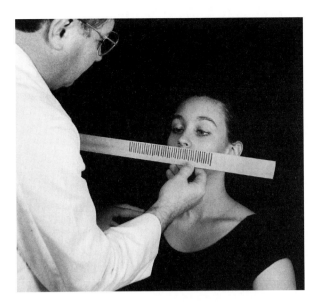

FIG. 13-66 The patient is seated. The examiner instructs the patient to keep the eyes open. A ruler or a tape measure is held approximately 10 inches in front of the patient's face. The examiner holds the ruler still and observes the patient's eyes for slight pupil constriction, indicating the attempt of the eyes to focus on the ruler markings.

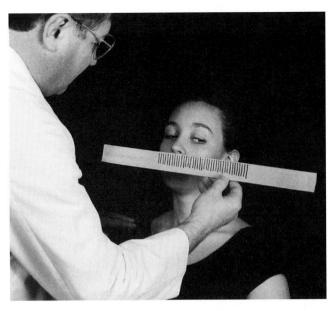

FIG. 13-67 The ruler is moved from left to right, across the patient's field of vision. A patient who can see the ruler will fix the vision on the vertical markings, and develop an involuntary eye movement, called *optokinetic nystagmus.* This test is used when routine eye examination reveals a normal fundus and intact pupillary reactions to light. Optokinetic nystagmus suggests a lack of organic basis for the blindness.

Assessment for Feigned Loss of Position Sense

Comment

Hereditary spastic paraplegia is familiar, but it may be present without a history of cases in previous generations because sporadic cases do occur. The symptoms are those of a slowly progressive degeneration of the pyramidal tracts, starting between 3 and 15 years of age but rarely at older ages. For a time, there is only a spastic paraplegia, but gradually spastic weakness spreads to the upper limbs and ultimately to the bulbar muscles. There is no sensory loss, but optic atrophy may occur. The disease takes many years to run its course and is one of the heredofamilial groups, of which Friedreich's ataxia is the best known. With the latter disease, symptoms usually come on in childhood or adolescence, and the earliest complaints are of weakness and clumsiness of the legs. Ataxia of gait is apt to obscure the presence of weakness because of pyramidal degeneration. This is more so as tendon reflexes are diminished or absent and tone is reduced. The ataxia is partly caused by degeneration of the spinocerebellar tracts and partly by loss of position sense.

PROCEDURE

- If a patient claims that the position of a body part cannot be differentiated, the patient is directed to close the eyes, and the examiner bends the patient's fingers or toes up or down (Fig. 13-68).
- The patient is instructed to state what direction the examiner is bending the digit.
- A patient may report contrary findings by saying "up" when the examiner is bringing the digit down, and vice versa (Fig. 13-69).
- With organic sensory loss, the patient has a 50% chance of correctly guessing the digit position.
- The malingerer's reporting average is always contrary to the actual digit position and therefore incorrect a majority of the time.

Confirmation Procedures

Coordination-disturbance testing, limb-dropping test (upper extremities), and Romberg test

---

DIAGNOSTIC STATEMENT

Position-sense testing is positive on the right. This result indicates feigned loss of position sense.

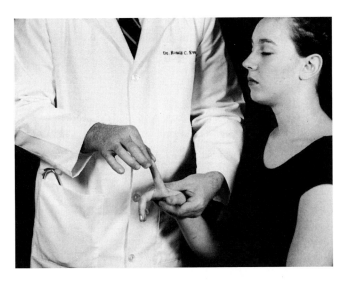

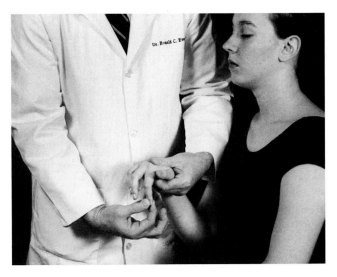

FIG. 13-68   The patient may be seated or recumbent. The patient is instructed to close the eyes. The examiner bends the patient's finger (or toe) up.

FIG. 13-69   The finger or toe is then bent down. The patient is instructed to identify the direction of the digit movement. The patient may report contrary findings to the actual position of the digit. In organic sensory loss, the patient has a 50% chance of success rate at guessing the digit position. The test is positive when the patient is consistently wrong. This result suggests malingering.

REGIONAL ANESTHESIA TESTING

Assessment for Feigned Anesthesia

Comment

Conversion of anxiety into symptoms of dysfunction of various organs or parts of the body is a common characteristic of conversion hysteria. The emotional conflict, instead of being experienced consciously, is converted into physical symptoms involving voluntary muscles or special sense organs. The patient often appears unconcerned about the sensory or motor paralysis (la belle indifference). The reaction not only serves to allay anxiety, but also may provide some secondary gain. The conversion symptom does not always follow the anatomic distribution of the sensorimotor nerves, but it is determined symbolically (glove or stocking anesthesia, tunnel vision). These reactions help in understanding the nature of the unconscious conflict.

PROCEDURE

- To define a regional complaint of numbness, the examiner uses a straight pin or a Wartenberg pinwheel and delineates the areas where the claimed numbness ceases.
- The usual organic cause of anesthesia or paresthesia is peripheral neuritis.
- With peripheral neuritis, the upper border of the anesthesia is blurry and usually different for each different sensation tested, such as pain, touch, heat, and vibration.

- In the hysterical or malingering patient, the border of anesthesia is extremely abrupt, stopping at a wrist crease, or some other external anatomic area that is unrelated to the dermatome pattern (Fig. 13-70).
- This numbness landmark may even vary from examination to examination.
- Most malingerers claim a simultaneous loss of all forms of sensation, including touch, pain, temperature, and vibratory sensation.
- All losses are identical as to extent and accurate neural distribution or dermatome patterns are not present.

Confirmation Procedures

Janet's test and midline tuning-fork test

DIAGNOSTIC STATEMENT

Regional anesthesia testing indicates a loss of all sensory modalities that do not follow known anatomic distributions. This loss indicates a lack of organic basis for the patient's complaint of anesthesia.

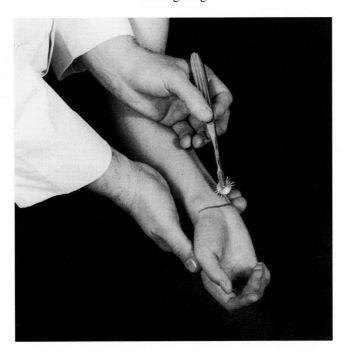

FIG. 13-70   The patient may be seated or recumbent for this test. The patient identifies the area of numbness. The examiner, using a pin or Wartenberg pinwheel, delineates the boundaries of the numbness. The test is positive when the borders of the anesthesia are extremely abrupt, stopping at some anatomic landmark unrelated to the dermatome involved. Such a sensory deficit distribution suggests malingering or hysteria.

ROMBERG'S SIGN

ALSO KNOWN AS STATION TEST

Assessment for Nonorganic Ataxia

Comment
Tabetic or ataxic gait is characteristic of posterior column disease and results from the loss of proprioceptive sense in the extremities. The patient walks on a wide base, slapping the feet, and usually watches the legs to know where they are. When the eyes are closed or the patient is in the dark, the ataxia is much worse. Clumsiness and uncertainty are characteristic. The feet are placed too widely apart, and in taking a step, the patient lifts the advancing leg abruptly and too high and then stamps or slaps the foot solidly to the ground. Uneven spacing of steps, tottering, and swaying occur, usually with deviation to one side or the other.

PROCEDURE
- With this disorder of balance loss, the patient is instructed to stand with the feet together, first with the eyes open, then with the eyes closed (Fig. 13-71).

- With organic sensory ataxia, the patient will sway the body from the ankles (Fig. 13-72).
- Swaying from the hips, toward a wall to catch one's self in the nick of time, suggests malingering (Fig. 13-73).

Confirmation Procedures
Coordination-disturbance testing, limb-dropping test (upper extremities), and position-sense testing

> ### DIAGNOSTIC STATEMENT
> Romberg's sign is absent. The patient sways from the hips. The absence of this sign indicates a lack of organic basis for the patient's ataxia.

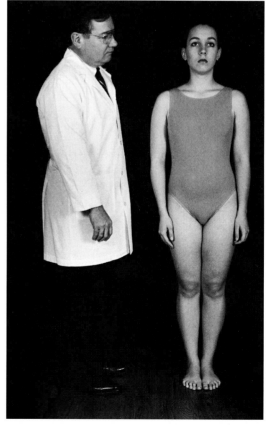

FIG. 13-71 The patient is standing and instructed to place the feet close together. The patient's eyes are open.

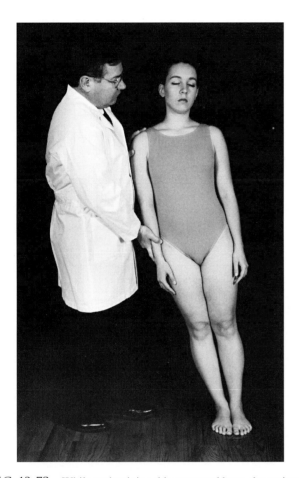

FIG. 13-72   While maintaining this narrowed base, the patient is instructed to close the eyes. In organic ataxia, the patient will lose balance, usually by falling from the ankles toward the side of the cerebellar lesion. The examiner maintains proximity to the patient for safety.

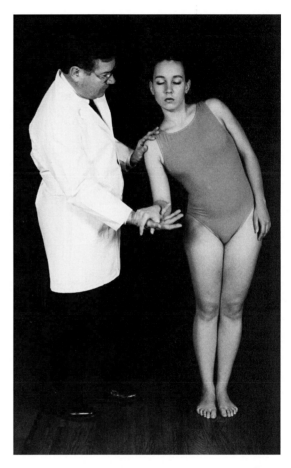

FIG. 13-73   The malingering patient will sway from the pelvis, usually toward a wall, catching the fall in the nick of time. In this instance, the sign is absent and indicates a lack of organic basis for the patient's loss of balance.

Assessment for Feigned Color Blindness

Comment

ORTHOPEDIC GAMUT 13-19

COLOR BLINDNESS

Color blindness may be hereditary or acquired. Hereditary types are transmitted as recessive characteristics, sometimes X-linked. These include the following:

1. Achromatopsia (total color blindness)
2. Monochromatism (partial color blindness, with ability to recognize one of the three basic colors remaining)
3. Dichromatism (ability to recognize two of the three basic colors)

In normal (trichromatic) vision, the eye can perceive three light primaries (red, blue, and green) and can mix these in suitable portions, so white or any color of the spectrum can be matched. Color blindness can result from a lessened capacity to match three primary colors. It can be dichromatic vision, in which only one pair of the primary colors is perceived, the two colors being complimentary to each other. Most dichromats are red-green blind and confuse red, yellow, and green.

PROCEDURE

- For pretended color blindness in one eye, the patient is requested to look at alternate red and green letters (Fig. 13-74).
- The admittedly good eye is covered with a red glass (Fig. 13-75).
- If the green letters are read, evidence of fraud is present.

Confirmation Procedures

Cuignet's test, Marcus Gunn's sign, and optokinetic nystagmus testing

---

DIAGNOSTIC STATEMENT

Snellen's test is positive on the right. This result indicates feigned color blindness on that side.

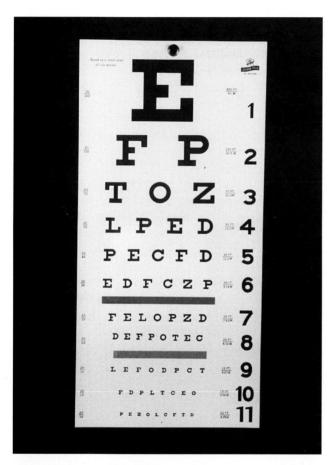

FIG. 13-74 The seated patient is placed an appropriate distance from a Snellen eye chart. The patient is instructed to read the red and green letters, using one eye at a time. The patient will state that the colorblind eye cannot read the chart.

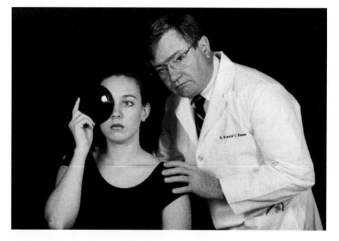

FIG. 13-75 The vision of the good eye is obscured with a red lens, and the patient is instructed to reread the chart. If the green letters are read, the test is positive. A positive test indicates that the vision of the alleged blind eye is preserved. This suggests malingering.

STOICISM INDEXING

Assessment for Congenital Insensitivity to Pain

Comment

Although it is rare, some patients are born with a lack of any pain appreciation. This is a congenital indifference to pain or an inability to perceive it at all. Whether the patient feels the pain but is indifferent to it or whether the patient lacks any pain sensation is difficult to determine. The patient does not suffer. The cause of this congenital absence of pain perception is unknown. As children, these patients undergo falls and bumps but never cry. The defect is central rather than peripheral because the child recognizes the stimulus without exhibiting signs of pain. Normal nerve endings, which subserve pain sensibilities, are found in the skin and periosteum. Free nerve endings are also found in the glandular tissue. Progressive degenerative changes of the Charcot type are observed in the adult joints of these patients.

PROCEDURE

- The interval between eye blinks in the average patient is 25 to 30 seconds (Fig. 13-76).

- A 60-second lapse between blinks, while staring straight ahead, indicates a patient who is stoic (Fig. 13-77).
- A stoic patient can be described as impassive and calm in the face of pain and discomfort.
- They may also be cool and indifferent to the sensations elicited in testing.

Confirmation Procedures

Libman's sign, Mannkopf's sign, marked part pain-suggestibility test, and related joint motion test

---

DIAGNOSTIC STATEMENT

The stoicism index for this patient is greater than 60 seconds. This result indicates a congenital insensitivity to pain.

The stoicism index for the patient is 10. This result indicates hypersensitivity to pain.

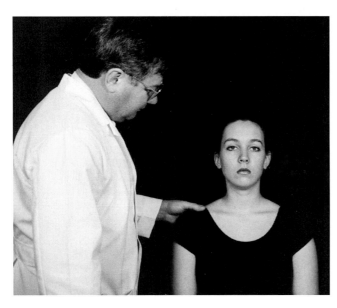

FIG. 13-76   The patient is seated, and the examiner observes the interval between blinks as the patient stares straight ahead.

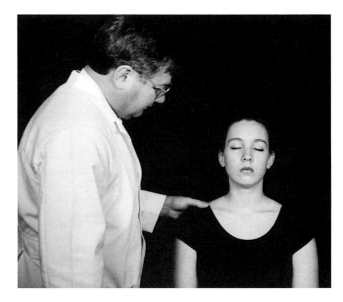

FIG. 13-77   A lapse of 60 seconds or more between blinks indicates decreased sensitivity to pain. A lapse of less than 20 seconds indicates a patient hypersensitive to pain.

PARALYSIS QUALIFICATION AND QUANTIFICATION

Overview

Motion is a fundamental property of most animal life. The lowest multicellular animals possess rudimentary neuromuscular mechanisms. In higher forms, motion is based on the transmission of impulses from a receptor through an afferent neuron and ganglion cell to muscle. This same principle is found in the reflex arc of higher animals, including humans, in whom the anterior spinal cord has developed into a central regulating mechanism. This central regulating mechanism is concerned with initiating and integrating movements.

Motor disturbances include weakness and paralysis, which may result from lesions of the voluntary motor pathways or of the muscles themselves. Impaired motor functioning may result from involvement of muscle, myoneural junction, peripheral nerve, or the central nervous system.

The types of paralysis or paresis are based on the location. Hemiplegia is a spastic or flaccid paralysis of one side of the body and extremities, limited by the median line sagittally.

Monoplegia is a paralysis of one extremity only. Diplegia is a paralysis of any two corresponding extremities, both of which are usually lower extremities, but may be upper extremities. Paraplegia is a symmetric paralysis of both lower extremities. Quadriplegia, or tetraplegia, is a paralysis of all four extremities. Hemiplegia alternans (crossed paralysis) is a paralysis of one or more ipsilateral cranial nerves and contralateral paralysis of the arm and leg.

Paralyses occur in many patients with hysteria, and they may be spastic or flaccid. With hysterical contracture, the affected muscles are not atrophied, except in severe cases of long duration. The deep tendon reflexes are increased and a spurious ankle-clonus may be present, but the Babinski sign is not observed. The limbs are most affected, as is the case with hemiplegia, monoplegia, or paraplegia. Less often, the muscles of the face are affected. Certain attitudes are characteristic of hysterical paralyses. The elbows, wrists, and fingers are kept flexed, and the arms are adducted. The hip and knee are extended, and the foot is held in a position of talipes equinovarus. Ptosis of the face may be simulated by spasm of the orbicularis palpebrarum, torticollis by contracture of the sternomastoid. In the less severe cases, the stiffness and paresis are neither complete nor marked enough for the condition to be called a *contracture*. The deformity produced is the result of active muscular spasm. In severe and longstanding cases, a true contracture results and the limb cannot be straightened by ordinary mechanical means. Highly characteristic of hysterical contracture is the patient's use of antagonistic muscles to prevent passive or active correction of the deformity exhibited.

CLINICAL PEARL (PARALYSIS ASSESSMENT)

Abnormalities of the motor system, which may be manifestations of both hysteria and malingering, include disturbances of muscle strength and power; disorders of tone; dyskinesia; and abnormalities of coordination, station, and gait. There are rarely changes in volume or contour (except for wasting from disuse), and no abnormalities are found on EMG. These motor changes of psychic etiology may resemble almost any type of motor disturbance that is brought about by organic disease of the nervous system.

In both hysterical and malingered paralyses, the patient makes little effort to contract the muscles necessary for executing the desired movement. The patient may remain calm and indifferent while demonstrating the lack of strength. The patient may also show little sign of alarm at the presence of complete paralysis and may smile cheerfully during the examination. Reliable evidence that the patient is not exerting all available power in an attempt to carry out a voluntary movement can be elicited by watching and palpating the contraction of the antagonists as well as the agonists.

BILATERAL LIMB-DROPPING TEST (LOWER EXTREMITIES)

Assessment for Feigned Paresis of Lower Extremity

Comment
Muscle imbalance at the hip encourages subluxation and dislocation. When the equilibrium between the flexor-adductor group and the abductor-extensor group is altered, so the former overpowers the latter, the femoral neck is pulled medially to a more vertical position.

Disproportionate muscle forces necessary for producing subluxation and dislocation occur most often in children with myelomeningocele. Paralysis or paresis in one or both lower extremities is present at birth in more than 90% of the infants with thoracolumbar or lumbar myelomeningocele and in more than 50% with lumbosacral or sacral myelomeningocele. The peculiar muscle imbalance is also found—but this is uncommon—in cerebral palsy, poliomyelitis, and diseases and injuries of the cauda equina.

PROCEDURE
- Lower extremities are usually portrayed to be either weak or completely paralyzed.
- To determine whether the patient has a weak hip or leg, the patient is placed on the examination table in a supine position.
- The examiner flexes the legs at the hip, keeping the knees straight.
- The examiner holds the legs in an elevated position by cradling the patient's feet in a hand and instructs the patient to push the legs downward and hard against the examiner's hand (Fig. 13-78).
- The examiner suddenly pulls the hand away (Fig. 13-79).
- If leg weakness is of an organic origin, the affected leg will fall to the examination table.
- If the weakness is faked, the leg may move up or hang in midair for a moment before falling because of hip muscle flexor actuation.

Confirmation Procedures
Hoover's sign, simulated foot-drop testing, and tripod test (bilateral leg-fluttering test)

DIAGNOSTIC STATEMENT
Lower extremity limb-dropping test indicates feigned paresis of the right leg.

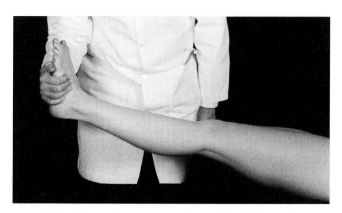

FIG. 13-78 The patient is lying supine on the examination table. The examiner performs a bilateral straight-leg-raising test. As the legs are in the elevated position, the examiner instructs the patient to push the heels of the legs downward, against the examiner's resistance.

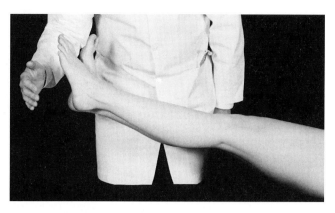

FIG. 13-79 The examiner unexpectedly pulls the supporting hand away from the legs. The leg affected with simulated paralysis will hang in the air momentarily before falling to the table. This result represents a positive test and indicates hysteria or malingering.

HEMIPLEGIC POSTURING

Assessment for Nonorganic Hemiplegia

Comment

Intracerebral hemorrhage destroys the parenchyma. Cerebral thrombosis or embolism causes necrosis of the parenchyma (infarction, encephalomalacia) in the area supplied by the occluded vessel. If the embolus is septic and infection spreads beyond the vessel wall, encephalitis, brain abscess, or meningitis may result.

The site of the lesion determines specific symptoms. Cerebral hemorrhage is most common in the region of the thalamus and internal capsule and is usually accompanied by severe hemiplegia, hemianesthesia, speech disturbance, and sometimes hemianopsia. Because the middle cerebral artery or its branches are often the site of thrombosis or embolism, common symptoms are hemiplegia (affecting the arm more than the leg) and cortical sensory loss in the affected limbs. Various disturbances (aphasia and apraxia) may follow damage to the dominant hemisphere.

PROCEDURE

- Paralysis is yet another symptom presentation from the repertoire of the hysteric, psychogenic, rheumatic, or malingering patient.
- A patient with a feigned paralyzed leg and arm may incorrectly assume there also will be difficulty in turning the head toward the paralyzed side (Fig. 13-80).
- Pronation drift (the inability to hold the pronated arms still) is absent on station and gait.

DIAGNOSTIC STATEMENT

Hemiplegic posturing is present and is inconsistent with organic hemiplegia.

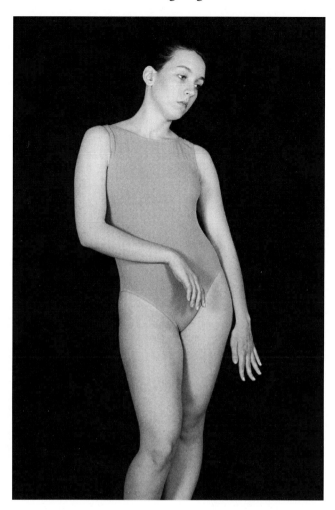

FIG. 13-80 The patient is standing, and the examiner assesses the patient's posture. In feigned paralysis, the paralyzed arm and leg are held in typical flexion contractures. The patient incorrectly assumes that the head cannot be turned toward the paralyzed side. Pronation drift is absent. This behavior indicates malingering or hysteria.

HOOVER'S SIGN

Assessment for Feigned Leg Paresis

Comment

Neurologic loss is usually described as a sensory or motor deficit. The sensory loss may produce hypoesthesia, paresthesia, or hyperesthesia and may manifest as pain or numbness over a specific area. The motor deficits may be described as a weakness, as stiffness, or more commonly, as difficulty in walking far, running, or jumping. If there is outright paralysis, the onset may have been sudden or insidious. The paralysis may be flaccid or spastic. Flaccidity is associated with lower motor neuron disorders and spasticity with upper motor neuron disorders. The examiner must determine whether the symptoms have increased or decreased and to what degree the patient is disabled. The examiner must also determine whether there has been a loss of sphincter control of the bladder and rectum.

PROCEDURE

- Hoover's sign is helpful in differentiating between organic and hysterical paralysis.
- When a supine patient is directed to lift the paralyzed or affected one leg, it is normal for the patient to unconsciously press the heel of the unaffected leg against the examination table.
- In organic hemiplegia, this downward pressure is accentuated on the healthy side as the patient attempts to raise the paretic leg.
- If the examiner places a hand under the heel, this pressure can be felt (Fig. 13-81).
- In malingering, there will be no, or very little, pressure on the opposite side of the affection as the patient attempts to raise the involved extremity.

Confirmation Procedures

Bilateral limb-dropping test (lower extremities), simulated foot-drop testing, and tripod test (bilateral leg-fluttering test)

DIAGNOSTIC STATEMENT

Hoover's sign is present on the right. The presence of this sign indicates feigned leg paresis.

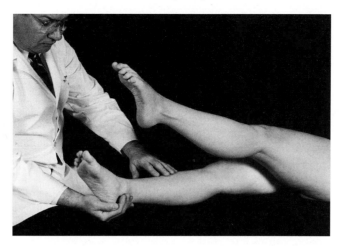

FIG. 13-81   The patient is lying supine on the examination table. The examiner places one hand under the heel of the unaffected leg. The patient attempts to lift the paralyzed leg off the table. The organically paralyzed patient presses the unaffected leg firmly downward, when attempting to flex the paralyzed hip. Because the malingerer is not trying, this synergistic action does not occur. The sign is present when the counterpressure is absent on the unaffected side. The sign indicates malingering or hysteria.

SIMULATED FOOT-DROP TESTING

Assessment for Feigned Steppage Gait or Foot Drop

Comment

Complicated, coordinated movements are examined by observing the patient's manner of walking. Paresis will produce a slow, guarded, short-stepped, and shuffling gait. Paralysis of the anterior tibial muscles, especially by anterior horn or peripheral nerve lesion, causes a drop foot and produces a steppage gait. To avoid tripping over the plantar flexed foot, the extremity is advanced with the knee and hip flexed. With spasticity, the legs are advanced slowly with shortened steps, and the toes scrape the ground. Adductor tightness produces a scissors gait, by which the legs are alternately crossed. With the ataxic, or tabetic, gait, the patient must constantly observe the placement of the feet because of the absence of deep position sense. The hip is flexed and externally rotated, and the forefoot is strongly dorsiflexed before being thrown down with the heel striking first. The patient is unable to stand with the eyes closed. In contrast, cerebellar ataxia is not aided by visual assistance. The gait appears stumbling and drunken, because the patient sways from side to side, and there is a tendency to fall toward the side of the lesion.

PROCEDURE

- With feigned total leg weakness/paralysis, a patient may pretend to be unable to raise the forefoot while walking.

- This complaint must be separated from organic foot drop.
- The patient is standing, and the examiner is positioned behind the patient (Fig. 13-82).
- The patient is instructed to maintain a rigid and narrow-based posture, with the feet close together.
- In a surprise move, the examiner grasps the shoulders of the patient and pulls the patient's body backward (Fig. 13-83).
- The examiner notes the movement of the toes and forefoot.
- If the forefoot rises, the test is positive.
- A positive test indicates feigned foot drop.

Confirmation Procedures

Bilateral limb-dropping test (lower extremities), Hoover's sign, and tripod test (bilateral leg-fluttering test)

DIAGNOSTIC STATEMENT

Simulated foot-drop testing is positive. This result indicates a feigned steppage gait or foot drop.

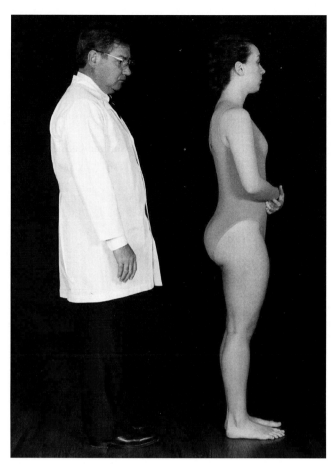

FIG. 13-82 The patient is standing, and the examiner is positioned behind the patient. The patient is instructed to maintain a rigid and narrow-based posture with the feet close together.

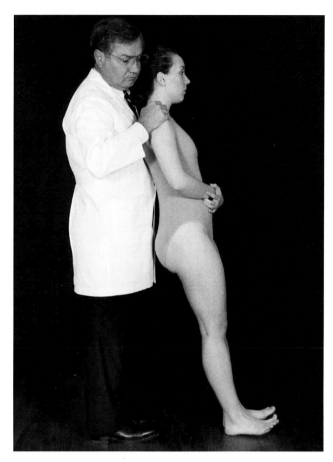

FIG. 13-83 In a surprise move, the examiner grasps the shoulders of the patient and pulls the patient's body backward. The examiner notes the movement of the toes and forefoot. If the forefoot rises, the test is positive. The positive test indicates feigned foot drop.

SIMULATED FOREARM-AND-WRIST-WEAKNESS TESTING

Assessment for Simulated Weakness of Forearm and Wrist

Comment
Although the function of one hand may be assessed, the impairment of function in one hand may clearly affect many activities that normally involve both hands performing together. The degree of overall functional impairment may be investigated by inquiring about or testing the patient's ability to perform certain tasks. This can be assessed efficiently with the Lamb Bilateral Hand Activity Index illustrated in the following box.

PROCEDURE
- If the complaint is persisting forearm or wrist weakness that is not associated with grip strength loss, the patient is directed to dorsiflex the wrist, usually by making a fist.

- If this cannot be done, the patient is then asked to squeeze a dynamometer while the examiner palpates the patient's forearm (Fig. 13-84).
- In functional or feigned weakness, the examiner will feel the patient's forearm extensors contract synergistically and will see the wrist extend when the patient squeezes.

Confirmation Procedure
Simulated grip-strength-loss testing

DIAGNOSTIC STATEMENT
Testing for simulated weakness of the forearm and wrist is positive on the right. This result indicates feigned muscular weakness.

ORTHOPEDIC GAMUT 13-20

LAMB BILATERAL HAND ACTIVITY INDEX

Lamb bilateral hand activity index of activities performed with both hands acting together*
Unscrew the top from a bottle.
Fill a cup or glass and drink.
Open a can with a manual can-opener.
Remove a match from a box or book and light it.
Use a knife and fork for eating.
Apply toothpaste to a toothbrush and clean teeth.
Put on a jacket.
Close buttons on clothing.
Fasten a belt around the waist.
Tie shoelaces.

Sharpen a pencil in a manual sharpener.
Write messages.
Use a dial telephone.
Staple papers together.
Wrap string around a package.
Use playing cards.

When progress is being measured, each of these items listed in the box below may be scored on a scale of 0 to 5, or 0 to 10, and added. A total score of 80 or 160, respectively, represents a return to normal bilateral hand functions.

*Modified from McRae R: *Clinical orthopaedic examination,* ed 3, Edinburgh, 1990, Churchill Livingstone.

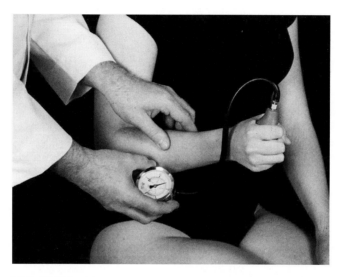

FIG. 13-84   The patient is seated and is directed to dorsiflex the wrist. If this move cannot be accomplished, the examiner instructs the patient to grip and squeeze a dynamometer. As the patient squeezes, the examiner palpates the forearm musculature. The test is positive when the examiner notes synergistic contraction of the forearm extensors and observes slight wrist dorsiflexion. The test is significant for feigned muscular weakness.

SIMULATED GRIP-STRENGTH-LOSS TESTING

Assessment for Simulated Grip Strength Loss

Comment

When a patient complains of weakness, the physician must consider many possible causes. There is such a wide range of differential diagnosis that an evaluation for all the possible causes of weakness not only would be cumbersome but also costly for the patient and time-consuming for the examiner. Perhaps even more important, the patient is exposed to potentially hazardous and painful tests that might be unnecessary. Therefore it is desirable to ascertain the anatomic locus of the patient's weakness.

When a weak patient presents with evidence of motor unit disease and the cause is not myopathic, the patient probably has a neuropathy.

PROCEDURE

- When grip strength loss is the complaint, the patient is directed to squeeze the examiner's fingers with the paralyzed hand as hard as possible (Fig. 13-85).
- While the patient does this, the examiner suddenly tears the fingers away.
- If grip weakness is caused by organic disease, a sudden tug will break the grasp easily.
- If the weakness is being faked, strong resistance is likely to be encountered before the malingerer realizes the error or contradiction and releases the grip (Fig. 13-86).

Confirmation Procedure
Simulated forearm-and-wrist-weakness testing

ORTHOPEDIC GAMUT 13-21

NEUROPATHY

The differential diagnosis of neuropathy includes many diseases that present with similar symptoms (symmetric distal sensory losses). However, patients with neuropathy occasionally may complain of the following symptoms:

1. Thickened nerves (hypertrophic neuropathy)
2. Mononeuritis
3. Radiculopathy
4. Cranial nerve involvement
5. Autonomic disturbances
6. Ascending neuritis
7. Weakness without sensory findings

DIAGNOSTIC STATEMENT

Simulated grip-strength-loss testing is positive on the right. This result indicates feigned loss of strength.

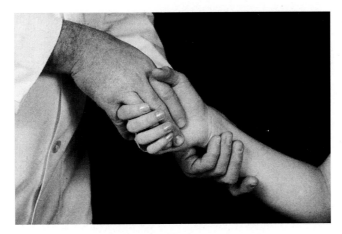

FIG. 13-85   The seated patient is instructed to grip and squeeze the examiner's fingers with the paralyzed hand as hard as possible.

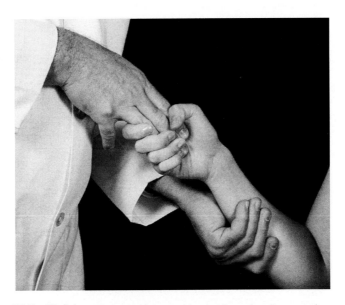

FIG. 13-86   As the patient continues the grip, the examiner unexpectedly tears the fingers from the grip. Strong resistance is likely to be encountered before the patient realizes the error and releases the grip. In organic disease, the sudden tug will break the grasp easily. The test is positive for feigned loss of grip.

TRIPOD TEST (BILATERAL LEG-FLUTTERING TEST)

Assessment for Simulated Lumbar Pain

Comment

Lesions of the lower motor neurons may be located in the ventral gray column of the spinal cord or brainstem or in their axons, which constitute the ventral roots of the spinal nerves or the cranial nerves. Lesions may result from trauma, toxins, infections, vascular disorders, congenital malformations, degenerative processes, or neoplasms. Signs of lower motor neuron lesions include flaccid paralysis of the involved muscles, muscle atrophy, and a degeneration reaction. Reflexes of the involved muscle are diminished or absent and no pathologic reflexes are obtainable.

PROCEDURE

- A patient may attempt to fake a leg paralysis as the result of a further faked lumbar intervertebral disc syndrome.
- In this instance, the patient is instructed to sit on the examination table with the knees flexed at 90 degrees and the legs hanging dependent (Fig. 13-87).
- The patient is directed to rapidly and repeatedly extend and relax, or flex, the legs (Fig. 13-88).

- If lumbar disc involvement exists, the patient will need to lean back to perform this maneuver, if able to do it at all (Fig. 13-89).
- The patient feigning disc involvement can accomplish the maneuver without assuming such a tripod posture (Fig. 13-90).

Confirmation Procedures

Bilateral limb-dropping test (lower extremities), Hoover's sign, and simulated foot-drop testing

---

DIAGNOSTIC STATEMENT

Tripod testing is negative, and simulated lumbar pain is indicated.

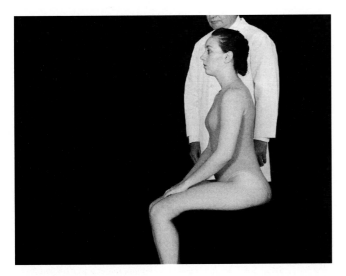

FIG. 13-87   The patient is instructed to sit on the examining table with the knees flexed at 90 degrees and the legs hanging dependent.

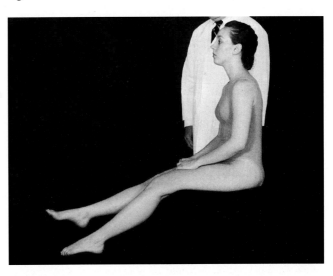

FIG. 13-88   The patient is directed to rapidly and repeatedly extend the legs, in a flutter maneuver.

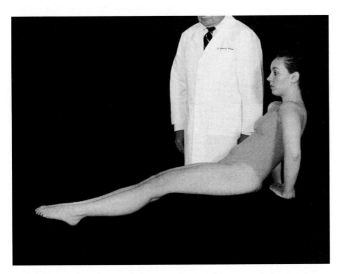

FIG. 13-89   If a lumbar disc involvement exists, the patient will need to lean back to perform this maneuver, if the patient is even able to perform the maneuver at all.

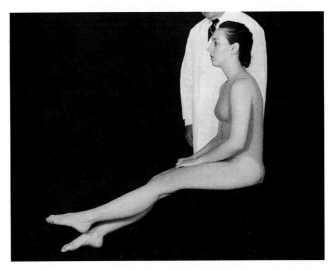

FIG. 13-90   The patient who is feigning disc involvement can accomplish the maneuver without assuming such a tripod posture.

BIBLIOGRAPHY

Abenhaim L, et al: The prognostic consequences in the making of the initial medical diagnosis of work-related back injuries, *Spine* 20:791, 1994.

Abrams WB, Berkow R: *The Merck manual of geriatrics,* Rahway, NJ, 1990, Merck Sharp & Dohme Research Laboratories.

Adams JC, Hamblen DL: *Outline of orthopaedics,* ed 11, Edinburgh, 1990, Churchill Livingstone.

Agnew LRC, editor: *Dorland's illustrated medical dictionary,* ed 27, Philadelphia, 1988, WB Saunders.

Alario AJ: *Practical guide to the care of the pediatric patient,* St Louis, 1997, Mosby.

Allaire SH, et al: Management of work disability, resources for vocational rehabilitation, *Arthritis Rheum* 36:1663, 1993.

Allison D, Strickland N: *Acronyms & synonyms in medical imaging,* Oxford, 1996, ISIS Medical Media.

American College of Sports Medicine: *Guidelines for exercise testing and prescription,* ed 4, Philadelphia, 1991, Lea & Febiger.

American Medical Association: *Guides to the evaluation of permanent impairment,* ed 4, Chicago, 1993, The Association.

American Medical Association: *How to use guides to the evaluation of permanent impairment,* ed 4, Falmouth, Conn, 1993, SEAK.

American Psychiatric Association: *Diagnostic and statistical manual of mental disorders,* ed 3, Washington, 1980, The Association.

Anderson KN, Anderson LE: *Mosby's pocket dictionary of medicine, nursing, & allied health,* ed 2, St Louis, 1994, Mosby.

Apley AG, Solomon L: *Concise system of orthopaedics and fractures,* London, 1988, Butterworth-Heinemann.

Aronoff GM: *Evaluation and treatment of chronic pain,* Baltimore, 1985, Urban and Schwartzenberg.

Aronoff GM, et al: Pain treatment programs: do they run workers to the workplace? *Spine* 2:123, 1987.

Ballinger PW: *Merrill's atlas of radiographic positions and radiologic procedures,* vol 1-3, ed 8, St Louis, 1995, Mosby.

Barkauskas VH, et al: *Health & physical assessment,* ed 2, St Louis, 1998, Mosby.

Battie MC, et al: Managing low back pain: attitudes and treatment preferences of physical therapist, *Phys Ther* 74:219, 1994.

Benson DF, Blumer D: *Psychiatric aspect of neurologic disease,* New York, 1975, Grune & Stratton.

Black HC: *Black's law dictionary,* St Paul, 1990, West Publishing.

Bongers PM, et al: Psychosocial factors at work and musculoskeletal disease, *Scand J Work Environ Health* 19:297, 1993.

Borenstein DG, Wiesel SW: *Low back pain, medical diagnosis and comprehensive management,* Philadelphia, 1987, WB Saunders.

Borg G: Psychophysical bases of perceived exertion, *Med Sci Sport Exercise* 14:377, 1982.

Bradley LA: Multivariate analysis of the MMPI profiles of low back pain patients, *J Behav Med* 1:253, 1978.

Brena SF, Chapman SL: *Pain and litigation, textbook of pain,* Edinburgh, 1984, Churchill Livingstone.

Brooks M, Evans R, Fairclough J: *Sports injuries,* ed 2, London, 1992, Gower Medical.

Brotzman SB: *Clinical orthopaedic rehabilitation,* St Louis, 1996, Mosby.

Brown DE, Neumann RD: *Orthopedic secrets,* Philadelphia, 1995, Hanley & Belfus.

Bucholz RW: *Orthopaedic decision making,* ed 2, St Louis, 1996, Mosby.

Buschbacher RM: *Musculoskeletal disorders, a practical guide for diagnosis and rehabilitation,* Boston, 1994, Andover Medical Publishers.

Campbell JB, Campbell JM: *Mosby's survival guide to medical abbreviations & acronyms prefixes & suffixes symbols Greek alphabet,* St Louis, 1995, Mosby.

Canale ST: *Campbell's operative orthopaedics,* vol 1-4, ed 9, St Louis, 1998, Mosby.

Cassidy JD, et al: Quebec task force on whiplash-associated disorders, redefining "whiplash" and its management (abridged), *Spine* 20(suppl):S1, 1995.

Cipriano JJ: *Photographic manual of regional orthopaedic and neurological test,* ed 3, Baltimore, 1997, Williams & Wilkins.

Cohn RE: *Impairment rating examination and disability evaluation,* ed 3, Wilkesboro, NC, 1994, R Ernest Cohn.

Cole AJ, Herring SA: *The low back pain handbook: a practical guide for the primary care clinician,* Philadelphia, 1997, Hanley & Belfus.

Conwell TD: *Documenting patient progress "daily office charting seminar" thorough accurate quick procedures,* ed 11, Lakewood, Colo, 1990, Clinical Advancement Plus Seminars.

Cousins MJ, Phillips GD: *Acute pain management,* New York, 1986, Churchill Livingstone.

Cramer GD, Darby SA: *Basic and clinical anatomy of the spine, spinal cord, and ans,* St Louis, 1995, Mosby.

Dambro MR, Griffith JA: *Griffith's 5 minute clinical consult,* Baltimore, 1997, Williams & Wilkins.

D'Ambrosia RD: *Musculoskeletal disorders regional examination and differential diagnosis,* Philadelphia, 1977, JB Lippincott.

Dandy DJ: *Essential orthopaedics and trauma,* Edinburgh, 1989, Churchill Livingstone.

Demeter SL, Andersson GBJ, Smith GM: *Disability evaluation,* St Louis, 1996, Mosby.

DeMeyer W: *Technique of the neurologic examination: a programmed text,* New York, 1969, McGraw-Hill.

Deshpande JK, Tobias JD: *The pediatric pain handbook,* St Louis, 1996, Mosby.

DeVellis B: The psychological impact of arthritis: prevalence of depression, *Arthritis Care Res* 8:284, 1995.

Doherty M: *Color atlas and text of osteoarthritis,* London, 1994, Wolfe.

Doherty M, Doherty J: *Clinical examination in rheumatology,* London, 1992, Wolfe.

Doherty M, George E: *Self-assessment picture tests in rheumatology,* London, 1995, Mosby-Wolfe.

Ellard J: Psychological reactions to compensable injury, *Med J Aust* 8:349, 1970.

Epstein O, et al: *Clinical examination,* ed 2, London, 1997, Mosby.

Evans RC: *Overview of orthopedic malingering, CAPIT homecoming and educational symposium,* Rotorura, New Zealand, 1986, Phillip Institute of Science and Technology.

Evans RC: Malingering/symptoms exaggeration. In Sweere JJ, editor: *Chiropractic family practice, a clinical manual,* Gaithersburg, Md, 1992, Aspen.

Fairbank JTC: The Oswestry low back pain disability questionnaire, *Physiotherapy* 8:66, 1980.

Farrar WE: *Atlas of infections of the nervous system,* London, 1993, Wolfe.

Feldmann E: *Current diagnosis in neurology,* St Louis, 1994, Mosby.

Ferezy JS: *The chiropractic neurological examination,* Gaithersburg, Md, 1992, Aspen.

Ferraz MB, et al: EPM-ROM scale: an evaluative instrument to be used in rheumatoid arthritis trials, *Clin Exp Rheumatol* 8:491, 1990.

Finneson BE: *Low back pain,* ed 2, Philadelphia, 1981, JB Lippincott.

Foreman SM, Stahl MJ, Sportelli L: *Medical-legal issues in chiropractic,* Palmerton, Pa, 1993, PracticeMakers Products.

Fries JF: *Arthritis, a take care of yourself health guide for understanding your arthritis,* ed 4, 1995, Addison-Wesley.

Garcia JH: *Neuropathology: the diagnostic approach,* St Louis, 1997, Mosby.

Goldie BS: *Orthopaedic diagnosis and management: a guide to the care of orthopaedic patients,* ed 2, Oxford, 1998, ISIS Medical Media.

Goldner JL: Volkmann's ischemia contracture. In Flynn JE, editor: *Hand surgery,* ed 2, Baltimore, 1975, Williams & Wilkins.

Goldner JL: Musculoskeletal aspects of emotional problems, editorial, *South Med J* 69:1, 1976.

Goldner JL, Bright DS: The effect of extremity blood flow on pain and cold tolerance. In Omer G, Spinner M, editors: *Peripheral nerve injuries,* Philadelphia, 1979, WB Saunders.

Greenstein GM: *Clinical assessment of neuromusculoskeletal disorders,* St Louis, 1997, Mosby.

Gunn CC, Bilbrandt WE: Early and subtle signs in low back sprain, *Spine* 3:267, 1978.

Guyton AC: *Structure and function of the nervous system,* Philadelphia, 1972, WB Saunders.

Hart FD: *French's index of differential diagnosis,* ed 10, Baltimore, 1973, Williams & Wilkins.

Hartley A: *Practical joint assessment lower quadrant,* ed 2, St Louis, 1995, Mosby.

Hawkins RJ: *An organized approach to musculoskeletal examination and history taking,* St Louis, 1995, Mosby.

Heilman KM, Watson RT, Greer M: *Handbook for differential diagnosis of neurologic signs and symptoms,* New York, 1977, Appleton-Century-Crofts.

Holvey DN, Talbott JH: *The Merck manual of diagnosis and therapy,* ed 12, New Jersey, 1972, Merck.

Iowa Trial Lawyers Association: *Medical damages,* Des Moines, 1995, Iowa Trial Lawyers Association.

Jabaley ME, et al: Comparison of histologic and functional recovery after peripheral nerve repair, *J Hand Surg* (Am)1:119, 1976.

Jablonski S: *Dictionary of medical acronyms & abbreviations,* ed 3, Philadelphia, 1998, Hanley & Belfus.

Jacobs JW: Screening for organic mental syndromes in the medically ill, *Ann Intern Med* 86:40, 1977.

Kanner R: *Pain management secrets,* Philadelphia, 1997, Hanley & Belfus.

Kasdan ML: *Occupational hand & upper extremity injuries & diseases,* ed 2, Philadelphia, 1998, Hanley & Belfus.

Katirji B: *Electromyography in clinical practice: a case study approach,* St Louis, 1998, Mosby.

Katz JN, et al: Stability and responsiveness of utility measures, *Med Care* 32:183, 1994.

Katz WA: *Rheumatic diseases diagnosis and management,* Philadelphia, 1977, JB Lippincott.

Keefe FJ: Behavioral assessment and treatment of chronic pain: current status and future directions, *J Consult Clin Psychol* 50:896, 1982.

Kelsey JL: An epidemiological study of acute herniated lumbar intervertebral disc, *Rheum Rehab* 14:144, 1975.

Kendall HO, Kendall FP, Wadsworth GE: *Muscles testing and function,* ed 2, Baltimore, 1971, Williams & Wilkins.

Klippel JH, Dieppe PA: *Rheumatology,* vol 1-2, ed 2, London, 1998, Mosby.

Koenigsberg R: *Churchill's illustrated medical dictionary,* New York, 1989, Churchill Livingstone.

Lavy CBD, Barrett DS: *Questions and answers on Apley's concise system of orthopaedics and fractures,* Oxford, 1991, Butterworth-Heinemann.

Lephart SM, Henry TJ: Functional rehabilitation for the upper and lower extremity, *Orthop Clin North Am* 26:579, 1995.

Lerner AJ: *The little black book of neurology,* ed 3, St Louis, 1995, Mosby.

Lewis CB, Knortz KA: *Orthopedic assessment and treatment of the geriatric patient,* St Louis, 1993, Mosby.

Lorish DK, et al: Disease and psychosocial factors related to physical functioning in rheumatoid arthritis, *J Rheumatol* 18:1150, 1991.

Loth TS: *Orthopedic boards review II: a case study approach,* St Louis, 1996, Mosby.

Magee DJ: *Orthopedic physical assessment,* ed 3, Philadelphia, 1997, WB Saunders.

Malone TR, McPoil TG, Nitz AJ: *Orthopedic and sports physical therapy,* ed 3, St Louis, 1997, Mosby.

Mayer TG: A prospective two year study of functional restoration in industrial low back injury: an objective assessment procedure, *JAMA* 258:1763, 1987.

Mayo Clinic and Mayo Foundation: *Clinical examinations in neurology,* ed 5, Philadelphia, 1981, WB Saunders.

Mazion JM: *Illustrated manual of neurological/reflexes/signs/tests, part I, orthopedic signs/tests/maneuvers for office procedure, part II,* Orlando, 1980, Daniels Publishing.

McBride ED: *Disability evaluation and principles of treatment of compensable injuries,* ed 6, Philadelphia, 1963, JB Lippincott.

McKechnie B: Low back pain in the 1990's. In McKechnie B, McRae R, editors: *Clinical orthopaedic examination,* ed 3, Edinburgh, 1990, Churchill Livingstone.

Medical Economics Books: *Patient care flow chart manual,* ed 3, Oradell, NJ, 1982, Medical Economics Books.

Mellion MB: *Sports medicine secrets,* Philadelphia, 1994, Hanley & Belfus.

Mellion MB: *Office sports medicine,* ed 2, St Louis, 1996, Mosby.

Melzack R: *The McGill pain questionnaire: pain measurement and assessment,* New York, 1983, Raven.

Mengel MB, Schwiebert LP: *Ambulatory medicine the primary care of families,* ed 2, Stamford, Conn, 1996, Appleton & Lange.

Mennell JM: *The musculoskeletal system differential diagnosis from symptoms and physical signs,* Gaithersburg, Md, 1992, Aspen.

Mercier LR, Pettid FJ: *Practical orthopedics,* ed 4, St Louis, 1995, Mosby.

Merskey H: *Pain and psychological medicine, textbook of pain,* Edinburgh, 1984, Churchill Livingstone.

Million T, Green CJ, Meagher RB: *Million behavioral health inventory,* ed 3, Minneapolis, 1982, Interpretive Scoring System.

Mosby-Year Book, Inc: *Expert 10-minute physical examination,* St Louis, 1997, Mosby.

Mountcastle VB: The view from within: pathways to the study of perception, *Johns Hopkins Med J* 136:109, 1975.

Nachemson AL: The lumbar spine: an orthopaedic challenge, *Spine* 1:59, 1976.

Nelson EC: Using outcome measures to improve care delivered by physicians and hospitals. In Heithoff KA, Lohr KN, editors: *Effectiveness and outcomes in healthcare,* Washington DC, Institute of Medicine, 1990, National Academy Press.

Nettina SM: *The Lippincott manual of nursing practice,* ed 6, Philadelphia, 1996, Lippincott.

Newton RW: *Color atlas of pediatric neurology,* St Louis, 1995, Mosby-Wolfe.

Nicholas JA, Hershman EB: *The lower extremity & spine in sports medicine,* vol 1-2, ed 2, St Louis, 1995, Mosby.

Nicholas JA, Hershman EB: *The upper extremity in sports medicine,* ed 2, St Louis, 1995, Mosby.

Nordin M, Andersson GBJ, Pope MH: *Musculoskeletal disorders in the workplace: principles and practice,* St Louis, 1997, Mosby.

O'Donoghue DH: *Treatment of injuries to athletes,* ed 3, Philadelphia, 1976, WB Saunders.

Olson WH, Brumback RA: *Handbook of symptom-oriented neurology,* Chicago, 1989, Mosby.

1012

Bibliography

Omer GE, Spinner M: *Management of peripheral nerve problems,* Philadelphia, 1980, WB Saunders.

Osterweis M, Kleinman A, Mechanic D: *Pain and disability: clinical, behavioral and public policy perspectives, report of the Institute of Medicine Committee on Pain, Disability and Chronic Illness Behavior,* Washington, DC, 1987, National Academy Press.

O'Young B, Young MA, Stiens SA: *PM&R secrets,* Philadelphia, 1997, Hanley & Belfus.

Parker JC, Wright GE: The implications of depression for pain and disability in rheumatoid arthritis, *Arthritis Care Res* 8:279, 1995.

Patten J: *Neurological differential diagnosis,* ed 2, London, 1996, Springer.

Pilling LF, Brannick TL, Swenson WM: Psychological characteristics of patients having pain as a presenting symptom, *Can Med Assoc J* 97:287, 1967.

Pope AM, Tarlov AR: *Disability in America: toward a national agenda for prevention,* Washington, DC, 1991, National Academy Press.

Pope MH, et al: *Occupational low back pain assessment, treatment and prevention,* St Louis, 1991, Mosby.

Reed R: *Malingering, symposium papers,* Los Angeles, 1986, American College of Chiropractic Orthopedists.

Rockwood CA Jr, Eilbert RE: Camptocormia, *J Bone Joint Surg* 51A:533, 1969.

Rolak LA: *Neurology secrets,* ed 2, Philadelphia, 1998, Hanley & Belfus.

Rotes-Querol J: The syndrome of psychogenic rheumatism, *Clin Rheum Dis* 5:797, 1979.

Saidoff DC, McDonough AL: *Critical pathways in therapeutic intervention,* St Louis, 1997, Mosby.

Schram S, Taylor T: Tension signs in lumber disc prolapse, *Clin Orthop* 75:195, 1971.

Schumacher HR, Klippel JH, Koopman WJ: *Primer on the rheumatic diseases,* ed 10, Atlanta, 1993, Arthritis Foundation.

Shankman GA: *Fundamental orthopedic management for the physical therapist assistant,* St Louis, 1997, Mosby.

Sherman MS: The nerves of bones, *J Bone Joint Surg* 45A:522, 1963.

Sledge CB, Poss R: *The year book of orthopedics 1997,* St Louis, 1997, Mosby.

Stedman TL: *Stedman's medical dictionary,* ed 25, Baltimore, 1990, Williams & Wilkins.

Stewart DL, Abeln SH: *Documenting functional outcomes in physical therapy,* St Louis, 1993, Mosby.

Sweere JJ: *Chiropractic family practice: a clinical manual,* Gaithersburg, Md, 1992, Aspen.

Thompson JM: *Clinical outlines for health assessment,* St Louis, 1997, Mosby.

Toghill PJ: *Examining patients: an introduction to clinical medicine,* London, 1990, Edward Arnold.

Tollison CD, Satterthwaite JR, Tollison JW: *Handbook of pain management,* ed 2, Baltimore, 1994, Williams & Wilkins.

Torg JS, Shepard RJ: *Current therapy in sports medicine,* ed 3, St Louis, 1995, Mosby.

Truex RC, Carpenter MB: *Human neuroanatomy,* ed 6, Baltimore, 1969, Williams & Wilkins.

Turek SL: *Orthopaedics principles and their application,* ed 3, Philadelphia, 1977, JB Lippincott.

Waddell G: An approach to backache, *Br J Hosp Med* 28:187, 1982.

Waddell G: A new clinical model for the treatment of low back pain, *Spine* 12:632, 1987.

Wakefield TS, Frank RG: *The clinician's guide to neuro musculoskeletal practice,* Abbotsford, Wisc, 1995, Allied Health of Wisconsin, SC.

Walshe FMR: *Diseases of the nervous system,* ed 11, Baltimore, 1970, Williams & Wilkins.

Walters A: Psychogenic regional pain alias-hysterical pain, *Brain* 84:1, 1961.

Watkins RG: *The spine in sports,* St Louis, 1996, Mosby.

Weineck J: *Functional anatomy in sports,* ed 2, St Louis, 1990, Mosby.

Weinstein SL, Buckwalter JA: *Turek's orthopaedics principles and their application,* ed 5, Philadelphia, 1994, JB Lippincott.

White AH, Schofferman JA: *Spine care,* vol 1-2, St Louis, 1995, Mosby.

Whitmore I, Willan PLT: *Multiple choice questions in human anatomy,* London, 1995, Mosby.

Windsor RE, Lox DM: *Soft tissue injuries: diagnosis and treatment,* Philadelphia, 1998, Hanley & Belfus.

Wing PC, Wilfling FJ, Kokan PJ: *Comprehensive analysis of disability following lumbar intervertebral fusion: medical diagnosis and management,* Philadelphia, 1987, WB Saunders.

Yelin E: Musculoskeletal conditions and employment, *Arthritis Care Res* 8:311, 1995.

Zatouroff M: *Diagnosis in color physical signs in general medicine,* ed 2, London, 1996, Mosby-Wolfe.

Zitelli BJ, Davis HW: *Atlas of pediatric physical diagnosis,* ed 2, London, 1992, Wolfe.

GLOSSARY
OF ABBREVIATIONS

A	Assessment
Abd. hall.	Abductor hallucis
Abd. dig. V	Abductor digiti five
Abd. poll. brev.	Abductor pollicis brevis
Abd. poll. long.	Abductor pollicis longus
abnl	Abnormal
AC	Acrocyanosis
ACJ	Acromioclavicular joint
A & D	Amplitude & duration
Abd. long.	Abductor longus
ADL	Activities of daily living
AE	Above elbow
AJ	Ankle jerk
AK	Above knee
AKA	Above-knee amputation
ALS	Amyotrophic lateral sclerosis
amb	Ambulate
AMP	Amputation
Amp. sl	Amplitude slightly increased
Ampl, dur & n	Amplitude, duration, & number
ANA	Antinuclear antibody
Anc	Anconeus
ANF	Antinuclear factor
ant	Anterior
Ant. tib.	Anterior tibialis
AP and lat.	Anteroposterior and lateral
ARM	Active range of motion
AS	Left ear
AU	Both ears
A&W	Alive and Well
ax	Axillary
B	Brisk
Bic	Biceps
Biceps fem.	Biceps femoris
BJ	Biceps jerk
BJM	Bones, joints, & muscles
BK	Below knee
BKA	Below-knee amputation
BP	Blood pressure
Brachiorad	Brachioradialis
Bru	Bruised
C/O	Complaint of
c/o	Complaining of

C1-C8	Cervical first root through cervical eighth root
C1-C2	First cervical vertebra through second cervical vertebra
Ca	Carcinoma
CAT	Computed axial tomography
CC	Chief complaint
cm	Centimeter(s)
CM	Costal margin
CMC	Carpometacarpal
CNS	Central nervous system
cond	Condition
cont	Continue
Dr.	Doctor
DRG	Diagnosis-related groups
DTR	Deep tendon reflexes
dur	duration
Dx	Diagnosis
e.r.	Evoked response
EBV	Epstein-Barr virus
ECG	Electrocardiogram
ECU	Extensor carpi ulnaris
edx	Electrodiagnosis
EEG	Electroencephalogram
EJ	Elbow jerk
EMG	Electromyogram
Enc	Encourage
EPS	Extraparametal symptoms
ESR	Erythrocyte sedimentation rate
eval	Evaluation
Evoked pot.	Evoked potential
Exam	Examination
ext	External
Ext. ind	Extensor indices
Ext. c. rad. B	Extensor carpi radialis brevis
Ext. c. rad. L	Extensor carpi radialis longus
Ext. dig. brev.	Extensor digitorum brevis
Ext. dig. comm.	Extensor digitorum communis
Ext. dig. long.	Extensor digitorum longus
Ext. hall. long.	Extensor hallucis longus
Ext. poll. brev.	Extensor pollicis brevis
Ext. poll. long.	Extensor pollicus longus
extr	Extremity
FB	Foreign body
FHx	Family history
FLEX	Flexion
Flex. c. rad.	Flexor carpi radialis
Flex. c. uln.	Flexor carpi ulnaris
Flex. dig. prof.	Flexor digitorum profundus
Flex. dig. subl.	Flexor digitorum sublimis
ft	Foot
FUO	Fever of undetermined origin
FWB	Full weight bearing
FX	Fracture
Gastroc	Gastrocnemius

Glut. max.	Gluteus maximus
Glut. med.	Gluteus medius
GP	General practitioner
GSW	Gunshot wound
H&P	History and physical
Ha	Headache
HBP	High blood pressure
HEENT	Head, eyes, ears, nose, & throat
ht	Height
Hx	History
ICS	Intercostal space
IM	Intramuscular
Inf. glut.	Inferior gluteal
Infraspin.	Infraspinatus
Instr	Instruction
IP	Interphalangeal
IPJ	Interphalangeal joint
JRA	Juvenile rheumatoid arthritis
jt	Joint
KJ	Knee jerk
Lab	Laboratory
LBP	Low blood pressure
LMN	Lower motor neuron
LMP	Last menstrual period
LOA	Left occiput anterior
LOC	Loss of consciousness
LOM	Limitation of motion
LOP	Left occiput posterior
med	Median
ML	Midline
mp	Metacarpophalangeal
MPJ	Metacarpophalangeal joint
MRI	Magnetic resonance imaging
MS	Multiple sclerosis
MTP	Metatarsophalangeal
MUAPs	Motor unit action potentials
N	Nerve
N&V	Nausea and vomiting
N/A	Not applicable
NAD	No acute distress
NCV	Nerve conduction velocity
NKA	No known allergies
NR	Normal range
NRC	Nerve root compression
N/V	Nausea/vomiting
NVD	Nausea, vomiting, and diarrhea
NWB	Non–weight bearing
OA	Osteoarthritis
obt	Obturator
Ortho	Orthopedic
O.T.	Occupational therapy
OTC	Over the counter
PA	Posteroanterior

palp	Palpate, palpated, palpable
PE	Physical examination
pect. maj.	Pectoralis major
pect. min.	Pectoralis minor
Periph	Peripheral
Peron. brevis	Peroneus brevis
Peron. long.	Peroneus longus
PERRLA	Pupils equal, round, reactive to light and accommodation
PH	Past history, personal history
PI	Present illness
PID	Pelvic inflammatory disease
PIP	Proximal interphalangeal
PIPJ	Proximal interphalangeal joint
PM&R	Physical medicine and rehabilitation
po	Phone order
pos	Positive
post	Posterior
post	After
PP	Proximal phalanx
PR	Pulse rate
PRIND	Partial residual ischemic neurovascular deficit
prn	As the occasion arises (pro re nata)
prod	Productive
Pron. quad.	Pronator quadratus
Pron. ter.	Pronator teres
prox	Proximal
P.T.	Physical therapy
pt	Patient
PVD	Peripheral vascular disease
PWB	Partial weight bearing
RA	Rheumatoid arthritis
Rehab	Rehabilitation
RF	Rheumatic fever
Rhomb	Rhomboids
RIND	Reversible ischemic neurologic deficit
RLE	Right lower extremity
R/O	Rule out
ROM	Range of motion
ROS	Review of systems
rp	Radial pulse
RPO	Right posterior oblique
R.T.	Recreation therapy
RTO	Return to office
RUE	Right upper extremity
S&S	Signs and symptoms
S1-S5	Sacral first root through sacral fifth root
S1-S2	First, second heart sounds
Sciat	Sciatic
SCM	Sternocleidomastoid
SD	Standard deviation
Sed. rate	Sedimentation rate
Semi. memb.	Semimembranosus
Sens	Sensory

Ser. ant.	Serratus anterior
SF	Spinal fluid
SHx	Social history
SI	Sacroiliac
SIJ	Sacroiliac joint
SLE	Systemic lupus erythematosus
SLR	Straight leg raises
SMA-12	Sequential multiple analysis (12-channel biochemical profile)
SOAP	Subjective, objective, assessment, plan
SOB	Short of breath
sol.	Soleus
St	Strong
Strep	Streptococcus
Sup. glut.	Superior gluteal
Suprascap	Suprascapular
Supraspin	Supraspinatus
Sx	Symptoms
T	Temperature
T1-T12	First thoracic root through twelfth thoracic root
Tc	Transcutaneous
thor	Thoracic
Ther	Therapy
THR	Total hip replacement
TIA	Transient ischemic attack
tib	Tibial
ting	Tingling
TJ	Triceps jerk
TMJ	Temporomandibular joint
tol	Tolerated
tp	Treatment plan
TPR	Temperature, pulse, and respiration
Trap	Trapezius
Tric	Triceps
Tx	Treatment
UMN	Upper motor neuron
UA	Urinalysis
vib	Vibration
Vig	Vigorous

LISTING OF TESTS, ALPHABETICALLY AND ANATOMICALLY

APPENDIX B

LISTING OF TESTS ACCORDING TO THE POSITION OF THE PATIENT

INDEX

Page numbers in italics indicate illustrations;
t indicates tables.